Nutrition, Immunity, and Infection

Nutrition, Immunity, and Infection

Edited By
Philip C. Calder and Anil D. Kulkarni

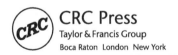

CRC Press
Taylor & Francis Group
Boca Raton London New York

CRC Press is an imprint of the
Taylor & Francis Group, an **informa** business

CRC Press
Taylor & Francis Group
6000 Broken Sound Parkway NW, Suite 300
Boca Raton, FL 33487-2742

Printed on acid-free paper

International Standard Book Number-13: 978-1-4822-5397-9 (Hardback)

Library of Congress Cataloging-in-Publication Data

Names: Calder, Philip C., editor. | Kulkarni, Anil D. (Anil Digambar), editor.
Title: Nutrition, immunity, and infection / editors, Philip C. Calder and Anil D. Kulkarni.
Other titles: Nutrition, immunity, and infection (Calder)
Description: Boca Raton : Taylor & Francis, 2018. | Includes bibliographical references.
Identifiers: LCCN 2017017013 | ISBN 9781482253979 (hardback : alk. paper)
Subjects: | MESH: Nutritional Physiological Phenomena--immunology | Immune
System--physiology | Nutrition Disorders--immunology |
Immunity--physiology | Infection--immunology
Classification: LCC QR181 | NLM QU 145 | DDC 616.07/9--dc23
LC record available at https://lccn.loc.gov/2017017013

Visit the Taylor & Francis Web site at
http://www.taylorandfrancis.com

and the CRC Press Web site at
http://www.crcpress.com

Contents

Preface..ix
About the Editors...xi
Contributors xiii

Chapter 1   Introduction to the Immune System..1

   Philip C. Calder and Gerald Sonnenfeld

Chapter 2   The Gut-Associated Lymphoid System..19

   Marie C. Lewis

Chapter 3   Obesity, Immunity, and Infection..33

   Scott D. Neidich and Melinda A. Beck

Chapter 4   Role of Immune Cells in Adipose Tissue..43

   Jack Warburton and Fátima Pérez de Heredia

Chapter 5   Influence of Infection and Inflammation on Nutrient Status 57

   David I. Thurnham and Christine A. Northrop-Clewes

Chapter 6   Undernutrition, Infection, and Poor Growth in Infants and Children 83

   D. Joe Millward

Chapter 7   Immunity in Anorexia Nervosa.. 111

   Esther Nova and Ascensión Marcos

Chapter 8   Prebiotics, Probiotics, and Response to Vaccination 125

   Caroline E. Childs

Chapter 9   The Immunological Benefits of Complex Oligosaccharides in Human Milk..........145

   *Ling Xiao, Bernd Stahl, Gert Folkerts, Johan Garssen,
   Leon Knippels, and Belinda van't Land*

Chapter 10 Mechanisms of Immune Regulation by Vitamin A and Its Metabolites 159

   *Randi Larsen Indrevær, Agnete Bratsberg Eriksen,
   and Heidi Kiil Blomhoff*

Chapter 11 Vitamin A, Immunity, and Infection..181

   Charles B. Stephensen

Chapter 12 Vitamin E, Immunity, and Infection 197

Dayong Wu and Simin Nikbin Meydani

Chapter 13 Iron, Immunity, and Infection 213

Hal Drakesmith

Chapter 14 Selenium as a Regulator of Inflammation and Immunity 231

Aaron H. Rose and Peter R. Hoffmann

Chapter 15 Zinc Regulation of the Immune Response 245

Veronika Kloubert and Lothar Rink

Chapter 16 Short-Chain Fatty Acids, G Protein-Coupled Receptors, and Immune Cells 279

*José Luís Fachi, Renan O. Corrêa, Fabio T. Sato, Angélica T. Vieira,
Hosana G. Rodrigues, and Marco Aurélio R. Vinolo*

Chapter 17 Omega-3 Fatty Acids and T-Cell Responses 295

Tim Y. Hou, David N. McMurray, and Robert S. Chapkin

Chapter 18 Novel Immunoregulatory Mediators Produced from Omega-3 Fatty Acids 315

Patricia R. Souza, Hefin R. Jones, and Lucy V. Norling

Chapter 19 Roles of Arginine in Cell-Mediated and Humoral Immunity 335

Wenkai Ren, Yulong Yin, Beiyan Zhou, Fuller W. Bazer, and Guoyao Wu

Chapter 20 Nitric Oxide and the Immune System 349

*Fernanda Salomao Costa, Anil Kulkarni, Alamelu Sundaresan,
Davide Cattano, and Marie-Francoise Doursout*

Chapter 21 Glutamine and the Immune System 357

Vinicius Fernandes Cruzat and Philip Newsholme

Chapter 22 Glutathione, Immunity, and Infection 375

Enrique Vera Tudela, Manpreet Singh, and Vishwanath Venketaraman

Chapter 23 Dietary Nucleotides and Immunity 387

Luis Fontana, Olga Martínez-Augustin, and Ángel Gil

Chapter 24 Gangliosides and Immune Regulation 405

Ricardo Rueda, Esther Castanys-Muñoz, and Enrique Vázquez

Chapter 25 AHCC Nutritional Supplement and the Immune Response....................................427

Takehito Miura and Anil D. Kulkarni

Chapter 26 Environmental Stressors, Immunity, and Nutrition 435

L. Olamigoke, E. Mansoor, D. Grimm, J. Bauer, V. Mann, and A. Sundaresan

Chapter 27 Nutrition, Immunity, and Infection: Ayurvedic and Conventional Perspectives 443

Kavita D. Chandwani, Shinil K. Shah, Erik B. Wilson, and Anil D. Kulkarni

Chapter 28 Poor Maternal Nutritional Status or HIV Infection and Infant Outcomes:
Evidence from India and Africa...453

Sarah Helen Kehoe and Marie-Louise Newell

Chapter 29 Postpregnancy Ethnic Nutritional Practices in India:
A Critical Perspective of Immunity and Infection 465

P. R. Janci Rani, N. Tharani Devi, and Murali Rangarajan

Index..521

Preface

The immune system is the core of defense against pathogenic organisms. It includes barrier functions, multiple cell types with specialized defense roles, and a myriad of chemicals, some involved directly in defense and others in regulation of the immune response. It is evident that a well-functioning immune system is central to protection against becoming infected and to the body's response to being infected. But the immune system does more than that: it is involved in surveillance against tumor cells, in the response to injury, and in the tolerance of foods, commensal organisms, and, in pregnancy, the fetus, each of which is foreign to the individual. Failure of the immune system to respond properly predisposes to infection and makes infections more severe, increases risk of cancer, diminishes the ability to heal wounds, and can result in adverse reactions to foods and to normally benign environmental exposures including harmless microorganisms. Such immune failures underlie immune-mediated conditions that can be pathological and in some cases fatal.

Nutrition is one of the determinants of immune competence, and the immune system is adversely affected by malnutrition. Malnutrition may come in several forms; one of these is sometimes called protein-energy malnutrition; this is frank undernutrition and is caused by inadequate access to food. The second form of malnutrition is specific essential nutrient deficiencies, such as deficiency of zinc, iron, or vitamin A. Such nutrient deficiencies may be multiple in a single individual and may coincide with protein-energy malnutrition. The immune system has a high demand for energy, so requiring fuels, and for biosynthesis and cell replication, so requiring the substrates that act as building blocks. Such intense metabolic activity requires cofactors and regulators; these are often vitamins and minerals. Thus, it is easy to see that either protein-energy malnutrition or essential nutrient deficiencies will impair the immune response, making the individual more susceptible to infection. The third form of malnutrition is overnutrition, principally in the form of an excessive intake of macronutrients resulting in overweight and obesity. It is now known that obesity is also linked to immune impairments. Billions of individuals worldwide, many of them children, suffer from each of protein-energy malnutrition, essential nutrient deficiencies, and overweight and obesity. Research has shown that reversing malnutrition improves immune competence with a subsequent improvement in resistance to infection. Thus, poor nutrition impacting the immune system is a global public health problem with immense consequences on childhood growth and development, on morbidity and mortality, and on social structures and health economies. In order to properly address this problem, a detailed understanding of the nutrition–immunity–infection interaction is required.

This book addresses different aspects of the nutrition–immunity–infection triad. It brings together the state of the art descriptions of different components of that triad with the aim of providing an integrated view overall. Life-course considerations are included and there is recognition that nutrition is culture and context specific, which may have an overall impact on the outcome of dietary exposures and particular interventions.

We are indebted to the authors of the individual chapters for their contributions to this important book, and we thank the publishers for their continued support throughout this project.

Philip C. Calder and Anil D. Kulkarni

About the Editors

Philip C. Calder is Professor of Nutritional Immunology within the Human Development and Health Academic Unit of the Faculty of Medicine at the University of Southampton in the United Kingdom. He has a PhD in biochemistry from the University of Auckland (New Zealand) and a DPhil in biochemistry from the University of Oxford (UK). He is a registered nutritionist and a fellow of both the Royal Society of Biology and the Association for Nutrition. He has broad-ranging research interests. Much of his research has focused on the metabolism and functionality of fatty acids with an emphasis on the roles of omega-3 fatty acids in immunity, inflammation, and cardiometabolic disease. He has received several awards for his work including the Sir David Cuthbertson Medal (1995), the Belgian Danone Institute Chair (2004), the Nutricia International Award (2007), the European Society for Clinical Nutrition and Metabolism's Cuthbertson Lecture (2008), the Muriel Bell Award (2009), the Louisiana State University Chancellor's Award in Neuroscience and Medicine (2011), the Normann Medal from the German Society for Fat Science (2012), the Ralph Holman Lifetime Achievement Award from the American Oil Chemists' Society (2015), the British Association for Parenteral & Enteral Nutrition's Pennington Lecture (2015), the British Nutrition Foundation Prize (2015), and the Danone International Prize for Nutrition (2016). He has served on many committees of professional societies and was for three years president of the International Society for the Study of Fatty Acids and Lipids (2009–2012). In 2016, he completed a three-year term as chair of the Scientific Committee of the European Society for Clinical Nutrition and Metabolism and started a three-year term as president of the Nutrition Society. Dr. Calder was editor-in-chief of the *British Journal of Nutrition* from 2006 to 2013, and he is currently an associate editor of *Clinical Science*, *Journal of Nutrition*, *Clinical Nutrition*, *Lipids*, and *Nutrition Research*. He is a member of the several other editorial boards of journals in the nutrition, clinical science, and lipidology fields. Professor Calder has more than 500 research publications (excluding abstracts), including more than 250 peer-reviewed research papers, and more than 150 review articles in journals. His work has been cited over 22,000 times and he is listed by Thomson Reuters as a Highly Cited Researcher.

Dr. Anil D. Kulkarni received his doctorate degree (faculty of medicine) from the Queen's University of Belfast, N. Ireland. He is currently Professor of Surgery in the Department of Surgery at the University of Texas McGovern Medical School in the world's largest medical center in Houston, Texas. His research specialization is in the role of nutrition in immune system function in health and disease and he has extensive in applied, basic, and translational research. He has a background in research and development and technology development. He has received two U.S. Patents on nutritional product development for modulation immune system function and nutritional formulations for wound healing. He also teaches medical students and mentors students from high school to graduate and medical students. He has traveled internationally extensively with numerous research collaborations in several countries in Asia, Europe, and Latin America. He is known internationally for his work in immunonutrition and functional foods and has been invited frequently to be a keynote speaker. He mentors medical students for their global health curriculum and their projects. Students are assigned a Leviticus project when they go abroad during their senior year rotations. He has been on the editorial boards of international journals and serves as a peer reviewer. One of his current active interests is in global health activities and education. Most of the current academic global health initiatives have largely ignored or not focused on nutrition—cultural or ethnic—in prevention or therapeutic applications to improve global health and education. He also develops international exchange programs for faculty, staff, and students.

He has trained several international and domestic graduate and medical students. Recently he was a recipient of two international awards as recognition for his contributions of global work: the "Hind Rattan Award" at the 33rd International Congress of Association of Non-resident Indians and the "Fulbright-Nehru Scholarship 2014 for Professional and Teaching Excellence." He is Honorary Professor at the Qingdao Municipal Hospital of Qingdao University, China. He is also a Member of ARTOI (Associazione Ricerca Terapie Oncologiche Integrate) in Italy.

Contributors

J. Bauer
Max-Planck Institute for Biochemistry
Martinsried, Germany

Fuller W. Bazer
Department of Animal Science
Texas A&M University
College Station, Texas

Melinda A. Beck
Department of Nutrition
Gillings School of Global Public Health
University of North Carolina
Chapel Hill, North Carolina

Agnete Bratsberg Eriksen
Department of Molecular Medicine
Institute of Basic Medical Science
University of Oslo
Oslo, Norway

Esther Castanys-Muñoz
Discovery R&D Department
Granada University Science Park
Abbott Nutrition
Granada, Spain

Davide Cattano
Department of Anesthesiology
University of Texas Medical School
   at Houston
Houston, Texas

Kavita D. Chandwani
Department of Surgery, Minimally Invasive
   Surgery/Bariatric Surgery
University of Texas Health Science Center
McGovern Medical School
Houston, Texas

Robert S. Chapkin
Department of Biochemistry and Biophysics
and
Department of Nutrition and Food Science
and
Program in Integrative Nutrition & Complex
   Diseases
and
Department of Microbial Pathogenesis &
   Immunology
Texas A&M University
College Station, Texas

Caroline E. Childs
Human Development & Health
   Academic Unit
Faculty of Medicine
University of Southampton
Southampton General Hospital
Southampton, United Kingdom

Renan O. Corrêa
Department of Genetics and Evolution and
   Bioagents
Institute of Biology
University of Campinas
São Paulo, Brazil

Fernanda Salomao Costa
Departments of Anesthesiology and Surgery
University of Texas Medical School at Houston
Houston, Texas

Vinicius Fernandes Cruzat
School of Biomedical Sciences
Curtin Health Innovation Research Institute
Biosciences
Curtin University
Perth, Western Australia, Australia

N. Tharani Devi
Food, Nutrition and Health Education Center
Amrita School of Engineering
Amrita University
Coimbatore, India

Marie-Francoise Doursout
Department of Anesthesiology
University of Texas Medical School
    at Houston
Houston, Texas

Hal Drakesmith
MRC Human Immunology Unit
Weatherall Institute of Molecular Medicine
University of Oxford
Oxford, United Kingdom

José Luís Fachi
Department of Genetics and Evolution and
    Bioagents
Institute of Biology
University of Campinas
São Paulo, Brazil

Gert Folkerts
Faculty of Science
Department of Pharmaceutical
    Sciences
Division of Pharmacology
Utrecht University
Utrecht, the Netherlands

Luis Fontana
Department of Biochemistry and Molecular
    Biology II
School of Pharmacy
University of Granada, Spain
and
Institute of Nutrition and Food Technology
    "José Mataix"
Biomedical Research Center
Parque Tecnológico Ciencias de la Salud
and
Instituto de Investigación
    Biosanitaria (ibs.GRANADA)
Granada, Spain

Johan Garssen
Faculty of Science
Department of Pharmaceutical Sciences
Division of Pharmacology
Utrecht University
and
Nutricia Research
Utrecht, the Netherlands

Ángel Gil
Department of Biochemistry and Molecular
    Biology II
School of Pharmacy
University of Granada, Spain
and
Institute of Nutrition and Food Technology
    "José Mataix"
Biomedical Research Center
Parque Tecnológico Ciencias de la Salud
and
Instituto de Investigación Biosanitaria (ibs.
    GRANADA)
Granada, Spain

D. Grimm
Department of Biomedicine
Aarhus, Denmark

Peter R. Hoffmann
John A. Burns School of Medicine
Department of Cell and Molecular Biology
University of Hawaii
Honolulu, Hawaii

Tim Y. Hou
Department of Biochemistry and Biophysics
and
Department of Nutrition and Food Science
Program in Integrative Nutrition & Complex
    Diseases
Texas A&M University
College Station, Texas

Hefin R. Jones
The William Harvey Research Institute
Barts and The London School of Medicine and
    Dentistry
Charterhouse Square
London, United Kingdom

Sarah Helen Kehoe
MRC Lifecourse Epidemiology Unit
Human Development and Health
    Academic Unit
Faculty of Medicine
University of Southampton
Southampton, United Kingdom

Heidi Kiil Blomhoff
Department of Molecular Medicine
Institute of Basic Medical Science
University of Oslo
Oslo, Norway

Veronika Kloubert
Institute of Immunology
Medical Faculty
RWTH Aachen University
Aachen, Germany

Leon Knippels
Faculty of Science
Department of Pharmaceutical
    Sciences
Division of Pharmacology
Utrecht University
and
Nutricia Research
Utrecht, the Netherlands

Randi Larsen Indrevær
Department of Molecular Medicine
Institute of Basic Medical Science
University of Oslo
Oslo, Norway

Marie C. Lewis
Food Microbial Sciences Unit
Department of Food & Nutritional
    Science
University of Reading
Reading, United Kingdom

Vivek Mann
Department of Environmental and
    Interdisciplinary Sciences
Texas Southern University
Houston, Texas

Elvedina Mansoor
Department of Environmental and
    Interdisciplinary Sciences
Texas Southern University
Houston, Texas

Ascensión Marcos
Institute of Food Science, Technology and
    Nutrition
Spanish National Research Council
Madrid, Spain

Olga Martínez-Augustin
Department of Biochemistry and Molecular
    Biology II
School of Pharmacy
University of Granada
and
Institute of Nutrition and Food Technology
    "José Mataix"
Biomedical Research Center
Parque Tecnológico Ciencias de la Salud
Granada, Spain
and
Centro de Investigación Biomédica en Red
    de Enfermedades Hepáticas y Digestivas
    (CIBERehd)
Granada, Spain

David N. McMurray
Program in Integrative Nutrition & Complex
    Diseases
Department of Microbial Pathogenesis &
    Immunology
Texas A&M University
College Station, Texas

Simin Nikbin Meydani
Nutritional Immunology Laboratory
Jean Mayer USDA Human Nutrition Research
    Center on Aging at Tufts University
Boston, Massachusetts

D. Joe Millward
Department of Nutritional Sciences
School of Biosciences and Medicine
Faculty of Health and Medical Sciences
University of Surrey
Guildford, United Kingdom

Takehito Miura
Amino Up Chemical Company
Researh Division
Sapporo, Japan

Scott D. Neidich
Human Vaccine Institute
Duke University
Durham, North Carolina

Marie-Louise Newell
Human Development and Health
    Academic Unit
Faculty of Medicine
University of Southampton
Southampton, United Kingdom

Philip Newsholme
School of Biomedical Sciences
Curtin Health Innovation Research
    Institute
Biosciences
Curtin University
Perth, Western Australia, Australia

Lucy V. Norling
The William Harvey Research Institute
Barts and The London School of Medicine
    and Dentistry
Charterhouse Square
London, United Kingdom

Christine A. Northrop-Clewes
Independent Consultant
Cambridge, United Kingdom

Esther Nova
Institute of Food Science, Technology and
    Nutrition
Spanish National Research Council
Madrid, Spain

Loretta Olamigoke
Department of Environmental and
    Interdisciplinary Sciences
Texas Southern University
Houston, Texas

Fátima Pérez de Heredia
Liverpool John Moores University
Liverpool, United Kingdom

Murali Rangarajan
Department of Chemical Engineering and
    Materials Science
Amrita School of Engineering
Amrita University
Coimbatore, India

P. R. Janci Rani
Food, Nutrition and Health Education
    Center
Amrita School of Engineering
Amrita University
Coimbatore, India

Wenkai Ren
Scientific Observing and Experimental Station
    of Animal Nutrition and Feed Science in
    South-Central
Ministry of Agriculture
Hunan Provincial Engineering Research Center
    of Healthy Livestock Key Laboratory of
    Agro-ecological Processes in Subtropical
    Region
Institute of Subtropical Agriculture
Chinese Academy of Sciences
Changsha, China

Lothar Rink
Institute of Immunology
Medical Faculty
RWTH Aachen University
Aachen, Germany

Hosana G. Rodrigues
Faculty of Applied Sciences
University of Campinas
São Paulo, Brazil

Aaron H. Rose
University of Hawaii
John A. Burns School of Medicine
Department of Cell and Molecular Biology
Honolulu, Hawaii

Ricardo Rueda
Discovery R&D Department
Abbott Nutrition
Granada, Spain

Fabio T. Sato
Department of Genetics and Evolution and
    Bioagents
Institute of Biology
University of Campinas
São Paulo, Brazil

Shinil K. Shah
University of Texas Health Science Center
McGovern Medical School
Department of Surgery, Minimally Invasive
    Surgery/Bariatric Surgery
Houston, Texas

Manpreet Singh
College of Osteopathic
    Medicine of the Pacific
Western University of
    Health Sciences
Pomona, California

Gerald Sonnenfeld
Department of Cell and Molecular Biology
The University of Rhode Island
Kingston, Rhode Island

Patricia R. Souza
The William Harvey Research Institute
Barts and The London
    School of Medicine and Dentistry
Charterhouse Square
London, United Kingdom

Bernd Stahl
Nutricia Research
Utrect, the Netherlands

Charles B. Stephensen
USDA Western Human
    Nutrition Research Center
University of California
Davis, California

Alamelu Sundaresan
Department of Biology
Texas Sourthern University
Houston, Texas

David I. Thurnham
Northern Ireland Centre for Food and Health
School of Biomedical Sciences
University of Ulster
Nothern Ireland, United Kingdom

Enrique Vera Tudela
College of Osteopathic Medicine of the Pacific
Western University of Health Sciences
Pomona, California

Belinda van't Land
Nutricia Research
and
The Wilhelmina Children's Hospital
University Medical Center
Laboratory of Translational Immunology
Utrecht, the Netherlands

Enrique Vázquez
Discovery R&D Department
Abbott Nutrition
Granada, Spain

Vishwanath Venketaraman
College of Osteopathic Medicine of the Pacific
Western University of Health Sciences
Pomona, California

Angélica T. Vieira
Department of Biochemistry and
    Immunology
Institute of Biological Sciences
Federal University of Minas Berais
Belo Horizonte, Brazil

Marco Aurélio R. Vinolo
Department of Genetics and Evolution and
    Bioagents
Institute of Biology
University of Campinas
São Paulo, Brazil

Jack Warburton
Liverpool John Moores University
Liverpool, United Kingdom

Erik B. Wilson
University of Texas Health Science Center
McGovern Medical School
Department of Surgery, Minimally Invasive
    Surgery/Bariatric Surgery
Houston, Texas

Dayong Wu
Nutritional Immunology Laboratory
Jean Mayer USDA Human
    Nutrition Research Center on Aging
Tufts University
Boston, Massachusetts

Guoyao Wu
Department of Animal Science
Texas A&M University
College Station, Texas

Ling Xiao
Faculty of Science
Department of Pharmaceutical Sciences
Division of Pharmacology
Utrecht University
Utrecht, the Netherlands

Yulong Yin
Scientific Observing and Experimental Station
    of Animal Nutrition and Feed Science in
    South-Central
Ministry of Agriculture
Hunan Provincial Engineering Research Center
    of Healthy Livestock Key Laboratory of
    Agro-ecological Processes in Subtropical
    Region
Institute of Subtropical Agriculture
Chinese Academy of Sciences
Changsha, China

Beiyan Zhou
Department of Immunology
UConn Health
Farmington, Connecticut

1 Introduction to the Immune System

Philip C. Calder and Gerald Sonnenfeld

CONTENTS

1.1   Introduction 2
1.2   Innate Immunity 2
    1.2.1   Barriers 2
    1.2.2   Pattern Recognition Receptors 2
    1.2.3   Cellular Components of Innate Immunity 3
        1.2.3.1   Neutrophils 3
        1.2.3.2   Monocytes and Macrophages 5
        1.2.3.3   Eosinophils 6
        1.2.3.4   Basophils and Mast Cells 6
        1.2.3.5   Natural Killer Cells 6
    1.2.4   Soluble Factors Involved in Innate Immunity 6
        1.2.4.1   Complement 7
        1.2.4.2   Acute Phase Proteins 7
        1.2.4.3   Cytokines 7
1.3   Adhesion Molecules and Chemokines 7
    1.3.1   Adhesion Molecules 7
    1.3.2   Chemokines 8
1.4   Adaptive Immunity 9
    1.4.1   Overview 9
    1.4.2   Antigen Presentation and Recognition by T-Lymphocytes 10
        1.4.2.1   Class I and II MHC Molecules 11
        1.4.2.2   HLA-Independent Presentation of Antigen 11
    1.4.3   T-Lymphocytes 11
        1.4.3.1   T-Cell Development 11
        1.4.3.2   T-Cell–Antigen Receptor Complex 12
        1.4.3.3   T-Cell Subpopulations 12
    1.4.4   B-Lymphocytes 13
        1.4.4.1   B-Cell Development 13
        1.4.4.2   Establishing the B-Cell Repertoire 14
        1.4.4.3   T-Cell-Dependent B-Cell Responses 14
        1.4.4.4   T-Cell-Independent B-Cell Responses 14
1.5   Other Immune Cell Types 15
1.6   Lymphoid Tissue and Cellular Communication 15
1.7   Regulatory T-Cells and Immune Tolerance 15
Further Reading 16

1.1   INTRODUCTION

The immune system is concerned with defense of the host against pathogenic organisms. It consists of a complex network of molecules and cells that have precise roles. The immune response may be divided into innate (sometimes called natural) and adaptive (sometimes called acquired) components. The innate immune response is rapid and nonspecific; it uses receptors encoded in the germ line. In contrast, the adaptive immune response is slower to react and specific; it uses receptors that are generated by somatic DNA rearrangement. Cells involved in the innate response include various phagocytic cells (neutrophils, monocytes, and macrophages), inflammatory cells (basophils, mast cells, and eosinophils), and natural killer (NK) cells. Molecules involved in innate immunity include complement, acute-phase proteins, and cytokines. The barrier function is also part of the innate immune response. The adaptive response involves the binding of antigen to surface receptors of antigen-specific B- and T-lymphocytes (also called B- and T-cells) via an antigen presenting cell (APC) and the subsequent activation and proliferation of the B- or T-cell. In response to the activation, B-cells secrete antibodies; these are antigen-specific immunoglobulins (Ig). The key role of antibodies is to identify and aid in the destruction of extracellular microorganisms. T-cells help B-cells to produce antibodies, therefore participating in adaptive immune defense against extracellular microorganisms. T-cells also play a key role in adaptive immune defense against intracellular microorganisms either directly, for example by killing virally infected cells, or indirectly, through activation of macrophages. The innate and adaptive immune responses work together in an integrated way to effectively eliminate organisms, toxins, and allergens. This chapter will provide an overview of the components and activities of the immune system. Further detail may be found in any immunology textbook.

1.2   INNATE IMMUNITY

1.2.1   Barriers

Barriers form a part of innate immune defense by acting to exclude pathogens and toxins. Barriers include the skin and the gastrointestinal, respiratory, and genitourinary tracts. These provide a physical impediment to entry. However, there are additional barrier functions. An example is mucosal secretions, which can trap microorganisms, and the acidic pH of the stomach, which can kill many invading bacteria.

1.2.2   Pattern Recognition Receptors

It is essential for the innate immune system to recognize pathogens. This is achieved through pattern recognition receptors (PRRs) that recognize molecular structures that are broadly shared by pathogens. Researchers term these structures pathogen-associated molecular patterns (PAMPs), but since they also exist on nonpathogenic organisms, they are more correctly described as microbial-associated molecular patterns (MAMPs). When PRRs recognize MAMPs, several signaling pathways are initiated to activate the first line of host defensive responses necessary for killing infectious microbes. In addition, PRR signaling induces maturation of dendritic cells (DCs), which are responsible for antigen processing and presentation, so initiating the second line of host defense, adaptive immunity.

Toll-like receptors (TLRs) were the first PRRs to be identified. They are expressed either on the cell surface or associated with intracellular vesicles (Figure 1.1). More than ten functional TLRs have been identified in humans. Each TLR detects distinct MAMPs derived from viruses, bacteria, mycobacteria, fungi, and parasites (Table 1.1). These include lipopolysaccharide (LPS) from gram-negative bacteria, peptidoglycan, lipoteichoic acid, bacterial flagellar proteins, viral double-stranded RNA, and unmethylated DNA with CpG motifs characteristic of microbial DNA. Other classes of cytosolic PRRs also exist, including RIG-I-like receptors (RLRs) and Nod-like receptors (NLRs).

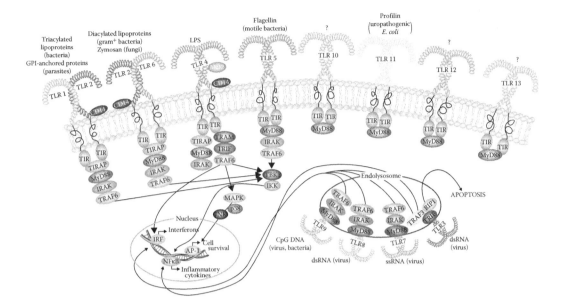

FIGURE 1.1 (See color insert.) Toll-like receptor (TLR) signaling. Individual TLRs initiate overlapping and distinct signaling pathways in various cell types such as macrophages, dendritic cells, and inflammatory monocytes. Engagement of TLRs with their ligands induces conformational changes of TLRs that lead to recruitment of adaptor proteins such as MyD88, TIRAP, TRIF, TRAF, and TRAM. TLR4, TLR5, TLR10, TLR11, TLR12, and TR13 exist as surface-bound homodimers, while TLR2 can form surface-bound heterodimers with TLR1 or TLR6. TLR3, TLR7, TLR8, and TLR9 are homodimers bound to the endolysosome membrane. All TLRs are capable of activating nuclear factor kappa B (NFκB) and inducing inflammatory cytokine production. Some TLRs also signal to promote production of type-1 interferon (interferon-α). Reproduced with permission from Cayman Chemical Company.

1.2.3 Cellular Components of Innate Immunity

All cells of the immune system derive from pluripotent stem cells in the bone marrow (Figure 1.2). A pluripotent stem cell can give rise to either a lymphoid stem cell or myeloid stem cell. Lymphoid stem cells can differentiate further into the four major populations of mature lymphocytes: T-cells, B-cells, NK cells, and NK-T cells. Myeloid stem cells (also termed common myeloid progenitors) give rise to granulocytes, monocytes, megakaryocytes and platelets, and erythrocytes.

1.2.3.1 Neutrophils

Neutrophils are the most numerous granulocyte in the bloodstream. Early in the innate immune response, neutrophils are recruited to the site of infection or tissue injury and become activated. Neutrophils make their way to a site of infection via many steps involving proinflammatory mediators, adhesion molecules, chemoattractants, and chemokines (this process is described in Section 1.3). Once at the site, neutrophils phagocytose (engulf) organisms by extending pseudopodia (projections of cytoplasmic membranes), which form a membranous vesicle (phagosome) around the organism. The phagosome fuses with neutrophil cytoplasmic granules forming a phagolysosome. In this enclosed compartment, killing occurs via two mechanisms. The first is an oxygen dependent response referred to as the respiratory burst. This involves the reduction of oxygen by an NADPH oxidase enzyme leading to the production of toxic oxygen metabolites such as singlet oxygen, hydrogen peroxide, and hydroxyl radicals. The second mechanism is oxygen independent. This uses highly toxic cationic proteins and enzymes such as myeloperoxidase and lysozyme, which are contained in the cytoplasmic granules. The phagocytic ingestion and killing of an organism is

TABLE 1.1

Toll-Like Receptors (TLRs) and the Microbial-Associated Molecular Patterns (MAMPs) That They Recognize

TLR	Cellular Location	MAMPs Recognized	Organisms the MAMPs Represent	Cell Types Expressing the TLR
TLR1	Cell surface	Lipopeptides	Bacteria	Monocytes and macrophages Some dendritic cells B-lymphocytes
TLR2	Cell surface	Glycolipids Lipopeptides Lipoproteins Lipoteichoic acid Zymosan	Bacteria Bacteria Bacteria Gram positive bacteria Fungi	Monocytes and macrophages Myeloid dendritic cells Mast cells
TLR3	Intracellular	Double-stranded RNA	Viruses	Dendritic cells B-lymphocytes
TLR4	Cell surface	Lipopolysaccharides	Gram negative bacteria	Monocytes and macrophages Neutrophils Myeloid dendritic cells B-lymphocytes Mast cells Intestinal epithelial cells
TLR5	Cell surface	Bacterial flagellin Profillin	Bacteria *Toxoplasma gondii*	Monocytes and macrophages Some dendritic cells Intestinal epithelial cells
TLR6	Cell surface	Diacyl lipopeptides	Mycoplasma	Monocytes and macrophages B-lymphocytes Mast cells
TLR7	Intracellular	Single-stranded RNA	Viruses	Monocytes and macrophages Plasmacytoid dendritic cells B-lymphocytes
TLR8	Intracellular	Single-stranded RNA	Viruses	Monocytes and macrophages Some dendritic cells Mast cells
TLR9	Intracellular	Unmethylated CpG oligonucleotide DNA	Viruses	Monocytes and macrophages Plasmacytoid dendritic cells B-lymphocytes
TLR10	-	Not known	-	-
TLR11	Intracellular	Profillin	*Toxoplasma gondii*	Monocytes and macrophages Liver cells Kidney Bladder epithelial cells

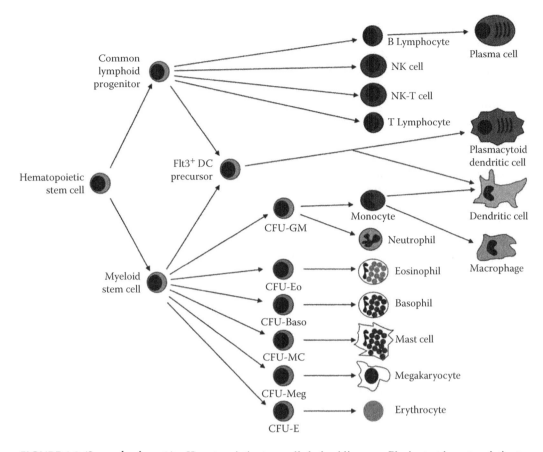

FIGURE 1.2 (See color insert.) Hematopoietic stem cell-derived lineages. Pluripotent hematopoietic stem cells differentiate in bone marrow into common lymphoid progenitor cells or myeloid stem cells. Lymphoid stem cells give rise to B-cell, T-cell, and natural killer (NK) cell lineages. Myeloid stem cells give rise to a second level of lineage-specific colony-forming unit (CFU) cells that go on to produce neutrophils and monocytes (granulocyte macrophage [GM]), eosinophils (Eo), basophils (Baso), mast cells (MC), megakaryocytes (Meg), and erythrocytes (E). Monocytes differentiate further into macrophages in peripheral tissue compartments. Dendritic cells (DC) appear to develop primarily from a dendritic cell precursor that is distinguished by its expression of the Fms-like tyrosine kinase 3 (Flt3) receptor. This precursor can derive from either lymphoid or myeloid stem cells, and gives rise to both classical and plasmacytoid dendritic cells. Classical dendritic cells can also derive from differentiation of monocytoid precursor cells. (Reprinted from *J. Allergy Clin. Immunol.*, 125, Chaplin, D. D. (2010) Overview of the immune response, S3–S23, with permission from Elsevier.)

more effective if it is opsonized (coated) with a specific antibody or complement. These molecules bind to Fc and complement receptors on the neutrophil, increasing adhesion between the organism and the phagocyte.

1.2.3.2 Monocytes and Macrophages

Monocytes circulate in the bloodstream; like neutrophils, they are attracted to sites of infection or tissue injury. After infiltration to the site of infection or injury, monocytes can differentiate into macrophages according to the cytokine milieu. Macrophages can be long lived—they can remain resident in tissues for prolonged periods of time. Scientists often give tissue-resident macrophages specific names such as microglia (within the central nervous system) and Kupffer cells (in the liver). Like neutrophils, macrophages have receptors for antibodies and complement, and as such, microorganisms coated with antibodies and/or complement enhance phagocytosis. Once ingested, the microorganisms are destroyed using the same mechanisms described for neutrophils. Macrophages can produce large numbers of cytokines, such as interleukin (IL)-12, IL-1, IL-6, tumor necrosis factor (TNF), and interferon (IFN)-γ. Since these cytokines affect the activity of other cell types, macrophages have an important regulatory role in immune responses.

1.2.3.3 Eosinophils

Large numbers of intracellular granules characterize eosinophils. These contain preformed proteins such as cationic proteins, eosinophil cationic proteins, and a wide range of cytokines, chemokines, and growth factors. Eosinophils are very important for host defense against helminthic parasites (i.e., worms). Eosinophils are only weakly phagocytic. Instead, they kill parasites by releasing cationic proteins and reactive oxygen metabolites into the extracellular fluid; they also secrete leukotrienes, prostaglandins, and various cytokines as well as intact membrane-bound organelles. These organelles express receptors, for example for cysteinyl-leukotrienes, and release their contents in the presence of receptor ligands.

1.2.3.4 Basophils and Mast Cells

Basophils and mast cells are morphologically similar to one another, although they come from distinct lineages. They have high affinity cell surface receptors for IgE (FcϵRI). Therefore, basophils and mast cells are the key initiators of immediate hypersensitivity responses and of the host response to helminthic parasites. They release histamine and other preformed mediators from their granules and they produce significant numbers of lipid mediators that stimulate tissue inflammation, edema, and smooth muscle contraction. Basophils can release substantial amounts of IL-4 and IL-13, although mast cells produce much less.

1.2.3.5 Natural Killer Cells

NK cells are large granular lymphocytes. They do not possess either the T-cell receptor (TCR) or surface immunoglobulin. NK cells can kill infected and malignant cells using a complex array of activating and inhibitory cell surface receptors (Jonsson and Yokoyama 2009). They can bind the Fc receptors that bind IgG (FcγR) and initiate antibody-dependent cellular cytotoxicity of the target cell. Alternatively, killer-activating receptors and killer-inhibitory receptors of NK cells may be used to bind target cells and shape the subsequent NK cell response. The killer-activating receptors recognize several different molecules present on the surface of all nucleated cells, whereas the killer-inhibitory receptors recognize major histocompatibility complex (MHC) class I molecules on all nucleated cells. If the killer-activating signal is released, then the NK cell destroys the target cell unless overridden by the killer-inhibitory signal upon recognition of the target cell MHC class I molecules. The lack of MHC class I receptor expression (due to infection or malignancy) ensures there is no inhibitory signal via the killer-inhibitory receptor and thus the NK cell will eliminate the cell with the abnormal phenotype. NK cells act by releasing the pore-forming molecule, perforin, and inserting it into the membrane of the target cell; subsequently the NK cell releases cytotoxic granzymes through the pore it has produced.

1.2.4 Soluble Factors Involved in Innate Immunity

The innate immune response involves the release of products such as complement (C), acute phase proteins, cytokines, reactive molecules such as those produced during the respiratory burst, and proinflammatory mediators such as leukotrienes and histamine. Other soluble factors are also involved in innate immunity.

1.2.4.1 Complement

The complement cascade can be activated in three different ways. The first is by antigen-antibody complexes, and this is referred to as the classic pathway. The second is by microbial cell walls, and this is referred to as the alternative pathway. The third is the lectin pathway, which involves the interaction of microbial carbohydrates with mannose-binding proteins in the plasma. Once the cascade is initiated, many immunologically active substances are released. Complement component C3, via its proteolytic-cleavage fragment C3b, binds to the surface of microorganisms, and this initiates phagocytosis of the microbe. The other complement fragments C3a, C4a, and C5a induce the release of inflammatory mediators from mast cells. C5a also attracts neutrophils to inflamed tissues. Complement components C5b, C6, C7, C8, and C9 finally form what is termed the membrane-attack complex, which perforates target cell membranes and thereby promotes death of the target cell.

1.2.4.2 Acute Phase Proteins

There are a number of acute phase proteins. Examples include C-reactive protein, serum amyloid A protein, and various proteinase inhibitors and coagulation proteins. They have different roles in host defense and in promoting the repair of damage caused during an immune response.

1.2.4.3 Cytokines

Cytokines are small molecular-weight proteins that act as soluble mediators; they are secreted by one cell to alter its own behavior or that of another cell. As such, they are regulators of immune responses, working within the immune system and between the immune system and other cellular networks within the body (Table 1.2). Cytokines are produced by all cells and have a wide variety of functions. They bind to specific cell surface receptors initiating intracellular signals. The biological effect depends on the cytokine and the cell involved, but normally cytokines affect cell activation, division, apoptosis, or movement. They act as autocrine, paracrine, or endocrine messengers. Cytokines produced by leukocytes that have effects mainly on other leukocytes are called interleukins. Cytokines that have a chemoattractant activity are called chemokines (see Section 1.3.2). Cytokines that cause differentiation and proliferation of stem cells are called colony-stimulating factors. Some cytokines also have a role in defense by interfering with viral replication; they are called interferons (IFNs).

1.3 ADHESION MOLECULES AND CHEMOKINES

1.3.1 ADHESION MOLECULES

Immune cells must be recruited from the bloodstream to sites of infection, inflammation, and injury, where they are subsequently activated. Their recruitment occurs through the interplay between cell-adhesion molecules and signaling molecules like cytokines and chemokines. Adhesion molecules are surface-bound molecules involved in cell-to-cell interactions. Their main function is in facilitating processes where close contact of cells is required (e.g., cell migration, phagocytosis, and cellular cytotoxicity). Adhesion molecule expression may be constitutive or may be induced by exposure to an inflammatory signal; such signals include cytokines, chemokines, microbial products (e.g., LPS), and activated complement proteins. Adhesion molecules are expressed on both leukocytes and endothelial cells enabling interaction between the two (Figure 1.3).

Based on structure and function, scientists classify adhesion molecules into several families (Table 1.3). The main families are the intercellular adhesion molecules, integrins, selectins, and cadherins (calcium-dependent adherins). In addition to adhesion molecules on leukocytes and the vascular endothelium, there are tissue-specific adhesion molecules called addressins. These target lymphocytes to a specific tissue location, such as the gut mucosa, lung, skin, peripheral lymph nodes, brain, and synovium.

TABLE 1.2

Selected Cytokines, Their Main Sources, and Their Functions

Cytokine	Main Sources	Main Function
Interleukin-1	Macrophages, endothelial cells	Immune activation
Interleukin-2	T-cells	Supports T-cell and NK cell function
Interleukin-3	T-cells	Growth of hemopoietic stem cells
Interleukin-4	T helper cells	T helper 2 lymphocyte growth factor; involved in IgE responses
Interleukin-5	T helper cells	Promotes growth of B-cells and eosinophils
Interleukin-6	Fibroblasts, macrophages	Promotes B-cell growth and antibody production. Induces acute phase responses
Interleukin-7	Stromal cells	Lymphocyte growth factor; important in the development of immature cells
Interleukin-8	Macrophages	Chemoattractant
Interleukin-10	CD4+ T-cells, monocytes, macrophages	Inhibits the production of interferon-α, interleukin-1, interleukin-6, and tumor necrosis factor-α, and stops antigen presentation
Interleukin-12	Monocytes, macrophages	Augments T helper 1 responses and induces interferon-γ
Interleukin-13	Activated T-cells	Stimulates B-cells
Interleukin-18	Macrophages, Kupffer cells	Augments T helper 1 responses and induces interferon-γ
Granulocyte colony stimulating factor	Monocytes	Promotes growth of myeloid cells
Monocyte colony stimulating factor	Monocytes	Promotes growth of macrophages
Granulocyte-macrophage colony stimulating factor	T-cells	Promotes growth of monomyelocytic cells
Interferon-α	Leukocytes	Immune activation and modulation; inhibits viral replication
Interferon-β	Fibroblasts	Immune activation and modulation
Interferon-γ	T-cells and natural killer cells	Immune activation and modulation
Tumor necrosis factor-α	Monocytes and macrophages	Stimulates generalized immune activation as well as tumor necrosis. Also known as cachectin
Tumor necrosis factor-β	T-cells	Stimulates immune activation; also known as lymphotoxin
Transforming growth factor-β	Platelets	Immunoinhibitory but stimulates connective tissue growth and collagen formation

1.3.2 CHEMOKINES

Chemokines are members of the cytokine family that play a key role in leukocyte migration (Table 1.4). They have a chemotactic (i.e., they attract cells) function and are named by the position of the two cysteine (C) residues compared with the other amino acids (X) within the peptide sequence. The two main subgroups are the CXC and CC chemokines, also known as α- and β-chemokines. Chemokines are produced by most cells upon stimulation with proinflammatory cytokines or bacterial products, while chemokine receptors are found on all leukocytes.

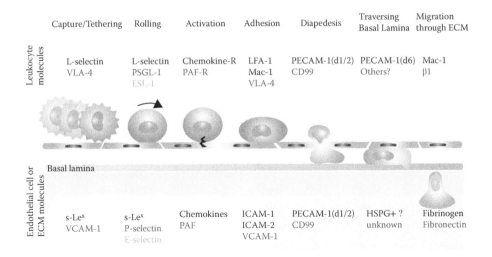

	Capture/Tethering	Rolling	Activation	Adhesion	Diapedesis	Traversing Basal Lamina	Migration through ECM
Leukocyte molecules	L-selectin VLA-4	L-selectin PSGL-1 ESL-1	Chemokine-R PAF-R	LFA-1 Mac-1 VLA-4	PECAM-1(d1/2) CD99	PECAM-1(d6) Others?	Mac-1 β1
Endothelial cell or ECM molecules	s-Le^x VCAM-1	s-Le^x P-selectin E-selectin	Chemokines PAF	ICAM-1 ICAM-2 VCAM-1	PECAM-1(d1/2) CD99	HSPG+ ? unknown	Fibrinogen Fibronectin

Basal lamina

FIGURE 1.3 (See color insert.) Leukocyte–endothelial cell interactions. Leukocyte recruitment is a multistep process involving initial attachment and rolling, tight binding, and transmigration across the vascular endothelium. Steps in leukocyte emigration are controlled by specific adhesion molecules on leukocytes and endothelial cells (see Table 1.3). The various steps of leukocyte emigration are depicted schematically here; interacting pairs of molecules are shown in the same color. The activated endothelium expresses selectins, which when binding to leukocytes initiate a rolling adhesion of leukocytes to the vessel's luminal wall. Integrins become activated by chemokines and bind to endothelial intercellular adhesion molecules (ICAMs) and vascular cell adhesion molecules (VCAMs), permitting a firmer adhesion. Transmigration across the vascular endothelium may be guided by further adhesive interactions, perhaps involving molecules such as platelet-endothelial cell adhesion molecule (PECAM)-1, which endothelial cells express at intercellular junctions. ESL, E-selectin ligand; HSPG, heparin sulfate proteoglycan; LFA, leukocyte function-associated antigen; PAF, platelet activating factor; PECAM-1 (d1/2), interaction involves immunoglobulin domains 1 and/or 2 of PECAM-1; PECAM-1 (d6), interaction involves immunoglobulin domain 6 of PECAM-1; PSGL, P-selectin glycoprotein ligand; s-Lex, sialyl-Lewisx carbohydrate antigen; VLA, very late (activation) antigen. (Reprinted with permission from Macmillan Publishers Ltd: Laboratory Investigation. Muller, W. A. (2002) *Lab. Invest.*, 82, 521–533, 2002.)

The effects of chemokines are more prolonged than other chemoattractants, such as complement activation products.

1.4 ADAPTIVE IMMUNITY

1.4.1 OVERVIEW

Adaptive immunity against pathogens involves the clonal expansion of antigen-specific T-lymphocytes that recognize their antigen presented on the surface of DCs in secondary lymphoid organs (e.g., lymph nodes). Once activated in this way, CD4$^+$ T-cells (these are helper T-cells) migrate to follicles within the lymphoid organ to provide help to B-cells in producing antibodies (i.e., antigen-specific immunoglobulins). They also migrate to peripheral sites of antigen exposure to attempt to eliminate incoming pathogens by ensuring the appropriate type of effector cell function. Type 1 helper T-cells (Th1 cells) produce IFN-γ that promotes clearance of viruses and intracellular bacteria, while type 2 helper T-cells (Th2 cells) produce IL-4, IL-5, and IL-13, which promote clearance of extracellular parasites. Once the source of antigen is eliminated, central memory and effector memory T-cells persist and provide immune surveillance in lymphoid organs and in peripheral nonlymphoid tissues enabling the host to react quickly if there is re-exposure to the pathogen.

TABLE 1.3

Adhesion Molecules, Their Ligands, and Cell and Tissue Distribution

Adhesion Molecule	Ligand	Cellular Distribution
Immunoglobulin superfamily	–	–
ICAM-1 (CD54)	LFA-1	Endothelial cells, monocytes, T- and B-cells, dendritic cells, keratinocytes, chondrocytes, epithelial cells
ICAM-2 (CD102)	LFA-1	Endothelial cells, monocytes, dendritic cells, subpopulations of lymphocytes
ICAM-3 (CD50)	LFA-1, Mac-1	Lymphocytes
VCAM-1 (CD106)	VLA-4	Endothelial cells, kidney epithelium, macrophages, dendritic cells, myoblasts, bone marrow fibroblasts
PECAM-1 (CD31)	$\alpha_v\beta_3$ integrin, HSPG	Platelets, T-cells, endothelial cells, monocytes, granulocytes
MAdCAM-1	$\alpha 4\beta 7$ integrin, L-selectin	Endothelial venules in mucosal lymph nodes
Selectin family	–	–
E-selectin (CD62E)	CD65, CD66	Endothelial cells
L-selectin (CD62L)	CD34, MAdCAM-1, GlyCAM-1, s-Le^x, Sgp200	Lymphocytes, neutrophils, monocytes
P-selectin (CD62P)	PSGL-1 (CD162)	Megakaryocytes, platelets, endothelial cells
Integrin family	–	–
VLA subfamily	–	–
VLA-1 to VLA-4 (CD49a,b,c,d/29)	Various molecules including laminin, fibronectin, collagen, VCAM-1	Endothelial cells, resting T-cells, monocytes, platelets, epithelial cells
VLA-5 (CD49e/29)	Fibronectin	Endothelial cells, monocytes, platelets
VLA-6 (CD49f/29)	Laminin	Endothelial cells, monocytes, platelets
Leucam subfamily	–	–
LFA-1 (CD11a/18)	ICAM-1, ICAM-2, ICAM-3	Leucocytes
Mac-1 (CD11b/18)	ICAM-1, fibrinogen, C3bi	Endothelial cells, megakaryocytes
Cytoadhesin subfamily	–	–
Vitronectin receptor (CD51/61)	Laminin, vitronectin, fibrinogen, fibronectin, von Willebrand factor, thrombospondin	Platelets, megakaryocytes

Abbreviations used: cluster of differentiation (CD); glycosylation-dependent cell adhesion molecule-1 (GlyCAM 1); intercellular adhesion molecule (ICAM); leukocyte function-associated antigen (LFA); macrophage-1 antigen (Mac-1); mucosal addressin cell adhesion molecule-1 (MAdCAM-1); platelet-endothelial cell adhesion molecule (PECAM); P-selectin glycoprotein ligand-1 (PSGL-1); sulfated glycoprotein 200 (Sgp200); vascular cell adhesion molecule (VCAM); very late (activation) antigen (VLA).

1.4.2 Antigen Presentation and Recognition by T-Lymphocytes

The basis for antigen recognition by T-cells is the presence of major histocompatibility (MHC) molecules. MHC molecules are cell-surface glycoproteins that bind peptide fragments of proteins that either have been synthesized within the cell (class I MHC molecules) or have been ingested by the cells (through phagocytosis) and proteolytically processed (class II MHC molecules). In humans, MHC molecules are referred to as human leukocyte antigens (HLAs).

TABLE 1.4

Selected Chemokines, Their Sources, and Their Target Cells

Chemokine	Other Name	Sources	Target Cells	Receptors
Monocyte chemoattractant protein-1 (MCP-1)	CCL2	Macrophages, fibroblasts, keratinocytes	Monocytes, dendritic cells, memory T-cells	CCR2
Macrophage inflammatory protein-1α (MIP-1α)	CCL3	Macrophages	Monocytes, neutrophils. T-cells	CCR1, CCR5
Macrophage inflammatory protein-1β (MIP-1β)	CCL4	Monocytes, macrophages, endothelial cells, T- and B-cells	Monocytes, CD8+ T-cells, natural killer cells	CCR5
Regulated on activation, normal T-cell expressed and secreted (RANTES)	CCL5	Platelets, T-cells	Monocytes, T-cells, eosinophils, basophils	CCR1, CCR3, CCR5
Interleukin-8	CXCL8	Macrophages	Neutrophils, other granulocytes, naive T-cells	CXCR1, CXCR2

1.4.2.1 Class I and II MHC Molecules

Class I MHC molecules (HLA-A, HLA-B, HLA-C) are composed of a variant chain that is noncovalently associated with a non-MHC invariant chain, β_2-microglobulin. Class II MHC molecules (HLA-DR, HLA-DQ, HLA-DP) are composed of an α-variant chain noncovalently associated with a β-variant chain. The role of the MHC molecules is to display ("present") antigenic peptides that enable the appropriate (i.e., the antigen-specific) T-cell receptors (TCRs) to bind them. Class I MHC molecules present endogenously derived antigenic peptides after antigen processing, such as viral epitopes, to CD8+ T-cells, whereas class II MHC molecules present exogenously derived antigenic peptides, such as soluble bacterial protein-derived antigenic peptides, to CD4+ T-cells. Class I MHC molecules are expressed on all nucleated cells. In contrast, class II MHC molecules are expressed constitutively on B-cells, DCs, monocytes, and macrophages, and can be induced on many additional cell types, including epithelial and endothelial cells after stimulation with IFN-γ.

1.4.2.2 HLA-Independent Presentation of Antigen

Class I and class II MHC molecules present protein-derived peptide antigens to T-cells. Some T-cells can recognize bacterial lipid antigens that are presented bound to CD1 molecules. Human CD1 molecules bind and present lipid and glycolipid antigens derived from mycobacteria for recognition by T-cells. Presentation requires uptake of antigen into endosomes, where it binds to CD1.

1.4.3 T-Lymphocytes

1.4.3.1 T-Cell Development

T-cells develop in the thymus where they undergo a process of selection that is aimed at ensuring the output of T-cells bearing rearranged αβ TCRs. This is a complex process. CD4−CD8− thymocytes undergo recombination activation gene (RAG)-mediated TCRβ gene rearrangement. Generation of a functional TCRβ-chain induces proliferation and CD4 and CD8 co-receptor expression. At this CD4$^+$CD8$^+$ double-positive stage, a second wave of RAG-dependent rearrangement occurs but now at the TCRα locus. This generates rearrangements that encode TCRα-chains that pair with the already available TCRβ-chains, and these TCRαβ pairs are tested for interactions with self-MHC molecules. Good affinity for self-MHC class II and class I molecules drives positive selection, upregulation of TCR surface expression, and commitment to the CD4 and CD8 T-cell lineages, respectively. Poor interactions with MHC result in cell death. Positively selected CD4 single-positive and CD8 single-positive thymocytes test their TCRs against a broad array of self-MHC–self-peptide ligands for self-reactivity, and those cells that recognize self are removed by apoptosis. Thus, thymic output is of CD4 or CD8 single-positive T-cells that should not exhibit self-reactivity. Most (90%–95%) circulating T-cells use the αβ TCR. The other 5%–10% use an alternate heterodimeric TCR composed of γ and δ chains. The γ and δ chains also assemble by means of RAG1/RAG2-mediated rearrangement of V, D (for the δ chain only), and J elements. However, only some γδ T-cells are generated in the thymus. Most are generated in an extrathymic compartment, and they populate the gut-associated lymphoid tissue.

1.4.3.2   T-Cell–Antigen Receptor Complex

The antigen-specific α and β chains of the TCR associate with invariant accessory chains that transduce signals when the TCR binds to antigen-MHC complexes. These accessory chains make up the CD3 complex, consisting of the transmembrane CD3γ, CD3δ, and CD3ε chains plus a largely intracytoplasmic homodimer of two CD3ζ chains. It appears that each TCR αβ pair associates with a CD3γε heterodimer, a CD3δε heterodimer, and a CD3ζ homodimer. Interaction of the TCR/CD3 complex with an antigenic peptide presented on an HLA molecule provides only a partial signal for cell activation. Full activation requires additional signals. These include interaction of a costimulatory molecule, such as CD28 on the T-cell and CD80 (also called B7.1) or CD86 (B7.2) on the APC, and cytokine/cytokine receptor interaction. Interaction of peptide-MHC with the TCR without the costimulatory signals can lead to prolonged nonresponsiveness of T-cells. Signaling events initiated as a consequence of the combination of signals mentioned above lead to T-cell activation, proliferation, and differentiation.

1.4.3.3   T-Cell Subpopulations

After exposure to antigen, both CD4$^+$ and CD8$^+$ T-cells differentiate into functionally distinct subsets determined by the precise environment that is present (Figure 1.4). For example, upon activation by TCR and cytokine mediated signaling, naive CD4$^+$ T-cells can differentiate into at least four major types of T helper (Th) cells, Th1, Th2, Th17, and inducible T regulatory (iTreg) cells, which play a critical role in orchestrating adaptive immune responses to various microorganisms. These subpopulations can be distinguished according to their cytokine-production profiles and their functions. Th1 cells secrete IFN-γ and are involved in combating intracellular bacteria and viruses. They do this by activating antiviral effector cells like macrophages and NK cells and by inducing proliferation of cytotoxic T-cells (CTLs). In contrast, Th2 cells, which produce cytokines like IL-4, IL-5 and IL-13, induce immunoglobulin E (IgE) and eosinophil-mediated destruction of helminths. Th17 cells are responsible for controlling extracellular bacteria and fungi through the production of IL-17a, IL-17f, and IL-22, while iTregs, together with naturally occurring T regulatory (nTreg) cells, are important in maintaining immune tolerance (see Section 1.7).

The major determinant for Thelper cell differentiation is the cytokine milieu at the time of antigen encounter. IL-12 and IFN-γ are two important cytokines driving Th1 differentiation. For Th2 differentiation, many cytokines including IL-4, IL-7, and thymic stromal lymphopoietin (TSLP) are involved. Transforming growth factor (TGF)-β induces Th17 differentiation in the presence of IL-6 but promotes iTreg cell differentiation when IL-2, but not IL-6, is also available. In general, more than one cytokine is required for differentiation to any particular phenotype and cytokines that promote differentiation to one lineage may suppress that to others.

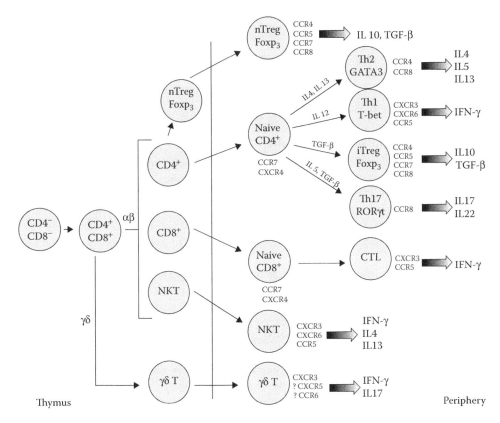

FIGURE 1.4 Development of T-cell subsets. CD4⁻CD8⁻ double-negative T-cells develop into CD4⁺, CD8⁺, NKT, and γδ T-cell subsets in the thymus. A subpopulation of CD4⁺ cells develops into natural Tregs (nTreg) in the thymus. After emigrating from the thymus, upon antigen presentation and activation, naive CD4⁺ cells further differentiate into effector subsets, such as Th1, Th2, inducible Tregs (iTregs), or Th17, in secondary lymphoid organs depending on the cytokine milieu. Encounter with antigen-loaded dendritic cells in secondary lymphoid organs and peripheral tissue also stimulates naive CD8⁺ cells to proliferate and differentiate into cytotoxic T-cells. Activation of different T-cell subsets results in the migration of the cells via chemokine receptors and subsequent production of the indicated cytokines. (Reprinted from Afshar, R., Medoff, B.D., and Luster, A.D., *Clin. Exp. Allergy* 38, 1847–1857, 2008. Copyright Wiley-VCH Verlag GmbH & Co. KGaA. With permission.)

Transcription factors are critical for helper T-cell differentiation and cytokine production. Cell fate determination in each lineage requires at least two types of transcription factors, the master regulators and the signal transducer and activator of transcription (STAT) proteins. The activity of the master regulators is controlled by their expression, whereas STAT proteins are activated by cytokines through posttranscriptional modifications such as phosphorylation. The essential transcription factors of Th lineages are T-bet/STAT4 (Th1), GATA-3/STAT5 (Th2), RORγt/STAT3 (Th17), and Foxp3/STAT5 (iTreg).

1.4.4 B-Lymphocytes

1.4.4.1 B-Cell Development

B-cells mature in the bone marrow and are defined by the immunoglobulins they produce. During B-cell maturation, rearrangements of the immunoglobulin heavy-chain and light-chain genes occur; these are independent of antigen exposure. However, the activation of mature B-cells into immunoglobulin-secreting B-cells or long-lived memory B-cells and then final differentiation into plasma cells depend on antigen interaction.

As with T-cells, the maturation and differentiation of B-cells is under the control of cytokines. IL-1 and IL-2 promote B-cell activation and growth; IL-4 induces switching to the IgE isotype; IL-5 enhances B-cell growth and differentiation; IL-6 increases the rate of secretion of Ig by B-cells; and IL-7 promotes proliferation of pre-B cells.

1.4.4.2   Establishing the B-Cell Repertoire

B-cell development follows a program of differential surface antigen expression and sequential heavy- and light-chain gene rearrangement. These processes result in the assembly of the antigen-binding component of the B-cell receptor. Like the TCR, the fully mature B-cell receptor includes additional transmembrane proteins designated Igα and Igβ that activate intracellular signals after receptor binding to antigen. B-cells also have a coreceptor complex consisting of CD19, CD81, and CD21 (complement receptor 2), which is activated by binding to the activated complement protein C3d.

Naive B-cells express IgM and IgD on their cell surfaces. As B-cells mature under the influence ("help") of Th cells, T-cell-derived cytokines induce isotype switching. This is the process of DNA rearrangement enabling the production of antibodies of different isotypes but the same antigenic specificity. T-cell-derived IL-10 causes switching to IgG1 and IgG3, IL-4 and IL-13 cause switching to IgE, and TGF-β causes switching to IgA. IFN-γ or other products of Th1 cells induce switching to IgG2. At the same time as B-cells undergo isotype switching, an active process produces mutations, apparently randomly, in the antigen-binding portions of the heavy and light chains. If the mutations result in increased affinity of antibody for the antigen, then the cell producing that antibody has a proliferative advantage in response to antigen and grows to dominate the pool of responding cells. The mutations and subsequent clonal expansion of mutated cells occurs in the germinal centers of secondary lymphoid tissues (e.g., lymph nodes).

1.4.4.3   T-Cell-Dependent B-Cell Responses

Antigens that activate T-cells and B-cells generate immunoglobulin responses in which T-cells provide "help" for the B-cells to mature. This maturation includes both induction of isotype switching, in which the cytokines derived from T-cells control the isotype of immunoglobulin produced, and activation of somatic mutation, as described in Section 1.4.4.2. The cellular interactions underlying T-cell help are driven by the specific antigen and take advantage of the ability of B-cells to serve as APCs. B-cells that capture their antigen through their membrane immunoglobulins can internalize the antigen and process it intracellularly for presentation on the cell surface using class II HLA proteins. Uptake of antigen induces increased class II expression and expression of CD80 and CD86. T-cells activated by this combination of costimulator and antigen–class II complex on the B-cell then signal reciprocally to the B-cell through the interaction of the T-cell CD40 ligand with B-cell CD40. Isotype switching and somatic mutations are strongly associated with the development of B-cell memory. Memory responses (i.e., rapid induction of high levels of high-affinity antibody after secondary antigen challenge) are characterized by production of IgG, IgA, or IgE.

1.4.4.4   T-Cell-Independent B-Cell Responses

B-cells can be activated without T-cell help. In the absence of costimulators (from T-cells), monomeric antigens are unable to activate B-cells. In contrast, polymeric antigens with a repeating structure are able to activate B-cells, probably because they can cross-link and cluster immunoglobulin molecules on the B-cell surface. T cell-independent antigens include bacterial LPS, and some polymeric polysaccharides and proteins. Somatic mutation does not occur in most T-cell–independent antibody responses, and as a consequence immune memory to T-cell–independent antigens is generally weak.

1.5 OTHER IMMUNE CELL TYPES

The distinction of a cell type being part of the innate or adaptive arm of the immune system is not clear for several cell types. These include B-1 cells, marginal zone (MZ) B-cells, certain subsets of γδ T-cells, CD8αα-expressing T-cells in the gut, mucosal-associated invariant T (MAIT) cells, and invariant natural killer T (iNKT) cells. Each of these cell types express an antigen-specific receptor, either a B-cell receptor or a TCR, that is generated by V(D)J recombination. However, the repertoire of specificities of these receptors is strongly limited, so that the cells react with a limited diversity of antigens. Hence, the receptors expressed by these so-called innate B- and T-lymphocytes bear similarities with the PRRs expressed by cells of the innate immune system. CD1d-dependent iNKT cells are a conserved subset of T-lymphocytes that recognize exogenous and endogenous glycolipid antigens presented by CD1d. They are considered innate lymphocytes. MAITs have emerged as a potentially important immunoregulatory cell type especially in mucosal systems. Although MAIT cells are present predominantly in the gut mucosa, they comprise 1% to 8% of circulating T-cells.

1.6 LYMPHOID TISSUE AND CELLULAR COMMUNICATION

It is obvious that cellular interactions are essential for a normally regulated, protective immune response. A major challenge for the immune system is to bring rare antigen-specific B-cells together with rare antigen-specific T-cells and antigen-charged APCs. The primary role of the secondary lymphoid tissues is to facilitate these interactions. Secondary lymphoid tissues include the lymph nodes, spleen, and tonsils. Generally, the secondary lymphoid tissues contain zones enriched for B-cells (follicles) and other zones enriched for T-cells. The B-cell zones contain clusters of follicular DCs that bind antigen-antibody complexes and provide sites adapted to efficient B-cell maturation, somatic mutation, and selection of high-affinity B-cells. The T-cell zones contain large numbers of DCs that are potent APCs for T-cell activation.

Recruitment of lymphocytes to secondary lymphoid tissues and also to peripheral tissue sites of microbial invasion is essential for intact host defense. The traffic of lymphocytes from blood to tissues occurs via a series of lymphocyte-endothelial interactions that are dependent on binding between lymphocyte surface molecules and endothelial molecules together with an interaction between tissue-specific chemokines and the corresponding chemokine receptors on lymphocytes. The combination of L-selectin (CD62L) and the chemokine receptor CCR7 expressed on naive T-cells allows them to migrate into secondary lymphoid tissues. Upon stimulation with antigen, naive T-cells become activated and acquire a new profile of tissue-specific homing receptors guiding them to peripheral tissues drained by the lymph node. Thus, T-cells activated in mesenteric lymph nodes or in Peyer's patches start to express the gut-homing intergrin α4β7 that binds to mucosal addressin cell adhesion molecule-1 (MAdCAM-1), which is only expressed on high-endothelial venules in gut-associated lymphoid tissues (GALT) and postcapillary venules in the gut. T-cells activated in cutaneous lymph nodes instead commence to express cutaneous lymphocyte-associated antigen that mediates localization to the skin via interaction with vascular ligand E-selectin. Moreover, the chemokine receptor CCR9 directs T-cells to the small intestinal mucosa, while CCR4 seems to attract T-cells to nongastrointestinal tissues, such as the skin and the lung.

1.7 REGULATORY T-CELLS AND IMMUNE TOLERANCE

CD4$^+$ regulatory T-cells (Treg) suppress effector T-cells and prevent or limit reactivity to self-antigens and to some pathogens, to blunt inflammation and to maintain antigen-specific T-cell homeostasis. Multiple populations of Treg cells have been reported, with natural Treg cells being the best characterized. Natural Treg cells constitutively express CD25 (IL-2-receptor α-chain), cytotoxic T lymphocyte-associated antigen 4 (CTLA-4 or CD152), and the forkhead/winged helix transcription factor Foxp3, which is a key control gene in their development and function. Thus, natural Treg cells are often defined as CD3⁺CD4⁺CD25⁺FoxP3⁺ cells. More recent studies demonstrated that Treg cells also express a low level of CD127 (IL-7 receptor) and are negative for CD49d (α-chain of intergrin VLA-4; α4β1). In addition to CD3⁺CD4⁺CD25⁺Foxp3⁺ Treg cells, other T-cells also possess regulatory activity. Most of these cells, which include IL-10–secreting T regulatory type 1 (Tr1) cells, TGFβ-secreting T helper 3 (Th3) cells, and certain CD4⁻CD8⁻ T cells and CD8⁺CD28⁻ T cells, are adaptively regulatory: that is, they acquire regulatory functions following specific antigenic stimulation in particular cytokine milieus. They therefore contrast with the naturally occurring CD4⁺Foxp3⁺ Treg cells, most of which are developmentally determined in the thymus as a distinct T-cell subpopulation that is specialized for suppressive function.

FURTHER READING

Overview of the Immune System

Chaplin DD (2010) Overview of the immune response. *J. Allergy Clin. Immunol.* 125, S3–23.

Parkin J and Cohen B (2001) An overview of the immune system. *Lancet.* 357, 1777–89.

Barriers

Daneman R and Rescigno M (2009) The gut immune barrier and the blood-brain barrier: Are they so different? *Immunity.* 31, 722–35.

Pattern Recognition Receptors

Akira S, Takeda K and Kaisho T (2001) Toll-like receptors: Critical proteins linking innate and acquired immunity. *Nat. Immunol.* 2, 675–80.

Kawai T and Akira S (2010) The role of pattern-recognition receptors in innate immunity: Update on Toll-like receptors. *Nat. Immunol.* 11, 373–84.

Kawai T and Akira S (2011) Toll-like receptors and their crosstalk with other innate receptors in infection and immunity. *Immunity.* 34, 637–50.

Mackey D and McFall AJ (2006) MAMPs and MIMPs: Proposed classifications for inducers of innate immunity. *Mol. Microbiol.* 61, 1365–71.

Neutrophils

Teng TS, Ji AL, Ji XY and Li YZ (2017) Neutrophils and immunity: From bactericidal action to being conquered. *J. Immunol. Res.* 2017, 9671604.

Witko-Sarsat V, Rieu P, Descamps-Latscha B, Lesavre P and Halbwachs-Mecarelli L (2000) Neutrophils: Molecules, functions and pathophysiological aspects. *Lab. Invest.* 80, 617–53.

Monocytes and Macrophages

Lauvau G, Loke P and Hohl TM (2015) Monocyte-mediated defense against bacteria, fungi, and parasites. *Semin. Immunol.* 27, 397–409.

Okabe Y and Medzhitov R (2016) Tissue biology perspective on macrophages. *Nat. Immunol.* 17, 9–17.

Eosinophils

Long H, Liao W, Wang L and Lu Q (2016) A player and coordinator: The versatile roles of eosinophils in the immune system. *Transfus. Med. Hemother.* 43, 96–108.

Ravin KA and Loy M (2016) The eosinophil in infection. *Clin. Rev. Allergy Immunol.* 50, 214–27.

Basophils

Karasuyama H and Yamanishi Y (2014) Basophils have emerged as a key player in immunity. *Curr. Opin. Immunol.* 31, 1–7.

Steiner M, Huber S, Harrer A and Himly M (2016) The evolution of human basophil biology from neglect towards understanding of their immune functions. *Biomed. Res Int.* 2016, 8232830.

Mast Cells

Mekori YA, Hershko AY, Frossi B, Mion F and Pucillo CE (2016) Integrating innate and adaptive immune cells: Mast cells as crossroads between regulatory and effector B and T cells. *Eur. J. Pharmacol.* 778, 84–9.

Morita H, Saito H, Matsumoto K and Nakae S (2016) Regulatory roles of mast cells in immune responses. *Semin. Immunopathol.* 38, 623–9.

Natural Killer Cells

Bendelac A, Savage PB and Teyton L (2007) The biology of NKT cells. *Annu. Rev. Immunol.* 25, 297–336.

Jonsson AH and Yokoyama WM (2009) Natural killer cell tolerance licensing and other mechanisms. *Adv. Immunol.* 101, 27–79.

Complement

Barnum SR (2017) Complement: A primer for the coming therapeutic revolution. *Pharmacol. Ther.* 172, 63–72.

Ghebrehiwet B (2016) The complement system: An evolution in progress. *F1000Res.* 5, 2840.

Adhesion and Adhesion Molecules

Muller WA (2002) Leukocyte-endothelial cell interactions in the inflammatory response. *Lab. Invest.* 82, 521–33.

Chemokines

Proudfoot AE and Uguccioni M (2016) Modulation of chemokine responses: Synergy and cooperativity. *Front. Immunol.* 7, 183.

Dendritic Cells

Patel VI and Metcalf JP (2016) Identification and characterization of human dendritic cell subsets in the steady state: A review of our current knowledge. *J. Investig. Med.* 64, 833–47.

MHC and Antigen Presentation

Bjorkman PJ (1997) MHC restriction in three dimensions: A view of T cell receptor/ligand interactions. *Cell.* 89, 167–70.

Bjorkman PJ, Saper MA, Samraoui B, Bennett WS, Strominger JL and Wiley DC (2005) Structure of the human class I histocompatibility antigen, HLA-A2. *J. Immunol.* 174, 6–19.

Brigl M and Brenner MB (2004) CD1: Antigen presentation and T cell function. *Annu. Rev. Immunol.* 22, 817–90.

Brown JH, Jardetzky TS, Gorga JC, Stern LJ, Urban RG, Strominger JL and Wiley DC (1993) Three-dimensional structure of the human class II histocompatibility antigen HLA-DR1. *Nature.* 364, 33–9.

Goldberg AC and Rizzo LV (2015) MHC structure and function–antigen presentation. Part 1. *Einstein (Sao Paulo).* 13, 153–6.

Klein J and Sato A (2000) The HLA system (in two parts). *N. Engl. J. Med.* 343, 702–9, 782–6.

T-Cell Development

Starr TK, Jameson SC and Hogquist KA (2003) Positive and negative selection of T cells. *Annu. Rev. Immunol.* 21, 139–76.

T-Cell Subsets

Afshar R, Medoff BD and Luster AD (2008) Allergic asthma: A tale of many T cells. *Clin. Exp. Allergy.* 38, 1847–57.

Fields PE, Kim ST and Flavell RA (2002) Cutting edge: Changes in histone acetylation at the IL-4 and IFN-gamma loci accompany Th1/Th2 differentiation. *J. Immunol.* 169, 647–50.

Lee DU, Agarwal S and Rao A (2002) Th2 lineage commitment and efficient IL-4 production involves extended demethylation of the IL-4 gene. *Immunity.* 16, 649–60.

Lee GR, Kim ST, Spilianakis CG, Fields PE and Flavell RA (2006) T helper cell differentiation: Regulation by cis elements and epigenetics. *Immunity.* 24, 369–79.

T-Cell Function

Seddon B and Zamoyska R (2003) Regulation of peripheral T-cell homeostasis by receptor signalling. *Curr. Opin. Immunol.* 15, 321–4.

Von Andrian UH and Mackay CR (2000) T-cell function and migration. Two sides of the same coin. *N. Engl. J. Med.* 343, 1020–34.

B-Cell Development and Function

Fillatreau S (2016) Regulatory roles of B cells in infectious diseases. *Clin. Exp. Rheumatol.* 34(4 Suppl. 98), 1–5.

Lebien TW and Tedder TF (2008) B lymphocytes: How they develop and function. *Blood.* 112, 1570–80.

Pupovac A and Good-Jacobson KL (2017) An antigen to remember: Regulation of B cell memory in health and disease. *Curr. Opin. Immunol.* 45, 89–96.

Lymphoid Tissues

Fu YX and Chaplin DD (1999) Development and maturation of secondary lymphoid tissues. *Annu. Rev. Immunol.* 17, 399–433.

Gasteiger G, Ataide M and Kastenmüller W (2016) Lymph node—An organ for T-cell activation and pathogen defense. *Immunol. Rev.* 271, 200–20.

Regulatory T-Cells

Fontenot JD, Gavin MA and Rudensky AY (2003) Foxp3 programs the development and function of CD4+CD25+ regulatory T cells. *Nat. Immunol.* 4, 330–6.

Janson PC, Winerdal ME, Marits P, Thorn M, Ohlsson R and Winqvist O. (2008) FOXP3 promoter demethylation reveals the committed Treg population in humans. *PLOS ONE* 3, e1612.

O'Garra A and Vieira P (2004) Regulatory T cells and mechanisms of immune system control. *Nat. Med.* 10, 801–5.

Sakaguchi, S. (2005) Naturally arising Foxp3-expressing CD25+CD4+ regulatory T cells in immunological tolerance to self and non-self. *Nat. Immunol.* 6, 345–52.

Sakaguchi S, Miyara M, Constantino CM and Hafler DA (2010) FOXP3+ regulatory T cells in the human immune system. *Nat. Rev. Immunol.* 10, 490–500.

2 The Gut-Associated Lymphoid System

Marie C. Lewis

CONTENTS

2.1 Introduction 19
2.2 Inductor Sites 19
    2.2.1 Peyer's Patches 20
    2.2.2 Isolated Lymphoid Follicles 21
    2.2.3 Mesenteric Lymph Nodes 21
2.3 Effector Sites 21
    2.3.1 Immunoglobulin A 22
2.4 Oral Tolerance 22
2.5 Antigen Presentation in Nonlymphoid Tissues 24
2.6 Immune Cell Trafficking 25
2.7 The Intestinal Microbiota and Immune Development 26
2.8 Conclusions 27
References 27

2.1 INTRODUCTION

The gut-associated lymphoid tissue, or GALT, comprises the largest immune organ in the mammal and functions as part of both the adaptive and innate arms of the immune system. Since it is the primary interface between the host and outside world, and it is continually exposed to the intestinal microbiota and to food antigens, it must make essential decisions regarding effector function and tolerance to maintain the health of the host.[1] As the primary site of antigen exposure, it also forms the first line of defense against invading pathogens. Tight cell junction (TCJ) proteins hold the cells of the epithelial layer together. TCJs include zonula occludens (ZO)-1, which control the permeability of the intestinal barrier. A layer of glycoprotein, called mucin, protects the epithelium. Goblet cells within the capillary endothelium secrete mucin.[2] GALT has a critical role in the development of systemic immunity and functions as an inductor site to other effector prime naive T- and B-lymphocytes that develop into effector cells. These activated cells then migrate to effector sites throughout the host to protect against immune challenge.

2.2 INDUCTOR SITES

GALT is composed of several areas of organized secondary lymphoid architecture called Peyer's patches (PPs), isolated lymphoid follicles (ILFs), and mesenteric lymph nodes (MLNs), and these primarily function as inductor sites (Figure 2.1). At these sites, professional antigen presenting cells, including dendritic cells (DCs), prime naïve T-cells, and T-cells, induce B-cell clonal expansion and IgA class switching in an antigen-specific manner. Once activated, T-cells and B-cells migrate to effector sites throughout the host, but primarily to more diffuse areas within the intestinal lamina propria where they exhibit the effector or suppressor function.[3]

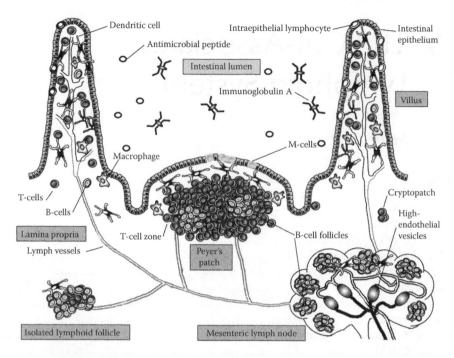

FIGURE 2.1   Organization of the gut-associated lymphoid tissue

2.2.1   Peyer's Patches

The first detailed description of Peyer's patches was by Johann Conrad Peyer in 1677. He defined them as aggregated, oval areas of lymphoid follicles located along the antimesenteric side of the gut and curbed by follicle-associated epithelium (FAE). This specialized epithelium contains microfold cells (M-cells) through which intact luminal antigen is transported to the underlying immune cells.[4] In order to aid this translocation, the subepithelial myofibroblast sheath is absent from the FAE, glycosylation patterns of the brush border glycocalyx are altered, mucus production is low,[5] and the basal lamina is considerably more porous than elsewhere in the gut.[6] The number of PPs varies according to species, and humans exhibit a great deal of individual variation.[7] However, more than half of the approximately 250 PPs are contained within the distal ileum, and in humans the number peaks between 15 and 25 years of age before declining with the age of the host.[8] During fetal development localized mesenchymal organizing centers composed of various chemokines and chemokine receptors initiate PP development by recruiting a specialized CD4+ T-cell subset to the locale.[9] These lymphocyte tissue inducer (LTi) CD4+ cells promote a cascade of lymphotoxin alpha/beta heterodimer (LTα/β) receptor-dependent events, which result in upregulation of the integrins intercellular adhesion molecule-1 (ICAM-1) and vascular cell adhesion molecule (VCAM-1) on any stromal cells nearby. Consequently, positive feedback recruits both T-cells and B-cells to the area, as well as LTi cells. The cell clusters then reorganize to form the early PPs.[9] These rudimentary PPs contain distinct corpora of T-cells and B-cells, but are void of germinal centers, which develop rapidly in response to antigenic stimulation following birth and continue to expand until around 35 years.[10] During this early stage, the number of resident B-cells and T-cells expands to fill the available space and become the T-cell zones and germinal centers at the core of each follicle, thus generating the distinctive domed appearance of PPs.[4] It is these germinal centers that promote the T-cell–B-cell interactions necessary for the diversification of immunoglobulin genes through class-switch DNA recombination and somatic hypermutation.[11] The process is facilitated by the plentiful supply of the IgA-inducing cytokine transforming growth factor beta (TGF-β) within PPs.[12] The expansion of IgA-expressing B-cell populations and their differentiation into IgA-secreting plasma cells is then promoted by the abundance of interleukin-4 (IL-4), IL-6, and IL-10 within the microenvironment.[13] With age, the proliferative capacity of lymphocytes within the PPs declines, and the number of T-cells in the interfollicular and parafollicular regions,[14] and Ig-A plasma cells,[15] start to fall.

2.2.2 ISOLATED LYMPHOID FOLLICLES

Isolated lymphoid follicles (ILFs) are small B-cell-rich areas of lymphoid tissue dispersed throughout the small and large intestine. In contrast to the PPs and MLNs, which are present at birth in nascent form, ILFs develop postnatally in response to stimulation from the intestinal microbiota, also in a LTα1β2-LTbR–dependent manner,[16] and in adults their numbers increase distally as the concentration of the microbiota intensifies.[17] Cryptopatch precursors, which contain small numbers of B220+ B-cells, CD3+ T-cells, and CD11c+ DCs, initiate ILFs. Like PPs, ILFs develop following the recruitment of LTi cells to the area[18] and contain CD4+ T-cells, macrophages, and other DC phenotypes, but in much lower numbers than in PPs.[19] As development continues, further B-cells are recruited to create the germinal centers and architecture forms, which is reminiscent of that seen in PPs, including the presence of M-cells.[20] It is this architecture which suggests that ILFs are inductor as opposed to effector sites. There is evidence to suggest that as well as being the precursors to ILFs, intestinal cryptopatches are also the primary site of the development of progenitor T9-cells for extrathymic descendants, which later migrate to the intraepithelial leukocyte (IEL) compartments.[21]

2.2.3 MESENTERIC LYMPH NODES

Professional antigen-presenting cells, particularly DCs, sequester antigen that enters the PPs and ILFs through M-cells. The antigen-presenting cells then migrate via the lymph to the MLNs and subsequently drain the PPs and ILFs, where they educate naive T-cells. MLNs are the interface between the gut and the peripheral immune system and first appear during fetal development in much the same way as PPs.[9] The well-defined architecture of the MLNs consists of multiple, distinct masses of fibrovascular tissue surrounded by lymph-filled sinuses enclosed by a capsule.[22] The cortical region contains mainly B-cells, but also macrophages and FDCs, arranged into densely packed lymphoid follicles. A deep paracortical region contains mainly T-cells and DCs, while the medullary region contains cellular cords of macrophages and plasma cells. A constant stream of lymph travels from the gut to the subcapsular sinus over each lobule of the MLNs via a single afferent lymphatic vessel. Lymph then spreads throughout the apex of the lobule and flows down the sides through transverse sinuses and into the medullary sinuses.[23] Lymph drains from all the lobules into a single efferent lymphatic vessel that exits the node at the hilus and carries the lymph, which now contains immune cells and secreted immunoglobulins, to the venous blood system.[24] Each lobule is potentially exposed to different antigens, APCs, and inflammatory mediators because each afferent vessel drains from a different point in the gut. As a result, diverse levels of immunological activity can occur within each lobule of the same lymph node, which gives rise to their irregular appearance.[25]

As well as being the major site of lymphocyte activation, MLNs are also the location where lymphocytes are primed to express surface molecules, which drive gut-specific homing. These molecules, specifically CCR9 and the integrin α4β7, facilitate cell entry into effector sites where they undergo further maturation and differentiation.

2.3 EFFECTOR SITES

Once APCs have interacted with naive lymphocytes in the PPs, ILFs, and MLNs, the now primed cells migrate through the periphery and other effector sites before the majority home to the LP and epithelium of the gut mucosa. These are the primary effector sites of the GALT since most cells that enter are antigen mature, phenotypic memory cells that are primed to respond to foreign antigens.

The LP is composed of CD4$^+$ T-helper cells (50%), cytotoxic CD8$^+$ T-cells (30%), DC subsets, macrophages, and IgA-plasma cells, but also contains some IgG- and IgM-plasma cells[26] and many small groups of specialized immune cells, which are less well characterized. The epithelial layer contains dispersed intraepithelial leukocytes (IELs), a large population of mainly CD8$^+$CD45RO$^+$ (activated) cells, which are functionally distinct from other peripheral T-cells. This population varies between species and disease states, but IELs are relatively abundant, with approximately one lymphocyte for every five epithelial cells.[19] These cells express the integrin αEβ7, which is important in sequestering them within the epithelium,[27] and also generally express either αβ T-cell receptors and drive IgA synthesis, or γδT-cell receptors and appear to be involved in both active immune responses and tolerance.[26]

2.3.1 IMMUNOGLOBULIN A

A primary characteristic of the intestinal humoral immune system is immunoglobulin A (IgA), which is secreted by IgA-plasmoblasts and serves as a component of the first line of defense against intestinal pathogens. It is the most abundant immunoglobulin in the mammalian intestine, and several grams are secreted daily into the gut lumen.[28] IgA functions primarily by blocking toxins and pathogens from adhering to the intestinal epithelium by direct recognition of receptor-binding domains.[29] Indeed a deficiency in IgA synthesis, caused by impaired B-cell development or poor B-cell response to T-cell signals, results in frequent intestinal infections.[30] IgA is a dimer bound by a J-chain and attached to an epithelial cell membrane receptor, the secretory component (SC). Once the plasma cells have migrated to an effector site, the SC functions to allow IgA to transverse the mucosal epithelium via the polymeric Ig receptor (pIgR) and enter the gut lumen, thus becoming secretory IgA (SIgA).[31] IgA eliminates microbial pathogens which have breached the intestinal epithelium by either transporting them back into the lumen using this pIgR,[11] or by promoting phagocytosis by DCs and neutrophils through activation of their IgA surface receptor FcαRI (CD89).[32]

Once within the intestinal lumen, in addition to its neutralizing effects, IgA appears to eliminate bacterial pathogens through a series of actions including agglutination, entrapment in the mucus, and clearance through peristalsis.[33] IgA-mediated cross-linking through polyvalent surface antigens results in the formation of macroscopic clumps of bacteria in a process called agglutination. This process facilitates the removal of the pathogens by host peristalsis. Although agglutination is not thought to have a direct detrimental effect on virulence, recent evidence suggests that some agglutinating antibodies may have immediate effects on bacterial-membrane integrity and gene expression, depending on the specific epitope recognized.[34] IgA has the capacity to entrap bacterial pathogens in the mucus layer overlying intestinal epithelia *in vitro* in both mouse[35] and rabbit[36] model systems. This activity was enhanced by the presence of SC because the oligosaccharide side chains associated with mucus. However, the molecular composition of mucus is complex, and the specific molecular interactions involved remain to be defined.[29] In specific cases, the binding of IgA to the O antigen of some bacterial species has been demonstrated to directly affect the bacterial type 3 secretion systems necessary for entry into intestinal epithelial cells. In addition, IgA binding also resulted in a partial reduction in the bacterial membrane potential and intracellular ATP levels.[37] Although IgA has been shown to exhibit quenching capacity in the above studies, it is unclear to what extent immune exclusion contributes to protective immunity outside model systems, especially with regard to viral agents.

2.4 ORAL TOLERANCE

Innocuous antigens, such as food proteins and molecular components of the commensal bacteria, constantly stimulate the intestinal immune system.[20] It is essential that these immune responses are either tolerogenic or anergic in nature to prevent the development of acute inflammation. Failure to induce tolerance against the intestinal microbiota can trigger inflammatory bowel diseases including ulcerative colitis and Crohn's disease,[38] while generating protective immunity against food protein results in allergy and celiac disease.[39] The process of negative selection eliminates developing self-reactive T-cells and B-cells from the repertoire. In addition, high-affinity self-reactive T-cells that escape this process often become natural regulatory T-cells (T-regs) with suppressor function. However, both these processes require that the specific antigen to which the T-cells are responding is expressed thymically.[20] Since most antigenic exposure in the gut originates orally, or from the microbiota, thymic expression does not occur, and an additional level of tolerance induction is required.

Oral tolerance describes the process by which active immune responses to orally administered antigen are suppressed. The generation of oral tolerance is complex and the mechanisms are not fully understood. However, in humans it appears to be initiated, in part, by a population of specialized DCs expressing CD103 surface molecules located in the intestinal LP. Following migration to the MLNs, these DCs have a unique capacity to induce the expression of the surface molecules on T-cells necessary for intestinal homing (CCR9 and $\alpha_4\beta_7$),[40] and strongly promote the induction of IL-10–secreting T-regs expressing the transcription factor forkhead box p3 (Foxp3).[41] Both these functions are dependent on dietary retinoic acid, a cofactor for TGF-β, which is essential for the differentiation of naive CD4$^+$ T-cells into Foxp3$^+$ T-regs.[41] Upon returning to the LP Foxp3$^+$ T-regs, which now have the capacity to suppress active immune responses in an antigen-specific manner, undergo secondary expansion and promote immune homeostasis.[20] It is thought that this secondary expansion may be driven by DC-like cells within the LP which express the chemokine receptor CX3CR. These cells are loaded with antigen, but do not migrate to MLNs and do not have naive T-cell priming capacity. They appear to sample antigen directly from the lumen without disrupting intestinal integrity through the production of transepithelial dendrites.[42] As mentioned above, a subpopulation of CD8$^+$ IELs could also play a crucial role in oral tolerance induction. In both *in vivo* and *in vitro* mouse models, loss of function, or total abolition of these $\gamma\delta$T-cells, can result in failure to generate oral tolerance and even the loss of established tolerance. Moreover, oral tolerance to specific antigens can be generated in naive recipients through adoptive transfer of splenic $\gamma\delta$T-cells from tolerant mice.[43] However, these poorly understood cells defined loosely by their $\gamma\delta$ receptor (as opposed to $\alpha\beta$) also appear to have a major role in protecting the host against pathogens through the spontaneous production of the inflammatory cytokines interferon gamma (IFN-γ) and IL-17 and the induction of IgE secretion from plasmoblasts, and can also trigger lysis in infected cells.[44] Since these initial findings, it has become apparent that $\gamma\delta$T-cell is an umbrella term describing a unique group of divergent cells that seem to bridge the gap between innate and adaptive immunity during both homeostatic and infection conditions, and that more evidence is required to understand the mechanisms of their contribution to oral tolerance.

Oral tolerance thus far has described processes that originate in effector sites. However, orally administered inert particles appear to localize preferentially to the organized tissues of the GALT rather than the villous LP.[45] The role of M-cell–mediated antigen uptake in the generation of oral tolerance is not clear. On the one hand, the development of oral tolerance can be reduced by inhibiting PP development during gestation,[46] while on the other hand, tolerance can be induced in spliced-out intestinal loops irrespective of the presence of PPs.[47] Moreover, specifically targeting M-cell facilitated uptake of ovalbumin (OVA) can induce tolerance through increased production of TGF-β1 and IL-10 from a considerably increased population of OVA-specific Foxp3$^+$ Tregs.[48]

To add to the uncertainty encompassing the mechanisms behind oral tolerance, it appears the dose and timing of the initial exposure to orally derived antigen is pivotal to its development. A single dose of antigen can produce lymphocyte anergy in a mouse model, while continuous low-dose exposure has been shown to drive the differentiation of activated T-cells towards a regulatory phenotype.[49] However, in a rat model, a daily dose of OVA administered by gavage resulted in the production of OVA-specific IgG and IgE, and delayed-type hypersensitivity developed within 42 days.[50] With regard to timing, oral tolerance can be generated by feeding mice antigen at 7–10 days, whereas feeding during the first few days of life induced allergic sensitization.[51]

This is inconsistent with the results of epidemiological studies, which linked delayed introduction of wheat[52] and peanuts[53] with the increased prevalence of allergy to these specific antigens. There is currently insufficient high-quality evidence to support weaning strategies for potentially allergic foods, especially for high allergy risk infants, since results have been somewhat contradictory. However, emerging evidence is consistent with exposure to an adequate dose of antigen occurring during a critical window in early life being necessary to generate an immune system that responds appropriately to that food.[54]

Tolerance to food proteins and tolerance to gut bacteria differ in the additional induction of systemic tolerance, and therefore probably occur through different mechanisms. Unresponsiveness to food proteins is thought to be induced primarily via the small intestine and in addition to local effects, this type of tolerance extends to the systemic immune system. However, unresponsiveness to gut bacteria appears colonic in origin and does not lead to attenuated systemic responses.[20] On balance, gut homeostasis is fundamental to host health, and it is likely that it is not reliant on a single mechanism, rather a series of processes, and the weight of the contribution of each process to functioning oral tolerance may differ between individuals, strains, and species.

2.5 ANTIGEN PRESENTATION IN NONLYMPHOID TISSUES

Prior to the appearance of the mammals, organized lymphoid structures including PPs and MLNs were effectively absent. This invites questions regarding where immune responses are initiated in fish, reptiles, and birds. In addition, do remnants of this ancient process still occur in mammals, and if so, do they have a significant role in immune development and function? A clue to extra-lymphoid tissue antigen presentation may lie with a subset of DCs isolated from human intestinal lamina propria that possess both macrophage and dendritic cell markers (CD14 and CD209 respectively). Under *in vitro* conditions, these cells have the capacity to expand naive T-cell populations to the same extent as monocyte-derived DCs,[55] which are known to activate naive T-cells in the MLNs. Similarly, a subpopulation of murine DCs which also express macrophage surface markers (F4/80) as well as DC markers (CD11c/CD11b) can induce naive T-cell differentiation towards inflammatory T-cell phenotypes (Th1 and Th17), and naive B-cells to become IgA-secreting plasma cells.[56] In both these cases, although the DCs were isolated from the LP, it is unclear whether they acquired the ability to activate naive T-cells prior to the potential to migrate to the MLNs, or if this ability was an artefact of the *in vitro* setting, or indeed if the main function of these unusual cells is to activate naive T-cells outside the organized lymphoid tissues.

Although much of the research focuses on professional antigen presentation by DCs, there is evidence for the importance of nonprofessional antigen presentation by stromal cells outside the lymph nodes in rodents, pigs, and humans.[57–61] *In vitro* experiments show that initial T-cell polarization in lymph nodes, which results in the expression of signature cytokines and transcription factors, can be reversed in response to conditions within the immediate environment.[5] In addition, immature DCs isolated from jejunal LP in the pig are capable of triggering unprimed T-cell responses in addition to their phagocytitic activities.[62] This is reflected *in vivo* by the observation of preferential interactions between T-cells and several DC subsets in the jejunal mucosa in both pigs and mice. Capillary endothelium constitutively expresses MHCII molecules in both these species[58,60] and of particular interest is the 3-way interactions that occur between T-cells, DCs, and capillary endothelial cells in the jejunal LP in neonates, but not in normal adult intestines.[63] This may be because the neonatal immune system is poory developed and the presence of organized lymphoid architecture is limited, or these interactions could be involved in driving tolerance, which is preferentially generated in the nonatal gut. Nonetheless, these findings do question whether the intestinal mucosa is limited to effector activity, and the importance of classical lymphoid tissue-limited naive T-cell activation during critical stages in the development of an effective immune system.

2.6   IMMUNE CELL TRAFFICKING

Complex signals present in both inductive and effector sites are essential in driving immune development and generating an appropriate balance between effector function and tolerance, thus avoiding the development of inflammatory and autoimmune diseases, and susceptibility to enteric infection. Since the activation of naive lymphocytes appears to occur primarily in organized lymphoid tissues, and effector function usually occurs at distant peripheral sites, cell trafficking and migration are clearly an essential component of appropriate immune function.

Initial understanding of the patterns of lymphocyte migration was established in rats and sheep.[64,65] In these studies, naive T-cells appeared to drain *from* the MLN since they were found primarily in the efferent lymph, whereas memory T-cells appeared to drain *to* the MLN since they were found in the afferent lymph. Divergent pathways of lymphocyte migration were suggested, where naive T-cells are restricted to blood and lymph, while effector memory T-cells (T_{EM}), capable of rapid cytokine production and kinetics, can in addition migrate through nonlymphoid tissues. The expression of specific surface molecules by T_{EM} cells is thought to permit access to those nonlymphoid tissues that express the corresponding ligand.[66] For example, under normal conditions, T_{EM} cells that express the chemokine receptor CCR9 and the integrin $\alpha_4\beta_7$ have been shown to preferentially home to intestinal capillary endothelium, which expresses the corresponding ligands CCL25, and the mucosal addressin MAdCAM.[67] Since these surface molecules are absent from naive T-cells, it has been suggested that they have no means by which to access nonlymphoid tissue. This paradigm of divergent migratory pathways of naive and T_{EM} cells was honed by the later discovery of high endothelial venules (HEVs). These are specialized postcapillary vessels found exclusively in lymph nodes and other secondary lymphoid tissues,[68] which allow blood-borne naive T-cells to navigate the lymph node/efferent lymph/blood pathway. Molecules on the surface of naive T-cells, including CCR7 and CD62L, permit homing to HEVs, which express the corresponding ligands, peripheral lymph node addressin (PNAd), and CCL21, respectively.[69] Since HEVs are absent from nonlymphoid tissues, it follows that naive T-cells are unable to transverse nonlymphoid endothelium and reside in or migrate through these tissues. Central memory T-cells (T_{CM}), with generally reduced functional capacity, appear to follow similar nonlymphoid tissue trafficking routes to naive T-cells since they also express the HEV-specific homing molecules CCR7 and CD62L at elevated levels.[70]

Despite the paradigm of differential T-cell trafficking, it is becoming increasingly apparent that naive T-cells do access nonlymphoid tissues in numbers approaching those of T_{EM} cells. Studies in fetal sheep[71] and mice[72] demonstrate that naive T-cells circulate throughout the nonlymphoid tissue, and this appears to be a function of the parenchymal tissue itself, as opposed to phenotypic or functional property of the naive T-cells. It would seem that the fetus is not a special case, and phenotypically naive CD8[+73] and CD4[+74–76] T-cells have been detected in the lungs of normal adult mice and rats respectively, and naive CD4+ T-cells have additionally been isolated from the thymic medulla of rats. Furthermore, naive CD4+ and CD8+ T-cells have been shown to reside in the human lung[77] and in the aortic wall of mice,[78] and naive CD8+ T-cells have also been identified in the mouse liver.[73] Histological techniques were used to demonstrate that these naive T-cells were resident in the nonlymphoid tissues, and not simply blood-borne contaminants.[74–76,79] The overall numbers of naive cells in these nonlymphoid tissues are on par with T_{EM} cell numbers, approximating 1.5% of the naive T-cell population, and therefore represent a significant reservoir. It is important to note that in all these cases, T-cell activation status was determined by phenotype and not function, and there is some evidence consistent with memory cells reverting to appear phenotypically naive, especially with regard to the expression of some surface molecules including CD44, CD62L, and the CD45 isoforms.[80,81] However, other surface molecules which define the memory phenotype, including CD11a, are stable.[79,82] For this reason, care should be taken while determining T-cell activation status if using phenotype alone due to the complexity of the issue, and multiple surface markers should be assessed. A further study took this point into consideration and isolated phenotypically and functionally naive CD4+ and CD8+ T-cells from various murine parenchymal tissues including the gut, brain, pancreas, lung, kidney, liver, skin, and testis, at numbers between 20% and 80% of the total T-cell population in these tissues.[79] If, as the evidence suggests, naive T-cells are circulating throughout nonlymphoid tissues including the gut, the purpose remains a mystery.

2.7 THE INTESTINAL MICROBIOTA AND IMMUNE DEVELOPMENT

Until recently, most microbe-host studies have focused on pathogen-host interactions since these relationships often result in clear phenotypes and promote understanding of the pathogenesis of infectious disease. However, in recent years it has become increasingly apparent that the commensal microorganisms that reside in both the lumen and mucosa of the intestinal tract have more influence over host health and disease than previously thought.[83] Consequently, the study of the intestinal microbiota and its interaction with the host is rapidly becoming an area of intense scrutiny. Bacteria are the predominant group within the microbiota, accounting for more than 100 different species[84] and somewhere in the region of 1,000 times more genes than the human genome,[85] thus providing enormous potential for host-microbe interactions. In addition, pathogens must outcompete the well-adapted and entrenched resident microbes for the resources available within metabolic and physical niches to colonize the gut and cause disease.

In addition to its crucial role in nutrient absorption[86] and biosynthesis of vitamins[87] and its influence in complex processes such as lipid[88] and carbohydrate[89] metabolism by the host, and tissue repair[90] and angiogenesis,[91] the gut microbiota has a direct role in the development and function of humoral and cellular immune systems.[92,93] In turn, host immunity has evolved to maintain the symbiotic relationship in order to promote homeostasis.[94] Evidence for the pivotal role of the gut microbiota in driving immune development is based on the study of germ-free (GF) animals, which have markedly altered gut morphology and physiology and fail to generate competent and effective immune defenses.[95] Specifically, such animals present with underdeveloped PP, ILF, and MLN architecture at inductor sites, which encompass inadequate germinal centers containing considerably reduced APC, B-cell, and CD4+ and CD8+ T-cell populations.[96] Additionally, the effector site LP contains limited numbers of myeloid and lymphoid cell phenotypes, especially IgA plasmablasts,[97] and the generation of oral tolerance is variable.[98] The fundamental role of the microbiota in immune development is demonstrated by the addition of microbes to previously germ-free animals in which immunity is restored,[99,100] albeit in an anomalous manner. It appears that different bacterial members of the microbiota drive the expansion of specific arms of the immune system. For example, monocolonization of germ-free mice with segmented filamentous bacteria (SFB) has been demonstrated to increase IgA-plasmablast and lymphoid cell populations in both the ileal and caecal LP.[99] Similarly, *Bacteroides fragilis* has been shown to induce anti-inflammatory cytokine production exclusively from an increased population of Foxp3+ Tregs.[101] However, this is somewhat of an oversimplification and multifactorial disorders associated with immune dysregulation, including obesity, diabetes,[102] and inflammatory bowel disease,[103] often correlate with a shift in the microbial population as opposed to the presence or absence of a single species, although the direction of causality is not always clear. What is clear is that the pattern of colonization of bacterial species in the neonatal intestine represents a programming event[104,105] that shapes the developing immune system and can therefore have long-term consequences for immune health. A range of noncommunicable twenty-first-century conditions, such as allergy and inflammation, can be traced back to early immune development, which was disrupted by alterations in the pattern of microbial colonization caused by, amongst other factors, early antibiotic use, caesarean delivery, and formula feeding. These early-life events have the potential to transform microbial allies into potential liabilities that stimulate an immune system that responds erroneously to harmless antigen while failing to protect against dangerous pathogens.

2.8 CONCLUSIONS

The gut-associated lymphoid system is the largest immune organ in the body and appears essential to both enteric and systemic protection against dangerous pathogens, while remaining tolerant to harmless antigens. It first appears during embryogenesis, but its expansion into a fully functioning protective immune system that responds appropriately to each encountered challenge occurs following birth and in response to antigenic stimulation, primarily from the intestinal microbiota but also from food antigens. The incidence of noncommunicable, allergic, and inflammatory diseases is rapidly increasing and current evidence suggests these conditions can originate from aberrant immune development in early life. However, developing effective preventative strategies to tackle these conditions will continue to present difficulties, while understanding of the fundamental mechanisms underlying effective gut-associated lymphoid system function remains limited.

REFERENCES

1. Wershil BK, Furuta GT. 4. Gastrointestinal mucosal immunity. *Journal of Allergy and Clinical Immunology* 2008, **121**(2 Suppl): S380–S383.
2. Turner JR. Intestinal mucosal barrier function in health and disease. *Nature Reviews Immunology* 2009, **9**: 799–809.
3. Yan Z, Wang J-B, Gong S-S, Huang X. Cell proliferation in the endolymphatic sac in situ after the rat Waldeyer ring equivalent immunostimulation. *Laryngoscope* 2003, **113**: 1609–1614.
4. Jung C, Hugot J-P, Barreau F. Peyer's patches: The immune sensors of the intestine. *International Journal of Inflammation* 2010, **2010**: 823710.
5. Sierro F, Pringault E, Assman PS, Kraehenbuhl JP, Debard N. Transient expression of M-cell phenotype by enterocyte-like cells of the follicle-associated epithelium of mouse Peyer's patches. *Gastroenterology* 2000, **119**: 734–743.
6. Takeuchi T, Gonda T. Distribution of the pores of epithelial basement membrane in the rat small intestine. *Journal of Veterinary Medical Science / Japanese Society of Veterinary Science* 2004, **66**: 695–700.
7. Van Kruiningen HJ, West AB, Freda BJ, Holmes KA. Distribution of Peyer's patches in the distal ileum. *Inflammatory Bowel Diseases* 2002, **8**: 180–185.
8. Cornes JS. Number, size, and distribution of Peyer's patches in the human small intestine: Part I The development of Peyer's patches. *Gut* 1965, **6**: 225–229.
9. Mebius RE, Rennert P, Weissman IL. Developing lymph nodes collect CD4+CD3–LTβ+ cells that can differentiate to APC, NK cells, and follicular cells but not T or B cells. *Immunity* 1997, **7**: 493–504.
10. Van Kruiningen HJ, Ganley LM, Freda BJ. The role of Peyer's patches in the age-related incidence of Crohn's disease. *Journal of Clinical Gastroenterology* 1997, **25**: 470–475.
11. Cerutti A, Rescigno M. The biology of intestinal immunoglobulin A responses. *Immunity* 2008, **28**: 740–750.
12. Gonnella PA, Chen Y, Inobe J, Komagata Y, Quartulli M, Weiner HL. In situ immune response in gut-associated lymphoid tissue (GALT) following oral antigen in TCR-transgenic mice. *Journal of Immunology* 1998, **160**: 4708–4718.
13. Sato A, Hashiguchi M, Toda E, Iwasaki A, Hachimura S, Kaminogawa S. CD11b+ Peyer's patch dendritic cells secrete IL-6 and induce IgA secretion from naive B cells. *Journal of Immunology* 2003, **171**: 3684–3690.
14. Schmucker DL. Intestinal mucosal immunosenescence in rats. *Experimental Gerontology* 2002, **37**: 197–203.
15. Taylor LD, Daniels CK, Schmucker DL. Aging compromises gastrointestinal mucosal immune-response in the rhesus-monkey. *Immunology* 1992, **75**: 614–618.
16. Lorenz RG, Chaplin DD, McDonald KG, McDonough JS, Newberry RD. Isolated lymphoid follicle formation is inducible and dependent upon lymphotoxin-sufficient B lymphocytes, lymphotoxin beta receptor, and TNF receptor I function. *Journal of Immunology* 2003, **170**: 5475–5482.
17. Knoop KA, Newberry RD. Isolated lymphoid follicles are dynamic reservoirs for the induction of intestinal IgA. *Frontiers in Immunology* 2012, **3**: 84.
18. Lügering A, Ross M, Sieker M, Heidemann J, Williams IR, Domschke W et al. CCR6 identifies lymphoid tissue inducer cells within cryptopatches. *Clinical and Experimental Immunology* 2010, **160**: 440–449.

19. Pabst O, Herbrand H, Worbs T, Friedrichsen M, Yan S, Hoffmann MW et al. Cryptopatches and isolated lymphoid follicles: Dynamic lymphoid tissues dispensable for the generation of intraepithelial lymphocytes. *European Journal of Immunology* 2005, **35**: 98–107.

20. Pabst O, Mowat AM. Oral tolerance to food protein. *Mucosal Immunology* 2012, **5**: 232–239.

21. Mebius RE. Organogenesis of lymphoid tissues. *Nature Reviews Immunology* 2003, **3**: 292–303.

22. von Andrian UH, Mempel TR. Homing and cellular traffic in lymph nodes. *Nature Reviews Immunology* 2003, **3**: 867–878.

23. Willard-Mack CL. Normal structure, function, and histology of lymph nodes. *Toxicologic Pathology* 2006, **34**: 409–424.

24. Randolph GJ, Angeli V, Swartz MA. Dendritic-cell trafficking to lymph nodes through lymphatic vessels. *Nature Reviews Immunology* 2005, **5**: 617–628.

25. Saintemarie G, Peng FS, Belisle C. Overall architecture and pattern of lymph-flow in the rat lymph-node. *American Journal of Anatomy* 1982, **164**: 275–309.

26. Ruth MR, Field CJ. The immune modifying effects of amino acids on gut-associated lymphoid tissue. *Journal of Animal Science and Biotechnology* 2013, **4**: 27.

27. Macdonald TT. The mucosal immune system. *Parasite Immunology* 2003, **25**: 235–246.

28. Pabst O. New concepts in the generation and functions of IgA. *Nature Reviews Immunology* 2012, **12**: 821–832.

29. Mantis NJ, Rol N, Corthesy B. Secretory IgA's complex roles in immunity and mucosal homeostasis in the gut. *Mucosal Immunology* 2011, **4**: 603–611.

30. Agarwal S, Mayer L. Pathogenesis and treatment of gastrointestinal disease in antibody deficiency syndromes. *Journal of Allergy and Clinical Immunology* 2009, **124**: 658–664.

31. Pabst R. The anatomical basis for the immune function of the gut. *Anatomny and Embryology* 1987, **176**: 135–144.

32. Wehrli M, Cortinas-Elizondo F, Hlushchuk R, Daudel F, Villiger PM, Miescher S et al. Human IgA Fc receptor FcalphaRI (CD89) triggers different forms of neutrophil death depending on the inflammatory microenvironment. *Journal of Immunology* 2014, **193**: 5649–5659.

33. Mantis NJ, Forbes SJ. Secretory IgA: Arresting microbial pathogens at epithelial borders. *Immunological Investigations* 2010, **39**: 383–406.

34. Forbes SJ, Martinelli D, Hsieh C, Ault JG, Marko M, Mannella CA et al. Association of a protective monoclonal IgA with the O antigen of Salmonella enterica serovar Typhimurium impacts type 3 secretion and outer membrane integrity. *Infection and Immunity* 2012, **80**: 2454–2463.

35. Phalipon A, Cardona A, Kraehenbuhl J-P, Edelman L, Sansonetti PJ, Corthésy B. Secretory component: A new role in secretory IgA-mediated immune exclusion in vivo. *Immunity* 2002, **17**: 107–115.

36. Boullier S, Tanguy M, Kadaoui KA, Caubet C, Sansonetti P, Corthésy B et al. Secretory IgA-mediated neutralization of Shigella flexneri prevents intestinal tissue destruction by down-regulating inflammatory circuits. *Journal of Immunology* 2009, **183**: 5879–5885.

37. Forbes SJ, Bumpus T, McCarthy EA, Corthesy B, Mantis NJ. Transient suppression of Shigella flexner type 3 secretion by a protective O-antigen-specific monoclonal IgA. *MBio* 2011, **2**: e00042–e00011.

38. Molodecky NA, Soon IS, Rabi DM, Ghali WA, Ferris M, Chernoff G et al. Increasing incidence and prevalence of the inflammatory bowel diseases with time, based on systematic review. *Gastroenterology* 2012, **142**: 46–54. e42.

39. Meresse B, Ripoche J, Heyman M, Cerf-Bensussan N. Celiac disease: From oral tolerance to intestinal inflammation, autoimmunity and lymphomagenesis. *Mucosal Immunology* 2008, **2**: 8–23.

40. Jaensson E, Uronen-Hansson H, Pabst O, Eksteen B, Tian J, Coombes JL et al. Small intestinal CD103+ dendritic cells display unique functional properties that are conserved between mice and humans. *Journal of Experimental Medicine* 2008, **205**: 2139–2149.

41. Sun CM, Hall JA, Blank RB, Bouladoux N, Oukka M, Mora JR et al. Small intestine lamina propria dendritic cells promote de novo generation of Foxp3 T reg cells via retinoic acid. *Journal of Experimental Medicine* 2007, **204**: 1775–1785.

42. Niess JH, Brand S, Gu X, Landsman L, Jung S, McCormick BA et al. CX3CR1-mediated dendritic cell access to the intestinal lumen and bacterial clearance. *Science* 2005, **307**: 254–258.

43. Mengel J, Cardillo F, Aroeira LS, Williams O, Russo M, Vaz NM. Anti-γδ T cell antibody blocks the induction and maintenance of oral tolerance to ovalbumin in mice. *Immunology Letters* 1995, **48**: 97–102.

44. Paul S, Singh AK, Shilpi, Lal G. Phenotypic and functional plasticity of gamma-delta (gammadelta) T cells in inflammation and tolerance. *International Reviews of Immunology* 2014, **33**: 537–558.

45. Shreedhar VK, Kelsall BL, Neutra MR. Cholera toxin induces migration of dendritic cells from the subepithelial dome region to T- and B-cell areas of Peyer's patches. *Infection and Immunity* 2003, **71**: 504–509.
46. Fujihashi K, Dohi T, Rennert PD, Yamamoto M, Koga T, Kiyono H et al. Peyer's patches are required for oral tolerance to proteins. *Proceedings of the National Academy of Sciences of the United States of America* 2001, **98**: 3310–3315.
47. Kraus TA, Brimnes J, Muong C, Liu JH, Moran TM, Tappenden KA et al. Induction of mucosal tolerance in Peyer's patch-deficient, ligated small bowel loops. *Journal of Clinical Investigation* 2005, **115**: 2234–2243.
48. Suzuki H, Sekine S, Kataoka K, Pascual DW, Maddaloni M, Kobayashi R et al. Ovalbumin-protein sigma 1 M-cell targeting facilitates oral tolerance with reduction of antigen-specific CD4+ T cells. *Gastroenterology* 2008, **135**: 917–925.
49. Burks AW, Laubach S, Jones SM. Oral tolerance, food allergy, and immunotherapy: Implications for future treatment. *Journal of Allergy and Clinical Immunology* 2008, **121**: 1344–1350.
50. Knippels LM, Penninks AH, Spanhaak S, Houben GF. Oral sensitization to food proteins: A Brown Norway rat model. *Clinical and Experimental Allergy* 1998, **28**: 368–375.
51. Strobel S, Ferguson A. Immune responses to fed protein antigens in mice. 3. Systemic tolerance or priming is related to age at which antigen is first encountered. *Pediatric Research* 1984, **18**: 588–594.
52. Poole JA, Barriga K, Leung DY, Hoffman M, Eisenbarth GS, Rewers M et al. Timing of initial exposure to cereal grains and the risk of wheat allergy. *Pediatrics* 2006, **117**: 2175–2182.
53. Fox AT, Sasieni P, du Toit G, Syed H, Lack G. Household peanut consumption as a risk factor for the development of peanut allergy. *Journal of Allergy and Clinical Immunology* 2009, **123**: 417–423.
54. Vickery BP, Scurlock AM, Jones SM, Burks AW. Mechanisms of immune tolerance relevant to food allergy. *Journal of Allergy and Clinical Immunology* 2011, **127**: 576–584.
55. Kamada N, Hisamatsu T, Honda H, Kobayashi T, Chinen H, Kitazume MT et al. Human CD14+ macrophages in intestinal lamina propria exhibit potent antigen-presenting ability. *Journal of Immunology* 2009, **183**: 1724–1731.
56. Uematsu S, Fujimoto K, Jang MH, Yang BG, Jung YJ, Nishiyama M et al. Regulation of humoral and cellular gut immunity by lamina propria dendritic cells expressing Toll-like receptor 5. *Nature Immunology* 2008, **9**: 769–776.
57. Bland PW. Antigen presentation by gut epithelial cells: Secretion by rat enterocytes of a factor with IL-1-like activity. *Advances in Experimental Medicine and Biology* 1987, **216A**: 219–225.
58. Haraldsen G, Sollid LM, Bakke O, Farstad IN, Kvale D, Molberg et al. Major histocompatibility complex class II-dependent antigen presentation by human intestinal endothelial cells. *Gastroenterology* 1998, **114**: 649–656.
59. Saada JI, Pinchuk IV, Barrera CA, Adegboyega PA, Suarez G, Mifflin RC et al. Subepithelial myofibroblasts are novel nonprofessional APCs in the human colonic mucosa. *Journal of Immunology* 2006, **177**: 5968–5979.
60. Wilson AD, Haverson K, Southgate K, Bland PW, Stokes CR, Bailey M. Expression of major histocompatibility complex class II antigens on normal porcine intestinal endothelium. *Immunology* 1996, **88**: 98–103.
61. Zimmer KP, Buning J, Weber P, Kaiserlian D, Strobel S. Modulation of antigen trafficking to MHC class II-positive late endosomes of enterocytes. *Gastroenterology* 2000, **118**: 128–137.
62. Haverson K, Singha S, Stokes CR, Bailey M. Professional and non-professional antigen-presenting cells in the porcine small intestine. *Immunology* 2000, **101**: 492–500.
63. Inman CF, Singha S, Lewis M, Bradley B, Stokes C, Bailey M. Dendritic cells interact with CD4 T cells in intestinal mucosa. *Journal of Leukocyte Biology* 2010, **88**: 571–578.
64. Mackay CR, Marston WL, Dudler L. Naive and memory T cells show distinct pathways of lymphocyte recirculation. *Journal of Experimental Medicine* 1990, **171**: 801–817.
65. Gowans JL, Knight EJ. The route of re-circulation of lymphocytes in the rat. *Proceedings of the Royal Society of London. Series B, Biological Sciences* 1964, **159**: 257–282.
66. Manes TD, Pober JS. Polarized granzyme release is required for antigen-driven transendothelial migration of human effector memory CD4 T cells. *Journal of Immunology* 2014, **193**: 5809–5815.
67. Hart AL, Ng SC, Mann E, Al-Hassi HO, Bernardo D, Knight SC. Homing of immune cells: Role in homeostasis and intestinal inflammation. *Inflammatory Bowel Diseases* 2010, **16**: 1969–1977.
68. Weninger W, Carlsen HS, Goodarzi M, Moazed F, Crowley MA, Baekkevold ES et al. Naive T cell recruitment to nonlymphoid tissues: A role for endothelium-expressed CC chemokine ligand 21 in autoimmune disease and lymphoid neogenesis. *Journal of Immunology* 2003, **170**: 4638–4648.

69. Miyasaka M, Tanaka T. Lymphocyte trafficking across high endothelial venules: Dogmas and enigmas. *Nature Reviews Immunology* 2004, **4**: 360–370.

70. Bingaman AW, Patke DS, Mane VR, Ahmadzadeh M, Ndejembi M, Bartlett ST et al. Novel phenotypes and migratory properties distinguish memory CD4 T cell subsets in lymphoid and lung tissue. *European Journal of Immunology* 2005, **35**: 3173–3186.

71. Kimpton WG, Washington EA, Cahill RN. Virgin alpha beta and gamma delta T cells recirculate extensively through peripheral tissues and skin during normal development of the fetal immune system. *International Immunology* 1995, **7**: 1567–1577.

72. Alferink J, Tafuri A, Vestweber D, Hallmann R, Hammerling GJ, Arnold B. Control of neonatal tolerance to tissue antigens by peripheral T cell trafficking. *Science* 1998, **282**: 1338–1341.

73. Bertolino P, Bowen DG, McCaughan GW, Fazekas de St Groth B. Antigen-specific primary activation of CD8+ T cells within the liver. *Journal of Immunology* 2001, **166**: 5430–5438.

74. Luettig B, Kaiser M, Bode U, Bell EB, Sparshott SM, Bette M et al. Naive and memory T cells migrate in comparable numbers through the normal rat lung: Only effector T cells accumulate and proliferate in the lamina propria of the bronchi. *American Journal of Respiratory Cell and Molecular Biology* 2001, **25**: 69–77.

75. Westermann J, Smith T, Peters U, Tschernig T, Pabst R, Steinhoff G et al. Both activated and nonactivated leukocytes from the periphery continuously enter the thymic medulla of adult rats: Phenotypes, sources and magnitude of traffic. *European Journal of Immunology* 1996, **26**: 1866–1874.

76. Luettig B, Pape L, Bode U, Bell EB, Sparshott SM, Wagner S et al. Naive and memory T lymphocytes migrate in comparable numbers through normal rat liver: Activated T cells accumulate in the periportal field. *Journal of Immunology* 1999, **163**: 4300–4307.

77. Saltini C, Kirby M, Trapnell BC, Tamura N, Crystal RG. Biased accumulation of T lymphocytes with "memory"-type CD45 leukocyte common antigen gene expression on the epithelial surface of the human lung. *Journal of Experimental Medicine* 1990, **171**: 1123–1140.

78. Galkina E, Kadl A, Sanders J, Varughese D, Sarembock IJ, Ley K. Lymphocyte recruitment into the aortic wall before and during development of atherosclerosis is partially L-selectin dependent. *Journal of Experimental Medicine* 2006, **203**: 1273–1282.

79. Cose S, Brammer C, Khanna KM, Masopust D, Lefrancois L. Evidence that a significant number of naive T cells enter non-lymphoid organs as part of a normal migratory pathway. *European Journal of Immunology* 2006, **36**: 1423–1433.

80. Bell EB, Sparshott SM. Interconversion of CD45R subsets of CD4 T cells in vivo. *Nature* 1990, **348**: 163–166.

81. Tough DF, Sprent J. Turnover of naive-and memory-phenotype T cells. *Journal of Experimental Medicine* 1994, **179**: 1127–1135.

82. Masopust D, Vezys V, Marzo AL, Lefrancois L. Preferential localization of effector memory cells in nonlymphoid tissue. *Science* 2001, **291**: 2413–2417.

83. Kelly D, King T, Aminov R. Importance of microbial colonization of the gut in early life to the development of immunity. *Mutation Research* 2007, **622**: 58–69.

84. Eckburg PB, Bik EM, Bernstein CN, Purdom E, Dethlefsen L, Sargent M et al. Diversity of the human intestinal microbial flora. *Science* 2005, **308**: 1635–1638.

85. Hsiao WW, Metz C, Singh DP, Roth J. The microbes of the intestine: An introduction to their metabolic and signaling capabilities. *Endocrinology and Metabolism Clinics of North America* 2008, **37**: 857–871.

86. Hooper LV, Midtvedt T, Gordon JI. How host-microbial interactions shape the nutrient environment of the mammalian intestine. *Annual Reviews in Nutrition* 2002, **22**: 283–307.

87. Hooper LV, Bry L, Falk PG, Gordon JI. Host-microbial symbiosis in the mammalian intestine: Exploring an internal ecosystem. *Bioessays* 1998, **20**: 336–343.

88. Backhed F, Ding H, Wang T, Hooper LV, Koh GY, Nagy A et al. The gut microbiota as an environmental factor that regulates fat storage. *Proceedings of the National Academy of Sciences USA* 2004, **101**: 15718–15723.

89. Underwood MA, Salzman NH, Bennett SH, Barman M, Mills DA, Marcobal A et al. A randomized placebo-controlled comparison of 2 prebiotic/probiotic combinations in preterm infants: Impact on weight gain, intestinal microbiota, and fecal short-chain fatty acids. *Journal of Pediatric Gastroenterology and Nutrition* 2009, **48**: 216–225.

90. Thompson-Chagoyán OC, Maldonado J, Gil A. Aetiology of inflammatory bowel disease (IBD): Role of intestinal microbiota and gut-associated lymphoid tissue immune response. *Clinical Nutrition* 2005, **24**: 339–352.

91. Bjorkholm B, Bok CM, Lundin A, Rafter J, Hibberd ML, Pettersson S. Intestinal microbiota regulate xenobiotic metabolism in the liver. *PLOS ONE* 2009, **4**: e6958.

92. Carter PB, Pollard M. Host responses to normal microbial flora in germ-free mice. *Journal of the Reticuloendothelial Society* 1971, **9**: 580–587.

93. Kabat AM, Srinivasan N, Maloy KJ. Modulation of immune development and function by intestinal microbiota. *Trends in Immunology* 2014, **35**: 507–517.

94. Round JL, Mazmanian SK. The gut microbiome shapes intestinal immune responses during health and disease. *Nature Reviews Immunology* 2009, **9**: 313–323.

95. Butler JE, Weber P, Sinkora M, Sun J, Ford SJ, Christenson RK. Antibody repertoire development in fetal and neonatal piglets. II. Characterization of heavy chain complementarity-determining region 3 diversity in the developing fetus. *Journal of Immunology* 2000, **165**: 6999–7010.

96. Cebra JJ, Periwal SB, Lee G, Lee F, Shroff KE. Development and maintenance of the gut-associated lymphoid tissue (GALT): The roles of enteric bacteria and viruses. *Developmental Immunology* 1998, **6**: 13–18.

97. Cebra JJ. Influences of microbiota on intestinal immune system development. *American Journal of Clinical Nutrition* 1999, **69**: 1046S–1051S.

98. Walton KLW, Galanko JA, Balfour Sartor R, Fisher NC. T cell-mediated oral tolerance is intact in germ-free mice. *Clinical and Experimental Immunology* 2006, **143**: 503–512.

99. Meyerholz DK, Stabel TJ, Cheville NF. Segmented filamentous bacteria interact with intraepithelial mononuclear cells. *Infection and Immunity* 2002, **70**: 3277–3280.

100. Talham GL, Jiang HQ, Bos NA, Cebra JJ. Segmented filamentous bacteria are potent stimuli of a physiologically normal state of the murine gut mucosal immune system. *Infection and Immunity* 1999, **67**: 1992–2000.

101. Round JL, Mazmanian SK. Inducible Foxp3+ regulatory T-cell development by a commensal bacterium of the intestinal microbiota. *Proceedings of the National Academy of Sciences USA* 2010, **107**: 12204–12209.

102. Duca FA, Sakar Y, Lepage P, Devime F, Langelier B, Dore J et al. Replication of obesity and associated signaling pathways through transfer of microbiota from obese-prone rats. *Diabetes* 2014, **63**: 1624–1636.

103. Huttenhower C, Kostic Aleksandar D, Xavier Ramnik J. Inflammatory bowel disease as a model for translating the microbiome. *Immunity* 2014, **40**: 843–854.

104. Munyaka PM, Kahfipour E, Ghia J-E. External influence of early childhood establishment of gut microbiota and subsequent health implications. *Frontiers in Pediatrics* 2014, **2**: 109.

105. Cox Laura M, Yamanishi S, Sohn J, Alekseyenko Alexander V, Leung Jacqueline M, Cho I et al. Altering the intestinal microbiota during a critical developmental window has lasting metabolic consequences. *Cell* 2014, **158**: 705–721.

3 Obesity, Immunity, and Infection

Scott D. Neidich and Melinda A. Beck

CONTENTS

3.1 Introduction 33
3.2 Direct Effects of Obesity on the Immune System 33
    3.2.1 Adipose Tissue as an Immunomodulatory Endocrine Organ 33
        3.2.1.1 Leptin 34
        3.2.1.2 Adiponectin 35
        3.2.1.3 Other Adipokines 35
    3.2.2 Innate Immune Cells: Local and Systemic Effects of Obesity 36
    3.2.3 Adaptive Immunity: Local and Systemic Effects of Obesity 36
3.3 Obesity and Infection 37
    3.3.1 Viral Infection in Obesity 37
    3.3.2 Bacterial Infection in Obesity 38
3.4 The Infectious Origin of Obesity Hypothesis 39
    3.4.1 Evidence Supporting the Hypothesis 39
    3.4.2 Arguments Against the Hypothesis 39
3.5 Summary 39
References 40

3.1 INTRODUCTION

Obesity is characterized by excessive adiposity resulting from prolonged positive energy balance due to consuming more calories than expended. Obesity is an increasingly prevalent problem with 13% of the worldwide population[1,2] (35% in the United States) classified as obese in 2014. Most individuals now live in countries where obesity is responsible for more deaths than underweight. This chapter will discuss the current literature on the impact of obesity on the immune system, both within the adipose tissue and systemically. It will discuss obesity's interactions with specific diseases, chiefly influenza. Lastly, the chapter will explore the relatively new idea that obesity may have an infectious origin.

3.2 DIRECT EFFECTS OF OBESITY ON THE IMMUNE SYSTEM

3.2.1 ADIPOSE TISSUE AS AN IMMUNOMODULATORY ENDOCRINE ORGAN

An excess amount of adipose tissue characterizes obesity; the tissue is composed largely of adipocytes but also includes macrophages, lymphocytes, fibroblasts, and endothelial cells. Obesity occurs through a combination of increased adipocyte number and increased adipocyte size. Immune cell infiltration into adipose tissue is also increased in obesity, further adding to the adipose-tissue cell population. Many of the infiltrating immune cells have a proinflammatory phenotype, secreting cytokines that promote insulin resistance.[3] Thus there is a link between adipose tissue inflammation and metabolic disturbances. Although the exact timing and series of events leading to adipose tissue inflammation in obese humans is not known, work in animal models has demonstrated that, as fat deposition increases, neutrophils enter the adipose tissue first, followed by macrophages, and then T- and B-cells.[4] How much of the inflammation is induced by feeding a high fat diet vs. the actual obesity is unresolved, although it is likely that both contribute to the inflammation. Indeed, mice that gain weight on a chow diet develop similar immune dysfunction (i.e., inflammation) compared with mice fed a high fat diet.[5] In addition to increased cellular infiltrate into the adipose tissue in obesity, the phenotype of the immune cells alters. Macrophages of the M2 type (anti-inflammatory, tissue repairing) become more M1 like (proinflammatory). T-cells infiltrating the adipose tissue display activation markers,[6] and regulatory T-cell populations increase within adipose tissue.

In addition to their role as a storage site for lipids, adipocytes secrete a variety of factors, termed adipokines, including leptin and adiponectin. Although leptin and adiponectin are primarily known for their roles in regulating food intake, body weight, and metabolism, it has recently become clear that they also play a role in regulation of T-cell function.

3.2.1.1 Leptin

Leptin is a 16 kD adipokine secreted directly in proportion to adipocyte mass, therefore increasing adiposity leads to increasing leptin levels. Leptin is a well-known regulator of food intake and energy expenditure, and more recently has received attention for its proinflammatory characteristics[7]. Leptin concentration in the blood of healthy-weight adults typically ranges between 10 and 20 ng/mL and can fluctuate within this range based on food intake. In obesity, however, the greater mass of adipose tissue alters serum leptin levels. Studies show average leptin concentration to be more than 30 ng/mL in obese humans, and the concentration is less responsive to dietary fluctuations.[8] Obese humans are in a constant state of hyperleptinemia. Hyperleptinemia promotes T-cell effector function while inhibiting T regulatory cell function,[9] whereas absence of leptin prevents T-cell activation. B-cells live longer in the presence of leptin and are more resistant to apoptosis.[10] Dendritic cells activate T-cells more strongly in the presence of leptin,[11] and natural killer (NK) cells experience greater metabolism and are more cytotoxic with increasing leptin.[12]

Leptin induces effects within a cell by binding to a specific cellular receptor, the OB-R leptin receptor, and transducing a signal into the cell through protein kinase and phosphatase cascades.[13] Which cascades activate determines the cell's response to leptin; however, it is important to note that multiple isoforms of the OB receptor exist, each with specific effects. Expression of different OB receptors on different cell types allow each type to respond distinctly from others.[10] There are six known isoforms including four short, cell-embedded isoforms (OB-Ra, OB-Rc, OB-Rd, and OB-Rf) and one long, cell-embedded isoform (OB-Rb), and even one that is not attached to the cell surface (OB-Re). The soluble OB-Re regulates circulating concentrations of leptin and cannot transduce signals into the cell. The short form leptin receptors are involved in leptin transport throughout the body, although researchers have observed some intracellular signaling from these isoforms. The long-chain OB-Rb is the primary receptor involved in signal transduction, thanks to an enlarged intracellular region of the protein which facilitates signal transduction through multiple kinase pathways reviewed in Allison and Myers.[14]

OB-Rb appears not only on the cells of the hypothalamus involved in satiety signaling, but in multiple immune cell populations including T- and B-cells, dendritic cells, monocytes, neutrophils, macrophages, and NK cells. Given the wide variety of cell types that are responsive to leptin, it should come as no surprise that the effects of leptin signaling on different cell types vary. For this reason, researchers consider leptin's function pleiotropic.

Regulatory T-cells (Tregs) express the OB-Rb receptor, and their activity is diminished by leptin signaling.[15] Dendritic cells, monocytes, B-cells, and NK cells are all dependent upon leptin signaling for their formation prior to activation, and inflammatory conditions including obesity have been shown to divert production of some of these cell types from the bone marrow to the periphery.[16] This shift in origin may lead to a shift in immune population favoring macrophages "primed" to become M1. While Tregs increase in number in adipose tissue, Treg frequency is reduced with leptin concentration in humans with autoimmune diseases such as multiple sclerosis.[17] The antiapoptotic effects of leptin observed in B-cells occurs similarly in neutrophils, albeit through different signaling cascades.[18] Leptin can also alter the metabolism of macrophages, which will be discussed later.

3.2.1.2 Adiponectin

Adiponectin behaves in a manner opposite to leptin.[19] Adipocytes also secrete it, but it is released during low-insulin, high-glucagon states such as fasting. Despite adipose tissue like leptin secreting it, adiponectin concentration significantly decreases in obese humans. Studies show healthy-weight humans have serum concentrations around 12 ng/mL, whereas in obese humans in the same study concentrations were closer to 4 ng/mL. Adiponectin triggers orexigenic pathways in the hypothalamus, inducing hunger and food-seeking behavior. It plays a role in generation of adipocytes, and can alter metabolism by decreasing gluconeogenesis and increasing glucose uptake. This alteration of metabolism may be involved in adiponectin's ability to reverse insulin resistance in mice,[19] an effect observed independently of obesity and weight loss.

Just as adiponectin's function is opposed to leptin's on satiety, they share an antagonistic relationship for several immune cell types. Interestingly, when at rest, only 1% of T-cells express adiponectin receptor (Adipo-R) on their surface, retaining the receptor in intracellular vesicles, where it is inactive.[20] Upon activation, the Adipo-R migrates to the cell surface, allowing the T-cells to respond to adiponectin. When adiponectin signaling occurs, T-cell activity is dampened by enhancing apoptosis of T effector cells and inhibiting their proliferation.[21] In contrast, 47% of B-cells, 93% of monocytes, and 21% of NK cells express Adipo-R on their surfaces.[22] When stimulated through this receptor, B-cells secrete a soluble factor that impairs T-cell migration into inflamed tissues, further diminishing inflammatory responses.[22] Monocytes undergo a greater degree of apoptosis, and secrete fewer proinflammatory cytokines when stimulated with adiponectin.[23]

Given the general effects of adiponectin on immune cell types, adiponectin induces anti-inflammatory effects. It is important to note that, while many of these effects are in opposition to leptin, the balance struck between adiponectin and leptin in the behavior of the immune system is nonsymmetrical. Unlike a game of chess, where two identical but opposing forces vie for dominance, adiponectin and leptin each produce effects that counter each other in indirect ways. Whether this brings the immune system to a proinflammatory or anti-inflammatory state is dependent not only on the relative abundance of these adipokines, but on innumerable other factors including presence of infection, availability of metabolic substrate, and likely many others.

3.2.1.3 Other Adipokines

Adiponectin and leptin are far from the only adipokines secreted from adipose tissue, although they are the only ones regulated by energy balance. Proinflammatory adipokines including IL-6, MCP-1, chemerin, and TNF-α are also produced by adipose tissue. While each of these is associated with obesity, IL-6 is very strongly correlated with obesity, and has a very important immunomodulatory role involving Tregs. Tregs are a special subset of T-cell that play an important anti-inflammatory role. A prolonged inflammation period induces Tregs, and the predominant cytokine causing their induction is TGF-β. Following induction, Tregs will dampen inflammatory signals in other CD4+ T-cells (Th1, Th2, and Th17), suppressing the T-cell response. Many other immune cells, including B-cells, dendritic cells, and macrophages, depend upon T-cell signaling for their inflammatory response, placing Tregs at a crucial point in inflammation progression. In combination with the adipokine IL-6, naive T-cells exposed to TGF-β will undergo differentiation into the proinflammatory Th17 cell type, depriving the inflammation site of anti-inflammatory Tregs[24] and adding to inflammation in a "1–2 punch."

The adipokines MCP-1 and chemerin play important roles in monocyte recruitment to adipose tissue. MCP-1[25] and chemerin[26] are both associated positively with human obesity. Recruitment of monocytes is the first step of adipose-tissue macrophage generation. Adipose-tissue macrophages have a tremendous impact on the microenvironment of adipose tissue.

TNF-α is associated with obesity,[27] although it is secreted from proinflammatory M1 macrophages[28] resident in the adipose tissue. TNF-α stimulates phagocytosis,[29] as well as M1 polarization and angiogenesis.

From leptin's proinflammatory effects, to the lack of adiponectin to dampen inflammation, obesity triggers a proinflammatory cytokine secretion that results in a persistent low-grade inflammatory state. This long-term, chronic inflammatory state is thought to have a tremendous impact on the response to pathogens, although the precise mechanism remains to be determined. Leading theories on the interaction between inflammation and infection outcome include damage from an excessive immune response and a delayed immune response resulting in greater pathogen replication.

3.2.2 Innate Immune Cells: Local and Systemic Effects of Obesity

While the precise origin of obesity's immunological consequences remains open to debate, researchers believe that cells of the innate immune system mediate physiological changes present in obesity. In the microenvironment of adipose tissue, macrophage infiltration and polarization to a proinflammatory subtype (M1 macrophage) is increased. It remains unclear whether increased presence of M1 macrophages is the cause, or merely a key step in the creation of the low-grade inflammation characteristic of metabolic syndrome. What is clear is the difference in macrophage phenotype. Lean adipose tissues include a relatively small number of anti-inflammatory M2 macrophages, which metabolize fatty acids and dampen immune activation through secretion of IL-10 and TGF-β. M2 macrophages tend to disperse throughout the adipose tissue, and may play a role in wound healing in the event of injury. However, the obese adipose environment recruits and polarizes M1 macrophages to five times[30] the level of M2 macrophages in lean adipose tissue. M1 macrophages utilize glucose as their fuel source, and secrete proinflammatory molecules including TNF-α, IL-1β, and MCP-1. Using glucose as a fuel source allows M1 macrophages to generate greater amounts of energy without consuming as much oxygen, which may be necessary considering the way M1 macrophages distribute. Unlike M2 macrophages, M1 macrophages tend to cluster around a specific feature, called a crown-like structure (CLS). CLS are cellular, inflammatory hurricanes, the eye of which is a dying or dead adipocyte. Whether due to hypoxia, inflammation, or unmanageable hypertrophy, each dying adipocyte recruits dozens of M1 macrophages, which degrade the damaged cell and consume its fat content. The M1 macrophages that facilitate this process share many morphological characteristics with foam cells in atherosclerosis, and they contribute to inflammation in a similar feed-forward mechanism. To clear lipids from the dead adipocyte, M1 macrophages secrete fatty acids into the tissue surrounding the CLS. Paradoxically considering their fuel sources, this may then facilitate conversion of M2 macrophages to M1, further shifting the adipocyte macrophage population toward the M1 phenotype.[4] This shift in macrophage population is not without consequence. M2 macrophage secretion of IL-4 and IL-10 promotes insulin sensitivity in adipocytes, whereas TNF-α secretion by M1 macrophages acts locally, diminishing insulin sensitivity in adipocytes. In addition to its feed-forward loop role in recruiting monocytes, MCP-1 also acts to recruit other immune cells including neutrophils, basophils, and mast cells. While these effects are pronounced within the adipose tissue, many of the adipokines generated have systemic effects when they leave the adipose tissue. As previously discussed, leptin and adiponectin's endocrine have an effect on satiety, but TNF-α and IL-6 also escape adipose tissue into the bloodstream, contributing to systemic insulin resistance.[31,32]

3.2.3 Adaptive Immunity: Local and Systemic Effects of Obesity

Cells from the adaptive immune system play roles in both lean and obese conditions. In lean adipose tissue, Th2 and Treg cells provide anti-inflammatory cytokine signals to infiltrating monocytes, promoting anti-inflammatory M2 cells. It is the action of these anti-inflammatory T-cells that maintains the inflammation-free environment of lean adipose tissue, which promotes insulin sensitivity and a healthy function of the endocrine organ. In obesity, however, Tregs and Th2 cells do not form as readily, and instead Th1, Th17, CD8+ T effector cells, and B-cells are the predominant adaptive immune cells, which give rise to M1 macrophage polarization, greater inflammation, and the pro-inflammatory state. While the mechanism of this transition from anti-inflammatory to proinflammatory adipose phenotype in obesity remains to be determined, the only question of the adaptive immunity's role is whether it is the cause, or merely a significant contributor.

Both in adipose tissue and systemically, Th1 cells act in concert with macrophages and CD8 T-cells to combat intracellular bacteria and viruses, whereas Th2 cells promote B-cell, eosinophil, and mast cell activation, prompting a wide response to a wide array of extracellular pathogens including viruses, bacteria, and fungi. Th17 cells are proinflammatory and aid in clearing pathogens.

Obesity affects the adaptive immune system beyond its changes to the adipose tissue microenvironment as well, which may be attributable, in part, to nutrient availability. CD4+ T-cell subtypes Th1, Th2, and Th17 are glycolytic cell types, and increasing glucose availability causes greater T effector cell function.[33] While each of these T-cell subtypes causes a distinct inflammatory response, together they all contribute to inflammation. Conversely, Treg cells depend on fatty acid oxidation for their metabolism, and do not increase their anti-inflammatory effects during increased glucose availability.[34]

Given T-cell function dependency upon glucose availability, it should come as no surprise that T-cell activation includes upregulation of glucose transporters. Specifically, T-cells will become insulin sensitive during activation, and use insulin signaling in a classical manner to activate the Glut-1 glucose transporter. Indeed, activated T-cells from hyperglycemic subjects produce greater levels of proinflammatory cytokines *in vitro*[35] and *in vivo*. Insulin deficiency due to poor diet or genetic defect results in poor T-cell function, increasing susceptibility to infection.[36] The extent this is attributable to insulin resistance remains unclear.

While relatively little has been characterized about B-cell metabolism and obesity, numerous studies have pointed to B-cell alterations related to obesity, including greater infiltration of mature, class-switched B-cells into visceral adipose tissue[37,38] and increasing B-regulatory cell activity in obese mice reducing inflammation.[37,39] It remains to be determined whether these are secondary effects from T-cell alterations, distinct effects brought on by obesity through B-cells directly, or a more complicated mechanism yet to be proposed.

3.3 OBESITY AND INFECTION

3.3.1 VIRAL INFECTION IN OBESITY

Researchers believe obesity has numerous synergistic interactions with viral infections. For example, hepatitis C infection combined with obesity induces a greater degree of hepatic steatosis:[40] while both obesity and hepatitis C can cause steatosis on their own, the combined effect is more pronounced than either disease individually. In HIV infection, obesity has a complicated relationship with the associated disease AIDS. Prior to the advent of antiretroviral therapy (ART), which has effectively turned HIV infection from near-certain mortality into a serious, chronic, but survivable viral infection, obesity was associated with prolonged lifespan following HIV infection. As mentioned earlier, obesity can lead to greater numbers of CD4+ T helper cells, which are also the cells HIV targets and therefore become depleted during infection. Unsurprisingly, obesity is positively associated with CD4+ T-cell levels in HIV-infected adults. Before ART, this also meant greater longevity.[41] However, ART has been shown to exacerbate dyslipidemia by damaging the mitochondria of adipocytes,[42] leading to greater occurrence of atherosclerosis in HIV positive adults, especially obese adults.[43] So while obesity may give some protections against HIV progression, it comes at a cost.

Obese humans are at a greater risk of hospitalization and death from influenza than healthy weight individuals,[44] and there are many hypotheses for this phenomenon. Chronic inflammation associated with obesity may delay the specific immune response, allowing the infection to become more virulent, or may cause the immune system to overreact to the infection and induce excessive tissue damage, paradoxically causing secondary infection and severe pneumonia. Or, there may be increased incidence of influenza infection in obese humans because of long-term, infection-preventing inflammation. Indeed, there is greater inflammation in lung tissues of obese mice infected with the influenza virus,[45] attributable to diminished Treg activity and increased systemic levels of CD4+ T-cells. Additionally, despite generating a normal response to influenza vaccination initially, higher weight correlates with a greater decrease in antibody concentrations 1 year post-vaccination in humans,[46] suggesting that although the immune system responds appropriately initially, it is unable to generate or maintain humoral memory toward influenza.

Influenza virus is not a single, immutable infectious agent: multiple strains that can infect humans do exist, and immunity—especially humoral immunity—to one strain may not equate to immunity to another due to differences in protein structure of the virus. Humoral immunity primarily targets external viral proteins, while T-cell immunity primarily responds to internal viral proteins, and proteins expressed during the virus's intracellular replication phase. For this reason, T-cells can produce cross-reactive immunity, as, in contrast to external viral proteins, internal influenza viral proteins are similar among strains. However, after priming obese mice with an influenza H3N2 strain and then reinfecting with what would otherwise be a lethal dose of influenza pandemic H1N1, 25% of obese mice died, with survivors experiencing 10–100 times greater viral titers in lung tissue, as well as higher concentrations of pro-inflammatory cytokines. In contrast, 100% of lean mice survived.[47] In humans, T-cells isolated from overweight and obese humans show diminished markers of activation, while dendritic cells express reduced MHC-II, the protein responsible for antigen presentation to T-cells.[48] Despite these deficits in T-cell responses, following vaccination, obese adults produce an antibody response equivalent to healthy-weight adults, however the antibody response declines more rapidly.[49]

Taken in sum, obesity exacerbates dyslipidemia associated with some infections, inhibits the immunologic memory response to infection, and contributes to a proinflammatory environment that licenses greater tissue damage from infection and inflammation.

3.3.2 Bacterial Infection in Obesity

Bacterial infections in the setting of obesity also alter in comparison with healthy weight. Periodontal disease[50] is more common in obese subjects across a wide range of age groups, although the mechanism for this link is undetermined. While it is possible the immune alterations linked to obesity cause increased susceptibility to bacterial infections, it is equally plausible that differences in diet account for greater chance of infection. Another proposed mechanism for the link between periodontal disease and obesity relates to alterations in bone homeostasis during obesity. Periodontal disease is in part brought on by resorption of bone tissue in the alveolar spacing of the teeth (i.e., under the gums near the jawbone). Studies have shown this resorption to increase in obese animals,[51] and to contribute to periodontal infection progression.

Another interesting finding is that obese, leptin-deficient mice are more susceptible to pneumococcal pneumonia;[52] however, this effect is not observed in leptin-sufficient obese animals.[53] While the specific mechanism remains to be determined, this may suggest that leptin may have lung-specific roles related to the immune response to pneumococcal pneumonia. This may be why obesity increases the severity of secondary bacterial infections,[54] although there may be other factors involved as well.

In a surgical context, obesity and bacterial infection correlate,[55] although to what extent this is an intrinsic characteristic of obesity remains hotly debated. Extrinsic factors explaining this correlation include increased hospital stays surrounding surgery, and longer hospital stays increase the risk of acquiring nosocomial infection. Intrinsic factors may also include the need for surgery: obese individuals are at greater risk for requiring cardiac, vascular, orthopedic, and gastrointestinal surgery, and surgical site infection was not associated with obesity in at least one study on elective surgery.[56] Perhaps it is that the severity of the underlying cause for hospitalization is greater in obese adults, and complications are more likely as a result.

3.4 THE INFECTIOUS ORIGIN OF OBESITY HYPOTHESIS

In 1988 canine distemper virus was found to have an interesting effect: it induced hyperinsulinemia[57] and obesity following infection in mice. Since that study, research has revealed similar findings in at least four different viral infections and one prion disease, although none of them has been shown to have the same impact in humans. Nevertheless, infection as a cause of obesity is a novel hypothesis.

3.4.1 Evidence Supporting the Hypothesis

Human adenovirus 36 (Ad-36) is a virus capable of infecting humans, chickens, mice, and nonhuman primates, among other organisms. This class of virus transmits via respiratory, sexual, and fecal-oral contact. Scientists have detected the virus in human visceral adipose tissue, and others have shown a similar virus induces weight gain in mice.[58] Additionally, researchers demonstrated epidemiological evidence that antibodies to Ad-36 were more prevalent in obese humans than in nonobese humans, correlating past exposure with current obesity.[59] A separate study showed that antibodies to Ad-36 and Ad-31 were associated with greater adiposity and elevated serum lipids, while Ad-5 (as a control) was not.[60,61] Yet another study found that this relationship had temporality, in that infection preceded the effects: a 10-year study assessing 1,400 Hispanic men and women found that subjects seropositive for Ad-36 at the start of the study had greater adiposity gain 10 years later than seronegative controls, although they also had better fasting glucose levels over time. These effects were modest, however, leading the authors to conclude that their study "strengthens the plausibility" that Ad-36 induces obesity and improves glycemic control, but is not a sole determiner of weight status.

3.4.2 Arguments Against the Hypothesis

Association does not prove causation. Although researchers have observed correlative and temporal effects in humans, confounding factors may still explain these effects. Based on the current evidence, at best, we can conclude that Ad-36 infection is an independent risk factor for obesity. But the poor penetrance of obesity in Ad-36 seropositive subjects, combined with a current lack of proposed biological mechanism and lack of control for confounding contributors make this hypothesis too early to accept. Furthermore, doctors widely accept that obesity is a multifactorial state dependent upon caloric intake, genetics, activity, and a slew of other factors that contribute to weight status. Even if Ad-36 infection impacts obesity, the relative contribution of this infection may be insignificant or minor.

3.5 SUMMARY

While excess adipose tissue characterizes obesity, that definition alone does not begin to cover the depth of impact of this state. Obesity causes changes in adipose tissues' endocrine behavior, chiefly increasing leptin and decreasing adiponectin output. In turn, this alters immune cell activity, contributing to a systemic, chronic, low-grade inflammatory state. Obesity shifts populations of immune cells to proinflammatory subtypes, and permits greater severity of certain viral infections. It increases the risk of bacterial infection following viral infection and following surgery, while decreasing the speed of recovery from these illnesses and procedures. As the average waistline of our world continues to grow, we will continue to see greater impacts of obesity on immunity and infection.

REFERENCES

1. WHO Media Centre. 2013. *Obesity and overweight.* http://www.who.int/mediacentre/factsheets/fs311/en/ (Accessed June 30, 2014).
2. Centers for Disease Control and Prevention. 2015. *Adult obesity facts.* http://www.cdc.gov/obesity/data/adult.html (Accessed June 30, 2014).
3. Sarvetnick N, Liggit D, Pitts, SL et al. 1988. Insulin-dependent diabetes mellitus induced in transgenic mice by ectopic expression of class II MHC and interferon-gamma. *Cell* 52:773–782.
4. Johnson AR, Milner JJ, Makowski L 2012. The inflammation highway: Metabolism accelerates inflammatory traffic in obesity. *Immunol Rev* 249:218–238.
5. Milner JJ, Rebeles J, Dhungana S et al. 2015. Obesity increases mortality and modulates the lung metabolome during pandemic H1N1 influenza virus infection in mice. *J Immunol* 194:4846–4859.
6. Travers RL, Motta AC, Betts JA et al. 2015. The impact of obesity on adipose tissue-resident lymphocyte activation in humans. *Int J Obes (Lond)* 39:762–769.
7. Conde J, Scotece M, Abella V et al. 2014. An update on leptin as immunomodulator. *Expert Rev Clin Immunol* 10:1165–1170.
8. Considine RV, Sinha MK, Heiman ML et al. 1996. Serum immunoreactive-leptin concentrations in normal weight and obese humans. *N Engl J Med* 334:292–295.
9. Gerriets VA, MacIver NJ. 2014. Role of T cells in malnutrition and obesity. *Front Immunol* 11:379.
10. Kwan Lam QL, Wang S, Ko OH et al. 2010. Leptin signaling maintains B-cell homeostasis via induction of Bcl-2 and Cyclin D1. *Proc Natl Acad Sci USA* 107:13812–13817.
11. Ramirez O, Garza KM. 2014. Leptin deficiency in vivo enhances the ability of splenic dendritic cells to activate T cells. *Int Immunol* 25:627–636.
12. Lamas B, Concalves-Mendes N, Nachat-Kappes R et al. 2013. Leptin modulates dose-dependently the metabolic and cytolytic activities of NK-92 cells. *J Cell Physiol* 226:1202–1209.
13. Yang R, Barouch LA. 2007. Leptin signaling and obesity. *Circ Res* 101:545–559.
14. Allison MB, Myers MG Jr. 2014. 20 years of leptin: Connecting leptin signaling to biological function. *J Endocrinol* 223:T25–T35.
15. Chi H. 2012. Regulation and function of mTOR signaling in T cell fate decisions. *Nat Rev Immunol* 12:325–338.
16. Nahrendorf M, Swirski FK. 2015. Lifestyle effects on hematopoiesis and atherosclerosis. *Circ Res* 116:884–894.
17. Matarese G, Carrieri PB, La Cava A et al. 2005. Leptin increase in multiple sclerosis associates with reduced number of CD4(+)CD25+ regulatory T cells. *Proc Natl Acad Sci USA* 102:5150–5155.
18. Bruno A, Conus S, Schmid I and Simon H. 2005. Apoptotic pathways are inhibited by leptin receptor activation in neutrophils. *J Immunol* 174:8090–8096.
19. Yamauchi T, Kamon J, Waki H et al. 2001. The fat-derived hormone adiponectin reverses insulin resistance associated with both lipoatrophy and obesity. *Nat Med.* 7:941–946.
20. Pang TT, Naerendran P. 2008. The distribution of adiponectin receptors on human peripheral blood mononuclear cells. *Ann N Y Acad Sci* 1150:143–145.
21. Wilk S, Scheibenbogen C, Bauer S et al. 2011. Adiponectin is a negative regulator of antigen-activated T-cells. *Eur J Immunol* 41:2323–2332.
22. Kugelberg KE. 2015. T cell responses: B cells control T cell traffic. *Nat Rev Immunol* 15:332–333.
23. Neumeier M, Weigert J, Schafler A et al. 2006. Different effects of adiponectin isoforms in human monocytic cells. *J Leukoc Biol* 4:803–808.
24. Bertola A, Ciucci T, Rousseau D et al. 2012. Identification of adipose tissue dendritic cells correlated with obesity-associated insulin resistance and inducing Th17 responses in mice and patients. *Diabetes* 61:2238–2247.
25. Christiansen T, Richelsen B, Bruun JM. 2004. Monocyte chemoattractant protein-1 is produced in isolated adipocytes, associated with adiposity and reduced after weight loss in morbid obese subjects. *Int J Obes Relat Metab Disord* 29:146–150.
26. Bozaoglu K, Segal D, Shields KA. 2009. Chemerin is associated with metabolic syndrome phenotypes in a Mexican American population. *J Clin Endocrinol Metab* 8:3085–3088.
27. Cottam DR, Mattar SG, Barinas-Mitchell E et al. 2004. The chronic inflammatory hypothesis for the morbidity associated with morbid obesity: Implications and effects of weight loss. *Obes Surg* 5:589–600.
28. Weisberg SP, McCann D, Desai M et al. 2003. Obesity is associated with macrophage accumulation in adipose tissue. *J Clin Invest* 2:1796–1808.

29. Yeang CH, McCormick F, Levine A. 2008. Combinatorial patterns of somatic gene mutations in cancer. *FASEB J* 8:2605–2622.
30. Weisberg SP, Hunter D, Huber R et al. 2006. CCR2 modulates inflammatory and metabolic effects of high-fat feeding. *J Clin Invest* 116:115–124.
31. Tzanavari T, Giannogonas P, Karalis KP. 2010. TNF-alpha and obesity. *Curr Dir Autoimmun* 145:145–156.
32. Eder K, Baffy N, Falus A, Fulop A. 2006. The major inflammatory mediator interleukin-6 and obesity. *Inflamm Res* 5:727–736.
33. Palmer CS, Ostrowski M, Balderson B et al. 2015. Glucose metabolism regulates T cell activation differentiation and functions. *Front Immunol* 6:1.
34. Michalek RD, Gerreits VA, Jacobs SR et al. 2011. Cutting edge: Distinct glycolytic and lipid oxidative metabolic programs are essential for effector and regulatory CD4+ T cell subsets. *J Immunol* 186:3299–3303.
35. Stentz FB, Kitabchi AE. 2003. Activated T lymphocytes in type 2 diabetes: Implications from in vitro studies. *Curr Drug Targets* 4:493–503.
36. Denkers EY, Gazinelli RT. 1998. Regulation and function of T-cell mediated immunity during toxoplasma gondii infection. *Clin Microbiol* 4:569–588.
37. Shaikh SR, Haas KM, Beck MA, Teague H. 2015. The effects of diet-induced obesity on B cell function. *Clin Exp Immunol* 1:90–99.
38. Winer DA, Winer S, Shen L et al. 2011. B cells promote insulin resistance through modulation of T cells and production of pathogenic IgG antibodies. *Nat Med* 5:610–617.
39. Wang G, McCain ML, Yang L. 2014. Modeling the mitochondrial cardiomyopathy of Barth syndrome with induced pluripotent stem cell and heart-on-chip technologies. *Nat Med* 6:616–623.
40. Younossi ZM, McCullogh AJ, Ong JP et al. 2004. Obesity and non-alcoholic fatty liver disease in chronic hepatitis C. *J Clin Gastroenterol* 38:705–709.
41. Shah K, Alio AP, Hall WJ, Luque AE. 2012. The physiological effects of obesity in HIV-infected patients. *J AIDS Clinic Res* 3:151.
42. Villaroya F, Domingo P, Giralt M. 2005. Lipodystrophy associated with highly anti-retroviral therapy for HIV infection: The adipocyte as a target of anti-retroviral-induced mitochondrial toxicity. *Trends Pharmacol Sci* 26:88–93.
43. Guraldi G, Stentarelli C, Zona S et al. 2010. Lipodystrophy and anti-retroviral therapy as predictors of sub-clinical atherosclerosis in human immunodeficiency virus infected subjects. *Atherosclerosis* 208:222–227.
44. Jain S, Chaves SS. 2011. Obesity and influenza. *Clin Infect Dis* 53:422–424.
45. Milner JJ, Beck MA. 2014. Obesity and influenza infection severity. *Futur Virol* 9:223–225.
46. Sheridan PA, Paich HA, Handy J et al. 2012. Obesity is associated with impaired immune response to influenza vaccination in humans. *Int J Obes* 36:1072–1077.
47. Karlsson EA, Sheridan PA, Beck MA. 2010. Diet-induced obesity impairs the T cell memory response to influenza virus infection. *J Immun* 184:3127–3133.
48. Paich HA, Sheridan PA, Handy J et al. 2013. Overweight and obese adult humans have a defective cellular immune response to pandemic H1N1 influenza A virus. *Obesity* 21:2377–2386.
49. Sheridan PA, Paich HA, Handy J et al. 2012. Obesity is associated with impaired immune response to influenza vaccination in humans. *Int J Obesity* 36:1072–1077.
50. Al-Zahrani MS, Bissada NF, Borawskit EA. 2003. Obesity and periodontal disease in young, middle-aged, and older adults. *J Periodontol* 74:610–615.
51. Perlstein MI, Bassada NF. 1997. Influence of obesity and hypertension on the severity of periodontitis in rats. *Oral Surg Oral Med Oral Pathol* 43:707–719.
52. Mancuso P. 2013. Obesity and respiratory infections: Does excess adiposity weigh down host defense? *Pulm Pharmacol Ther* 26:412–419.
53. Mancuso P, Calleri A, Gregato G et al. 2014. A subpopulation of circulating endothelial cells express CD109 and is enriched in the blood of cancer patients. *PLOS ONE* 9:e114713.
54. Karlsson EA, van de Velde N, McCullers J, Schultz-Cherry S. 2013. Obesity increases the severity of secondary bacterial coinfection following influenza virus infection. *FASEB J* 27:123–124.
55. Huttunen R, Karppelin M, Syrjanen J. 2013. Obesity and nosocomial infections. *J Hosp Infect* 85:8–16.
56. Dindo D, Muller MK, Weber M, Clavien P. 2003. Obesity in general elective surgery. *Lancet* 361:2032–2035.
57. Bernard A, Zwingelstein G, Meister R, Wild TF. 1988. Hyperinsulinemia induced by canine distemper virus of mice and its correlation with the appearance of obesity. *Comp Biochem Physiol B* 4:691–696.

58. So PW, Herlihy AH, Bell JD. 2005. Adiposity induced by adenovirus 5 innoculation. *J Obesity* 29:603–606.
59. Ginneken V, Sitnyakowsky L, Jeffery JE. 2009. Infectobesity: Viral infections (especially with human adenovirus-36: AD-36) may be a cause of obesity. *Med Hypotheses* 72:383–388.
60. Bil-Lula I, Stapor S, Sochoka M et al. 2014. Infectobesity in the Polish population-evaluation of an association between adenoviruses type 5, 21, 36 and human obesity. *Int J Virol Mol Biol* 3:1–8.
61. Dhurandhar, NV. 2012. Is obesity caused by an adenovirus? *Expert Rev Anti Infect Ther* 10:521–524.

4 Role of Immune Cells in Adipose Tissue

Jack Warburton and Fátima Pérez de Heredia

CONTENTS

4.1 Introduction..43
4.2 Adipose Tissue and the Immune System: A Common
Developmental Origin?...44
4.3 Adipose Cells can Behave like Immune Cells 45
4.4 Adipose Tissue Is Populated by Immune Cells..46
4.5 Adipokine Regulation of Immune Function 46
    4.5.1 Leptin...46
    4.5.2 Adiponectin..47
    4.5.3 TNF-α 47
    4.5.4 IL-1β 47
    4.5.5 IL-6 47
    4.5.6 Proteins of the Complement System..47
    4.5.7 Chemerin..48
    4.5.8 Omentin 48
4.6 Types and Roles of Adipose Tissue–Resident Immune Cells 48
    4.6.1 Monocytes and Macrophages 48
    4.6.2 Mast Cells..49
    4.6.3 Neutrophils 50
    4.6.4 Eosinophils 50
    4.6.5 Natural Killer (NK) and Natural Killer T (NKT) Cells.................................50
    4.6.6 T Lymphocytes 50
    4.6.7 B Lymphocytes 51
4.7 Role of Adipose Tissue–Resident Immune Cells in Pathological
States..51
    4.7.1 Metabolic Syndrome..52
    4.7.2 Cardiovascular Risk 52
4.8 Summary and Conclusions 53
References..53

4.1 INTRODUCTION

The last two decades have witnessed a dramatic change of paradigm in adipose tissue physiology, from the classic passive fat-storage depot to the current view of the complex endocrine and immune organ. Today, it is evident that adipose tissue plays a key role in the development of a vast group of metabolic and chronic diseases that go beyond obesity, including diabetes, cardiovascular disease, liver disease, systemic inflammation, respiratory disorders, and cancer. Given this, it is surprising that it took so long for researchers to realize that adipose tissue could not be a mere fat-storing depot. The status of energy reserves in an organism must be a fundamental limiting factor for normal function of all the other bodily systems, particularly the most resource-consuming ones, like reproduction and immune defense. This alone would be enough to suggest the need for a network of communication between the adipose tissue and the rest of the organism, a network by which the adipose depots could inform the other organs of the availability of the resources required to perform their functions. It was not until the early 1990s that researchers discovered leptin (Zhang et al. 1994), but that discovery changed the understanding of adipose tissue and its function. Leptin is a hormone that can regulate fat stores and inform the hypothalamus of the state of such stores, and at the same time it can exert effects on other systems, modulating functions important for the survival of both the individual and the species. These realizations changed the focus of research on adipose tissue, resulting in the ongoing unraveling of a highly complex web of metabolic and endocrine functions and a fascinating network of communication between adipocytes and other cell types, tissues, and organs. This chapter presents an overview of adipose tissue as an immune organ, reviewing how the transition in our concept of adipose physiology occurred, and discussing the role of adipose tissue as part of the immune response and the presence and role of immune cells within adipose tissue. Finally, we will review the potential involvement of adipose tissue–resident immune cells in the etiopathology of certain chronic diseases.

4.2   ADIPOSE TISSUE AND THE IMMUNE SYSTEM: A COMMON DEVELOPMENTAL ORIGIN?

In a recent paper, van Niekerk and Engelbrecht (2015) presented the hypothesis that the evolutionary occurrence of adipose tissue was fundamental in the development of the adaptive (highly antigen-specific) immune response (see Table 4.1). The authors argued that this type of response is so energetically demanding that it could only be possible with the aid of associated specialized energy-providing cells (i.e., the adipocytes). Hence why, according to van Niekerk and Engelbrecht, this immune response has appeared, or succeeded, only in vertebrates but not in invertebrates (which, although able to store lipids, do not possess a specialized tissue for that purpose). The authors also reviewed how there is a location-specific functionality of adipose tissue, whereby depots associated with lymphoid tissue are unresponsive to fasting but sensitive to immune activation, implying that the primary function of these adipose depots would be to provide energy to meet the demands of an

TABLE 4.1
Immune Cells and Their Functions

Immune Cell Type	Main Function	Type of Immune Response
Monocytes/Macrophages	Phagocytosis	Innate/Nonspecific
Mast	–	Innate/Nonspecific
Granulocytes	–	–
Neutrophils	Phagocytosis	Innate/Nonspecific
Eosinophils	Exocytosis; defense against parasites	Innate/Nonspecific
Basophils	Exocytosis; allergic reactions	Innate/Nonspecific
Lymphocytes	–	–
Natural killer (NK)	Cytotoxicity; defense against tumor cells	Innate/Nonspecific
T Helper (Th)	Production of cytokines; regulation of other immune cells' functions	Adaptive/Specific
T Cytotoxic (Tc)	Cytotoxicity; defense against pathogens	Adaptive/Specific
T Regulatory (Treg)	Production of cytokines; regulation of other immune cells' functions	Adaptive/Specific
B	Production of antibodies; defense against pathogens	Adaptive/Specific

immune response. Based on their own conclusions and those of other authors (in particular, Pond 2005), van Niekerk and Engelbrecht (2015) suggested that adipocytes could have evolved from providing specific support to immune cells to gradually acquiring a more sophisticated immune role themselves. This is coherent with the idea of a common evolutionary origin for immune cells and adipocytes.

There is evidence that adipocyte precursors, or preadipocytes, can originate in bone marrow like immune cells and then migrate to adipose tissue (Crossno et al. 2006, as cited by Dani and Billon 2012). Also, a hematopoietic origin has been proposed where preadipocytes and adipocytes would derive from macrophage progenitors. Very interestingly, these origins may not apply to all adipocytes in adipose tissue, but only to restricted populations that would present a more inflammatory profile than adipose-derived ones (Cousin et al. 1999; Sera et al. 2009; Majka et al. 2010, as cited by Dani and Billon 2012).

4.3 ADIPOSE CELLS CAN BEHAVE LIKE IMMUNE CELLS

Later in the chapter, we will discuss the cross-talk between adipose and immune cells and how each cell type can modulate the other through paracrine messengers. Before that, it is worth briefly addressing a fascinating aspect of adipose cells, which supports the idea of a common developmental origin with immune cells. Direct immune actions have been described for both preadipocytes and adipocytes. Researchers acknowledged these actions firstly and primarily for preadipocytes, revealing that preadipocytes could exert phagocytic activity, and that preadipocytes lost this activity once they differentiated into adipocytes (Cousin et al. 1999). Furthermore, preadipocytes could differentiate into macrophage-like cells, and so become part of the innate immune response (Schäffler et al. 2007). Studies describe immune-like phenotypes for adipocytes: both preadipocytes and adipocytes express a family of membrane receptors typical of macrophages, known as toll-like receptors (TLRs) (Pietsch et al. 2006). Their main function is pattern recognition and the subsequent initiation of the inflammatory response, but some of these TLRs can modulate adipose function; for example, stimulation of TLR2 inhibits differentiation of preadipocytes into adipocytes (Pevsner-Fischer et al. 2007). Also, both preadipocytes and adipocytes can respond to lipopolysaccharide (LPS)-mediated stimulation of TLR4, and do so by releasing proinflammatory cytokines. Similarly, lactate stimulation of preadipocytes, alone or in combination with LPS, can also result in secretion of proinflammatory signals (Pérez de Heredia et al. 2010), and TLR4 could mediate this response, as observed in macrophages (Samuvel et al. 2009). This inflammatory activity in response to TLR4 ligands is enhanced in preadipocytes compared to adipocytes (Poulain-Godefroy and Froguel 2007; Pérez de Heredia et al. 2010). Finally, some studies have highlighted the importance of macrophage TLR4 in mediating insulin resistance in adipose tissue (Schäffler et al. 2007), and it could be hypothesized that a similar process might take place in preadipocytes.

In addition, adipocytes express molecules of other components of the innate immune response—specifically, of the complement system and the family of tumor necrosis factor (TNF) ligands; these molecules are collectively known as the C1q- and TNF-related protein (CTRP) superfamily. Furthermore, adiponectin, one of the most important adipokines, shares a high degree of structural similarity with the CTRP superfamily, both at the gene and protein levels (Schäffler et al. 2007).

The expression of these proteins in preadipocytes and adipocytes is a strong argument in favor of considering adipose tissue as an immune organ and a very important part of the innate immune system, due to its potential capacity to respond to microbial antigens. But recent evidence reinforces this view: adipocytes can secrete antimicrobial substances directly in response to bacterial infections (Zhang et al. 2015).

This body of evidence suggests that specific activation of adipocytes and preadipocytes under conditions of adipose tissue stress could also cause metabolic alterations usually observed following infectious states, such as insulin resistance and elevated levels of free fatty acids.

4.4   ADIPOSE TISSUE IS POPULATED BY IMMUNE CELLS

Studies have identified many types of immune cells, belonging to both the innate and the adaptive immune responses, within adipose tissue (Grant and Dixit 2015). Those involved in innate immunity include macrophages, neutrophils, eosinophils, mast cells, and natural killer (NK) cells, and those involved in the adaptive immunity are B-cells and T-cells (Table 4.1).

Weisberg et al. (2003) reported macrophages as the most abundant immune cells present in adipose tissue. Although we have discussed the similarities between macrophages and adipocytes, and we have raised the capacity of preadipocytes to differentiate into macrophages, these cell types are distinct. Studies using bone marrow chimeric mice demonstrated that macrophages found in adipose tissue were primarily derived from bone marrow, indicating that they originated from circulating monocytes infiltrating adipose tissue (Weisberg et al. 2003). However, there is also evidence of macrophages transdifferentiated locally from preadipocytes and mesenchymal stem cells in adipose tissue (Schäffler et al. 2007). Lymphocytes constitute another important adipose-tissue resident immune cell population. Caspar-Bauguil et al. (2005) characterized the lymphocyte population in adipose tissue of lean and obese mice, and found that lymphocytes comprised up to 10% of the stromal-vascular fraction of the subcutaneous inguinal and the visceral epididymal depots. B- and T-cells were more abundant in subcutaneous adipose tissue (SAT), while NK and NKT cells were more abundant in the visceral depot (VAT). They also found a higher proportion of γδ-T cells, which are a more primitive type of T lymphocytes. These findings led the authors to suggest that white adipose tissue had the profile of an ancestral immune organ when compared to blood and lymph nodes, and that it could represent a link between the innate and the adaptive immune systems (Caspar-Bauguil et al. 2005), in agreement with the evolutionary hypotheses presented at the beginning of this chapter.

4.5   ADIPOKINE REGULATION OF IMMUNE FUNCTION

Since the discovery of adipose tissue as an active endocrine organ, studies have revealed a vast number of bioactive molecules produced by it. Over the past few years no less than 600 molecules have been recognized as adipokines (Lehr et al. 2012). Adipokines play specific roles in a diverse range of biological processes, including the immune response (Fasshauer and Blüher 2015), control of immune cell migration into adipose tissue, and induction of an inflammatory response. While this is the case for cytokines and chemokines such as interleukin (IL)-6, TNF-α, and monocyte chemoattractant protein (MCP)-1 (Schäffler et al. 2007; Kloting and Blüher 2014), traditional adipokines like leptin, adiponectin, and resistin also have important immunomodulatory actions.

4.5.1   LEPTIN

Although the primary role of leptin is the regulation of body weight through control of appetite and energy expenditure, it has been demonstrated that this adipokine has an important role in innate and adaptive immunity (Sánchez-Margalet et al. 2003). Studies have shown that leptin acts as a proinflammatory cytokine. It stimulates the innate immune response by promoting the production of IL-1, IL-6, IL-12, and TNF-α, and it also activates neutrophil chemotaxis, to stimulate the production of reactive oxygen species (ROS) and to promote the activation of phagocytosis by macrophages and their secretion of mediators like leukotriene B_4 (LTB_4), cyclooxygenase 2 (COX2), and nitric oxide (Zhao et al. 2003). Leptin has been characterized as a recruiter of immune cells into adipose tissue. Bartra et al. (2010) have identified the long leptin receptor isoform (LepRb) on most immune cells including monocytes and macrophages; it is responsible for leptin's physiological activities. Leptin deficient (*ob/ob*) and leptin-receptor deficient (*db/db*) mice display reduced macrophage infiltration and inflammatory gene expression in adipose tissue, regardless of increased weight gain and adiposity (Xu et al. 2003). Additionally, Curat et al. (2004) have shown that high concentrations of leptin can increase endothelial cell adhesion molecule expression and promote macrophage adherence. Leptin is also necessary for the normal development and cytotoxic function of NK cells (Tian et al. 2002; Wrann et al. 2012). This is supported by the observation that mice that are leptin receptor–deficient, present impaired NK cell development (Zhao et al. 2003).

4.5.2 ADIPONECTIN

Adiponectin is an adipocyte-specific adipokine, the levels of which decrease in obesity (Maeda et al. 2002), and which is capable of exerting anti-inflammatory properties. It can modulate the function and phenotype of macrophages and thus play a critical role in chronic inflammation (Ouchi et al. 2001). Adiponectin can promote the macrophage phenotype linked with anti-inflammatory states, known as M2 type, stimulating the expression of M2 markers, including arginase-1 and IL-10 (Ohashi et al. 2010), and it can also suppress the production of interferon (IFN)-γ by LPS-stimulated macrophages (Wolf et al. 2004). Further to this, adiponectin can downregulate the activation of NK cells mediated by IL-2, through inhibition of the nuclear factor kappa beta (NF κB)–light chain enhancer. In addition, adiponectin activates adenosine monophosphate-activated protein kinase (AMPK), which also suppresses IL-2-enhanced NF-κB activity and thus NK cytotoxicity (Kim et al. 2006).

4.5.3 TNF-α

Tumor necrosis factor alpha (TNF-α) is a cytokine with pleiotropic functions, regulating immune function, cell differentiation, proliferation, apoptosis, and energy metabolism, among others. Studies have shown TNF-α to be highly expressed in adipose tissue, and therefore qualifies as an adipokine (Sopasakis et al. 2005). TNF-α has proinflammatory effects on adipocytes through its promotion of increased leptin secretion (Trujillo et al. 2006) and an inverse relation with adiponectin (Maeda et al. 2002). Further to this, TNF-α modulates the secretion of other proinflammatory adipokines such as MCP-1 and IL-6 (Cawthorn and Sethi 2008).

4.5.4 IL-1β

IL-1β is another proinflammatory cytokine produced by immune cells, but also secreted from adipose tissue. It has been suggested that its presence in this tissue could contribute to defense against infection or injury (Fernandez-Real and Ricart 1999; Klein et al. 2007). There seems to be a connection between lipogenesis in macrophages and IL-1β production, as evidenced by the observation that cells from mice lacking the sterol-regulatory element-binding protein-1a (SREBP-1a), and therefore unable to activate lipogenesis, failed to release IL-1β after an LPS challenge; this suggests a role for IL-1β as a mediator between lipid metabolism and the innate immune response (Im et al. 2011).

4.5.5 IL-6

Fain et al. (2004) have shown adipose tissue of obese subjects to produce large amounts of IL-6, likely contributing to its elevated circulating levels. IL-6 has been shown to exert both pro-and anti-inflammatory actions. On the one hand, it stimulates neutrophil proliferation and the differentiation of T helper cells, and inhibits regulatory T-cell (Treg) differentiation (Covarrubias and Horng 2014); on the other hand, Mauer et al. (2014) found that IL-6 is a critical instigator of M2 polarization of macrophages, therefore presenting an important inflammation-limiting role.

4.5.6 PROTEINS OF THE COMPLEMENT SYSTEM

The complement system is part of the innate immune response, and consists of the sequential activation of enzymes and factors, resulting in the formation of the membrane attack complex—a structure that opens pores in the membrane of the target cell, leading to its destruction. Studies have found adipose tissue expresses at least three members of the complement system. Adipsin is expressed by adipocytes in mice and by adipocytes and monocytes in humans (White et al. 1992; Gabrielsson et al. 2003). It is identical to the complement factor D (Choy et al. 1992), one of the enzymes of the alternative pathway of complement activation. In addition, adipose tissue expresses the proteins C3 and complement factor B (Choy et al. 1992). Deleting and/or blocking C3a activity seems to confer protection against obesity, adipose tissue inflammation, and insulin resistance (Mamane et al. 2009; Lim et al. 2013).

4.5.7 CHEMERIN

Chemerin regulates the chemotaxis and activation of dendritic cells and macrophages (Wittamer et al. 2003). In adipose tissue, it can also regulate the differentiation of adipocytes in an autocrine/paracrine manner and modulate the expression of genes involved in the metabolism of lipids and glucose (Bozaoglu et al. 2007; Goralski et al. 2007), in lipogenesis (Huang et al. 2010), and in insulin signaling (Takahashi et al. 2008). Studies in humans have found that circulating levels of chemerin are associated with body mass index (BMI), serum triglycerides, and blood pressure (Bozaoglu et al. 2007; Goralski et al. 2007), and with TNF-α, IL-6, and C-reactive protein (CRP) (Lehrke et al. 2009; Weigert et al. 2010).

4.5.8 OMENTIN

Omentin was first identified in adipose tissue in 2005 (Schäffler et al. 2005), and is expressed by the stromal fraction of the visceral depot (Yang et al. 2006). Its expression is inversely associated with obesity and insulin resistance (Tan et al. 2010; Sitticharoon et al. 2014), whereas its circulating levels are negatively correlated with BMI, CRP, insulin, LDL-cholesterol, triglycerides, and leptin, but positively with HDL-cholesterol (Urbanova et al. 2014). It has been suggested that omentin is an anti-inflammatory mediator that acts upon several signaling pathways, including those involving cyclooxygenase-2, AMPK, and endothelial nitric oxide synthase (Tan et al. 2010; Yamawaki et al. 2011).

4.6 TYPES AND ROLES OF ADIPOSE TISSUE–RESIDENT IMMUNE CELLS

As mentioned earlier, several types of immune cells have been reported to be present in adipose tissue, but not all of them are found at the same time or under the same conditions. Although immune cells are normal constituents of the stromal vascular (nonadipose) fraction of the tissue under physiological conditions, their numbers increase in response to challenges such as nutrient overload (e.g., during high-fat diets), obesity, or adipose tissue inflammation. Then, immune cells seem to infiltrate adipose tissue sequentially, promoting in turns the migration and activation of other type(s); the first to arrive would be neutrophils, followed by macrophages, and then lymphocytes (Grant and Dixit 2015). Cytokines and other bioactive molecules secreted by the different cell populations will continue stimulating each other's migration and activation in a typical inflammatory loop.

4.6.1 MONOCYTES AND MACROPHAGES

Adipose tissue–resident macrophages can occur as a consequence of the greater survival and proliferation of this macrophage population, the inhibition of macrophage migration out of adipose tissue, or an increased trafficking of circulating monocytes toward adipose tissue (Bourlier and Bouloumie 2009). Their functions comprise a variety of roles, including scavenging cellular debris derived from apoptotic cells, regulating angiogenesis, and remodeling the extracellular matrix (Chawla et al. 2011). TNF-α secreted by adipose tissue macrophages inhibits preadipocyte differentiation and stimulates lipolysis in adipocytes; in turn, saturated fatty acids released from adipocytes can activate macrophages through binding to TLR4 (Schäffler et al. 2007). This initiates an inflammatory feedback loop—normally in response to nutrient overload—that will ultimately lead to insulin resistance and impaired fat storage within adipose tissue. Under physiological conditions, adipose tissue–resident macrophages express IL-10, which is able to sustain insulin sensitivity through the suppression of proinflammatory mediators such as TNF-α (Lumeng et al. 2007). However, the situation is different in obesity; populations of adipose tissue macrophages in obese mice and humans are greater than in their lean counterparts (Weisberg et al. 2003; Xu et al. 2003). This increase in the population of macrophages within adipose tissue in obesity is a result of greater monocyte recruitment, which is initiated through the chemokine receptor pathways CCR2/CCL2, CCR1/CCL5, and others (Huber et al. 2008). Once in adipose tissue, monocytes differentiate into the classical forms of macrophages, M1 and M2, upon stimulation. The majority of macrophages resident in adipose tissue of lean individuals are M2, which express high levels of anti-inflammatory cytokines (Chawla et al. 2011). Macrophages of lean mice express the marker galactose/n-acetyl-galactosamine-specific lectin 1 (MGL1), and other characteristic genes such as ARG1, IL-10, and MGL2 (Lumeng et al. 2007), and are in the interstitial spaces between adipocytes (Lumeng et al. 2008). Alternatively, in obese mice and humans, most adipose tissue–resident macrophages are the phenotype M1, which secrete proinflammatory cytokines, leading to an inflammatory response in the adipose tissue and then to tissue destruction (Xu et al. 2003). In diet-induced obese mice, MGL1$^-$CCR2$^+$ (M1) macrophages accumulate in clusters surrounding necrotic adipocytes (Lumeng et al. 2008). IFN-γ and LPS cause the polarization of macrophages in obese individuals toward the proinflammatory phenotype M1 (Mathis 2013), but it can also originate at the recruitment of monocytes into adipose tissue (Westcott et al. 2009). In mice, the monocytes normally recruited to a site of inflammation are 7/4^{hi} CCR2$^+$ Ly-6C^{hi} CX$_3$CR1^{lo}, and turn into classically activated M1 macrophages (Gordon 2007), whereas those monocytes responsible for patrolling noninflamed tissue are 7/4^{mid} CCR2$^-$ Ly-6C^{lo} CX$_3$CR1^{hi}, and will become the adipose tissue–resident M2 macrophages under normal conditions. The presence of 7/4^{hi} monocytes is increased in obesity, suggesting that they may be specific mediators of the associated inflammation (Westcott et al. 2009).

4.6.2 Mast Cells

Mast cells are phenotypically and functionally versatile cells. Mature mast cells are found in connective and mucosal tissues, where they inform the immune system of infection or injury. Their cytoplasmic granules contain mediators such as histamine, serotonin, heparin, serine proteases, eicosanoids, and cytokines, which the granules release upon activation, promoting the recruitment of inflammatory cells to the site (Mathis 2013). Mast cells also release large amounts of IL-6, IL-8, TNF-α, and growth factors (Theoharides et al. 2007). Through the expression of IL-6 and IFN-γ, adipose tissue–resident mast cells can promote angiogenesis (Lui et al. 2009); induction of angiogenesis is part of the local inflammatory response associated with adipose tissue hypertrophy (reviewed in Pérez de Heredia et al. 2012). The presence of mast cells is higher in subcutaneous adipose tissue than in the visceral, at least in mice (Altintas et al. 2011). The reason for this could be the closer proximity of subcutaneous fat to the skin; mast cells would provide support to the skin's immune system, and/or contribute to neutralize inflammatory signals present in the microenvironment (Metz et al. 2008). However, the population of mast cells increases in obesity in mice (Liu et al. 2009; Altintas et al. 2011), and this increase is more dramatic in the visceral depot compared to the subcutaneous one (Altintas et al. 2011). Also, studies show mice genetically modified to be mast cell deficient gain less visceral adipose tissue on a high-fat diet than their wild-type counterparts (Liu et al. 2009). In addition, these mice had fewer visceral adipose tissue–resident macrophages, lower levels of both adipose tissue and circulatory inflammatory mediators, and higher insulin sensitivity (Liu et al. 2009). This suggests that mast cells have proinflammatory roles in obesity.

4.6.3 NEUTROPHILS

Neutrophils are part of the innate immune system (Table 4.1) and are early participants in the inflammatory response, typically being the first immune cells that arrive to the site of inflammation. Endothelium- and/or tissue-resident macrophages and mast cells recruit them from the circulation, and in turn neutrophils promote the recruitment of monocytes and other immune cells through the release of cytokines and chemokines, including TNF-α, MCP-1, IL-1β, and IL-8 (Soehnlein et al. 2008; Amulic et al. 2012). Activated neutrophils also release reactive oxygen species (ROS), which support the function of phagocytic immune cells (Sakai et al. 2012). Research has linked high-fat diets with enhanced recruitment of neutrophils in the visceral adipose tissue of mice (Talukdar et al. 2012). Similar to what was observed with mast cells, loss of function of the neutrophil protease elastase led to a 90% reduction in the numbers of adipose tissue–resident neutrophils, the amelioration of the inflammatory state, and the improvement of metabolic indices in mice fed on high-fat diets, regardless of changes in body weight status or adiposity (Talukdar et al. 2012).

4.6.4 EOSINOPHILS

Eosinophils circulate in an immature state, and once mature they are restricted to a limited number of tissues, which can be extended in the event of a parasitic infection. They play a critical role in controlling helminthic and parasitic infections and in allergic responses. The eosinophil population within adipose tissue is inversely correlated with adiposity (reviewed by Mathis 2013). There, eosinophils are responsible for up to 90% of IL-4 expression and for accelerated M2-phenotype macrophage polarization by secreting cytokines such as IL-4 and IL-3 (Fulkerson and Rothenberg 2013). Mice with reduced numbers of eosinophils in their visceral adipose tissue also exhibit a reduction in M2 macrophages, greater body weight, and visceral adipose tissue accumulation, and increased insulin resistance when fed a high-fat diet, whereas mice enriched with eosinophils showed a reversion in all these variables (Mathis 2013).

4.6.5 NATURAL KILLER (NK) AND NATURAL KILLER T (NKT) CELLS

NK cells are part of the innate immune system, despite being a type of lymphocyte, and their main function is to identify and eliminate tumor cells. They can comprise up to 30% of the lymphocytes present in visceral adipose tissue in mice (Caspar-Bauguil et al. 2005). In humans, they are more abundant, and express higher levels of proinflammatory IFN-γ, in the visceral depot than in the subcutaneous one (Caspar-Bauguil et al. 2005; O'Rourke et al. 2009). Some studies have shown NK cells protect against the development of metabolic syndrome in obese humans (Lynch et al. 2009). NKT cells express markers typical of both T lymphocytes and NK cells; they may constitute a bridge between the innate and the adaptive immune systems (Bendelac et al. 2007). They occur as well in adipose tissue, where lipid antigens presented by adipocytes themselves could trigger their activity, and it has been proposed that adipose tissue–resident NKT cells can be the first line of defense against adipocyte dysfunction, adipose tissue inflammation, and insulin resistance (Schipper et al. 2012b).

4.6.6 T LYMPHOCYTES

Specific T-cell subsets, such as CD8$^+$, IFN-γ^+CD4$^+$ (Th1), and Foxp3$^+$ regulatory T (Treg) cells, have been proposed to have distinct roles in adipose tissue immune homeostasis (Feuerer et al. 2009). The infiltration of the CD8$^+$ or cytotoxic T-cells has been demonstrated to precede the influx of macrophages in obesity, and they are likely to be involved in the recruitment of monocytes into adipose tissue and in their polarization toward the M1 phenotype, as indicated by both *in vitro* and *in vivo* studies. Interestingly, CD8$^+$ T-cell–deficient mice also present improved insulin sensitivity

(Schipper et al. 2012a). This suggests that CD8⁺ T-cells contribute to the initiation of adipose tissue inflammation and insulin resistance, through recruitment and polarization of macrophages towards the proinflammatory phenotype M1. T helper 1 (Th1) or IFN-γ⁺CD4⁺ cells have been implicated as well in adipose tissue inflammation and insulin resistance. Studies have demonstrated that mice deficient in these cells show reduced adipose tissue inflammation, and that antibody-mediated skewing of Th1 cells to Treg cells within adipose tissue improves insulin sensitivity (Schipper et al. 2012a).

In contrast to CD8⁺ T and Th1 cells, Foxp3⁺ regulatory T-cells (Treg) decrease in the presence of obesity, and studies demonstrate they prevent the onset of adipose tissue inflammation and insulin resistance (Feuerer et al. 2009). Researchers have proposed two potential explanations for these effects. First, Treg cells seem to improve glucose uptake of adipocytes *in vitro* (Feuerer et al. 2009). Secondly, Treg cells resident within human adipose tissue show an inverse correlation with the polarization of macrophages to the M1 phenotype (Schipper et al. 2012a).

4.6.7 B LYMPHOCYTES

Researchers have found B lymphocytes in adipose tissue—particularly the B-2 subtype, which is the most abundant type in the spleen and lymph nodes (Schipper et al. 2012a). B-2 lymphocytes produce and release IgG2c antibodies, which studies show are elevated in obesity and could mediate insulin resistance, at least in mice; transferring IgG2c antibodies to lean mice results in adipose tissue inflammation and insulin resistance (Winer et al. 2011). Antibody-driven M1 switch of macrophages likely mediates this outcome, because B-cell infiltration into adipose tissue has been observed to precede macrophage polarization (Schipper et al. 2012a). Additionally, adipose tissue–resident macrophages presented decreased M1 polarization in mice that were B-cell deficient (Winer et al. 2011). Furthermore, research has identified more than one hundred IgG targets that are associated with insulin resistance, expressed in a variety of tissues, including adipose tissue. These findings therefore indicate a proinflammatory effect for B-cells within adipose tissue, and their involvement in the obesity-associated inflammation.

4.7 ROLE OF ADIPOSE TISSUE–RESIDENT IMMUNE CELLS IN PATHOLOGICAL STATES

In 1997, Dong and colleagues reported that loss of function of the intercellular cell adhesion molecule (ICAM)-1 could lead to obesity under a high-fat diet, suggesting that the control of fat deposition requires the presence of immune cells in adipose tissue (Dong et al. 1997). Later, the classic works by Weisberg and colleagues and by Xu and colleagues demonstrated increased macrophage infiltration in adipose tissue of obese mice (Weisberg et al. 2003; Xu et al. 2003). Obesity therefore favors immune cell migration toward adipose tissue, and it also promotes a phenotypic switch in resident immune cells. For example, as mentioned previously, M2 macrophages will progressively adopt a more proinflammatory M1 phenotype (Lumeng et al. 2007). Conversely, absence of the M2 phenotype has been associated with a higher susceptibility to obesity, inflammation, and insulin resistance (Odegaard et al. 2007). Furthermore, obesity leads to changes in the lymphocyte population. The content of NK cells in the visceral depots reduces, whereas that of primitive γδ lymphocytes increases, which could lead to further activation of macrophage recruitment and activity (Caspar-Bauguil et al. 2005). Also, adipose tissue in obesity experiences a loss of IL-10-secreting Treg cells (Feuerer et al. 2009) and an increase in the presence of activated memory T-cells (Yang et al. 2010) All these changes, consequently, will lead to an increased ratio of proinflammatory/anti-inflammatory mediators, further amplifying the inflammatory status in the adipose tissue. The objective of these changes is to induce a state of insulin resistance in adipocytes, to reduce lipid storage, and to stimulate lipolysis, so as to control adipose tissue expansion. However, under a situation of chronic positive energy imbalance, where the flux of nutrients into the adipose tissue exceeds their oxidation, the result is a nonresolved inflammatory response and defective insulin signaling, which may develop into the well-known metabolic alterations associated with obesity, such as systemic insulin resistance, diabetes, and metabolic syndrome.

4.7.1 Metabolic Syndrome

Mathis (2013) implicated innate immune cells, whether of a pro- or anti-inflammatory nature, in the development of metabolic syndrome. In overweight and obese subjects with a diagnosis of incipient metabolic syndrome (but in the absence of diabetes or cardiovascular disease), samples of subcutaneous adipose tissue presented higher levels of the macrophage marker CD68 and no detectable CD3 and CD5, when compared to subjects without metabolic syndrome risk factors (Bremer and Jialal 2013). This suggests a specific increase of macrophage infiltration but no T-cell infiltration in adipose tissue associated with the establishment of metabolic syndrome. In addition, the number of crown-like structures (CLS) formed by macrophages in the adipose tissue was three times greater when metabolic syndrome was present. Also, the levels of MCP-1 were higher in subjects with signs of metabolic syndrome and correlated positively with levels of CRP (used by the authors as a marker for inflammation) and HOMA index (used as a marker for insulin resistance). Finally, concentrations of the chemoattractant chemerin were higher in the metabolic syndrome group (Bremer and Jialal 2013). These results indicate that increased macrophage infiltration in adipose tissue is linked to the development of metabolic syndrome, inflammation, and insulin resistance, independent of obesity. However, although both groups compared in the study had average BMIs in the range of overweight and obesity, the metabolic syndrome group was significantly heavier (34 vs 29 kg/m^2), and it is difficult to detach a diagnosis of metabolic syndrome from obesity. Therefore, the question remains whether immune cells in adipose tissue can promote adipose dysfunction in the absence of excess body fat accumulation.

4.7.2 Cardiovascular Risk

A study in obese subjects analyzed samples of abdominal subcutaneous adipose tissue and found CLS in 65% of them (CLS$^+$ group), and no indication of such structures or inflammatory activity in the rest (CLS$^-$ group) (Apovian et al. 2008). Total macrophage count was positively associated with insulin concentrations and insulin resistance (represented by the HOMA-IR index), and negatively with adiponectin levels. When researchers compared the CLS$^+$ and CLS$^-$ groups, the CLS$^+$ group presented higher values for insulin and HOMA-IR, despite a similar prevalence of metabolic syndrome. In addition, vascular endothelial function seemed impaired in the CLS$^+$ group, as suggested by lower flow-mediated dilation capacity in the brachial artery, indicating higher arteriosclerotic risk and consequently higher cardiovascular risk. Interestingly, no differences were found between groups for indices of adiposity, which supports an obesity-independent role of macrophage-induced inflammation in the development of cardiovascular disease. Similarly, instances of bariatric surgery performed on morbidly obese patients improved markers of vascular function, particularly arterial stiffness (Samaras et al. 2012). However, this improvement was not correlated with observed reductions in body weight or indices of adiposity, although it did correlate with amelioration of insulin resistance. More interestingly, arterial stiffness was negatively correlated with expression of the lymphocyte chemoattractant CCL20 in subcutaneous adipose tissue of the patients, and positively with MCP-1 expression in the visceral tissue, and improvement of arterial stiffness after bariatric surgery was inversely associated with visceral adipose tissue expression of MCP-1 and IFN-γ (Samaras et al. 2012). In a different study, researchers analyzed samples of epicardial adipose tissue in normal weight subjects with or without coronary artery disease (CAD) (Zhou et al. 2011). Epicardial fat is a visceral depot that shares properties with intra-abdominal fat, and as such it produces proinflammatory factors potentially contributing to the development of cardiovascular disease (Matsuda et al. 2002; Iacobellis et al. 2005). Apart from lower adiponectin levels in CAD patients, researchers found higher expression of IL-6, TNF-α, and TLR4, and increased CD68[+] positive cells, meaning macrophage presence, in these subjects. Another study researched subcutaneous adipose tissue from patients with severe heart failure, and compared it with samples from subjects without cardiovascular disease (Khan et al. 2012). Patients with heart failure were of lower BMI than healthy donors, and their adipocytes were of smaller size, despite which their adipose tissue presented increased macrophage infiltration and signs of inflammation. Implantation of ventricular assist devices (a step prior to heart transplant) resulted in reduced macrophage presence in adipose tissue, even when the adipocytes increased in size, compared to before implantation of the devices, and those changes paralleled improvement of insulin sensitivity. These results confirm the participation of adipose tissue–resident macrophages in the establishment of an inflammatory environment that promotes insulin resistance and cardiovascular disease, independently of obesity.

4.8 SUMMARY AND CONCLUSIONS

Adipose tissue and the immune system are intimately related, and research suggests a common developmental origin. Research has found many different subsets of immune cells populating adipose tissue, and they are key for maintaining homeostasis within this organ. M1-type macrophages, mast cells, neutrophils, T cytotoxic, T memory, and B lymphocytes exert proinflammatory effects in the tissue, contributing to the development of adipose tissue inflammation and insulin resistance associated with obesity. On the other hand, M2-type macrophages, eosinophils, NK, NKT, and T regulatory cells could constitute protective populations in the face of adipose tissue dysfunction. Macrophages have been the most extensively studied population so far, and they are closely involved in the chain of events that connect adipocyte dysfunction with metabolic syndrome and cardiovascular disease, even independently of obesity. Further research into the phenotypes and actions of adipose tissue–resident immune cells will be of great help for a better understanding of adipose tissue pathophysiology, obesity, and its related comorbidities.

REFERENCES

Altintas, M., Azad, A., Nayer, B. et al. 2011. Mast cells, macrophages, and crown-like structures distinguish subcutaneous from visceral fat in mice. *J Lipid Res* 52:480–8.

Amulic, B., Cazalet, C., Hayes, G. et al. 2012. Neutrophil function: From mechanisms to disease. *Ann Rev Immunol* 30:459–89.

Apovian, C. M. Bigornia, S., Mott, M. et al. 2008. Adipose macrophage infiltration is associated with insulin resistance and vascular endothelial dysfunction in obese subjects. *Arterioscler Thromb Vasc Biol* 28:1654–9.

Batra, A., Okur, B., Glauben, R. et al. 2010. Leptin: A critical regulator of CD4+ T-cell polarization in vitro and in vivo. *Endocrinology* 151:56–62.

Bendelac, A., Savage, P. and Teyton, L. 2007. The biology of NKT cells. *Ann Rev Immunol* 25:297–336.

Bourlier, V. and Bouloumie, A. 2009. Role of macrophage tissue infiltration in obesity and insulin resistance. *Diabetes Metab* 35:251–60.

Bozaoglu, K., Bolton, K., McMillan, J. et al. 2007. Chemerin is a novel adipokine associated with obesity and metabolic syndrome. *Endocrinology* 148:4687–94.

Bremer, A.A. and Jialal, I. 2013. Adipose tissue dysfunction in nascent metabolic syndrome. *J Obes.* 2013:393192.

Caspar-Bauguil, S., Cousin, B., Galinier, A. et al. 2005. Adipose tissues as an ancestral immune organ: Site-specific change in obesity. *FEBS Lett* 579:3487–92.

Cawthorn, W. and Sethi, J. 2008. TNF-alpha and adipocyte biology. *FEBS Lett* 582:117–31.

Chawla, A., Nguyen, K. and Goh, Y. 2011. Macrophage-mediated inflammation in metabolic disease. *Nat Rev Immunol* 11:738–49.

Choy, L., Rosen, B. and Spiegelman, B. 1992. Adipsin and endogenous pathway of complement from adipose cells. *J Biol Chem* 267:12736–41.

Cousin, B., Munoz, O., Andre, M. et al. 1999. A role for preadipocytes as macrophage-like cells. *FASEB J* 13:305–12.

Covarrubias, A.J. and Horng, T. 2014. IL-6 strikes a balance in metabolic inflammation. *Cell Metab* 19:898–9.

Crossno, J.T. Jr, Majka, S.M., Grazia, T. et al. 2006. Rosiglitazone promotes development of a novel adipocyte population from bone marrow-derived circulating progenitor cells. *J Clin Invest* 116:3220–8.

Curat, C., Miranville, A., Sengenès, C. et al. 2004. From blood monocytes to adipose tissue-resident macrophages: Induction of diapedesis by human mature adipocytes. *Diabetes* 53:1285–92.

Dani, C. and Billon, N. 2012. Adipocyte precursors: Developmental origins, self-renewal, and plasticity. In: *Adipose Tissue Biology*, ed. M. E. Symonds, 1–16. New York: Springer.

Dong, Z.M., Gutierrez-Ramos, J.C., Coxon, A. et al. 1997. A new class of obesity genes encodes leukocyte adhesion receptors. *Proc Natl Acad Sci USA* 94:7526–30.

Fain, J.N., Madan, A.K., Hiler, M.L. et al. 2004. Comparison of the release of adipokines by adipose tissue, adipose tissue matrix, and adipocytes from visceral and subcutaneous abdominal adipose tissues of obese humans. *Endocrinology* 145:2273–82.

Fasshauer, M. and Blüher, M. 2015. Adipokines in health and disease. *Trends Pharmacol Sci* 36:461–70.

Fernandez-Real, J. and Ricart, W. 1999. Insulin resistance and inflammation in an evolutionary perspective: The contribution of cytokine genotype/phenotype to thriftiness. *Diabetologia* 42:1367–74.

Feuerer, M., Herrero, L., Cipolletta, D. et al. 2009. Lean, but not obese, fat is enriched for a unique population of regulatory T cells that affect metabolic parameters. *Nat Med* 15:930–9.

Fulkerson, P. and Rothenberg, M. 2013. Targeting eosinophils in allergy, inflammation and beyond. *Nat Rev Drug Discov* 12:117–29.

Gabrielsson, B., Johansson, J., Lonn, M. et al. 2003. High expression of complement components in omental adipose tissue in obese men. *Obes Res Clin Pract* 11:699–708.

Goralski, K., McCarthy, T., Hanniman, E. et al. 2007. Chemerin, a novel adipokine that regulates adipogenesis and adipocyte metabolism. *J Biol Chem* 282:28175–88.

Gordon, S. 2007. Macrophage heterogeneity and tissue lipids. *J Clin Invest* 117:89–93.

Grant, R.W. and Dixit V.D. 2015. Adipose tissue as an immunological organ. *Obesity* 23:512–8.

Huang, J., Zhang, J., Lei, T. et al. 2010. Cloning of porcine chemerin, ChemR23 and GPR1 and their involvement in regulation of lipogenesis. *BMB Rep* 43:491–8.

Huber, J., Kiefer, F., Zeyda, M. et al. 2008. CC chemokine and CC chemokine receptor profiles in visceral and subcutaneous adipose tissue are altered in human obesity. *J Clin Endocrinol Metab* 93:3215–21.

Iacobellis, G., Corradi, D. and Sharma, A.M. 2005. Epicardial adipose tissue: Anatomic, biomolecular and clinical relationships with the heart. *Nat Clin Pract Cardiovasc Med* 2:536–43.

Im, S., Yousef, L., Blaschitz, C. et al. 2011. Linking lipid metabolism to the innate immune response in macrophages through sterol regulatory element binding protein-1a. *Cell Metab* 13:540–9.

Khan, R.S., Kato, T.S., Chokshi, A. et al. 2012. Adipose tissue inflammation and adiponectin resistance in patients with advanced heart failure: Correction after ventricular assist device implantation. *Circ Heart Fail* 5:340–8.

Kim, K.Y., Kim, J.K., Han, S.H. et al. 2006. Adiponectin is a negative regulator of NK cell cytotoxicity. *J Immunol* 176:5958–64.

Klein, J., Permana, P., Owecki, M. et al. 2007. What are subcutaneous adipocytes really good for? *Exp Dermatol* 16:45–70.

Kloting, N. and Blüher, M. 2014. Adipocyte dysfunction, inflammation and metabolic syndrome. *Rev Endocr Metab Disord* 15:277–87.

Lehr, S., Hartwig, S. and Sell, H. 2012. Adipokines: A treasure trove for the discovery of biomarkers for metabolic disorders. *Proteomics Clin Appl* 6:91–101.

Lehrke, M., Becker, A., Greif, M. et al. 2009. Chemerin is associated with markers of inflammation and components of the metabolic syndrome but does not predict coronary atherosclerosis. *Eur J Endocrinol* 161:339–44.

Lim, J., Iyer, A., Suen, J. et al. 2013. C5aR and C3aR antagonists each inhibit diet-induced obesity, metabolic dysfunction, and adipocyte and macrophage signalling. *FASEB J* 27:822–31.

Liu, J., Divoux, A., Sun, J. et al. 2009. Genetic deficiency and pharmacological stabilization of mast cells reduce diet-induced obesity and diabetes in mice. *Nat Med* 15:940–5.

Lumeng, C., Bodzin, J. and Saltiel, A. 2007. Obesity induces a phenotypic switch in adipose tissue macrophage polarization. *J Clin Invest* 117:175–84.

Lumeng, C., DelProposto, J., Westcott, D. et al. 2008. Phenotypic switching of adipose tissue macrophages with obesity is generated by spatiotemporal differences in macrophage subtypes. *Diabetes* 57:3239–46.

Lynch, L., O'Connell, J., Kwasnik, A. et al. 2009. Are natural killer cells protecting the metabolically healthy obese patients? *Obesity (Silver Spring)* 17:601–5.

Maeda, N., Shimomura, I., Kishida, K. et al. (2002). Diet-induced insulin resistance in mice lacking adiponectin/ACRP30. *Nat Med* 8: 731–7.

Majka, S.M., Fox, K.E., Psilas, J.C. et al. 2010. De novo generation of white adipocytes from the myeloid lineage via mesenchymal intermediates is age, adipose depot, and gender specific. *Proc Natl Acad Sci USA* 107:14781–6.

Mamane, Y., Chung Chan, C., Lavallee, G. et al. 2009. The C3a anaphylatoxin receptor is a key mediator of insulin resistance and functions by modulating adipose tissue macrophage infiltration and activation. *Diabetes* 58:2006–17.

Mathis, D. 2013. Immunological goings-on in visceral adipose tissue. *Cell Metab* 17:851–9.

Matsuda, M., Shimomura, I., Sata, M. et al. 2002. Role of adiponectin in preventing vascular stenosis. The missing link of adipo-vascular axis. *J Biol Chem* 277:37487–91.

Mauer, J., Chaurasia, B., Goldau, J. et al. 2014. Signaling by IL-6 promotes alternative activation of macrophages to limit endotoxemia and obesity-associated resistance to insulin. *Nat Immunol* 15:423–30.

Metz, M., Siebenhaar, F. and Maurer, M. 2008. Mast cell functions in the innate skin immune system. *Immunobiology* 213:251–60.

O'Rourke, R., Metcalf, M., White, A. et al. 2009. Depot-specific differences in inflammatory mediators and a role for NK cells and IFN-gamma in inflammation in human adipose tissue. *Int J Obes (Lond)* 33:978–90.

Odegaard, J., Ricardo-Gonzalez, R., Goforth, M. et al. 2007. Macrophage-specific PPARgamma controls alternative activation and improves insulin resistance. *Nature* 447:1116–20.

Ohashi, K., Parker, J.L., Ouchi, N. et al. (2010). Adiponectin promotes macrophage polarization toward an anti-inflammatory phenotype. *J Biol Chem* 285(9):6153-60. doi: 10.1074/jbc.M109.088708.

Ouchi, N., Kihara, S., Arita, Y. et al. 2001. Adipocyte-derived plasma protein, adiponectin, suppresses lipid accumulation and class A scavenger receptor expression in human monocyte-derived macrophages. *Circulation* 103:1057–63.

Pérez de Heredia, F., Gómez-Martínez, S. and Marcos, A. 2012. Obesity, inflammation and the immune system. *Proc Nutr Soc* 71:332–8.

Pérez de Heredia, F., Wood, I.S. and Trayhurn, P. 2010. Lactate enhances the inflammatory response in human preadipocytes in vitro. *Obes Rev* 11 (Suppl. 1):122.

Pevsner-Fischer, M., Morad, V., Cohen-Sfady, M. et al. 2007. Toll-like receptors and their ligands control mesenchymal stem cell functions. *Blood* 109:1422–32.

Pietsch, J., Batra, A., Stroh, T. et al. 2006. Toll-like receptor expression and response to specific stimulation in adipocytes and preadipocytes: On the role of fat in inflammation. *Ann NY Acad Sci* 1072:407–9.

Pond, C.M. 2005. Adipose tissue and the immune system. *Prostaglandins Leukot Essent Fatty Acids* 73:17–30.

Poulain-Godefroy, O. and Froguel, P. 2007. Preadipocyte response and impairment of differentiation in an inflammatory environment. *Biochem Biophys Res Commun* 356:662–7.

Sakai, J., Li, J., Kulandayan, S. et al. 2012. Reactive oxygen species-induced actin glutathionylation controls actin dynamics in neutrophils. *Immunity* 37:1037–49.

Samaras, K., Viardot, A., Lee, P.N. et al. 2012. Reduced arterial stiffness after weight loss in obese type 2 diabetes and impaired glucose tolerance: The role of immune cell activation and insulin resistance. *Diab Vasc Dis Res* 10:40–8.

Samuvel, D.J., Sundararaj, K.P., Nareika, A. et al. 2009. Lactate boosts TLR4 signaling and NF-κB pathway-mediated gene transcription in macrophages via monocarboxylate transporters and MD-2 up-regulation. *J Immunol* 182:2476–84.

Sánchez-Margalet, V., Marin-Romero, C., Santos-Alvarez, J. et al. 2003. Role of leptin as an immunomodulator of blood monocular cells: Mechanisms of action. *Clin Exp Immunol* 133:11–9.

Schäffler, A., Neumeier, M., Herfarth, H. et al. 2005. Genomic structure of human omentin, a new adipocytokine expressed in omental adipose tissue. *Biochim Biophys Acta* 1732:96–102.

Schäffler, A., Schölmerich, J. and Salzberger, B. 2007. Adipose tissue as an immunological organ: Toll-like receptors, C1q/TNFs and CTRPs. *Trends Immunol* 28:393–9.

Schipper, H., Prakken, B., Kalkhoven, E. et al. 2012a. Adipose tissue-resident immune cells: Key players in immunometabolism. *Trends Enocrinol Metab* 23:407–15.

Schipper, H., Rakhshandehroo, M., van de Graaf, S. et al. 2012b. Natural killer T cells in adipose tissue prevent insulin resistance. *J Clin Invest* 122:3343–54.

Sera, Y., LaRue, A.C., Moussa, O. et al. 2009. Hematopoietic stem cell origin of adipocytes. *Exp Hematol* 37:1108–20, e1101–4.

Sitticharoon, C., Nway, N., Chatree, S. et al. 2014. Interactions between adiponectin, visfatin, and omentin in subcutaneous and visceral adipose tissues and serum, and correlations with clinical and peripheral metabolic factors. *Peptides* 62:164–75.

Soehnlein, O., Zernecke, A., Eriksson, E. et al. 2008. Neutrophil secretion products pave the way for inflammatory monocytes. *Blood* 112:1461–71.

Sopasakis, V., Nagaev, I. and Smith, U. 2005. Cytokine release from adipose tissue of no obese individuals. *Int J Obes (Lond)* 29:1144–7.

Takahashi, M., Takahashi, Y., Takahashi, K. et al. 2008. Chemerin enhances insulin signalling and potentiates insulin-stimulated glucose uptake in 3T3-L1 adipocytes. *FEBS Lett* 582:573–8.

Talukdar, S., Oh D.Y., Bandyopadhyay, G. et al. 2012. Neutrophils medicate insulin resistance in mice fed a high fat diet through secreted elastase. *Nat Med* 18:1407–12.

Tan, B., Adya, R. and Randeva, H. 2010. Omentin: A novel link between inflammation, diabesity, and cardiovascular disease. *Trends Cardiovasc Med* 20:143–8.

Theoharides, T., Kempuraj, D., Tagen, M. et al. 2007. Differential release of mast cell mediators and the pathogenesis of inflammation. *Immunol Rev* 217:65–78.

Tian, Z., Sun, R., Wei, H. et al. 2002. Impaired natural (NK) cell activity in leptin receptor deficient mice: Leptin as a critical regulator in NK cell development and activation. *Biochem Biophys Res Commun* 298:297–302.

Trujillo, M., Lee, M., Sullivan, S. et al. 2006. Tumour necrosis factor and glucocorticoid synergistically increase leptin production in human adipose tissue: Role for p38 mitogen-activated protein kinase. *J Clin Endocrinol Metab* 91:1484–90.

Urbanova, M., Dostalova, I., Trachta, P. et al. 2014. Serum concentrations and subcutaneous adipose tissue mRNA expression of omentin in morbid obesity and type 2 diabetes mellitus: The effect of very-low-calorie diet, physical activity and laparoscopic sleeve gastrectomy. *Physiol Res* 63:207–18.

Van Niekerk, G. and Engelbrecht, A.M. 2015. On the evolutionary origin of the adaptive immune system—The adipocyte hypothesis. *Immunol Lett* 164:81–7.

Weigert, J., Neumeier, M., Wanninger, J. et al. 2010. Systemic chemerin is related to inflammation rather than obesity in type 2 diabetes. *Clin Endocrinol (Oxford)* 72:342–8.

Weisberg, S.P., McCann, D., Desai, M. et al. 2003. Obesity is associated with macrophage accumulation in adipose tissue. *J Clin Invest* 112:1785–8.

Westcott, D., DelProposto, J., Geletka, L. et al. 2009. MGL1 promotes adipose tissue inflammation and insulin resistance by regulating 7/4[hi] monocytes in obesity. *J Exp Med* 13:3143–56.

White, R., Damm, D., Hancock, N. et al. 1992. Human adipsin is identical to complement factor D and is expressed at high levels in adipose tissue. *J Biol Chem* 267:9210–3.

Winer, D., Winer, S., Shen, L. et al. 2011. B cells promote insulin resistance through modulation of T cells and production of pathogenic IgG antibodies. *Nat Med* 17:610–7.

Wittamer, V., Franssen, J.D., Vulcano, M. et al. 2003. Specific recruitment of antigen-presenting cells by chemerin, a novel processed ligand from human inflammatory fluids. *J Exp Med* 198:977–85.

Wolf, A., Wolf, D., Rumpold, H. et al. 2004. Adiponectin induces the anti-inflammatory cytokines IL-10 and IL-I RA in human leukocytes. *Biochem Biophys Res Commun* 323:630–5.

Wrann, C., Laue, T., Hubner, L. et al. 2012. Short-term and long-term exposure differentially affect human natural killer cell immune function. *Am J Physiol Endocrinol Metab* 302:108–16.

Xu, H., Barnes, G., Quing, Y. et al. 2003. Chronic inflammation in fat plays a crucial role in the development of obesity-related insulin resistance. *J Clin Invest* 112:1821–30.

Yamawaki, H., Kuramoto, J., Kameshima, S. et al. 2011. Omentin, a novel adipocytokine inhibits TNF-induced vascular inflammation in human endothelial cells. *Biochem Biophys Res Commun* 408:339–43.

Yang, R., Lee, M., Hu, H. et al. 2006. Identification of omentin as a novel depot-specific adipokine in human adipose tissue: Possible role in modulating insulin action. *Am J Physiol Endocrinol Metab* 290:1253–61.

Yang, H., Youm, Y.H., Vandanmagsar, B. et al. 2010. Obesity increases the production of proinflammatory mediators from adipose tissue T cells and compromises TCR repertoire diversity: Implications for systemic inflammation and insulin resistance. *J Immunol* 185:1836–45.

Zhang, L., Guerrero-Juarez, C.F., Hata, T. et al. 2015. Dermal adipocytes protect against invasive Staphylococcus aureus skin infection. *Science* 347:67–71.

Zhang, Y., Proenca, R., Maffei, M. et al. 1994. Positional cloning of the mouse obese gene and its human homologue. *Nature* 372:425–32.

Zhao, Y., Sun, R., You, L. et al. 2003. Expression of leptin receptors and response to leptin stimulation of human natural killer cell lines. *Biochem Biophys Res Commun* 300:247–52.

Zhou, Y., Wei, Y., Wang, L. et al. 2011. Decreased adiponectin and increased inflammation expression in epicardial adipose tissue in coronary artery disease. *Cardiovasc Diabetol* 10:2.

5 Influence of Infection and Inflammation on Nutrient Status

David I. Thurnham and Christine A. Northrop-Clewes

CONTENTS

5.1 Introduction..57
5.2 The Inflammatory Response and Serum Nutrient Concentrations...........................59
5.3 Use of Meta-Analysis to Calculate Adjustment Factors 60
5.4 Specific Nutrients and The Effects Of Inflammation...62
    5.4.1 Fat-Soluble Vitamins..62
        5.4.1.1 Vitamin A 62
        5.4.1.2 Vitamin D (Cholecalciferol) 64
        5.4.1.3 Vitamin E (α-Tocopherol)...66
        5.4.1.4 Vitamin K (Phylloquinone; K1)..68
    5.4.2 Water-Soluble Vitamins 68
        5.4.2.1 Vitamin C (Ascorbic Acid) 68
        5.4.2.2 Thiamin (Vitamin B_1) 70
        5.4.2.3 Riboflavin (Vitamin B_2) 70
        5.4.2.4 Niacin (Nicotinic Acid, Vitamin B_3) 71
        5.4.2.5 Pyridoxine (Vitamin B_6) 71
        5.4.2.6 Folic Acid..72
        5.4.2.7 Vitamin B_{12} (Cyanocobalamin)..73
    5.4.3 Carotenoids 74
    5.4.4 Minerals 74
        5.4.4.1 Iron (Fe)..74
        5.4.4.2 Zinc (Zn)...75
        5.4.4.3 Selenium (Se)..76
        5.4.4.4 Copper..77
References..77

5.1 INTRODUCTION

Nutrient status is assessed using biomarkers and, of these, the biomarkers most commonly used are the concentrations of the specific nutrient of interest in blood or urine. In a person who is healthy, nutrient concentrations in serum or urine will reflect the dietary intake. Serum nutrients may also be controlled by physiological factors including nutritional status. Standard criteria to assess nutritional status derived from depletion and repletion experiments in healthy volunteers, enable researchers to interpret status in individuals and population groups from nutrient concentrations in blood.[1] However, when a person suffers trauma or an infection, there is an inflammatory response which includes a number of metabolic changes in blood nutrient concentrations. These changes may be deliberate strategies by the body to withhold nutrients from an invading organism, may indicate increased catabolism or utilization of the nutrient or may simply reflect the consequences of anorexia. The changes induced by the immune or inflammatory response to infection are usually transitory and limited to the clinical and sub-clinical phases of an infection or period of trauma. However, during this period, blood nutrient concentrations are unlikely to reflect true nutritional status and if the presence of sub-clinical inflammation is overlooked, status will probably be misinterpreted. In the case of most serum nutrients there is a depression in concentration so if a researcher is unaware of the presence of sub-clinical inflammation, the prevalence of nutritional deficiencies can be exaggerated. In some cases, an increase in urinary metabolites may indicate increased nutrient utilization. This chapter will summarize what is known of many of the common blood nutrients and nutritional biomarkers during the inflammatory response and the potential effects on nutritional status. Blood nutrients may share common properties with one another, e.g. fat or water-solubility, but they are nevertheless unique substances with specific roles in metabolism. It is therefore important that each nutrient is examined separately in order to understand its response in infection and the impact of infection on status.

For most nutrients the principal populations at risk of nutritional deficiency are women of reproductive age and children less than 5 years of age, due to the higher nutrient requirements imposed by pregnancy, lactation and/or growth. The primary objective of this chapter will be to assist the reader to interpret nutritional status in apparently-healthy people using acute phase proteins[2,3] and/or cytokines[4] as biomarkers of inflammation. Interpreting nutritional status during infection is more difficult as duration and severity of illness will both influence nutritional biomarkers as indicated by the multiple factors associated with severe anemia in Malawian preschool children.[5] Duration and severity of disease can be assessed using acute phase proteins, particularly C-reactive protein (CRP). Workers in Burkina Faso investigated iron status biomarkers in 1564 children (6–23 m) with moderate acute malnutrition suggested regression analysis using CRP could be used to adjust serum ferritin in research settings.[6] In addition, workers in hospitals have assessed the influence of disease and trauma on a number of nutritional biomarkers by comparison with the degree of elevation in CRP and albumin.[7] Their observations will be reported in the sections on specific nutrients. The effects of inflammation in apparently-healthy people however, will be more comparable between individuals than that between hospital patients, so regression analysis is less useful and a single cut off to identify inflammation is sufficient. By definition, the clinical signs of disease will have disappeared in apparently-healthy subjects.[2,3] In addition, where surgical evidence is available in previously-healthy subjects, longitudinal data on inflammation and nutritional biomarkers can be examined.[8,9] In the case of vitamin A and iron, methods will be described to adjust nutrient concentrations to remove the effects of inflammation.[2,3] In other chapters in this book the roles of specific vitamins and minerals in the host response to infection will be addressed in greater depth.

Readers may also want to consult the report on Inflammation and Nutritional Science for Programs/Policies and Interpretation of Research Evidence (INSPIRE) published in 2015.[10] The main objectives of this study were to better understand the bidirectional relationship between nutritional status and the function of the immune and inflammatory response and the specific impact of the inflammatory response on the selection, use and interpretation of nutrient biomarkers. The purpose of the work was to provide guidance to users in all fields of nutrition enterprise in evaluating programs and generating evidence-based policy. In addition during 2017, a supplement in the American Journal of Clinical Nutrition will summarize the work of the Biomarkers Reflecting Inflammation and Nutrition Determinants of Anemia (BRINDA) group, who have looked at various approaches to correcting concentrations of ferritin, retinol, retinol binding protein (RBP) and transferrin receptors (sTfR) in the presence of inflammation in apparently-healthy people, using for the most part, national survey data.[11–13]

5.2 THE INFLAMMATORY RESPONSE AND SERUM NUTRIENT CONCENTRATIONS

The sequential production of different inflammatory proteins during the incubation period and following an infection or traumatic episode has been used to provide adjustment factors with which to correct blood nutrient or biomarker concentrations for the influence of inflammation. The inflammatory response is typically initiated by tissue macrophages or blood monocytes.[14] Activated macrophages release a broad spectrum of protein mediators of which the cytokines of the interleukin 1 (IL-1) and tumor necrosis factor (TNF) families trigger the next series of reactions both locally and distally. In the second wave of inflammatory mediators, IL-6 is produced which has particularly important effects in the hypothalamus and liver. Within the hypothalamus, temperature set points may be altered generating a fever and, in the liver, there are alterations in most metabolic pathways and gene regulation to produce essential metabolites for defense, damage limitation and the repair of tissues following recovery. In particular the liver response is characterized by the coordination and stimulation of the acute phase proteins (APP).

Three APP are particularly useful to characterize the stages of inflammation in apparently-healthy persons. Whereas, the increase in cytokine concentrations takes place within minutes, may reach maximum concentrations within 0.5–4.0 hours and have disappeared by 24 hours (Figure 5.1),[15,16] changes in APP concentrations can be monitored during the incubation period of infection and during convalescence.[13] We have used two acutely responding APP to monitor the initial response to infection, CRP and α1-antichymotrypsin (ACT), and one other, α1-acid glycoprotein (AGP), to monitor the later stages, namely convalescence. CRP and ACT both increase within the first 6 hours of infection or trauma, rise to a maximum within 24–48 hours and decline as the clinical signs of the disease diminish. In contrast, AGP rises more slowly; it remains within the normal range during the first 48 hours, may take 3–5 days to reach a plateau and remains elevated during the convalescent period.[17]

In an apparently-healthy population, four groups of people can be identified using CRP and AGP.[18–20] ACT can be used instead of CRP, but as CRP is more commonly used than ACT, we will restrict the discussions in this chapter to CRP. In the population, there will be those with no elevated APP who are healthy and can be described as the reference group. There will be those who have recently been exposed to trauma or infection and will show the very early signs of inflammation (group 2, raised CRP and normal AGP; incubation group) but are not yet showing signs of clinical disease. Then there will be those who have recently recovered from infection and who are in early or late convalescence stages (groups 3 and 4 respectively). In

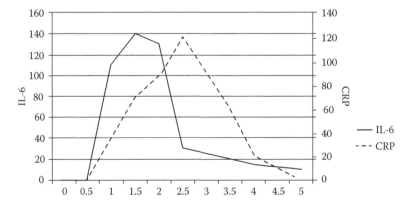

FIGURE 5.1 Time course of interleukin (IL) 6 and C-reactive protein (CRP) concentrations after surgery. The increase in IL-6 precedes the rise in CRP and has almost disappeared at 2.5 days when CRP peaked (concentrations are shown in arbitrary units); x-axis is days. (From Engler R., *Rev fr Allergol.*, 36, 903–913; Thurnham DI and McCabe GP. In LM Rogers [ed.], *Priorities in the Assessment of Vitamin A and Iron Status in Populations*, Panama City, Panama, Geneva, World Health Organisation, 2012.)[16,19]

TABLE 5.1

Nutritional Biomarkers Influenced by Inflammation

Serum Biomarkers (unless otherwise indicated)	Direction of Change	Acute Response (24–48 hours) %	Chronic or Long-Term Response (3–10 days) %	Reference
Retinol	↓	40–70	10–15	2,8,9,21
Retinol binding protein	↓	40–70	10–15	2,8,9,21
Carotenoids	↓	20–50	40–60	22–25
Zinc	↓	70	10–15	7,26
Iron	↓	50		26
Ferritin	↑	100% or more	100% or more	15
Transferrin receptor	(↓)↑	Small fall	~50 increase	27
25-Hydroxy-cholecalciferol	↓	40	20–30	28
Pyridoxine	↓	No information	Negative association with inflammation	29,30
Selenium	↓	No information	40–60	7
Leukocyte ascorbic acid	↓	~40	Normalized at 5 days	31
Vitamin C	↓	10–80	Variable fall	7,32

Source: Thurnham DI., *Sight and Life*, 1, 59–66. With permission.

group 3, both CRP and AGP are raised while in group 4, only the AGP concentration is above the normal range. The changes in serum nutrient concentrations that follow the onset of infection or trauma (Table 5.1), closely parallel the behavior of CRP.[9,15] That is, most serum nutrient concentrations fall rapidly during the initial period, may plateau or continue to fall during sickness and then return to normal more gradually during the period of convalescence. The interrelationship between the changing APP concentrations and serum retinol following infection is shown in Figure 5.2. The initial changes in serum nutrient concentrations following infection will be detectable by elevated serum CRP (>5 mg/L; or ACT>0.6 g/L) and normal AGP (≤ 1 g/L) concentrations. This period lasts 24–48 hours before the appearance of clinical signs of disease. People with clinical signs of trauma or disease will not be recruited in an apparently-healthy population so the remaining subjects will be in convalescence which can be divided into two periods as described above.

5.3   USE OF META-ANALYSIS TO CALCULATE ADJUSTMENT FACTORS

The model shown in Figure 5.2 was used to calculate adjustment factors for retinol[2] and ferritin.[3] The principle was the same for both but serum retinol concentrations are reduced by infection while ferritin concentrations are increased. The studies used for the two meta-analyses are shown in Table 5.2. In order that adjustment factors could be calculated for the 3 groups exhibiting inflammation, studies had to include measurements of both an acute and chronic APP and subjects with inflammation had to be present in the 3 inflammation groups. All of the studies included measurements of CRP and AGP except a study of Pakistani pre-school children[34] where ACT were used instead of CRP. Performing the meta-analyses with and without the Pakistani children made no difference to the adjustment factors calculated for either retinol or ferritin. To calculate adjustment factors we calculated mean log nutrient concentrations for all four groups and compared each group with all other groups for each study separately. Using 4 groups there are 6 pairs of comparisons for each

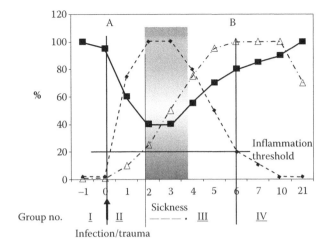

FIGURE 5.2   Model of the behavior of the plasma acute phase proteins CRP and AGP and retinol concentrations following an infection or trauma. The ordinate axis indicates arbitrary % values where zero represents normal, 20% represents the inflammation threshold of CRP (>5 mg/L) and AGP (>1 g/L), and 100% represents a normal serum retinol concentration or the maximum increase in CRP or AGP concentrations. The figure shows the rapid rise in C-reactive protein (CRP, short dashes) and fall in retinol concentrations (solid line) following an infection stimulus at time zero (A). The CRP concentration plateaus when clinical evidence of sickness appears and retinol reaches its nadir. Alpha-1-acid glycoprotein (AGP; long dashes) concentrations rise more slowly from time zero and only pass the inflammation threshold 2–5 days later. As sickness wanes, concentrations of CRP fall, retinol rises, and AGP plateaus. In the final stage of convalescence, CRP concentrations return to normal (B) leaving only AGP elevated. The model is used to categorize subjects in the following groups; I), reference, no raised acute phase proteins; II), incubation, only CRP increased; III), early convalescence, CRP and AGP both above the inflammation threshold; and IV), late convalescence only AGP is raised. (Modified from Thurnham DI. et al., *Proc Nutr Soc.*, 502–509, 2005, With permission.)[18]

TABLE 5.2

Summary of Studies Used for the Two Meta-analyses to Calculate Adjustment Factors for Retinol and Ferritin[a]

	Retinol	Ferritin (Iron status)
Total number of studies	15	30
Total number of subjects	9914	8796
Studies eligible for 4-group analysis[b]	7	22
Subjects (number)	4975	7848
Infant studies (number)	1	5
Pre-school age children studies (number)	5[c]	3[d]
Non-pregnant women studies (number)	0	5
Pregnant and lactating women studies (number)	1	6
Men studies (number)	0	3

[a]   Values are numbers of studies or subjects used for the 4-group retinol[2] and ferritin[3] meta-analyses.

[b]   4-Group analyses indicated that a study included subjects in the reference (no raised acute phase proteins) and the 3 inflammation groups namely; incubation (raised C-reactive protein (CRP) only), early convalescence (both CRP and α1-acid glycoprotein (AGP) raised) and late-convalescent groups (raised AGP only).

[c]   All subjects were apparently healthy although one study included pre-school age children from Papua New Guinea[35] where malaria was endemic but there was no information on parasite positivity.

[d]   Included both pre-school age and older children.

TABLE 5.3

Adjustment Factors from the Retinol[2] and Ferritin[3] 4-group Meta-Analyses[a]

Group comparison	Serum Retinol (n = 7)			Serum Ferritin (n = 22)		
	Mean	95%CI	P =	Mean	95%CI	P
Reference vs incubation	1.15	1.07, 1.24	0.001	1.30	1.15, 1.47	<0.001
Reference vs early convalescence	1.31	1.09, 1.58	0.005	1.90	1.51, 2.37	<0.001
Reference vs late convalescence	1.12	0.96, 1.31	0.16	1.36	1.19, 1.55	<0.001

[a] Values are mean (95%CI) of the geometric mean nutrient biomarker concentrations for the respective pairs from the 4-group analyses. See Table 5.2 for more details.

study however only 3 are relevant to calculate adjustment factors i.e. the ratios between the reference group and each of the 3 inflammation groups.

The adjustment factors were calculated from the summary statistic (effect size) which was the difference (ratio) between 2 log means, and the variability associated with each summary statistic was related to sample sizes. In general, studies with a large number of samples will have smaller variability than those with smaller numbers; therefore traditional weights were calculated on the basis of the inverse of the study variance. Thus studies with a large variance, and therefore a relatively imprecise estimate of the study summary, received less weight than a study with a smaller variance. In the 4-group analysis, weights were computed from the sum of the variances for the 4 groups and on the total size for the 4 groups. To estimate the variability of the overall summary statistic and to provide study-to-study variation, the random effect model was used for all of the analyses reported because it allowed for small differences between studies and enabled the generation of valid standard deviations (SD).

The data obtained for the group comparisons for all studies combined are summarized in Table 5.3. For retinol there were 7 studies that provided data for the 4-group analysis and for ferritin there were 22 studies. The mean ratios (summary statistics) are the values used to adjust data in the inflammation groups to remove the influence of that inflammation. So for retinol, mean concentrations in the reference group are 1.15 times greater than in the incubation group. That is, values in the incubation, early and late convalescent groups need to be increased by factors of 1.15, 1.32 and 1.12 respectively to remove the influence of inflammation. For ferritin the inverse of the ratio is used to calculate the adjustment factor as ferritin concentrations increase following infection. Ferritin adjustment factors in the three groups with inflammation were 0.77, 0.53 and 0.74 respectively.

The cut-off for serum retinol concentrations to indicate a risk of vitamin A deficiency is <0.7 µmol/L[36] and for ferritin concentrations indicating iron deficiency are <12 or <15 µg/L for subjects ≥ 5 years of age respectively.[37] That is, the net effect of correction for vitamin A is to reduce the number of subjects with retinol values <0.7 µmol/L and, for iron deficiency, to increase the number of subjects below the ferritin cut-off values shown above.

5.4 SPECIFIC NUTRIENTS AND THE EFFECTS OF INFLAMMATION

5.4.1 FAT-SOLUBLE VITAMINS

5.4.1.1 Vitamin A

In 2001, a working group (Annecy Accords) recommended and revised the criteria to assess vitamin A status. The working group set standards for both clinical and blood measurements of status, but serum retinol and retinol binding protein concentrations are the most frequently used methods.

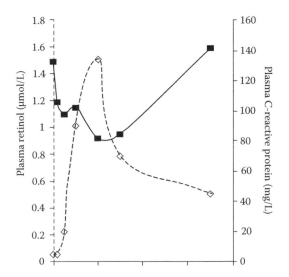

FIGURE 5.3 Changes in plasma retinol and C-reactive protein concentrations over 7 days in a group of nutritionally-adequate patients in response to uncomplicated orthopedic surgery. A rapid decrease in plasma retinol concentration (solid line) coincides with an increase in C-reactive protein (dashed line) in the first 48 hours following surgery. (Data are taken from Louw JA., *Crit Care Med.*, 20, 934–941.)[9]

In children a concentration of <0.7 μmol/L (<20 μg/dL) indicates a risk of vitamin A deficiency (VAD) and a prevalence of 15% or more in a community, indicates a public health problem.[38] Serum retinol concentrations are physiologically controlled and only when the store of retinol in the liver falls to very low concentrations (<0.07 μmol/g liver)[36], does the concentration of retinol in blood fall. A normal serum retinol concentration in young children is approximately 1 μmol/L and this rises to approximately 2 μmol/Lin adults (Figure 5.3). Low serum retinol concentrations may therefore be an indicator of low stores of liver retinol and poor vitamin A status but it may also be depressed by inflammation.[2,39] Unfortunately, the working group[38] made no mention of the dramatic effects which inflammation has on serum retinol concentrations. The depression caused by the trauma of surgery on serum retinol concentrations had been shown as early as 1978[8] and again in 1992[9] and a paper published in 1998 had reported that Bangladeshi children admitted to hospital with shigellosis had a mean (SD) serum retinol concentration of 0.36 (0.22) μmol/L which had normalized at discharge to 1.15 (0.5) μmol/L without any vitamin A treatment during hospitalisation.[21] As the prevalence of disease is often high in developing countries where most VAD occurs, the risk of exaggerating the prevalence of deficiency through effects of inflammation on serum retinol concentrations alone is high. Therefore, to obtain correct estimates of VAD it is important to identify inflammation and use the adjustment factors described above.

Surgery provides an opportunity to examine the influence of an altered inflammatory state on serum nutrient concentrations without the complications of disease.[28] The data shown in Figure 5.3 illustrate the rapidity with which plasma retinol concentrations fall in previously well-nourished adults following uncomplicated orthopedic surgery.[9] Mean plasma retinol concentrations fell by 40% in the 48 hours following surgery, plateaued for a day and then returned to pre-surgical concentrations by day 7. In contrast mean plasma CRP concentrations rose to a maximum in the first 48 hours and then initially declined rapidly but concentrations still indicated sub-clinical inflammation at day 7. It is important to note that a fall of 40% in plasma retinol concentration would take many months to achieve by withholding vitamin A from the diet alone.

The cut-off of 0.7 μmol/L is only 30% below the normal mean retinol concentration in healthy children and therefore a fall in the retinol concentration of 40% obtained in the patients above would categorize many children as at risk of VAD. Therefore concentrations <0.7 μmol retinol/L only indicate a risk of VAD, especially in countries where there is a high prevalence of disease. For this reason many researchers will measure an acute phase protein, commonly CRP, at the same time as retinol in order to determine the prevalence of inflammation. Where inflammation is detected, researchers often exclude those subjects with inflammation or ignore the inflammation if the prevalence is low.

The problem with using only one acute-reacting protein like CRP, serum amyloid A (SAA) or ACT to detect inflammation is that it underestimates the prevalence of inflammation. As indicated above, the APP which rise acutely in response to infection or other traumas, fall rapidly as the clinical signs diminish. Sub-clinical inflammation however continues and needs to be monitored with AGP.[40,41] Figure 5.1 shows the rapid rise in CRP concentrations at the onset of trauma but as soon as clinical signs of the trauma wane or disappear, concentrations of CRP rapidly return to near normal.[17,42] This was also demonstrated in a study on 2519 Pakistani pre-school children where, of the 274 children with an elevated ACT concentration, most ($n = 260$) also had an elevated AGP suggesting that they were only recently recovered from illness. In this group (early convalescence) there was a greater depression in the mean retinol concentration (0.73 µmol/L) than in those where there was elevated ACT or AGP alone (0.81; 0.83 µmol/L respectively.[34] Most children with inflammation ($n = 881$, 35%) were in late convalescence (raised AGP only). The mean retinol concentration in those without inflammation was 0.9 µmol/L, and this figure probably represents the best estimate of serum retinol concentration in the healthy Pakistani pre-school children and 54% of the sample was present in this group.

5.4.1.2   Vitamin D (Cholecalciferol)

Vitamin D exists in two forms, vitamin D3 (cholecalciferol) and vitamin D2 (ergocalciferol). Some of the D3 form is obtained from the diet (dairy foods, eggs and fish) but the main source is probably endogenous synthesis through the action of short wavelength, ultra-violet light (290–315 nm) on human skin. The D2 form is produced from yeast and principally obtained from vitamin D supplements. The action of sunlight on human skin converts 7-dehydrocholecalciferol into cholecalciferol. Cholecalciferol is fat-soluble and stores of this compound are found in adipose tissue. Some undergoes hydroxylation in the liver to 25-hydroxy-vitamin D (25-OHD). Adipose tissue stores of vitamin D are in equilibrium with plasma 25-OHD concentrations hence 25-OHD concentrations are a useful measure of vitamin D status.[43] Plasma 25-OHD has a half-life of approximately 3 weeks and this is longer than all other vitamin D metabolites.[44] Deficiency is generally regarded at <30 nmol/L (12 ng/mL) but sufficiency is variously stated as >50, >80[45] or even >150[46] nmol/L.

In terms of the functional vitamin D concentration, it is widely considered that it is best to assess the free (i.e. unbound) concentration in plasma.[47] Most (80%–90%) plasma vitamin D metabolites circulate bound to vitamin D-binding protein (VDBP) and most of the remainder (10%–20%) is bound to albumin. Very little 25-OHD remains free i.e. biologically active in plasma (0.02%–0.05%).[48,49] The relative affinity of VDBP for 1,25-$(OH)_2$D is 10-fold less than for 25-OHD so free plasma concentrations of 1,25-$(OH)_2$D are 10 fold higher than those of 25-OHD (0.2%–0.6%). However, the concentration of VDBP in plasma is 20-fold higher than the total amount of vitamin D metabolites and the physiological consequence of the large molar excess of circulating VDBP is unclear. Only 5% of the total VDBP capacity is usually occupied by vitamin D compounds; therefore most, if not all, circulating vitamin D compounds are protein bound and will have little access to target cells. Thus, concentrations of free rather than total forms of 25-OHD and 1,25-(OH)2D are likely to provide a better assessment of functional vitamin D status.[50]

Further metabolism of 25-OHD is mostly determined by the best-known function of vitamin D, namely the control of calcium metabolism. A fall in plasma calcium concentrations stimulates the formation of another hydroxylase enzyme in the kidney which converts 25-OHD to 1,25 dihydroxy-vitamin D (1,25-$(OH)_2$D). 1,25-$(OH)_2$D controls a number of metabolic process that raise plasma calcium concentrations either by increasing calcium absorption and/or releasing calcium from bone. However, the 1α-hydroxylase enzyme and the 1,25 vitamin D receptor are also found in many immune and other cells throughout the body.[51] The important functions of $1,25(OH)_2D$ necessitate a much tighter control over its plasma concentration than of the 25-OHD metabolite and the half life is only 4 hours.[44]

Beyond its critical function in calcium homeostasis, vitamin D has been found to play an important role in the modulation of the immune/inflammation system via regulating the production of inflammatory cytokines and inhibiting the proliferation of pro-inflammatory cells, both of which are crucial for the pathogenesis of inflammatory diseases.[52] This important secondary function of vitamin D may explain why serum concentrations of 25-OHD fell by more than 40% within 24 hours of elective knee surgery (arthroplasty) and were still 20% lower than pre-operative values 3 months after the operation.[28] This study provided an opportunity to examine the influence of an altered inflammatory state on vitamin D status without the complication of accompanying disease.[28] In fact, similar observations to those of Reid et al. were first reported by Louw et al.[9] almost 20 years ago. Louw et al. showed that a transient depression in plasma 25-OHD concentrations of ~16% followed uncomplicated orthopedic surgery in 25 volunteers of both sexes. In almost all cases, concentrations of 25-OHD had normalized by day six when CRP had almost returned to normal. The authors pointed out that the nutritional status of the group prior to surgery was good and no patient fasted more than 12 hours post-operatively. The authors also monitored hydration and concluded that the patients had a normal fluid intake and this made hemodilution very unlikely. The authors concluded that the self-correcting nature of the decreased values in the study argued against the low values representing true nutritional status.[9]

In contrast to the study of Louw et al. however, plasma 25-OHD concentrations following the surgery described by Reid et al. remained low for several months suggesting that vitamin D status was reduced by the surgery. Reid and colleagues measured plasma 25-OHD, 25-OHD:VDBP ratio and free 25-OHD concentrations in the immediate post-operative period. The depression in concentrations was large (~40%) (Table 5.4) and consistent with the reports of the previously observed effects of inflammation on plasma retinol,[8,9] many other nutrients[23] and the increase in ferritin (Table 5.1).[15] Not only were concentrations of 25-OHD depressed but also the 25-OHD:VDBP ratio and free 25-OHD concentrations. Furthermore, in blood samples taken at three months, the three markers of vitamin D status were no different from those observed in the samples collected on day 5 postoperatively but CRP concentrations had returned to the preoperative value. The authors concluded that plasma concentrations of 25-OHD decrease after an inflammatory insult and therefore are unlikely to be a reliable measure of 25-OHD status in subjects with evidence of a significant systemic inflammatory response.

TABLE 5.4
Peri-operative Measurements in Patients Following Elective Knee Surgery

	Pre-Operative	6–12 hr	Day 1	Day 2	Day 3	Day 4	Day 5	P
CRP (mg/L)	2.8	–	56	164	189	136	113	<0.001
25-OHD (nmol/L)	40	26	23	23	25	28	29	<0.001
Albumin (g/L)	39	–	33	32	31	30	31	<0.001
VDBP (μmol/L)	7.5	6.6	6.9	7.1	–	–	7.9	<0.001
Molar ratio 25-OHD:VDBP	6.9	5.4	4.2	4.8	–	–	4.0	<0.001
Free 25-OHD (pmol/L)	9.04	–	5.41	6.40	–	–	6.09	<0.001

Source: Reid D. et al., *Am J Clin Nutr.*, 91,1006–1011.[28]
Note: All values are medians.

Reid et al. considered what might have contributed to the apparent loss of 25-OHD from the blood. The possibility that the fall in the binding protein and albumin concentrations may have contributed to the loss of 25-OHD was considered but the fall in the protein concentrations (albumin and VDBP) was only ~20% while 25-OHD concentrations fell by 40%. However, it is interesting to compare the behavior of 25-OHD with that of plasma retinol about which more is known. Early changes in epithelial permeability and vasodilatation stimulated by inflammation may well facilitate the movement of plasma retinol into to the extracellular fluid compartment contributing to initial decline in plasma retinol concentrations. Furthermore, losses of the retinol:RBP complex into the urine during fever have been shown[53] and there is inhibition of the liver RBP synthesis from 12 hours following experimental infection in rats.[54]

Similar movements between the blood and extracellular fluid in the 25-OHD:VDBP complex to those of retinol may also follow the onset of trauma, and inflammation may also depress VDBP synthesis since a fall in VDBP concentrations is associated with multiple trauma,[48] organ dysfunction and sepsis.[49] However, there does not appear to be any direct evidence for an effect of inflammation on VDBP synthesis and the fall in the serum concentration may be a consequence of the increased 'leakiness' of the vasculature which affects several other plasma proteins such as albumin, transferrin and thyroxin-binding protein at the onset of the acute phase response.[17] There is evidence that the 25-OHD:VDBP complex can be found in urine. Patients with uremia can excrete considerable amounts (0.27–10 nmol/day (average 3.7 (SD 3.5)) nmol/day),[55] but glomerular filtration in the arthroplasty patients was unaltered throughout the five post-operative days. Reid and colleagues would appear to dismiss the idea that turnover and cellular uptake of 25-OHD could explain the large decrease in plasma concentrations but the increase in CRP in the patients indicated a considerable inflammatory response. This inflammation will also have increased the activity of macrophages in body tissues and the uptake of 25-OHD by stimulated macrophages can also be considerable.[56]

The long-term nature of the effects of inflammation from the arthroplasty on plasma 25-OHD concentrations appear to indicate that surgery depressed vitamin D status.[28] Their results contrasted with those of Louw et al.[9] where the transient depression in 25-OHD suggested that status was unaffected by surgery. The difference may be attributable to differences in surgical severity or in sunlight exposure following surgery but these possibilities have not been examined. However, there are many reports of low 25-OHD concentrations associated with chronic inflammatory diseases such as those of heart, bowel and lung and vitamin D may play a pleiotropic role in the pathology of these diseases.[57] However, interpretation of causality is difficult. Low concentrations of 25-OHD may be due to low exposure to sunlight which may increase disease risk but may also be a consequence of the inflammation associated with increased disease risk. Two hospital studies on the blood of 3677[58] and 5327[59] patients referred for nutritional assessment concluded that concentrations of 25-OHD were independently associated with CRP and albumin concentrations consistent with a systemic immune response as a major confounding factor in determining vitamin D status. The authors concluded that a reliable clinical interpretation of vitamin D status can be made only if the CRP concentration is <10 mg/L (Table 5.5). Heart disease has been associated with low concentrations of 25-OHD.[60,61] Cardiovascular and cancer mortality are higher in persons with lower 25-OHD concentrations [68] but data from recent randomized controlled trials designed to assess the impact of vitamin D supplements on cardiovascular outcomes are conflicting.[69] The discrepancy between observational and intervention studies suggests that low 25-OHD concentrations are just a marker of ill health.[60]

5.4.1.3 Vitamin E (α-Tocopherol)

Vitamin E circulates in the blood predominantly with low density lipoproteins;[70] hence the concentration in blood is correlated with the lipid load and it is usual to measure the ratio of vitamin E to the cholesterol or fatty acid concentration. Most vitamin E in the blood is in the form of α-tocopherol with approximately 10% as γ-tocopherol. Status is commonly assessed from the concentration of α-tocopherol in serum when concentrations <11.6 μmol/L are indicators of vitamin E deficiency.

TABLE 5.5

Impact of Inflammation on Measurements of Micronutrient Status in Hospital Patients

Micronutrient	Biomarker	Concentration of CRP with Measureable Impact on Biomarkers	Reference
Vitamin A	Serum retinol or retinol-binding protein	Depressed when CRP>5 mg/L	2,7
Vitamin E	Serum α-tocopherol	Unaffected by inflammation	58
Vitamin D	Serum 25 hydroxycholecalciferol	Depressed when CRP>10 mg/L	58
Vitamin K	Serum phylloquinone:triglyceride ratio	Unaffected by inflammation	62
Carotenoids	Serum carotenoids Serum carotenoid:lipid ratio	Serum carotenoids are depressed but carotenoid:lipid ratio is unaffected by inflammation	7,23,63
Thiamin (Vitamin B_1)	Red cell thiamin diphosphate	Unaffected by inflammation	64
Riboflavin (Vitamin B_2)	Red cell flavin adenine dinucleotide phosphate	Transient depression when CRP increased	64
Niacin (Vitamin B_3)	Red cell niacin or urinary metabolites	No reports of influence of inflammation	
Pyridoxine (Vitamin B_6)	Serum pyridoxal-5-phosphate	Transient depression when CRP>5-7 mg/L	29,58,64,65
Folic acid	Serum or red cell folate	Unaffected by inflammation	7
Vitamin B_{12}	Serum cyanocobalamin	Unaffected by inflammation	7
Iron	Serum iron and ferritin but other biomarkers also influenced at some stage	CRP>5 mg/L	3
Zinc	Serum zinc	CRP≥20 mg/L CRP>5 mg/L	58 66
Selenium	Whole blood selenium	CRP>10 mg/L	58
Copper	Serum ceruloplasmin	Serum ceruloplasmin increases but copper:ceruloplasmin ratio is unaffected by inflammation	67

However, to correct for variations in serum lipids the tocopherol:cholesterol (T:C) ratio had best sensitivity and specificity, and deficiency was indicated by values for a T:C ratio <2.22 μmol:mmol.[71]

α-Tocopherol is the most reactive, free-radical, chain-breaking phenolic antioxidant known[72] and it is widely distributed in all biological membranes to protect and repair membrane fatty acids. The antioxidant properties of the fat-soluble vitamin E are supported by water-soluble vitamin C. Vitamin E reduces lipid radicals in biological membranes to non-radical products by donating its hydrogen atom and becomes transiently an α-tocopheroxyl radical. The α-tocopheroxyl radical probably regains the missing hydrogen atom from circulating vitamin C, converting the latter to dehydroascorbate. Dehydroascorbate can be absorbed by circulating red cells where vitamin C is regenerated by reaction with reduced glutathione (GSH).[73] Red cell GSH concentrations are maintained through the activity of glutathione reductase.

Infection and inflammation increase oxidant stress; thus demands for the antioxidant vitamin E are probably increased in disease and trauma. Low circulating concentration of vitamin E have been reported in developing countries, in the elderly and in smokers, that is situations where there is increased evidence of disease or of oxidant load.[74,75] However, serum lipid levels are often not taken into account and increased capillary permeability in acute infection can contribute to a fall in plasma lipoproteins.[76] So low vitamin E concentrations may be due to low concentrations of plasma lipids. In our own studies on apparently-healthy, HIV-positive Kenyan adults α-tocopherol concentrations were no different between subjects with and without inflammation.[23] Likewise Duncan et al. who categorized CRP concentrations from 1303 patients on their hospital database by severity, found no association between the CRP categories and vitamin E (Table 5.5).[58] However, a longitudinal study of vitamin E concentrations in 11 patients who underwent elective hip arthroplasty reported that α-tocopherol concentrations fell by 36% in the 3 days following the operation proportional with the systemic immune response but cholesterol also fell by 40%. When the vitamin E:cholesterol ratios were compared before and after arthroplasty there was no association with the systemic immune response.[32] Thus, in the case of vitamin E there is little evidence that the vitamin E status is reduced by inflammation but where low concentrations of serum vitamin E are found, it is important always to take the serum lipid or cholesterol concentration into account when assessing status.

5.4.1.4   Vitamin K (Phylloquinone; K1)

The plasma concentration of vitamin K1 is the most reliable index for assessing vitamin K status. Vitamin K1 can be measured using high performance liquid chromatography (HPLC) and evidence suggests that concentrations are influenced both by plasma triglyceride concentrations and inflammation.[62] In a reference population, the correlation coefficient (r) between plasma phylloquinone and triglyceride concentrations was $r = 0.7$ and the 95% reference interval for the phylloquinone:triglyceride ratio was 0.20–2.20 nmol/mmol. Following surgery, plasma concentrations of triglyceride and phylloquinone but not the phylloquinone:triglyceride ratio were transiently decreased >50%. The authors suggested that the phylloquinone population reference intervals should be expressed as a ratio to the triglyceride concentration. Phylloquinone concentrations in plasma are decreased in the acute-phase response and, unless corrected for by using the plasma triglyceride concentration, are unlikely to be a reliable index of vitamin K status. Therefore, in the presence of a systemic inflammatory response, plasma phylloquinone concentrations are unlikely to be a reliable measure of status, and during such a response the plasma phylloquinone:triglyceride ratio may provide a more reliable measurement of phylloquinone status (Table 5.5).

5.4.2   Water-Soluble Vitamins

5.4.2.1   Vitamin C (Ascorbic Acid)

Vitamin C status is usually assessed by the concentration of ascorbate in plasma or leukocytes (LAA). A high risk of deficiency is indicated by a plasma ascorbate concentration of <11.4 μmol/L(<2 mg/dL) or <45 nmol (8 μg)/10^8 leukocytes in the blood buffy coat[77] when the total body pool of ascorbate has fallen to ~300 mg.[78] Depletion studies in the 1970s showed that as little as 6.5 mg vitamin C per day was sufficient to fully replete vitamin C stores and prevent scurvy in human volunteers.[78] Collagen synthesis is dependent on vitamin C and urinary excretion of hydroxyproline showed a significant rise during depletion which normalized during repletion. Experimental wound repair was not influenced by vitamin C supplements during repletion.[79] Inflammation is accompanied by reductions in both plasma ascorbate[32,58] and LAA concentrations.[9,31]

The fall in plasma vitamin C concentrations following surgery can be large. A study of 11 patients who underwent hip arthroplasty reported a 76% reduction in the 3 days following the surgery proportional with the systemic immune response.[32] Surgery was also associated with a reduction in the LAA concentration and this was first observed in the 1970s[80] when it was also noted that the postoperative changes in the LAA concentration were unrelated to the extent of surgical trauma or the volume of blood transfused during operation. These workers reported a 42% reduction in circulating LAA levels on the third postoperative day and suggested the findings created an argument for the use of ascorbic acid supplements in surgical patients.[80] However, it was previously shown by American workers in human volunteers that amounts of vitamin C from 4 to 38 mg/d had no significant effects on wound repair.[79] Instead, the fall LAA concentration is probably the result of the postoperative release of leukocytes from the bone marrow[81] since these are low in ascorbic acid content.[80]

The release of leukocytes from the bone marrow is one of the early events occurring in an acute phase response.[81] On entering the blood, they initially dilute the LAA concentrations but the nascent leukocytes rapidly take up ascorbate from the plasma. Workers studying the sequence of events in patients with the common cold noted that the LAA fell on day 1, remained low during days 2–3 but had normalized by day 5.[31] The authors also reported they had observed similar changes in patients following a myocardial infarction and Louw and colleagues reported the same phenomenon in 26 adult patients who underwent uncomplicated orthopedic surgery.[9] They reported a transient reduction in plasma vitamin C concentrations in men (40%) at 48 hours when CRP concentrations were at their peak.[9] Similar results were obtained in another hospital study which examined cross-sectional, hospital data from 516 patients on plasma vitamin C and CRP concentrations.[58] Their data suggested that plasma ascorbate concentrations are reduced by approximately 25% even when CRP concentrations ranged from 5 to 10 mg/L and observed that median plasma ascorbate concentrations fell below 11.4 μmol/L when CRP concentrations were >20 mg/L.[58] These data suggest that nascent leukocytes released into the blood start taking up plasma ascorbate early in the inflammatory response.

The endothelium plays a critical role in communicating between the site of trauma or infection and circulating leukocytes. The inflammatory cytokines interleukin-1 (IL-1) and tumor necrosis factor (TNF) up-regulate surface expression of adhesion and integrin molecules including intercellular adhesion molecule (ICAM). These molecules interact specifically with circulating leukocytes, slowing their flow and initiating trans-endothelial migration into infected or damaged tissues.

Circulating leukocytes will phagocytize bacteria as well as scavenging cell debris. The uptake of vitamin C by the newly emerging leukocytes or its presence in plasma may make them more efficient scavengers and ascorbate may serve as an important physiological protecting agent against oxygen radical damage in inflammation.[82] Alternatively, lowering the concentration of plasma ascorbate in the blood reduces the risk of its reaction with iron. Damaged tissue will release iron into the circulation which is potentially able to react with ascorbate to generate hydroxyl radicals (OH). Tissue iron is normally in the ferric state but reaction with ascorbate generates ferrous iron which is a potent catalyst of the Haber-Weiss reaction in which peroxide and superoxide react to generate hydroxyl radical.

$$H_2O_2 + O_2^{\cdot} \rightarrow O_2 + HO^- + HO^{\cdot}$$

The hydroxyl radical is the most powerful of free radicals potentially formed in tissues. It will instantly oxidize any organic material in the immediate surroundings.

The fall in plasma vitamin C during inflammation certainly represents redistribution of the vitamin but it is more difficult to say whether it also indicates an increased requirement. Vitamin C is an anti-oxidant and oxidative stress will be increased during inflammation potentially destroying the vitamin. However, partially oxidized ascorbate (i.e. dehydro-ascorbate) can be regenerated to the reduced form by reduced glutathione (GSH). There is adequate enzymic capacity in tissues to regenerate GSH. The studies of Baker and colleagues found that wound healing was not influenced by vitamin C supplements and LAA concentrations normalize when health returns without vitamin C supplementation. Therefore, the reductions in plasma and leukocyte ascorbate observed in inflammation would appear to be transitory and not affecting vitamin C status. There is equivocal evidence that vitamin C supplements assists humans in some way against the common cold but no clear mechanism has been demonstrated. However, there is clear evidence that changes in circulating vitamin C concentrations take place during inflammation with the consequence that vitamin C status cannot be assessed from plasma ascorbate or LAA concentrations. Cross-sectional hospital studies suggest that a reliable assessment of status can only be achieved if plasma CRP concentrations are <5 mg/L.[58]

5.4.2.2   Thiamin (Vitamin B$_1$)

Thiamin is the essential precursor of the co-enzymes thiamin diphosphate (TDP) and thiamin triphosphate (TTP). Both coenzymes are involved in intermediary metabolism, TDP in the Krebs and Embden-Myerhof cycles and TTP in nerve function.[83] The assessment of thiamin status is based on the concentration of TDP in the red cell measured by HPLC or the activation coefficient (AC) obtained from the ratio of the red cell transketolase activity in the red cell haemolysate measured with or without TDP.[84,85] The transketolase AC method is a functional test of status which quantifies both the total TDP in the red cell as well as the degree of unsaturation in the enzyme. However, the direct red cell TDP measurement by HPLC is a more sensitive and specific assessment of thiamin status and is probably the method of choice as almost all the red cell TDP is present in the enzyme.[84,86]

Inflammation is often associated with a large increase in energy requirements, especially if accompanied by fever, since a 1°C rise in temperature increases basal metabolism 10%–13%.[87] Red cell TDP concentrations remained stable following uncomplicated surgery.[64] In 10 patients 60–83 years old who underwent elective knee arthroplasty, the median (25, 75% quartiles) red cell TDP increased from 411 (351–540) to 462 (305–552; P = 0.015) at the peak time as monitored by CRP, but in fact both values were within the laboratory reference range.[64] Inflammation was monitored in the study using CRP and median concentrations increased from <6 to 170 (peak) and was 31 mg/L at day 7. The lack of any significant elevation in red cell TDP concentrations suggests that inflammation does not interfere with this measurement of thiamin status (Table 5.5).[64]

5.4.2.3   Riboflavin (Vitamin B$_2$)

Riboflavin is the precursor for two important co-enzymes flavin mononucleotide (FMN) and flavin adenine dinucleotide (FAD) which play important roles in intermediary metabolism. Nutritional status is commonly assessed using a functional test based on the FAD-dependant red cell enzyme glutathione reductase (EGR).[88] Washed red cells are prepared and stored at –20°C. Riboflavin status is obtained from the ratio of EGR enzyme activity measured with and without additional FAD. The ratio is expressed as the EGR activity coefficient or EGRAC.[89] Other measurements of status include urinary riboflavin (per unit creatinine) and red cell riboflavin.[77,90]

Mobilization of riboflavin from a labile tissue pool during infections may produce artifactual changes in the biochemical indices of riboflavin status. Indian workers who studied pre-school children suffering from either measles or other upper respiratory infections and matched controls, reported significantly higher levels of urinary and erythrocyte riboflavin and EGR activity and lower EGRAC values. That is, riboflavin mobilization from the tissues appeared to increase measures of riboflavin status; higher urinary and erythrocyte riboflavin and increased EGR saturation and lower EGRAC values.[90] The observations on EGRAC during infection are not unique. Bates and colleagues reported an apparent increase in riboflavin status as reflected by EGRAC during periods of infection in pregnant Gambian women.[91]

However, studies done on 10 previously-healthy, apparently well-nourished men and women who underwent elective knee arthroplasty reported no change in red cell FAD expressed per g hemoglobin and a 37% decrease in median plasma FAD (P<0.001) concentration around 48 hour when plasma CRP was maximum. The change in plasma FAD was transient and returned to the pre-operation values by day 7.[64]

It is obvious that there are conflicting results between the observational field studies and the surgical study. In the surgical study the only effect of inflammation was a transient fall in circulating FAD coinciding with the maximum increase in CRP i.e. the period of greatest effect on vascular permeability.[17] In contrast, the field studies suggest that tissue riboflavin was being mobilized into the circulation and into red cells but also being lost in the urine. No urine measurements were done in the surgical study but both sets of results indicate that measurements of riboflavin status during inflammation are unreliable. In addition, the Indian field studies suggest that nutritional status may be adversely affected by infection but this may be a specific observation linked to the infection. Measles is well known to have devastating effects on biological membranes[92] and may be responsible for the increase in urinary riboflavin. Mild trauma or infection has minimal effects on riboflavin status but in severe infection, riboflavin status may be impaired due to urinary losses of riboflavin.

5.4.2.4 Niacin (Nicotinic Acid, Vitamin B₃)

Niacin is obtained from food mainly as nicotinic acid and nicotinamide but the body can also synthesize it from the amino acid tryptophan. Synthesis from tryptophan is quite inefficient since 60 mg are required to produce 1.0 mg niacin and dietary tryptophan is preferentially used to incorporate into proteins and the neurotransmitter serotonin. However, tryptophan makes up about 1% of mixed dietary proteins so a protein intake of 70 g is equivalent to about 12 mg niacin. Red cell niacin concentration is probably the simplest measurement of nutritional status but status can also be obtained by measuring one of the two urinary metabolites, N'-methylnicotinamide or N'-methyl-2-pyridine-5-carboxamide in relation to the creatinine concentration or in a 24 hour sample.[93]

Niacin is principally used to synthesize the coenzymes nicotinamide adenine dinucleotide (NAD) and the compound with the extra phosphate group, NADP. NAD plays a central role in energy metabolism as it is the first hydrogen receptor in the mitochondrial electron transport chain during oxidative phosphorylation. Hence, niacin requirements are proportional to energy expenditure and recommended intakes are expressed as 6.6 mg niacin equivalents (NE) per 1000 kcal (1.6 mg NE per 1000 kjoule) which in absolute numbers is about 14 mg in adult women and 16 mg in men.[72] As previously described there is a 10%–13% increased energy expenditure associated with inflammation[65] so some redistribution of tissue niacin concentrations would be expected in association with trauma and inflammation. However, we can find no reports on the effects of infection or inflammation on niacin status as measured by the concentrations of plasma niacin or its urinary metabolites. There are reports that tryptophan degradation into kynurenine by immune cells plays a crucial role in the regulation of immune response during infections and inflammation.[94] There are also reports that niacin inhibits vascular inflammation, i.e. plasma concentrations of IL-6 and TNF-α in vivo and in vitro via down-regulating the NF-κB signaling pathway. Furthermore, niacin also modulates plasma lipid by up-regulating the expression of factors involved in the process of reverse cholesterol transport but these effects are linked to the use of niacin as a treatment of vascular inflammation and are not a product of inflammation.[95]

It is probable that the response of niacin to inflammation is minimal and similar to some of the other B vitamins (e.g. thiamin, folic acid and cyanocobalamin, Table 5.5).

5.4.2.5 Pyridoxine (Vitamin B₆)

There are 3 main vitamers of vitamin B₆ in blood, pyridoxal-5'-phosphate (PLP), pyridoxal and 4-pyridoxic acid (4PA). PLP is the active co-enzyme form and its concentration is the metabolite most frequently used to measure of vitamin B₆ status.[65] A number of indirect methods were used previously including urinary excretion of 4-pyridoxic acid (4PA) or of xanthurenic acid following a tryptophan load and two red cell stimulation tests involving the erythrocyte enzymes aspartate and alanine aminotransferases.[77] The latter enzymes formed the basis of functional tests by measuring the enzyme activity with and without PLP however with the advent of improved liquid chromatography techniques, the direct measure of plasma PLP concentrations is now considered the most relevant to status.[96]

Over the past 60 years there has been an increased awareness of the importance of vitamin B_6 in human nutrition. Vitamin B_6 is involved in more than 100 enzymatic reactions including the metabolism of amino acids, neurotransmitters, nucleic acids, heme and lipids. It is also involved in energy homeostasis through glycogen degradation and gluconeogenesis.[29] In cross-sectional survey studies of apparently-healthy people, low concentrations of plasma PLP[97] and high aspartate aminotransferase activity coefficients were correlated with concentrations of the acute phase protein ACT.[30] Others have reported low plasma PLP in various diseases.[29] Measurements of plasma and red cell PLP concentrations in 10 pre-operatively healthy patients who underwent elective knee arthroplasty reported a strong inverse relationship between plasma PLP and CRP but no change in red cell PLP concentrations over 7 days. At the peak CRP concentration, the median plasma PLP concentration was half pre-operative values[64] suggesting the plasma PLP concentrations are transiently lowered during the inflammatory response although the red cell PLP concentrations suggest that tissue vitamin B_6 status remained unaltered. Based on hospital data from 1303 patients, Duncan and colleagues suggest that the clinical interpretation of plasma B_6 status can be made only when the CRP concentration is <5 mg/L.[58]

There is an increased need for energy and protein during inflammation. Muscle protein catabolism is a source of amino acids for APP synthesis and gluconeogenesis, and lipolysis of body fat supplies fatty acids to meet demands for extra energy.[87,98] As indicated above many of the enzymes needed for these functions are PLP dependent[99] so it is possible that when inflammation is severe, extended or mildly chronic that some PLP is utilized and lost. The principal catabolite of PLP is 4PA and Ulvik and colleagues reported a small increase (P = 0.04) in a Norwegian trial of ~1000 patients with stable angina pectoris which increased after pyridoxine supplementation for 28 days ($p = 0.01$).[29] The authors noted that plasma 4PA was positively associated with two plasma biomarkers of T-helper cell type-1 immune activation namely neopterin and the kynurenine:tryptophan ratio both before and after the 28 days vitamin B_6 treatment. These results suggested an increased catabolism of vitamin B_6 to the main metabolite 4PA during activated cellular immunity. The positive associations between 4PA and the biomarkers of immune activation indicate an increased depletion of vitamin B_6 associated with the inflammatory response. Dose response curves for the plasma concentrations of the 3 vitamin B_6 vitamers, PLP, pyridoxal and 4PA, suggest the effects take place when plasma CRP concentrations rise above 7 mg/L.[29,65] Thus, the results were similar to that obtained from clinical records that plasma B_6 status can only be evaluated when plasma CRP concentrations are below 5 mg/L (Table 5.5).[58]

In the Norwegian studies, the authors excluded patients with acute coronary syndrome from the analyses and suggested that their results may extend to a healthy population of a similar age.[65] However, Bates and colleagues did not find any increase in plasma 4PA in a similar sized survey even though plasma PLP concentrations were inversely related with ACT.[30] Unfortunately plasma 4PA concentrations were not measured in the previously-healthy arthroplasty patients[64] and although plasma PLP concentrations fell, red cell PLP remained stable during the inflammation. The evidence suggests therefore that in an apparently-healthy population the effects of inflammation on vitamin B_6 vitamers are mainly due to altered tissue distribution but there is increased catabolism in more acute and chronic disease with a concomitant increase in vitamin B_6 requirements.

5.4.2.6 Folic Acid

Folate functions as a donor of one-carbon units and is essential for the re-methylation of homocysteine to methionine, which is a precursor of S-adenosylmethionine, the primary methyl group donor for most biological methylations. Methylation of DNA is an important epigenetic determinant in gene expression, in the maintenance of DNA integrity and stability as well as nucleotide and DNA synthesis, stability and repair.[86] Thus, folate is necessary to support growth and cell replication and the earliest signs of deficiency are the appearance of hyper-segmented neutrophilic polymorphonuclear leukocytes followed by a gradual increase in red cell size (mean corpuscular volume) and the appearance of macrocytic anemia.[77] Folate status is assessed using either the concentration of the vitamin in serum or red cells. Serum folate concentrations respond more rapidly to changes in the dietary intake, while the red cell concentration is a more stable biomarker of longer-term intake.

There is very little evidence that either serum or red cell folate concentrations are affected by inflammation. Galloway and colleagues reviewed the literature in 2000 on the changes occurring in commonly-measured vitamins in clinical settings where there was a high risk of inflammation. In patients with major inflammation (CRP 100–200 mg/L) there were no changes in serum folate concentrations. They found no studies looking at minor inflammation (CRP<15 mg/L) and concluded that serum folate concentrations were a reliable measure of nutritional status in the presence of inflammation (Table 5.5).[7] People who smoke have been observed to show evidence of mild inflammation[100] but a review of the literature on vitamin status in smokers found no evidence that serum folate concentrations were influenced by smoking.[101] More recently a group of smokers in Bangalore in India were found to have low folate concentration which displayed an inverse correlation with inflammation.[102] However, a much larger Asian study of 1000 children 6–8 years from Nepal reported inflammation in 31% and a very weak positive correlation with CRP (r 0.07, $P<0.05$) but not with AGP (r 0.00).[103] Similar sized studies in Western countries have reported no correlation between serum folate concentrations and inflammation; e.g. the Italian CHIANTI study in over 1000 men and women[97] and the Womens' Health Initiative Observational Study (WHIOS) in the USA.[104] In the WHIOS, workers measured one-carbon metabolism biomarkers in 988 women who later developed colorectal cancer and a similar number of age- (and other factors) matched controls. Plasma PLP was the only one-carbon metabolism biomarker to show a correlation with inflammation biomarkers. In conclusion, serum folate does not appear to be influenced by inflammation.

5.4.2.7 Vitamin B$_{12}$ (Cyanocobalamin)

Vitamin B$_{12}$ status is assessed by measuring the serum concentration of the vitamin usually by microbiological techniques.[105] In vitamin B$_{12}$ deficiency, serum levels of the vitamin are usually less than 100 µg/L. The vitamin is widely distributed in foods of animal origin so deficiencies are usually restricted to countries where there is poverty and the diet is predominantly vegetarian. Likewise, vegetarians and especially vegans have a high risk of deficiency. Deficiency of vitamin B$_{12}$ results in megaloblastic anemia and there is a close interrelationship between vitamin B$_{12}$ and folate as both deficiencies are associated with megaloblastic bone marrow changes and hyper-segmented polymorphonuclear neutrophils in the peripheral blood.[77] Independently of folate, a deficiency vitamin B$_{12}$ can cause neurological symptoms but usual body stores of vitamin B$_{12}$ are large enough to last for 5 or more years. Pernicious anemia is due to a deficiency of vitamin B$_{12}$ but the cause is a defect in the intestinal absorption of the vitamin. There is a lack of an intrinsic factor which is normally secreted by the parietal cells in the stomach to bind to the vitamin and protect it from degradation during its passage through the gut to the distal portion of the ilium where it is absorbed. At high intakes some vitamin B$_{12}$ can be taken up by passive absorption.[93]

Published reports on serum vitamin B$_{12}$ and inflammation provide a very similar picture to that of folate. The review by Galloway and colleagues found no evidence that serum vitamin B$_{12}$ concentrations were influenced by inflammation in hospital patients (Table 5.5).[7] Likewise the review by Northrop-Clewes and Thurnham found no evidence that serum vitamin B$_{12}$ concentrations were influenced by inflammation in smokers.[101] In the WHIOS, workers measured serum vitamin B$_{12}$ in ~2000 women but found no relationship with inflammation.[104] Two studies have reported weak positive associations between vitamin B$_{12}$ concentrations and CRP; a study on 1000 Nepalese children 6–8 years[103] and a study on 98 seriously ill Australian patients.[106] There is no evidence to suggest that these observations are due to anything other than chance. In conclusion, inflammation does not adversely affect vitamin B$_{12}$ status and the serum concentration appears to be a reliable biomarker of nutritional status in the presence of inflammation.

5.4.3 CAROTENOIDS

The carotenoids are tetraterpenoid compounds responsible for the vivid colors of many fruits, vegetables and flowers. Although there are many hundreds in nature only about 20 are found in human blood[107] and of these, the ones most commonly measured, are lutein, zeaxanthin, lycopene, α- and β-cryptoxanthin, and α- and β-carotene. The compounds are transported by lipoproteins in the blood and widely distributed in the body especially in fatty tissues. They are anti-oxidants and this property may be important in the macula of the eye where lutein and zeaxanthin are concentrated.[108] However, the most widely recognized function of the carotenoids is to supply vitamin A for which β-carotene and to a lesser extent α-carotene and β-cryptoxanthin are precursors. [109]

In studies on apparently-healthy HIV-positive Kenyan adults we found all the main blood carotenoid concentrations were depressed in those with inflammation[23] suggesting that carotenoids may be consumed or metabolized in the presence of enhanced free-radical activity.[7] However, the increase in microvascular permeability which accompanies inflammation[17] can lead to transient falls in blood lipids and the associated carotenoids.[63] Other workers have also noted that carotenoids were reduced by infection and trauma[7] and in a separate study, Gray and colleagues measured blood carotenoids in previously healthy patients who underwent elective knee arthroplasty. They showed that when the blood carotenoid concentrations were adjusted for cholesterol or triglycerides, the changes in the post-operative period were no longer significant.[63] These results suggest that the reductions in blood carotenoids associated with inflammation are mainly due to a redistribution within the tissues and not a change in nutritional status.

There have however been some interesting reports concerning lutein and components of the complement system. The complement system is part of the innate immune defense system and workers have shown that lutein supplements markedly decrease circulating concentrations of some complement end-products in blood of patients with early age-related macular degeneration (AMD).[110,111] The pathogenesis of AMD is not well understood, but a hallmark of the early disease is the appearance of drusen deposits which accumulate in the space between the retinal pigment epithelium and Bruche's membrane in the eye. Studies on the molecular composition of drusen have implicated inflammation and particularly the activation of the alternative pathway of complement activation in the retina.[112] The complement system plays an important role in the defense against microbial pathogens by the classical stimulation route,[113] but there is also a mechanism whereby systemic activation through the alternative pathway can occur and this is implicated in the pathology of AMD.[111,113] Raised concentrations of pathogenic complement end-products in the blood of patients with early AMD is further evidence of activation of the alternative pathway and the fact that lutein supplements markedly decrease the complement end-products suggests that lutein may have a biological role in preventing over-stimulation of the complement system.[110,111]

In conclusion, there is evidence for both redistribution and metabolism of carotenoids in inflammation Therefore to measure status, carotenoid concentrations should be adjusted for serum cholesterol or triglyceride concentrations. Low carotenoid:lipid ratios may indicate metabolism within the tissues but dietary carotenoid intakes should also be assessed to exclude dietary deficiencies as the cause of a low serum carotenoid concentration.

5.4.4 MINERALS

5.4.4.1 IRON (FE)

Iron is essential for the synthesis of hemoglobin and because of the high prevalence of anemia in both the developed and developing world there has been enormous effort to investigate markers of iron status. Frequently blood hemoglobin concentrations are used as a proxy biomarker of iron status, but this is inappropriate as there are a number of vitamin deficiencies,[114] genetic, environmental (altitude)and physiological (smoking) factors which can affect hemoglobin synthesis.[115]

Biomarkers of iron status include serum iron and its transport proteins namely transferrin, total iron binding capacity (TIBC) and ferritin. Experiments in human volunteers more than 50 years ago showed the rapid influence of infection on serum iron. Concentrations of serum iron and TIBC fell early on exposure of volunteers to virulent *Francisela tularsis*. Serum iron fell significantly below normal variations or the differences between individuals. There were two phases of hypoferremia. The 'exposure' phase was a consistent fall of modest magnitude early in the incubation period and was independent of the subsequent illness or its absence. The 'febrile' phase hypoferremia was an exaggerated superimposed response related to the severity and timing of the illness. In severe fever; mean serum iron concentrations fell from 1.35 to 0.5 mg/L (−63%). Authors suggested that a endogenous mediating factor was released from neutrophilic leucocytes. [116]

Serum iron and transferrin display similar characteristics in certain types of cancer and in patients with rheumatoid arthritis. That is, the relationship between the inflammatory response and iron and other trace elements, including zinc and selenium concentrations, appears to persist when the condition is chronic. The data suggest that trace element responses are similar in acute and chronic illness and these biomarkers cannot be reliably used as measures of nutritional status. [7]

The most important biomarker of nutritional iron status is the concentration of serum ferritin[117] but this too is influenced by inflammation.[15] In healthy people, low concentrations of serum ferritin are a biomarker for storage iron in the liver. Concentrations below 12 µg/L in children <5 years or 15 µg/L in everyone else indicate very low stores of iron and a high risk of anemia.[118] In an apparently-healthy population any increase in ferritin due to covert inflammation distorts the true interpretation of iron status; however it was shown earlier how it is possible to correct serum ferritin concentrations and remove the influence of inflammation (see Section 5.3).[3]

The changes occurring in iron biomarkers accompanying inflammation initially reflect a redistribution of iron and are orchestrated through the actions of a small protein known as hepcidin.[119] The protein is a small cysteine-rich peptide hormone which is homeostatically increased by inflammation and iron-loading and decreased by anemia.[120] An increase in hepcidin blocks iron absorption and prevents the release of iron from the reticulo-endothelial system. Apo-ferritin is released into the circulation and presumably scavenges any iron that is released from damaged tissues. The objective of these actions is believed to withhold iron from invading pathogens and assist the host to overcome an infection. Thus, in a short, acute infection or traumatic event, nutritional status with respect to iron is protected. However, where inflammation is chronic, elevated hepcidin concentration will depress iron absorption and iron stores will eventually be depleted, hemoglobin synthesis reduced and anemia of chronic infection (ACD) will result. ACD is well recognized and is a frequent accompaniment of chronic diseases.[121] Thus, short infections are unlikely to seriously reduce iron status but where infections are more frequent or become chronic, iron status is likely to fall. Thus, in hospital patients and apparently-healthy subjects, concentrations of serum CRP >5 mg/L will interfere with iron biomarkers and the interpretation of iron status.[3]

5.4.4.2   ZINC (ZN)

The clinical consequences of zinc deficiency include growth delay, diarrhea, pneumonia, other infections, disturbed neuropsychological performance and abnormalities of fetal development but there is a lack of ideal biomarkers to assess milder zinc deficiency states.[122] Less than 1% of total body zinc is found in the blood,[123] but nevertheless serum zinc concentration is the only biomarker recommended to assess zinc status by the international organizations such as the World Health Organization (WHO). Zinc is transported in the serum bound principally to albumin (70%). The remainder is bound tightly to α-2-macroglobulin (18%), and other proteins such as transferrin and ceruloplasmin. A very small amount (i.e. 0·01%) is complexed with amino acids, especially histidine and cystine. Homeostatic mechanisms, regulated by two families of zinc transporters, maintain serum zinc concentrations in healthy persons within a narrow range (about 12–15 mmol/L; 78–98 mg/dL), even in the presence of markedly varying zinc intakes.[124] One family, ZnT (Solute-linked carrier (SLC) 30) promote zinc efflux from cells or into intracellular vesicles while the second group (Zip, SLC39) promote extracellular zinc uptake and, perhaps, vesicular zinc release into the cytoplasm. Both the ZnT and Zip transporter families exhibit unique tissue-specific expression, differential responsiveness to dietary zinc deficiency and excess, and differential responsiveness to physiologic stimuli via hormones and cytokines.[125]

It has been known for more than 40 years that generalized infections cause rapid falls in serum zinc concentrations with a general movement of zinc to the liver.[26] For example, mean plasma zinc concentrations fell from 17 to 11 µmol/L (−35%) in human volunteers given *F. tularencis* infection or live attenuated Venezuelan equine encephalomyelitis virus vaccine; the fall in zinc coinciding with the fever.[126] Likewise, after major surgery serum zinc concentrations fall 40%–50% within 6 hours but with lesser degrees of trauma the reduction in zinc may only be 10% (CRP concentrations 20–30 mg/L).[7] Part of the fall in zinc concentration will be due to the fall in serum albumin concentration during inflammation. The fall in zinc concentration is mediated by cytokines which promote the uptake of zinc into the liver where it is bound to metallothioneins involved in the production of new proteins.[7] In addition, studies using radio-labeled zinc showed increased tissue concentration at sites of inflammation which suggests a localized role in tissue regeneration.[127]

The effects of inflammation on serum zinc concentrations of apparently-healthy people in the community are less than those seen following major trauma. Brown et al. reported marginally lower zinc (7.0 cf 7.5 µmol/l; not significant) concentrations in children with evidence of inflammation. There were153 Peruvian children aged 11–19 months of whom 52 (34.7%) had some reported sign of infection and 43 (28.3%) had elevated CRP or leucocytosis.[128] Likewise, in our own studies on 163 apparently-healthy, HIV-positive Kenyan adults, we found slightly lower mean zinc concentrations (9.52 cf 8.43 µmol/L, 11%; $P<0.015$) in those with inflammation (n 97, 60%).[66] By identifying those with inflammation, we were able to show that only the adults without inflammation responded to a zinc supplement. In both these studies there appeared to be a far greater effect of dietary zinc deficiency than inflammation on the serum zinc concentrations.

In a recently reported nutritional screen of zinc status in 743 hospital patients there were strong correlations between plasma zinc concentrations and CRP ($r^2 = -0.404$, $p < 0.001$) and albumin ($r^2 = 0.588$, $p < 0.001$) and concluded the impact of the systemic immune response could be largely adjusted for by albumin concentrations.[129] Previously, workers from the same laboratory suggested, that the clinical interpretation of plasma zinc concentrations can only be made where CRP concentrations are <20 mg/L.[58] In fact in the two community examples given above, CRP concentrations were below this cut off but the inflammation still had residual effects on serum zinc and results could be improved even when mild inflammation was taken into account.[66] The effect of trauma on zinc metabolism would appear to be one of redistribution and one report suggests that zinc supplements during inflammation worsen the febrile response.[130] Community studies suggest that a dietary deficiency of zinc has a greater effect on serum zinc concentrations than inflammation but that inflammatory markers may assist interpretation of results.[66]

5.4.4.3 SELENIUM (SE)

Dietary selenium is found as seleno-proteins in both plant and animal foods but wheat and meat are probably the most important sources. In general, seleno-proteins serve as enzymes that catalyze redox reactions. On the basis of response to selenium supplementation, the data from 18 studies indicated that plasma, erythrocyte, and whole-blood selenium, plasma selenoprotein P, and plasma, platelet, and whole-blood glutathione peroxidase (GPX) activity respond to changes in selenium intake.[131] Plasma Se, while easily measured, is not a single entity. It has several components, which, with our current knowledge, are currently defined as: two selenoproteins (selenoprotein P and the extracellular GPX3), which specifically contain selenocysteine (SeCys); Se incorporated non-specifically as seleno-methionine in lieu of methionine in albumin and other proteins; and a small amount of non-protein bound Se.[132]

Selenium is a negative acute phase reactant and in intensive-care, selenium concentrations were 40%–60% lower in patients admitted for various conditions than those in healthy individuals.[7] The effects of inflammation on serum selenium would appear to be initially a redistribution of the element within the body but a positive clinical response to supplements[133] by some patients may suggest that status is impaired in critical illness. A study of 833 patients referred for nutritional assessment of selenium status reported plasma selenium was significantly and independently associated with CRP ($r^2 = -0.489$, $p < 0.001$) and albumin ($r^2 = 0.600$, $p < 0.001$) but, in contrast to zinc, the impact of the systemic immune response could not reasonably be adjusted for by albumin alone.[129] This is presumably because selenium is bound by a number of proteins in plasma and not just albumin. Concentrations of selenium are depressed by quite mild inflammation and workers suggest that a reliable clinical interpretation of selenium status can only be made when CRP concentrations are <10 mg/L.[58]

5.4.4.4 COPPER

Copper in blood is bound to the protein caeruloplasmin, so measurements of plasma copper concentrations are influenced by the binding protein and the ratio does not change during injury or infection.[67] Observations on blood copper concentrations and inflammation were first reported more than 40 years ago. In experiments with human volunteers infected with *F. Tularencis* or given live attenuated Venezuelan equine encephalomyelitis virus vaccine, the authors reported mean plasma copper concentrations increased 2–3 days later from 0.85 to 1.05 mg/L (+24%).[116,126]

Surgery has also been shown to be followed by increases in blood copper concentrations.[134] Galloway and colleagues reported that after major surgery serum copper concentrations increased steadily and after one week were 30% higher or after less radical surgery, the increase was 12%.[7] Community studies on 153 young Peruvian children 1–1.5 years of age found significantly greater serum copper concentration associated with infection.[128] The children were recruited to assess rotavirus antibody titers and study diarrhea and other infections following vaccination at 2 months so were not necessarily 'apparently-healthy'. Evidence of inflammation was present in ~35% of children and their mean copper concentration was ~9% higher than those without inflammation. The authors assessed the effect of the inflammation-associated rise in blood copper concentrations and suggested that inflammation resulted in low copper status being reported only 1% fewer children.

The increase in the carrier protein caeruloplasmin during illness is part of the hypoferremic response to infection, for the ferroxidase properties of caeruloplasmin promote conversion of ferrous to ferric iron.[135] Iron is normally stored in the ferric state so the increase in ceruloplasmin during inflammation may assist the uptake of free ferrous iron to protein-bound ferric iron in transferrin and ferritin.[136] However, the increase in ceruloplasmin in inflammation is a slow response unlike that of ferritin and its main role may be in the restoration of homeostasis following the acute febrile response of infection or trauma.[136] There is no indication that nutritional copper status is affected by inflammation.

REFERENCES

1. Thurnham DI, Northrop-Clewes CA. Inflammation and biomarkers of micronutrient status. *Curr Opin Clin Nutr Metab Care* 2016; 19: 458–463.
2. Thurnham DI, McCabe GP, Northrop-Clewes CA et al. Effect of subclinical infection on plasma retinol concentrations and assessment of prevalence of vitamin A deficiency: Meta-analysis. *Lancet* 2003; 362: 2052–2058.
3. Thurnham DI, McCabe LD, Haldar S et al. Adjusting plasma ferritin concentrations to remove the effects of subclinical inflammation in the assessment of iron deficiency: A meta-analysis. *Am J Clin Nutr* 2010; 92: 546–555.
4. Tabone MD, Muanza K, Lyagoubi M et al. The role of interleukin-6 in vitamin A deficiency during Plasmodium falciparum malaria and possible consequences for vitamin A supplementation. *Immunol* 1992; 75: 553–554.

5. Calis JC, Phiri KS, Faragher EB et al. Severe anemia in Malawian children. *New Engl J Med* 2008; 358: 899.
6. Cichon B, Ritz C, Fabiansen C et al. Assessment of Regression Models for Adjustment of Iron Status Biomarkers for Inflammation in Children with Moderate Acute Malnutrition in Burkina Faso. *J Nutr* 2017; 147: 125–132.
7. Galloway P, McMillan DC, Sattar N. Effect of the inflammatory response on trace element and vitamin status. *Ann Clin Biochem* 2000; 37: 289–297.
8. Ramsden DB, Prince HP, Burr WA et al. The inter-relationship of thyroid hormones, vitamin A and their binding proteins following acute stress. *Clin Endocrinol (Oxf)* 1978; 8: 109–122.
9. Louw JA, Werbeck A, Louw MEJ et al. Blood vitamin concentrations during the acute-phase response. *Critical Care Med* 1992; 20: 934–941.
10. Raiten DJ, Sakr Ashour FA, Ross AC et al. Inflammation and nutritional science for programs/policies and interpretation of research evidence (INSPIRE). *J Nutr* 2015; 145: 1039S-1108S.
11. Merrill RD, Burke RM, Northrop-Clewes CA et al. Factors associated with inflammation in preschool children and women of reproductive age: Biomarkers reflecting inflammation and nutritional determinants of anemia (BRINDA) project. *Am J Clin Nutr* 2017;ajcn142315.
12. NamasteSM, RohnerF, HuangJ et al. Adjusting ferritin concentrations for inflammation: Biomarkers reflecting inflammation and nutritional determinants of anemia (BRINDA) project. *Am J Clin Nutr* 2017;ajcn141762.
13. Namaste SM, Aaron GJ, Varadhan R et al. Methodologic approach for the biomarkers reflecting inflammation and nutritional determinants of anemia (BRINDA) project. *Am J Clin Nutr* 2017;ajcn142273.
14. Baumann H, Gauldie J. The acute phase response. *Immunol Today* 1994; 15: 74–80.
15. Feelders RA, Vreugdenhil G, Eggermont AMM et al. Regulation of iron metabolism in the acute-phase response: Interferon-γ and tumor necrosis factor-α induce hypoferraemia, ferritin production and a decrease in circulating transferrin receptors in cancer patients. *Eur J Clin Invest* 1998; 28: 520–527.
16. Engler R. Concept moderne de la résponse systématique de las phase aiguë de l'inflammation. *Rev fr Allergol* 1996; 36: 903–913.
17. Fleck A, Myers MA. Diagnostic and prognostic significance of acute phase proteins. In: Gordon AH, Koj A, editors. *The Acute Phase Response to Injury and Infection.* 1 ed. Amsterdam, the Netherlands: Elsevier Scientific Publishers; 1985. 249–271.
18. Thurnham DI, Mburu ASW, Mwaniki DL et al. Micronutrients in childhood and the influence of subclinical inflammation. *Proc Nutr Soc* 2005; 64: 502–509.
19. Thurnham DI, McCabe GP. Influence of infection and inflammation on biomarkers of nutritional status with an emphasis on vitamin A and iron. In: RogersLM, editor. *Priorities in the Assessment of Vitamin A and Iron Status in Populations, Panama City, Panama 15-17 September 2010.* Geneva: World Health Organisation; 2012. 63–80.
20. Thurnham DI, Northrop-Clewes CA, Knowles JM. The use of adjustment factors to address the impact of inflammation on vitamin A and iron status in humans. *J Nutr* 2015; 253: 1231–1243.
21. Mitra AK, Alvarez JO, Wahed MA et al. Predictors of serum retinol in children with shigellosis. *Am J Clin Nutr* 1998; 68: 1088–1094.
22. Cser MA, Majchrzak D, Rust P et al. Serum carotenoid and retinol levels during childhood infections. *Ann Nutr Metab* 2004; 48: 156–162.
23. Thurnham DI, Mburu ASW, Mwaniki DL et al. Using plasma acute-phase protein concentrations to interpret nutritional biomarkers in apparently healthy HIV-1-seropositive Kenyan adults. *Brit J Nutr* 2008; 100: 174–182.
24. Thurnham DI. Bioequivalence of β-carotene and retinol. *J Sci Fd Agric* 2007; 87: 13–39.
25. Erlinger TP, Guallar E, Miller ER et al. Relationship between systemic markers of inflammation and serum β-carotene levels. *Arch Intern Med* 2001; 161: 1903–1908.
26. Beisel WR. Trace elements in infectious processes. *Med Clin North Am* 1976; 60: 831–849.
27. Knowles JM, Thurnham DI, Phengdy B et al. Impact of inflammation on biomarkers of iron status in a cross-sectional survey of Lao women and children. *Brit J Nutr* 2013; 110: 2285–2297.
28. Reid D, Toole BJ, Knox S et al. The relation between acute changes in the systemic inflammatory response and plasma 25-hydroxyvitamin D concentrations after elective knee arthroplasty. *Am J Clin Nutr* 2011; 93: 1006–1011.
29. Ulvik A, Midttun Ø, Pedersen ER et al. Association of plasma B-6 vitamers with systemic markers of inflammation before and after pyridoxine treatment in patients with stable angina pectoris. *Am J Clin Nutr* 2012; 95: 1072–1078.

30. Bates CJ, Pentieva KD, Prentice A et al. Plasma pyridoxal phosphate and pyridoxic acid and their relationship to plasma homocysteine in a representative sample of British men and women aged 65 years and over. *Brit J Nutr* 1999; 81: 191–201.
31. Hume R, Weyers E. Changes in leucocyte ascorbic acid during the common cold. *Scot Med J* 1973; 18: 3–7.
32. Conway FJ, Talwar D, McMillan DC. The relationship between acute changes in the systemic inflammatory response and plasma ascorbic acid, alpha-tocopherol and lipid peroxidation after elective hip arthroplasty. *Clin Nutr* 2015; 34: 642–646.
33. Thurnham DI. Inflammation and biomarkers of nutrition. *Sight and Life* 2015; 1: 59–66.
34. Paracha PI, Jamil A, Northrop-Clewes CA et al. Interpretation of vitamin A status in apparently-healthy Pakistani children using markers of sub-clinical infection. *Am J Clin Nutr* 2000; 72: 1164–1169.
35. Shankar AH, Genton B, Semba RA et al. Effect of vitamin A supplementation on morbidity due to Plasmodium falciparum in young children in Papua New Guinea: A randomised trial. *Lancet* 1999; 354: 203–209.
36. WHO. Serum retinol concentrations for determining the prevalence of vitamin A deficiency in populations. *Vitamin and mineral nutrition information system.* WHO/NMH/NHD/MNM/11.3. Geneva: World Health Organisation http://www.who.int/vmnis/indicators/retinol.pdf accessed July 2015; 2011.
37. WHO. Serum ferritin concentrations for the assessment of iron status and iron deficiency in populations. *Vitamin and mineral nutrition information system, (WHO/NMH/NHD/MNM/11.2).* Geneva: World Health Organisation http://www.who.int/vmnis/indicators/serum_ferritin.pdf accessed July 2015; 2011.
38. Sommer A, Davidson FR. Assessment of control and vitamin A deficiency: The Annecy accords. *J Nutr* 2002; 132: 2845S–2851S.
39. Schweigert FS. Inflammation-induced changes in the nutritional biomarkers serum retinol and carotenoids. *Curr Opin Clin Nutr Metab Care* 2001; 4: 477–481.
40. Thompson D, Milford-Ward A, Whicher JT. The value of acute phase protein measurements in clinical practice. *Ann Clin Biochem* 1992; 29: 123–131.
41. Northrop-Clewes CA. Interpreting indicators of iron status during an acute phase response - lessons from malaria and HIV. *Ann Clin Biochem* 2008; 45: 18–32.
42. Calvin J, Neale G,Fotherby KJ et al. The relative merits of acute phase proteins in the recognition of inflammatory conditions. *Ann Clin Biochem* 1988; 25: 60–66.
43. Lenders CM, Feldman HA, Von SchevenE et al. Relation of body fat indexes to vitamin D status and deficiency among obese adolescents. *Am J Clin Nutr* 2009; 90: 459–467.
44. Zerwekh JE. Blood biomarkers of vitamin D status. *Am J Clin Nutr* 2008; 87: 1087S–1091S.
45. Heaney RP. The Vitamin D requirement in health and disease. *J Steroid Biochem Mol Biol* 2005; 97: 13–19.
46. Holick MF. The role of vitamin D for bone health and fracture prevention. *Curr Osteoporos Rep* 2006; 4: 96–102.
47. van Hoof HJ, de Sévaux RG, van BaelenH et al. Relationship between free and total 1, 25-dihydroxyvitamin D in conditions of modified binding. *Eur J Endocrinol* 2001; 144:391–396.
48. Dahl B, Schiødt FV, Kiaer T et al. Serum Gc-globulin in the early course of multiple trauma. *Crit Care Med* 1998; 26: 285–289.
49. Dahl B, Schiødt FV, Ott P et al. Plasma concentration of Gc-globulin is associated with organ dysfunction and sepsis after injury. *Crit Care Med* 2003; 31: 152–156.
50. Al-oanzi ZH, Tuck SP, RajN et al. Assessment of vitamin D status in male osteoporosis. *Clin Chem* 2006; 52: 248–254.
51. Bikle DD. *Nonclassic actions of vitamin D. J Clin Endocrinol Metab* 2009; 94: 26–34.
52. Zerwekh JE. Blood biomarkers of vitamin D status. *Am J Clin Nutr* 2008; 87: 1087S–1091S.
53. Stephensen CB, Alvarez JO, Kohatsu J et al. Vitamin A is excreted in the urine during acute infection. *Am J Clin Nutr* 1994; 60: 388–392.
54. Rosales FJ, Ritter SJ, Zolfaghari R et al. Effects of acute inflammation on plasma retinol, retinol-binding protein, and its messenger RNA in the liver and kidneys of vitamin A sufficient rats. *J Lipid Res* 1996; 37: 962–971.
55. Sato KA, Gray RW, Lemann JJr. Urinary excretion of 25-hydroxyvitamin D in health and the nephrotic syndrome. *J Lab Clin Med* 1982; 99: 325–330.
56. Reichel H, Koeffler HP, Bishop JE et al. 25-Hydroxyvitamin D_3 metabolism by lipopolysaccharide-stimulated normal human macrophages. *J Clin Endocrinol Metab* 1987; 64: 1–9.
57. Louw JA, Werbeck A, Louw MEJ et al. Blood vitamin concentrations during the acute-phase response. *Crit Care Med* 1992; 20: 934–941.

58. Duncan A, Talwar D, McMillan DC et al. Quantitative data on the magnitude of the systemic inflammatory response and its effect on micronutrient status based on plasma measurements. *Am J Clin Nutr* 2012; 95: 64–71.

59. Ghashut RA, Talwar D, Kinsella J et al. The effect of the systemic inflammatory response on plasma vitamin 25 (OH) D concentrations adjusted for albumin. *PLOS ONE* 2014; 9: e92614.

60. Autier P, Boniol M, Pizot C et al. Vitamin D status and ill health: A systematic review. *Lancet Diabetes Endocrinol* 2014; 2: 76–89.

61. Brøndum-Jacobsen P, Benn M, Jensen GB et al. 25-hydroxyvitamin D levels and risk of ischemic heart disease, myocardial infarction, and early death: Population-based study and meta-analyses of 18 and 17 studies. *Arterioscler Thromb Vasc Biol August 30*, 2012. [Epub ahead of print].

62. Azharuddin MK, O'Reilly DS, Gray A et al. HPLC method for plasma vitamin K1: Effect of plasma triglyceride and acute-phase response on circulating concentrations. *Clin Chem* 2007; 53: 1706–1713.

63. Gray A, McMillan DC, Wilson C et al. The relationship between the acute changes in the systemic inflammatory response, lipid soluble antioxidant vitamins and lipid peroxidation following elective knee arthroplasty. *Clin Nutr* 2005; 24: 746–750.

64. Gray A, McMillan DC, Wilson C et al. The relationship between plasma and red cell concentrations of vitamins thiamine diphosphate, flavin adenine dinucleotide and pyridoxal 5-phosphate following elective knee arthroplasty. *Clin Nutr* 2004; 23: 1080–1083.

65. Ulvik A, Midttun O, Pedersen ER et al. Evidence for increased catabolism of vitamin B-6 during systemic inflammation. *Am J Clin Nutr* 2014; 100: 250–255.

66. Mburu ASW, Thurnham DI, Mwaniki DL et al. The influence of inflammation on plasma zinc concentration in apparently-healthy, HIV+ Kenyan adults and zinc responses after a multi-micronutrient supplement. *Eur J Clin Nutr* 2010; 64: 510–517.

67. Taggart DP, Fraser WD, Shenkin A et al. The effects of intraoperative hypothermia and cardiopulmonary bypass on trace metals and their protein binding ratios. *Eur J Cardiothorac Surg* 1990; 4: 587–594.

68. Chowdhury R, Kunutsor S, Vitezova A et al. Vitamin D and risk of cause specific death: Systematic review and meta-analysis of observational cohort and randomised intervention studies. *BMJ* 2014; 348: g1903.

69. Chowdhury R, Kunutsor S, Vitezova A et al. Vitamin D and risk of cause specific death: Systematic review and meta-analysis of observational cohort and randomised intervention studies. *BMJ* 2014; 348: g1903.

70. Davies T, Kelleher J, Losowsky MS. Interrelation of serum lipoprotein and tocopherol levels. *Clin Chim Acta* 1969; 24: 431–436.

71. Thurnham DI, Davies JA, Crump BJ et al. The use of different lipids to express serum tocopherol:lipid ratios for the measurement of vitamin E status. *Ann Clin Biochem* 1986; 23: 514–520.

72. Burton GW, Ingold KU. Autoxidation of biological molecules. 1. The antioxidant activity of vitamin E and related chain-breaking phenolic antioxidants in vitro. *J Am Chem Soc* 1981; 103: 6472–6477.

73. Niki E, Tsuchiya J, Tanimura R et al. *Regeneration of vitamin E from α-chromanoxyl radical by glutathione and vitamin C. Chem Lett* 1982; 27: 789–792.

74. Dror DK, Allen LH. Vitamin E deficiency in developing countries. *Food Nutr Bull* 2011; 32: 124–143.

75. Anderson R. Assessment of the roles of vitamin C, vitamin E, and β-carotene in the modulation of oxidant stress mediated by cigarette smoke-activated phagocytes. *Am J Clin Nutr* 1991; 53: 358–361.

76. Nilsson-Ehlel, Nilsson-Ehle P. Changes in plasma lipoproteins in acute malaria. *J Int Med* 1990; 227: 151–155.

77. Sauberlich HE, Dowdy L, Skala JH. *Laboratory Tests for the Assessment of Nutritional Status*. Boca Raton, FL: CRC Press; 1974.

78. Baker EM, Hodges RE, Hood J et al. Metabolism of ascorbic-1-^{14}C acid in experimental human scurvy. *Am J Clin Nutr* 1969; 22: 549–558.

79. Hodges RE, Baker EM, Hood J et al. Experimental scurvy in man. *Am J Clin Nutr* 1969; 22: 535–548.

80. IrvinTT, ChattopadhyayK, Smythe A. Ascorbic acid requirements in postoperative patients. *Surg Gynecol Obstet* 1978; 147: 49–55.

81. Sipe JD. Cellular and humoral components of the early inflammatory reaction. In: GordonAH, Koj A, editors. *The Acute Phase Response to Injury and Infection*. 1 ed. London: Elsevier; 1985. 3–21.

82. Hemila H, Roberts P, Wikstrom M. Activated polymorphonuclear leukocytes consume vitamin C. *FEBS Lett* 1984; 178: 25–30.

83. Thurnham DI. Thiamin, physiology. In: Allen LH, Prentice A, Caballero B, editors. *Encyclopedia of Human Nutrition*. 3nd ed, volume 4. Waltham, MA: Academic Press; 2013. 274–279.

84. Herve C, Beyne P, Letteron Ph et al. Comparison of erythrocyte transketolase activity with thiamine and thiamine phosphate ester levels in chronic alcoholic patients. *Clin Chim Acta* 1995; 234: 91–100.

85. Mount JN, Heduan E, Herd C et al. Adaptation of coenzyme stimulation assays for the nutritional assessment of vitamins B1, B2 and B6 using the Cobas Bio centrifugal analyser. *Ann Clin Biochem* 1987; 24:41–46.
86. Talwar D, Davidson H, Cooney J et al. Vitamin B(1) status assessed by direct measurement of thiamin pyrophosphate in erythrocytes or whole blood by HPLC: Comparison with erythrocyte transketolase activation assay. *Clin Chem* 2000; 46: 704–710.
87. Keusch GT. Infection, fever and nutrition. In: Macrae R, Robinson RK, Sadler MJ, editors. *Encyclopaedia of Food Science, Food Technology and Nutrition*. Academic Press; 1993. 2522–2526.
88. Glatzle D, Körner WF, Christeller S et al. Method for the detection of biochemical riboflavin deficiency. *Int J Vit Nutr Res* 1970; 40: 166–183.
89. Thurnham DI, Rathakette P. Incubation of NAD(P)H$_2$:glutathione oxidoreductase (EC 1.6.4.2) with flavin adenine dinucleotide for maximal stimulation in the measurement of riboflavin status. *Brit J Nutr* 1982; 48: 459–466.
90. Bamji MS, Bhaskaram P, Jacob CM. Urinary riboflavin excretion and erythrocyte glutathione reductase activity in pre-school children suffering from upper respiratory tract infections and measles. *Ann Nutr Metab* 1987; 31: 191–196.
91. Bates CJ, Prentice AM, Paul AA et al. Riboflavin status in Gambian pregnant and lactating women and its implications for recommended dietary allowances. *Am J Clin Nutr* 1981; 34: 928–935.
92. Morley D. Severe measles in the tropics. I. *Br Med J* 1969; 1: 297–300.
93. Truswell AS. The B vitamins. In: MannJ, TruswellAS, editors. *Essential of Human Nutrition*. 3 ed. Oxford: Oxford University Press; 2007. 184–200.
94. Le Floc'hN, OttenW, MerlotE. Tryptophan metabolism, from nutrition to potential therapeutic applications. *Amino Acids* 2011; 41: 1195–1205.
95. SiY, Zhang Y, Zhao J et al. Niacin inhibits vascular inflammation via downregulating nuclear transcription factor-kappaB signaling pathway. *Mediators Inflamm* 2014; 2014: 263786.
96. Leklem JE. Vitamin B-6: A status report. *J Nutr* 1990; 120: 1503–1507.
97. Gori AM, Sofi F, Corsi AM et al. Predictors of vitamin B6 and folate concentrations in older persons: The InCHIANTI study. *Clin Chem* 2006; 52: 1318–1324.
98. Koj A. Definition and classification of acute-phase proteins. In: GordonAH, KojA, editors. *The Acute-Phase Response to Injury and Infection*. 1 ed. Amsterdam, the Netherlands: Elsevier Science Publishers; 1985. 139–144.
99. Xu X, Zhang L, Shao B et al. Safety evaluation of meso-zeaxanthin. *Food Control* 2013; 32: 678–686.
100. Das I. Raised C-reactive protein levels in serum from smokers. *Clin Chim Acta* 1985; 153: 9–13.
101. Northrop-Clewes CA, Thurnham DI. Monitoring micronutrients in cigarette smokers. *Clin Chim Acta* 2007; 377: 14–38.
102. Warad S, Kalburgi NB, Manak M et al. Determining the Effect of Gutkha on Serum Levels of Vitamin B12 and Folic Acid as Compared to Smoking among Chronic Periodontitis Subjects: A Cross-Sectional Study. *J Clin Diagn Res* 2014; 8:ZC85–ZC89.
103. Schulze KJ, Christian P, Wu LS et al. Micronutrient deficiencies are common in 6- to 8-year-old children of rural Nepal, with prevalence estimates modestly affected by inflammation. *J Nutr* 2014; 144: 979–987.
104. Abbenhardt C, Miller JW, Song X et al. Biomarkers of one-carbon metabolism are associated with biomarkers of inflammation in women. *J Nutr* 2014; 144: 714–721.
105. Kelleher BP, Broin SD. Microbiological assay for vitamin B12 performed in 96-well microtitre plates. *J Clin Pathol* 1991; 44: 592–595.
106. Corcoran TB, O'Neill MP, Webb SA et al. Inflammation, vitamin deficiencies and organ failure in critically ill patients. *Anaesth Intensive Care* 2009; 37: 740–747.
107. Khachik F, Beecher GR, Smith JC Jr. Lutein, lycopene, and their oxidative metabolites in chemoprevention of cancer. *J Cell Biochem* 1995; 22 (Suppl.):236–246.
108. O'Connell E, Neelam K, Nolan JM et al. Macular carotenoids and age-related maculopathy. *Ann Acad Med Singapore* 2006; 35: 821–830.
109. Thurnham DI. Carotenoids: Functions and fallacies. *Proc Nutr Soc* 1994; 53: 77–87.
110. Tian Y, Kijlstra A, van der Veen RL et al. The effect of lutein supplementation on blood plasma levels of complement factor D, C5a and C3d. *PLOS ONE* 2013; 8: e73387.
111. Tian Y, Kijlstra A, van der Veen RL et al. Lutein supplementation leads to decreased soluble complement membrane attack complex sC5b-9 plasma levels. *Acta Ophthalmol* 2015; 93: 141–145.
112. Hageman GS, Luthert PJ, Victor Chong NH et al. An integrated hypothesis that considers drusen as biomarkers of immune-mediated processes at the RPE-Bruch's membrane interface in aging and age-related macular degeneration. *Prog Retin Eye Res* 2001; 20: 705–732.

113. Sjoberg AP, Trouw LA, Blom AM. Complement activation and inhibition: A delicate balance. *Trends Immunol* 2009; 30: 83–90.

114. Fishman SM, Christian P, West KP Jr. Role of vitamins in the prevention and control of anaemia. *Pub Hlth Nutr* 2000; 3: 125–150.

115. Sanchaisuriya K, Fucharoen S, Ratanasiri T et al. Thalassemia and hemoglobinopathies rather than iron deficiency are major causes of pregnancy-related anemia in northeast Thailand. *Blood Cells Mol Dis* 2006; 37: 8–11.

116. Pekarek RS, Bostian KA, Bartonelli PJ et al. The effect of Francisella tularensis on iron metabolism in man. *Am J Med Sci* 1969; 258: 14–25.

117. World Health Organisation, Centres for Disease Control and Prevention (CDC). *Assessing the iron status of populations.* 2 ed. Geneva: WHO Press; 2007.

118. UNICEF, UNU, WHO. Iron deficiency anaemia. *Assessment, prevention and control. A Guide for Programme Managers.* IDA Consultation G1, editor. WHO/NHD/01.3, 1–114. 2001. Geneva, Switzerland, World Health Organisation.

119. Ganz T. Hepcidin, a key regulator of iron metabolism and mediator of anemia of inflammation. *Blood* 2003; 102: 783–788.

120. Nemeth E, Ganz T. Regulation of iron metabolism by hepcidin. *Ann Rev Nutr* 2006; 26: 323–342.

121. Thurnham DI, Northrop-Clewes CA. Infection in the etiology of anemia. In: KraemerK, ZimmermannMB, editors. *Nutritional Anemia.* Basel: Sight & LIfe Press; 2007. 231–256.

122. Hambidge KM. Human Zinc Deficiency. *J Nutr* 2000; 130: 1344S-1349S.

123. Aggett PJ, Favier A. Zinc. *Int J Vit Nutr Res* 1993; 63: 301–307.

124. Gibson RS, Hess SY, Hotz C et al. Indicators of zinc status at the population level: A review of the evidence. *Brit J Nutr* 2008; 99: S14–S23.

125. Liuzzi JP, Cousins RJ. Mammalian zinc transporters. *Annu Rev Nutr* 2004; 24: 151–172.

126. Pekarek RS, Burghen GA, Bartelloni PJ et al. The effect of live attenuated Venezuelan equine encephalomyelitis virus vaccine on serum iron, zinc, and copper concentrations in man. *J Lab Clin Med* 1969; 76: 293–303.

127. Savlov ED, Strain WH, Huegin F. Radio zinc studies in experimental wound healing. *J Surg Res* 1962; 2: 209–212.

128. Brown KH, Lanata CF, Yuen ML et al. Potential magnitude of misclassification of a population's trace element status due to infection: Example from a survey of young Peruvian children. *Am J Clin Nutr* 1993; 58: 549–554.

129. Ghashut RA, McMillan DC, KinsellaJ et al. The effect of the systemic inflammatory response on plasma zinc and selenium adjusted for albumin. *Clin Nutr* 2016; 35: 381–387.

130. Braunschweig CL, Sowers M, KovacevichDS et al. Parental zinc supplementation in adult humans during the acute phase response increases the febrile response. *J Nutr* 1997; 127: 70–74.

131. Ashton K, Hooper L, Harvey LJ et al. Methods of assessment of selenium status in humans: A systematic review. *Am J Clin Nutr* 2009; 89: 2025S–2039S.

132. Combs GF, Jr., Watts JC, Jackson MI et al. Determinants of selenium status in healthy adults. *Nutr J* 2011; 10: 75–10.

133. Berger M, Chiolero R. Antioxidant supplementation in sepsis and systemic inflammatory response syndrome. *Crit Care Med* 2007; 35: S584–S590.

134. Shenkin A. Trace elements and inflammatory response: Implications for nutritional support. *Nutrition* 1995; 11: 100–105.

135. Gutteridge JMC. Plasma ascorbate levels and inhibition of the antioxidant activity of caeruloplasmin. *Clin Sci* 1991; 81: 413–417.

136. Koj A. Biological functions of acute phase proteins. In: Gordon AH, Koj A, editors. *The Acute Phase Response to Injury and Infection.* 1 ed. Amsterdam, the Netherlands: Elsevier Science Publishers; 1985. 145–160

6 Undernutrition, Infection, and Poor Growth in Infants and Children

D. Joe Millward

CONTENTS

6.1   Introduction 83
6.2   The Physiology and Cellular Biology of Bone Growth Regulation 85
    6.2.1   Endochondral Ossification 86
    6.2.2   Endocrine Regulation 87
    6.2.3   Paracrine Signaling within the Growth Plate 87
    6.2.4   Direct Anabolic Influences of Amino Acids and Zinc 88
6.3   Nutrition and Growth 89
    6.3.1   Growth Regulation as Observed in Animal Models 89
        6.3.1.1   Protein 89
        6.3.1.2   Zinc 91
    6.3.2   Human Studies of Nutrition and Growth 92
        6.3.2.1   Energy Intake 93
        6.3.2.2   Protein Intake 95
        6.3.2.3   Zinc Intake 96
        6.3.2.4   Iodine Intake 97
        6.3.2.5   Animal Source Foods and Growth 98
6.4   Infection and Poor Growth in Children 101
    6.4.1   Environmental Enteric Dysfunction 102
    6.4.2   Inflammation and Endochondral Ossification 103
6.5   Conclusions 104
References 105

6.1   INTRODUCTION

The stature of human adults reflects individual genotype and those environmental factors that influence child growth and limit the phenotypic expression of the genotype. In describing the changes in the growth of children in Britain since the early nineteenth century, Tanner identified growth as a "mirror of the conditions of society" referring to the "nutritional and hygienic status" of the population (Tanner, 1992). In fact, the industrial revolution and urbanization of the population during Victorian Britain had resulted in very poor conditions for much of British society. This influenced child growth and adult height to such an extent that at the outbreak of the Boer War in 1899 military recruitment standards in terms of acceptable height had to be lowered to find enough men to enlist: the new minimum height for recruits was reduced to five feet. These changes occurred even though the period had seen extensive improvements in public health, especially in "sanitary science," largely prompted by the series of cholera epidemics starting in the UK in 1831. Thus, both sewage disposal and water supplies improved in the large cities and it may be that without this, child growth and adult height would have fallen even more than it did. A 1904 government report (Great Britain. Inter-departmental Committee on Physical Deterioration, 1904), identified "urban poverty leading to insufficient food and malnutrition" as a main cause of "ill health, poor physical and mental performance and a general deterioration of the race." This report is credited with the subsequent introduction of free school meals and other benefits for poor children and their families. The result was an increase in adult height in British men born between 1900 and 1946 of about 1.25 cm/decade, a secular trend in height which continued in those born between 1946 and 1960, albeit at a lower rate of 0.6 cm/decade (Tanner, 1992). Unfortunately, the dreadful conditions in the English cities in the nineteenth century still exist throughout the developing world today with reduced growth a consequence.

Poor growth in children is currently defined as inadequate height, weight, and weight in proportion to height, based on growth standards. Since 2006, WHO has recommended its own Child Growth Standards (WHO, 2006), especially when discussing the issue in global terms. The current terminology is stunting, underweight, and wasting which describe a height-for-age, weight-for-age, and weight-for-height at or greater than 2 standard deviations (SDs) below the median of the relevant standard. Severe stunting or wasting reflects growth failure greater than 3 SDs below the median. Because underweight can reflect either a short stature with normal body composition or actual body weight loss, stunting and wasting are the most informative terms. In practice, the entire spectrum of growth deficits can be expressed as a Z score of the height-for-age or weight-for-height (i.e., HAZ and WHZ). These are values calculated as the differences between the observed values and the growth standards as a fraction or multiple of the SD of the mean values of the standards. Thus, children with negative values of HAZ or WHZ have growth deficits, and values of −2 or more are stunted or wasted.

Globally more children are stunted than wasted, with prevalence rates and burdens in 2012 of 25% or 162 million stunted preschool children compared with 8% or 51 million wasted (UNICEF, WHO, World Bank, 2012; de Onis et al., 2012). Prevalence rates are particularly high in sub-Saharan Africa and South Asia, but some 7% or 5 million children in the developed world are also stunted.

Although it has long been accepted that growth failure can result from multiple environmental influences of which poor nutrition and infection are important, the complexity of the interactions between environmental adverse influences has been recently reviewed by Prendergast and Humphrey (2014) in terms of a "stunting syndrome." Thus, the multiple pathological changes marked by linear growth retardation in early life are associated with increased morbidity and mortality; reduced physical, neurodevelopmental, and economic capacity; and an elevated risk of metabolic disease into adulthood. This concept also includes the cyclical process connecting maternal nutrition to an intergenerational cycle of growth failure which explains how growth failure is transmitted across generations through the mother (see United Nations System Standing Committee on Nutrition, 2011). This is because small adult women are more likely to have low-birth-weight babies, in part because maternal size has an statistically significant influence on birth weight. Furthermore, children born with a low birth weight are more likely to have growth failure during childhood so that girls born with a low birth weight are more likely to become small adult women. This cycle is accentuated by high rates of teenage pregnancy, as adolescent girls are even more likely to have low-birth-weight babies. A somewhat simplified version of the stunting syndrome is shown in Figure 6.1.

As for the details of the nutritional deficiencies and of the infectious and inflammatory insults which inhibit height growth, in their review of the pathogenesis of stunting, Prendergast and Humphrey (2014) argue that the pathogenesis underlying linear growth failure is surprisingly poorly understood. In this chapter, the intention is to attempt to examine the importance of both nutritional deficiencies and infectious-inflammatory insults in the context of what might be described as a first principles model of growth regulation.

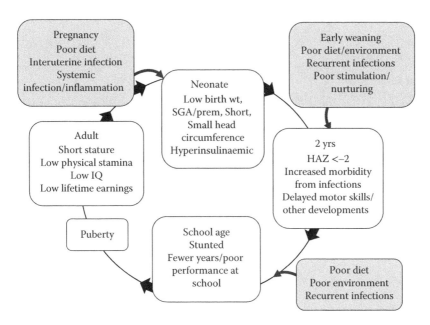

FIGURE 6.1 The stunting syndrome. The shaded boxes indicate adverse influences while the unshaded boxes indicate outcomes. (Modified from Prendergast AJ and Humphrey JH, *Paed Int Child Health,* 34, 250–265, 2014.)

6.2 THE PHYSIOLOGY AND CELLULAR BIOLOGY OF BONE GROWTH REGULATION

The growth potential of an individual in height and overall shape, mainly a function of bone growth, is genetically determined, and each individual will follow a growth curve canalized in terms of both extent and time if conditions are favorable (Tanner, 1979). In the context of this review, favorable conditions include a diet that can exert an appropriate regulatory anabolic drive on growth (Millward and Rivers, 1988, 1989), and provide necessary substrates, in an environment which presents minimal inflammatory challenges. From a detailed analysis of the pattern and associated systemic hormonal changes, Karlberg (1989) identified three additive and partly superimposed phases of postnatal growth from birth to maturity, the ICP model, involving *infancy*, a continuation of the insulin-dependent fetal phase, *childhood*, mainly growth hormone dependent and *puberty*, mainly sex steroid dependent. When interrupted by malnutrition or infection there is usually some period of catch-up growth in weight-for-height (Ashworth, 1974; Ashworth and Millward, 1986; Waterlow, 2006) and in height-for-age (Golden, 1994), i.e., a self-correcting response returning the growth pattern to the individual growth channel.

The nature of the genetic programming is quite complex. Genetic factors are often estimated to account for 80% of the variation in height and genome-wide association studies in adults of recent European origin indicate hundreds of single nucleotide polymorphisms clustered in genomic loci and biological pathways that affect human height (Allen et al., 2010). Nevertheless, these identified variants explain only ~10% of the phenotypic variance with unidentified common variants of similar effect sizes possibly increasing the overall influence to ~20% of heritable variation. The genetic programming of the time course of growth, especially in relation to events in the growth plate which mediate the slowing down of the initial very rapid fetal, early infancy growth phase with eventual cessation of linear growth after puberty, is particularly complex (see Lui and Baron, 2011). Furthermore, the mechanisms that link linear growth to the growth of other organs and tissues are

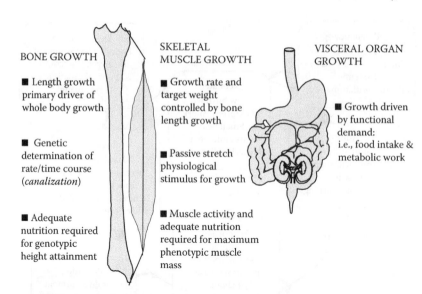

FIGURE 6.2 Physiological control of long bone growth. Growth of the long bones is the primary driver of growth with skeletal muscle growth linked to bone growth through the passive stretch mechanism (see Millward,1995).

also complex. It is suggested that the progressive decline in cellular proliferation throughout the organism results from a genetic program involving the downregulation of a large set of growth-promoting genes (Lui and Baron, 2011).

However nongenetic mechanisms also exist to coordinate growth throughout the organism. Because growth can be considered to be the accumulation of protein-containing structures, with dietary protein also providing a key regulatory and permissive (substrate) role, a protein-stat model of growth control was developed (Millward, 1995). Within this model the overall metabolic demand for amino acids is linked to dietary intake through an aminostatic appetite mechanism that enables protein intake to meet the demand. The demand itself is regulated through a mechanism in which amino acid intake exerts an anabolic drive on the growth plate of the long bones. Lean tissue growth, especially that of skeletal muscle, is also subject to this anabolic drive but this is also linked to linear growth through the specific activation of the synthesis of muscle connective tissue and myofibrillar protein deposition by passive stretching of skeletal muscle by the length growth of the bones to which they are attached. This ensures that skeletal muscle growth occurs at a rate and time course that ensures sufficient muscle mass and strength to allow function to develop with increasing bone length and associated height. With sufficient and appropriate dietary protein and other type II nutrients (see below), which mediate the anabolic drive on the growth plate of the long bones and permit the linked muscle growth, the genetically programmed postnatal growth pattern is enabled. This linkage of long bone growth to the growth of muscle and the rest of the organism is shown schematically in Figure 6.2.

6.2.1 Endochondral Ossification

The target of the anabolic drive as far as the majority of bone growth which directly influences height (limb bones, ribs, and vertebrae), is endochondral ossification within the growth plate (see Kronenberg, 2003; Long and Ornitz, 2013; Xian, 2014). This starts with the differentiation cascade initiated by stem cell clonal expansion as proliferative chondrocytes, followed by hypertrophy, cartilage matrix secretion, and cell death (probably apoptosis). This forms the mineralized cartilaginous templates, which are in turn replaced by bone tissues through osteogenesis and associated vascularization. The bone growth which ensues can be envisaged as the combined influence of those systemic endocrine and local paracrine/autocrine anabolic influences, acting together with small molecules which include specific amino acids, such as leucine (see Millward, 2012) and zinc, which mediate signaling cascades via a variety of pathways.

6.2.2 ENDOCRINE REGULATION

The endocrine signals of the dietary anabolic drive include insulin, the GH-IGF-1 axis (a mixed endocrine-paracrine-autocrine system), the T4/T3 axis, glucocorticoids, androgens, estrogens, vitamin D, and possibly leptin (Nilsson et al., 2005; Wit and Camacho-Hübner, 2011). Both insulin and IGF-1 act directly on chondrocytes through their specific receptors, although it is likely that they have overlapping functions (Zhang et al., 2014). IGF-1 activity is also modulated through both inhibitory (IGFBP-3) and stimulatory (IGFBP-5) binding proteins, the synthesis of which it controls, at least in cultured rat growth-plate chondrocytes (Kiepe et al., 2005). T3 acts through at least two nuclear receptors, TR-β1 and the splice variant TR-α2 (Abu et al., 1997), and is thought to play an important role in the maturation of new chondrocytes after they have been formed from the appropriate stem cells. Glucocorticoids, androgens, estrogens, and vitamin D all act through nuclear receptors.

One of the principal apparent functions of the endocrine system is to allow rapid growth only when the organism is able to consume abundant and appropriate nutrients, with dietary amino acids and zinc regulating insulin and systemic (and probably local) IGF-1 levels. Thus, during the GH-driven growth phase, growth can only occur when GH can activate the various paracrine growth factors as a result of the appropriate dietary signaling. In the growing rat it has long been known that circulating levels of insulin, IGF-1, and free T_3 fall markedly in response to protein deficiency (Jepson et al., 1988; Yahya et al., 1990). The observation that muscle growth and protein synthesis was shown to be directly related to changes in these circulating hormone levels gave rise to the concept of the anabolic drive in which dietary protein stimulates growth through endocrine mediators as well as direct influences of key amino acids (Millward and Rivers, 1988, 1989). Furthermore, in the growing rat, the reduced insulin levels in response to a low protein meal are thought to be a mediator of lower T3 and IGF-1 synthesis rates in the liver. Thus, very marked systemic hormonal and metabolic changes explain much of the slow growth induced by protein deficiency. Zinc deficiency is also involved in changes in these hormones although as discussed below the responses are more difficult to evaluate (see MacDonald, 2000).

However, two points need to be made about these responses. First, in the growing rat, changes in IGF-1 within the epiphyseal cartilage do not show a simple relationship with either protein or proteoglycan synthesis or actual length growth of bone (Yahya et al., 1990). This probably reflects the complexity of the IGF-1, IGFBP, growth factor-paracrine system. Secondly, in children hormonal changes in response to variation in dietary protein and zinc intake are much less marked than in the growing rat, with insulin in particular much less sensitive to amino acid intake. This means that the way in which the dietary anabolic drive on growth operates in children will be much more difficult to unravel.

6.2.3 PARACRINE SIGNALING WITHIN THE GROWTH PLATE

This is quite complex (see Kronenberg, 2003; Long and Ornitz, 2013; Lui et al., 2014; Xie et al., 2014) and includes the involvement of IGFs, parathyroid hormone-related peptide (PTHrP), indian hedgehog (IHH), bone morphogenetic proteins (BMPs), wingless/integrated proteins (Wnts), fibroblast growth factors (FGFs), epidermal growth factor (EGF), vascular endothelial growth factor (VEGF), and transforming growth factor (TGF)-β. Vitamin D also acts in an anabolic way within the growth plate (Nilsson et al., 2005) exhibiting an endocrine feedback loop between 1.25 $(OH)_2$VitD and parathyroid hormone (PTH) and through a functional paracrine feedback loop between 1.25

(OH)$_2$VitD and PTH-related protein (PTHrP) in the growth plate. Thus, 1.25 (OH)$_2$VitD decreases PTHrP production, while PTHrP increases chondrocyte sensitivity to 1.25 (OH)$_2$VitD by increasing VDR production (Bach et al., 2014).

6.2.4 Direct Anabolic Influences of Amino Acids and Zinc

Although the endocrine system can mediate nutritional influences on the growth plate, the extent and nature of direct anabolic influences of nutrients such as amino acids or zinc on endochondral ossification is poorly understood. For example, chondrocyte development in cell culture has long been known to be sensitive to amino acid levels (Ishikawa et al., 1986), but whether such direct effects of amino acids involve leucine, which acts through the mTOR/S6 signaling pathway to regulate protein synthesis in muscle (see Millward, 2012), mediating similar changes within the chondrocyte, is not known. However, Chen and Long (2015) have recently reported that mTORC1 signaling does promote osteoblast differentiation from preosteoblasts in mouse primary calvarial cells, so it might be expected that similar signal-transduction pathways operate in chondrocytes.

A role for zinc within the growth plate would be expected from the growing understanding of zinc's structural, catalytic, and regulatory functions throughout the organism. As much as 10% of the human genome codes for proteins with zinc-binding domains (see Cousins et al., 2006). Zn^{2+} acts as an activator or coactivator of a variety of proteins by providing a structural scaffold, for example in the form of zinc fingers and zinc clusters (Prasad, 1995). In fact, there are more than 100 Zn^{2+}-dependent enzymes and more than 2,000 Zn^{2+}-dependent transcription factors in mammals (Andreini et al., 2006). Labile Zn^{2+}, in extra and intracellular compartments, exerts a wide range of influences on cellular functions with an imbalance in Zn^{2+} homeostasis linked to dysfunction; a role of the Zn^{2+} in growth-related signaling is emerging.

Because Zn^{2+} may also be overtly toxic when accumulated in excess in cells, the organism has evolved specific pathways to homeostatically regulate its availability through a complex array of transporters which mediate intracellular zinc trafficking as well as Zn-binding proteins, the metallothioneins (MTs), through which zinc signaling occurs.

Zn transporters are from either the ZnT family (ZnT1-10), which reduce intracellular zinc availability by mediating Zn^{2+} efflux from cells or influx into intracellular vesicles, or the ZIP family (ZIP1-14), which increase intracellular zinc availability by promoting Zn^{2+} influx from the extracellular fluid or intracellular vesicles into the cytoplasm. The most clearly defined evidence for transporter-mediated signaling roles for Zn has been derived for the ZIP family. Children affected by the recessive condition acrodermatitis enteropathica (AE) have low serum concentrations of Zn because of mutations in the intestinal Zn transporter ZIP4 (see Fukada et al., 2008). Cousins et al. (2010) identified ZIPs 6, 8, and 10 with signaling processes, and ZIP13 and 14 are also now known to be involved. For example, in human osteoarthritis cartilage, ZIP8 is specifically upregulated resulting in increased levels of intracellular Zn^{2+} in chondrocytes, which upregulates expression of matrix-degrading enzymes as a result of Zn activation of the metal-regulatory transcription factor-1 (MTF1; Kim et al., 2014). Fukada et al. (2008) have shown that ZIP13 knockout mice show changes in bone, teeth, and connective tissue reminiscent of the clinical spectrum of human Ehlers-Danlos syndrome (EDS), which are a group of genetic disorders affecting connective tissues. Importantly, the ZIP13 knockout mice show defects in the maturation of osteoblasts, chondrocytes, odontoblasts, and fibroblasts, which reflect impairment in bone morphogenic protein (BMP) and TGF-β signaling. Furthermore, homozygosity for a ZIP13 loss of function mutation has been detected in siblings affected by a unique variant of EDS that recapitulates the phenotype observed in ZIP13-KO mice, of which short stature is a component.

ZIP14, which controls G-protein coupled receptor (GPCR)-mediated signaling, has also been implicated in growth regulation at the level of GPCR-cAMP-CREB signaling (Hojyo et al., 2011). Thus ZIP14 knockout mice exhibit growth retardation and impaired gluconeogenesis, which are attributable to disrupted GPCR signaling in the growth plate, pituitary gland, and liver. In this case, the decreased signaling is a consequence of the reduced basal level of cyclic AMP caused by increased phosphodiesterase (PDE) activity in ZIP14-KO cells. This suggests that ZIP14 facilitates GPCR-mediated cAMP-CREB signaling by suppressing the basal PDE activity.

Taken together, these examples show that the availability of Zn^{2+} could influence the regulation of growth in diverse ways, although much remains to be learned about the level of zinc transport and signaling within the growth plate.

6.3 NUTRITION AND GROWTH

Golden (1988, 1991) introduced the concept of classifying nutrients according to their influence on growth. In this system, Type I nutrients, the largest group, have specific functions in one or a limited number of biological pathways. Their deficiency can be easily identified through a failure of the process with which they are uniquely involved (e.g., vitamin C and scurvy, iron and anemia, iodine and thyroid hormone deficiency, and so on). Although the deficiency of type I nutrients may influence growth, such as with iron or iodine deficiency, this is usually a late response to their deficiency and their deficiency is easily identified. Type II nutrients, a smaller group, are those involved in a widespread range of pathways and functions. Their deficiency is difficult to identify because apart from growth failure there are no other specific indicators of this. However, growth inhibition is an immediate response to their deficiency. Golden identifies type II nutrients as protein (specifically nitrogen and indispensable amino acids), zinc, phosphorus, and the main electrolytes potassium, sodium, and magnesium. Of these, there is evidence that deficiencies of protein and zinc can occur in the human diet, and there is very limited evidence for phosphate deficiency occurring through a dietary lack (see Waterlow, 2006), although it is generally believed that phosphate deficiency is likely to be very rare. Protein and zinc deficiency are particularly important for populations consuming diets based on starchy roots with little or no animal source foods as discussed below.

6.3.1 Growth Regulation as Observed in Animal Models

6.3.1.1 Protein

The protein-stat model was developed from a detailed study of the nutritional regulation of bone length growth in the rat, a species for which the consequences of undernutrition and protein deficiency are well understood (Yahya and Millward, 1994; Tirapegui et al., 1994; Yahya et al., 1994). The specific effects of dietary protein on bone growth in the rat are shown in Figure 6.3. There is a marked slowing of length growth in response to protein deficiency although this response is delayed for at least 3 days. However, after this time there are graded reductions with reduced protein intakes. A similar dependence on dietary protein levels was observed during refeeding. Catch-up growth in weight commences immediately in most dietary groups, but bone growth recovers slowly at a rate that reflects the dietary protein intake over a wide range of protein intakes. Most importantly, differences in length growth occur between the three highest intakes (9%, 12%, and 20% protein), even though the rate of body weight and muscle growth is maximal at 9% protein and does not differ markedly between these levels. Thus, the influence of dietary amino acids on bone length growth can be observed at intakes above those necessary to ensure maximal rates of whole body protein accretion.

These influences of dietary protein on linear bone growth seem more powerful than influences exerted by energy intake. While food restriction has long been known to inhibit linear growth (Dickerson and McCance, 1961), the specific effects of energy deficiency, independently from protein deficiency, are more difficult to evaluate. Figure 6.4a shows experiments in which energy restriction was imposed either by feeding 25% of normal intakes or by total starvation. While weight loss occurred in both groups, the length of the tibia continued to increase in the energy-restricted

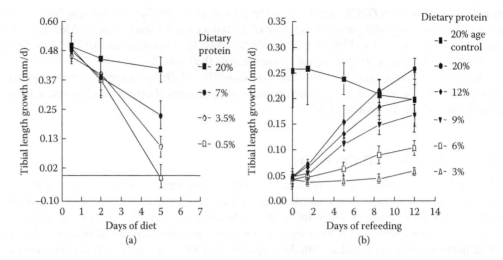

FIGURE 6.3 Effects of dietary protein on bone growth. Total tibia length was measured radiographically (a) in rats in which growth inhibition was induced by ad libitum feeding of low protein diets for up to 7 d, and (b) in rats during catch-up growth on increasing dietary protein levels after complete growth inhibition (21 d of a 0.5% protein diet). (Data are from Yahya ZAH and Millward DJ, *Clin Sci.*, 87, 213–224, 1994.)

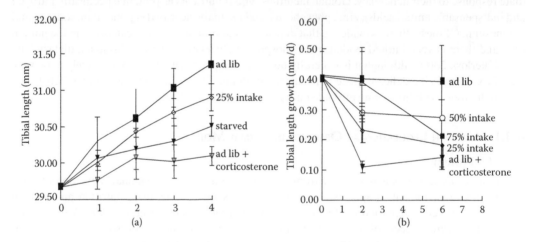

FIGURE 6.4 Effects of dietary energy restriction and corticosterone (CS) on bone growth. (a) Experiment 1. Energy restriction imposed either by feeding 25% of normal intake or by total starvation. Corticosterone treatment, 100 mg/kg daily, resulted in plasma levels observed in rats after prolonged starvation (b) Experiment 2. Energy restricted diets included increased protein concentrations to maintain constant protein intakes of the ad lib diet (12% protein). (Data are from Tirapegui JO et al., *Clin Sci.*, 87, 599–606, 1994.)

and starved groups, albeit at reduced rates. Only with corticosterone treatment at doses that resulted in plasma levels observed after prolonged starvation was linear growth inhibited immediately. In Figure 6.4b the effect of progressive food restriction with constant protein intakes (i.e., diets containing increasing concentrations of protein) is shown. Although body weight growth was arrested in all groups, with weight loss in the severely restricted rats, some tibial length growth continued at all levels of energy restriction with a slow development of inhibition. A comparison of the relative influences of protein as opposed to energy deficiency on bone growth in these studies indicates that protein deficiency is the most powerful influence. Thus, in the most severely energy-restricted group (25% *ad libitum* intake), while body weight fell by 20% (Tirapegui et al., 1994), tibial length growth was similar to or even greater than in rats that were maintaining body weight and fed protein-deficient diets (7% or 3.5% protein) for a similar period. Taken together, these experimental data strongly support a dietary control mechanism for linear growth in which protein intake is the most powerful macronutrient influence. They also show how one of the components of inflammation (i.e., high levels of corticosteroids) is a powerful inhibitory factor.

As indicated above, the cellular mechanisms of these changes in bone length growth involve complex paracrine signaling systems, but little is known about how amino acids and other nutritional signals activate the pathways. However, protein synthesis is ultimately a target. The delayed inhibition of linear growth by protein deficiency, as indicated in Figure 6.4a, reflects the parallel inhibition of both growth plate protein synthesis, through reductions in both ribosomal capacity (RNA/protein ratio) and activity (protein synthesis/RNA) and in proteoglycan sulfation (Yahya et al., 1994). In contrast, the inhibition of length growth by energy deficiency or corticosteroids was dissociated from and preceded inhibition of protein synthesis and ^{35}S uptake. These responses were only observed in the most severely restricted groups or after prolonged corticosterone treatment. It is possible that this reflects an elevation of rates of proteolysis and proteoglycan degradation associated with elevated corticosterone levels.

To summarize then, while dietary protein has a clear, specific regulatory influence on bone growth, the cellular mechanisms of that influence remain to be discovered.

6.3.1.2 Zinc

Hambidge and Krebs (2007) reviewed the challenges associated with zinc deficiency and identified zinc as a micronutrient of exceptional biologic and public health importance, especially in relation to prenatal and postnatal development. This view is consistent with Golden's identification of zinc as a type II nutrient likely to be important in the control of growth. The growth of skeletal muscle is dependent on the zinc supply because it has been shown repeatedly that the zinc concentration of muscle never falls when the dietary zinc supply is limited. This was shown in rat studies which involved feeding diets in which there was a complete absence of dietary zinc (Giugliano and Millward, 1984). Some limited muscle growth occurred, with zinc supplied from bone which showed a marked fall in zinc content. Also during the rapid catch-up growth of malnourished children in the recovery phase on a high-energy soy-based formula, unless additional zinc is added growth eventually slows, fat is mainly deposited, and the energy cost of growth increases. With added dietary zinc, growth is more rapid with a lower energy cost per gram of weight gain, because increased lean tissue deposition occurs (Golden and Golden, 1981). As for longitudinal growth, the challenge is in demonstrating this type II nutrient role of zinc from the perspectives of both the identification of the extent of zinc deficiency in stunted children and of the cellular mechanisms through which zinc acts to mediate linear growth.

From the outset, animal studies clearly showed that the inhibition of growth is a cardinal symptom of zinc deficiency (Williams and Mills, 1970). Subsequent studies have suggested that reduced growth factor levels and reduced anabolic signaling within the growth plate are a feature of zinc deficiency, although it has proved extremely difficult to demonstrate this, yet alone dissect the mechanisms in any detail. For example, Rossi et al. (2001) showed after 28 d of a very low zinc (ZD) diet, when compared with both well fed and pair fed (PF) animals, there were reductions in ponderal growth, femur weight and length, and circulating IGF-1, altered bone mechanical properties, markedly lowered bone zinc, and reduced thicknesses of both the overall growth plate and hypertrophic cartilage. However, apart from the markedly reduced bone zinc content and a different bone histology of the ZD and PF rats, the differences between the ZD and PF animals were in fact generally small. The authors' interpretation of this is that the bone growth failure in the ZD animals reflected a severe reduction in bone growth mediated by growth plate dysfunction compared with a less severe reduction of bone growth coupled with an increase in bone remodeling in the PF rats (more osteoclasts per unit of trabecular surface). However, a detailed examination of the behavior of the severely zinc-deficient rat shows it to be a generally unsatisfactory model for investigating the role of zinc in growth regulation and how zinc-poor human diets might limit growth. The marked inhibitory effect of a severely zinc-deficient diet on appetite and the characteristic feeding behavior raises problems that simple pair feeding studies do not overcome. As we (Giugliano and Millward, 1984) and others have shown, zinc-deficient rats exhibit cyclic changes in food intake and body weight mediated in part by cycles of catabolism associated with elevated corticosterone (Giugliano and Millward, 1987). These cyclic gains and losses of body and organ weight result in a redistribution of zinc from bone to muscle and some other tissues allowing some limited muscle growth to occur. However, the detection of an influence of the zinc deficiency *per se* requires careful studies throughout the anabolic and catabolic phases of the food intake cycling. When this was done, it was clear that during the period when the appetite was transiently restored and food intake occurred, insulin secretion remained low so that plasma insulin levels were unresponsive to changes in food intake. Consequently, the insulin-dependent ribosomal translation phase of protein synthesis in skeletal muscle was markedly lower than observed in Zn-replete well-fed rats. Thus, although a major part of the growth failure in this zinc-deficient rat model involves a corticosteroid-induced blockade due to anorexia and reduced food intake, the inability of the animal to respond to food intake when appetite returns, with sufficient insulin to fully activate the translational phase of protein synthesis, constitutes an important additional reason for the impaired growth. This shows that there is a zinc deficiency–induced impairment of the anabolic drive at the key initial step of insulin production.

One attempt to overcome this anorexia problem in the zinc-deficient rat model has involved the use of megestrol acetate, a synthetic progestin used clinically to correct anorexia in patients with cancer or AIDS. Browning et al. (1998) showed that for rats treated with this compound and fed a zinc-deficient diet, although food intake and serum IGF-I levels were maintained, growth inhibition persisted in the zinc-deficient rats. This is a relatively unambiguous demonstration of the inhibition of the anabolic signaling by IGF-I with zinc deficiency. Further investigations by these workers (MacDonald et al., 1998) demonstrated the need for zinc in the IGF-1 mediation of cell division in cultured 3T3 cells, but the localization of the zinc-dependent step in this pathway has proved to be difficult. One possibility is a specific step in calcium-dependent mitogenic signal transduction through the IGF-I receptor protein kinase C (PKC) pathway (MacDonald, 2000), which is significant because PKC is a zinc metalloenzyme.

The regulatory systems which maintain zinc availability over a wide range of intakes mean that the detection of zinc deficiency in terms of Zn concentrations in plasma, serum, and other tissues is very difficult. Furthermore, the very complexity of intracellular zinc metabolism especially in terms of its multiple signaling functions as briefly summarized above means that the identification of its role in the regulation of endochondral ossification within the growth plate at the level of stem cell recruitment, active proliferation, differentiation, apoptosis, and mineralization is only slowly becoming apparent.

6.3.2 HUMAN STUDIES OF NUTRITION AND GROWTH

As would be expected from Figure 6.1, in many communities where growth failure occurs, it can be difficult to disentangle poor nutrition from other adverse environmental influences, such as infections or environmental enteric dysfunction (discussed in detail below). The main nutritional feature of the diets of stunted children in developing societies is that they are plant based and often limited to staples, of which starchy root crops are nutritionally poor, with few vegetables or pulses and often little or no animal source foods. However, plant-based diets can be nutritionally adequate. Thus, studies of child growth in developed countries within vegetarian communities (e.g., O'Connell et al., 1989) have indicated that for vegans who strictly avoid animal foods, growth may be near normal among educated communities in which the principles of protein complementation are observed and children are supplemented with known limiting nutrients (e.g., with vitamins A, D, and B12). With diets where supplementation does not occur and when foods are restricted, as with the macrobiotic diet, retarded growth is observed (Dwyer et al., 1983). In fact, the children within a Netherlands macrobiotic community raised in sanitary environments and relatively good socioeconomic conditions are a widely quoted example of stunting as a consequence of poor nutrition alone. The macrobiotic diet is a vegan diet based on cereals (mainly rice), vegetables, legumes, and marine algae; small amounts of cooked fruit; and occasional fish but no meat or dairy products. The height growth of these children falters after 4 months to a rate which is 3.5 cm/yr less than normal (Dagnelie et al., 1994). Some catch-up occurs in adolescence, and importantly the extent of this reflects divergence from the strict macrobiotic regime in terms of the amount of dairy foods consumed (Van Dusseldorp et al., 1996). Which aspect of the macrobiotic diet is responsible for the growth failure has not been identified, however.

Most studies of growth failure in the developing world are more difficult to interpret in terms of an uncomplicated, nutritionally poor diet. Thus, longitudinal studies in severely stunted infants and preschool children in Guatemala showed no benefit of supplementation with good quality protein (such as atole, dried skim milk, and cereal) or energy alone even though many of them consumed more energy and much more protein than their requirements (Martorell and Klein, 1980). Malcolm's studies of the Bundi children in Papua New Guinea (Malcolm, 1970a; Lampl et al., 1978, discussed in detail below) indicated very severe stunting and small adult height associated with a nutrient-poor, bulky diet of mainly sweet potato and taro providing protein at only 3% dietary energy and low levels of most other nutrients. Malcolm argued that with the establishment of a mission school and health services in the 1950s, prevalence of severe malnutrition had fallen markedly and there were few signs of overt deficiency or morbidity other than stunting. Malaria rates were low at 3%–7% but diarrhea and dysentery did occur and accounted for a quarter of the admissions to the mission hospital. However, given this evidence of infection, Malcolm's assertion, "It is unlikely that disease is a significant factor in the slow growth rates in Bundi," has been challenged (Garn, 1972).

Thus interventions, rather than observational studies, are more likely to be informative and many nutritional interventions aimed at stimulating height growth in children have been reported, as well as observational studies of height growth in relation to a range of dietary and other factors (for reviews see Golden, 1988, 1994; Waterlow, 1992; Allen and Gilliard, 2001; Hoppe et al., 2006; Allen and Dror, 2011). Here the purpose is to identify the extent to which stunting in children reflects deficiency of energy and other specific nutrients, especially protein and zinc as indicated by animal studies.

6.3.2.1 Energy Intake

As discussed by Allen and Gilliard (2001), it is difficult to interpret associations between energy intake and growth because when food energy intake is low, intakes of many other nutrients will also be inadequate. However, the introduction of the term protein-calorie malnutrition in the 1960s resulted in a debate into the extent of a protein as opposed to a food or energy gap (e.g., Hegsted, 1972) and this was examined with intervention studies. Gopalan et al. (1973) reported an intervention with an energy-rich, low-protein supplement (310 kcal and 3 g protein/day), given to undernourished children in India. They were consuming a cereal-based diet with some buffalo milk, judged to provide sufficient protein but inadequate energy. The intervention increased both height and weight gain over 14 months. This is shown in Figure 6.5a. Furthermore, during the study there was an outbreak of measles enabling the interaction between measles and the supplement to be examined over 6–8 weeks after the infective episode. The changes in height are shown in Figure 6.5b. In the unsupplemented group, height gain was considerably depressed, with some weight loss, in children who had developed measles compared with the noninfected children. In marked contrast, in supplemented children, gain in height and weight were similar, whether or not they had developed measles, and these increases were similar to those of the 50th percentile of American children. The authors commented that although their results may be generally applicable to poor communities

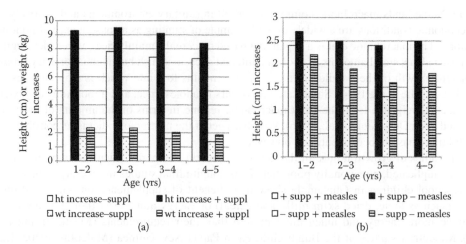

FIGURE 6.5 The effect of supplements of energy on growth of undernourished children in India. The supplement was an energy-rich low-protein supplement (310 kcal and 3 g protein/day) given to undernourished Indian children consuming a cereal-based diet with some buffalo milk for 14 months. (a) shows height and weight increases over 14 months in the various age groups. (b) shows growth over 6–8 weeks in the various age groups during which time there was a measles outbreak. (Data are from Gopalan C et al., *Am J Clin Nutr.*, 26, 563–536, 1973.)

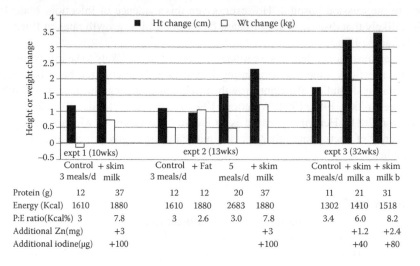

FIGURE 6.6 Data from Malcolm's supplementation trials with the Bundi children. Experiments 1 and 2 from Malcolm, 1970; Experiment 3 from Lampl et al., 1978. The additional zinc and iodine intakes are estimates from the published composition of skimmed milk powder.

consuming mainly cereals and some legumes and pulses, they may not be applicable to children where the staples, such as plantains, are less nutrient dense.

The Bundi children in Papua New Guinea studied by Malcolm, all severely stunted, may have been energy deficient to some extent (Malcolm, 1970a, b). The diet of the community was very bulky and low fat, comprising mainly sweet potato and taro, providing only 3% dietary protein calories, and children in the mission school with restricted meal times may have eaten less food and were more stunted than village children who ate continuously. He observed a small increase in height growth when the children ate 60% more food (a lower increase than observed with skim milk; see below) but no increase with additional fat energy (see Figure 6.6, Experiment 2).

In an INCAP longitudinal study of infants and preschool children in Guatemala provided with a good-quality protein (such as atole) or energy alone, energy intake was the strongest predictor of both linear growth and weight increase (Martorell and Klein, 1980). However, the supplements did contain some micronutrients and thus their intake covaried with energy intake. That said, the supplemented children remained severely stunted, even though many of them consumed more energy than their requirements, and their protein intakes were two to three times higher than recommendations.

6.3.2.2 Protein Intake

Contrary to popular belief, the protein requirements of young children are low in terms of the P:E ratio of the requirement: the safe level is about 5% energy for preschool children, although energy requirements are high (WHO, 2007a) so that absolute protein requirements per kilogram are higher than for older children and adults. This means that with the exception of some very low-protein starchy-root staples like plantain, cassava, taro, and sweet potato, most diets and especially cereal-based diets provide more than adequate amounts of protein if a sufficient amount is consumed to meet the energy requirement. The challenge is to define the lower and upper limits of the range of P:E ratios of intakes, which ensures that the genotype in relation to stature can be expressed.

During exclusive breast feeding, length growth is generally considered to be optimal with protein intakes much lower (about 6%–7% P:E) than at any other stage during childhood. Furthermore, in what is probably the most thorough and detailed analysis of the growth and nutritional intakes of healthy, breast fed (BF) or formula fed (FF) infants in the US during the first year of life by Dewy and her colleagues, linear growth did not differ between BF and FF infants and was independent of protein intake for both groups. However, the much lower protein intakes of the BF infants were associated with lower weight, lean body mass, and fat mass gain (Heinig et al., 1993). Thus, the BF infants were the same length but leaner than FF infants at one year of age. Furthermore, the BF infants had lower morbidity than the heavier FF infants implying that the higher weights carried no advantage. Räihä et al. (2002) also found no difference in length growth in infants fed either breast milk or experimental formulae with protein intakes either higher than or similar to breast milk. Whether this means that during the infancy insulin-dependent growth phase (as defined by Karlberg, 1989) linear growth is insensitive to dietary signals or that the threshold for dietary proteins' influence is below the lowest level of intake observed in healthy breast or formula-fed infants is not known.

In developed societies, the change to a diet based on family foods at weaning involves a dramatic increase in protein intake to levels considerably in excess of requirements. For example, Hoppe et al. (2004) report dietary P:E ratios of 13% in Danish infants at 9 months. This is at least twice the P:E ratio of breast milk and these and even higher values appear to be maintained among children in the Nordic countries up to puberty (Hörnell et al., 2013). The consequences of this increase in protein intake for linear growth and whether any influence is desirable is a controversial and complicated issue. This is mainly because of the possibility of a link between higher protein intakes, fat gain, and obesity, and because there are currently inexplicable links between the food sources of the higher protein intakes and height growth. In their systematic review of protein intakes and growth of children in the Nordic countries up to puberty Hörnell et al. (2013) concluded that a higher protein intake in infancy and early childhood is convincingly associated with increased growth and higher body mass index in childhood, and that increased intake of animal protein in childhood is probably related to earlier puberty, outcomes not viewed as desirable. However, the review is not entirely satisfactory since little attempt was made to disentangle weight gain associated with height gain from increased BMI and fat mass. For example, a study in healthy Danish children examined at 9 months and followed up at 10 years, showing that protein intakes at 9 months were significantly correlated with infant length and with weight and length at 10 years, was included as a study "seeing a positive association between protein intake and growth, and/or BMI." In fact, in this study there was no relationship between protein intake at either age and body fatness at 10 years expressed as

%BF or BMI (Hoppe et al., 2004). This group also reported that in healthy Danish preschool children, height was positively associated with total protein intakes (Hoppe et al., 2004), of which milk but not meat protein was the main dietary correlate with height. As discussed below this may be an example of the "milk effect" on growth. The issue of excess protein intakes and obesity in late childhood and adult life requires further clarification.

For cereal-based diets with minimal animal source foods it is not clear how well linear growth can occur in the best circumstances given the often occurring dietary limitations of micronutrients and minerals, as well as the suboptimal protein quality. The high P:E ratio of cereals, especially that of wheat, means that the lysine limitation is to some extent offset by the higher protein intakes, although digestibility may limit the protein quality of cereals like millet. However, there is evidence that improving the protein quality of cereals can increase height growth, the example being maize. Like all cereals, maize protein has low levels of lysine but uniquely zein, the main storage protein of maize, is also low in tryptophan, hence its association with pellagra (niacin deficiency). However, with selective breeding, maize varieties have been developed with much higher levels of lysine and tryptophan. They also have agronomic properties, which make them viable alternatives to the traditional maize variety. The best known is Quality Protein Maize (QPM), developed in the 1960s and shown with studies on young men to have a biological value of its protein comparable to that of most animal proteins (Young et al., 1971). In fact, while the protein content is unchanged, the concentrations of lysine, tryptophan, the sulfur amino acids, and threonine are increased by 50, 75, 90, and 40% respectively. Graham and colleagues in Lima, Peru, showed that QPM would support height growth comparable to that observed with a cow milk formula, when fed as the sole source of dietary protein, fat, and energy for rapidly growing young children (Graham et al., 1990). It should be noted that the QPM was fed with micronutrient and mineral supplements so that this study evaluated only the quantity and quality of the dietary protein, not the overall nutritional quality of the maize. Since these initial studies, the introduction of QPM has been relatively slow, but trials comparing QPM and normal maize have now been reported with a recent meta-analysis of community-based studies (Nilupa et al., 2010). Although the reported studies vary in quality and few were peer reviewed, the meta-analysis of nine studies that reported on both weight and height indicated a positive effect of QPM on growth of young children. Specifically, consumption of QPM instead of conventional maize resulted in a 12% increase in weight gain and a 9% increase in height gain in infants and young children with mild-to-moderate undernutrition from populations in which maize is a significant part of the diet.

These growth effects are small but they reinforce the evidence from the studies of Danish infants that dietary protein and specifically dietary indispensable amino acids are important regulators of human height growth as in the animal models. On the other hand, sufficient or even excess dietary protein intake may not be able to prevent the stunting observed in poor communities. Thus, the Nutrition Collaborative Research Support Program (CRSP) found that linear-growth faltering was prevalent in preschool children in Egypt, Kenya, and Mexico, even though their intakes of protein and essential amino acids were adequate (Beaton et al., 1992).

6.3.2.3   Zinc Intake

The prevalence of zinc deficiency is difficult to assess because of a lack of simple status indicators (Hambidge and Krebs, 2007). However, it is widely believed to be widespread in developing countries because of low intakes of zinc-rich animal products; diets high in phytates, which inhibit zinc absorption; and zinc losses due to diarrhea. Wessells and Brown (2012) estimated the country-specific prevalence of inadequate zinc intake, from absorbable zinc content of the national food supply (from national food balance sheet data), and estimates of physiological requirements for absorbed zinc. They estimated 17.3% of the world's population to be at risk of inadequate zinc intake, with prevalence of inadequate zinc intake ranging from 7.5% in high-income regions to 30% in South Asia, and with countries in South and Southeast Asia, sub-Saharan Africa, and Central America having the greatest risk of inadequate zinc intake. Within 138 low- and middle-income countries, the prevalence of inadequate zinc intake was correlated with the prevalence of stunting in children under 5 years of age and explained almost a quarter of the between-country variation in stunting. Clearly the best evidence of dietary zinc deficiency contributing to stunting will come from supplementation trials which have been reviewed by several authors. Allen and Gilliard (2001) commented that in terms of pregnancy and birthweight, evidence for the efficacy of zinc supplements was mixed with the majority of studies identifying no influence. For children, benefits of zinc supplementation include reductions in the duration and severity of both diarrhea and dysentery and of acute lower respiratory infections (Allen and Gilliard, 2001), all of which may indirectly influence height growth. Randomized, controlled trials of zinc supplementation for children have produced varying degrees of growth response. A 1997 meta-analysis of twenty-five studies revealed that there was an overall small, but highly significant impact of zinc supplements on height, but only in children with initial HA Z-scores less than –2.0 (Brown et al., 1997). Because of this, the *Lancet* series on Maternal and Child Undernutrition recommended zinc supplementation as an effective intervention to reduce morbidity and prevent stunting (Bhutta et al., 2008). However, a more recent meta-analysis of the influence of micronutrient supplementation (vitamin A, iron, or zinc) on growth of preschool children, which for zinc included most of the studies assessed in 1997 and 32 additional data sets, found that for a total of 53 data sets, changes in height were positive for 30 studies and statistically significant for 11, but the overall weighted mean effect of zinc was small and not statistically significant, as was also the case for vitamin A and iron (Ramakrishnan et al., 2006). Only in the case of multiple supplementation of at least three micronutrients (27 data sets from 20 studies) was there a significant change in height, albeit quite small (mean effect size of 0.09 [95% CI: 0.008, 0.17]). Eighty percent of these data sets involved vitamin A, iron, and zinc, with some also containing iodine, selenium, and copper. As the authors comment, it would appear from the literature to date that micronutrient interventions, whether single or multi-nutrient, appear to do little to prevent stunting *per se*. An intervention in 6-month-old peri-urban infants in Guatemala, many of them (22%) stunted, involving small amounts of bovine serum concentrate, with or without zinc, iron, iodine, selenium, and a range of vitamins given for 2–8 months, did not affect growth velocity or rates of infection (Begin et al., 2008). In fact, the prevalence of stunting increased to 50%.

6.3.2.4 Iodine Intake

Iodine deficiency is seldom included in discussions of the nutritional etiology of stunting, yet globally, it is estimated that 2 billion individuals have an insufficient iodine intake, with South Asia and sub-Saharan Africa particularly affected. Even after the widespread introduction of salt-iodination programs, globally, 30% (241 million) of school-age children are estimated to have insufficient iodine intakes (Zimmermann, 2009; Andersson et al., 2012). As discussed below it may well be that the Bundi children studied by Malcolm in Papua New Guinea were iodine deficient. Given the importance of the T4/T3 axis for growth and development, and the fact that severe iodine deficiency results in severe growth retardation, it might be expected that in otherwise unsymptomatic iodine deficiency, growth faltering would occur. However, evidence that this is the case is scarce. Most RCTs of iodine supplementation have involved pregnancy and generally aim to prevent irreversible brain damage associated with cretinism (Zimmermann, 2012), and of these, a recent systematic review identified only two studies that reported on child growth observing no improvements (Zhou et al., 2013). However, inadequate iodine intake in infants and children is the key concern as far as growth is concerned. In this case, iodine repletion in school-age children who were severely iodine-deficient (7- to 10- year-old Moroccan children), moderately iodine-deficient (10- to 12-year-old Albanian children), or mildly iodine-deficient (5- to 14-year-old South African children) increased IGF-1 levels in each case and also increased TT4, IGFBP-3, and both weight-for-age and height-for-age Z scores in the Moroccan and Albanian children (Zimmermann et al., 2007). This means that in communities of low iodine availability, and where use of iodized salt is limited, if stunting is prevalent, iodine deficiency must be included as a potential part of any nutritional etiology.

6.3.2.5 Animal Source Foods and Growth

Several observational studies, for example, the Nutrition Collaborative Research Support Program (NCRSP) in Egypt, Kenya, and Mexico, show obvious associations between intakes of animal source foods (ASFs) and better growth, which remain positive even after controlling for covariates and confounders, such as socioeconomic status, morbidity, parental literacy, and nutritional status (Neumann et al., 2002). In these studies, the greatest deficits in linear growth were found in those with little or no ASFs in their diet. Based on these studies, Allen and colleagues have widely promoted the strategy of increasing consumption of ASFs (i.e., meat, fish, eggs, and milk) for improving the amount and bioavailability of micronutrients available to children in the developing world. It is the case that for many population groups of children, ASFs often comprise only a very small part of their diet, if any at all. The obvious reasons for this strategy is that animal products are high in most micronutrients, which are better absorbed than from plant-derived foods. Also, ASFs may contain more fat, making them more energy dense, as well as being a good source of fat-soluble vitamins and essential fatty acids, and the only source of vitamin B12. As discussed above, diets free of animal products can support near normal growth when they contain a wide variety of plant food sources and are supplemented with key micronutrients. However, in poor communities in much of the developing world, diets are much less varied and often contain few ASFs or energy-dense foods. Indeed, ASFs may be culturally unacceptable in some communities.

6.3.2.5.1 Meat

Although Allen and Gilliard (2001) report some evidence that animal products are associated with better growth in several countries, few involve meat as such. In healthy Danish preschool children, height was not associated with meat but was with milk intake (Hoppe et al., 2004a). In fact, specific interventions of increased intakes of meat on its own have generally failed to increase height growth and reduce stunting. In a Kenyan trial that supplied schoolchildren daily snacks of a local dish (maize, beans, and greens) for 2 years with additions of meat, milk, or equivalent energy, while all children increased weight compared with no snacks, there was little effect on height, although meat did improve muscle mass and cognitive function more than milk (Neumann et al., 2003, 2007). A more recent 12-month intervention compared the effect of meat (lyophilized beef) with that of an equicaloric micronutrient-fortified cereal, starting at 6 months of age in rural communities in the Democratic Republic of the Congo and Zambia, semirural communities in the Western Highlands of Guatemala, and urban communities in Karachi, Pakistan (Krebs et al., 2012). Inclusion criteria in this study was an estimated prevalence of stunting of $\geq 20\%$. At baseline (6 months) there was a low length-for-age Z score of -1.4 with one-third of the infants stunted. The extent of stunting worsened by 18 months, Z score of -1.9, with no difference between the two groups. In fact, only maternal height and education emerged as (positive) influences on length growth and the authors commented that this may be a surrogate for better socioeconomic status and favorable practices such as hygiene and medical care. Thus, these findings are illustrative of the principles of the stunting syndrome shown in Figure 6.1 and it may well be that environmental enteropathy (see Figure 6.7) was a determinant of the stunting and prevented any benefit of the nutritional supplementations.

6.3.2.5.2 Milk

Nutrition and linear growth were first investigated with studies focusing on milk (i.e., in the 1920–30s in the United Kingdom and India, and in the 1950s in the United States). Increased milk intake has been the main feature of most cross-sectional, observational, or intervention studies in which ASFs have been associated with increased height growth. Pollock (2006) has reviewed some of these

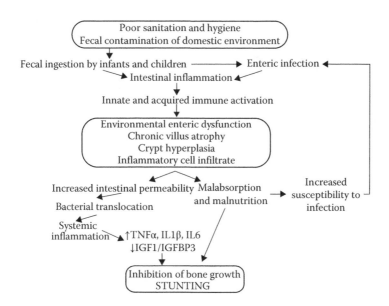

FIGURE 6.7 Stunting as a predominantly inflammatory disease resulting from poor hygiene and environmental enteric dysfunction. See Humphrey (2009), Keusch et al. (2013), and Prendergast and Humphrey (2014).

early studies, especially the interventions in institutionalized children in the 1920s by McCollum in the United States and Corry Mann in the United Kingdom, and the subsequent community-based work of Orr, Leighton, and Clark in Scotland and Belfast, Northern Ireland. While all the studies leave much to be desired in terms of their design and analyses, they resulted in the identification of milk as an important determinant of height growth in children, and of legislation in the United Kingdom in 1934, in 1940, and in 1945 when free school milk was introduced (Atkins, 2005). Since these early studies, the influence of cows' milk intake on height growth post-weaning has been repeatedly confirmed in a large variety of cross-sectional, observational, and intervention studies in both stunted children in developing societies and in healthy children in the UK, Denmark, United States, and Japan (see Takahashi, 1971, 1984; Bogin, 1988, 1998; Wiley, 2005; Hoppe et al., 2006). Some examples of these studies are discussed here.

Regarding children in developing countries, data on preschool children from seven countries in Central and South America indicate that milk intake was significantly associated with higher height-for-age Z scores in all countries, whereas meat and egg/fish/poultry intakes were only associated with height in one of the countries (Ruel, 2003). Rutishauser and Whitehead (1969) reported on Ugandan children's heights and weights, comparing the Karamoja, a cattle-herding, milk-consuming people with the Buganda, farmers growing plantain, sweet potatoes, and cassava. The Karamoja children showed normal height growth but were thin, while the Bugandan children were stunted but of normal weight-for-height.

Malcolm's intervention in stunted schoolchildren (1970a) is probably the best known. He describes the growth and development of children living in the highlands of Papua New Guinea and performed a number of dietary interventions, which increased their height (Malcolm, 1970b; Lampl et al., 1978). According to Malcolm's measurements (1970a), the growth rate of the Bundi children was slower than that of any other reported population in the world with markedly delayed puberty and small adults (i.e., adult men and women were typically 1.56 m and 1.48 m tall with BMIs of 22 and 20 kg/m^2 respectively). The diet of the community was mainly sweet potato and taro providing 3% dietary protein calories. Malcolm was able to compare the growth of children in a Catholic boarding school showing it was slightly slower than village children possibly because in the school the children may have eaten less from their strict three meals per day compared with the continuous eating of the village children, and because of less opportunity to forage in the forest for some animal source foods (e.g., insects, frogs, rodents, etc.). The interventions are shown in Figure 6.6. In Experiment 1, 8-year-olds consumed either the usual taro and sweet potato diet without or with a daily supplement of skim-milk powder (25 g protein) 5/7 days/week for 10 weeks. In Experiment 2, 8-year-olds were given skim milk, similar extra energy such as margarine, or extra taro and sweet potato (5 meals/d as compared to 3) for 13 weeks. In Experiment 3, 8–13-year-olds were given supplements of skim milk powder providing either 10 or 20 g protein 5/7 days a week compared with their school diet for 8 months. In all three studies, some linear growth was observed with the usual diet, which was slightly increased by more of the usual diet in Experiment 2. However, the growth rate in length was doubled by the skim milk in all three experiments with no difference between the two doses, although weight increased more with the higher dose. In Experiment 3, measurements were also made of periosteal bone breadth, and of skeletal maturation, which each increased with the skimmed milk supplements. Clearly, given the previous interventions with milk, the outcome of these studies is not surprising.

As with all such interventions with milk, although the studies are discussed by their authors in terms of protein supplementation, they provide increases in minerals, phosphate, and other key nutrients. The extra zinc and iodine intakes are shown in Figure 6.6. For zinc, this ranges from additions of 1.2–3 mg per day, not insignificant amounts given that most zinc supplementation studies involve 5 mg/d. For iodine, the additions range from 40 to 100 µg/d. Given that WHO (2007b) recommends a daily intake of iodine of 120 µg for schoolchildren, if these children were iodine deficient, the milk intervention would have met their iodine requirements. Malcolm makes no mention of iodine deficiency in his monograph on the Bundi people (Malcolm, 1970b). However, the highlands of New Guinea were known to be an area of iodine deficiency from the 1960s and were where the now classic iodized oil supplementation study by Pharoah, Buttfield, and Hetzel occurred, aiming to prevent endemic cretinism (Pharoah et al., 1971). This means that the growth response observed by Malcolm could have reflected an improvement of their protein, zinc, and iodine status.

As for experiences in developed societies, for healthy Danish preschoolers all with protein intakes more than 60% of which came from ASFs, and well above current protein requirements, height was positively associated with intakes of total animal protein and milk, but not with intakes of vegetable protein or meat (Hoppe et al., 2004a). In New Zealand, long-term avoidance of cow's milk was associated with small stature in prepubertal schoolchildren, which the authors argued reflects the simple chronic avoidance of milk, rather than health problems associated with milk allergy or intolerance (Black et al., 2002). In the United States, analysis of NHANES 1999–2002 indicated that adult height was positively associated with milk consumption at ages 5–12 and 13–17, after controlling for sex, education, and ethnicity (Wiley, 2005). Clearly, given the complexity of height-growth regulation, it would be very surprising if milk intake explained all the variation and Wiley reports on five intervention studies in the United Kingdom, Switzerland, New Zealand, and the United States, which report no significant effect on height in mainly adolescent girls. However, it is undeniable that milk, which has the function of supporting rapid postnatal growth, can also influence growth throughout childhood and is a determinant of adult height.

At the outset of these studies, milk was viewed simply as a nutrient-rich food providing for growth in stature, with elaborations of this view into a "milk hypothesis" predicting that a greater consumption of milk during infancy and childhood will result in greater stature in adult life (Bogin, 1998). It is the case that milk consumption and lactose digestion after weaning are exclusively human traits made possible by lactase persistence (LP), the continued production of the enzyme in the post-weaning period into adulthood. LP post-weaning is not an ancestral condition in humans but is made possible by a relatively recent single nucleotide polymorphism (SNP) of the LPH gene. This is probably of western Eurasian origin and is inherited in a dominant Mendelian fashion and accounts for much of observed lactase persistence in northern Europe, Arabia, and northwestern India (see Romero et al., 2012). LP is also present at moderately high frequencies in some milk-consuming pastoralists from sub-Saharan Africa, the Middle East, and the Mongolian Plateau, as a result of one of several separate SNPs. While the emergence of LP was advantageous among early pastoralists with a constant source of fresh milk, consumption in industrialized urban societies was very limited until the pasteurization of the milk supply to cities in the late nineteenth to early twentieth century and the widespread use of refrigeration. This means that the marked increase in milk consumption by populations in northern Europe and North America is a twentieth-century phenomenon.

It has certainly become clear in recent years that because the specific biological function of milk is to enable rapid postnatal growth, it differs in many ways from all other human foods in having growth-promoting properties not found in meat or other ASFs. However, these properties are by no means understood. Also, the widely assumed beneficial role of milk in the human diet after weaning is being questioned (see Hoppe et al., 2006). Melnik et al. (2013) identifies the presence of microR-NAs in milk exosomes, which could possibly act as anabolic signals for the stimulation of cellular growth and proliferation. Also, milk has uniquely high levels of amino acids, which are known to be involved in anabolic signaling. The caseins and lactoglobulins contain high concentrations of leucine, although this is not unique to milk with higher levels in maize and sorghum. However, tryptophan concentrations in milk proteins are uniquely high, 40% higher than egg and double that of meat. Tryptophan is said to activate the GH-IGF-1-mTORC1 pathway either directly or through gastrointestinal GIP production, while leucine activates the insulin-mTORC1 pathway, with the mTORC1 signaling pathway important for cell replication and growth. These features may explain why Hoppe et al. (2004a) showed in a cross-sectional study of Danish preschoolers that serum IGF-1 levels and overall height were significantly related to milk but not meat intake. They also showed in an intervention study with a high protein supplement of either milk or beef in 8-year-olds that milk and not meat increased concentrations of s-IGF-1 and the s-IGF-1/s-IGFBP-3 ratio significantly (Hoppe et al., 2004b) and that fasting insulin levels and consequently insulin resistance (calculated with the homeostasis model assessment) were higher in the milk but not meat-supplemented children (Hoppe et al., 2005). This combination of increased growth and insulin resistance raises the question of whether these effects of milk in these otherwise healthy children are of benefit or not (see Hoppe et al., 2006). Furthermore, it has been known for some time that societies with high rates of milk consumption and with tall adults generally exhibit poor bone health in old age with higher fracture rates compared with less-developed countries with much less milk consumption (see Hegsted, 2001). Why this should occur is not known, but the possibility that the more rapid growth of childhood and earlier puberty results in a bone architecture that becomes more fragile in old age deserves investigation. Ecological studies also suggest higher mortality rates from ischemic heart disease in countries with high milk consumption (Segall, 2008). Recently two large cohort studies in men and women in Sweden have shown that liquid milk consumption is associated with increased mortality from CVD and cancer in men and women, and a higher fracture incidence in women (Michaëlsson et al., 2014). While the authors recommend that the observational study designs and the inherent possibility of residual confounding and reverse causation phenomena necessitate a cautious interpretation of the results, studies have generated considerable criticisms. Nevertheless, they propose that increased intakes of galactose could explain their findings, given that galactose feeding is an established animal model of aging by induction of oxidative stress and inflammation. They did report a positive association between milk intake and both urine 8-iso-PGF2α (a biomarker of oxidative stress) and serum interleukin 6 (an inflammatory biomarker).

6.4   INFECTION AND POOR GROWTH IN CHILDREN

The role of infections and environmental factors as possible determinants of stunting in children has long been thought to be of great importance (e.g., Nabarro et al., 1988). The stunting syndrome as illustrated in Figure 6.1 identifies interactions between malnutrition and infection throughout the maternal, infant, and child life cycle inhibiting growth. These interactions are mutually reinforcing through infection exacerbating any malnutrition because of appetite suppression and reduced food intake, and any malabsorption reducing nutrient intake, while malnutrition reduces immune defense systems, thereby worsening the adverse influence of infections. However, it is clear that infection and the associated inflammation has direct inhibitory influences on anabolic processes throughout the organism, including the growth plate, which are additional to growth inhibition through malnutrition. We showed some years ago that in response to either endotoxemia or parasitic infection in the rat (Jepson et al., 1986; Omwega et al., 1988), muscle protein synthesis is profoundly inhibited to a much greater extent than the influence of the reduced food intake. Furthermore, this response involved a profound insulin resistance, partly due to the elevated glucocorticoid levels, which exert a direct inhibitory influence on both muscle (Odedra et al., 1982) and bone growth (see Figure 6.4; Tirapegui et al., 1994), in addition to direct inhibitory influences of the proinflammatory cytokines.

6.4.1 Environmental Enteric Dysfunction

In the context of the stunting syndrome as illustrated in Figure 6.1, infection includes parasitic infections, especially malaria and intestinal helminths, and diarrhea, particularly in conditions of poor sanitation and hygiene. One study suggested that 25% of stunting was attributed to five or more episodes of diarrhea (Checkley et al., 2008). However, while all agree that diarrhea is implicated as a cause of poor growth, there has been a debate about its relative importance (Solomons et al., 1993; Bhutta et al., 2008). For example, in Gambian infants in which growth faltering in terms of weight and height growth was reported to become apparent in the second year of life, although diarrhea did occur, its frequency was insufficient to explain the growth faltering. Direct measurements of an enteropathy associated with increased intestinal permeability (as indicated by the handling of oral lactulose and mannitol) was a much better predictor of impaired weight and height gain (Lunn et al., 1991). Increased gut permeability implies a failure of normal gut barrier function, which normally prevents translocation of pathogenic organisms and endotoxins, and which can, in extreme cases, be a route to the development of sepsis in patients in intensive care. Subsequent studies in Gambian infants indicated endotoxin translocation in terms of increased plasma concentrations of total IgG and IgG-endotoxin-core antibody (EndoCAb), and these responses were correlated with increased intestinal permeability. In fact, intestinal permeability, plasma IgG concentration, and EndoCAb together accounted for 56% of the growth inhibition (Campbell et al., 2003a). Mucosal biopsies of these children indicated chronic T-cell-mediated enteropathy with crypt hyperplasia, villous stunting, and high numbers of intraepithelial lymphocytes in all Gambian children, regardless of nutritional status (Campbell et al., 2003b). However, with worsening nutrition mucosal cytokine production became biased toward a proinflammatory response (i.e., a dominance of IFN-γ over TGF-β expression and with increased TNF-α producing cells in the mucosa). These authors concluded that in these Gambian children translocation of immunogenic luminal macromolecules across a compromised gut mucosa had resulted in stimulation of systemic immune/inflammatory processes and subsequent growth impairment. On the basis of this and other evidence, Prendergast and Humphrey (2014) argue that subclinical infection with enteric pathogens is common, even in the absence of diarrhea (Kotloff et al., 2013). Humphrey (2009) identified this subclinical infection with enteric pathogens as tropical enteropathy, characterized by villous atrophy, crypt hyperplasia, increased permeability, inflammatory cell infiltrate, and modest malabsorption. It is caused by fecal bacteria ingested in large quantities by young children living in conditions of poor sanitation and hygiene, and is the primary causal pathway from poor sanitation and hygiene to undernutrition (and by implication stunting), rather than diarrhea. Korpe and Petri (2012) have reviewed the distinction between this environmental enteropathy and other noninfectious tropical malabsorption syndromes such as tropical sprue, celiac sprue, and Crohn's disease, while Keusch et al. (2013) use the term "environmental enteric dysfunction." Importantly in the context of this review, Prendergast and Humphrey (2014) write, "We therefore view stunting as an inflammatory disease arising, in part, from primary gut pathology. Since gut damage also occurs with recurrent (especially persistent) diarrhea, severe acute malnutrition, HIV infection and micronutrient deficiencies, there are multiple overlapping causes of enteropathy in settings of poverty which may exacerbate the growth failure arising from EED (environmental enteric dysfunction)." Recently, Prendergast et al. (2014) have reported an association between low-grade inflammation in the first year of life and perturbation of the growth hormone-IGF axis, which is associated with stunting in apparently healthy Zimbabwean infants. Their longitudinal measurements over 18 months showed that the stunting at 18 months reflected both impaired intrauterine growth, implicating poor maternal health and low in-utero IGF-1 levels, and impaired postnatal growth associated with chronic inflammation, starting very early in infancy. The pathway between the poor environment and stunting as discussed above is illustrated in Figure 6.7.

6.4.2 INFLAMMATION AND ENDOCHONDRAL OSSIFICATION

At the cellular level, the mechanisms by which endochondral ossification is inhibited in children remains poorly understood. However, Sederquist et al. (2014) have recently reviewed what is known about the impact of inflammatory cytokines on longitudinal bone growth mainly from the perspective of children suffering from specific inflammatory diseases such as inflammatory bowel disease, Crohn's disease, ulcerative colitis, and juvenile idiopathic arthritis. Such children usually display abnormal growth patterns as well as delayed puberty, with growth suppressed by the use

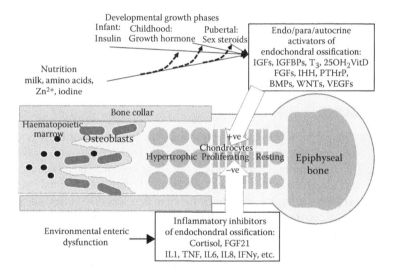

FIGURE 6.8 The role of nutrition and inflammation on the regulation of endochondral ossification. The primary endocrine activators of growth according to the ICP model of Karlberg (1989) are insulin (infant stage), growth hormone (childhood stage), and the sex steroids during puberty. These act on the paracrine/autocrine system within the growth plate, which mediates endochondral ossification. However, a suitable nutritional anabolic drive is necessary for this process to occur involving both Type I nutrients like iodine and Type II nutrients of which amino acids and zinc are particularly important in both stimulating the endocrine/ paracrine system and having direct regulatory influences, although this is poorly understood. Milk also appears to have a specific influence not observed with other animal source foods. Elevated levels of glucocorticoids, inhibitory fibroblast growth factors (e.g., FGF21), and proinflammatory cytokines associated with infection and inflammation caused by environmental enteric dysfunction as in Figure 6.7 block the nutritional anabolic drive and inhibit endochondral ossification. How these interactions between nutrition and infection occur at the cellular and molecular level is very poorly understood.

of glucocorticoids as anti-inflammatory drugs, and by physiologically elevated levels of glucocorticoids in nontreated children as well as proinflammatory cytokines, such as TNF-α, IL-1α, and IL-6. These contribute to growth retardation through both systemic actions on the GH/IGF1 axis, reducing IGF-1 and IGFBP3 levels, and local direct inhibitory actions on the growth plate. High concentrations of these cytokines suppress growth in a dose-dependent manner by decreasing chondrocyte proliferation and hypertrophy while increasing apoptosis. In these patients, the inhibition of these cytokines, with for example a recombinant protein derived from a TNF receptor and part of human IgG1, which acts as a soluble TNF receptor, reduces inflammation and increases growth.

One important consequence of a widespread occurrence of EED is that it would explain the largely disappointing nature of nutritional intervention trials (i.e., the fact that only in a few studies has the provision of supplements of either specific nutrients or foods been shown to restore growth to normal or to the increased rates that might be expected if catch-up was occurring). While a review by Dewey and Adu-Afarwuah (2008) of 38 reports of such supplementation trials indicated both weight and height gain, the latter in the range of an increase in 0.0–0.64 length-for-age Z score by 12–24 months, Humphrey (2009) commented that none of children studied in these various interventions achieved normal growth. In fact, the height growth achieved in the most successful of these studies was equivalent to only about a third of the average deficit of Asian and African children. Dewey and Adu-Afarwuah (2008) did argue that although changes in mean HAZ scores were small, nevertheless the impact on the lower tail of the distribution—that is, on stunting rates *per se*—could be considerably larger (e.g., a fall from 15.8% to 4.7% in the intervention group). However, they concluded that complementary feeding interventions, by themselves, cannot change the underlying conditions of poverty and poor sanitation that contribute to poor child growth. A typical recent example of the failure of a nutritional intervention is the RCT of a meat supplement undertaken by Krebs et al. (2012) discussed above. The rural, semirural, and urban communities involved in that study were all likely to be exposed to poor hygiene and suffer from EED. The role of nutrition and inflammation on the regulation of endochondral ossification incorporating what has been discussed in this chapter is illustrated in Figure 6.8.

6.5 CONCLUSIONS

As commented by Onis et al. (2012) even though more than a quarter of the world's children are stunted, stunting often goes unrecognized in children who live in communities where short stature is so common that it seems normal. Nevertheless, for these communities, because of the cycle of adverse consequences identified in the stunting syndrome (Figure 6.1), few will be able to experience the same sense of wellbeing experienced by many in developed societies. Clearly, appropriate child growth requires adequate nutrition involving sufficient amounts of all those nutrients influencing growth by activating endochondral ossification within the growth plate, of which iodine, amino acids, and zinc have been discussed here. It remains to be discovered what the minimum requirements are for acceptable growth and whether the plant-based diets of the most deprived communities can be sufficiently improved to meet such requirements. As for the nutritional interventions that have improved growth, milk stands out from all other ASFs in its growth-promoting actions. The evidence of more rapid growth and earlier puberty with high milk intakes during childhood suggested by the studies on Scandinavian children raise important but as yet unanswerable questions about the long-term consequences for health within milk-drinking developed communities. However, it is clear that the dietary anabolic drive on growth cannot occur or is at best seriously compromised in the presence of inflammation. While the outlook for many children in less developed countries is bleak, it is encouraging and informative that there are success stories. Thus, de Onis et al. (2012) point out the dramatic improvements in northeastern Brazil, where stunting decreased from 34% in 1986 to 6% in 2006 as a result of rising incomes and increased access to schools, clean water, sanitation, and basic health care. This would reinforce the views of

Prendergast and Humphrey (2014) that stunting is an inflammatory disease with the public health programs most likely to be successful being those focusing on improved water supplies, sanitation, and hygiene, reducing environmental enteric dysfunction.

REFERENCES

Abu EO, Bord S, Horner A, Chatterjee VKK, and Compston JE (1997) The expression of thyroid hormone receptors in human bone. *Bone* 21: 137–142.

Allen HL, Estrada K, Lettre G et al. (2010) Hundreds of variants clustered in genomic loci and biological pathways affect human height. *Nature* 467: 832–838.

Allen LH and Dror DK (2011) Effects of animal source foods, with emphasis on milk, in the diet of children in low-income countries In: *Milk and Milk Products in Human Nutrition. Nestlé Nutrition Institute Workshop Series Pediatric Program*, Eds. RA Clemens, O Hernell, KF Michaelsen, vol. 67, pp. 113–130, Basel: Nestec Ltd., Vevey/S. Karger AG.

Allen LH and Gilliard D (2001) *What Works? A Review of the Efficacy and Effectiveness of Nutrition Interventions*. Asian Development Bank, Manila: ACC/SCN, Geneva.

Andersson M, Karumbunathan V, and Zimmermann MB (2012) Global iodine status in 2011 and trends over the past decade. *J Nutr* 142: 744–750.

Andreini C, Banci L, Bertini I, and Rosato A (2006) Counting the zinc-proteins encoded in the human genome. *J Proteome Res* 5: 196–201.

Ashworth A (1974) Ad lib. feeding during recovery from malnutrition. *Brit J Nutr* 31: 109–112.

Ashworth A and Millward DJ (1986) Catch-up growth in children. *Nutr Rev* 44: 157–163.

Atkins PJ (2005) The milk in schools scheme, 1934–45: 'Nationalization' and resistance. *Hist Edu* 34: 1–21.

Bach FC, Rutten KR, Hendriks K et al. (2014) The paracrine feedback loop between vitamin D3 (1,25(OH)2 D3) and PTHrP in prehypertrophic chondrocytes. *J Cell Physiol* 229: 1999–2014.

Beaton GH, Calloway D, and Murphy SP (1992) Estimated protein intakes of toddlers: Predicted prevalence of inadequate intakes in village populations in Egypt, Kenya, and Mexico. *Am J Clin Nutr* 55: 902–911.

Begin F, Santizo M-C, Peerson JM et al. (2008) Effects of bovine serum concentrate, with or without supplemental micronutrients, on the growth, morbidity, and micronutrient status of young children in a low-income, peri-urban Guatemalan community *Eur J Clin Nutr* 62: 39–50.

Bhutta ZA, Ahmed T, Black RE et al. (2008) Maternal and child undernutrition 3: What works? Interventions for maternal and child undernutrition and survival. *Lancet* 371: 417–440.

Black RE, Williams SM, Jones IE et al. (2002) Children who avoid drinking cow milk have low dietary calcium intakes and poor bone health. *Am J Clin Nutr* 76: 675–680.

Bogin B (1988) *Patterns of Human Growth*. New York, NY: Cambridge University Press.

Bogin B (1998) Milk and human development: An essay on the "milk hypothesis." *Antropol Port* 15: 23–36.

Brown KH, Peerson JM, and Allen LH (1997) Effect of zinc supplementation on children's growth: A meta-analysis of intervention trials. *Biblio Nutr Diet* 54: 76–83.

Browning JD, MacDonald RS, Thornton WH et al. (1998) Reduced food intake in zinc deficient rats is normalized by megestrol acetate but not by insulin-like growth factor-I. *J Nutr* 128: 136–142.

Campbell DI, Elia M, and Lunn PG (2003a) Growth faltering in rural Gambian infants is associated with impaired small intestinal barrier function, leading to endotoxemia and systemic inflammation. *J Nutr* 133: 1332–1338.

Campbell DI, Murch SH, Elia M. et al. (2003b) Chronic T cell–mediated enteropathy in rural west African children: Relationship with nutritional status and small bowel function. *Pediatr Res* 54:306–311.

Checkley W, Buckley G, Gilman RH et al. (2008) Multi-country analysis of the effects of diarrhoea on childhood stunting. *Int J Epidemiol* 37:816–830.

Chen J and Long F (2015) mTORC1 signaling promotes osteoblast differentiation from preosteoblasts. *PLOS ONE* 10: e0130627.

Cousins RJ, Aydemir TB, and Lichten LA (2010) Transcription factors, regulatory elements and nutrient–gene communication. *Proc Nutr Soc* 69: 91–94.

Cousins RJ, Liuzzi JP, and Lichten LA (2006) Mammalian zinc transport, trafficking, and signals. *J Biol Chem* 281: 24085–24089.

Dagnelie PC, van Dusseldorp M, van Staveren WA et al. (1994) Effects of macrobiotic diets on linear growth in infants and children until 10 years of age. *Eur J Clin Nutr* 48 (Suppl. 1): S103–S111.

de Onis M, Blössner M, and Borgh E (2012) Prevalence and trends of stunting among pre-school children, 1990–2020. *Public Health Nutr* 15: 142–148.

Dewey KG and Adu-Afarwuah S (2008) Systematic review of the effcacy and effectiveness of complementary feeding interventions in developing countries. *Matern Child Nutr* 4:24–85. Blackwell Publishing Ltd: Program in International and Community Nutrition, University of California, Davis, CA, pp 24–85.

Dickerson JWT and McCance RA (1961) Severe undernutrition in growing and adult animals. 8. The dimensions and chemistry of the long bones. *Brit J Nutr* 15: 567–576.

Dwyer JT, Andrew EM, Berkey C et al. (1983) Growth in "new" vegetarian preschool children using the Jenss-Bayley curve fitting technique. *Am J Clin Nutr* 37: 815–827.

Fukada T, Civic N, Furuichi T et al. (2008) The zinc transporter SLC39A13/ZIP13 is required for connective tissue development; its involvement in BMP/TGF-b signaling pathways. *PLOS ONE* 3: e3642.

Garn SM (1972) Growth and development in New Guinea—A study of the Bundi people of the Madang district. *By L. A. Malcolm.* (Book review) *Am J Phys Anthropol* 37: 157–159.

Giugliano R and Millward DJ (1984) Growth and zinc homeostasis in the severely zinc deficient rat. *Brit J Nutr* 52: 545–560.

Giugliano R and Millward DJ (1987) The effects of severe zinc deficiency on protein turnover in muscle and thymus. *Brit J Nutr* 51: 139–155.

Golden MHN and Golden BE (1981) Effect of zinc supplementation on the dietary intake, rate of weight gain and energy cost of tissue deposition in children recovering from severe malnutrition. *Am J Clin Nutr* 34: 900–905.

Golden MHN (1994) Is complete catch-up possible for stunted malnourished children? *Eur J Clin Nutr* 48: S58–S71.

Golden MH (1988) The role of individual nutrient deficiencies in growth retardation of children as exemplified by zinc and protein. In: *Linear Growth Retardation in Less Developed Countries*, Ed. JC Waterlow, pp. 143–163. New York, NY: Raven Press.

Golden MH (1991) The nature of nutritional deficiency in relation to growth failure and poverty. *Acta Paed Scand* 374: 95–110.

Gopalan C, Swaminathan MC, Krishna Kumari VK et al. (1973) Effect of calorie supplementation on growth of undernourished children. *Am J Clin Nutr* 26: 563–536.

Graham GG, Lembcke J, and Morales E (1990). Quality-protein maize as the sole source of dietary protein and fat for rapidly growing young children. *Pediatrics* 85: 85–91.

Great Britain. Inter-departmental Committee on Physical Deterioration. (1904). *Report of the Inter-Departmental Committee on Physical Deterioration*. London: Printed for H.M. Stationery Office.

Hambidge KM and Krebs NF (2007) Zinc deficiency: A special challenge. *J Nutr* 137: 1101–1105.

Hegsted DM (2001) Fractures, calcium, and the modern diet. *Am J Clin Nutr* 74: 571–573.

Hegsted DM (1972). Deprivation syndrome or protein-calorie malnutrition. *Nutr Rev* 30: 51–54.

Heinig MJ, Nommsen LA, Peerson JM et al. (1993) Energy and protein intakes of breast-fed and formula-fed infants during the first year of life and their association with growth velocity: The DARLING Study. *Am J Clin Nutr* 58: 152–161.

Hojyo S, Fukada T, Shimoda et al. (2011) The zinc transporter SLC39A14/ZIP14 controls G-protein coupled receptor-mediated signaling required for systemic growth. *PLOS ONE* 6: e18059.

Hoppe C, Mølgaard C, and Michaelsen KF (2006) Cow's milk and linear growth in industrialized and developing countries. *Annu Rev Nutr* 26: 131–173.

Hoppe C, Molgaard C, Thomsen BL. et al. (2004) Protein intake at 9 mo of age is associated with body size but not with body fat in 10-y-old Danish children. *Am J Clin Nutr* 79: 494–501.

Hoppe C, Udam TR, Lauritzen L et al. (2004a) Animal protein intake, serum insulin-like growth factor I, and growth in healthy 2.5-y-old Danish children. *Am J Clin Nutr* 80: 447–452.

Hoppe C, Mølgaard C, Juul A et al. (2004b) High intakes of skimmed milk, but not meat, increase serum IGF-I and IGFBP-3 in eight-year-old boys. *Eur J Clin Nutr* 58: 1211–1216.

Hoppe C, Mølgaard C, Vaag A et al. (2005) High intakes of milk, but not meat, increases s-insulin and insulin resistance in 8-year-old boys. *Eur J Clin Nutr* 59: 393–398.

Hörnell A, Lagström H, Lande B et al. (2013) Protein intake from 0 to 18 years of age and its relation to health: A systematic literature review for the 5th Nordic Nutrition Recommendations. *Food Nutr Res 57.* doi:10.3402/fnr.v57i0.21083.

Humphrey JH (2009) Child undernutrition, tropical enteropathy, toilets, and handwashing. *Lancet* 374: 1032–1035.

Ishikawa Y, Chin JE, Schalk EM et al. (1986) Effect of amino acid levels on matrix vesicle formation by epiphyseal growth plate chondrocytes in primary culture. *J Cell Physiol* 126: 399–406.

Jepson MM, Bates PC, and Millward DJ (1988) The role of insulin and thyroid hormones in the regulation of muscle growth and protein turnover in response to dietary protein. *Brit J Nutr* 59: 397–415.

Jepson MM, Pell J, Bates PC et al. (1986) The effects of endotoxaemia on protein metabolism in skeletal muscle and liver of fed and fasted rats. *Biochem J* 235: 329–336.

Karlberg J (1989) A biologically-oriented mathematical model (ICP) for human growth. *Acta Paediatr Scand Suppl* 350: 70–94.

Keusch GT, Rosenberg IH, Denno DM et al. (2013) Implications of acquired environmentalenteric dysfunction for growth and stunting in infants and children living in low- and middle-income countries. *Food Nutr Bull* 34: 357–364.

Kiepe D, Ciarmatori S, Hoeflich A et al. (2005) Insulin-like growth factor (IGF)-I stimulates cell proliferation and induces IGF binding protein (IGFBP)- 3 and IGFBP-5 gene expression in cultured growth plate chondrocytes via distinct signaling pathways. *Endocrinology* 146: 3096–3104.

Kim J-H, Jeon J, Shin M et al (2014) Regulation of the catabolic c-ascade in osteoarthritis by the zinc-ZIP8-MTF1 axis. *Cell* 156: 730–743.

Korpe PS and Petri WA Jr. (2012) Environmental enteropathy: Critical implications of a poorly understood condition. *Trends Mol Med* 18: 328–336.

Kotloff KL, Nataro JP, Blackwelder WC et al. (2013) Burden and aetiology of diarrhoeal disease in infants and young children in developing countries (the Global Enteric Multicenter Study, GEMS): A prospective, case-control study. *Lancet* 382: 209–222.

Krebs NF, Mazariegos M, Chomba E et al. (2012) Randomized controlled trial of meat compared with multimicronutrient-fortified cereal in infants and toddlers with high stunting rates in diverse settings. *Am J Clin Nutr* 96: 840–847.

Kronenberg HM (2003) Developmental regulation of the growth plate. *Nature* 423: 332–336.

Lampl M, Johnston FE, and Malcolm LA (1978) The effects of protein supplementation on the growth and skeletal maturation of New Guinean school children. *Ann Human Biol* 5: 219–227.

Long F and Ornitz DM (2013) Development of the endochondral skeleton. *Cold Spring Harb Perspect Biol* 5: a008334.

Lui JC and Baron J (2011). Mechanisms limiting body growth in mammals. *Endocrine Rev* 32: 422–440.

Lui JC, Nilsson O, and Baron J (2014) Recent insights into the regulation of the growth plate. *J Mol Endocrinol* 53: T1–T9.

Lunn PG, Northrop-Clewes CA, and Downes RM (1991) Intestinal permeability, mucosal injury, and growth faltering in Gambian infants. *Lancet* 338: 907–910.

MacDonald RS (2000) The role of zinc in growth and cell proliferation. *J Nutr* 130: 1500S–1508S.

MacDonald RS, Wollard-Biddle LC, Browning JD et al (1998) Zinc deprivation of murine 3T3 cells by use of diethylenetrinitrilopentaacetate impairs DNA synthesis upon stimulation with insulin-like growth factor-I (IGF-I). *J Nutr* 128: 1600–1605.

Malcolm LA (1970a) Growth retardation in a New Guinea boarding school and its response to supplementary feeding. *Brit J Nutr* 24: 297–305.

Malcolm LA (1970b) *Growth and Development in New Guinea. A Study of the Bundi People of the Madang District. Monograph Series No. 1.* Madang: Institute of Human Biology.

Martorell R and Klein RE (1980) Food supplement and growth rates in preschool children. *Nutr Rep Int* 21: 447–454.

Melnik BC, Malte S, and Schmitz G (2013) Milk is not just food but most likely a genetic transfection system activating mTORC1 signaling for postnatal growth. *Nutr J* 12:103.

Michaëlsson K, Wolk A, Langenskiöld S et al. (2014) Milk intake and risk of mortality and fractures in women and men: Cohort studies. *BMJ* 349: g6015.

Millward DJ and Rivers JPW (1989) The need for indispensable amino acids: The concept of the anabolic drive. *Diabet Metab Rev* 5: 191–212.

Millward DJ (2012) Knowledge gained from studies of leucine consumption in animals and humans. *J Nutr* 142: 2212S–2219S.

Millward DJ (1995) A protein-stat mechanism for the regulation of growth and maintenance of the lean-body mass. *Nutr Res Rev* 8: 93–120.

Millward DJ and Rivers J (1988) The nutritional role of indispensible amino acids and the metabolic basis for their requirements. *Eur J Clin Nutr* 42: 367–393.

Nabarro D, Howard P, Cassels C et al. (1988) The importance of infections and environmental factors as possible determinants of growth retardation in children. In: *Linear Growth Retardation in Less Developed Countries*, Ed. JC Waterlow, pp. 165–184. Vevey: Nestlé Nutrition/New York, NY: Raven Press.

Neumann CG, Bwibo NO, Murphy SP et al. (2003) Animal source foods improve dietary quality, micronutrient status, growth and cognitive function in Kenyan school children: Background, study design and baseline findings. *J Nutr* 133:3941S–3949S.

Neumann CG, Murphy SP, Gewa C et al. (2007) Meat supplementation improves growth, cognitive, and behavioral outcomes in Kenyan children. *J Nutr* 137: 1119–1123.

Neumann CG, Harris DM, and Rogers LM (2002) Contribution of animal source foods in improving diet quality and function in children in the developing world. *Nutr Res* 22: 193–220.

Nilsson O, Marino R, De Luca F et al. (2005) Endocrine regulation of the growth plate. *Horm Res* 64: 157–165.

Nilupa S. Gunaratna H. and De Groote P et al. (2010) A meta-analysis of community-based studies on quality protein maize. *Food Policy* 35: 202–210.

O'Connell JM, Dibley MJ, Sierra J et al. (1989) Growth of vegetarian children: The farm study. *Pediatrics* 84: 475–481.

Odedra BR and Millward DJ (1982) Effect of corticosterone treatment on muscle protein turnover in adrenalectomised rats and diabetic rats maintained on insulin. *Biochem J* 204: 663–672.

Omwega AM, Bates PC, and Millward DJ (1988) Vitamin E deficiency in the rat and the response to malarial infection. *Proc Nutr Soc* 47: 12A.

Pharoah POD, Buttfield IH, and Hetzel BS (1971) Neurological damage to the fetus resulting from severe iodine deficiency during pregnancy. *Lancet* 297: 308–310.

Pollock JI (2006). Two controlled trials of supplementary feeding of British school children in the 1920s. *J R Soc Med* 99: 323–327.

Prasad AS (1995) Zinc: An overview. *Nutrition* 11(1 Suppl): 93–99.

Prendergast AJ and Humphrey JH (2014) The stunting syndrome in developing countries. *Paed Int Child Health* 34: 250–265.

Prendergast AJ, Rukobo S, Chasekwa B et al. (2014) Stunting is characterized by chronic inflammation in zimbabwean infants. *PLOS ONE* 9: e86928.

Räihä NC, Fazzolari-Nesci A, Cajozzo C et al. (2002) Whey predominant, whey modified infant formula with protein/energy ratio of 1.8 g/100 kcal: Adequate and safe for term infants from birth to four months. *J Ped Gastroenterol Nutr* 35: 275–281.

Ramakrishnan U, Nguyen P, and Martorell R (2009) Effects of micronutrients on growth of children under 5 y of age:meta-analyses of single and multiple nutrient interventions. *Am J Clin Nutr* 89: 191–203.

Romero IG, Mallick CB, Liebert A et al. (2012) Herders of Indian and European cattle share their predominant allele for lactase persistence. *Mol Biol Evol* 29: 249–260.

Rossi L, Migliaccio S, Corsi A et al. (2001) Reduced growth and skeletal changes in zinc-deficient growing rats are due to impaired growth plate activity and inanition. *J Nutr* 131: 1142–1146.

Ruel MT (2003) Milk intake is associated with better growth in Latin America: Evidence from the Demographic and Health Surveys. *FASEB J* 17: A1199.

Rutishauser IHE and Whitehead RG (1969) Nutritional status assessed by biological tests. *Br J Nutr* 23: 1–13.

Sederquist B, Fernandez-Vojvodich P, Zaman F et al. (2014) Impact of inflammatory cytokines on longitudinal bone growth. *J Mol Endoc* 53: T35–T44.

Segall JJ (2008). Hypothesis: Is lactose a dietary risk factor for ischaemic heart disease? *Int J Epidemiol* 37: 1204–1208.

Solomons NW, Mazariegos M, Brown KH et al. (1993) The underprivileged, developing country child: Environmental contamination and growth failure revisited. *Nutr Rev* 51: 327–332.

Takahashi E (1971) Geographic distribution of human stature and environmental factors—An ecologic study. *J Anthropol Soc Nippon* 76: 259–285.

Takahashi E (1984) Secular trend in milk consumption and growth in Japan. *Hum Biol* 56: 427–437.

Tanner JM (1992) Growth as a measure of the nutritional and hygienic status of a population. *Horm Res* 38 (Suppl. 1): 106–115.

Tanner JM (1979) A concise history of growth studies from Buffon to Boas. In: *Human Growth: A Comprehensive Treatise*, vol. 3, Neurobiology and Nutrition, Eds. F Faulkner and JM Tanner, pp. 515–593. New York, NY: Plenum Press.

Tirapegui JO, Yayha ZAH, Bates PC et al. (1994) Dietary energy, glucocorticoids, and the regulation of long bone and muscle growth in the rat. *Clin Sci* 87: 599–606.

UNICEF, WHO, World Bank (2012) Levels and Trends in Child Malnutrition. *Joint Child Malnutrition Estimates*. New York, NY: United Nations International Children's Fund; Geneva: WHO; Washington, DC: World Bank, Available from: http://www.who.int/nutgrowthdb/jme_2012_summary_note_v2.pdf

United Nations System Standing Committee on Nutrition (2011) 6th Report on the World Nutrition Situation: Progress in Nutrition. United Nations Standing Committee on Nutrition, Geneva, Switzerland.

Van Dusseldorp M, Arts ICW, Bergsma JS et al. (1996) Catch-up growth in children fed a macrobiotic diet in early childhood. *J Nutr* 126: 2977–2983.

Waterlow JC (2006) *Protein Energy Malnutrition*. London: Smith–Gordon.

Wessells KR and Brown KH (2012) Estimating the global prevalence of zinc deficiency: Results based on zinc availability in national food supplies and the prevalence of stunting. *PLOS ONE* 7: e50568.

WHO (2006) Multicentre Growth Reference Study Group. *WHO Child Growth Standards: Length/Height-for-Age, Weight-for-Age, Weight-for-Length, Weight-for-Height and Body Mass Index-for-Age: Methods and Development*. Geneva: WHO, Available from: http://www.who.int/childgrowth/publications/technical_report_pub/en/index.html

Wiley AS (2005). Does milk make children grow? Relationships between milk consumption and height in NHANES 1999–2002. *Am J Hum Biol* 17: 425–441.

Williams RB and Mills CF (1970) The experimental production of zinc deficiency in the rat. *Br J Nutr* 24: 989–1003.

Wit JM and Camacho-Hübner C (2011) Endocrine regulation of longitudinal bone growth In: *Cartilage and Bone Development and Its Disorders, Eds. C Camacho-Hübner, O Nilsson, L Savendahl, vol. 21, pp. 30-41*. Basel: Karger

World Health Organization/Food and Agriculture Organization/United Nations University (2007a) Protein and Amino Acid Requirements in Human Nutrition Report of a Joint WHO/FAO/UNU Expert Consultation. *WHO Technical Report Series no. 935*. WHO, Geneva, Switzerland.

World Health Organization, United Nations Children's Fund, International Council for the Control of Iodine Deficiency Disorders (2007b) *Assessment of Iodine Deficiency Disorders and Monitoring their Elimination*. 3rd ed. Geneva: WHO.

Xian CJ (2014) Recent research on the growth plate: Regulation, bone growth defects, and potential treatments. *J Mol Endoc* 53: E1–E2.

Xie Y, Zhou S, Chen H et al. (2014) Advances in fibroblast growth factor signalling in growth plate development and disorders. *J Mol Endoc* 53: T11–T34.

Yahya ZAH. and Millward DJ (1994) Dietary protein and the regulation of long bone and muscle growth in the rat. *Clin Sci* 87: 213–224.

Yahya ZAH, Bates PC, and Millward DJ (1990) Responses to protein deficiency of plasma and tissue insulin-like growth factor-I levels and proteoglycan synthesis rates in rat skeletal muscle and bone. *J Endocr* 127: 497–503.

Yahya ZAH, Tirapegui JO, Bates PC et al. (1994) Influence of dietary protein, energy and corticosteroids on protein turnover, proteoglycan sulphation and growth of long bone and skeletal muscle in the rat. *Clin Sci* 87: 607–618.

Young VR, Ozalp I, Chalakos B et al. (1971) Protein value of Colombian opaque-2 corn for young adult men. *J Nutr* 101: 1475–1481.

Zhang F, He Q, Tsang WP et al. (2014) Insulin exerts direct, IGF-1 independent actions in growth plate chondrocytes. *Bone Res* 2: 14012.

Zhou SJ, Anderson AJ, Gibson RA et al. (2013) Effect of iodine supplementation in pregnancy on child development and other clinical outcomes: A systematic review of randomized controlled trials. *Am J Clin Nutr* 98: 1241–1254.

Zimmermann MB (2009) Iodine deficiency in pregnancy and the effects of maternal iodine supplementation on the offspring: A review. *Am J Clin Nutr* 89 (Suppl): 668S–672S.

Zimmermann MB (2012) The effects of iodine deficiency in pregnancy and infancy. *Paediatr Perinat Epidemiol* 26 (Suppl. 1): 108–117.

Zimmermann MB, Jooste PL, Mabapa NS et al. (2007) Treatment of iodine deficiency in school-age children increases insulin-like growth factor (IGF)-I and IGF binding protein-3 concentrations and improves somatic growth. *J Clin Endocrinol Metab* 92: 437–442.

7 Immunity in Anorexia Nervosa

Esther Nova and Ascensión Marcos

CONTENTS

7.1 Anorexia Nervosa—The Eating Disorder 111
7.2 Immune System Characteristics in Anorexia Nervosa.. 111
7.3 Lymphocyte Subsets: Preserved or Compromised?.. 112
7.4 Why Do Anorexia Nervosa Patients Seem Refractory to Infections?................................. 113
7.5 Adipocytokine Involvement in Eating Disorders Etiology and Adaptation Mechanisms..... 114
    7.5.1 Role of Cytokines... 114
    7.5.2 Role of Adipokines... 117
7.6 Are There Immunological Markers to Follow Up Disease Progress toward Recovery or
    Relapse?... 118
7.7 Involvement of Perinatal Immune Factors in Disease Etiology.. 119
7.8 Conclusions... 120
References.. 120

7.1 ANOREXIA NERVOSA—THE EATING DISORDER

Anorexia nervosa (AN) and bulimia nervosa (BN) are clear examples of malnutrition in developed countries, with a prevalence that approaches 2% for young females in western societies (Hoek and van Hoeken, 2003). These two eating disorders (ED) are very much related regarding psychopathological traits. In addition, clinical features in patients may change over time, often switching from anorexia to bulimia, making diagnosis difficult (Fairburn and Harrison, 2003). AN is a serious psychiatric syndrome characterized by a restriction of energy intake relative to requirements and an intense fear of fatness. This leads to a significantly low body weight, which is usually accompanied by a disturbance in the way that weight status is experienced. Some patients with AN exhibit binge/ purging behaviors; however, these are diagnostic characteristics of BN when both episodes of binge eating and compensatory mechanisms (physical exercise, vomiting, or abuse of laxatives and/or diuretics) occur at least once per week for more than 3 months (APA, 2013). As a result, the weight of patients with BN presents in a large range from low to excessive but is usually normal in contrast with the extremely slim or emaciated AN patient. Eating behavior in these syndromes is deeply influenced by aesthetic patterns, and an undue influence of body weight and shape on self-evaluation is common to AN and BN. Eating behavior dominates the life of such patients to the point that severe situations of malnutrition develop over time and notable mortality rates are associated with these eating disorders, particularly with AN (Arcelus et al., 2011; Marcos, 2000).

7.2 IMMUNE SYSTEM CHARACTERISTICS IN ANOREXIA NERVOSA

Semistarvation, overeating, purges—all these behaviors that can be part of the presentation signs of AN/BN lead the patient to particular situations of malnutrition, which may or may not be evidenced by their weight and body composition. The impact of this nontypical malnutrition on the immune system has received little attention, and the scientific literature that has been published has not always offered consistent findings. There seems to be consensus accepting that, overall, immunocompromised state of patients with ED is less severe than in the classical protein-energy malnutrition (Silber and Chan, 1996). Frequent findings described in AN are leukopenia with relative lymphocytosis, thrombocytopenia, and a decreased delayed hypersensitivity skin test (DHST) response (Cason et al., 1986; Varela et al., 1988; Marcos et al., 1993a; Devuyst et al., 1993). These findings are not as frequent in BN, and only when the disease in not diagnosed early enough is a decrease in neutrophil or monocyte counts potentially observed, as well as relative lymphocytosis. Nevertheless, blood lymphocyte counts are lower in patients with AN or BN than in controls. This suggests that factors other than weight loss might have a role in the immune system adaptations occurring in eating disorders (Marcos et al., 1997a). Moreover, in anorexic patients in a low-weight stage, a decrease in bone marrow cellularity and the appearance of an acidic mucopolysaccharide substance are also frequently found (Van de Berg et al., 1994).

When analyzing immune parameters it is necessary to bear in mind the complex interactions and reciprocal control among the immune system, the endocrine system, and the central nervous system (Marcos, 2000). The association of psychological and neuroendocrine changes in patients with AN has led investigators to speculate that abnormalities of neurotransmission may be involved in the pathogenesis of the syndrome. Epinephrine and norepinephrine, beta-endorphin, and gut peptides may have a mediating role in the abnormalities in eating behaviors observed in AN and BN (Warren and Locke, 2008). On the other hand, malnutrition may impact the communication between the immune, endocrine, and nervous systems, and thus perpetuate pathologic eating behaviors and be responsible for several comorbid psychiatric symptoms including stress, anxiety, and depression (Brambilla et al., 1996), which are usually associated with immunological alterations. The primary and secondary roles of the neurochemical alterations remain to be established.

7.3   LYMPHOCYTE SUBSETS: PRESERVED OR COMPROMISED?

In eating disorders, as in more classical forms of malnutrition, cell-mediated immunity is generally affected while humoral immunity is fairly well preserved (Marcos, 2000). Despite this general presumption, the studies published in the literature regarding lymphocyte subsets, and especially T lymphocytes, are inconsistent. The disparity of findings might arise from subject variability among studies and even within studies. Lack of stringency in recruitment criteria in terms of age and duration of the disease (Mustafa et al., 1997), nutritional status (mixing patients recently diagnosed with refed patients) (Allende et al., 1998), or subtype of AN (restricting type mixed with binge-purging type) (Fink et al., 1996) results in much heterogeneity in the subjects studied and can account for the variable results reported. Nevertheless, a reduction in both percentage and absolute number of CD8+ T-cells in patients with AN has been described by several authors (Fink et al., 1996; Mustafa et al., 1997; Nagata et al., 1999a), which has been attributed to the CD45RO+RA-CD8+ (memory) T-cell population (Mustafa et al., 1997). This is in contrast with Allende et al. (1998) who found a reduction in naïve T helper cells (CD4+CD45RA+) together with an increase of CD8+ cells. However, these last results refer to percentage values of total lymphocytes and absolute numbers were not given. In addition, high variability in disease duration at time of study might be an issue. However, a different study also found increased percentage and number of CD8+ cells in AN patients (Marcos et al., 1993a). Regarding helper T-cells (CD4+), some consistency has been found for a trend to increase the percentage, perhaps in an attempt to preserve absolute numbers of CD4+ cells (Nagata et al., 1999a; Mustafa et al., 1997). However, it is not clear how such a compensatory mechanism might work in relation to the degree of malnutrition. In the study of Mustafa et al. (1997) it seems to be successful only after refeeding, while CD4+ numbers are found below control values in the malnourished state. Nagata et al. (1999a) found CD4+ counts to be slightly but not significantly decreased compared to controls. The increased proportion of CD4+ cells as total lymphocytes decrease has been observed in Japanese women with AN (Saito et al., 2007). Although the authors argue that this is an attempt to counteract the effects of malnutrition, they observe that the adaptation does not avoid that patients with severe malnutrition (serum zinc < 40 µg/dL) present critically low CD4+ counts of less than 200 cells/µL. A recent study investigated lymphocyte subsets in patients with three different diagnosis of ED: the restricting type of AN (AN-R), the binge/purging type (AN-BP), and patients with Feeding or eating disorders not elsewhere classified (FED-NEC). All of them were suffering their first episode of the ED. There was a relative lymphocytosis with significantly increased CD4$^+$ percentage but no differences in CD4$^+$ cell numbers versus the control group in all three ED groups (Elegido et al., 2017). There was also decreased memory CD8$^+$ percentage and counts in all three groups although the AN-BP group showed the lowest values. An increased percentage of CD4$^+$ cells and decreased CD8$^+$ counts were also found by Nagata et al. (1999a) in six patients with AN-BP compared to controls and a similar nonsignificant trend in seven patients with AN-R. Thus, the findings seem to be similar in AN-R and AN-BP, although the acquisition of binge-compensatory habits is probably working as a strain on the already stressed body. Regarding the diminished number of memory CD8$^+$ cells, a decrease in the capacity of dendritic cells to expand memory T-cell clones might be an explanation, according to the results that have also been observed in animal models of starvation (Abe et al., 2003).

In a one-year follow-up study carried out in 16 restricting-type AN patients (age range 12–19 years) on recent admission for hospital treatment, all T lymphocyte subsets (CD2$^+$, CD3$^+$, CD4$^+$, and CD8$^+$) and also NK cells (CD57$^+$) were significantly lower than in the control group (Marcos et al., 1997b). B lymphocytes, on the contrary, were similar in both groups. After inpatient treatment (mean duration of 2 months), all lymphocyte subsets were significantly increased and were no longer different from controls; however, a progressive decrease was observed at subsequent measures after discharge (outpatient treatment period), which suggests that lymphocyte subsets might have an early response to changes in eating behavior after partial nutritional recovery. It is generally agreed that risk of relapse is high during the first year after patients are discharged from hospital. This might be related with a resumption of restrictive behaviors when the anthropometrical recovery interferes with the acceptance of self-body image (Nova et al., 2001).

The CD4$^+$/CD8$^+$ ratio, which is known to decrease in PEM, is usually found unaffected in AN, although occasionally there have been reports of both decreased (Marcos et al., 1993a) and increased values (Nagata et al., 1999a) with respect to the control group.

Regarding cell-mediated immune function evaluated by the DHST, a poor response (number of positive responses and sum of their diameters) was very frequent in the patients during the one-year follow-up mentioned above, in comparison to controls (Marcos et al., 1997b). Conversely, the effect on the mitogen-stimulated lymphoproliferation response remains uncertain, since it has been reported both unaffected (Golla et al., 1981; Brambilla et al., 1996; Nagata et al., 1999b) and impaired (Cason et al., 1986; Polack et al., 1993) in AN patients. Overall, the evidence suggests that, similar to other starvation states, even in animal models (Freitag et al., 2000), immunocompetence and particularly T-cell subsets are a useful tool to follow up the nutritional status in patients with ED. This applies also to BN patients, since T-cell subsets seem to reflect their state of malnutrition, which is not evidenced by weight measures. Patients with long duration of the disease have a more serious distortion of the lymphocyte subset profile, and the CD4$^+$/CD8$^+$ ratio is decreased as a result of diminished CD4$^+$ cell counts (Marcos et al., 1993b). Vomiting as a purging strategy is associated with a more deleterious effect on T-cells, as evidenced by the comparatively lower values of CD2$^+$, CD3$^+$, CD4$^+$, and CD8$^+$ cells in vomiting versus nonvomiting BN patients. Only the vomiting group showed significantly lower values than the control group for the mentioned T-cell subsets (Marcos et al., 1997a).

7.4   WHY DO ANOREXIA NERVOSA PATIENTS SEEM REFRACTORY TO INFECTIONS?

Typically, malnourished subjects suffer from an increased risk of infections; however, this is not the case for ED patients. They seem to be surprisingly free from infectious complications despite their undernourished state, at least until the late stages of debilitation (Dally, 1969; Bowers and Eckert, 1978; Wade et al., 1985). From our experience, despite the patients being admitted to the hospital for long periods, they seem to be protected against nosocomial infections and in general against any common viral infections (Marcos, 2000; Nova et al., 2002b). There is, so far, no clear answer for this observation, but it could result from the adaptation mechanisms of the immune system to the particular eating pattern of AN patients. This is characterized by a large reduction of energy intake but the food choice practiced by anorexic patients grants them a diet with relatively well-preserved protein and vitamin intakes. This seems to be true at least until the very advanced stages of the disease (Marcos, 1997). These findings are in contrast with the nutrient deficiencies common in typical malnutrition. In ED, several authors have found that the relative protein contribution to energy intake is increased versus a control group and allows for physiological compensation despite the overall food deprivation (Beaumont et al., 1981; Fernstrom et al., 1994). According to Beaumont et al. (1981) a mean intake of 701 kcal/d corresponds to the stage of disease onset and is found reduced to a mean of 296 kcal/d at an advanced stage. Rock and Yager (1987) have reported mean intakes in patients with AN before treatment in the range of 600–900 kcal/d. Thus, as the illness advances and these critical levels of restriction are achieved, the probability increases that some nutrient requirements, even protein, are not conveniently met through diet (Schebendach and Nussbaum, 1992). On the other hand, it has been speculated that the marked reduction in the percentage and absolute number of memory CD8$^+$ T-cells found in AN patients could lead to a reduced frequency of lymphocytes capable of recall responses, and thus to a reduced intensity of antiviral responses; it is argued that the symptoms of common viral infections might be absent to some extent in underweight anorexic patients (Mustafa et al., 1997). In fact, immune processes seem to return to normal after refeeding and weight recovery (Hart, 1990). However, there is still no evidence establishing a cause-and-effect relationship between the pattern of eating behavior of these patients and lymphocyte subset changes. It is difficult to analyze it with independence of other factors that affect patients with ED such as the neuroendocrine-immune interactions. However, various studies in calorie or dietary restriction animal models have shown a preservation of naive T-cells over the memory T-cell subsets (Messaoudi et al., 2006; Jolly, 2004) with benefits such as delayed aging and delayed onset of autoimmune disease.

Not only T-cells, but also innate immunity might be involved in the absence of symptoms of infection (fever, etc.). In particular, a suppressed capacity to mount the stereotypical acute phase response during the first steps of defense against pathogen infection has been suggested. In this respect, a reduced febrile response to bacterial infection has been described in four AN patients (Birmingham et al., 2003), and this has been related to the impaired cytokine profiles that are exhibited by patients with ED, both *in vivo* and *in vitro*.

A fourth hypothesis has also been considered regarding the possibility that starvation might reduce the number of T regulatory cells (Tregs) in AN patients and this led in turn to an enhanced T-cell effector function abolishing the usual effects of malnutrition on the immune defense system. Although this hypothesis aimed to explain why AN patients do not suffer more infections as opposed to other types of malnourished patients, this was not supported by experimental data since no relevant changes were found in the number of Tregs, nor in dendritic cells, in AN patients compared to controls (Pászthy et al., 2007a).

7.5 ADIPOCYTOKINE INVOLVEMENT IN ED ETIOLOGY AND ADAPTATION MECHANISMS

7.5.1 ROLE OF CYTOKINES

Cytokines are soluble proteins secreted mainly by immune cells that act as signaling molecules in the intercellular communications among the cells of the immune system. Many other cell types also have receptors for cytokines, which is evidence for their involvement in the regulation of multiple metabolic and neuroendocrine pathways.

Pro-inflammatory cytokines such as TNF-α, IL-1, and IL-6 are involved in the initiation of the acute-phase reaction, which is stereotypical and includes fever, loss of appetite, decreased food intake, cellular hypermetabolism, and multiple endocrine and enzyme responses (Grimble, 1994). These cytokines are capable of activating the hypothalamic-pituitary-adrenal axis (HPAA) and have a direct stimulatory effect on ACTH secretion. In turn, glucocorticoids alter the production of these cytokines in a feedback regulation. These cytokines may be fundamental regulators of body metabolism in AN and BN (Holden and Pakula, 1996; Emeric-Sauval et al., 1989). Elevated plasma levels of pro-inflammatory cytokines (IL-1, IL-6, and TNF-α) have been reported in some studies (Allende et al., 1998; Emeric-Sauval et al., 1989; Pomeroy et al., 1994; Nakai et al., 1999). Another study found activation of the TNF-α axis in AN patients, with elevated TNF-α and TNF-α receptor levels in blood. The latter were negatively correlated with BMI and positively with disease duration (Agnello et al., 2012). The authors suggest that pro-inflammatory cytokines could have a role in the evolution of eating disorders. However, since this is a study with high variability in patients' age and duration of disease, it would be worthwhile to try to discern the precise role of pro-inflammatory cytokines at disease onset and during the first episode as compared to their role in chronic patients. More so because there is no full consistency among studies and many have found no alteration in cytokine levels in comparison with healthy adolescents (Vaisman et al., 1996; Brambilla et al., 1998, 2001; Monteleone et al., 1999; Nagata et al., 1999b; Corcos et al., 2001).

An elevated spontaneous production of pro-inflammatory cytokines (IL-1, IL-6, and TNF-α) has also been observed when peripheral blood mononuclear cells (PBMCs) from patients with AN have been cultured *in vitro* (Allende et al., 1998; Schattner et al., 1990a; Limone et al., 2000). This basally high level of pro-inflammatory cytokine production has been suggested to be linked to a deficient response to an extra stimulus, which might explain the impaired capacity to mount an acute-phase response to an infection (Figure 7.1). In support of this hypothesis, we have found a decreased PHA-stimulated TNF-α and IL-6 production by PBMCs from a group of AN patients admitted to hospital for refeeding, in comparison with matched controls (Nova et al., 2002a). This blunted cytokine response to mitogen stimulation might be the consequence of an alteration in the regulatory pathways between pro-inflammatory cytokines and cortisol. Cortisol, the stress response hormone, has been found to be elevated in serum of AN patients and a positive correlation with the *in vitro* secretion of IL-1β by PBMCs has also been reported (Limone et al., 2000), which suggests that the negative feedback by cortisol on this cytokine synthesis is deranged in AN patients. On the other hand, it is not known if the maintenance of high cortisol levels could result, *in vivo*, in an impaired IL-1β production in response to an infection (Nova et al., 2002a) (Figure 7.1). In this case, a blunted cytokine (IL-1) response to bacterial challenge might be linked to an impaired febrile response (Yirmiya et al., 1998), and the absence of infection symptoms in patients with ED. Despite

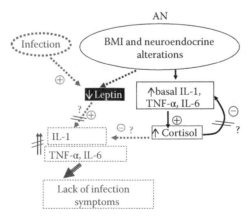

FIGURE 7.1 Pro-inflammatory cytokines and their relationships with cortisol and leptin alterations in anorexia nervosa: hypothetical implications during infection. (Reproduced from Marcos A, Nova E, Lopez-Varela S. In R. Fuller, G. Perdigon [eds.], *Gut Flora, Nutrition, Immunity and Health*, Oxford, Blackwell Publishing, 2003.)

this discussion, the importance of cytokine involvement in the pathogenesis of ED is difficult to establish since many different results have been described. There is an extensive review on this topic by Corcos et al. (2003). One aspect worth mentioning refers to cytokines produced by Th-1 (T helper 1) cells. It has been reported that the *in vitro* IL-2 production (Allende et al., 1998; Bessler et al., 1993) and serum levels (Corcos et al., 2001; Licinio et al., 1990) are lower in anorexics than in healthy controls. Also the percentage of IL-2-producing CD4⁺ cells after activation was found decreased in AN patients together with delayed maximal intracellular calcium levels compared to controls (Pászthy et al., 2007b). There may be several explanations for this depressed Th-1-like activity. In the first place, circulating levels of IL-2 correlate with white blood cells, which are lower than in controls (Licinio et al., 1991), but also, the capacity to produce Th-1 type cytokines might be suppressed by glucocorticoids, which are known to be increased in these conditions, as already mentioned, and finally, the reduced IL-2 production could be due to the reduction of CD4⁺ T-cells (Allende et al., 1998; Savendhal and Underwood, 1997).

Cytokines have been related not only to immune function but also to the neuroendocrine abnormalities in eating disorders. An interesting question posed by Corcos et al. (2003) is whether cytokines from the central or from the peripheral compartment alter neurotransmission in the brain. Whatever the source, the increase in IL-1β in the central nervous system would be associated with an increase in catecholamines (Shintani et al., 1993; Smagin et al., 1996) and an inhibition of neuropeptide-Y production in the hypothalamus (McCarthy et al., 1995; Reyes and Sawchenko, 2000; Konsman et al., 2001) that would induce anorexia. Pro-inflammatory cytokines also interact with proopiomelanocortin (POMC) derived peptides such as β-endorphins, which are involved in eating behavior.

Although an etiologic role has been considered for cytokine deregulation in ED, it might be only secondary to other alterations such as the impaired nutritional status or associated psychopathology, including stress, anxiety, or depression. Many of the studies found that refeeding normalizes cytokine levels when compared to the control group (Pomeroy et al., 1994; Vaisman et al., 1996; Schattner et al., 1990a, b; Kahl et al., 2004; Vaisman and Hahn, 1991). According to Nagata et al. (1999b) the capacity of PBMCs to produce IL-1, IL-6, and TNF-α is recovered even with the start of refeeding, when patients reach only 65% of the standard body weight. This makes them suggest that this capacity depends on something else than the absolute weight gain, such as the start of refeeding, the neuroendocrine system, or the autonomic nervous system. However, this recovery in cytokine production with refeeding was not confirmed in another study, in which there was decreased *in vitro* production of IL-6 and TNF-α by PBMCs from restrictive AN patients both on admission to hospital and at discharge, with an 84% of their ideal body weight (Nova et al., 2002a). Since complex interactions occur between cytokines and the central nervous system, differences in the capacity of AN patients to evoke a compensatory mechanism through either the neuroendocrine system or the autonomic nervous system could explain the variability of the results found among different patients. Recently, the macrophage inhibitory cytokine (MIC-1) measured in a group of previously untreated AN patients was found inversely related to Buzby nutritional risk index, serum insulin-like growth factor-1, serum glucose, serum total protein, serum albumin, and lumbar bone mineral density, and did not normalize completely after 2 months of treatment (Dostálová et al., 2010).

It is worth noting that there can be methodological difficulty in the measurement of circulating plasma levels of some cytokines (i.e., IFN-γ, TNF-α, IL-2), which are often below the detection limit of the available enzyme-linked immunosorbent assays (ELISA). Moreover, some of the discrepant findings regarding cytokine levels measured in anorexic patients could be related to the methods used to measure them (ELISA, radioimmunoassay [RIA], bioassay). While bioassays specifically detect biologically active cytokines, immunoassays (ELISA, RIA) also measure inactive fragments (Corcos et al., 2003). Depending on the equilibrium as a function of synthesis, release, and catabolism, different methodologies might show different findings. Moreover a recent study that included only ten AN patients (subtype not specified) and ten controls found that culture conditions upon stimulation of PBMCs are significant modifiers of experimental results (Omodei et al., 2015).

Particularly, using autologous serum (AS) instead of heterologous serum (HS) to complement culture medium greatly changed the findings. IL-6 and TNF-α were higher in HS-cultured AN PBMCs than in controls. However, this secretion was abolished in AS-cultured PBMCs. The authors suggested that the high levels of adiponectin present in serum affect IL-6 and TNF-α secretion.

7.5.2 ROLE OF ADIPOKINES

Leptin is a protein encoded by the *ob* gene that is known to regulate appetite, weight, and energy expenditure. Leptin has been recognized as a longer-term adiposity signal, secreted in proportion to body fat stores. Therefore, it is not surprising that this hormone is usually positively correlated with BMI in obese, normal, and slim individuals and also in AN and BN patients (Monteleone et al., 2000). Low-serum leptin levels in AN patients compared to controls have been reported in numerous studies (Terra et al., 2013; Dostálová et al., 2007; Modan-Moses et al., 2007; Omodei et al., 2015; Janas-Kozik et al., 2011) and these increase after refeeding. Under physiological conditions, low leptin levels increase energy intake and decrease expenditure; however, this function seems to be deranged in AN patients. Leptin has also been suggested to function as a prominent regulator of immune system activity, linking the function of T lymphocytes to nutritional status. In starvation, the dramatic reduction in leptin seems to be a key mediator of thymic atrophy and immune suppression, involving for instance, an inhibitory effect on CD4$^+$ T lymphocyte activation (Matarese, 2000; Matarese et al., 2005). In addition, exogenous leptin has been reported to stimulate phagocytic function and activate macrophages to produce pro-inflammatory cytokines, such as TNF-α, IL-6, and IL-12, in *ob/ob* mice (Loffreda et al., 1998). Therefore, there is a function for leptin as an up-regulator of inflammatory immune responses. Moreover, leptin production is acutely increased during infection and inflammation (Fantuzzi, 2005). Thus, impairment in this acute increase in leptin production in AN patients might be related to the lack of infection symptoms (Nova et al., 2002b) (Figure 7.1). In BN patients, whose weight does not usually differ from age-matched controls, basal leptin concentrations are decreased as well (Monteleone et al., 2000). Therefore, factors other than body weight may play a role in leptin changes in ED. Another aspect to consider is the relationship between leptin and cortisol, because an alteration in their temporal coupling has been observed in the semistarvation state of AN (Herpertz et al., 2000).

Adiponectin and its role as a marker of nutritional status in AN has received special attention. Adiponectin is a hormone secreted by adipose tissue that enhances insulin sensitivity, controls body weight, prevents atherosclerosis, and negatively regulates hematopoiesis and immune functions, decreasing the production of pro-inflammatory cytokines (Diez and Iglesias, 2003; Yokota et al., 2000; Ouchi et al., 2011). The circulating level of adiponectin falls in obesity and insulin resistant states, but is increased in AN patients in comparison with a control group (Brichard et al., 2003; Pannacciulli et al., 2003; Omodei et al., 2015; Alberti et al., 2007). Total adiponectin and also high molecular weight adiponectin have both been found increased in AN (Terra et al., 2013). However, this increase has not always been consistent (Iwahashi et al., 2003; Tagami et al., 2004; Nogueira et al., 2013) or has been restricted to the binge-purge subtype of the AN patients studied (Nogueira et al., 2010). The physiological state at the time of analysis, whether this is at a moment of steady restriction, acute restriction, recent renourishment treatment, stabilized target weight, etc., might influence the findings. In this sense, several authors have observed an increase during the initial phase of weight restoration under refeeding treatment and a decrease associated to subsequent weight gain after a critical threshold of fat mass has been reached (Modan-Moses et al., 2007; Iwahashi et al., 2003). Adiponectin levels have been suggested to have an effect on immune cell responses through changes in cellular metabolism. Extracellular acidification rate and oxygen conversion rate were studied in PBMCs of AN patients as markers of the two major energy-producing pathways of cellular metabolism, glycolysis, and mitochondrial respiration, respectively. These analyses showed low levels of both processes compared to controls, which suggest that in AN, immune cells are metabolically less active. This situation is consistent with the enhancement of the antioxidant status found in these patients, as assessed by the expression of genes encoding antioxidant enzymes in PBMCs and in fibroblasts cultured with AN patient's sera (Omodei et al., 2015). In addition, AN serum protects fibroblasts from the cytotoxic effect of hydrogen peroxide. The authors suggest that further studies are required in order to elucidate whether the high plasma adiponectin levels in AN patients are responsible for the enhanced antioxidant status. It is also interesting to note that an association has been observed in outpatient anorexic subjects between adiponectin level and carbohydrate intake (Misra et al., 2006). Since these patients show a higher intake of carbohydrate and fiber than controls (Misra et al., 2006), an increased complex carbohydrate and antioxidant intake derived from fruit and vegetables might be a connection between adiponectin and the enhanced antioxidant status.

Finally, resistin is another fat-mass derived molecule with a role in insulin resistance and actions on immune cells. Resistin expression has been found in human monocytes and is increased by the action of pro-inflammatory cytokines (IL-1, IL-6, and TNF-α) (Patel et al., 2003). In anorexic patients, resistin levels have been found decreased (Ziora et al., 2011) or unchanged (Terra et al., 2013; Dolezalova et al., 2007) compared to control subjects. However, it seems that resistin levels are not as much associated to the inflammatory status as to insulin sensitivity, at least in the hyperactive subtypes of the disease (Nogueira et al., 2010).

Further studies are needed to examine the links between adipokine alterations and pro-inflammatory cytokine impairments in the particular case of ED patients. The studies are scarce and have a limited number of subjects. Nogueira et al. did not find associations between adipokines, IL-1β, and TNF-α (Nogueira et al., 2010), and in addition, the local perturbations in the expression of adipokine and cytokine genes found in subcutaneous adipose tissue of anorexic patients compared to controls seem not to be reflected in their circulating levels (Dolezalova et al., 2007).

7.6   ARE THERE IMMUNOLOGICAL MARKERS TO FOLLOW UP DISEASE PROGRESS TOWARD RECOVERY OR RELAPSE?

As the restrictive behavior of the AN patient progresses, metabolic adaptations seem to occur that counteract energy shortage and evade serious metabolic imbalances. Thus, abnormalities in blood biochemistry are rare during long periods of the evolution of the disease despite changes in neurochemical signaling and hormone levels. In these disorders, seeking medical assistance is sometimes delayed because negation of the disease by the patient is common and the family is not able to perceive the magnitude of the problem. Thus, a variable amount of time elapses until a correct diagnosis is made and adequate treatment implemented. In this situation, finding biomarkers that can discriminate between the different stages of the disease and also be associated to the probability to fully recover or the risk to suffer relapses would be very useful. In our experience, molecules that are involved simultaneously in functions related to weight and appetite control, energy balance, and immune functions, such as cytokines, adipokines, and other molecules that have a relationship with fat deposits might play this role. However, to date, there is not a clear biomarker that is already routinely used for monitoring of treatment progression and disease remission, which relies on BMI deviation from the ideal for patient's age and height (BMI Z-score) to follow up the patient's evolution. However, some molecules might show associations with BMI change at the end of treatment as shown in a recent study (Terra et al., 2013). This included 28 AN patients measured at week 3.2 ± 0.6 of their inpatient treatment. Both subtypes were included in the study and the disease duration was long (8.3 ± 1.4 y.). Ghrelin and the TNF-α receptor II (TNFRII) levels were associated negatively with BMI change at the end of treatment. No differences in ghrelin or TNFRII were observed compared to healthy women. The authors, thus, suggest that changes in adipocytokines could serve as weight restoration biomarkers. However, these results should be interpreted having in mind that the biomarker values are already under the effect of partial weight and fat mass recovery and the associations might not exist with the biomarker levels at the beginning of treatment.

Proteins of hepatic synthesis might also be good biomarkers for disease outcome. In this sense, we observed in a one-year follow-up study of restrictive AN girls entering hospital treatment that the complement factor C3 and transferrin were the best biomarkers among a set of 15 serum biomarkers including liver-synthesized hormones and minerals (Nova et al., 2004). C3 has shown an independent association with waist circumference in adolescents (Wärnberg et al., 2006) and has shown a correlation with transferrin in AN patients (Pomeroy et al., 1997). Both biomarkers decreased during the last 6 months of follow-up, when findings in anthropometric variables and diet assessment showed an increased risk of relapse in a subset of the patients studied (Nova et al., 2001, 2004). Transferrin, in particular, decreased in that period only in those patients who did not gain further weight or lost weight after discharge from hospital, and the change was significantly different from the change in the group of girls who gained weight (Nova et al., 2004). In addition, Flierl et al. (2011) found decreased C3 levels in AN patients with a BMI < 14 kg/m² compared to healthy subjects and a strong correlation with BMI; however, no differences in activation fragments or the 50% hemolytic complement activity (CH50) were observed, which suggests that complement function is preserved.

Another study performed in a homogenous group of short-duration restricting-type AN patients (n = 11) (Nogueira et al., 2013) provided interesting data from changes in growth hormone (GH) concentration during refeeding. The AN patients in remission (BMI > 17.5 kg/m²) 6 months after discharge showed a significantly greater decrease in GH between basal and discharge measurements and showed a significantly greater BMI increase compared to the AN nonremission group. In addition, in multiple regression analysis, the change in GH observed between admission and discharge (discharge-basal) was associated negatively with BMI measured 6 months after discharge. This factor together with the change in leptin and BMI in the hospitalization period explained 88% of BMI variability 6 months after discharge. The authors concluded that a low GH level at admission and the absence of its decrease after weight recovery could predict short-term relapse in women suffering from a restrictive form of AN.

7.7 INVOLVEMENT OF PERINATAL IMMUNE FACTORS IN DISEASE ETIOLOGY

Some epidemiological data in AN have been pointed out as suggesting a link to the hygiene hypothesis. These factors are the disease being more common in females than in males, peak incidence in teenage years and in the higher socioeconomic groups, and seasonal variation in birth. According to these authors' hypothesis, AN is an autoimmune disease caused by delayed exposure to common microorganisms in which autoantibodies to regulatory peptides and hypothalamic neurons, which cross-react with microbial antigens, disturb appetite, and lead to decreased intake of food. Since the hypothesis and preliminary evidence exist, and serum autoantibodies against regulatory peptides have also been pointed out as contributing to the etiology, a trial of pooled immunoglobulin therapy in patients with life-threatening AN has been proposed (Acres, Heath, and Morris, 2012).

Additionally, a hypothesis has been put forward linking AN and pathogenic microorganisms, suggesting that *in utero* viral infections might be an etiological factor of AN onset later in life. Peak exposure to chickenpox and rubella (ecological measures, not direct measures) was associated to a higher odds ratio to develop AN in an epidemiological study performed in the Padua region of Italy among the female population born between 1970 and 1984 in that area (Favaro et al., 2011). However, the authors suggest that it is necessary to confirm the results with serologically demonstrated maternal infections. The pathogenic mechanisms of the prenatal viral infection might include both neurodevelopmental interference for those viruses crossing the placenta and the high exposure of the brain to corticosteroids and cytokines during the maternal immunological response to infection.

7.8 CONCLUSIONS

EDs, including AN, are a challenge to the immune system, which has to face nutrient shortage and altered brain neurochemistry. Some immune parameters seem to be affected by the nutritional status, which is impaired through variable total weight and fat mass loss and depleted nutrient reservoirs. Thus, cells of the immune system (lymphocyte subsets) and soluble mediators (cytokines) show alterations compared to control subjects. However, it is still necessary to add new insights on the determinants of the changes observed. In order to gain that insight, it is relevant to perform studies that take into consideration disease duration (the time from onset to entering treatment) and the grade of psychopathological comorbidity, body dissatisfaction, and disordered eating. Delays in diagnosis and treatment will lead to more severe malnutrition and psychopathology, and hence, more severe disruption of the communication between the nervous, endocrine, and immune systems. The involvement of mediators such as cortisol, leptin, adiponectin, and cytokines, in the communication between these systems, seems to be relevant in AN. Researchers in this field should never lose sight of the complex interactions between nutrients and mediators/signaling molecules involved in the control of weight and appetite, mood and psychiatric comorbidities, and the homeostasis/active immune response mechanisms. New experimental tools should be used to advance understanding of these interactions in patients with AN in order to better understand the condition and its comorbidities and to design better therapeutic strategies. The precise impact of AN on immune responses, infection risk, and on inflammation-driven morbidities needs to be better defined. This needs to be done within the context of interactions of the immune system with the endocrine and neuroendocrine systems.

REFERENCES

Abe M, Akbar F, Matsuura B, Horiike N, Onji M. 2003. Defective antigen-presenting capacity of murine dendritic cells during starvation. *Nutrition* 19:265–9.

Acres MJ, Heath JJ, Morris JA. 2012. Anorexia nervosa, autoimmunity and the hygiene hypothesis. *Med Hypotheses* 78:772–5.

Agnello E, Malfi G, Costantino AM. 2012. Tumour necrosis factor alpha and oxidative stress as maintaining factors in the evolution of anorexia nervosa. *Eat Weight Disord* 17:e194–9.

Alberti L, Gilardini L, Girola A et al. 2007. Adiponectin receptors gene expression in lymphocytes of obese and anorexic patients. *Diabetes Obes Metab* 9:344–9.

Allende LM, Corell A, Manzanares J et al. 1998. Immunodeficiency associated with anorexia nervosa is secondary and improves after refeeding. *Immunology* 94:543–51.

American Psychiatric Association. 2013. *Diagnostic and Statistical Manual of Mental Disorders* (5th ed.). Washington, DC: American Psychiatric Association.

Arcelus J, Mitchell AJ, Wales J, Nielsen S. 2011. Mortality rates in patients with anorexia nervosa and other eating disorders. A meta-analysis of 36 studies. *Arch Gen Psychiatry* 68:724–31.

Beaumont PJV, Chambers TL, Rouse L, Abraham SF. 1981. The diet composition and nutritional knowledge of patients with anorexia nervosa. *J Hum Nutr* 35:265–73.

Bessler H, Karp L, Notti I et al. 1993. Cytokine production in anorexia nervosa. *Clin Neuropharmacol* 16:237–43.

Birmingham CL, Hodgson DM, Fung J et al. 2003. Reduced febrile response to bacterial infection in anorexia nervosa patients. *Int J Eat Disord* 34:269–72.

Bowers TK, Eckert E. 1978. Leukopenia in anorexia nervosa: Lack of risk of increased infection. *Arch Intern Med* 138:1520–3.

Brambilla F, Bellodi L, Brunetta M, Perna G. 1998. Plasma concentrations of interleukin-1 beta, interleukin-6 and tumor necrosis factor-alpha in anorexia and bulimia nervosa. *Psychoneuroendocrinology* 23:439–47.

Brambilla F, Ferrari E, Brunetta M et al. 1996. Immunoendocrine aspects of anorexia nervosa. *Psychiatry Res* 62:97–104.

Brambilla F, Monti D, Franceschi C. 2001. Plasma concentrations of interleukin-1-beta, interleukin 6 and tumor necrosis factor-alpha, and of their soluble receptors and receptor antagonist in anorexia nervosa. *Psychiatry Res* 103:107–14.

Brichard SM, Delporte ML, Lambert M. 2003. Adipocytokines in anorexia nervosa: A review focusing on leptin and adiponectin. *Horm Metab Res* 35:337–42.

Cason J, Ainley CC, Volstencroft RA, Norton KRW, Thompson RPH. 1986. Cell mediated immunity in anorexia nervosa. *Clin Exp Immunol* 64:370–5.

Corcos M, Guilbaud O, Chaouat G et al. 2001. Cytokines and anorexia nervosa. *Psychosom Med* 63:502–4.

Corcos M, Guilbaud O, Paterniti S et al. 2003. Involvement of cytokines in eating disorders: A critical review of the human literature. *Psychoneuroendocrinology* 28:229–49.

Dally P. 1969. *Anorexia Nervosa*. London, UK: William Heinemann Medical Books Ltd, pp. 30–46.

Devuyst O, Lambert M, Rodhain J, Lefebvre C, Coche E. 1993. Haematological changes and infectious complications in anorexia nervosa: A case-control study. *Q J Med* 86:791–9.

Diez JJ, Iglesias P. 2003. The role of the novel adipocyte-derived hormone adiponectin in human disease. *Eur J Endocrinol* 148:293–300.

Dolezalová R, Lacinova Z, Dolinkova M et al. 2007. Changes of endocrine function of adipose tissue in anorexia nervosa: Comparison of circulating levels versus subcutaneous mRNA expression. *Clin Endocrinol (Oxf)* 67:674–8.

Dostálová I, Kaválková P, Papezová H, Domluvilová D, Zikán V, Haluzík M. 2010. Association of macrophage inhibitory cytokine-1 with nutritional status, body composition and bone mineral density in patients with anorexia nervosa: The influence of partial realimentation. *Nutr Metab (Lond)* 23:34.

Dostálová I, Smitka K, Papezová H, Kvasničková H, Nedvídková J. 2007. Increased insulin sensitivity in patients with anorexia nervosa: The role of adipocytokines. *Physiol Res* 56(5):587–94.

Elegido A, Graell M, Andrés P, Gheorghe A, Marcos A, Nova E. 2017. Increased naïve CD4(+) and B lymphocyte subsets are associated with body mass loss and drive relative lymphocytosis in anorexia nervosa patients. *Nutr Res* 39:43–50.

Emeric-Sauval E, Polack E, Bello M et al. 1989. Anorexia nervosa y bulimia-un modelo para el estudio de las interaciones immunoneuroendocrinas en respecto al CRH humano. *Rev Argent Endocrinol Metab* 26:72–3.

Fairburn CG, Harrison PJ. 2003. Eating disorders. *Lancet* 361:407–16.

Fantuzzi G. 2005. Adipose tissue, adipokines and inflammation. *J Allergy Clin Immunol* 115:911–9.

Favaro A, Tenconi E, Ceschin L, Zanetti T, Bosello R, Santonastaso P. 2011. In utero exposure to virus infections and the risk of developing anorexia nervosa. *Psychol Med* 41:2193–9.

Fernstrom MH, Weltzin TE, Neuberger S, Srinivasagam N, Kaye WH. 1994. Twenty-four-hour food intake in patients with anorexia nervosa and in healthy control subjects. *Biol Psychiatry* 36:696–702.

Fink S, Eckert E, Mitchell J, Crosby R, Pomeroy C. 1996. T-lymphocyte subsets in patients with abnormal body weight: Longitudinal studies in anorexia nervosa and obesity. *Int J Eat Disord* 20:295–305.

Flierl MA, Gaudiani JL, Sabel AL, Long CS, Stahel PF, Mehler PS. 2011. Complement C3 serum levels in anorexia nervosa: A potential biomarker for the severity of disease? *Ann Gen Psychiatry* 10:16.

Freitag KA, Saker KE, Thomas E, Kalnitsky J. 2000. Acute starvation and subsequent refeeding affect lymphocyte subsets and proliferation in cats. *J Nutr* 130:2444–9.

Golla AG, Larson LA, Anderson CF, Lucas AR, Wilson WR, Tomasi TB. 1981. Immunological assessment of patients with anorexia nervosa. *Am J Clin Nutr* 34:2756–62.

Grimble RF. 1994. Malnutrition and the immune response. 2. Impact of nutrients on cytokine biology in infection. *Trans R Soc Trop Med Hyg* 88:615–9.

Hart BL. 1990. Behavioral adaptations to pathogens and parasites: Five strategies. *Neurosci Biobehav Rev* 14:273–94.

Herpertz S, Norbert A, Richard W et al. 2000. Longitudinal changes of circadian leptin, insulin and cortisol plasma levels and their correlation during refeeding in patients with anorexia nervosa. *Eur J Endocrinol* 142:373–9.

Hoek HW, van Hoeken D. 2003. Review of the prevalence and incidence of eating disorders. *Int J Eat Disord* 34:383–96.

Holden RJ, Pakula IS. 1996. The role of tumour necrosis factor-α in the pathogenesis of anorexia and bulimia nervosa, cancer cachexia and obesity. *Med Hypotheses* 47:423–38.

Iwahashi H, Funahashi T, Kurokawa N et al. 2003. Plasma adiponectin levels in women with anorexia nervosa. *Horm Metab Res* 35:537–40.

Janas-Kozik M, Stachowicz M, Krupka-Matuszczyk I et al. 2011. Plasma levels of leptin and orexin A in the restrictive type of anorexia nervosa. *Regul Pept* 168:5–9.

Jolly CA. 2004. Dietary restriction and immune function. *J Nutr* 134:1853–6.

Kahl KG, Kruse N, Rieekmann P, Schmidt MH. 2004. Cytokine mRNA expression patterns in the disease course of female adolescents with anorexia nervosa. *Psychoneuroendocrinology* 29:13–20.

Konsman JP, Dantzer R. 2001. How the immune and nervous systems interact during disease-associated anorexia. *Nutrition* 17:664–8.

Licinio J, Altemus ME, Wong M, Gold PW. 1991. Circulating levels of interleukin-2 in patients with anorexia nervosa. *Biol Psychiatry* 29 (Suppl. 9A), 56A (Abstract).

Licinio J, Litsvak S, Altemus ME et al. 1990. Serum and CSF interleukin-1 in bulimia nervosa. *Biol Psychiatry* 27 (Suppl. 9A), 147A (Abstract).

Limone P, Biglino A, Bottino F et al. 2000. Evidence for a positive correlation between serum cortisol levels and IL-1beta production by peripheral mononuclear cells in anorexia nervosa. *J Endocrinol Invest* 23:422–7.

Loffreda S, Yang SQ, Lin HZ et al. 1998. Leptin regulates proinflammatory immune responses. *FASEB J* 12:57–65.

Marcos A. 1997. The immune system in eating disorders: An overview. *Nutrition* 13:853–62.

Marcos A. 2000. Eating disorders: A situation of malnutrition with peculiar changes in the immune system. *Eur J Clin Nutr* 54 (Suppl 1):S61–4.

Marcos A, Nova E, Lopez-Varela S. 2003. The immune system in eating disorders. In: Fuller R, Perdigon G (eds.),. *Gut Flora, Nutrition, Immunity and Health*. Oxford, UK: Blackwell Publishing, pp. 137–54. ISBN 1-4051-0000-1.

Marcos A, Varela P, Santacruz I, Muñoz-Velez A, Morandé G. 1993a. Nutritional status and immunocompetence in eating disorders. A comparative study. *Eur J Clin Nutr* 47:787–93.

Marcos A, Varela P, Santacruz I, Muñoz-Vélez A. 1993b. Evaluation of immunocompetence and nutritional status in patients with bulimia nervosa. *Am J Clin Nutr* 57:65–9.

Marcos A, Varela P, Toro O, Nova E, López-Vidriero I, Morandé G. 1997a. Evaluation of nutritional status by immunological assessment in bulimia nervosa. Influence of BMI and vomiting episodes. *Am J Clin Nutr* 66:S491–S7.

Marcos A, Varela P, Toro O et al. 1997b. Interactions between nutrition and immunity in anorexia nervosa. A one year follow-up. *Am J Clin Nutr* 66:S485–S90.

Matarese G. 2000. Leptin and the immune system: How nutritional status influences the immune response. *Eur Cytokine Netw* 11:7–13.

Matarese G, Moschos S, Mantzoros CS. 2005. Leptin in immunology. *J Immunol* 174:3137–42.

McCarthy HD, Dryden S, Williams G. 1995. Interleukin-1 beta induced anorexia and pyrexia in rats: Relationship to hypothalamic neuropeptide Y. *Am J Physiol* 269:E852–7.

Messaoudi I, Warner J, Fischer M et al. 2006. Delay of T cell senescence by caloric restriction in aged long-lived nonhuman primates. *Proc Natl Acad Sci U S A* 103:19448–53.

Misra M, Tsai P, Anderson EJ et al. 2006. Nutrient intake in community-dwelling adolescent girls with anorexia nervosa and in healthy adolescents. *Am J Clin Nutr* 84:698–706.

Modan-Moses D, Stein D, Pariente C et al. 2007. Modulation of adiponectin and leptin during refeeding of female anorexia nervosa patients. *J Clin Endocrinol Metab* 92:1843–7.

Monteleone P, Di Lieto A, Tortorella A, Longobardi N, Maj M. 2000. Circulating leptin in patients with anorexia nervosa, bulimia nervosa or binge eating disorder: Relationship to body weight, eating patterns, psychopathology and endocrine changes. *Psychiatry Res* 94:121–9.

Monteleone P, Maes M, Fabrazzo M et al. 1999. Immunoendocrine findings in patients with eating disorders. *Neuropsychobiology* 40:115–20.

Mustafa A, Ward A, Treasure J, Peakman M. 1997. T lymphocyte subpopulations in anorexia nervosa and refeeding. *Clin Immunol Immunopathol* 82:282–9.

Nagata T, Kiriike N, Tobitani W, Kawarada Y, Matsunaga H, Yagamami S. 1999a. Lymphocyte subset, lymphocyte proliferative response and soluble interleukin-2 receptor in anorexic patients. *Biol Psychiatry* 45:471–4.

Nagata T, Tobitani W, Kiriike N, Iketani T, Yamagami S. 1999b. Capacity to produce cytokines during weight restoration in patients with anorexia nervosa. *Psychosom Med* 61:371–7.

Nakai Y, Hamagaki S, Tagaki R, Taniguchi A, Kurimoto F. 1999. Plasma concentrations of tumor necrosis factor α (TNF-α) and soluble TNF receptors in patients with anorexia nervosa. *J Clin Endocrinol Metab* 84:1226–8.

Nogueira JP, Maraninchi M, Lorec AM et al. 2010. Specific adipocytokines profiles in patients with hyperactive and/or binge/purge form of anorexia nervosa. *Eur J Clin Nutr* 64:840–4.

Nogueira JP, Valéro R, Maraninchi M et al. 2013. Growth hormone level at admission and its evolution during refeeding are predictive of short-term outcome in restrictive anorexia nervosa. *Br J Nutr* 109:2175–81.

Nova E, Gómez-Martínez S, Morandé G, Marcos A. 2002a. Cytokine production by blood mononuclear cells from in-patients with anorexia nervosa. *Br J Nutr* 88:183–8.

Nova E, Lopez-Vidriero I, Varela P, Toro O, Casas J, Marcos A. 2004. Indicators of nutritional status in restrict-ing-type anorexia nervosa patients. A one-year follow-up study. *Clin Nutr* 23:1353–9.

Nova E, Samartín S, Gómez S, Morandé G, Marcos A. 2002b. The adaptive response of the immune system to the particular malnutrition of eating disorders. *Eur J Clin Nutr* 56:34S–7S.

Nova E, Varela P, López-Vidriero I et al. 2001. A one-year follow-up study in anorexia nervosa. Dietary pattern and anthropometrical evolution. *Eur J Clin Nutr* 55:547–54.

Omodei D, Pucino V, Labruna G et al. 2015. Immune-metabolic profiling of anorexic patients reveals an anti-oxidant and anti-inflammatory phenotype. *Metabolism* 64:396–405.

Ouchi N, Parker JL, Lugus JJ, Walsh K. 2011. Adipokines in inflammation and metabolic disease. *Nat Rev Immunol* 11:85–97.

Pannacciulli N, Vettor R, Milan G et al. 2003. Anorexia nervosa is characterized by increased adiponectin plasma levels and reduced nonoxidative glucose metabolism. *J Clin Endocrinol Metab* 88:1748–52.

Pászthy B, Svec P, Túry F et al. 2007b. Impact of anorexia nervosa on activation characteristics of lymphocytes. *Neuro Endocrinol Lett* 28:422–6.

Pászthy B, Svec P, Vásárhelyi B et al. 2007a. Investigation of regulatory T cells in anorexia nervosa. *Eur J Clin Nutr* 61:1245–9.

Patel L, Buckels AC, Kinghorn IJ et al. 2003. Resistin is expressed in human macrophages and directly regu-lated by PPAR gamma activators. *Biochem Biophys Res Commun* 300:472–6.

Polack E, Nahmod VE, Emeric Sauval E et al. 1993. Low lymphocyte interferon-gamma production and vari-able proliferative response in anorexia nervosa patients. *J Clin Immunol* 13:445–51.

Pomeroy C, Eckert E, Shuxian H et al. 1994. Role of interleukine-6 and transforming growth factor-α in anorexia nervosa. *Soc Biol Psychiatry* 36:836–9.

Pomeroy C, Mitchell J, Eckert E, Raymond N, Crosby R, Dalmasso AP. 1997. Effect of body weight and caloric restriction on serum complement proteins, including Factor D/adipsin: Studies in anorexia nervosa and obesity. *Clin Exp Immunol* 108:507–15.

Reyes TM, Sawchenko PE. 2000. Is the arcuate nucleus involved in cytokine-induced anorexia? *Soc Neurosci Abstr* 26:4413.

Rock CL, Yager J. 1987. Nutrition and eating disorders: A primer for clinicians. *Int J Eat Disord* 6:267–80.

Saito H, Nomura K, Hotta M, Takano K. 2007. Malnutrition induces dissociated changes in lymphocyte count and subset proportion in patients with anorexia nervosa. *Int J Eat Disord* 40:575–9.

Savendhal L, Underwood LE. 1997. Decreased interleukin-2 production from cultured peripheral blood mono-nuclear cells in human acute starvation. *J Clin Endocrinol Metab* 82:1177–80.

Schattner A, Steinbock M, Tepper R, Schonfeld A, Vaisman N, Hahn T. 1990b. Tumour necrosis factor produc-tion and cell-mediated immunity in anorexia nervosa. *Clin Exp Immunol* 79:62–6.

Schattner A, Tepper R, Steinbock M, Vaisman N, Hahn T, Schonfeld A. 1990a. TNF, interferon-gamma, and cell-mediated cytotoxicity in anorexia nervosa; effect of refeeding. *J Clin Lab Immunol* 32:183–4.

Schebendach J, Nussbaum MP. 1992. Nutrition management in adolescents with eating disorders. *Adolesc Med* 3:541–58.

Shintani F, Kanba S, Nakaki T et al. 1993. Interleukin-1 beta augments release of norepinephrine, dopamine, and serotonin in the rat anterior hypothalamus. *J Neurosci* 13:3574–81.

Silber TJ, Chan M. 1996. Immunologic fluorometric studies in adolescents with anorexia nervosa. *Int J Eat Disord* 19:415–8.

Smagin GN, Swiergiel AH, Dunn AJ. 1996. Peripheral administration of interleukin-1 increases extracellular concentrations of norepinephrine in rat hypothalamus: Comparison with plasma corticosterone. *Psychoneuroendocrinology* 21:83–93.

Tagami T, Satoh N, Usui T, Yamada K, Shimatsu A, Kuzuya H. 2004. Adiponectin in anorexia nervosa and bulimia nervosa. *J Clin Endocrinol Metab* 89:1833–7.

Terra X, Auguet T, Agüera Z et al. 2013. Adipocytokine levels in women with anorexia nervosa. Relationship with weight restoration and disease duration. *Int J Eat Disord* 46:855–61.

Vaisman N, Barak Y, Hahn T, Karov Y, Malach L, Barak V. 1996. Defective in vitro granulopoiesis in patients with anorexia nervosa. *Pediatr Res* 40:108–11.

Vaisman N, Hahn T. 1991. Tumor necrosis factor-α and anorexia-cause or effect? *Metabolism* 40:720–3.

Van de Berg BC, Malghem J, Devuyst O, Maldague BE, Lambert MJ. 1994. Anorexia nervosa: Correlation between MR appearance of bone marrow and severity of disease. *Radiology* 193:859–64.

Varela P, Marcos A, Muñoz Velez A, Santacruz I, Requejo A. 1988. Delayed hypersensitivity skin test in anorexia nervosa and bulimia. *Med Sci Res* 16:1135.

Wade S, Bleiberg F, Mossé A et al. 1985. Thymulin (Zn-facteur thymique serique) activity in anorexia nervosa patients. *Am J Clin Nutr* 42:275–80.

Wärnberg J, Nova E, Moreno LA et al. 2006. Inflammatory proteins are related to total and abdominal adiposity in a healthy adolescent population: The AVENA Study. *Am J Clin Nutr* 84:505–12.

Warren M, Locke R. 2008. *Anorexia Nervosa and Bulimia*. In: Arulkumaran S. (ed.). The Global Library of Women's Health. On-line text book. (ISSN: 1756-2228). doi:10.3843/GLOWM.10300.

Yirmiya R, Chiappelli F, Tio DL, Tritt SH, Taylor AN. 1998. Effects of prenatal alcohol and pair feeding on lipopolysaccharide-induced secretion of TNF-alpha and corticosterone. *Alcohol* 15:327–35.

Yokota T, Oritani K, Takahashi I et al. 2000. Adiponectin, a new member of the family of soluble defense collagens, negatively regulates the growth of myelomonocytic progenitors and the functions of macrophages. *Blood* 96:1723–32.

Ziora KT, Oswiecimska JM, Swietochowska E et al. 2011. Assessment of serum levels resistin in girls with anorexia nervosa. Part I. Relationship between resistin and body mass index. *Neuro Endocrinol Lett* 32:691–6.

8 Prebiotics, Probiotics, and Response to Vaccination

Caroline E. Childs

CONTENTS

8.1 Introduction 125
8.2 Probiotics and Vaccine Responses in Infants and Children 127
8.3 Probiotics and Vaccine Responses in Adults 128
8.4 Probiotics and Vaccine Responses in Older Adults 133
8.5 Prebiotics and Vaccine Responses 135
8.6 Synbiotics and Vaccine Responses 138
8.7 Discussion and Conclusions 140
References 142

8.1 INTRODUCTION

The human body is host to a varied and significant community of microbes, with the large intestine being the location of the vast majority of bacteria. Studies of the gut microbiota have revealed that both diet and the presence or absence of several diseases can significantly influence the number and diversity of bacterial species (Human Microbiome Project Consortium, 2012). In addition to hosting the largest quantity of microbes in the human body, the gut is also the largest site of immune tissue (see also Chapter 2), and the numerous links between nutrition, the gut microbiota, and immune function are the focus of significant research (Kau et al., 2011). Prebiotics, probiotics, and synbiotics are dietary ingredients with the potential to act as "functional foods," influencing health and/or mucosal and systemic immune function via alterations in the gut microbiota composition.

Prebiotics are "a selectively fermented ingredient that results in specific changes, in the composition and/or activity of the gastrointestinal microbiota, thus conferring benefit(s) upon host health" (Gibson et al., 2010). Nutrients with widely reported prebiotic functions include fructo-oligosaccharides and galacto-oligosaccharides, although any nondigestible dietary component that enters the large intestine is a candidate prebiotic (Gibson et al., 2010). Probiotics are defined as "live microorganisms that, when administered in adequate amounts, confer a health benefit on the host" (Food and Agriculture Organization of the United Nations, 2001, 2002). Probiotic products typically contain bifidobacteria or lactobacilli, often contained within fermented milk products, or provided as lyophilized powder in capsule form. The term synbiotic refers to a dietary intervention that combines prebiotics and probiotics. This may confer advantages, such as increasing probiotic survival after consumption (a true "synergy") or simply provide the additive benefits of each individual component (Rastall and Maitin, 2002).

It is possible to assess immune function in humans using a wide variety of techniques, ranging from observations of mortality rates following infection, to *in vitro* experiments assessing intracellular production of individual immune signaling molecules. One of the challenges of investigating the effect of foods, nutrients, or dietary ingredients upon the human immune system is the selection of appropriate assay(s), which is both logistically feasible and representative of clinically relevant changes in immune function. A review was undertaken to assess the clinical relevance, biological sensitivity, and feasibility of immune assays that can be used to investigate the effect of nutrition interventions upon immune function (Albers et al., 2013). This review concluded that the markers that provide the most useful indication of immune function were the assessment of symptoms of common infections or allergies, and the response to vaccination or allergen testing.

Using vaccination responses as a proxy for assessing changes in immune function provides insight into the overall efficacy of the coordinated function of a wide range of immune processes. A comprehensive overview of the immunology of vaccine responses is available elsewhere (Siegrist, 2008) describing the cellular mechanisms involved in orchestration of a successful immune response to challenge via vaccination. In brief, vaccination provides long-term protection against pathogens by inducing vaccine-specific antibody production and/or the induction of immune memory cells. Vaccination responses can therefore be assessed via measurement of the quantity of vaccine-specific serum antibodies. Vaccination schedules across the life course provide ample opportunity to use vaccination to assess immune function in nutrition studies. Studies of infants and children can be scheduled in tandem with routine childhood vaccinations; oral vaccinations such as rotavirus, cholera, or polio can be used to gain insight into mucosal immunity in children and adults; and influenza vaccinations recommended for older adults provide annual windows to assess immune responses against a background of declining immune function. Levels of antibody titers, which have been found to correlate to rates of protection against infection, are used as thresholds to define whether an individual is "seroprotected" postvaccination (Table 8.1). Rates of protection achieved postvaccination will vary between specific vaccinations and according to the population studied. Older adults, for example, often exhibit significantly lower rates of seroprotection after influenza vaccination than observed in younger adults.

This review details the available data from human studies, reporting the effects of dietary prebiotics, probiotics, and synbiotics upon responses to vaccination. Only those studies which report vaccine-specific antibody antibody titres or rates of seroprotection or seroconversion are included, and summary tables detail any statistically significant effects observed ($p<0.05$). Where data on clinical outcomes are available (clinically confirmed rates of infections, participant-reported

---

TABLE 8.1

Published Antibody Titers Associated with Clinical Protection

Vaccination	Titer Associated with Clinical Protection
Pertussis	20 EU/ml
Diphtheria	0.01 IU/ml
Tetanus	0.01 IU/ml
Hib	0.15 µg/mL (protective against short-term invasive disease)
	1 µg/mL (protective against long-term invasive disease)
	5 µg/mL (protective against colonization)
9-valent pneumococcal conjugate vaccine	≥0.35 µg/ml
Meningococcal C conjugate vaccine	Rabbit complement serum bactericidal assay (rSBA) titers ≥128, human complement serum bactericidal assay (hSBA) titers ≥4 or fourfold increase in rSBA postvaccination; rSBA cutoff of 8 at one month postvaccination.
Hepatitis B (HepB)	10 IU/L
Measles	Pertactin (PRN) >120 mIU/mL
Trivalent influenza	Seroprotection: hemagglutination inhibition assay (HAI) titer >1:40
	Seroconversion: influenza-specific titer mean fold increase 2.5

Note: EU = endotoxin units; IU = international units

Source: The European Agency for the Evaluation of Medicinal Products Committee for Proprietary Medicinal Products (EMA CPMP). Note for Guidance on Harmonisation of Requirements for Influenza Vaccines. 12 March 1997. CPMP/BWP/214/96; van den Berg JP. et al., *PLOS ONE*, 8, e70904, 2013; World Health Organization (WHO), *Correlates of Vaccine-Induced Protection: Methods and Implications*, Geneva, WHO, 2013.

symptoms), these are also discussed. Studies that investigated the effects of probiotics or prebiotics as part of a multinutrient intervention are not included in this review.

8.2 PROBIOTICS AND VACCINE RESPONSES IN INFANTS AND CHILDREN

Five studies were identified, which assessed the effects of probiotics on vaccine responses in infants and children (Table 8.2). These include studies of healthy-term infants (Isolauri et al., 1995; West et al., 2008), infants identified as being at high risk of developing atopic disease (Soh et al., 2010), infants who had previously be hospitalized with acute illness (Youngster et al., 2011), and children within a developing country (Matsuda et al., 2011). A minority of study designs provided very short-term probiotic supplementation in the days before and after vaccination (Isolauri et al., 1995; Matsuda et al., 2011), with the majority of studies providing supplementation for several months (Soh et al., 2010; West et al., 2008; Youngster et al., 2011). A variety of probiotic organisms was used, but these were typically lactobacilli or bifidobacteria (Table 8.2). The majority of studies conducted in infants and young children reported no significant improvement in vaccine-specific antibody responses (Isolauri et al., 1995; Soh et al., 2010; West et al., 2008; Youngster et al., 2011), and one study reported a significantly impaired response to oral cholera vaccination (Matsuda et al., 2011). Interestingly, the study by West et al. (2008) identified a significant effect upon vaccine-specific antibody responses when a subgroup analysis was performed on those infants who had been breastfed for less than 6 months, indicating that there might be variation in the ability of probiotics to influence immune function dependent upon other nutritional or lifestyle influences. The currently available data therefore do not support a beneficial effect of probiotics upon vaccine responses in infants or young children.

TABLE 8.2
Studies Investigating the Effects of Probiotics on Vaccine Responses in Infants and Children

Reference	Probiotic, Dose, and Matrix	Vaccine	Study Design	Outcomes
Isolauri et al. (1995)	*Lactobacillus casei* strain GG; 5×10^{10} cfu in 0.1 g powder reconstituted in 5 ml water.	Single dose of oral human-rhesus reassortant rotavirus vaccine (DxRRV).	Randomized, placebo-controlled study of $n = 60$ infants aged 2–5 months (Finland). Probiotic administered immediately prior to vaccination and twice daily for 5 days postvaccinati on. Blood samples collected at baseline, 8 days postvaccination (subset), and 30 days postvaccination.	No significant effects upon rates of seroconversion or postvaccination vaccine-specific antibody titers. No change in postvaccination symptoms or incidence of fever, vomiting, or loose stools during 7-day follow-up.
West et al. (2008)	*Lactobacillus paracasei ssp. paracasei* strain F19; 10^8 cfu in cereal.	Parenteral diphtheria, tetanus toxoid and acellular pertussis (DTaP), polio, and Hib vaccines at 3, 5, and 12 months.	Randomized, double-blind placebo-controlled study of $n = 180$ infants aged 4 months (Sweden). Probiotics given in cereal at least once per day until age 13 months. Blood collected at 5, 6, 12, and 13 months.	No significant differences in vaccine-specific antibody titers between groups. Probiotic resulted in significantly higher antidiphtheria and anti-Hib capsular polysaccharide antibody titers in infants breastfed for < 6 months. Infants in the probiotic group had significantly fewer days with antibiotics.

(Continued)

TABLE 8.2 (*Continued*)
Studies Investigating the Effects of Probiotics on Vaccine Responses in Infants and Children

Reference	Probiotic, Dose, and Matrix	Vaccine	Study Design	Outcomes
Soh et al. (2010)	Infant formula containing *Bifidobacterium longum* BL999 and *Lactobacillus rhamnosus* LPR; minimum dose of 2.8×10^8 cfu in 60 ml infant formula.	Two schedules of Hepatitis B (HepB) at age 0, 1, and 6 months, either monovalent HepB at dose 1 and 2, and diphtheria, tetanus, and pertussis (DTaP) vaccine containing HepB component at dose 3, or monovalent HepB vaccine for all doses.	Randomized, double-blind controlled study of $n = 253$ infants at risk of eczema (Singapore). Newborn infants given minimum of 60 ml/day infant formula containing probiotics for 6 months. Blood sample collected at 12 months.	No significant effects of probiotic on HepB antibody titers.
Matsuda et al. (2011)	Bifidobacterium breve strain Yakult; 4×10^9 cfu in 1 g.	Two doses of oral cholera vaccine Dukoral® 14 days apart.	Randomized, double-blind placebo-controlled study of $n = 128$ children aged 2–5 years (Bangladesh). Probiotic given from first vaccination until 7 days post second vaccination. Blood samples collected prevaccination, day of vaccinations, and 2 weeks post second vaccination.	Significantly lower proportion of responders in the probiotic group for viral cholera toxin B subunit specific IgA.
Youngster et al. (2011)	*Lactobacillus acidophilus* strain ATCC4356, *Bifidobacterium bifidum* DSMZ20082, *Bifidobacterium longum* ATCC157078, *Bifidobacterium infantis* ATCC15697 (Altman Probiotic Kid Powder); 3×10^9 cfu of each microorganism in sachet of powder.	Parenteral mumps, measles, rubella, and varicella (MMRV) vaccine at age 12 months.	Randomized, placebo-controlled double-blind study of $n = 47$ infants aged 8–10 months admitted to the pediatric ward with acute illness (Israel). Probiotic given daily for 2 months prevaccination and 3 months postvaccination. Blood samples collected 3 months postvaccination.	No significant effect of probiotic on participants reaching protective IgG antibody titers.

8.3 PROBIOTICS AND VACCINE RESPONSES IN ADULTS

Nine studies of probiotics and vaccine responses in adults were identified (Table 8.3), which included studies of oral (de Vrese et al., 2005; Fang et al., 2000; Link-Amster et al., 1994; Ouwehand et al., 2014; Paineau et al., 2008), nasal (Davidson et al., 2011), and parenteral vaccinations (Jespersen et al., 2015; Olivares et al., 2007; Rizzardini et al., 2012). Six of these studies identified significant

TABLE 8.3

Studies Investigating the Effects of Probiotics on Vaccine Responses in Adults

Reference	Probiotic, Dose, and Matrix	Vaccine	Study Design	Outcomes
Link-Amster et al. (1994)	*Lactobacillus acidophilus* La1 and Bifidobacteria Bb12; 10^7–10^8 cfu/g in 125 g fermented milk.	Oral attenuated *Salmonella typhi* Ty21a vaccine capsule on day 8, 10, and 12.	Preliminary group: Randomized study of $n = 10$ healthy male volunteers (Switzerland). Probiotic proved three times per day for 3 weeks, starting one week before vaccination. Blood samples collected at baseline and 14, 24, and 42 days after first vaccination.	Preliminary group: No significant differences in vaccine-specific antibody responses.
			Main group: Randomized study of $n = 30$ healthy adults aged 19–59 years (Switzerland). Probiotics proved three times per day for 3 weeks, starting one week before vaccination. Blood samples collected 3 days prior to probiotic treatment and 14 and 24 days after first vaccination.	Main group: Significantly greater fold increase in vaccine-specific serum IgA antibody titer in probiotic group
Fang et al. (2000)	*Lactobacillus* GG 4×10^{10} cfu or *Lactococcus lactis* 3.4×10^{10} cfu as lyophilized powder.	Three doses of oral attenuated *Salmonella typhi* Ty21a vaccine (day 1, 3, and 5).	Randomized, placebo-controlled study of $n = 30$ healthy adult volunteers aged 20–50 years (Finland). Probiotics provided from day of first vaccination for 7 days. Blood samples collected prior to vaccination and 7 days postvaccination.	No significant difference in vaccine-specific IgA, IgG, or IgM antibody secreting cells between groups.

(Continued)

TABLE 8.3 (*Continued*)
Studies Investigating the Effects of Probiotics on Vaccine Responses in Adults

Reference	Probiotic, Dose, and Matrix	Vaccine	Study Design	Outcomes
de Vrese et al. (2005)	*Lactobacillus rhamnosus* GG or *Lactobacillus paracasei* ssp. *paracasei* strain CRL431; 1×10^{10} cfu in 100 g acidified milk product.	Oral attenuated poliomyelitis virus types 1, 2, and 3 vaccine.	Randomized, placebo-controlled, double-blind study of $n = 64$ healthy males aged 20–30 years (Germany). Probiotics provided for 5 weeks starting 1 week prior to vaccination. Blood samples collected 4 weeks prior to vaccination, day of vaccination, and 2, 4, and 7 weeks postvaccination.	No significant effect of probiotics upon rates of seroprotection to any of the three virus types. *Lactobacillus rhamnosus* GG group had significantly greater increase in neutralizing antibody responses to poliomyelitis virus types 1, 2 compared to placebo and significantly greater increase in poliomyelitis virus type 1 specific IgA titre compared to placebo. *Lactobacillus paracasei* ssp. *paracasei* strain CRL431 had significantly greater increase in poliomyelitis virus type 2 specific IgM titer compared to placebo.
Olivares et al. (2007)	*Lactobacillus fermentum* (CECT5716); 10^{10} cfu in a capsule.	Parenteral inactivated trivalent influenza vaccine for the campaign of 2004/2005.	Parallel, randomized, double-blind, placebo-controlled study of $n = 50$ healthy adults aged 22–56 years (Spain). Probiotic provided for 2 weeks pre- and postvaccination. Blood samples collected 2 weeks prior to vaccination, immediately prior to vaccination and 2 weeks postvaccination.	Significantly higher vaccine-specific IgM 2 weeks postvaccination in probiotic-treated group. Significantly lower participant reported incidence of influenza-like illnesses 5 months postvaccination in probiotic-treated group.

(Continued)

TABLE 8.3 (*Continued*)
Studies Investigating the Effects of Probiotics on Vaccine Responses in Adults

Reference	Probiotic, Dose, and Matrix	Vaccine	Study Design	Outcomes
Paineau et al. (2008)	*Lactibacillus acidophilus* La-14, *Lactibacillus acidophilus* NCFM®, *Lactibacillus plantarum* Lp-115, *Lactibacillus paracasei* Lpc-37, *Lactibacillus salivarius* Ls-33, *Bifidobacterium lactis* Bl-04, *Bifidobacterium lactis* Bi-07 each provided at 1×10^{10} cfu in capsules	Two doses of oral cholera vaccine Dukoral® 7 days apart.	Parallel, randomized, double-blind controlled study of n = 83 healthy adults aged 18–62 years (France). Probiotics taken twice daily for 3 weeks, starting one week prior to vaccination. Blood samples collected 7 days prior to vaccination, and at 7 and 14 days after second vaccination.	Significantly higher increase in vaccine-specific serum IgG on day 21 in subjects given probiotics *Bifidobacterium lactis* Bl-04 and those given *Lactobacillus acidophilus* La-14 compared to placebo. Significantly lower levels of vaccine-specific IgM on day 28 in subjects given *Bifidobacterium lactis* Bl-04 compared to placebo.
Davidson et al. (2011)	*Lactobacillus casei* strain GG (LGG) 10^{10} cfu and 295 mg inulin in gelatin capsule. Placebo = 355mg inulin in gelatin capsule.	Nasally administered live attenuated trivalent influenza vaccine for the campaign of 2007/2008.	Randomised, double-blind placebo controlled study of n = 42 healthy adults aged 18–49 (USA). Probiotic provided twice daily for 28 days, starting on the day of vaccination. Blood samples collected at baseline, day 14, 28, and 56.	No significant differences in seroconversion rates for H1N1 and B strains. Probiotic significantly increased seroprotection rate to the H3N2 strain at day 28. No significant differences in seroconversion rates at day 56.
Rizzardini et al. (2012)	*Bifidobacterium animalis* ssp. *lactis* (BB-12®) 10^9 cfu in a capsule or *Lactobacillus paracasei* ssp. *paracasei* (L. casei 431®) 10^9 cfu in 110 ml of acidified dairy drink.	Parenteral attenuated trivalent influenza vaccine for the campaign of 2008/2009.	Parallel, randomized, placebo-controlled study of n = 211 healthy adults aged 19–60 years (Italy). Probiotics were provided for 6 weeks, starting 2 weeks prior to vaccination. Blood samples collected at baseline and after 6 weeks of probiotic supplementation.	Significantly greater increase in vaccine-specific IgG antibody titer with both probiotic treatments compared to placebo.

(*Continued*)

TABLE 8.3 (*Continued*)
Studies Investigating the Effects of Probiotics on Vaccine Responses in Adults

Reference	Probiotic, Dose, and Matrix	Vaccine	Study Design	Outcomes
Ouwehand et al. (2014)	*Lactobacillus acidophilus* ATCC 700396; 10^9 cfu as capsulated powder to be mixed with 150 ml soya milk products.	Oral challenge with attenuated *Escherichia coli*.	Parallel, double-blind, placebo-controlled study of $n = 40$ healthy men, mean age 24 years (The Netherlands). Probiotics were provided twice daily for 4 weeks, starting 2 weeks prior to vaccination. Blood samples collected 9 and 15 days postvaccination oral challenge.	No significant differences between probiotic and placebo in antigen-specific serum IgG, IgM, or IgA. Clinical measures (fever, headache, nausea, loose stools) more often reported in probiotic group.
Jespersen et al. (2015)	*Lactobacillus paracasei* subsp. paracasei, L. casei431 (Chr. Hansen A/S); $\geq 10^9$ cfu in 100 ml acidified milk drink.	Parenteral inactivated trivalent influenza virus vaccine for the 2011/2012 campaign.	Randomized, double-blind, placebo-controlled trial of $n = 1104$ healthy adults aged 18–60 years (Germany, Denmark). Probiotic provided for 42 days, starting 3 weeks prior to vaccination. Blood samples collected 21 days postvaccination.	No significant effect upon vaccine-specific seroprotection, seroconversion, or geometric mean titer. Significantly shorter duration of common cold and influenza-like illness on day 21–42 of probiotic treatment.

differences in vaccine-specific antibody production (Davidson et al., 2011; de Vrese et al., 2005; Link-Amster et al., 1994; Olivares et al., 2007; Paineau et al., 2008; Rizzardini et al., 2012). Vaccination via the oral or nasal routes is anticipated to directly influence mucosal immune responses. Four of the six studies using oral or nasal vaccinations identified significant positive effects upon vaccine-specific antibody titers (Davidson et al., 2011; de Vrese et al., 2005; Link-Amster et al., 1994; Paineau et al., 2008), and two reported no significant effect of probiotic supplementation (Fang et al., 2000; Ouwehand et al., 2014). Of the studies reporting no significant effects, it is noteworthy that these included the study with the shortest intervention period (7 days, Fang et al., 2000). Strain-specific effects may also account for some variations between studies, as evidenced by the data presented by Paineau et al. (2008), where significant positive effects were only observed for two of the seven probiotic treatments tested. Among studies that assessed the influence of probiotics upon influenza vaccination responses, two identified significant increases in vaccine-specific IgG (Olivares et al., 2007; Rizzardini et al., 2012). The third and largest study identified no significant effect on vaccine-specific antibody responses (Jespersen et al., 2015).

Within healthy adults, significant positive effects of probiotics upon vaccination responses are therefore supported by the available data. Where other clinically relevant outcomes were reported, a mixed picture was seen. Two studies indicated that providing probiotics as an adjuvant to influenza vaccination led to significant reductions in participant-reported days with influenza-like illness (Olivares et al., 2007; Jespersen et al., 2015). In contrast, Ouwehand et al. (2014) noted that adverse vaccine side effects (fever, headache, nausea, loose stools) were more prevalent among participants receiving probiotic supplementation after an oral *Escherichia coli* challenge.

8.4 PROBIOTICS AND VACCINE RESPONSES IN OLDER ADULTS

Six studies of probiotics used concurrently with parenteral influenza vaccination in older adults were identified (Table 8.4). These studies were conducted in nursing home residents (Akatsu

TABLE 8.4
Studies Investigating the Effects of Probiotics on Vaccine Responses in Older Adults

Reference	Probiotic, Dose, and Matrix	Vaccine	Study Design	Outcomes
Boge et al. (2009)	*Lactobacillus paracasei* ssp. *paracasei* (Actimel ®); 10^{10} cfu in 100 g sweetened, flavored, fermented dairy drink.	Parenteral inactivated trivalent influenza virus vaccine (pilot study 2005–2006; confirmatory study 2006–2007).	Pilot study: Randomized, controlled, double-blind study of $n = 86$ healthy nursing home residents aged ≥ 70 years (France). Probiotic provided twice daily for 7 weeks, starting 4 weeks prior to vaccination. Blood samples collected at baseline and 3 weeks, 3 months, and 5 months postvaccination. Confirmatory study: Randomized, controlled, double-blind study of $n = 222$ healthy nursing home residents aged ≥ 70 years (France). Probiotic provided twice daily for 13 weeks, starting 4 weeks prior to vaccination. Blood samples collected at baseline and 3 weeks, 6 weeks, 9 weeks, and 5 months postvaccination.	Pilot study: No significant differences in strain-specific antibody titers, seroprotection rates, or seroconversion rates 3 weeks postvaccination. Confirmatory study: Significantly higher B/Malaysia/2506/2004 antibody titers in probiotic group at 3, 6, and 9 weeks postvaccination, and associated significantly higher seroconversion rates at 6 and 9 weeks postvaccination. Significantly higher seroconversion to B/Malaysia/2506/2004 and A/Wisconsin/67/2005(H3N2) 5 months postvaccination in probiotic group.
Bosch et al. (2012)	*Lactobacillus plantarum* CECT7315/7316 at 5×10^9 cfu or 5×10^8 cfu in 20 g powdered skim milk to be dissolved in water or other cold drink.	Parenteral inactivated trivalent influenza virus vaccine for the 2006/2007 campaign.	Randomized, double-blind, placebo-controlled study of $n = 60$ institutionalized volunteers aged 65–85 (Spain). Probiotics provided for 3 months, starting 3–4 months postvaccination. Blood samples collected at baseline of probiotic treatment and after 3 months probiotic treatment.	Significant increase in vaccine-specific IgG in high-dose probiotic group. Significant increase in vaccine-specific IgA in probiotic-treated groups.

(Continued)

TABLE 8.4 (*Continued*)
Studies Investigating the Effects of Probiotics on Vaccine Responses in Older Adults

Reference	Probiotic, Dose, and Matrix	Vaccine	Study Design	Outcomes
van Puyenbroeck et al. (2012)	*Lactobacilluscasei* Shirota (*Lc*S); 6.5 x 10^9 cfu in a fermented milk product.	Parenteral inactivated trivalent influenza virus vaccine for the 2007/2008 campaign.	Randomized, double-blind, placebo-controlled trial of $n = 737$ healthy nursing home residents aged ≥ 65 (Belgium). Probiotic provided twice daily for 176 days, starting 3 weeks prior to vaccination. Blood samples collected prior to probiotic treatment, 4 weeks after vaccination and at the end of the study (day 176).	No significant effect upon influenza-specific titers, seroconversion, or seroprotection rates.
Akatsu et al. (2013a)	Heat-killed *Lactobacillus paracasei* MoLac-1; 10^9 cfu in jelly.	Parenteral inactivated trivalent influenza virus vaccine for the 2012/2013 campaign.	Randomized, placebo-controlled study of $n = 15$ nursing home residents, mean age 76 years (Japan). Probiotic provided for 12 weeks, starting 3 weeks prior to vaccination. Blood samples collected at baseline and 3 and 9 weeks postvaccination.	No significant differences between probiotic and placebo group in the change in haemagglutination inhibition (HAI) titers postvaccination compared to baseline. No significant differences in rates of seroconversion.
Akatsu et al. (2013b)	*Bifidobacterium-longum* BB536; 5 × 10^{10} cfu in 2 g powder mixed into enteral tube feeding formula one hour before feeding.	Parenteral inactivated trivalent influenza virus vaccine for the 2009/2010 campaign.	Parallel, double-blind, randomized, placebo-controlled study of $n = 45$ patients fed by enteral tube aged ≥ 65 yr (Japan). Probiotics provided for 12 weeks, starting 4 weeks prior to vaccination. Blood samples collected at baseline, day of vaccination, and 2, 4, 8, and 12 weeks postvaccination.	Significantly more patients receiving probiotic had A/H1N1 antibody titers >20 at week 6. No significant effect of probiotic upon seroprotection (antibody titer >40).
Maruyama et al. (2016)	Heat-killed *L. paracasei* MCC1849; 10^9 in jelly.	Parenteral inactivated trivalent influenza virus vaccine for the 2013–2014 campaign.	Parallel, double-blind, randomized, placebo-controlled study of $n = 45$ elderly nursing home residents (aged 72–99). Probiotics provided for 6 weeks, starting 3 weeks prior to vaccination. Blood samples collected at baseline and 3 weeks postvaccination.	No significant effects upon antibody titers with probiotic treatment. Seroprotection/seroconversion rates not reported. Subgroup analysis conducted on participants >85 years old: more participants with >twofold increase in antibody titers with probiotic treatment.

et al., 2013a; Boge et al., 2009; Maruyama et al., 2016; van Puyenbroeck et al., 2012), institutionalized older adults (Bosch et al., 2012) or those receiving enteral feeding (Akatsu et al., 2013b). While several identified significantly higher vaccine-specific antibody titers with probiotic treatment (Akatsu et al., 2013b; Boge et al., 2009; Bosch et al., 2012), in only one study was this associated with significantly increased rates of seroconversion (Boge et al., 2009). The study by Bosch et al. (2012) is of interest as this was the only study identified that did not provide probiotic supplementation before or immediately after vaccination: in this study, probiotic supplementation was commenced 3–4 months postvaccination, yet still significantly increased vaccine-specific IgA and IgG titers. Further studies that investigate the best time for dietary probiotic provision in relation to vaccination schedules are therefore warranted. The studies by Akatsu et al. (2013a) and Maruyama et al. (2016) are notable in that they provided heat-inactivated probiotics, and so would rely on mechanisms other than colonization to exert any immunomodulatory effect. No significant effect on vaccine responses was observed in either study, although a subgroup analysis in Maruyama et al. (2016) of those participants > 85 years old indicated that probiotic supplementation increased the likelihood of achieving a twofold increase in antibody titers.

8.5   PREBIOTICS AND VACCINE RESPONSES

Seven studies were identified where prebiotics were provided as adjuvants to vaccination (Table 8.5). These included studies of preterm (Van den Berg et al., 2013) and term infants (Duggan et al., 2003, Salvini et al., 2011, Stam et al., 2011), and middle-aged (Lomax et al., 2015) or older adults (Bunout et al., 2002; Akatsu et al., 2016), indicating a lack of available data on the effect that prebiotics might have upon vaccine responses in younger adults. Only two of these seven studies identified any significant effects of prebiotics upon vaccine responses, but it is of interest that those

---

TABLE 8.5
Studies Investigating the Effects of Prebiotics on Vaccine Responses

Reference	Prebiotic, Dose, and Matrix	Vaccine	Study Design	Outcomes
Bunout et al. (2002)	3 g of fructooligosaccharides (70% raftilose and 30% raftiline) to be mixed with a government-provided nutritional supplement.	Influenza and pneumococcal vaccination.	Randomized, double-blind, placebo-controlled study of $n = 66$ healthy, free-living older adults aged ≥ 70 yr (Chile). Prebiotics provided twice daily for 28 weeks, starting 2 weeks prior to vaccination. Blood samples collected at baseline, day of vaccination and 6 weeks postvaccination.	No significant differences in vaccine-specific antibody titers.

(Continued)

TABLE 8.5 (*Continued*)

Studies Investigating the Effects of Prebiotics on Vaccine Response

Reference	Prebiotic, Dose, and Matrix	Vaccine	Study Design	Outcomes
Duggan et al. (2003)	First trial: Infant cereal supplemented with oligofructose (0.55 g/ 15 g cereal) Second trial: Infant cereal supplemented with oligofructose (0.55 g/ 15 g cereal) and zinc (1mg/15 g cereal)	Haemophilus influenza type B (Hib) at 5–6 months age.	First trial: Randomized, double-blind study of $n = 282$ healthy, weaned infants aged 6–12 months (Peru). Prebiotic-enriched cereal provided for 6 months. Blood sample collected on enrollment and at 5 and 6 months after enrollment. Second trial: Randomized, double-blind study of $n = 349$ healthy, weaned infants aged 6–12 months (Peru). Prebiotic-enriched cereal provided for 6 months. Blood sample collected on enrollment and at 5 and 6 months after enrollment.	No significant differences in post-Hib vaccine antibody titer. No significant differences in post-Hib vaccine antibody titer.
Salvini et al. (2011)	Infant formula enriched with 8 g/L short-chain galactooligosaccharides and long-chain fructooligosaccharides (9:1).	HepB vaccine at 12 months age.	Randomized, placebo-controlled study of $n = 22$ full-term formula-fed newborns of hepatitis C–infected mothers (Italy). Prebiotic-enriched formula provided from day of birth for first 6 months of life. Blood samples collected for vaccine responses at 12 months.	No significant effect upon vaccine-specific antibody titers.

(*Continued*)

TABLE 8.5 (*Continued*)
Studies Investigating the Effects of Prebiotics on Vaccine Response

Reference	Prebiotic, Dose, and Matrix	Vaccine	Study Design	Outcomes
Stam et al. (2011)	6.8 g/L short-chain galactooligosaccharides/ long-chain fructooligosaccharides (9:1) and 1.2 g/L pectin-derived acidic oligosaccharides within infant formula.	Hib and tetanus immunization at 2, 3, 4, and 11 months age.	Randomized, placebo-controlled, double-blind study of $n = 164$ healthy, full term nonatopic infants (The Netherlands) who had received at least one formula feed prior to 8 weeks age. Prebiotic-enriched formula provided from enrollment until 12 months of age. Blood samples collected at 6 and 12 months old.	No significant effect of prebiotic treatment upon vaccine-specific antibody levels.
Van den Berg et al. (2013)	80% neutral oligosaccharides [small-chain galactooligosaccharides/ long-chain fructooligosaccharides] in combination with 20% pectin-derived acidic oligosaccharides in enteral supplementation at a maximum dose of 1.5 g/ kg/day.	DTaP, polio and Hib combination vaccine at 2, 3, and 4 months age.	Randomized trial of $n = 113$ preterm infants (gestational age <32 weeks and/or birth weight <1500 g) admitted to level III neonatal intensive care unit (The Netherlands). Prebiotics provided between day 3 and day 30 after birth. Blood samples collected within 48 hours of birth and at 5 and 12 months age.	No significant effect upon vaccination response.
Lomax et al. (2015)	Long-chain inulin and oligofructose, 8 g/day provided as powder to be mixed with water.	Parenteral inactivated trivalent influenza virus vaccine.	Parallel, randomized, double-blind, placebo-controlled study of $n = 49$ middle-aged adults (45–63 yr). Prebiotic provided 4 weeks prior to vaccination and 4 weeks postvaccination. Blood samples collected at baseline and at 2 and 4 weeks postvaccination.	No significant treatment effects observed upon rates of seroprotection or seroconversion. Significantly higher H3N2 antibody titers with prebiotic treatment.

(Continued)

TABLE 8.5 (*Continued*)
Studies Investigating the Effects of Prebiotics on Vaccine Response

Reference	Prebiotic, Dose, and Matrix	Vaccine	Study Design	Outcomes
Akatsu et al. (2016)	Galactooligosaccharides 4 g/day and a novel prebiotic (bifogenic growth stimulator) 0.4 g/day, dissolved in water and provided enterally.	Parenteral inactivated trivalent influenza virus vaccine.	Parallel, open label, randomized controlled study of n = 30 bedridden elderly subjects receiving enteral feeding by percutaneous endoscopic gastrostomy. Prebiotics were provided for 4 weeks prior to vaccination, and blood samples collected 2 and 6 weeks postvaccination.	Significantly higher rates of seroprotection to H3N2 strain 6 weeks postvaccination with prebiotic treatment. No significant differences in antibody titers observed.

which did were both studies of the parenteral inactivated trivalent influenza vaccine. These studies identified significant effects of prebiotic treatment on the response to the H3N2 strain, with a higher rate of seroprotection 6 weeks postvaccination among elderly adults (Akatsu et al., 2016), and a significant increase in H3N2 antibody titers among middle-aged adults (Lomax et al., 2015).

8.6 SYNBIOTICS AND VACCINE RESPONSES

Five studies of synbiotics and vaccine responses were identified (Table 8.6). These included studies of infants at risk of atopic disease (Kukkonen et al., 2006), healthy children (Firmansyah et al., 2011; Perez et al., 2010), healthy younger adults (Przemska-Kosicka et al., 2016), and older adults (Bunout et al., 2004; Przemska-Kosicka et al., 2016). The studies conducted in children indicated no significant effects upon vaccine responses (Firmansyah et al., 2011; Perez et al., 2010). Among infants identified as being at increased risk of atopic disease, there was an increased rate of protection against *Haemophilus influenzae* type B (Hib) after synbiotics were provided to mothers during late pregnancy and infants during the first 6 months of life. Among adults, a mixed picture is seen. Some data indicate an impaired influenza vaccine response with synbiotic treatment, particularly among older adults (Przemska-Kosicka et al., 2016), while another study of older adults that provided synbiotics over a longer duration identified no significant effects on vaccine-specific responses (Bunout et al., 2004). A similarly mixed picture was observed for studies reporting clinical outcomes, with a study in children identifying no significant effects of treatment upon days of fever or infectious episodes (Perez et al., 2010), while a study of older adults identified significantly lower incidence of subject reported infections during the 12-month supplementation period (Bunout et al., 2004). There is currently insufficient data to draw strong conclusions on the influence that synbiotics may have upon vaccine responses.

TABLE 8.6

Studies Investigating the Effects of Synbiotics on Vaccine Responses

Reference	Probiotic, Prebiotic, Dose, and Matrix	Vaccine	Study Design	Outcomes
Bunout et al. (2004)	*Lactobacillus paracasei* (NCC 2461) 10^9 cfu, 6 g fructooligosaccharides (raftilose: raftiline 2:1) within a 117 g powder-based nutritional drink	Influenza and pneumococcal vaccination.	Open label, parallel study of $n = 60$ healthy elderly subjects (≥ 70 years) (Chile). Synbiotic provided for one year, starting 4 months prior to vaccination. Blood sample collected 2 months postvaccination.	No significant differences in vaccine-specific antibodies 2 months postvaccination. Significantly lower incidence of subject reported infections during the 12-month supplementation period.
Kukkonen et al. (2006)	*Lactobacillus rhamnosus* GG (ATCC 53103) 5 × 10^9 cfu, *Lactobacillus rhamnosus* (LC705) 5 × 10^9 cfu, *Bifidobacterium breve* (Bbi99) 2 × 10^8 cfu, *Propionibacterium freudenreichii* ssp. *shermanii* JS 2 × 10^9 cfu in capsule form. 0.8 g galactooligosaccharides.	DTaP when infants 3, 4, and 5 months, Hib vaccines at 4 months.	Randomized, double-blind, placebo-controlled study of $n = 98$ pregnant women (35 weeks gestation) with a family history of atopic disease and their infants (Finland). Mothers take probiotic capsules twice daily until delivery. Infants take one capsule with 0.8 g galactooligosaccharide syrup until 6 months. Blood samples collected from infants at 6 months.	Higher frequency of protective Hib-specific IgG antibody responses in the synbiotic group ($p = 0.02$) No significant differences in diphtheria- and tetanus-specific titers.
Perez et al. (2010)	*Lactobacillus casei*, 95 × 10^6 cfu, *Lactobacillus acidophilus* 95 × 10^6 cfu, oligofructose (950 mg), and inulin (240 mg) within 95 g fermented milk.	DTaP-Hib at 18 months age or 23-valent antipneumococcal vaccine.	Double-blind, placebo-controlled trial of $n = 162$ low socioeconomic status children aged 9 months to 10 years who attended hospital outpatient facilities (Argentina). Synbiotic drink taken once daily for at least 4 months prior to vaccination. Blood samples collected prior to vaccination and 30—40 days postvaccination.	No significant effects upon antibody response, days of fever, or infectious episodes.

(Continued)

TABLE 8.6 (*Continued*)
Studies Investigating the Effects of Synbiotics on Vaccine Responses

Reference	Probiotic, Prebiotic, Dose, and Matrix	Vaccine	Study Design	Outcomes
Firmansyah et al. (2011)	*Bifidobacterium longum* (BL999), *Lactobacillus rhamonosus* (LPR), inulin, and fructooligosaccharides (30:70) in milk, minimum dose of 57.6 g of this combination in 400 ml milk.	Measles booster and primary hepatitis A vaccine at 14 months.	Parallel, randomized, double-blind, placebo-controlled study of $n = 393$ healthy toddlers aged 12 months (Indonesia). Synbiotic provided for 4 months. Blood samples collected at baseline and 2 months postvaccination.	No significant differences in vaccine-specific antibody responses.
Przemska-Kosicka et al. (2016)	*Bifidobacterium longum bv. infantis* CCUG 52,486 (10^9 CFU) and glucooligosaccharide (8 g), provided as powder for mixing with water or milk or with breakfast cereal	Parenteral-inactivated trivalent influenza virus vaccine.	Parallel, randomized, double-blind, placebo-controlled study of $n = 62$ younger adults (18–35 years old) and $n = 62$ older adults (60–85 years old). Synbiotic provided 4 weeks prior to vaccination and 4 weeks postvaccination. Blood samples collected at baseline and at 2 and 4 weeks postvaccination.	No significant differences in rates of seroprotection or seroconversion with synbiotic treatment in either age group. When data from all participants were combined, significantly lower H1N1 titers with synbiotic treatment. Amongst older adults, significantly lower H3N2 and Brisbane strain antibody titers with synbiotic treatment.

8.7 DISCUSSION AND CONCLUSIONS

This review details the available data from 32 studies of dietary prebiotics, probiotics, and synbiotics, as well as vaccine-specific immune responses in humans. These studies reflect a diverse field of research, with variations in cohort age, geographical population studied, intervention period, vaccination type, and vaccination route. While this presents challenges in drawing out patterns on the effect of prebiotics, probiotics, or synbiotics upon vaccination responses, some data trends are apparent. For probiotics, no available study of dietary supplementation demonstrated any improvement in the vaccine-specific immune responses of infants and children, and indeed one study identified impaired vaccine responses associated with probiotic treatment (Matsuda et al., 2011). Early life and infancy is a period where the immune system undergoes rapid development and change against a background of passive immunity provided by antibodies transferred from the mother during pregnancy and breastfeeding. It is of interest that the study by West et al. (2008) indicated positive effects of probiotic supplementation among a subset of infants who were breastfed for less than 6 months. This may suggest that breastfeeding provides such immune benefits to infants that there is little scope for further improvement in function via dietary probiotics. The picture for probiotics as vaccine adjuvants among adults was more positive, with nine of the fourteen identified publications indicating a significant benefit upon diverse vaccine responses, including upon responses to oral salmonella (Link-Amster et al., 1994), cholera (Paineau et al., 2008), and polio (de Vrese et al., 2005) vaccinations, and nasal (Davidson et al., 2011) and parenteral influenza vaccinations (Akatsu et al., 2013b; Boge et al., 2009; Bosch et al., 2012; Olivares et al., 2007; Rizzardini et al., 2012). However, the lack of significant effects upon vaccine-specific immune responses reported within the largest scale studies of probiotics ($n = 1104$, Jespersen et al., 2015; $n = 737$, van Puyenbroeck et al., 2012) cannot be ignored. One proposed explanation put forward by Jespersen et al. (2015) is that participants who are already capable of responding strongly to vaccination do not have the capacity for further improvement via dietary intervention. Work by Przemska-Kosicka et al. (2016) and Maruyama et al. (2016) highlights that variations in the degree of immunosenesence among older adults is a significant potential confounder. In addition, comparing results obtained in studies that have used influenza vaccination as a model of immune responses presents a challenge because the three strains included in this vaccine are subject to review each year. While this provides a research advantage in enabling repeated studies of immune responses among adults who have previously been vaccinated, it comes at the cost of variations in vaccine effectiveness year-to-year (Table 8.7),

TABLE 8.7

Northern Hemisphere Trivalent Seasonal Influenza Vaccine Effectiveness Estimates by Campaign Year

Campaign Year	WHO: Recommendations for Seasonal Influenza Vaccine Composition (Northern Hemisphere)[a]			Adjusted Overall Vaccine Effectiveness[b]	Studies of Probiotics, Prebiotics, or Synbiotics and the Response to Influenza Vaccination
	H1N1	H3N2	B-strain		
2004–05	A/New Caledonia/20/ 99	A/Fujian/411/ 2002	B/Shanghai/361/ 2002	10	Olivares et al. (2007)[c]
2005–06	A/New Caledonia/20/ 99	A/California/7/ 2004	B/Shanghai/361/ 2002	21	Boge et al. (2009) – pilot study
2006–07	A/New Caledonia/20/ 99	A/Wisconsin/67/ 2005	B/Malaysia/2506/ 2004	52	Boge et al. (2009) – confirmatory study,[c] Bosch et al. (2012)[c]
2007–08	A/Solomon Islands/3/ 2006	A/Wisconsin/67/ 2005[d]	B/Malaysia/2506/ 2004	37	Akatsu et al. (2016)[c], Davidson et al. (2011)[c], van Puyenbroeck et al. (2012)
2008–09	A/Brisbane/59/ 2007	A/Brisbane/10/ 2007	B/Florida/4/2006	41	Rizzardini et al. (2012),[c] Lomax et al. (2015)[c]
2009–10	A/Brisbane/59/ 2007	A/Brisbane/10/ 2007	B/Brisbane/60/ 2008	56	Akatsu et al. (2013b)[c]
2010–11	A/California/7/ 2009	A/Perth/16/ 2009	B/Brisbane/60/ 2008	60	Przemska-Kosicka et al. (2016)[c]
2011–12	A/California/7/ 2009	A/Perth/16/ 2009	B/Brisbane/60/ 2008	47	Jespersen et al. (2015)
2012–13	A/California/7/ 2009	A/Victoria/361/ 2011	B/Wisconsin/1/ 2010	49	Akatsu et al. (2013a)

(Continued)

TABLE 8.7 (*Continued*)
Northern Hemisphere Trivalent Seasonal Influenza Vaccine Effectiveness Estimates by Campaign Year

Campaign Year	WHO: Recommendations for Seasonal Influenza Vaccine Composition (Northern Hemisphere)[a]			Adjusted Overall Vaccine Effectiveness[b]	Studies of Probiotics, Prebiotics, or Synbiotics and the Response to Influenza Vaccination
	H1N1	H3N2	B-strain		
2013–14	A/California/7/ 2009	A/Victoria/361/ 2011	B/ Massachusetts/2/ 2012	51	–
2014–15	A/California/7/ 2009	A/Texas/50/ 2012	B/ Massachusetts/2/ 2012	19	Maruyama et al. (2016)[c]

Source: Centers for Disease Control and Prevention (CDC). Seasonal Influenza Vaccine Effectiveness, 2005–2016. http:// www.cdc.gov/flu/professionals/vaccination/effectiveness-studies.htm, accessed date 03/02/2017.

[a] http://www.who.int/influenza/vaccines/virus/recommendations/en/.
[b] The reduction in risk provided by the influenza vaccine (CDC, 2005–16).
[c] Significant effect of pre/probiotic treatment upon vaccine-specific antibody responses.
[d] Akatsu et al. (2016) used alternative H3N2 candidate vaccine virus A/Hiroshima/52/2005.

and altered responses among participants exposed to similar antigens in previous years, which may account for some of the differences in results between studies. While only limited data are available for the effects of prebiotics and synbiotics upon vaccination responses, only three of the eleven identified studies demonstrated a benefit of dietary supplementation (Akatsu et al., 2016; Kukkonen et al., 2006; Lomax et al., 2015) upon vaccination responses. Whether any positive effects that may arise from synbiotic supplementation are a result of the prebiotic or the probiotic, or are a truly synergistic effect of the combined ingredients, remains to be addressed.

In summary, available data indicate that treatment of adults with live probiotic strains can induce significant increases in vaccine-specific antibody responses to a wide range of vaccines, including seasonal influenza. This is of significant public health importance, given that annual influenza epidemics are estimated to cause 250,000–500,000 deaths (World Health Organization, 2014). However, available data also indicate that those individuals most vulnerable to severe consequences following impaired vaccination responses (children under 2 years of age, adults over 65 years of age) are not the most responsive populations to the vaccine-specific effects of dietary probiotics, limiting the clinical benefit of widespread probiotic supplementation. Further studies are required to fully assess the strain-specific effects of probiotics and the optimal timing and duration of interventions planned around vaccination schedules.

REFERENCES

Akatsu H, Arakawa K, Yamamoto T et al. Lactobacillus in jelly enhances the effect of influenza vaccination in elderly individuals. *J Am Geriatr Soc*. October 2013a;61(10):1828–30.

Akatsu H, Iwabuchi N, Xiao JZ et al. Clinical effects of probiotic Bifidobacterium longum BB536 on immune function and intestinal microbiota in elderly patients receiving enteral tube feeding. *J Parenter Enteral Nutr*. 2013b;37:631–40.

Akatsu H, Nagafuchi S, Kurihara R et al. Enhanced vaccination effect against influenza by prebiotics in elderly patients receiving enteral nutrition. *Geriatr Gerontol Int*. 2016; 16: 205–13.

Albers R, Bourdet-Sicard R, Braun D et al. Monitoring immune modulation by nutrition in the general population: Identifying and substantiating effects on human health. *Br J Nutr.* 2013;110:1–30.

Boge T, Rémigy M, Vaudaine S et al. A probiotic fermented dairy drink improves antibody response to influenza vaccination in the elderly in two randomised controlled trials. *Vaccine* 2009;27:5677–84.

Bosch M, Méndez M, Pérez M et al. Lactobacillus plantarum CECT7315 and CECT7316 stimulate immunoglobulin production after influenza vaccination in elderly. *Nutr Hosp.* 2012;27:504–9.

Bunout D, Barrera G, Hirsch S et al. Effects of a nutritional supplement on the immune response and cytokine production in free-living Chilean elderly. *JPEN J Parenter Enteral Nutr.* 2004;28:348–54.

Bunout D, Hirsch S, Pía de la Maza M et al. Effects of prebiotics on the immune response to vaccination in the elderly. *JPEN J Parenter Enteral Nutr.* 2002;26:372–6.

Centers for Disease Control and Prevention (CDC). *Seasonal Influenza Vaccine Effectiveness*, 2005–2016. http://www.cdc.gov/flu/professionals/vaccination/effectiveness-studies.htm, accessed date 03/02/2017.

Davidson LE, Fiorino AM, Snydman DR et al. Lactobacillus GG as an immune adjuvant for live-attenuated influenza vaccine in healthy adults: A randomized double-blind placebo-controlled trial. *Eur J Clin Nutr.* 2011;65:501–7.

de Vrese M, Rautenberg P, Laue C et al. Probiotic bacteria stimulate virus-specific neutralizing antibodies following a booster polio vaccination. *Eur J Nutr.* 2005;44:406–13.

Duggan C, Penny ME, Hibberd P et al. Oligofructose-supplemented infant cereal: 2 randomized, blinded, community-based trials in Peruvian infants. *Am J Clin Nutr.* 2003;77:937–42.

The European Agency for the Evaluation of Medicinal Products Committee for Proprietary Medicinal Products (EMA CPMP). Note for Guidance on Harmonisation of Requirements for Influenza Vaccines. 12 March 1997. CPMP/BWP/214/96.

Fang H, Elina T, Heikki A et al. Modulation of humoral immune response through probiotic intake. *FEMS Immunol Med Microbiol.* 2000;29:47–52.

Firmansyah A, Dwipoerwantoro PG, Kadim M et al. Improved growth of toddlers fed a milk containing synbiotics. *Asia Pac J Clin Nutr.* 2011;20:69–76.

Gibson GR, Scott KP, Rastall RA et al. Dietary prebiotics: Current status and new definition. *Food Sci Technol Bull: Funct Foods* 2010;7:1–19.

Human Microbiome Project Consortium. Structure, function and diversity of the healthy human microbiome. *Nature* 2012;486:207–14.

Isolauri E, Joensuu J, Suomalainen H et al. Improved immunogenicity of oral Dx RRV reassortant rotavirus vaccine by Lactobacillus casei GG. *Vaccine* 1995;13:310–2.

Jespersen L, Tarnow I, Eskesen D et al. Effect of Lactobacillus paracasei subsp. paracasei, L. casei 431 on immune response to influenza vaccination and upper respiratory tract infections in healthy adult volunteers: A randomized, double-blind, placebo-controlled, parallel-group study. *Am J Clin Nutr.* 2015;101:1188–96.

Kau AL, Ahern PP, Griffin NW et al. Human nutrition, the gut microbiome, and immune system: Envisioning the future. *Nature* 2011;474:327–336.

Kukkonen K, Nieminen T, Poussa T et al. Effect of probiotics on vaccine antibody responses in infancy—A randomized placebo-controlled double-blind trial. *Pediatr Allergy Immunol.* 2006;17:416–21.

Link-Amster H, Rochat F, Saudan KY et al. Modulation of a specific humoral immune response and changes in intestinal flora mediated through fermented milk intake. *FEMS Immunol Med Microbiol.* 1994;10:55–63.

Lomax AR, Cheung LV, Noakes PS et al. Inulin-type β2-1 fructans have some effect on the antibody response to seasonal influenza vaccination in healthy middle-aged humans. *Front Immunol.* 2015;6:490.

Maruyama M, Abe R, Shimono T et al. The effects of non-viable Lactobacillus on immune function in the elderly: A randomised, double-blind, placebo-controlled study. *Int J Food Sci Nutr.* 2016;67: 67–73.

Matsuda F, Chowdhury MI, Saha A et al. Evaluation of a probiotics, Bifidobacterium breve BBG-01, for enhancement of immunogenicity of an oral inactivated cholera vaccine and safety: A randomized, double-blind, placebo-controlled trial in Bangladeshi children under 5 years of age. *Vaccine* 2011; 29:1855–8.

Olivares M, Díaz-Ropero MP, Sierra S et al. Oral intake of Lactobacillus fermentum CECT5716 enhances the effects of influenza vaccination. *Nutrition* 2007;23:254–60.

Ouwehand AC, ten Bruggencate SJ, Schonewille AJ et al. Lactobacillus acidophilus supplementation in human subjects and their resistance to enterotoxigenic Escherichia coli infection. *Br J Nutr.* 2014;111:465–73.

Paineau D, Carcano D, Leyer G et al. Effects of seven potential probiotic strains on specific immune responses in healthy adults: A double-blind, randomized, controlled trial. *FEMS Immunol Med Microbiol.* 2008;53:107–13.

Perez N, Iannicelli JC, Girard-Bosch C et al. Effect of probiotic supplementation on immunoglobulins, isoagglutinins and antibody response in children of low socio-economic status. *Eur J Nutr.* 2010;49:173–9.

Przemska-Kosicka P, Childs CE, Enani S et al. Effect of a synbiotic on the response to seasonal influenza vaccination is strongly influenced by degree of immunosenescence. *Immun Ageing*. 2016;13:6.

Rastall RA, Maitin V. Prebiotics and synbiotics: Towards the next generation. *Curr Opin Biotechnol*. 2002;13:490–6.

Rizzardini G, Eskesen D, Calder PC et al. Evaluation of the immune benefits of two probiotic strains Bifidobacterium animalis ssp. lactis, BB-12® and Lactobacillus paracasei ssp. paracasei, L. casei 431® in an influenza vaccination model: A randomised, double-blind, placebo-controlled study. *Br J Nutr*. 2012;107:876–84.

Salvini F, Riva E, Salvatici E et al. A specific prebiotic mixture added to starting infant formula has long-lasting bifidogenic effects. *J Nutr*. 2011;141:1335–9.

Siegrist C-A. Vaccine immunology. In *Vaccines*, S Plotkin, W Orenstein, P Offit (Eds.), 5th ed, pp. 17–36. Philadelphia, PA: Saunders Elsevier, 2008.

Stam J, van Stuijvenberg M, Garssen J et al. A mixture of three prebiotics does not affect vaccine specific antibody responses in healthy term infants in the first year of life. *Vaccine* 2011;29:7766–72.

Soh SE, Ong DQ, Gerez I et al. Effect of probiotic supplementation in the first 6 months of life on specific antibody responses to infant Hepatitis B vaccination. *Vaccine* 2010; 28: 2577–9.

Food and Agriculture Organization of the United Nations (UNFAO). *Health and nutritional properties of probiotics in food including powder milk with live lactic acid bacteria*, 2001.http://www.fao.org/3/a-a0512e.pdf accessed 25/06/17.

Food and Agriculture Organization of the United Nations (UNFAO). *Guidelines for the evaluation of probiotics in food*, 2002.http://www.fao.org/3/a-a0512e.pdf accessed 25/06/17

van den Berg JP, Westerbeek EA, van der Klis FR et al. Neutral and acidic oligosaccharides supplementation does not increase the vaccine antibody response in preterm infants in a randomized clinical trial. *PLOS ONE* 2013;8:e70904.

Van Puyenbroeck K, Hens N, Coenen S et al. Efficacy of daily intake of Lactobacillus casei Shirota on respiratory symptoms and influenza vaccination immune response: A randomized, double-blind, placebo-controlled trial in healthy elderly nursing home residents. *Am J Clin Nutr*. 2012;95:1165–71.

West CE, Gothefors L, Granström M et al. Effects of feeding probiotics during weaning on infections and antibody responses to diphtheria, tetanus and Hib vaccines. *Pediatr Allergy Immunol*. 2008;19:53–60.

World Health Organization (WHO). *Correlates of Vaccine-Induced Protection: Methods and Implications*, Geneva : WHO, 2013.

WHO: Recommendations for Influenza Vaccine Composition. http://www.who.int/influenza/vaccines/vaccinerecommendations1/en/, accessed date 02/07/2015.

Youngster I, Kozer E, Lazarovitch Z et al. Probiotics and the immunological response to infant vaccinations: A prospective, placebo controlled pilot study. *Arch Dis Child*. 2011; 96: 345–9.

9 The Immunological Benefits of Complex Oligosaccharides in Human Milk

Ling Xiao, Bernd Stahl, Gert Folkerts, Johan Garssen,
Leon Knippels, and Belinda van't Land

CONTENTS

9.1 Introduction.. 145
9.2 Early Life Immune Development 146
9.3 Human Milk Oligosaccharides (HMOs).. 146
9.4 Breastfeeding Reduces the Risk for Infection 147
9.5 How Does Breastfeeding Reduce the Risk for Infection? 148
9.6 Effect of Breastfeeding on Vaccination-Induced Immune Responses 149
9.7 Breastfeeding Lowers Risk of Allergy Development 150
9.8 Breastfeeding and Development of Autoimmunity 151
9.9 What Is the Role of Immune Modulation by Oligosaccharides Including HMOs?............ 152
9.10 HMO-Induced Interplay between Gut Microbiota, Gut Permeability,
      and Immune Responses... 153
9.11 Oligosaccharides in Infant Formula.. 153
9.12 Conclusion 154
References... 154

9.1 INTRODUCTION

Human milk remains the preferred nutrition in early life for infant development. Infant formula has been developed over many decades into adequate nutrition for those infants who cannot receive human milk. However, even modern infant formulas lack components that are tailor-made by each mother for the immune imprinting of her baby, such as specific antibodies (based on the immunologic history of the mother) and human milk oligosaccharides (HMOs) (based on the mother's specific genetic makeup with regard to Lewis blood group and secretor status). The primary immune challenge after birth is infection, but secondary to this, the immune system should develop and mature in the most appropriate way to fight against the onset of immune disorders such as allergies and autoimmunity (i.e., learning to distinguish between self and nonself), which is pivotal for healthy development. Within this chapter, we will highlight the immunological importance of unique and specific oligosaccharides known to be present in human milk, focusing on their role in immune development. Moreover, the unique interactions between specific oligosaccharides on the microbiome and immune development will be discussed, as well as the impact of such interactions regarding specific immune-related diseases.

9.2 EARLY LIFE IMMUNE DEVELOPMENT

At birth the human immune system is invariably different from that of adults regarding immune responsiveness. Although competent and able to recognize most infections, the relative immunologic immaturity at birth is an important factor in the challenging fight against many infections. The limited antigen exposure as well as the natural biased immune status during pregnancy (in order to prevent adverse immunological reactions and rejection between mother and child) result in the immaturity of the immune system at birth [1]. For instance, immune responses elicited in response to infectious pathogens and vaccines are inefficient during the neonatal period [2,3]. In addition, the gastrointestinal (GI) tract is functionally underdeveloped and immature like the immune system of the newborn infant. Proper maturation of the GI mucosa tract requires not only the first colonization by microorganisms, but also a fully integrated balance between a functional microbial community and the nutritional and immunological requirements of the host [4–6]. The mucosal contact to the external microbiota plays a crucial role in establishing and maturing of the mucosal, as well as the systemic immune system [7]. The first postnatal year of life seems to be an essential period for programming the immune system leading to lifelong consequences. Factors that might influence development of the immune system include environmental exposures like feeding (i.e., preferably human milk), antigenic exposure, and the use of antibiotics. Emerging knowledge provides understanding of the protective and programming effects of nutritional components on healthy immune development, providing opportunities to improve health and, as a consequence, reduce the risk of diseases later in life. A better understanding of the biological mechanisms involved, including the relative contributions of individual dietary components, is important to understand early life development, leading to better strategies for prevention and/or treatment of -related disorders early and/ or later in life.

9.3 HUMAN MILK OLIGOSACCHARIDES (HMOs)

Within the first few months of life infants should receive preferably only human milk as their diet. This implies that during the most rapid growth phase, all essential nutrients need to be present. Indeed, human milk has evolved to contain all the nutrients necessary for the infant to thrive (Figure 9.1). In addition, on top of the essential (and nonessential) nutrients, human milk is known to contain unique molecules providing additional health benefits. HMOs are among these unique functional ingredients. More than one hundred different oligosaccharides have been identified in human milk; these are unique in their structural diversity and high amount. The actual variety is estimated to be in the range of approximately one thousand different structures. Although the composition of human milk varies extensively between individuals and time of feeding [8,9], on average the variety of complex oligosaccharides present in human milk exceeds the variety in cow's milk and consequently in infant milk formula. Currently, almost all major infant milk formula contains a limited number of nondigestible oligosaccharides. However, the main evidence with regard to oligosaccharide-based benefits on stool characteristics (pH, frequency, consistency, microbiota)

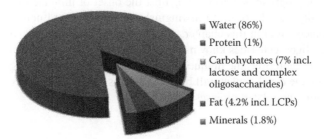

- Water (86%)
- Protein (1%)
- Carbohydrates (7% incl. lactose and complex oligosaccharides)
- Fat (4.2% incl. LCPs)
- Minerals (1.8%)

FIGURE 9.1 (See color insert.)   Summary of the composition of human milk.

and immunity is for a specific mixture of short-chain galactooligosaccharides (scGOS) and long-chain fructooligosaccharides (lcFOS) (in a ratio of 9:1). In addition, very recently a first study was reported on the use of specific HMOS 2'-fucosyllactose (2'FL) in infant formula: growth and 2'FL uptake were similar to what is seen in breastfed infants [10].

The largest carbohydrate component of human milk is lactose, a disaccharide which consists of galactose combined with glucose. Lactose serves as a fundamental building block for the larger oligosaccharides found in human milk. If fucose is linked to the lactose, the oligosaccharide structure that arises is termed a fucosyllactose (FL), whereas if N-acetylneuraminic acid is linked to lactose it generates a sialyllactose (SL). Depending on the binding site, different structures might arise. Recently the identification of different oligosaccharides in nonhuman milk revealed the presence of complex structures with fucose as well. 2'FL is present in about 20% of the oligosaccharides found in human milk [11]. In contrast only 0.3% of bovine oligosaccharides were found to be fucosylated, highlighting the differences between species. The more combinations produced between these building blocks, the more complex the oligosaccharide structures become. For instance, when combining N-acetylglucosamine with galactoses and N-acetylneuraminic acids with glucose, different HMOs including disialyllacto-N-tetraose are formed. This illustrates the possibilities of generating large panels of complex oligosaccharides, and implicates an important difference between human and nonhuman milk.

9.4 BREASTFEEDING REDUCES THE RISK FOR INFECTION

Both UNICEF and the World Health Organization (WHO) recommend exclusive breastfeeding up to the age of 6 months, with continued breastfeeding along with appropriate complementary foods up to the age of 2 years or even beyond. Numerous positive health benefits are associated with breastfeeding (Figure 9.2). Human milk is not only a comprehensive source of nutrition, it is also a well-established provider of immune factors helping immune maturation and defense against many different infectious diseases in infants [12]. Indeed, in both the neonatal period and after weaning, the clinical benefits of breastfeeding are well documented. Large cohort studies, in which

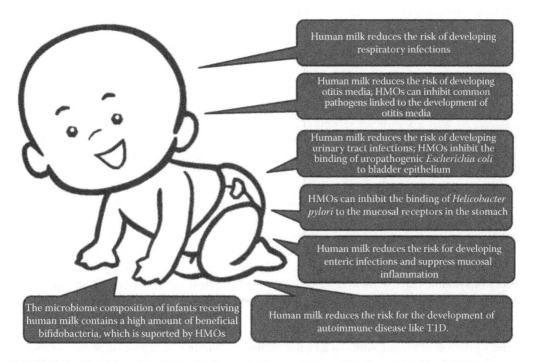

FIGURE 9.2 Health benefits of breastfeeding and of human breast milk oligosaccharides (HMOs).

mother-infant dyads are systematically studied, provide insights into differences related to mode of infant feeding and the impact on the incidence of different diseases generally known to occur during infancy. Infants consuming mother's milk were found to have a significantly lower risk for the development of infectious diarrhea and a lower risk for respiratory tract infections as well as other types of infectious diseases, including otitis media. Moreover, breastfeeding reduces the risk of hospitalization for lower respiratory tract infections during the first year of life [13]. The findings have been replicated by subsequent studies conducted over several decades and on different continents [12,14].

The protective effect of breastfeeding on infections can be explained by passive immunity provided by the mother through pathogen-specific antibodies present in milk. In addition, human milk contains a wide range of immune modulatory factors including HMOs, fatty acids, nucleotides, cytokines, lysozyme, and lactoferrin and even immune cells [15]. Moreover, perhaps for supporting early microbial colonization, human milk has been shown to contain bacteria as well, including staphylococci, streptococci, bifidobacteria, and lactic acid bacteria [16,17]. These microbes might play a significant role in supporting a balanced development of the infant's immune system. The composition of human milk changes in accordance to maternal nutritional status. Although it has been shown that nutritional deficiencies within the mother directly contribute to the deficiencies in their infants [18], it remains difficult to prove that there is a direct association between maternal nutritional status and the level of immune factors found in human milk [19]. In general, it is accepted that malnutrition leads to impaired immune responsiveness and consequently impairs the defense against infections. Observations from cohort studies have shown an association between maternal malnutrition and low birth weight, leading to an impaired response to vaccines [20,21]. This malnutrition-induced immunological impairment is multifactorial, including but not limited to a reduced complement activation, impaired mucosal barrier function, insufficient antibody production, and reduced numbers of circulating cells (including T lymphocytes [T-cells], natural killer [NK] cells, and dendritic cells [DCs]) in the neonate. In addition, increased numbers of infectious episodes will contribute to nutrient deficiencies via altered nutrient transport, decreased absorption, and increased energy requirements. Furthermore, impaired gut function and microbiota further impair the immune defense and increase susceptibility to infections ([22,23] and reviewed by Cunningham-Rundles et al.[24]).

9.5   HOW DOES BREASTFEEDING REDUCE THE RISK FOR INFECTION?

The development of a healthy and balanced immune response and robust microbiome composition are closely related, especially in early life. Breastfeeding seems to have an important role therein (Figure 9.2). Exclusive breastfeeding until the age of 4 months followed by partial breastfeeding is associated with a significant reduction in respiratory and gastrointestinal infectious diseases [25,26]. In addition, infants who were not exclusively breastfed at 6–8 weeks of age have a higher risk for hospitalization in early life in relation to a wide range of common infections [14]. The protective effect of breastfeeding has been shown to persist during childhood [27,28]. This indicates that human milk can provide passive immunity through, for instance, maternal antibodies, but also supports the development of the innate and adaptive immunity [29,30]. Although several studies have been performed to address the effect of human milk on innate immunity (i.e., the direct generic way of the immune system to respond to a pathogen), as well as the pathogen-specific adaptive immunity (providing long-lasting protection), the observations have not been consistent across studies. For instance, in some studies breastfeeding was found to be associated with a lower frequency of systemic naive (CD45RA+) T-cells in infants, whereas others showed higher numbers of these cells. Furthermore, an association was found with increasing numbers of peripheral CD4+ and CD8+ T-cells in infants and long-term breastfeeding [31–34]. Mainly due to the small sample size of these studies and the limitations in detection of memory T-cells, these studies remain inconclusive regarding the role of breastfeeding on adaptive immunity. Within a large population-based prospective cohort study (Gen R) the impact of breastfeeding on memory B- and T-cells was studied in infants and young children. Within a large number of healthy children, it was shown that the number of memory B-cells (CD27$^+$IgA$^+$, CD27$^+$IgM$^+$, and CD27$^-$IgG$^+$ memory B-cells) decreased with longer breastfeeding duration. In addition, the number of CD8$^+$ T-cells, and especially the central memory CD8$^+$ T-cells, was higher in breastfed children up to 6 months of age compared to exclusively formula-fed infants. Although the functional immunity to specific pathogens could not be studied, the previous findings within small studies (n < 40) (of increased CD8$^+$ T-cell frequency or decreased CD4/CD8 T-cell ratio) was confirmed. Infants who were breastfed until 3 months of age had a higher frequency of CD8$^+$ T-cells compared to infants who did not receive any human milk. This difference persisted over time when breastfeeding until 6 months was compared to nonbreast-fed infants. This indicates that the development of CD8$^+$ T-cells is supported by exposure to human milk, but no confirmed accumulation occurs over time. These results extend previous observations and suggest that on top of the protective effects of maternal pathogen-specific antibodies in breast milk, the CD8$^+$ T-cell support might contribute to the protective effect against infectious diseases in infancy as shown through breastfeeding [35].

The protective effect of breastfeeding against infections is suggested to be attributed at least in part to the presence of complex human milk specific oligosaccharides. The anti-rotavirus activity of HMOs in both *in vitro* and *in vivo* systems has demonstrated the potential of both neutral (LNnt) and acidic HMOs to effectively inhibit infection by specific rotavirus strains [36]. The possible mechanisms by which these specific HMOs exert their anti-infective properties might be inhibiting rotavirus binding to the host cells and/or blocking virus entry into the cell or blocking viral replication. In addition to direct blockage of viral infection by mimicking viral receptors, indirect modulation by HMOs has been hypothesized. Modulation of intestinal microbiota, through nurturing intestinal cells and/or intestinal microbiota directly with oligosaccharide-lectin interactions will have an impact on the immune responsiveness.

9.6 EFFECT OF BREASTFEEDING ON VACCINATION-INDUCED IMMUNE RESPONSES

Adaptive immune responses to specific antigens develop differently in infants receiving formula feeding or breastfeeding. Difference in responses to measles-mumps-rubella vaccine [37] as well as to *Haemophilus influenzae* type b (Hib) and pneumococcal vaccines [29,38] have been reported between breastfed infants and those who were not breastfed. Infants immunized with Hib-vaccine who were breastfed developed significantly higher vaccine-specific antibody responses at the age of 7 months [39]. In addition, this impact remained significant at later ages [40]. Moreover, Kanariou et al. showed that the level of IgA was positively correlated with breastfeeding [41]. Breastfeeding has also been associated with a decreased incidence of fever after immunizations [42]. More recently it was shown that breastfeeding around the time of rotavirus (RV1) vaccine administration tended to increase the antirotavirus IgA seroconversion compared to those temporarily withheld from breastfeeding [43].

It has been shown that early life immune modulating aspects have longer-term consequences regarding vaccination responsiveness [44]. In correlation to the finding of increased naive CD8$^+$ T-cells in breastfed infants compared to those fed formula, breastfed children show increased interferon-γ production, as well as an increase in frequencies of CD8$^+$ T-cells after vaccination for mumps, measles, and rubella. On a cellular level, it has been reported that 2 weeks after live viral vaccination, only the breastfed infants had increased percentages of CD56$^+$ and CD8$^+$ lymphocytes with increased production of virus-specific interferon-γ. The immunologic responses to vaccination were sustained over a longer period of time in subjects that were breastfed compared to the formula-fed group [40]. Moreover, beneficial effects on virus-specific immune responses to poliovirus, diphtheria toxoid, and tetanus toxoid have been indicated through breastfeeding, whereas the responses to rotavirus are not clearly enhanced [38,45,46]. These studies however were not designed to find differences between feeding type and may therefore not have been powered to take all confounding factors into account.

Recent studies showed that the effects of prebiotic oligosaccharides (produced by fermentation), mimicking the functional benefits of those present in human milk, could significantly enhance vaccine-specific cellular responses as measured by a delayed hypersensitivity response (DTH). However, the level of vaccine-specific IgG did not differ between the feeding groups at 12 months of age[47]. These studies explain in part some of the immune modulatory benefits of breast milk.

9.7   BREASTFEEDING LOWERS RISK OF ALLERGY DEVELOPMENT

Although the protection against infectious diseases among children receiving human milk is clearly observed, the possible benefit for the prevention of immune-related disorders such as allergy development remains controversial [25,48,49]. It is shown that the maternal allergic state affects composition of human milk [48]. Within the PATCH study (birth cohort study entitled Prediction of Allergies in Taiwanese Children), colostrum samples were analyzed from 98 lactating mothers and a positive association between maternal allergy status and level of inflammatory markers such as sIgA, IL-8, and sCD14 was found [50]. They also detected an increased level of fecal sIgA in infants receiving breastfeeding irrespective to the maternal allergic state. sIgA is an abundant immunoglobulin found in human milk and within the gastrointestinal tract of the infant. sIgA can bind to bacteria, toxins, and other components reducing their ability to bind to the intestinal epithelial cell modulating foreign antigen uptake by the intestine. This in turn may influence the risk for allergic sensitization. sIgA is known to be critical for the development of oral tolerance and a high level of intestinal IgA (possible induced by local low-grade inflammation) has been associated with a reduced risk for the development of IgE-associated allergic diseases [51]. In addition, since the level of sIgA has been validated as a marker for intestinal maturation and known to play an important role in the development of oral tolerance in infants, increase in fecal sIgA may suggest a potential mechanism to explain the protective effects of breastfeeding against the development of allergic manifestations.

Next to the inflammatory markers in breast milk, several food antigens can be detected in human milk as well. The presence of peanut, hen's egg, and cow's milk proteins has been described, as well as other lesser-known allergens like wheat and peach proteins [52]. Whether the presence of food allergens in human milk might lead to sensitization or tolerance induction to these foods in infants later on remains unknown and requires more in-depth studies. Early sensitization to food allergens through components in breast milk may occur and thereby might explain why some infants respond to proteins in an allergic way although they have never eaten them before. An additional influencing factor on the risk for allergy development is the time of solid food introduction. Although scientific evidence is limited, the timing of solid foods as well as formula has been associated with the development of allergic diseases [53]. Any discordance between the early developmental requirements for infant's immune development and the dynamic nature of human milk constituents may possibly contribute to the development of allergic diseases [49].

The mechanism of specific HMOs to reduce the risk for allergy development is currently not known, although recently some studies in mice may suggest an immune modulatory effect. Supplementation of the diet with 2'FL or 6'SL did not show any effect on the levels of allergen-specific IgE in sensitized or challenged mice This is in accordance with the earlier findings in the vaccination models and clinical studies [47,54,55]. Dietary supplementation with specific oligosaccharides has been shown to reduce the risk of developing allergies in infants [56–59]. The question however remains whether the observed effects are derived from direct interaction with immune cells or indirectly through the alteration in microbiome composition and change in derivatives thereof followed by immune changes. It is clear that the microbiota composition and activity has an influence on the development of allergy, more specifically regulatory T-cell development is strongly influenced by the microbial composition, and therefore subject to modulation by dietary intervention and specific oligosaccharides [60,61]. With *in vitro* assays, it has been shown that the addition of specific oligosaccharides during dendritic cell development induces a regulatory T-cell response potentially of benefit in an allergic setting [62]. Therefore, during the development of the immune system in early life it seems likely that via multiple direct and indirect pathways specific HMOs contribute to the development of a balanced immune system and reduce the risk of allergic manifestations.

9.8   BREASTFEEDING AND DEVELOPMENT OF AUTOIMMUNITY

Type 1 diabetes (T1D) is a multifactorial, immune-mediated disease, which is characterized by the progressive destruction of autologous insulin-producing beta cells in the pancreas. Environmental factors that have been correlated to the risk of developing T1D include delivery mode at birth [63,64], early life nutrition [65–68], and frequent usage of antibiotics [69,70]. These factors are known to impact the development of the microbiota directly, and directly or indirectly influence the immune system. Nutrition early in life has been suggested as the determinant of disease incidence by its effects on immune status (i.e., early childhood [≤3 month] introduction to cereals [65,66] was shown to promote beta cell autoimmunity). The increased T1D incidence in infants who were delivered by caesarean section has recently been associated with altered composition of gut microbiome [63,64]. Moreover, evidence that both biobreeding diabetic (BB-DP) and nonobese diabetic (NOD) rats were protected from diabetes onset by antibiotic use supports the crucial role that the gut microbiota plays in this type of immune-related disorder/disease [70]. However, it remains controversial whether breastfeeding is protective for the development of T1D. Breastfeeding has been shown to reduce the risk and/or prolonged the time to T1D onset [67,68], whereas other studies presented opposite findings [65,66]. Regardless, the beneficial effect of breastfeeding has been suggested to be attributed to the regulation of the (mucosal) immune system. Elevated levels of $CD4^+CD25^+Foxp3^+$ in the mesenteric lymph nodes of prolonged exclusive breastfed BBDP rat pups throughout life were observed as well as low cytokine secretion at weaning [71]. Additionally, some studies suggest that the protective effect is based on the effect on intestinal maturation and thus decreased intestinal permeability. Through degradation and fermentation of carbohydrates into short-chain fatty acids (SCFAs) in the mature gut, indirectly the HMOs can have an influence on intestinal mucosal immunity and stability. Butyrate, as one of the dominant SCFAs found in breastfed infants, has been shown to enhance the intestinal barrier by regulating the assembly of tight junctions [72]. In addition, SCFAs have been shown to be crucial for efficient mucin synthesis. The production of mucin is negatively influenced by nonbutyrate producers in autoimmune individuals, rendering them more susceptible to intestinal inflammation. In line with this concept is the observed decrease in abundance of *F. prausnitzii* (butyrate-producing bacterium) in children with detectable diabetes-related autoantibodies [73], suggesting an involvement of the microbiome. Temporary dietary exposure of nonobese diabetic (NOD/ShiLtJ) mice to HMOs in early life reduced the incidence of autoimmune diabetes later in life [74]. The data regarding splenic Tregs from NOD mice indicate that the alterations are induced in response to the severity of the disease process, rather than being a causal factor of the protective HMOs effect. These results indicate that benefits of breastfeeding may include changes in immune development by HMOs, leading to suppression of spontaneous autoimmune reactions later in life. However, it would be important to examine the regulation of intestinal immunity by HMO intervention, which may be related to their modulatory effects on gut microbiota, thus providing a possible mechanism underlying the protective effects.

9.9 WHAT IS THE ROLE OF IMMUNE MODULATION BY OLIGOSACCHARIDES INCLUDING HMOs?

With the progression of manufactured HMOs more and more becomes known about the functional benefits these oligosaccharides may elicit as depicted within Figure 9.2. For instance, among the most studied HMOs is the 2-linked-fucosylated oligosaccharides of human milk, which has been reported to control diarrhea caused by the heat-stable toxin of *E. coli* and inhibit the binding of *C. jejuni* to the colon wall [75–77]. An additional aspect of interest related to 2'FL is that it is not present in the milk from all lactating women, and the concentration varies significantly during lactation. The high variability of fucoses in human milk is dependent on the genetically determined expression of FUT2. The lack of this enzyme results in the inability to attach 2-linked fucoses during the glycosylation process, which is essential in protein folding, but also in the production of specific oligosaccharides. The presence or absence of α1,2-linked fucosylated epitopes in secretions, including saliva and milk, defines secretor and nonsecretors respectively. Consequently, the secretor-phenotype distribution differs among populations providing the opportunity to test efficacy of these pathogen inhibitors in a human population [78,79]. The protective capacity differences between the phenotypes has been studied by taking 93 breastfeeding mother-infant pairs and following them prospectively from birth up to 2 years of age with weekly infant feeding and diarrhea data collection. In this study, human milk of secretors of all blood group types was effective at blocking norovirus binding, whereas milk from nonsecretors did not block norovirus binding. Infants who received milk containing high levels of total 2-FL as a percentage of milk oligosaccharides less often showed moderate-to-severe diarrhea symptoms regardless of the pathogen causing the diarrhea. Within this study associations were found between levels of 2-FL, lacto-N-difucohexaose (LDFH-I) (a 2-linked fucosyloligosaccharide) and ratios between 2-linked to 3/4-linked oligosaccharide, with specific pathogens like *E. coli*, campylobacter, and norovirus [80]. In addition to the human oligosaccharides, human milk also contains hyaluronan (HA), a polymer from glycosaminoglycans. It has been found that the expression of antimicrobial peptides (like human defensin-2) in the intestinal epithelium can be stimulated with HA, enhancing the resistance to an infection by *Salmonella typhimurium*. This is thought to be mediated through CD44 receptor and Toll-like receptor-4 activation which enhanced the functional resistance of cultured epithelial cells [81]. In addition, glycosaminoglycans were found to be functional components of the human milk glycome, due to the demonstrated inhibition of HIV binding with its cognate receptor CD4. More specific cell interactions of HMOs with the immune system, in particular DC-SIGN, have been studied by Kooyk et al. [82]. Because C-type lectins are vital in immune modulation and in maintaining a balanced immune response, human milk prevents the interaction of specific pathogens like *Salmonella*, *Shigella*, *Vibriocholerae*, *Escherichia coli*, polioviruses, rotavirus, and respiratory syncytial virus (RSV) [83,84]. The glycosylated protein MUC1, which is abundantly present in human milk, was observed to interact with DC-SIGN on dendritic cells (DCs) via Lewis X, but not Lewis moieties. Moreover, it was specifically demonstrated that fucosylated milk components and in particular MUC1 interacted with DC-SIGN and inhibited DC-mediated transfer of HIV-1 [85,86]. Other human milk proteins have demonstrated potent protective effects through a diversity of mechanisms including soluble CD14, bile-salt-stimulated lipase (BSSL), lysozyme, lactoferrin, and of course pathogen-specific immunoglobulins, as reviewed elsewhere [15]. Although these milk proteins may exert their protective effect individually, synergistic interactions with specific oligosaccharide moieties are more likely to occur. The interaction between MUC1 and DC-SIGN is seen as a significant mechanism in the protective capacity of human milk. In particular, 2-linked fucoses seemed likely candidates for the interaction. Extensive glycan analysis on MUC1 derived from human milk reveals the presence of terminal fucoses that are not present in bovine milk, confirming the data that bovine milk does not bind DC-SIGN.

Interestingly the HMO composition is different in HIV-infected women compared with non-infected women. Specifically, the level of nonfucosylated HMOs (including LNT and 3'SL) have been found in higher concentrations in breast milk from HIV-infected women and this was suggested to be correlated to their CD4 count. This links to the immunological changes observed in a study where HAART-naive HIV-infected adults received specific prebiotic oligosaccharides [87]. As discussed, the HMO composition is highly variable in time and between individuals, determined in part by genetic characteristics like the Lewis and secretor status blood groups (i.e., preterm milk differs from term milk [88] and there is also geographic influence). In addition, an interesting association of HMO composition and the mortality rates by the age of 2 years in children born to HIV-infected mothers has been suggested. Although the effect cannot be associated to the level of specific HMOs directly, there are reports suggesting an association between higher levels of HMOs and the reduced risk of postnatal HIV transmission through breastfeeding [89–91].

9.10   HMO-INDUCED INTERPLAY BETWEEN GUT MICROBIOTA, GUT PERMEABILITY, AND IMMUNE RESPONSES

The concept that the indigenous gut microbiota play a crucial role in health and disease of the host may be particularly true during the early life of an individual, because the interaction with the mucosal immune system as well as intestinal mucosal barrier in infancy may have lifelong effects. As reviewed earlier, complete HMOs or specific human milk oligosaccharides are able to beneficially regulate gut microbiota composition, maintain gut integrity, and most importantly, enhance mucosal immunity. Therefore, it is suggested that HMOs may have a positive impact on different diseases through multiple pathways. These pathways include, but may not be limited to, the pathogen decoy capacity of specific HMOs, the prebiotic effect on the microbiome composition [92], the modulation of the production of SCFAs that in turn support gut barrier integrity, and/or through direct immune modulatory functions [93]. However, further studies are needed to support either one of the working mechanisms.

9.11   OLIGOSACCHARIDES IN INFANT FORMULA

Within the human gastrointestinal tract, the complex microbial ecosystem plays an essential role through its contributions to nutrient synthesis and digestion, protection from pathogens, and promoting maturation of innate and adaptive immune system. Disrupted microbiota development through the use of antibiotics in early life has been shown to have critical impact on immune development. Antibiotic use predisposes to the development of allergic diseases. Within the Avon Longitudinal Study of Parents and Children (ALSPAC) cohort, it was found that antibiotic use during the first 2 years of life increased the likelihood of developing asthma at the age of 7.5 years, with an increasing risk with a greater number of antibiotic courses [94]. However, this did not appear to be mediated through an association with atopic diseases, but may instead relate to alterations in gut microbiota; the role of HMOs in modulating the microbiota is reviewed elsewhere [95]. Specific individual HMOs are differentially digested by specific bacterial species including bifidobacteria and bacteroides. The major fucosylated milk oligosaccharides seem to be a strong driving factor in the development of the microbiome. Providing protection through HMOs can be generated directly through the occupation of pathogen-specific mucosal receptors, limiting the first step of pathogen invasion. In addition, the oligosaccharides serve as substrate for the generation of SCFAs and lactate by the microbiome. Fermentation products on their own can inhibit pathogens, but are also strong immune modulators, stimulating mucosal immunity [96].

The plant-derived oligosaccharides that are currently used in infant formula are known to stimulate the growth of health beneficial microbes (therefore they are termed prebiotics) but are structurally different from those in human milk. Examples of plant-derived oligosaccharides are inulin, lcFOS, scGOS, and pectin-derived acidic oligosaccharides; these share some characteristics with HMOs. Both clinical studies and experimental animal models have shown that specific mixtures of these prebiotics impact the immune response to infections. Early in life the addition of a specific prebiotic mixture to the infant formula (scGOS and lcFOS; 9:1 ratio) has been shown to reduce the number of infections [59,97]. Moreover, the protective effect against infections was still evident at the age of 2 years [98], suggesting a longer-term effect of the specific mixture of prebiotics beyond the intervention period. Recently it was shown that the SCFA butyrate (produced by commensal microorganisms) as well as propionate (another SCFA of microbial origin capable of histone deacetylase [HDAC] inhibition) induced the generation of regulatory T-cells. This suggests that these bacterial metabolites mediate communication between the commensal microbiota and the immune system [99]. Dietary nondigestible oligosaccharides can influence the function of regulatory T-cells, a process which has been demonstrated using both vaccination and allergy models in mice [55,100,101]. Although these plant-derived oligosaccharides have proven immunological benefits and recommended by the WAO for use in not-exclusively breastfed infants, they are still limited compared to the benefits provided by human milk and the complexity of the oligosaccharide structures found therein consisting of short and long chain HMOs [102].

9.12   CONCLUSION

The understanding of the whole complexity HMOs beyond single compounds and their benefits in the development of infant's immune system will provide new insights and possibly opportunities to support optimal development of the immune system and thereby lower the risk of inflammatory and infectious diseases.

REFERENCES

1. Levy O. Innate immunity of the newborn: Basic mechanisms and clinical correlates. *Nat Rev Immunol.* 2007;7(5):379–90.
2. Fadel S, Sarzotti M. Cellular immune responses in neonates. *Int Rev Immunol.* 2000;19(2–3):173–93.
3. Siegrist CA. Neonatal and early life vaccinology. *Vaccine* 2001;19(25–26):3331–46.
4. Backhed F, Ley RE, Sonnenburg JL, Peterson DA, Gordon JI. Host-bacterial mutualism in the human intestine. *Science* 2005;307(5717):1915–20.
5. van't Land B, Schijf MA, Martin R, Garssen J, van Bleek GM. Influencing mucosal homeostasis and immune responsiveness: The impact of nutrition and pharmaceuticals. *Eur J Pharmacol.* 2011;668(Suppl. 1): S101–7.
6. Palmer C, Bik EM, DiGiulio DB, Relman DA, Brown PO. Development of the human infant intestinal microbiota. *PLOS Biol.* 2007;5(7):e1771.
7. Martin R, Nauta AJ, Ben Amor K, Knippels LM, Knol J, Garssen J. Early life: Gut microbiota and immune development in infancy. *Benef Microbes.* 2010;1(4):367–82.
8. Thurl, S.; Munzert, M.; Henker, J.; Boehm, G.; Muller-Werner, B.; Jelinek, J.; Stahl, B. Variation of human milk oligosaccharides in relation to milk groups and lactational periods. *British J Nut.* 2010; 104: 1261–71.
9. Stahl B, Thurl S, Henker J, Siegel M, Finke B, Sawatzki G. Detection of four human milk groups with respect to Lewis-blood-group-dependent oligosaccharides by serologic and chromatographic analysis. *Adv Exp Med Biol.* 2001; 501:299–306.
10. Marriage BJ, Buck RH, Goehring KC, Oliver JS, Williams JA. Infants fed a lower calorie formula with 2'-fucosyllactose (2'FL) show growth and 2'FL uptake like breast-fed infants. *J Pediatr Gastroenterol Nutr.* 2015 Dec;61(6):649–58.
11. Mehra R, Barile D, Marotta M, Lebrilla CB, Chu C, German JB. Novel high-molecular weight fucosylated milk oligosaccharides identified in dairy streams. *PLOS ONE.* 2014;9(5):e96040.
12. Howie PW, Forsyth JS, Ogston SA, Clark A, Florey CD. Protective effect of breast feeding against infection. *BMJ.* 1990;300(6716):11–6.
13. Lanari M, Prinelli F, Adorni F, Di Santo S, Faldella G, Silvestri M et al. Maternal milk protects infants against bronchiolitis during the first year of life. Results from an Italian cohort of newborns. *Early Hum Dev.* 2013;89(Suppl. 1):S51–7.
14. Ajetunmobi OM, Whyte B, Chalmers J, Tappin DM, Wolfson L, Fleming M et al. Breastfeeding is associated with reduced childhood hospitalization: Evidence from a Scottish Birth Cohort (1997–2009). *J Pediatr.* 2015;166(3):620–5 e4.

15. van't Land B, Boehm G, Garssen J. Breast milk: Components with immune modulating potential and their possible role in immune mediated disease resistance. In: Watson RR, Zibadi S, Preedy VR, editors. *Dietary Components and Immune Function (Nutrition and Health)*. Humana Press; 2010. pp. 25–41.

16. Solis G, de Los Reyes-Gavilan CG, Fernandez N, Margolles A, Gueimonde M. Establishment and development of lactic acid bacteria and bifidobacteria microbiota in breast-milk and the infant gut. *Anaerobe*. 2010;16(3):307–10.

17. Tuzun F, Kumral A, Duman N, Ozkan H. Breast milk jaundice: Effect of bacteria present in breast milk and infant feces. *J Pediatr Gastroenterol Nutr*. 2013;56(3):328–32.

18. Allen LH. Multiple micronutrients in pregnancy and lactation: An overview. *Am J Clin Nutr*. 2005;81(5):1206S–12S.

19. Palmer AC. Nutritionally mediated programming of the developing immune system. *Adv Nutr*. 2011;2(5):377–95.

20. Moore SE, Jalil F, Ashraf R, Szu SC, Prentice AM, Hanson LA. Birth weight predicts response to vaccination in adults born in an urban slum in Lahore, Pakistan. *Am J Clin Nutr*. 2004;80(2):453–9.

21. McDade TW, Beck MA, Kuzawa C, Adair LS. Prenatal undernutrition, postnatal environments, and antibody response to vaccination in adolescence. *Am J Clin Nutr*. 2001;74(4):543–8.

22. Stephensen CB. Vitamin A, infection, and immune function. *Annu Rev Nutr*. 2001;21:167–92.

23. He CS, Handzlik M, Fraser WD, Muhamad A, Preston H, Richardson A et al. Influence of vitamin D status on respiratory infection incidence and immune function during 4 months of winter training in endurance sport athletes. *Exerc Immunol Rev*. 2013;19:86–101.

24. Cunningham-Rundles S, McNeeley DF, Moon A. Mechanisms of nutrient modulation of the immune response. *J Allergy Clin Immunol*. 2005;115(6):1119–28; quiz 29.

25. Walker WA, Iyengar RS. Breast milk, microbiota, and intestinal immune homeostasis. *Pediatr Res*. 2015;77(1–2):220–8.

26. Duijts L, Jaddoe VW, Hofman A, Moll HA. Prolonged and exclusive breastfeeding reduces the risk of infectious diseases in infancy. *Pediatrics* 2010;126(1):e18–25.

27. Wilson AC, Forsyth JS, Greene SA, Irvine L, Hau C, Howie PW. Relation of infant diet to childhood health: Seven year follow up of cohort of children in Dundee infant feeding study. *BMJ*. 1998;316(7124):21–5.

28. Silfverdal SA, Bodin L, Hugosson S, Garpenholt O, Werner B, Esbjorner E et al. Protective effect of breastfeeding on invasive Haemophilus influenzae infection: A case-control study in Swedish preschool children. *Int J Epidemiol*. 1997;26(2):443–50.

29. Silfverdal SA, Bodin L, Ulanova M, Hahn-Zoric M, Hanson LA, Olcen P. Long term enhancement of the IgG2 antibody response to Haemophilus influenzae type b by breast-feeding. *Pediatr Infect Dis J*. 2002;21(9):816–21.

30. Hanson LA, Korotkova M, Lundin S, Haversen L, Silfverdal SA, Mattsby-Baltzer I et al. The transfer of immunity from mother to child. *Ann N Y Acad Sci*. 2003;987:199–206.

31. Jeppesen DL, Hasselbalch H, Lisse IM, Ersboll AK, Engelmann MD. T-lymphocyte subsets, thymic size and breastfeeding in infancy. *Pediatr Allergy Immunol*. 2004;15(2):127–32.

32. Hawkes JS, Neumann MA, Gibson RA. The effect of breast feeding on lymphocyte subpopulations in healthy term infants at 6 months of age. *Pediatr Res*. 1999;45(5 Pt 1):648–51.

33. Carver JD, Pimentel B, Wiener DA, Lowell NE, Barness LA. Infant feeding effects on flow cytometric analysis of blood. *J Clin Lab Anal*. 1991;5(1):54–6.

34. Andersson Y, Hammarstrom ML, Lonnerdal B, Graverholt G, Falt H, Hernell O. Formula feeding skews immune cell composition toward adaptive immunity compared to breastfeeding. *J Immunol*. 2009;183(7):4322–8.

35. Jansen MA, van den Heuvel D, van Zelm MC, Jaddoe VW, Hofman A, de Jongste JC et al. Decreased memory B cells and increased CD8 memory T cells in blood of breastfed children: The generation R study. *PLOS ONE*. 2015;10(5):e0126019.

36. Hester SN, Chen X, Li M, Monaco MH, Comstock SS, Kuhlenschmidt TB et al. Human milk oligosaccharides inhibit rotavirus infectivity in vitro and in acutely infected piglets. *Br J Nutr*. 2013;110(7):1233–42.

37. Pabst HF, Spady DW, Pilarski LM, Carson MM, Beeler JA, Krezolek MP. Differential modulation of the immune response by breast- or formula-feeding of infants. *Acta Paediatr*. 1997;86(12):1291–7.

38. Pabst HF, Godel J, Grace M, Cho H, Spady DW. Effect of breast-feeding on immune response to BCG vaccination. *Lancet* 1989;1(8633):295–7.

39. Ogra SS, Weintraub D, Ogra PL. Immunologic aspects of human colostrum and milk. III. Fate and absorption of cellular and soluble components in the gastrointestinal tract of the newborn. *J Immunol*. 1977;119(1):245–8.

40. Pabst HF, Spady DW. Effect of breast-feeding on antibody response to conjugate vaccine. *Lancet* 1990;336(8710):269–70.
41. Kanariou M, Petridou E, Liatsis M, Revinthi K, Mandalenaki-Lambrou K, Trichopoulos D. Age patterns of immunoglobulins G, A & M in healthy children and the influence of breast feeding and vaccination status. *Pediatr Allergy Immunol.* 1995;6(1):24–9.
42. Pisacane A, Continisio P, Palma O, Cataldo S, De Michele F, Vairo U. Breastfeeding and risk for fever after immunization. *Pediatrics* 2010;125(6):e1448–52.
43. Ali A, Kazi AM, Cortese MM, Fleming JA, Moon S, Parashar UD et al. Impact of withholding breast-feeding at the time of vaccination on the immunogenicity of oral rotavirus vaccine—A randomized trial. *PLOS ONE.* 2015;10(6):e0127622.
44. Kleinnijenhuis J, van Crevel R, Netea MG. Trained immunity: Consequences for the heterologous effects of BCG vaccination. *Trans R Soc Trop Med Hyg.* 2015;109(1):29–35.
45. John TJ. Letter: The effect of breast feeding on the antibody response of infants to trivalent oral poliovirus vaccine. *J Pediatr.* 1974;84(2):307–8.
46. Rennels MB. Influence of breast-feeding and oral poliovirus vaccine on the immunogenicity and efficacy of rotavirus vaccines. *J Infect Dis.* 1996;174(Suppl. 1):S107–11.
47. Salvini F, Riva E, Salvatici E, Boehm G, Jelinek J, Banderali G, Giovannini M. A specific prebiotic mixture added to starting infant formula has long-lasting bifidogenic effects. *J of Nutrition.* 2011; doi:10.3945/jn.110.136747.
48. Snijders BE, Damoiseaux JG, Penders J, Kummeling I, Stelma FF, van Ree R et al. Cytokines and soluble CD14 in breast milk in relation with atopic manifestations in mother and infant (KOALA Study). *Clin Exp Allergy* 2006;36(12):1609–15.
49. Verhasselt V, Milcent V, Cazareth J, Kanda A, Fleury S, Dombrowicz D et al. Breast milk-mediated transfer of an antigen induces tolerance and protection from allergic asthma. *Nat Med* 2008;14(2):170–5.
50. Hua MC, Chen CC, Yao TC, Tsai MH, Liao SL, Lai SH et al. Role of maternal allergy on immune markers in colostrum and secretory immunoglobulin A in stools of breastfed infants. *J Hum Lact.* 2016 Feb; 32(1):160-7. doi: 10.1177/0890334415598783.
51. Kukkonen K, Kuitunen M, Haahtela T, Korpela R, Poussa T, Savilahti E. High intestinal IgA associates with reduced risk of IgE-associated allergic diseases. *Pediatr Allergy Immunol.* 2010;21(1 Pt 1):67–73.
52. Pastor-Vargas C, Maroto AS, Diaz-Perales A, Villaba M, Casillas Diaz N, Vivanco F et al. Sensitive detection of major food allergens in breast milk: First gateway for allergenic contact during breastfeeding. *Allergy.* 2015;70(8):1024–7.
53. Snijders BE, Thijs C, van Ree R, van den Brandt PA. Age at first introduction of cow milk products and other food products in relation to infant atopic manifestations in the first 2 years of life: The KOALA Birth Cohort Study. *Pediatrics* 2008;122(1):e115–22.
54. Schijf MA, Kruijsen D, Bastiaans J, Coenjaerts FE, Garssen J, van Bleek GM et al. Specific dietary oligosaccharides increase Th1 responses in a mouse respiratory syncytial virus infection model. *J Virol.* 2012;86(21):11472–82.
55. van't Land B, Schijf M, van Esch BC, van Bergenhenegouwen J, Bastiaans J, Schouten B et al. Regulatory T-cells have a prominent role in the immune modulated vaccine response by specific oligosaccharides. *Vaccine* 2010;28(35):5711–7.
56. van der Aa LB, van Aalderen WM, Heymans HS, Henk Sillevis Smitt J, Nauta AJ, Knippels LM et al. Synbiotics prevent asthma-like symptoms in infants with atopic dermatitis. *Allergy* 2011;66(2):170–7.
57. Moro G, Arslanoglu S, Stahl B, Jelinek J, Wahn U, Boehm G. A mixture of prebiotic oligosaccharides reduces the incidence of atopic dermatitis during the first six months of age. *Arch Dis Child* 2006;91(10):814–9.
58. Arslanoglu S, Moro GE, Boehm G, Wienz F, Stahl B, Bertino E. Early neutral prebiotic oligosaccharide supplementation reduces the incidence of some allergic manifestations in the first 5 years of life. *J Biol Regul Homeost Agents* 2012;26(Suppl. 3):49–59.
59. Arslanoglu S, Moro GE, Boehm G. Early supplementation of prebiotic oligosaccharides protects formula-fed infants against infections during the first 6 months of life. *J Nutr.* 2007;137(11):2420–4.
60. Round JL, Mazmanian SK. Inducible Foxp3+ regulatory T-cell development by a commensal bacterium of the intestinal microbiota. *Proc Natl Acad Sci USA* 2010;107(27):12204–9.
61. Atarashi K, Tanoue T, Oshima K, Suda W, Nagano Y, Nishikawa H et al. Treg induction by a rationally selected mixture of Clostridia strains from the human microbiota. *Nature* 2013;500(7461):232–6.
62. Lehmann S, Hiller J, van Bergenhenegouwen J, Knippels LM, Garssen J, Traidl-Hoffmann C. In vitro evidence for immune-modulatory properties of non-digestible oligosaccharides: Direct effect on human monocyte derived dendritic cells. *PLOS ONE.* 2015;10(7):e0132304.

63. Cardwell CR, Stene LC, Joner G, Cinek O, Svensson J, Goldacre MJ et al. Caesarean section is associated with an increased risk of childhood-onset type 1 diabetes mellitus: A meta-analysis of observational studies. *Diabetologia* 2008;51(5):726–35.

64. Khashan AS, Kenny LC, Lundholm C, Kearney PM, Gong T, Almqvist C. Mode of obstetrical delivery and type 1 diabetes: A sibling design study. *Pediatrics* 2014;134(3):e806–13.

65. Ziegler AG, Schmid S, Huber D, Hummel M, Bonifacio E. Early infant feeding and risk of developing type 1 diabetes-associated autoantibodies. *JAMA*. 2003;290(13):1721–8.

66. Norris JM, Barriga K, Klingensmith G, Hoffman M, Eisenbarth GS, Erlich HA et al. Timing of initial cereal exposure in infancy and risk of islet autoimmunity. *JAMA*. 2003;290(13):1713–20.

67. Holmberg H, Wahlberg J, Vaarala O, Ludvigsson J, Group AS. Short duration of breast-feeding as a risk-factor for beta-cell autoantibodies in 5-year-old children from the general population. *Br J Nutr*. 2007;97(1):111–6.

68. Kimpimaki T, Erkkola M, Korhonen S, Kupila A, Virtanen SM, Ilonen J et al. Short-term exclusive breastfeeding predisposes young children with increased genetic risk of Type I diabetes to progressive beta-cell autoimmunity. *Diabetologia* 2001;44(1):63–9.

69. Hansen CH, Krych L, Nielsen DS, Vogensen FK, Hansen LH, Sorensen SJ et al. Early life treatment with vancomycin propagates Akkermansia muciniphila and reduces diabetes incidence in the NOD mouse. *Diabetologia* 2012;55(8):2285–94.

70. Brugman S, Klatter FA, Visser JT, Wildeboer-Veloo AC, Harmsen HJ, Rozing J et al. Antibiotic treatment partially protects against type 1 diabetes in the Bio-Breeding diabetes-prone rat. *Is the gut flora involved in the development of type 1 diabetes? Diabetologia* 2006;49(9):2105–8.

71. Brugman S, Visser JT, Hillebrands JL, Bos NA, Rozing J. Prolonged exclusive breastfeeding reduces autoimmune diabetes incidence and increases regulatory T-cell frequency in bio-breeding diabetes-prone rats. *Diabetes Metab Res Rev*. 2009;25(4):380–7.

72. Wang HB, Wang PY, Wang X, Wan YL, Liu YC. Butyrate enhances intestinal epithelial barrier function via up-regulation of tight junction protein Claudin-1 transcription. *Dig Dis Sci*. 2012;57(12):3126–35.

73. Brown CT, Davis-Richardson AG, Giongo A, Gano KA, Crabb DB, Mukherjee N et al. Gut microbiome metagenomics analysis suggests a functional model for the development of autoimmunity for type 1 diabetes. *PLOS ONE*. 2011;6(10):e25792.

74. Xiao L, Vos AP, Nato A, Bastiaans J, Leusink-Muis A, Stahl B et al. Modulation and Programming of Immunity and Intestinal Microbiota through Early life Supplementation with Human Milk Oligosaccharides in an Autoimmune Mice Model. *Submitted*.

75. Cleary TG, Chambers JP, Pickering LK. Protection of suckling mice from the heat-stable enterotoxin of Escherichia coli by human milk. *J Infect Dis*. 1983;148(6):1114–9.

76. Newburg DS, Ruiz-Palacios GM, Morrow AL. Human milk glycans protect infants against enteric pathogens. *Annu Rev Nutr*. 2005;25:37–58.

77. Ruiz-Palacios GM, Cervantes LE, Ramos P, Chavez-Munguia B, Newburg DS. Campylobacter jejuni binds intestinal H(O) antigen (Fuc alpha 1, 2Gal beta 1, 4GlcNAc), and fucosyloligosaccharides of human milk inhibit its binding and infection. *J Biol Chem*. 2003;278(16):14112–20.

78. Erney RM, Malone WT, Skelding MB, Marcon AA, Kleman-Leyer KM, O'Ryan ML et al. Variability of human milk neutral oligosaccharides in a diverse population. *J Pediatr Gastroenterol Nutr*. 2000;30(2):181–92.

79. Chaturvedi P, Warren CD, Altaye M, Morrow AL, Ruiz-Palacios G, Pickering LK et al. Fucosylated human milk oligosaccharides vary between individuals and over the course of lactation. *Glycobiology* 2001;11(5):365–72.

80. Shang J, Piskarev VE, Xia M, Huang P, Jiang X, Likhosherstov LM et al. Identifying human milk glycans that inhibit norovirus binding using surface plasmon resonance. *Glycobiology* 2013;23(12):1491–8.

81. Hill DR, Rho HK, Kessler SP, Amin R, Homer CR, McDonald C et al. Human milk hyaluronan enhances innate defense of the intestinal epithelium. *J Biol Chem*. 2013;288(40):29090–104.

82. Koning N, Kessen SF, Van Der Voorn JP, Appelmelk BJ, Jeurink PV, Knippels LM et al. Human milk blocks DC-SIGN-pathogen interaction via MUC1. *Front Immunol*. 2015;6:112.

83. Goldman AS. The immune system in human milk and the developing infant. *Breastfeed Med*. 2007;2(4):195–204.

84. Turfkruyer M, Verhasselt V. Breast milk and its impact on maturation of the neonatal immune system. *Curr Opin Infect Dis*. 2015;28(3):199–206.

85. Saeland E, de Jong MA, Nabatov AA, Kalay H, Geijtenbeek TB, van Kooyk Y. MUC1 in human milk blocks transmission of human immunodeficiency virus from dendritic cells to T cells. *Mol Immunol*. 2009;46(11–12):2309–16.

86. Naarding MA, Ludwig IS, Groot F, Berkhout B, Geijtenbeek TB, Pollakis G et al. Lewis X component in human milk binds DC-SIGN and inhibits HIV-1 transfer to CD4+ T lymphocytes. *J Clin Invest.* 2005;115(11):3256–64.
87. Gori A, Rizzardini G, Van't Land B, Amor KB, van Schaik J, Torti C et al. Specific prebiotics modulate gut microbiota and immune activation in HAART-naive HIV-infected adults: Results of the "COPA" pilot randomized trial. *Mucosal Immunol.* 2011;4(5):554–63.
88. Filteau S. The HIV-exposed, uninfected African child. *Trop Med Int Health.* 2009;14(3):276–87.
89. Bode L, Kuhn L, Kim HY, Hsiao L, Nissan C, Sinkala M et al. Human milk oligosaccharide concentration and risk of postnatal transmission of HIV through breastfeeding. *Am J Clin Nutr.* 2012;96(4):831–9.
90. Kuhn L, Thea DM, Aldrovandi GM. Bystander effects: Children who escape infection but not harm. *J Acquir Immune Defic Syndr.* 2007;46(5):517–8.
91. Smilowitz JT, O'Sullivan A, Barile D, German JB, Lonnerdal B, Slupsky CM. The human milk metabolome reveals diverse oligosaccharide profiles. *J Nutr.* 2013;143(11):1709–18.
92. de Goffau MC, Luopajarvi K, Knip M, Ilonen J, Ruohtula T, Harkonen T et al. Fecal microbiota composition differs between children with beta-cell autoimmunity and those without. *Diabetes* 2013;62(4):1238–44.
93. Bollrath J, Powrie F. Immunology. Feed your Tregs more fiber. *Science* 2013;341(6145):463–4.
94. Hoskin-Parr L, Teyhan A, Blocker A, Henderson AJ. Antibiotic exposure in the first two years of life and development of asthma and other allergic diseases by 7.5 yr: A dose-dependent relationship. *Pediatr Allergy Immunol.* 2013;24(8):762–71.
95. Garrido D, Dallas DC, Mills DA. Consumption of human milk glycoconjugates by infant-associated bifidobacteria: Mechanisms and implications. *Microbiology* 2013;159(Pt 4):649–64.
96. Lange K, Hugenholtz F, Jonathan MC, Schols HA, Kleerebezem M, Smidt H et al. Comparison of the effects of five dietary fibers on mucosal transcriptional profiles, and luminal microbiota composition and SCFA concentrations in murine colon. *Mol Nutr Food Res.* 2015;59(8):1590–602.
97. Bruzzese E, Volpicelli M, Squeglia V, Bruzzese D, Salvini F, Bisceglia M et al. A formula containing galacto- and fructo-oligosaccharides prevents intestinal and extra-intestinal infections: An observational study. *Clin Nutr.* 2009;28(2):156–61.
98. Arslanoglu S, Moro GE, Schmitt J, Tandoi L, Rizzardi S, Boehm G. Early dietary intervention with a mixture of prebiotic oligosaccharides reduces the incidence of allergic manifestations and infections during the first two years of life. *J Nutr.* 2008;138(6):1091–5.
99. Arpaia N, Campbell C, Fan X, Dikiy S, van der Veeken J, deRoos P et al. Metabolites produced by commensal bacteria promote peripheral regulatory T-cell generation. *Nature* 2013;504(7480):451–5.
100. Schijf MA, Kerperien J, Bastiaans J, Szklany K, Meerding J, Hofman G et al. Alterations in regulatory T cells induced by specific oligosaccharides improve vaccine responsiveness in mice. *PLOS ONE.* 2013;8(9):e75148.
101. Schouten B, van Esch BC, Hofman GA, Boon L, Knippels LM, Willemsen LE et al. Oligosaccharide-induced whey-specific CD25(+) regulatory T-cells are involved in the suppression of cow milk allergy in mice. *J Nutr.* 2010;140(4):835–41.
102. Cuello-Garcia C, Fiocchi A, Pawankar R, Yepes-Nuñez J, Morgano G, Zhang Y, et al. World Allergy Organization-McMaster University guidelines for allergic disease prevention (GLAD-P): Prebiotics. *World Allergy Organ J.* 2016 Mar 1; 9:10. doi: 10.1186/s40413–016–0102–7.

10 Mechanisms of Immune Regulation by Vitamin A and Its Metabolites

Randi Larsen Indrevær, Agnete Bratsberg Eriksen, and Heidi Kiil Blomhoff

CONTENTS

10.1 Introduction 159
10.2 Vitamin A Metabolism and Mode of Action 160
    10.2.1 Retinoids and Dietary Intake of Vitamin A 160
    10.2.2 A Short Overview of Vitamin A Metabolism 161
    10.2.3 Retinoic Acid: Modes of Action 162
10.3 Vitamin A and Innate Immunity 162
    10.3.1 Mucosal Barriers and DCs 163
    10.3.2 Innate Lymphoid Cells 164
    10.3.3 Toll-Like Receptors 165
10.4 Vitamin A and Adaptive Immunity 165
    10.4.1 T-Cells 165
        10.4.1.1 The Role of Vitamin A in Regulating Th2 and Th1 Responses 166
        10.4.1.2 Retinoic Acid Regulates the Balance between Tregs and Th17 Cells 166
        10.4.1.3 Anti-versus Pro-Inflammatory Roles of Retinoic Acid 167
        10.4.1.4 Balancing T-Cell Death 167
    10.4.2 B-cells 169
        10.4.2.1 Retinoic Acid and B-Cell Development 169
        10.4.2.2 Proliferation of Mature B-Cells Regulated by RA 169
        10.4.2.3 The Role of RA in Antibody Production 171
    10.4.3 The Role of Retinol and Retro-Retinoids in Lymphocyte Functions 172
10.5 Clinical Aspects of Vitamin A in Immune-Related Diseases 172
10.6 Concluding Remarks 173
References 174

10.1 INTRODUCTION

Vitamin A and its active metabolites have crucial roles in vital processes in the body, such as in vision, embryonic development, and the nervous system (Niederreither and Dolle 2008; Blomhoff and Blomhoff 2006; Ross et al. 2000). The role of vitamin A as an important immune regulator was recognized in the 1920s with its reported anti-infective effects in animal models (Green and Mellanby 1928). Since then, numerous studies both in animal models and *in vitro* studies in isolated immune cells have revealed that vitamin A and its metabolites modulate both innate and adaptive immunity (Semba 1994, 1998; Stephensen 2001; Ross 2007). However, the substantial evidence supporting supplementation of vitamin A as a means to decrease childhood mortality related to infectious diseases has been even more important(WHO 2011; Barclay, Foster, and Sommer 1987;

Hussey and Klein 1990; Stephensen 2001). Today, therefore, the World Health Organization (WHO) supports vitamin A supplementation of children aged 6–59 months as a cost-effective strategy to improve child health in areas of the world with high risk of vitamin A deficiency—mainly in regions of Africa and Southeast Asia (WHO 2011).

This chapter will focus on the role of vitamin A in the various parts of the immune system, not only as an important factor in maintaining the integrity of mucosal epithelial barriers, but also its role in regulating the functions of the different immune cells. In particular, the molecular mechanisms whereby the vitamin A metabolites exert their immune modulatory effects will be highlighted.

10.2 VITAMIN A METABOLISM AND MODE OF ACTION

10.2.1 Retinoids and Dietary Intake of Vitamin A

Vitamin A is defined as any compound possessing the biological activity of all-trans retinol (Figure 10.1). The term "retinoids" was originally designated to include naturally occurring forms of vitamin A, as well as the many synthetic analogs of retinol, with or without biological activity. Today, most researchers define retinoids as natural or synthetic retinol analogs (with or without biological activity), and also include several compounds that are not closely related to retinol but elicit biological vitamin A or retinoid activity (Blomhoff and Blomhoff 2006).

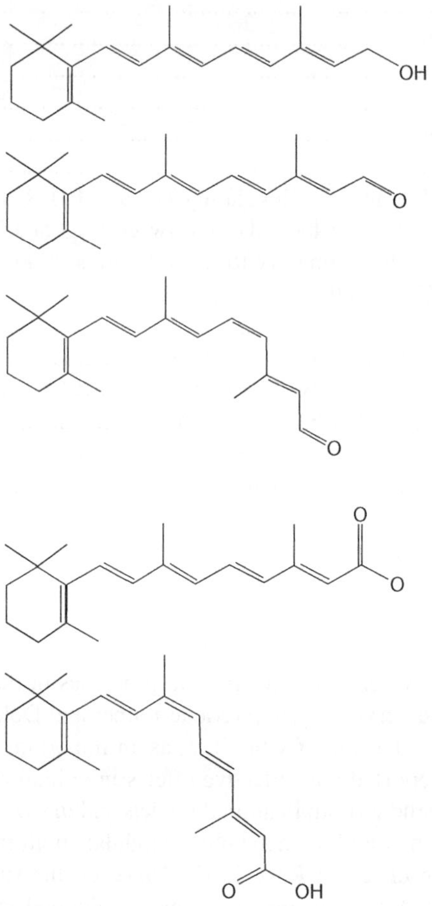

all-trans retinol

all-trans retinal

11-cis retinal

all-trans retinoic acid

9-cis retinoic acid

FIGURE 10.1 Structural formulas of some naturally occurring retinoids.

Animals do not have the capacity for *de novo* synthesis of vitamin A. However, plants and some microorganisms can synthesize carotenoids, and animals and plants can cleave carotenoids to various forms of retinoids (Nagao 2004). Animals, including humans, can therefore obtain compounds with vitamin A activity from diets rich in plants and plant materials. Alternatively, humans can obtain dietary vitamin A by eating tissues from animals that already have converted provitamin A carotenoids into retinoids, such as retinyl esters. Retinyl esters (and to a lesser extent retinol) accumulate in fish, birds, and mammalian livers as well as in other animal tissues. Retinyl esters will therefore also contribute to dietary intake of vitamin A. Clinical vitamin A deficiency is characterized by ocular features like xerophthalmia and a generalized impaired resistance to infections (Sommer 2008); this is a public health problem in many regions of the world, affecting as many as 190 million preschoolers (WHO 2011). It should, however, be emphasized that intakes of vitamin A only marginally above recommended dietary intake also may be harmful, in terms of increased risk of embryonic malformations (Rothman et al. 1995) and reduced bone mineral density (Melhus et al. 1998). The classical signs of hypervitaminosis A are related to the skin, nervous system, musculoskeletal system, circulation, and internal organs, and can be seen after excessive dietary intake of vitamin A or intake of drugs containing large doses of specific retinoids (Biesalski 1989; Hathcock et al. 1990).

10.2.2 A SHORT OVERVIEW OF VITAMIN A METABOLISM

Carotenoids are taken up by enterocytes in the small intestine, and β-carotene is enzymatically cleaved to form two molecules of retinal, which in turn are reduced to retinol (Blomhoff and Blomhoff 2006; D'Ambrosio, Clugston, and Blaner 2011). Dietary retinyl esters are hydrolyzed to retinol in the intestinal lumen, and un-esterified retinol is taken up by enterocytes (Blomhoff and Blomhoff 2006; Harrison 2005). In enterocytes, retinol is bound to the binding protein CRBP-II, and retinol is re-esterified with long-chain fatty acids. The majority of retinyl esters are then incorporated into chylomicrons, and these large lipoprotein complexes are subsequently secreted from the enterocytes into the intestinal lymph. Following secretion of chylomicrons into the lymph, these particles move into the circulation, resulting in the formation of chylomicron remnants (CR), which retain almost all of the retinyl esters. The CR are mainly taken up by parenchymal liver cells (hepatocytes) (Blomhoff et al. 1990), but extrahepatic uptake of CR may be important for the delivery of retinyl esters to tissues and organs important for the immune system, such as bone marrow, peripheral blood cells, and the spleen (Paik et al. 2004).

In hepatocytes, the retinyl esters are hydrolyzed, and un-esterified retinol will associate with the retinol binding protein (RBP). Binding to RBP will facilitate the secretion of retinol-RBP into plasma, but a large portion of un-esterified retinol will also be transferred to the perisinusoidal stellate cells in the liver for storage (Blomhoff et al. 1990). This extensive storage of retinyl esters in stellate cells contributes to a steady blood plasma retinol concentration of 1–2 µM despite normal fluctuations in daily intake of vitamin A. In addition to retinol and retinyl esters, nanomolar concentrations (5–10 nM) of a number of other retinoids are also found in the plasma, such as all-trans retinoic acid, 13-cis retinoic acid, 13-cis-4-oco retinoic acid, and all-trans 4-oxo retinoic acid (Wyss and Bucheli 1997; Barua and Sidell 2004), and these retinoic acids are transported in plasma bound to albumin.

Active retinoid metabolites are generally synthesized in target cells. Except for 11-cis retinal crucial in the vision process, the important active metabolite for most cells and tissues, including cells of the immune system, is all-trans retinoic acid. The major source for synthesis of all-trans retinoic acid is all-trans retinol taken up from plasma (Blomhoff and Blomhoff 2006). However, plasma-derived retinoic acids and lipoproteins containing retinyl esters may also contribute. In target cells, retinol is oxidized to retinoic acid in a two-step reaction, involving alcohol dehydrogenases (ADH) and retinal dehydrogenases (RALDH), respectively (Blomhoff and Blomhoff 2006). RALDH is expressed in a limited set of cell types, including activated dendritic cells (DCs) and gut epithelial cells (Iwata et al. 2004), as well as in thymic epithelial cells (Kiss et al. 2008). Lymphoid cells do not appear to express the enzymes required for producing retinoic acids from retinol, but such cells may still obtain retinoic acid from plasma or directly from neighboring cells (Kiss et al. 2008; Iwata et al. 2004).

It should also be emphasized that regulation of catabolism of all-trans retinoic acid is an equally important mechanism for controlling the levels of retinoic acid in various cells and tissues (Blomhoff and Blomhoff 2006). The cytochrome P450 enzymes CYP26A1/B1 and C1 show non-overlapping expressions in various tissues and can catabolize all-trans retinoic acid to water-soluble polar metabolites. The cellular retinoic acid binding protein type I (CRABP-1) seems to be involved in this process.

10.2.3 RETINOIC ACID: MODES OF ACTION

Being a lipophilic molecule, retinoic acid is in principle able to diffuse through membranes. In fact, retinoic acid was the first diffusible morphogen identified in vertebrates (Thaller and Eichele 1987). In 1987 the first member of the family of retinoic acid receptors (RARs) was cloned (Petkovich et al. 1987; Giguere et al. 1987). The RARs belong to the family of steroid/thyroid hormone receptors and act as ligand-dependent transcription factors. Later, a new subfamiliy of RARs (called RXRs) was identified (Szanto et al. 2004), and to date six different genes coding for nuclear RARs have been cloned (RARβ, γ and RXR α β, γ). The expression pattern of these receptors varies in different tissues, and it has been demonstrated that RAR α, RAR γ, and RXR α are expressed in lymphocytes (Lomo et al. 1998). RA primarily functions via RAR/RXR heterodimers (Wei 2003). The dimers bind to DNA sequences called retinoic acid response elements (RAREs) or retinoid X response elements (RXREs) located in the promoters of target genes (Blomhoff and Blomhoff 2006).

In vitro binding studies have identified all-trans retinoic acid and 9-cis retinoic acid as high-affinity ligands for RARs, whereas only 9-cis retinoic acid binds with high affinity to RXRs (Soprano, Qin, and Soprano 2004). However, the physiological role of 9-cis retinoic acid has been questioned, since it has not yet been possible to identify 9-cis retinoic acid as an endogenous compound (Blomhoff and Blomhoff 2006). Hence, the most important ligand for the RAR/RXR heterodimers appears to be all-trans retinoic acid binding to the RARs.

More than 500 genes have been suggested to be either direct targets of retinoic acid via RAR/RXR heterodimers binding to DNA response elements, or indirect targets via intermediate transcription factors or via other mechanisms (Balmer and Blomhoff 2002, 2005). Of these, 27 genes have been identified as unquestionably direct targets of the classical RAR/RXR pathway, whereas 100 other genes have been classified as good candidates for being such direct targets (Balmer and Blomhoff 2002). It should also be mentioned that retinoic acid–RAR/RXR complexes can regulate gene expression independently of RAREs, through transactivation of other transcription factors such as AP1 (Schule et al. 1991; Kamei et al. 1996) and NFκB (Na et al. 1999; Bayon et al. 2003). Even nongenomic modes of action of retinoic acids have been demonstrated. Hence, all-trans retinoic acid has been shown to bind directly to PKC and modulate its activity (Radominska-Pandya et al. 2000; Ochoa et al. 2003), and to induce autophagosome maturation through redistribution of the cation-independent mannose-6-phosphate receptor (Rajawat, Hilioti, and Bossis 2011).

10.3 VITAMIN A AND INNATE IMMUNITY

Innate immunity is our oldest defense system against infections. It comprises the epithelial barriers of the skin, as well as mucosal epithelial barriers found in the conjunctiva of the eyes and in the respiratory, intestinal, and urogenital tracts. Innate immune defense also includes circulating phagocytes and innate lymphoid cells (ILCs), including conventional natural killer (NK) cells, as well as complement proteins, acute-phase proteins, and pattern-recognizing receptors.

10.3.1 Mucosal Barriers and DCs

It has long been established that vitamin A deficiency leads to increased susceptibility to infections at mucosal sites (Semba 1994; Stephensen 2001). The mucosal epithelial barriers are significantly compromised in vitamin A–deficient animals, due to loss of mucus-producing goblet cells as well as squamous metaplasia in cases of infections (Stephensen 2001). As a result, vitamin A deficiency may reduce the clearance of pathogenic bacteria from the respiratory tract (Chandra 1988), and may allow easier penetration of pathogenic bacteria through gut mucosal barriers (Shoda et al. 1995; Wiedermann et al. 1995).

Mucosal immunity is closely linked to the production of IgA from plasma cells in the lamina propria and mesenteric lymph nodes adjacent to mucosal surfaces (see also Chapter 2). Here IgA is involved in the defense against both viral and bacterial infections. *In vitro* studies have demonstrated the ability of retinoic acid to enhance isotype switching to IgA in the presence of interleukin interleukin 5 (IL-5) (Tokuyama and Tokuyama 1996; Nikawa et al. 2001), and numerous *in vivo* studies have reported diminished levels of IgA in vitamin A–deficient animals (Mora and von Andrian 2009).

The role of retinoic acid for intestinal IgA production has been particularly well studied. Naive lymphocytes circulate in the blood and can occasionally enter lymphoid tissues such as lymph nodes and Peyer's patches (PP). To enter nonlymphoid tissues like the lamina propria of the gut, the cells need to be activated with cognate antigens in the secondary lymphoid tissues. Homing of lymphocytes refers to the migration of lymphocytes into lymphoid organs or to nonlymphoid tissues where they first encountered the antigens. Naive T-cells activated in gut-associated lymphoid tissues (GALT), PP, or mesenteric lymph nodes typically migrate to intestinal tissues (Iwata 2009). In secondary lymphoid organs, lymphocytes home at specifically developed postcapillary venules called high endothelial venules (HEV) (Miyasaka and Tanaka 2004). The homing relies on tissue-specific chemokines and adhesion molecules produced by the epithelial cells, and the lymphocytes require homing receptors. Thus, for homing to the small intestine, T-cells express integrin $\alpha4\beta7$ that binds to the adhesion molecule MAdCAM-1 and the chemokine receptor CCR9 that recognizes the ligand CCL25 (Hamann et al. 1994; Svensson et al. 2002). Later, generation of gut-homing IgA secreting B-cells was shown to require expression of the integrin $\alpha4\beta7$ on the surface of B-cells (Mora and von Andrian 2009; Mora et al. 2006). It was demonstrated that imprinting of the homing receptors on T-cells (Mora et al. 2003) and B-cells (Mora et al. 2006) was dependent on resident dendritic cells (DCs), and it was elegantly demonstrated that RA produced by the specific DCs was responsible for inducing the homing receptors (Iwata et al. 2004; Mora et al. 2006).

As discussed above, retinoic acid can be formed in target cells from plasma-derived retinol in a two-step process involving ADH and RALDH (Blomhoff and Blomhoff 2006). Lymphoid cells do not express the required enzymes for producing retinoic acids from retinol, and these cells may therefore depend on retinoic acid from plasma or directly from neighboring cells (Iwata et al. 2004; Kiss et al. 2008). Whereas DCs from all secondary lymphoid organs seem to express at least one ADH isoform, RALDH expression is limited to DCs in tissues like PP or mesenteric lymph nodes (Iwata et al. 2004). By converting all-trans retinol to all-trans retinoic acid, the local production of retinoic acid by DCs may enhance the expression of homing receptors on T-cells (Iwata et al. 2004) and B-cells (Mora et al. 2006). It should be mentioned that mucosal epithelial cells also have been known to express RALDH, and that these cells may contribute to homing of T-cells via production of retinoic acid (Iwata et al. 2004; Frota-Ruchon, Marcinkiewicz, and Bhat 2000; Westerlund et al. 2007). Retinoic acid itself upregulates the expression of RALDH and thereby engages in a positive feedback loop shown to correlate with vitamin A levels in the diet (Beijer, Kraal, and den Haan 2014). Interestingly, it was recently demonstrated that respiratory tract epithelial cells also express RALDH, and that such cells could support IgA production by activated B-cells in the presence of retinol (Rudraraju et al. 2014). These results may encourage clinical trials on nasal supplementation of vitamin A to fight respiratory tract infections in vitamin A–deficient populations.

Retinoic acid might not only be involved in regulating homing of lymphocytes, but also in immune tolerance. Hence, retinoic acid derived from intestinal DCs has been shown to promote the differentiation of naive T-cells into Foxp3+ regulatory T-cells (Tregs) and simultaneously suppress their differentiation into proinflammatory Th17 cells (Sun et al. 2007; Mucida et al. 2007; Kang et al. 2007). However, as *in vivo* studies on vitamin A–deficient mice demonstrate decreased frequencies of Th17 cells rather than of Treg cells (Cha et al. 2010; Kang et al. 2009), the role of retinoic acid in regulating the balance between Treg and Th17 cells is not yet fully established.

10.3.2 INNATE LYMPHOID CELLS

Some of the most exciting recent discoveries in the vitamin A field have been related to the function and distribution of ILCs and intestinal barrier functions. ILCs were initially linked to development of lymphoid tissues, but have later been given roles in inflammation at barrier surfaces in response to infection and tissue damages, and to participate in the transition from innate to adaptive immunity (McKenzie, Spits, and Eberl 2014). ILCs were previously considered to comprise only NK cells. However, the current view is that in addition to conventional NK (cNK) cells, three groups of ILCs (ILC1, ILC2, and ILC3) can be identified based on distinct transcriptional programs and functions (McKenzie, Spits, and Eberl 2014; Diefenbach, Colonna, and Koyasu 2014). The cNK cells represent a disparate lineage referred to as cytotoxic or killer ILCs, whereas ILC1, ILC2, and ILC3 can be grouped as helper ILCs (Diefenbach, Colonna, and Koyasu 2014). ILC1s predominantly express interferon-γ (IFN-γ); ILC2s primarily express IL-5, IL-9, and IL-13; and ILC3s mainly express IL-22 and/or IL-17 (McKenzie, Spits, and Eberl 2014). The various ILCs have distinct roles in protection against viruses (cNK cells), bacteria (ILC1s and ILC3s), intracellular parasites (ILC1s), fungi (ILC3s), and parasitic worms (ILC2s) (McKenzie, Spits, and Eberl 2014). Fighting a virus, a bacterium or a worm involves defined immune responses that are orchestrated by distinct T-cell subsets. Whereas it takes days for the right T-cells to be selected and respond in the lymph nodes, ILCs can do a similar job within hours due to direct responses to signaling molecules produced in the infected tissues (Spits and Di Santo 2011).

In an interesting study on intestinal barrier function, Spencer and coworkers observed that vitamin A deficiency in mice decreased the frequencies of ILC3s (and thereby of IL-17 and IL-22) and increased the frequency of IL-13–producing ILC2s (Spencer et al. 2014). The altered homeostasis resulted in profound defective immunity to acute bacterial infections, such as to *Citrobacter rodentium*. More interestingly, however, the vitamin A–deficient mice developed resistance to nematode infections, such as to the nutrient-consuming helminth *Trichuris muris*. Both ILC2s and ILC3s selectively express RAR α (Mielke et al. 2013). Whereas exogenous delivery of retinoic acid caused a dominant expression of ILC3, the pan-RAR inhibitor BMS493 or deletion of RARα-favored ILC2 accumulation (Spencer et al. 2014). Abrogating IL-7 signaling in mice treated with the pan-RAR inhibitor also diminished the accumulation of ILC2, suggesting that vitamin A deficiency is associated with an increased frequency of ILC2s, possibly involving increased responsiveness to IL-7. The study concluded that nutrient deficiency not necessarily causes general immunosuppression, but that it also may result in specific activation of distinct branches of barrier immunity. In this case, vitamin A deficiency would favor elimination of the nutrient-consuming helminthes by selectively increasing the frequency of ILC2s. ILC2s thereby act as primary sensors for nutrient deficiency and may compensate for the well-established malfunctions in adaptive immunity related to vitamin A deficiency.

ILC3s have been shown to have a vital function in development of lymph nodes (Eberl 2014). Taken together with the newly established role of vitamin A in formation of ILC3s (Spencer et al. 2014), the facts pointed to a more fundamental role of vitamin A in the immune system (i.e., in the development of lymphoid tissues). A distinct cell type, called lymphoid tissue inducer (LTi), accumulates in the developing lymph nodes in the fetus (Mebius, Rennert, and Weissman 1997). LTi cells are considered to be prototypical ILC3s, and their generation requires the RAR-related orphan receptor RORγt (Eberl et al. 2004). In the conceptually important paper by van de Pavert and colleagues, it was discovered that generation of LTi cells requires retinoic acid (van de Pavert et al. 2014). Retinoic acid was shown to induce maturation of LTi cells from precursor cells in the developing lymph nodes via RAR-mediated transcription of the Rorc gene–encoding RORγt. In mice lacking RARs, the number of mature LTi cells was reduced, the lymph nodes were signifi-cantly smaller, and the adaptive immune response to viral infections was diminished. The same features were seen when the pregnant mice were treated with a RAR antagonist. Having proven the role of retinoic acid in the development of lymph nodes in the fetus, the question emerged as to what was the source of retinoic acid. Van de Pavert and coworkers elegantly showed that the lymph node size and immune responses directly reflected the level of vitamin A in the diet of the mother during pregnancy (van de Pavert et al. 2014). Hence, in mice whose mothers were fed a vitamin A–deficient diet during pregnancy, the lymph nodes were small and the immune response impaired, suggest-ing that the mother was responsible both for the uptake of vitamin A and its conversion to retinoic acid. The intriguing implications of these results are that immune responses to infection might be predetermined in early life through the diet of the mother. This has wide implications for public health, emphasizing the importance of vitamin A supplementation in areas at risk of maternal and childhood vitamin A deficiency.

10.3.3 Toll-Like Receptors

Toll-like receptors (TLRs) recognize pathogen-associated molecular patterns (PAMPs) from micro-organisms or danger-associated molecular patterns (DAMPs) from damaged cells and tissues. Until the discoveries of TLRs throughout the 1980s and 1990s, innate immunity was considered as a primitive part of the immune system. The identification and characterization of the 10 human and 12 murine TLRs has provided molecular insight into key processes in innate immunity, and has also been key to understanding and bridging the innate and adaptive immune systems (O'Neill, Golenbock, and Bowie 2013; Paul 2011). There have been few studies addressing the role of vita-min A in TLR signaling and function. Liu and coworkers demonstrated that treatment of primary monocytes with retinoic acid downregulated TLR2 as well as its co-receptor CD14 (Liu et al. 2005). As inflammation in acne is partly due to the ability of *Propionibacterium acne* to activate TLR2 (Kim et al. 2002; Vowels, Yang, and Leyden 1995), it was suggested that the anti-inflammatory role of retinoic acid in acne could be attributed to its ability to inhibit the function of TLR2 (Liu et al. 2005). Yet, reduced expression of TLRs is not a general consequence of retinoic acid exposure. More recently, two independent studies concluded that retinoic acid increases the expression of TLR5 in macrophages (Cho et al. 2011) and mucosal DCs (Feng et al. 2012) respectively, to activate the macrophages and to maintain intestinal homeostasis and host defense against enterobacterial infections. RA-mediated stimulation of TLR9 and RP105 functions has also recently been docu-mented in human B-cells (Ertesvag et al. 2007; Eriksen et al. 2012; Indrevaer et al. 2013). However, as TLRs have important roles also in the regulation of adaptive immune responses, the impact of vitamin A and TLRs related to T- and B-cell functions will be addressed in later sections.

10.4 VITAMIN A AND ADAPTIVE IMMUNITY

10.4.1 T-Cells

T-cells play critical roles in the adaptive part of the immune system. In addition to mediating cellu-lar immune responses, they are also involved in humoral immunity as helpers of B-cell proliferation and differentiation (Mitchison 2004). T-cells develop from immature T-cell precursors in the bone marrow, and continue their maturation in the thymus as thymocytes. Two main types of mature T-cells are produced by the thymus: CD8+ and CD4+ T-cells. Upon activation, these cells will develop into cytotoxic and helper T-cells, respectively. CD8+ cytotoxic T-cells kill pathogen-infected cells, whereas CD4$^+$ helper T-cells provide help to B-cells and to CD8$^+$ cytotoxic T-cells. The naive CD4$^+$ T-cells can differentiate into several different subsets—Th1, Th2, Th17, and Treg cells—depending on the antigen stimulation and cytokine environment. The characteristics of the various subsets will be presented in the subsections below, in connection with discussions of the roles of vitamin A in regulating their development and function.

10.4.1.1   The Role of Vitamin A in Regulating Th2 and Th1 Responses

Naive T-cells can differentiate into effector T-cells such as Th1 and Th2 cells in response to antigenic stimulation in secondary lymphoid organs. Whereas Th1 cells produce IFN-γ and play important roles in mounting effective antimicrobial cellular immunity, Th2 cells produce IL-4, IL-5, and IL-13, and are required for effective clearance of helminths and extracellular pathogens. It has long been accepted that vitamin A favors Th2 responses at the expense of Th1 responses *in vivo* (Stephensen 2001). Hence, vitamin A deficiency was shown to result in excess production of IFN-γ and impaired antibody responses (Cantorna, Nashold, and Hayes 1994), whereas high levels of dietary vitamin A favored Th2 cytokine production and IgA responses (Racke et al. 1995). Iwata and coworkers later demonstrated a direct effect of RA (via RARs) to inhibit the differentiation of T-cells into Th1 cells by downregulating T-box expressed in T-cell (T-bet) expression, while favoring Th2 development via induced expression of the GATA-binding protein-3 (GATA3), MAF, and STAT6 (Iwata, Eshima, and Kagechika 2003). Retinoic acid has also been shown to indirectly induce differentiation into Th2 cells by enhancing the production of the Th2-stimulating cytokines IL-4 and IL-5 from Th2 cells (Hoag et al. 2002), and to enhance the proliferation of T-cells via enhanced production of IL-2 (Ertesvag et al. 2002; Engedal, Ertesvag, and Blomhoff 2004).

Despite the many studies suggesting that retinoic acid favors the formation of Th2 cells, there have also—as will be further discussed below—been studies supporting the notion that retinoic acid under certain circumstances may foster the balance toward Th1 cells (Pino-Lagos et al. 2011; Hall et al. 2011). In a recent review on vitamin A and the immune system, it was suggested that previously documented effects of retinoic acid on Th2 responses in VAD mice may be due to the expansion of ILC2 cells producing Th2-type cytokines (Brown and Noelle 2015). Furthermore, it was proposed that retinoic acid via RARα is critical for stabilizing the Th1 cell lineage (Brown and Noelle 2015), supported by recent studies on dnRara mice (Brown et al. 2015).

10.4.1.2   Retinoic Acid Regulates the Balance between Tregs and Th17 Cells

Th1 and Th2 cells are not the only T-cell subsets influenced by vitamin A levels. In the periphery, naive CD4$^+$ T-cells can develop into Th17 cells in a process that requires IL-6 and TGFβ (Bettelli et al. 2006; Veldhoen et al. 2006). Th17 cells are characterized by the expression of RORγt and production of IL-17, and whereas these cells are considered to exert pro-inflammatory responses and tissue damage linked to autoimmune diseases, their normal roles are to provide antimicrobial immunity at epithelial and mucosal barriers. In the presence of TGFβ, naive CD4$^+$ T-cells can also develop into regulatory T-cells (Tregs) characterized by expression of Foxp3 and CD25. These cells are called induced FoxP3$^+$ T-cells (iTregs) to distinguish them from the naturally occurring Tregs that develop from cells in the thymus (Piccirillo 2008). Tregs have evolved to enforce suppressive effects on T-cell responses and thereby to maintain tolerance to self-antigens and prevent autoimmune diseases. The groundbreaking findings by Iwata and coworkers (Iwata et al. 2004) that RA enhances the expression of the gut-homing molecules α4β7 and CCR9 on CD4$^+$ T-cells, was followed by other important discoveries related to the function of retinoic acid in maintaining intestinal homeostasis. Hence, local production of retinoic acid by DCs and macrophages in the intestine was shown to cooperate with TGFβ to convert naive CD4$^+$ T-cells into iTregs, and this conversion was largely mediated via RARα (Raverdeau and Mills 2014). Furthermore, retinoic acid was shown to promote the gut-homing properties of the Tregs by enhancing their expression of α4β7 and CCR9 (Raverdeau and Mills 2014).

Concomitant with the well-documented induction of Foxp3⁺ Treg cells by retinoic acid, numerous studies have shown that retinoic acid via RARs inhibits the formation of the pro-inflammatory Th17 cells (Kang et al. 2007; Mucida et al. 2007; Brown et al. 2015). Hence, it seems that retinoic acid is able to determine whether naive CD4⁺ T-cells will differentiate into iTregs or Th17 cells to maintain mucosal homeostasis (Mucida, Park, and Cheroutre 2009; Mucida et al. 2007; Xiao et al. 2008; Raverdeau and Mills 2014; Kim 2011). A key to understanding this balanced production of Th17 versus Treg cells is in the cooperation between retinoic acid, TGFβ, and IL-6. Whereas the formation of both Th17 cells and Tregs requires TGFβ, generation of Th17 cells also requires IL-6 (Mucida, Park, and Cheroutre 2009). Retinoic acid inhibits Th17 cell formation by inhibiting the expression of the transcription factor RORγt (Mucida, Park, and Cheroutre 2009), but also by downregulating IL-6Rα on naive T-cells (Raverdeau and Mills 2014). Since IL-6 on the other hand inhibits the expression of RARα (Nolting et al. 2009), retinoic acid–mediated inhibition of IL-6 will indirectly promote the RARα-mediated induction of Foxp3⁺ as well as activation of the TGFβ-regulated Smad3 and the transcription factor Stat5 to induce differentiation into Tregs (Mucida, Park, and Cheroutre 2009; Raverdeau and Mills 2014).

10.4.1.3 Anti-versus Pro-Inflammatory Roles of Retinoic Acid

The intestine forms a large entry surface for invading pathogens, and it is therefore crucial for the immune system to mount effective protection in this part of the body. However, the challenge of the immune system is to simultaneously maintain tolerance against resident harmless bacteria and absorbed nutrients that are also present in the intestine. Dietary vitamin A seems to have an important role in balancing these inflammatory and suppressive immune responses. Hence, the ability of the vitamin A metabolite retinoic acid to drive the differentiation to Foxp3⁺ Tregs, suppressing the formation of pro-inflammatory suppressive Th17 cells, and to promote the homing of effector T-cells to the gut, fits with a role of retinoic acid in maintaining the mucosal integrity of the intestine and to provide tolerance when protective immune responses are not required (Iwata 2009; Mucida, Park, and Cheroutre 2009; Raverdeau and Mills 2014). Importantly however, the role of retinoic acid might change in the context of inflammatory signals. Hall and colleagues discovered that Th1 and Th17 responses were impaired in vitamin A–deficient mice challenged with *T. gondii* infection, and that retinoic acid was able to restore the impaired immune responses *in vivo* in a RARα-dependent manner (Hall et al. 2011). Furthermore, retinoic acid signaling was shown to be enhanced in CD4⁺ T-cells in a pro-inflammatory context (Pino-Lagos et al. 2011), and retinoic acid–mediated formation of Tregs was reduced concomitant with enhanced conversion to Th1 responses in the presence of IL-15 in a mouse model of coeliac disease (DePaolo et al. 2011). Thus, in a microbe-rich environment such as the gut mucosa, retinoic acid may under certain circumstances enhance the inflammatory tone. Taken together it seems that retinoic acid helps to promote Treg generation and tolerance during steady state conditions in the body, whereas in the context of inflammation, infections, or autoimmunity, retinoic acid may have an opposite effect by promoting adaptive T-cell responses—fitting with VAD being associated with defective immune responses to infections or following vaccinations.

10.4.1.4 Balancing T-Cell Death

10.4.1.4.1 Role of Retinoic Acid in Death of Thymocytes

T-cell death is a crucial part of the positive and negative selection of developing T-cells in the thymus (for a review, see Klein et al. 2014). In the thymic cortex, thymocytes that express T-cell receptors (TCRs) with only low avidity for self-peptide-loaded MHC molecules will die by a process called death by neglect. The surviving positively selected thymocytes then move to the medulla, where thymocytes that recognize self-antigens will die by activation-induced cell death (AICD). Hence, only cells expressing TCRs with low avidity for self-antigens will survive. The mechanisms involved in the selective death of thymocytes are poorly understood. A role of glucocorticoids as well as lack of prosurvival Bcl-2 has been suggested in cortical "death by neglect" of thymocytes (Ashwell, Lu, and Vacchio 2000), whereas AICD of medullary thymocytes appears to involve the intrinsic apoptotic pathway by modifications of pro-apoptotic proteins like Bim and Nur77 (Siggs, Makaroff, and Liston 2006).

The role of vitamin A in "death by neglect" has primarily been studied in the context of spontaneous death of thymocytes in culture, and the general conclusion seems to be that retinoic acid enhances "death by neglect"—at least in the presence of glucocorticoids (Engedal 2011). In contrast, it appears that retinoic acid generally inhibits AICD of thymocytes, both *in vitro* and *in vivo*. Hence, retinoic acid was shown to inhibit specific antigen-driven AICD (Yang, Vacchio, and Ashwell 1993), AICD induced by crosslinking TCRs, or AICD induced by combining phorbol esters with calcium ionophores (Iwata et al. 1992). It was later demonstrated that a RARα-selective agonist (CD336) protected thymocytes from anti-CD3-mediated AICD *in vivo*, reversing the 50% thymic weight loss observed in mice one day after injection of anti-CD3 antibodies (Szondy et al. 1998). Interestingly however, CD336 did not mount any inhibiting effect on AICD induced by the superantigen staphylococcal enterotoxin A, and this difference was correlated to the diminished induction of Bim and Nurr77 in thymocytes from superantigen-treated mice (Szegezdi et al. 2003).

10.4.1.4.2 Role of Retinoic Acid in Death of Mature T-Cells

In contrast to thymocytes that readily undergo spontaneous apoptosis in culture, mature resting T-cells in culture are resistant to apoptosis due to their high expression of Bcl-2 proteins and low expression of death receptors like Fas (Ashwell, Lu, and Vacchio 2000; Marrack and Kappler 2004). Upon activation of mature T-cells, the cells can undergo apoptosis by two main mechanisms (i.e., by activated T-cell autonomous death [ACAD] or by AICD [Krammer, Arnold, and Lavrik 2007; Engedal 2011]). ACAD is the process that ensures the efficient contraction of clonally expanded T-cells that occurs when the antigen is cleared after antigen-induced proliferation. The process appears to involve induction of the intrinsic apoptotic pathway due to diminishing levels of cytokine-mediated survival signals (Hildeman et al. 2002). AICD is induced directly by TCR signaling, and occurs when already expanded mature T-cells are reactivated. The process involves Fas-mediated cell death and is considered to have a role in eliminating autoreactive T-cells as well as in limiting the clonal expansion of T-cells at the end of an acute immune response (Krammer, Arnold, and Lavrik 2007). During the primary activation of T-cells, both the death receptor Fas and its ligand (FasL) are induced, but rapid cell death is prevented by the concomitant anti-apoptotic signals induced by TCR signaling (Engedal 2011). AICD is induced upon reactivation of the cells, due to lack of these anti-apoptotic signals.

It is believed that long-term peripheral survival of mature T-cells requires continual low-affinity MHC interactions and cytokines, or else they will die by neglect (Hildeman et al. 2002). Our lab could show that whereas the slow rate of spontaneous death of cultured T-cells was unaffected by retinoic acid, retinoic acid prevented ACAD of stimulated T-cells via a RAR-dependent induction of IL-2 (Engedal, Ertesvag, and Blomhoff 2004). The retinoic acid–mediated inhibition of ACAD in normal T-cells supported earlier studies on the effects of oral administration of retinoic acid to HIV patients, showing that retinoic acid inhibited the *ex vivo* death of their cultured peripheral blood mononuclear cells (PBMCs) (Yang et al. 1995). However, PBMCs contain a significant fraction of B-cells, and retinoic acid has been shown to reduce the spontaneous death of B-cells (Lomo et al. 1998). It was therefore assuring that retinoic acid also was able to inhibit the spontaneous death of CD4+ T-cells from HIV-infected individuals (Szondy et al. 1998).

When it comes to elucidating the effects of vitamin A on AICD of normal mature T-cells, surprisingly little has been done. To our knowledge, only one study has addressed this issue. Hence, Yang and coworkers prestimulated PBMCs in a two-step procedure with concanavalin A and IL-2, followed by anti-CD3 stimulation to induce AICD. Retinoic acid was demonstrated to inhibit AICD in a concentration-dependent manner (Yang et al. 1995). Related studies on the effects of retinoic acid on AICD have been performed on either CD3-activated T-cell hybridoma cell lines or the T-cell leukemia cell line Jurkat. In a comprehensive summary of these studies, the conclusion was that 9-cis retinoic acid seems to be more efficient than all-trans retinoic acid to inhibit AICD (Engedal 2011). Furthermore, it has been shown that the retinoic acid–mediated inhibition of AICD involves downregulation of FasL (Yang et al. 1995; Szondy et al. 1998).

As noted, in many of the reports on retinoic acid and T-cell death, 9-cis retinoic acid appears to be more potent than all-trans retinoic acid. As mentioned earlier, it should however be emphasized that although 9-cis retinoic acid can easily be formed *in vitro*, the *in vivo* existence of this metabolite is yet to be conclusively proven. Furthermore, available data indicate that 9-cis retinoic acid is not likely to be the major physiological ligand for RXR (Wolf 2006; Blomhoff and Blomhoff 2006). Clearly, more studies are required before we can conclude whether or not the reported effects of 9-cis retinoic acid on T-cell death is of physiological relevance.

10.4.2   B-CELLS

B-cell progenitors arise from hematopoietic stem cells in the bone marrow and progress through well-defined stages of development before leaving the bone marrow as immature B-cells expressing cell surface IgM. The immature B-cells will in turn populate secondary lymphoid organs to develop into B-cell subsets that may respond to T-cell-dependent or independent antigens (LeBien 2000; LeBien and Tedder 2008). Upon proper stimulation, naive B-cells will evolve into memory B-cells populating secondary lymphoid organs or into long-lived plasma cells primarily residing in the bone marrow.

10.4.2.1   Retinoic Acid and B-Cell Development

Kincade and coworkers discovered that retinoids are rate limiting for B lymphopoiesis in adult bone marrow. Hence, they found that all-trans retinoic acid (hereafter named RA) accelerated B-cell development in adult bone marrow of C57BL/6 mice by shortening the maturation time concomitant with the enhanced expression of the transcription factors Pax5 and Ebf1 (Chen et al. 2008). The same group later showed that both VAD and a RAR antagonist tended to slow down B lymphopoiesis, consistent with contribution of RA to this process (Chen, Welner, and Kincade 2009). It was therefore surprising that adding RA to cultures of fetal lymphoid progenitors reduced the differentiation of these cells, possibly via a mechanism involving downregulation of the transcription factor Ebf1. The authors suggested that these somewhat conflicting results could be due to the well-established differences between fetal and adult B lymphopoiesis and also due to the fetal precursors being pre-exposed to RA during embryogenesis. However, in line with the previous finding that RA inhibits the expansion of normal human and murine B-cell precursors (Fahlman et al. 1995), the Kincade group had in their previous study shown that sustained high ($>10^{-7}$ M) levels of RA also inhibited the differentiation of adult B-cell progenitors (Chen et al. 2008). As suggested by Chen and coworkers, it therefore appears that RA concentrations should be kept within a critical range to support adult B lymphopoiesis (Chen, Welner, and Kincade 2009), and furthermore that any suppression of B lymphopoiesis in patients extensively treated with retinoids might be fully reversible.

10.4.2.2   Proliferation of Mature B-Cells Regulated by RA

Given the established view that vitamin A protects against infections and strengthens the immune system, it came as a surprise to the research field when it was demonstrated that RA inhibited B-cell receptor (BCR)–mediated stimulation of normal peripheral blood B-cells (Blomhoff et al. 1992; Naderi and Blomhoff 1999). The B-cells were arrested in the G0/G1 phase of the cell cycle via RA-mediated reduced levels of cyclin E and A concomitant with transient induction of the CDK inhibitor p21[cip] resulting in reduced phosphorylation of pRB (Naderi and Blomhoff 1999). Later, the inhibitory effect of RA on peripheral blood B-cells was confirmed on EBV-immortalized

B-cells (Dolcetti et al. 1998), as well as on human tonsillar B-cells and murine splenic B-cells *in vitro* (Morikawa and Nonaka 2005). Interestingly however, it was shown that although RA reduced the proliferation of B-cells stimulated via BCR, CD38, or CD40, RA simultaneously enriched the population of cells with more differentiated phenotypes like AID, Blimp1, CD138, and sIgG1 (Chen and Ross 2005, 2007).

It should be emphasized that not all B-cell proliferation is inhibited by RA. It was shown that, whereas RA diminishes proliferation of BCR-stimulated human peripheral blood B-cells, the proliferative response is enhanced by RA when the cells are stimulated via toll-like receptor (TLR) 9 in the presence or absence of another member of the TLR family, RP105 (Ertesvag et al. 2007; Eriksen et al. 2012). The proliferative effect of RA was particularly strong in CD27+ memory B-cells, and involved RAR-mediated induction of IL-10, as well as of cyclin D3 resulting in phosphorylation of pRB (Ertesvag et al. 2007). Thus, the effects of RA seem to depend on both the B-cell subset and the way the cells are stimulated (see Figure 10.2). Future studies are required to establish whether it is the B-cell subset (naive or memory B-cell compartment) *per se* or the stimulus itself that determines how RA will affect B-cell proliferation. However, our finding that stimulating the same purified subset of naive peripheral blood B-cells either via BCR or TLR9 results in inhibition versus stimulation of proliferation (Ertesvag et al. 2007) suggests that the mode of stimulation is particularly important.

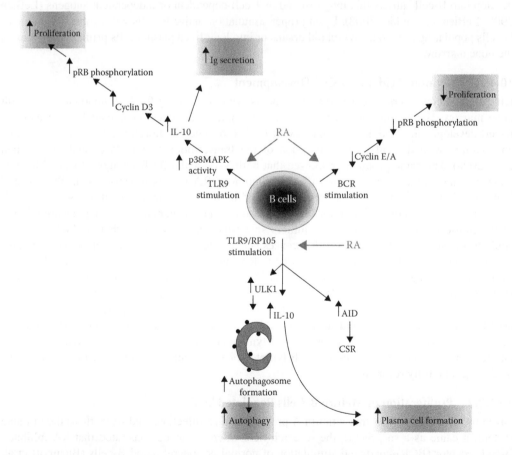

FIGURE 10.2 Vitamin A and B-cell functions. All-trans retinoic acid (RA) enhances or inhibits proliferation of primary human B-cells depending on whether the cells are stimulated via toll like receptor 9 (TLR9) and RP105 or via the B-cell receptor (BCR). RA will induce AID-mediated class switch recombination (CSR) in TLR9/RP105-stimulated B-cells, and it will also promote Ig production and plasma cell formation in a process that involves ULK1-mediated autophagy and IL-10.

10.4.2.3 The Role of RA in Antibody Production

10.4.2.3.1 In Vivo Antibody Responses

Antigens can be classified as either T-cell-dependent (TD) or T-cell-independent type 1 or 2 (TI-1 or TI-2). Most antigens are T-cell dependent, meaning that T-cell help is required for maximal antibody production. TI-1 responses are typically elicited by TLR ligands like LPS (for TLR4) and bacterial DNA (for TLR9), whereas TI-2 responses are provoked by repetitive forms of antigens on the surface of pathogens, typically polysaccharides crosslinking the BCRs. Numerous *in vivo* studies have demonstrated reduced antibody responses to TD- and TI-2 antigens in VAD animals, and that vitamin A supplementation can restore or increase the antibody responses in such animals (for a comprehensive review, see Ross, Chen, and Ma 2009). Optimal TD antibody responses require at least three signals generated by the pathogens: signals generated by binding of Ag to its receptor (signal 1), costimulatory signals provided by T-cells (signal 2), and TLR stimulation as signal 3 (Ruprecht and Lanzavecchia 2006). Interestingly, RA might provide a fourth signal for a stronger and longer-acting antibody response (Ross, Chen, and Ma 2009). Hence, studies by Ross and coworkers have demonstrated that antibody responses to TD antigens like tetanus toxoid (TT) can be greatly improved in adult mice by combining RA with the synthetic TLR3 ligand polyriboinosinic:polyribocytidylic acid (PIC) (Ma, Chen, and Ross 2005). Given the high susceptibility of neonates to developing VAD and infections (Adkins, Leclerc, and Marshall-Clarke 2004), the demonstrated benefit of early life treatment of neonatal mice with RA and PIC for eliciting anti-TT responses appears as particularly significant (Ma and Ross 2005).

10.4.2.3.2 In Vitro Activation and Differentiation of B-cells

The most described pathway of B-cell activation and differentiation is the germinal center (GC) reaction. During a primary immune response, cells challenged with a certain antigen will undergo a strong proliferative burst and receive signals from cells located in the GCs, such as follicular dendritic cells and T-cells. The B-cells will undergo somatic hypermutation (SHM) and class switch recombination (CSR) as part of the GC reaction. Eventually, some of the B-cells will undergo differentiation into high-affinity memory B-cells, or alternatively, the activated B-cells may differentiate into high-affinity, antibody-secreting plasma cells (Shapiro-Shelef and Calame 2005; Tarlinton et al. 2008). Cells of the memory B-cell compartment can persist for a long time after infection or vaccination, and the memory B-cell pool is maintained by the periodic reexposure to antigens and possibly also by polyclonal activation via TLRs like TLR9 (Bernasconi, Traggiai, and Lanzavecchia 2002). The ability of RA to enhance TLR9/RP105-mediated proliferation and Ig production in B-cells (Ertesvag et al. 2007; Eriksen et al. 2012; Indrevaer et al. 2013) might be important for keeping up a repertoire of circulating polyclonal memory B-cells.

The GC reactions and plasma cell development are most often sequential events, and they appear to involve two distinct regulatory protein networks (Shapiro-Shelef and Calame 2005; Tarlinton et al. 2008). Whereas the formation and function of plasma cells depend on a set of transcription factors that include IRF4, Blimp1, and XBP1 (Shapiro-Shelef and Calame 2005; Todd et al. 2009; Klein et al. 2006), the GC reactions require the transcription factors BCL6, Pax5, and BACH2, as well as the enzyme activation-induced deaminase (AID) (Shapiro-Shelef and Calame 2005). The transcription factors regulate the expression of each other in a complex regulatory network, functioning as transcriptional repressors or enhancers to stabilize one of the two cellular programs (Shapiro-Shelef and Calame 2005).

Upon stimulation of murine B-cells via BCR, CD38, or CD40, physiological levels of RA were shown to reduce the level of Pax5 concomitant with increased levels of Blimp1 and AID. Consequently, the cells expressed higher levels of sIgG1 and the plasma cell marker CD138 (Chen and Ross 2005, 2007). A similar increased expression of both AID and Igs was found when human peripheral blood B-cells were stimulated via the TLR9 and RP105 in the presence of RA (Indrevaer et al. 2013). The ability of RA to induce AID, and hence CSR, may not only regulate the magnitude of the antibody response, but it can also drive the production of antibodies towards certain Ig sub-classes. Hence, the important role of RA in mucosal immunity has been underlined by its ability to promote class switching to IgA in the presence of different stimuli (Tokuyama and Tokuyama 1999; Watanabe et al. 2010). Upon stimulation of B-cells with CD40 and IL-4, however, enhanced switching into IgG types of antibodies, concomitant with reduced production of IgE, was reported (Worm et al. 1998; Chen and Ross 2007; Scheffel et al. 2005), supporting the notion that RA has a role in balancing the production of specific Ig subclasses.

10.4.2.3.3 RA-Mediated Regulation of Autophagy

Autophagy is a self-digestive process aimed at degradation and recycling of cytoplasmic components. The process is highly conserved and involves bulk degradation of cytoplasmic elements like damaged organelles, microbes, and long-lived proteins through their sequestration into a double-membraned vesicle, the autophagosome. The role of autophagy in the immune system is an emerging field of research, involving immune responses like antigen presentation, microbe removal, and lymphocyte activation (Deretic 2011; Deretic, Saitoh, and Akira 2013; Levine, Mizushima, and Virgin 2011; Liu et al. 2013). A particularly crucial role for autophagy in humoral immunity has recently been linked to generation and maintenance of plasma cells (Pengo and Cenci 2013; Pengo et al. 2013; Conway et al. 2013). Hence, whereas Conway and coworkers concluded that antibody-specific responses to TNP-CGG or *H. polygyrus* larvae was severely impaired in autophagy-deficient murine B-cells, Pengo and coworkers demonstrated that both TD and TI antibody responses were reduced in autophagy-deficient (Atg5fl/fl CD19-Cre) mice. We recently revealed that physiological levels of RA noticeably enhance autophagy in TLR9/RP105-stimulated human peripheral blood B-cells (Eriksen et al. 2015a). The effect of RA on Ig production was at least partly exerted via increased transcription of the gene encoding the autophagy-inducing protein Unc-51-like kinase 1 (ULK1), and we identified a putative RARE/RXRE in the ULK1 gene. We believe that by demonstrating a critical role of RA in promoting autophagy in human peripheral blood B-cells, we have ident-ified a novel mechanism whereby vitamin A exerts its important role in the immune system (see Figure 10.2).

10.4.3 THE ROLE OF RETINOL AND RETRO-RETINOIDS IN LYMPHOCYTE FUNCTIONS

Although RA is considered the most important vitamin A metabolite in lymphoid cells, other vitamin A metabolites have also been reported to regulate immune cells. As for most retinoids, RA contains five double bonds between carbon atoms 5-6, 7-8, 9-19, 11-12, and 13-14. However, under certain conditions the positions of these double bonds may shift, forming biologically active retinoids called retro-retinoids. Anhydroretinol was the first retro-retinoid to be identified, and this compound is formed from retinol in various cell types (Bhat et al. 1979). 14-hydroxy-4,14-retro-retinol (14-HRR) was later identified as an essential cofactor for growth and activation of B- and T-cells (Buck et al. 1990, 1991; Garbe, Buck, and Hammerling 1992), and anhydroretinol was reported to inhibit the growth-promoting effects of 14-HRR (Buck et al. 1993). Interestingly, nearly all cell types have the ability to convert RA to HRR, and together with 13,14-dihydroxy-retinol, shown to support lymphocyte viability (Derguini et al. 1995), these retro-reinoids have been suggested to bind to and act via the serine/threonine kinases cRaf and PKC (Imam et al. 2001).

10.5 CLINICAL ASPECTS OF VITAMIN A IN IMMUNE-RELATED DISEASES

Vitamin A metabolites have been proven to be beneficial in inflammatory conditions like acne and neonatal bronchopulmonary dysplasia (Reifen 2002), as well as for psoriasis (van de Kerkhof 2006). There have also been promising results of synthetic retinoids for treatment of rheumatic diseases based on experimental animal models, but only a few incomplete studies have been performed on rheumatic patients (Miyabe, Miyabe, and Nanki 2015). It is well established that vitamin A supplementation decreases childhood mortality in areas of the world with widespread vitamin A deficiency, and that most of the deaths related to vitamin A deficiency are infectious diseases like measles and diarrhea (Stephensen 2001) (see also Chapter 11). On the other hand, it is also clear that infectious diseases like measles, diarrhea, respiratory infections, and HIV increase the risk of developing vitamin A deficiencies by decreasing intake and absorption and increasing excretion (Stephensen 2001). There have been attempts to correlate low serum retinol levels to HIV severity, but it appears that vitamin A supplementation does not directly improve HIV-specific immunity but rather diminishes the severity of opportunistic infections in HIV patients in populations at risk of vitamin A deficiency (Stephensen 2001).

Reduced serum levels of vitamin A have also been reported in patients with common variable immunodeficiency (CVID) (Aukrust et al. 2000; Kilic et al. 2005; dos Santos-Valente et al. 2012), and vitamin A supplementation to CVID patients was shown to improve IgG secretion from PBMCs collected from these patients (Aukrust et al. 2000). CVID patients are characterized by severely reduced levels of serum IgG and recurrent infections (Cunningham-Rundles 2010; Cunningham-Rundles and Bodian 1999), and it is therefore not established if the reduced vitamin A level in these patients is the cause of infections or vice versa. The etiology of CVID is not yet established, but several studies have attempted to elucidate the mechanisms causing CVID-derived symptoms. An interesting feature of CVID-derived B-cells is their impaired ability to respond to TLR9 and RP105 activation *in vitro* (Yu et al. 2009; Cunningham-Rundles et al. 2006; Yamazaki et al. 2010). Based on the previously demonstrated positive effects of RA on TLR9/RP105-activated B-cells (Ertesvag et al. 2007; Eriksen et al. 2012), we addressed the possibility of RA being able to improve defective immune responses in CVID-derived B-cells. It was shown that pharmacological concentrations (100 nM) of RA nearly restored defective TLR9/RP105-mediated proliferation and induction of IL-10 secretion in the patient-derived B-cells (Indrevaer et al. 2013). Furthermore, it was demonstrated that the diminished IgG production in CVID B-cells was linked to defective AID-mediated Ig switching, and the IgG levels in most of the patient-derived B-cells only were partially restored by RA (Indrevaer et al. 2013).

Interestingly, diminished TLR9-responses (Hirotani et al. 2010) and reduced serum levels of retinol (Besler, Comoglu, and Okcu 2002; Loken-Amsrud et al. 2013; Fragoso, Stoney, and McCaffery 2014) have also been associated with multiple sclerosis (MS) patients. There has been an increasing awareness of the role of B-cells in the pathogenesis of MS (Disanto et al. 2012), based for instance on the reduced ratio between the anti-inflammatory cytokine IL-10 and the proinflammatory cytokine TNF-α in MS-derived B-cells (Duddy et al. 2007; Hirotani et al. 2010; Knippenberg et al. 2011). Our recent observation that RA markedly enhances the IL-10/TNF-α ratio in B-cells from MS patients—even in patients receiving treatment with common anti-MS drugs like glatiramer acetate or IFN-β-1b (Eriksen et al. 2015b)—supports the growing attention to potential beneficial effects of vitamin A supplementation in treatment of MS (Fragoso, Stoney, and McCaffery 2014; Jafarirad et al. 2012; Torkildsen et al. 2013).

10.6 CONCLUDING REMARKS

It is evident that vitamin A has a vital role in the immune system, and that RA is important both for formation of an effective immune system—even influenced by the vitamin A status of the pregnant mother—and in prevention of inflammatory diseases. These differential functions of RA are mediated via distinct cells in the immune system, and it is still not known if graded concentrations of RA in the various lymphoid organs or target cells might contribute to the multitude of effects seen. Vitamin A supplementation of children 6–59 months in areas of the world with high risk of VAD is recommended by WHO to reduce morbidity and mortality due to infectious diseases. Although many open questions remain, vitamin A metabolites and synthetic retinoids have great potential in clinical settings to combat inflammatory diseases. The documented capacity of RA to direct gut-homing T- and B-cells to the intestine might aid in the development of strategies for mucosal vaccination, and intranasal vitamin A supplementation in vitamin A–deficient populations might improve mucosal immune responses towards respiratory pathogens and vaccines. The ability of RA to support TLR-mediated immune responses such as induction of IgG and anti-inflammatory IL-10 in B-cells supports clinical trials combining TLR-ligands and vitamin A metabolites to treat immune disorders. The TLR9 ligands CpG-ODNs have been extensively tested as vaccine adjuvants, and these synthetic oligonucleotides are also in clinical trials as adjuvants in cancer treatment. However, discrepancies between promising *in vitro/ex vivo* results and disappointing effects on patients when it comes to vitamin A supplementation should encourage more emphasis to be put on how—and in which form—vitamin A should be administered in clinical trials. At what dose and at which interval should the retinoid be administered? Therapeutic concentration of RA, as for instance used in treatment of acute promyelocytic leukemia, might cause "RA syndrome," as a result of toxic and even lethal levels of RA. Furthermore, it is not easy to predict which of the retinoic acid isomers, all-trans-, 13-cis, or 9-cis RA, will turn out to be most efficient in a certain clinical setting. Would perhaps one of the many synthetic forms of retinoids be preferable for the patients? Evidently, we lack a lot of knowledge to be able to conclude we have a comprehensive picture of how vitamin A supports immunity and how we can exploit this knowledge to combat inflammatory conditions and treat diseases related to the immune system.

REFERENCES

Adkins, B., C. Leclerc, and S. Marshall-Clarke. 2004. Neonatal adaptive immunity comes of age. *Nat Rev Immunol* 4 (7):553–64.

Ashwell, J. D., F. W. Lu, and M. S. Vacchio. 2000. Glucocorticoids in T cell development and function*. *Annu Rev Immunol* 18:309–45.

Aukrust, P., F. Muller, T. Ueland et al. 2000. Decreased vitamin A levels in common variable immunodeficiency: Vitamin A supplementation in vivo enhances immunoglobulin production and downregulates inflammatory responses. *Eur J Clin Invest* 30 (3):252–9.

Balmer, J. E. and R. Blomhoff. 2002. Gene expression regulation by retinoic acid. *J Lipid Res* 43 (11):1773–808.

Balmer, J. E. and R. Blomhoff. 2005. A robust characterization of retinoic acid response elements based on a comparison of sites in three species. *J Steroid Biochem Mol Biol* 96 (5):347–54.

Barclay, A. J., A. Foster, and A. Sommer. 1987. *Vitamin A supplements and mortality related to measles: A randomised clinical trial.* Br Med J (Clin Res Ed) 294 (6567):294–6.

Barua, A. B. and N. Sidell. 2004. Retinoyl beta-glucuronide: A biologically active interesting retinoid. *J Nutr* 134 (1):286S–9S.

Bayon, Y., M. A. Ortiz, F. J. Lopez-Hernandez et al. 2003. Inhibition of IkappaB kinase by a new class of retinoid-related anticancer agents that induce apoptosis. *Mol Cell Biol* 23 (3):1061–74.

Beijer, M. R., G. Kraal, and J. M. den Haan. 2014. Vitamin A and dendritic cell differentiation. *Immunology* 142 (1):39–45.

Bernasconi, N. L., E. Traggiai, and A. Lanzavecchia. 2002. Maintenance of serological memory by polyclonal activation of human memory B cells. *Science* 298 (5601):2199–202.

Besler, H. T., S. Comoglu, and Z. Okcu. 2002. Serum levels of antioxidant vitamins and lipid peroxidation in multiple sclerosis. *Nutr Neurosci* 5 (3):215–20.

Bettelli, E., Y. Carrier, W. Gao et al. 2006. Reciprocal developmental pathways for the generation of pathogenic effector TH17 and regulatory T cells. *Nature* 441 (7090):235–8.

Bhat, P. V., L. M. De Luca, S. Adamo et al. 1979. Retinoid metabolism in spontaneously transformed mouse fibroblasts (Balb/c 3T12-3 cells): Enzymatic conversion of retinol to anhydroretinol. *J Lipid Res* 20 (3):357–62.

Biesalski, H. K. 1989. Comparative assessment of the toxicology of vitamin A and retinoids in man. *Toxicology* 57 (2):117–61.

Blomhoff, R. and H. K. Blomhoff. 2006. Overview of retinoid metabolism and function. *J Neurobiol* 66 (7):606–30.

Blomhoff, R., M. H. Green, T. Berg et al. 1990. Transport and storage of vitamin A. *Science* 250 (4979):399–404.

Blomhoff, H. K., E. B. Smeland, B. Erikstein et al. 1992. Vitamin A is a key regulator for cell growth, cytokine production, and differentiation in normal B cells. *J Biol Chem* 267 (33):23988–92.

Brown, C. C., D. Esterhazy, A. Sarde et al. 2015. Retinoic acid is essential for Th1 cell lineage stability and prevents transition to a Th17 cell program. *Immunity* 42 (3):499–511.

Brown, C. C. and R. J. Noelle. 2015. Seeing through the dark: New insights into the immune regulatory functions of vitamin A. *Eur J Immunol* 45 (5):1287–95.

Buck, J., F. Derguini, E. Levi et al. 1991. Intracellular signaling by 14-hydroxy-4,14-retro-retinol. *Science* 254 (5038):1654–6.

Buck, J., F. Grun, F. Derguini et al. 1993. Anhydroretinol: A naturally occurring inhibitor of lymphocyte physiology. *J Exp Med* 178 (2):675–80.

Buck, J., G. Ritter, L. Dannecker et al. 1990. Retinol is essential for growth of activated human B cells. *J Exp Med* 171 (5):1613–24.

Cantorna, M. T., F. E. Nashold, and C. E. Hayes. 1994. In vitamin A deficiency multiple mechanisms establish a regulatory T helper cell imbalance with excess Th1 and insufficient Th2 function. *J Immunol* 152 (4):1515–22.

Cha, H. R., S. Y. Chang, J. H. Chang et al. 2010. Downregulation of Th17 cells in the small intestine by disruption of gut flora in the absence of retinoic acid. *J Immunol* 184 (12):6799–806.

Chandra, R. K. 1988. Increased bacterial binding to respiratory epithelial cells in vitamin A deficiency. *BMJ* 297 (6652):834–5.

Chen, X., B. L. Esplin, K. P. Garrett et al. 2008. Retinoids accelerate B lineage lymphoid differentiation. *J Immunol* 180 (1):138–45.

Chen, Q. and A. C. Ross. 2005. Vitamin A and immune function: Retinoic acid modulates population dynamics in antigen receptor and CD38-stimulated splenic B cells. *Proc Natl Acad Sci U S A* 102 (40):14142–9.

Chen, Q. and A. C. Ross. 2007. Retinoic acid promotes mouse splenic B cell surface IgG expression and maturation stimulated by CD40 and IL-4. *Cell Immunol* 249 (1):37–45.

Chen, X., R. S. Welner, and P. W. Kincade. 2009. A possible contribution of retinoids to regulation of fetal B lymphopoiesis. *Eur J Immunol* 39 (9):2515–24.

Cho, H. Y., E. K. Choi, S. W. Lee et al. 2011. All-trans retinoic acid induces TLR-5 expression and cell differentiation and promotes flagellin-mediated cell functions in human THP-1 cells. *Immunol Lett* 136 (1):97–107.

Conway, K. L., P. Kuballa, B. Khor et al. 2013. ATG5 regulates plasma cell differentiation. *Autophagy* 9 (4):528–37.

Cunningham-Rundles, C. 2010. How I treat common variable immune deficiency. *Blood* 116 (1):7–15.

Cunningham-Rundles, C. and C. Bodian. 1999. Common variable immunodeficiency: Clinical and immunological features of 248 patients. *Clin Immunol* 92 (1):34–48.

Cunningham-Rundles, C., L. Radigan, A. K. Knight et al. 2006. TLR9 activation is defective in common variable immune deficiency. *J Immunol* 176 (3):1978–87.

D'Ambrosio, D. N., R. D. Clugston, and W. S. Blaner. 2011. Vitamin A metabolism: An update. *Nutrients* 3 (1):63–103.

DePaolo, R. W., V. Abadie, F. Tang et al. 2011. Co-adjuvant effects of retinoic acid and IL-15 induce inflammatory immunity to dietary antigens. *Nature* 471 (7337):220–4.

Deretic, V. 2011. Autophagy in immunity and cell-autonomous defense against intracellular microbes. *Immunol Rev* 240 (1):92–104.

Deretic, V., T. Saitoh, and S. Akira. 2013. Autophagy in infection, inflammation and immunity. *Nat Rev Immunol* 13 (10):722–37.

Derguini, F., K. Nakanishi, U. Hammerling et al. 1995. 13,14-Dihydroxy-retinol, a new bioactive retinol metabolite. *J Biol Chem* 270 (32):18875–80.

Diefenbach, A., M. Colonna, and S. Koyasu. 2014. Development, differentiation, and diversity of innate lymphoid cells. *Immunity* 41 (3):354–65.

Disanto, G., J. M. Morahan, M. H. Barnett et al. 2012. The evidence for a role of B cells in multiple sclerosis. *Neurology* 78 (11):823–32.

Dolcetti, R., P. Zancai, R. Cariati et al. 1998. In vitro effects of retinoids on the proliferation and differentiation features of Epstein-Barr virus-immortalized B lymphocytes. *Leuk Lymphoma* 29 (3–4):269–81.

dos Santos-Valente, E. C., R. da Silva, M. I. de Moraes-Pinto et al. 2012. Assessment of nutritional status: Vitamin A and zinc in patients with common variable immunodeficiency. *J Investig Allergol Clin Immunol* 22 (6):427–31.

Duddy, M., M. Niino, F. Adatia et al. 2007. Distinct effector cytokine profiles of memory and naive human B cell subsets and implication in multiple sclerosis. *J Immunol* 178 (10):6092–9.

Eberl, G. 2014. Immunology: A is for immunity. *Nature* 508 (7494):47–8.

Eberl, G., S. Marmon, M. J. Sunshine et al. 2004. An essential function for the nuclear receptor RORgamma(t) in the generation of fetal lymphoid tissue inducer cells. *Nat Immunol* 5 (1):64–73.

Engedal, N. 2011. Immune regulator vitamin A and T cell death. *Vitam Horm* 86:153–78.

Engedal, N., A. Ertesvag, and H. K. Blomhoff. 2004. Survival of activated human T lymphocytes is promoted by retinoic acid via induction of IL-2. *Int Immunol* 16 (3):443–53.

Eriksen, A. B., T. Berge, M. W. Gustavsen et al. 2015b. Retinoic acid enhances the levels of IL-10 in TLR-stimulated B cells from patients with relapsing-remitting multiple sclerosis. *J Neuroimmunol* 278:11–8.

Eriksen, A. B., R. L. Indrevaer, K. L. Holm et al. 2012. TLR9-signaling is required for turning retinoic acid into a potent stimulator of RP105 (CD180)-mediated proliferation and IgG synthesis in human memory B cells. *Cell Immunol* 279 (1):87–95.

Eriksen, A. B., M. L. Torgersen, K. L. Holm et al. 2015a. Retinoic acid-induced IgG production in TLR-activated human primary B cells involves ULK1-mediated autophagy. *Autophagy* 11 (3):460–71.

Ertesvag, A., H. C. Aasheim, S. Naderi et al. 2007. Vitamin A potentiates CpG-mediated memory B-cell proliferation and differentiation: Involvement of early activation of p38MAPK. *Blood* 109 (9):3865–72.

Ertesvag, A., N. Engedal, S. Naderi et al. 2002. Retinoic acid stimulates the cell cycle machinery in normal T cells: Involvement of retinoic acid receptor-mediated IL-2 secretion. *J Immunol* 169 (10):5555–63.

Fahlman, C., S. E. Jacobsen, E. B. Smeland et al. 1995. All-trans- and 9-cis-retinoic acid inhibit growth of normal human and murine B cell precursors. *J Immunol* 155 (1):58–65.

Feng, T., Y. Cong, K. Alexander et al. 2012. Regulation of toll-like receptor 5 gene expression and function on mucosal dendritic cells. *PLOS ONE* 7 (4):e35918.

Fragoso, Y. D., P. N. Stoney, and P. J. McCaffery. 2014. The evidence for a beneficial role of vitamin A in multiple sclerosis. *CNS Drugs* 28 (4):291–9.

Frota-Ruchon, A., M. Marcinkiewicz, and P. V. Bhat. 2000. Localization of retinal dehydrogenase type 1 in the stomach and intestine. *Cell Tissue Res* 302 (3):397–400.

Garbe, A., J. Buck, and U. Hammerling. 1992. Retinoids are important cofactors in T cell activation. *J Exp Med* 176 (1):109–17.

Giguere, V., E. S. Ong, P. Segui et al. 1987. Identification of a receptor for the morphogen retinoic acid. *Nature* 330 (6149):624–9.

Green, H. N. and E. Mellanby. 1928. Vitamin a as an anti-infective agent. *Br Med J* 2 (3537):691–6.

Hall, J. A., J. L. Cannons, J. R. Grainger et al. 2011. Essential role for retinoic acid in the promotion of CD4(+) T cell effector responses via retinoic acid receptor alpha. *Immunity* 34 (3):435–47.

Hamann, A., D. P. Andrew, D. Jablonski-Westrich et al. 1994. Role of alpha 4-integrins in lymphocyte homing to mucosal tissues in vivo. *J Immunol* 152 (7):3282–93.

Harrison, E. H. 2005. Mechanisms of digestion and absorption of dietary vitamin A. *Annu Rev Nutr* 25:87–103.

Hathcock, J. N., D. G. Hattan, M. Y. Jenkins et al. 1990. Evaluation of vitamin A toxicity. *Am J Clin Nutr* 52 (2):183–202.

Hildeman, D. A., Y. Zhu, T. C. Mitchell et al. 2002. Molecular mechanisms of activated T cell death in vivo. *Curr Opin Immunol* 14 (3):354–9.

Hirotani, M., M. Niino, T. Fukazawa et al. 2010. Decreased IL-10 production mediated by toll-like receptor 9 in B cells in multiple sclerosis. *J Neuroimmunol* 221 (1–2):95–100.

Hoag, K. A., F. E. Nashold, J. Goverman et al. 2002. Retinoic acid enhances the T helper 2 cell development that is essential for robust antibody responses through its action on antigen-presenting cells. *J Nutr* 132 (12):3736–9.

Hussey, G. D. and M. Klein. 1990. A randomized, controlled trial of vitamin A in children with severe measles. *N Engl J Med* 323 (3):160–4.

Imam, A., B. Hoyos, C. Swenson et al. 2001. Retinoids as ligands and coactivators of protein kinase C alpha. *FASEB J* 15 (1):28–30.

Indrevaer, R. L., K. L. Holm, P. Aukrust et al. 2013. Retinoic acid improves defective TLR9/RP105-induced immune responses in common variable immunodeficiency-derived B cells. *J Immunol* 191 (7):3624–33.

Iwata, M. 2009. Retinoic acid production by intestinal dendritic cells and its role in T-cell trafficking. *Semin Immunol* 21 (1):8–13.

Iwata, M., Y. Eshima, and H. Kagechika. 2003. Retinoic acids exert direct effects on T cells to suppress Th1 development and enhance Th2 development via retinoic acid receptors. *Int Immunol* 15 (8):1017–25.

Iwata, M., A. Hirakiyama, Y. Eshima et al. 2004. Retinoic acid imprints gut-homing specificity on T cells. *Immunity* 21 (4):527–38.

Iwata, M., M. Mukai, Y. Nakai et al. 1992. Retinoic acids inhibit activation-induced apoptosis in T cell hybridomas and thymocytes. *J Immunol* 149 (10):3302–8.

Jafarirad, S., F. Siassi, M. H. Harirchian et al. 2012. The effect of vitamin A supplementation on stimulated T-cell proliferation with myelin oligodendrocyte glycoprotein in patients with multiple sclerosis. *J Neurosci Rural Pract* 3 (3):294–8.

Kamei, Y., L. Xu, T. Heinzel et al. 1996. A CBP integrator complex mediates transcriptional activation and AP-1 inhibition by nuclear receptors. *Cell* 85 (3):403–14.

Kang, S. G., H. W. Lim, O. M. Andrisani et al. 2007. Vitamin A metabolites induce gut-homing FoxP3+ regulatory T cells. *J Immunol* 179 (6):3724–33.

Kang, S. G., C. Wang, S. Matsumoto et al. 2009. High and low vitamin A therapies induce distinct FoxP3+ T-cell subsets and effectively control intestinal inflammation. *Gastroenterology* 137 (4):1391–402.

Kilic, S. S., E. Y. Kezer, Y. O. Ilcol et al. 2005. Vitamin A deficiency in patients with common variable immunodeficiency. *J Clin Immunol* 25 (3):275–80.

Kim, C. H. 2011. Retinoic acid, immunity, and inflammation. *Vitam Horm* 86:83–101.

Kim, J., M. T. Ochoa, S. R. Krutzik et al. 2002. Activation of toll-like receptor 2 in acne triggers inflammatory cytokine responses. *J Immunol* 169 (3):1535–41.

Kiss, I., R. Ruhl, E. Szegezdi et al. 2008. Retinoid receptor-activating ligands are produced within the mouse thymus during postnatal development. *Eur J Immunol* 38 (1):147–55.

Klein, U., S. Casola, G. Cattoretti et al. 2006. Transcription factor IRF4 controls plasma cell differentiation and class-switch recombination. *Nat Immunol* 7 (7):773–82.

Klein, L., B. Kyewski, P. M. Allen et al. 2014. Positive and negative selection of the T cell repertoire: What thymocytes see (and don't see). *Nat Rev Immunol* 14 (6):377–91.

Knippenberg, S., E. Peelen, J. Smolders et al. 2011. Reduction in IL-10 producing B cells (Breg) in multiple sclerosis is accompanied by a reduced naive/memory Breg ratio during a relapse but not in remission. *J Neuroimmunol* 239 (1–2):80–6.

Krammer, P. H., R. Arnold, and I. N. Lavrik. 2007. Life and death in peripheral T cells. *Nat Rev Immunol* 7 (7):532–42.

LeBien, T. W. 2000. Fates of human B-cell precursors. *Blood* 96 (1):9–23.

LeBien, T. W. and T. F. Tedder. 2008. B lymphocytes: How they develop and function. *Blood* 112 (5):1570–80.

Levine, B., N. Mizushima, and H. W. Virgin. 2011. Autophagy in immunity and inflammation. *Nature* 469 (7330):323–35.

Liu, G., Y. Bi, R. Wang, and X. Wang. 2013. Self-eating and self-defense: Autophagy controls innate immunity and adaptive immunity. *J Leukoc Biol* 93 (4):511–9.

Liu, P. T., S. R. Krutzik, J. Kim et al. 2005. Cutting edge: All-trans retinoic acid down-regulates TLR2 expression and function. *J Immunol* 174 (5):2467–70.

Loken-Amsrud, K. I., K. M. Myhr, S. J. Bakke et al. 2013. Retinol levels are associated with magnetic resonance imaging outcomes in multiple sclerosis. *Mult Scler* 19 (4):451–7.

Lomo, J., E. B. Smeland, S. Ulven et al. 1998. RAR-, not RXR, ligands inhibit cell activation and prevent apoptosis in B-lymphocytes. *J Cell Physiol* 175 (1):68–77.

Ma, Y., Q. Chen, and A. C. Ross. 2005. Retinoic acid and polyriboinosinic:polyribocytidylic acid stimulate robust anti-tetanus antibody production while differentially regulating type 1/type 2 cytokines and lymphocyte populations. *J Immunol* 174 (12):7961–9.

Ma, Y. and A. C. Ross. 2005. The anti-tetanus immune response of neonatal mice is augmented by retinoic acid combined with polyriboinosinic:polyribocytidylic acid. *Proc Natl Acad Sci U S A* 102 (38):13556–61.

Marrack, P. and J. Kappler. 2004. Control of T cell viability. *Annu Rev Immunol* 22:765–87.

McKenzie, A. N., H. Spits, and G. Eberl. 2014. Innate lymphoid cells in inflammation and immunity. *Immunity* 41 (3):366–74.

Mebius, R. E., P. Rennert, and I. L. Weissman. 1997. Developing lymph nodes collect CD4+CD3- LTbeta+ cells that can differentiate to APC, NK cells, and follicular cells but not T or B cells. *Immunity* 7 (4):493–504.

Melhus, H., K. Michaelsson, A. Kindmark et al. 1998. Excessive dietary intake of vitamin A is associated with reduced bone mineral density and increased risk for hip fracture. *Ann Intern Med* 129 (10):770–8.

Mielke, L. A., S. A. Jones, M. Raverdeau et al. 2013. Retinoic acid expression associates with enhanced IL-22 production by gammadelta T cells and innate lymphoid cells and attenuation of intestinal inflammation. *J Exp Med* 210 (6):1117–24.

Mitchison, N. A. 2004. T-cell-B-cell cooperation. *Nat Rev Immunol* 4 (4):308–12.

Miyabe, Y., C. Miyabe, and T. Nanki. 2015. Could retinoids be a potential treatment for rheumatic diseases? *Rheumatol Int* 35 (1):35–41.

Miyasaka, M. and T. Tanaka. 2004. Lymphocyte trafficking across high endothelial venules: Dogmas and enigmas. *Nat Rev Immunol* 4 (5):360–70.

Mora, J. R., M. R. Bono, N. Manjunath et al. 2003. Selective imprinting of gut-homing T cells by Peyer's patch dendritic cells. *Nature* 424 (6944):88–93.

Mora, J. R., M. Iwata, B. Eksteen et al. 2006. Generation of gut-homing IgA-secreting B cells by intestinal dendritic cells. *Science* 314 (5802):1157–60.

Mora, J. R. and U. H. von Andrian. 2009. Role of retinoic acid in the imprinting of gut-homing IgA-secreting cells. *Semin Immunol* 21 (1):28–35.

Morikawa, K. and M. Nonaka. 2005. All-trans-retinoic acid accelerates the differentiation of human B lymphocytes maturing into plasma cells. *Int Immunopharmacol* 5 (13–14):1830–8.

Mucida, D., Y. Park, and H. Cheroutre. 2009. From the diet to the nucleus: Vitamin A and TGF-beta join efforts at the mucosal interface of the intestine. *Semin Immunol* 21 (1):14–21.

Mucida, D., Y. Park, G. Kim et al. 2007. Reciprocal TH17 and regulatory T cell differentiation mediated by retinoic acid. *Science* 317 (5835):256–60.

Na, S. Y., B. Y. Kang, S. W. Chung et al. 1999. Retinoids inhibit interleukin-12 production in macrophages through physical associations of retinoid X receptor and NFkappaB. *J Biol Chem* 274 (12):7674–80.

Naderi, S. and H. K. Blomhoff. 1999. Retinoic acid prevents phosphorylation of pRB in normal human B lymphocytes: Regulation of cyclin E, cyclin A, and p21(Cip1). *Blood* 94 (4):1348–58.

Nagao, A. 2004. Oxidative conversion of carotenoids to retinoids and other products. *J Nutr* 134 (1):237S–40S.

Niederreither, K. and P. Dolle. 2008. Retinoic acid in development: Towards an integrated view. *Nat Rev Genet* 9 (7):541–53.

Nikawa, T., M. Ikemoto, M. Kano et al. 2001. Impaired vitamin A-mediated mucosal IgA response in IL-5 receptor-knockout mice. *Biochem Biophys Res Commun* 285 (2):546–9.

Nolting, J., C. Daniel, S. Reuter et al. 2009. Retinoic acid can enhance conversion of naive into regulatory T cells independently of secreted cytokines. *J Exp Med* 206 (10):2131–9.

Ochoa, W. F., A. Torrecillas, I. Fita et al. 2003. Retinoic acid binds to the C2-domain of protein kinase C(alpha). *Biochemistry* 42 (29):8774–9.

O'Neill, L. A., D. Golenbock, and A. G. Bowie. 2013. The history of toll-like receptors—redefining innate immunity. *Nat Rev Immunol* 13 (6):453–60.

Paik, J., S. Vogel, L. Quadro et al. 2004. Vitamin A: Overlapping delivery pathways to tissues from the circulation. *J Nutr* 134 (1):276S–80S.

Paul, W. E. 2011. Bridging innate and adaptive immunity. *Cell* 147 (6):1212–5.

Pengo, N. and S. Cenci. 2013. The role of autophagy in plasma cell ontogenesis. *Autophagy* 9 (6):942–4.

Pengo, N., M. Scolari, L. Oliva et al. 2013. Plasma cells require autophagy for sustainable immunoglobulin production. *Nat Immunol* 14 (3):298–305.

Petkovich, M., N. J. Brand, A. Krust et al. 1987. A human retinoic acid receptor which belongs to the family of nuclear receptors. *Nature* 330 (6147):444–50.

Piccirillo, C. A. 2008. Regulatory T cells in health and disease. *Cytokine* 43 (3):395–401.

Pino-Lagos, K., Y. Guo, C. Brown et al. 2011. A retinoic acid-dependent checkpoint in the development of CD4+ T cell-mediated immunity. *J Exp Med* 208 (9):1767–75.

Racke, M. K., D. Burnett, S. H. Pak et al. 1995. Retinoid treatment of experimental allergic encephalomyelitis. IL-4 production correlates with improved disease course. *J Immunol* 154 (1):450–8.

Radominska-Pandya, A., G. Chen, P. J. Czernik et al. 2000. Direct interaction of all-trans-retinoic acid with protein kinase C (PKC). Implications for PKC signaling and cancer therapy. *J Biol Chem* 275 (29):22324–30.

Rajawat, Y., Z. Hilioti, and I. Bossis. 2011. Retinoic acid induces autophagosome maturation through redistribution of the cation-independent mannose-6-phosphate receptor. *Antioxid Redox Signal* 14 (11):2165–77.

Raverdeau, M. and K. H. Mills. 2014. Modulation of T cell and innate immune responses by retinoic acid. *J Immunol* 192 (7):2953–8.

Reifen, R. 2002. Vitamin A as an anti-inflammatory agent. *Proc Nutr Soc* 61 (3):397–400.

Ross, A. C. 2007. Vitamin A supplementation and retinoic acid treatment in the regulation of antibody responses in vivo. *Vitam Horm* 75:197–222.

Ross, A. C., Q. Chen, and Y. Ma. 2009. Augmentation of antibody responses by retinoic acid and costimulatory molecules. *Semin Immunol* 21 (1):42–50.

Ross, S. A., P. J. McCaffery, U. C. Drager et al. 2000. Retinoids in embryonal development. *Physiol Rev* 80 (3):1021–54.

Rothman, K. J., L. L. Moore, M. R. Singer et al. 1995. Teratogenicity of high vitamin A intake. *N Engl J Med* 333 (21):1369–73.

Rudraraju, R., B. G. Jones, S. L. Surman et al. 2014. Respiratory tract epithelial cells express retinaldehyde dehydrogenase ALDH1A and enhance IgA production by stimulated B cells in the presence of vitamin A. *PLOS ONE* 9 (1):e86554.

Ruprecht, C. R. and A. Lanzavecchia. 2006. Toll-like receptor stimulation as a third signal required for activation of human naive B cells. *Eur J Immunol* 36 (4):810–6.

Scheffel, F., G. Heine, B. M. Henz et al. 2005. Retinoic acid inhibits CD40 plus IL-4 mediated IgE production through alterations of sCD23, sCD54 and IL-6 production. *Inflamm Res* 54 (3):113–8.

Schule, R., P. Rangarajan, N. Yang et al. 1991. Retinoic acid is a negative regulator of AP-1-responsive genes. *Proc Natl Acad Sci U S A* 88 (14):6092–6.

Semba, R. D. 1994. Vitamin A, immunity, and infection. *Clin Infect Dis* 19 (3):489–99.

Semba, R. D. 1998. The role of vitamin A and related retinoids in immune function. *Nutr Rev* 56 (1 Pt 2):S38–48.

Shapiro-Shelef, M. and K. Calame. 2005. Regulation of plasma-cell development. *Nat Rev Immunol* 5 (3):230–42.

Shoda, R., D. Mahalanabis, M. A. Wahed et al. 1995. Bacterial translocation in the rat model of lectin induced diarrhoea. *Gut* 36 (3):379–81.

Siggs, O. M., L. E. Makaroff, and A. Liston. 2006. The why and how of thymocyte negative selection. *Curr Opin Immunol* 18 (2):175–83.

Sommer, A. 2008. Vitamin A deficiency and clinical disease: An historical overview. *J Nutr* 138 (10):1835–9.

Soprano, D. R., P. Qin, and K. J. Soprano. 2004. Retinoic acid receptors and cancers. *Annu Rev Nutr* 24:201–21.

Spencer, S. P., C. Wilhelm, Q. Yang et al. 2014. Adaptation of innate lymphoid cells to a micronutrient deficiency promotes type 2 barrier immunity. *Science* 343 (6169):432–7.

Spits, H. and J. P. Di Santo. 2011. The expanding family of innate lymphoid cells: Regulators and effectors of immunity and tissue remodeling. *Nat Immunol* 12 (1):21–7.

Stephensen, C. B. 2001. Vitamin A, infection, and immune function. *Annu Rev Nutr* 21:167–92.

Sun, C. M., J. A. Hall, R. B. Blank, N et al. 2007. Small intestine lamina propria dendritic cells promote de novo generation of Foxp3 T reg cells via retinoic acid. *J Exp Med* 204 (8):1775–85.

Svensson, M., J. Marsal, A. Ericsson et al. 2002. CCL25 mediates the localization of recently activated CD8alphabeta(+) lymphocytes to the small-intestinal mucosa. *J Clin Invest* 110 (8):1113–21.

Szanto, A., V. Narkar, Q. Shen et al. 2004. Retinoid X receptors: X-ploring their (patho)physiological functions. *Cell Death Differ* 11 (Suppl 2):S1261–43.

Szegezdi, E., I. Kiss, A. Simon et al. 2003. Ligation of retinoic acid receptor alpha regulates negative selection of thymocytes by inhibiting both DNA binding of nur77 and synthesis of bim. *J Immunol* 170 (7):3577–84.

Szondy, Z., U. Reichert, J. M. Bernardon et al. 1998. Inhibition of activation-induced apoptosis of thymocytes by all-trans- and 9-cis-retinoic acid is mediated via retinoic acid receptor alpha. *Biochem J* 331 (Pt 3):767–74.

Tarlinton, D., A. Radbruch, F. Hiepe et al. 2008. Plasma cell differentiation and survival. *Curr Opin Immunol* 20 (2):162–9.

Thaller, C. and G. Eichele. 1987. Identification and spatial distribution of retinoids in the developing chick limb bud. *Nature* 327 (6123):625–8.

Todd, D. J., L. J. McHeyzer-Williams, C. Kowal et al. 2009. XBP1 governs late events in plasma cell differentiation and is not required for antigen-specific memory B cell development. *J Exp Med* 206 (10):2151–9.

Tokuyama, Y. and H. Tokuyama. 1996. Retinoids as Ig isotype-switch modulators. The role of retinoids in directing isotype switching to IgA and IgG1 (IgE) in association with IL-4 and IL-5. *Cell Immunol* 170 (2):230–4.

Tokuyama, H. and Y. Tokuyama. 1999. The regulatory effects of all-trans-retinoic acid on isotype switching: Retinoic acid induces IgA switch rearrangement in cooperation with IL-5 and inhibits IgG1 switching. *Cell Immunol* 192 (1):41–7.

Torkildsen, O., K. I. Loken-Amsrud, S. Wergeland et al. 2013. Fat-soluble vitamins as disease modulators in multiple sclerosis. *Acta Neurol Scand Suppl* 127(196):16–23.

van de Kerkhof, P. C. 2006. Update on retinoid therapy of psoriasis in: An update on the use of retinoids in dermatology. *Dermatol Ther* 19 (5):252–63.

van de Pavert, S. A., M. Ferreira, R. G. Domingues et al. 2014. Maternal retinoids control type 3 innate lymphoid cells and set the offspring immunity. *Nature* 508 (7494):123–7.

Veldhoen, M., R. J. Hocking, C. J. Atkins et al. 2006. TGFbeta in the context of an inflammatory cytokine milieu supports de novo differentiation of IL-17-producing T cells. *Immunity* 24 (2):179–89.

Vowels, B. R., S. Yang, and J. J. Leyden. 1995. Induction of proinflammatory cytokines by a soluble factor of Propionibacterium acnes: Implications for chronic inflammatory acne. *Infect Immun* 63 (8):3158–65.

Watanabe, K., M. Sugai, Y. Nambu et al. 2010. Requirement for Runx proteins in IgA class switching acting downstream of TGF-beta 1 and retinoic acid signaling. *J Immunol* 184 (6):2785–92.

Wei, L. N. 2003. Retinoid receptors and their coregulators. *Annu Rev Pharmacol Toxicol* 43:47–72.

Westerlund, M., A. C. Belin, M. R. Felder et al. 2007. High and complementary expression patterns of alcohol and aldehyde dehydrogenases in the gastrointestinal tract: Implications for Parkinson's disease. *FEBS J* 274 (5):1212–23.

WHO. 2011. *Guideline: Vitamin A Supplementation in Infants and Children 6–59 Months of Age*. Geneva: World Health Organization.

Wiedermann, U., L. A. Hanson, T. Bremell et al. 1995. Increased translocation of Escherichia coli and development of arthritis in vitamin A-deficient rats. *Infect Immun* 63 (8):3062–8.

Wolf, G. 2006. Is 9-cis-retinoic acid the endogenous ligand for the retinoic acid-X receptor? *Nutr Rev* 64 (12):532–8.

Worm, M., J. M. Krah, R. A. Manz et al. 1998. Retinoic acid inhibits CD40 + interleukin-4-mediated IgE production in vitro. *Blood* 92 (5):1713–20.

Wyss, R. and F. Bucheli. 1997. Determination of endogenous levels of 13-cis-retinoic acid (isotretinoin), all-trans-retinoic acid (tretinoin) and their 4-oxo metabolites in human and animal plasma by high-performance liquid chromatography with automated column switching and ultraviolet detection. *J Chromatogr B Biomed Sci Appl* 700 (1–2):31–47.

Xiao, S., H. Jin, T. Korn et al. 2008. Retinoic acid increases Foxp3+ regulatory T cells and inhibits development of Th17 cells by enhancing TGF-beta-driven Smad3 signaling and inhibiting IL-6 and IL-23 receptor expression. *J Immunol* 181 (4):2277–84.

Yamazaki, K., T. Yamazaki, S. Taki et al. 2010. Potentiation of TLR9 responses for human naive B-cell growth through RP105 signaling. *Clin Immunol* 135 (1):125–36.

Yang, Y., J. Bailey, M. S. Vacchio et al. 1995. Retinoic acid inhibition of ex vivo human immunodeficiency virus-associated apoptosis of peripheral blood cells. *Proc Natl Acad Sci U S A* 92 (7):3051–5.

Yang, Y., M. S. Vacchio, and J. D. Ashwell. 1993. 9-cis-retinoic acid inhibits activation-driven T-cell apoptosis: Implications for retinoid X receptor involvement in thymocyte development. *Proc Natl Acad Sci U S A* 90 (13):6170–4.

Yu, J. E., A. K. Knight, L. Radigan et al. 2009. Toll-like receptor 7 and 9 defects in common variable immunodeficiency. *J Allergy Clin Immunol* 124 (2):349–56.

11 Vitamin A, Immunity, and Infection

Charles B. Stephensen

CONTENTS

11.1 Historical Overview: Vitamin A in the Twentieth Century 181
11.2 Barriers to Infection: Vitamin A and Epithelial Surfaces... 182
11.3 Vitamin A and Innate Immune Cells... 183
    11.3.1 Overview.. 183
    11.3.2 Vitamin A and Granulocyte Development and Function 183
    11.3.3 Vitamin A and Macrophage Development and Function...................................... 184
    11.3.4 Vitamin A and Dendritic Cell Development and Function 186
    11.3.5 Vitamin A and Innate Lymphoid Cell Development and Function...................... 187
11.4 Vitamin A and Adaptive Immune Cells... 188
    11.4.1 Overview.. 188
    11.4.2 Vitamin A and Thymic Function.. 188
    11.4.3 Vitamin A and T-Cell Development and Function... 189
    11.4.4 Vitamin A, B-Cells, and Antibody Responses 190
    11.4.5 Vitamin A and Mucosal Targeting of Lymphocytes... 190
11.5 Conclusions.. 190
References... 191

11.1 HISTORICAL OVERVIEW: VITAMIN A IN THE TWENTIETH CENTURY

Vitamin A is essential for many biological functions, including maintaining growth and vision. These activities were first described as an "essential factor" in milk in 1913. This factor was eventually identified as vitamin A (Semba 2012b), and the vitamin was first synthesized in 1947 (Eggersdorfer et al. 2012). In 1928 vitamin A was also recognized as having anti-infective properties (Green and Mellanby 1928; Semba 2012c). This activity was of great interest to physicians concerned with the prevention and treatment of infectious diseases in the early twentieth century, particularly because antibiotics were not yet available. Clinical trials conducted at that time evaluated the use of vitamin A in treating infectious diseases of childhood, including measles, with mixed results. Interest in the anti-infective activity of vitamin A waned with the introduction of antibiotics (Semba 2012a, 1999).

Through most of the twentieth century, treatment of vitamin A deficiency in the clinical setting or in public health practice was focused on the treatment and prevention of blindness due to xerophthalmia, the principal clinical manifestation of vitamin A deficiency (Sommer 1982, 2014). It was well known for many decades that vitamin A deficiency was associated with an increased risk of death from infectious diseases, as described in a comprehensive review in 1968 (Scrimshaw, Taylor, and Gordon 1968). However, it was not until 1986 and later that community intervention trials demonstrated that vitamin A supplementation could substantially decrease mortality from infectious diseases, particularly deaths associated with diarrhea and measles, in young children at risk of vitamin A deficiency living in settings with high mortality rates from infectious diseases (Sommer et al. 1986; Imdad et al. 2010). These findings led to the formulation of guidelines by the World Health Organization for the use of vitamin A supplementation in children from 6 to 59 months of age to decrease mortality (WHO 2011a, b, c). More recently, vitamin A supplementation was assessed during the neonatal period in three additional community trials and similar benefits were not found in decreasing the risk of death from infectious diseases below 6 months of age (Edmond et al. 2015; Masanja et al. 2015; Mazumder et al. 2015; Haider and Bhutta 2015).

In 1986 when a decade of work examining the effects of vitamin A supplementation on preventing deaths from infectious diseases was just beginning, the molecular mechanism-of-action by which vitamin A improved survival was unknown. Vitamin A, or retinol, has no significant biological activity itself, and retinaldehyde was long known to be the key molecule mediating the action of vitamin A in the visual cycle but was not felt to have other significant biological activities (Sommer 1982). In 1987, however, two laboratories described how retinoic acid, the second principal metabolite of vitamin A, regulated gene transcription by binding to the retinoic acid receptor (RAR) (Benbrook et al. 2014; Giguere et al. 1987; Petkovich et al. 1987). This work enabled description at the molecular level of how vitamin A functioned in the immune system, as well as other tissues, by regulating the transcription of hundreds of genes (Benbrook et al. 2014). As discussed below, this finding led to a great deal of work on how vitamin A is metabolized to retinoic acid in the immune system where it acts as an autocrine and paracrine factor affecting the development, differentiation, function, and survival of many cell types in the immune system (Guo et al. 2015).

11.2 BARRIERS TO INFECTION: VITAMIN A AND EPITHELIAL SURFACES

Epithelial surfaces, including the skin and mucosal epithelium in the respiratory, intestinal, and urogenital tracts, are important barriers to infection. These surfaces also have innate immune capacities that allow active responses to microorganisms (Moens and Veldhoen 2012). Vitamin A deficiency does not have a pronounced effect on diminishing the barrier function of the skin and the normal keratinized, squamous epithelial surface of the skin develops without any activity of retinoic acid (at least in its late stages). Retinoic acid can inhibit keratinization of the skin and topical application of retinoic acid, and synthetic retinoids are used in dermatology for "reverse aging" by increasing the proliferation of basal cells (Hubbard, Unger, and Rohrich 2014; Sporn, Roberts, and Goodman 1994). Appropriate basal cell proliferation is, of course, needed to maintain the long-term integrity of the skin.

Vitamin A is required for prenatal lung development, including development of airway epithelium and normal alveolar and airway structure (Biesalski and Nohr 2003). Normal airway epithelium consists of ciliated columnar or cuboidal epithelium interspersed with mucus-secreting goblet cells. Premature birth occurring before the lung maturation process is complete can result in the development of a life-threatening lung disease, bronchopulmonary dysplasia (BPD). This disease is exacerbated by the typically low stores of vitamin A found in the liver of premature infants (Olson, Gunning, and Tilton 1984) and can be treated, to a degree, with vitamin A therapy (Guimaraes et al. 2012). Squamous metaplasia of the airways can develop postnatally in animals and humans with vitamin A deficiency and, in particular, when another environmental factor (e.g., respiratory infection, cigarette smoke) causes damage to the airway epithelium. This damage triggers repair and may thus unmask vitamin A deficiency by creating a higher demand for retinoic acid during tissue regeneration. The metaplasia resulting from this process in the presence of vitamin A deficiency is often localized, occurring at the site of the injury to the respiratory epithelium (Stephensen et al. 1993). Squamous metaplasia developing at these sites may increase the risk of opportunistic infections of the respiratory tract. For example, bacteria are typically removed from airways after being trapped in the mucus blanket that overlays the ciliated epithelial cells. Action of the cilia moves the mucus and bacteria up and out of the airways. Areas of squamous metaplasia lack this protective mechanism and may be colonized by bacteria. This process has been described in a previous review (Stephensen 2001).

Vitamin A deficiency has long been known to affect the eye, including its associated epithelial surfaces, resulting in the cardinal sign of deficiency, xerophthalmia (Sommer 1982). Xerophthalmia involves squamous metaplasia of the corneal and conjunctival epithelium, thus compromising the normal secretory function and production of a protective mucus layer by these tissues (Kim et al.

2012). Such corneal lesions may increase the risk or severity of corneal infections that could result in the loss of vision due to the development of punctate keratosis that can occur as a result of xerophthalmia (Bhaskaram et al. 1986).

Vitamin A deficiency also affects the intestinal epithelium. While squamous metaplasia is typically not seen, goblet cell number may be decreased though other histological aspects (e.g., crypt depth and villus length) may appear normal (Olson, Rojanapo, and Lamb 1981; Ahmed, Jones, and Jackson 1990). However, an infectious challenge may produce pathologic changes in vitamin A–deficient but not control animals. For example, during experimental rotavirus infection intestinal villi were severely damage by infection in the deficient but not control mice, suggesting regeneration is impaired by deficiency (Ahmed, Jones, and Jackson 1990). Translocation of intestinal bacteria from the gut lumen to other tissues may also be enhanced by vitamin A deficiency in some experimental models (Kozakova et al. 2003). Such changes may account for the apparent disruption of epithelial integrity seen in children living in settings with poor environmental hygiene that appears to be corrected by vitamin A supplementation (McCullough, Northrop-Clewes, and Thurnham 1999).

11.3 VITAMIN A AND INNATE IMMUNE CELLS

11.3.1 OVERVIEW

The innate immune system is comprised of barrier defenses that typically involve the response of a class of leukocytes termed myeloid cells, in contrast to the lymphoid cells, which comprise the principal cellular component of the adaptive immune system. Myeloid cells develop in the bone marrow and include neutrophils, eosinophils, and basophils (termed granulocytes), which are seen in peripheral blood and in tissues during inflammation. Monocytes are another myeloid cell type seen in blood. When monocytes enter tissues, they differentiate into macrophages. Dendritic cells are another myeloid cell found in blood and tissues.

11.3.2 VITAMIN A AND GRANULOCYTE DEVELOPMENT AND FUNCTION

Neutrophils are the most abundant granulocytes (and leukocytes) in peripheral blood. They develop in the bone marrow in response to innate and environmentally derived signals, with production increasing as a result of increased need. In response to a local infection, neutrophils leave the bloodstream to perform their essential effector function, killing microorganisms, typically bacteria and sometimes fungi, via phagocytosis and oxidative killing in phagocytic vesicles. Extracellular killing and the release of soluble mediators (e.g., IL-1β and leukotrienes) is also part of the neutrophil's response (Murphy et al. 2011).

During hematopoiesis in the bone marrow, the granulocytes (neutrophils, eosinophils, and basophils), and monocytes, which circulate in the blood before developing into macrophages in tissues, develop from a common progenitor cell. Retinoic acid acts via RARα (Kastner and Chan 2001) during this process to promote development of neutrophils rather than eosinophils and basophils (Paul et al. 1995; Leber and Denburg 1997; Kinoshita et al. 2000; Denburg, Sehmi, and Upham 2001; Upham et al. 2002), or monocytes (Lawson and Berliner 1999). However, vitamin A deficiency in animal models increases rather than decreases the concentration of neutrophils in peripheral blood (Nauss, Mark, and Suskind 1979; Twining et al. 1996a; Zhao and Ross 1995), though the neutrophils in blood appear to have been released from the bone marrow in an immature state, based on the hypersegmented appearance of their nuclei (Twining et al. 1996a). The function of neutrophils is also impaired by vitamin A deficiency, as shown by decreased production of factors involved in bacterial killing such as cathepsin G (Twining et al. 1996b), decreased chemotaxis, decreased phagocytic activity, decreased oxidative burst, and, as a result, a decreased ability to kill bacteria and clear them from the blood (Ongsakul, Sirisinha, and Lamb 1985; Twining et al. 1997; Wiedermann et al. 1996b). The net effect of vitamin A deficiency thus appears to be a decrease in the protective ability of the neutrophilic response to infection due to impaired development and function of neutrophils. The increased concentration of neutrophils in peripheral blood in vitamin A–deficient animals may result from the development of subclinical infections, the resulting increased inflammation relative to vitamin A adequate controls (Wiedermann et al. 1996a), and the likely increase in production of mediators (e.g., granulocyte colony-stimulating factor or perhaps IL-17A), which would act at the level of the bone marrow to increase production of neutrophils as a result of an increased need.

While eosinophil development is not enhanced and may be impeded by retinoic acid, as discussed above, eosinophilic inflammation may be enhanced by high dietary levels of vitamin A, as has been seen in the mouse ovalbumin-induced model of eosinophilic pulmonary inflammation (Schuster, Kenyon, and Stephensen 2008), a model used to examine some aspects of atopic asthma in humans. This enhancement could be due to the ability of retinoic acid to increase the expression of the receptor for eotaxin, CCR3, on eosinophils (Ueki et al. 2013), which could increase their chemotactic ability and thus their accumulation in tissue sites where eotaxin is produced (e.g., the lungs of mice treated with ovalbumin). Retinoic acid also inhibits eosinophil apoptosis (Ueki et al. 2008), which could prolong eosinophil residence in inflamed tissues. However, the accumulation of eosinophils in the ovalbumin model of asthma could be due to the underlying effects of vitamin A on enhancing the development of Th2 cells, which is discussed below, rather than to direct effects on eosinophils. The importance of T-cells is suggested by an experiment that stimulated pulmonary inflammation involving both neutrophils and eosinophils using inert particles, which would not induce a memory T-cell response (Torii et al. 2004). In this case, treatment of mice receiving normal dietary levels of vitamin A with additional vitamin A via injection reduced the eosinophilic and neutrophilic pulmonary inflammation in this model system. The authors speculate that inhibition of the NF-κB pathway in inflammatory cells in the lungs, which was also observed in the study, was the underlying reason for the anti-inflammatory effect of vitamin A treatment. These contrasting results with two different types of granulocytic inflammation in the lungs of mice demonstrate that it is difficult to predict the effect of vitamin A on inflammatory conditions, even ones that are quite similar, because vitamin A has many different activities in the immune system.

11.3.3 VITAMIN A AND MACROPHAGE DEVELOPMENT AND FUNCTION

Tissue macrophages are phagocytic cells that respond to microbial infections and other causes of tissue injury (e.g., autoimmune disease, cellular damage leading to development of plaque in coronaries). Macrophages may ingest and kill bacteria (e.g., *Mycobacterium tuberculosis*) but also play a role in clearing damaged host cells during inflammation. Macrophages may also act as antigen-presenting cells if they upregulate expression of proteins involved in presentation of antigen to T-cells, such as MHCI and MHCII. Tissue macrophages derive primarily from monocytes that enter tissues from the blood, but macrophage progenitor cells may also be found in some tissues (Murphy et al. 2011).

While neutrophil development is enhanced by vitamin A, macrophage development is not. Early work has shown that monocyte/macrophage development from progenitor cells is inhibited by retinoic acid (Januszewicz and Cooper 1984; Ozawa et al. 1984). In addition, retinoic acid treatment decreases the survival of peripheral blood monocytes *ex vivo* by decreasing macrophage colony-stimulating factor (MCSF) production by these cells, and also decreased differentiation of monocytes to macrophages (Kreutz et al. 1998). Retinoic acid also inhibits Fc-γ receptor expression on macrophages differentiated from peripheral blood monocytes (Rhodes and Oliver 1980). Expression of this receptor allows phagocytosis of IgG-coated microorganisms. In addition, retinoic acid inhibits the production of the oxidative metabolites superoxide anion (O_2-) and hydrogen peroxide (H_2O_2) by activated human macrophages, which are involved in killing microorganisms ingested by macrophages (Wolfson et al. 1988). Thus, the effects of retinoic acid treatment *ex vivo* can dampen the antimicrobial activity of macrophages.

In addition to decreasing some aspects of macrophage development and phagocytic activity, retinoic acid treatment of human skin has been shown to decrease expression of MHCII (HLA-DR) by macrophages following UV treatment, and also to decrease autologous and allogeneic T-cell reactivity, as would be expected as a result of decreased MHC expression (Meunier, Voorhees, and Cooper 1996). Retinoic acid also downregulates the expression of CD1d (Chen and Ross 2007), a surface molecule on macrophages that presents glycolipid antigens to T-cells, consistent with its downregulation of MHC expression, which presents classic peptide antigens. Thus, retinoic acid treatment can decrease the antigen-presenting function of macrophages, which could decrease the development of adaptive immune responses.

Retinoic acid can also decrease the production of pro-inflammatory cytokines by macrophages. Early work showed that retinoic acid inhibits the production of TNF-α and nitric oxide by murine peritoneal macrophages (Mehta et al. 1994). This same effect was seen in a human macrophage cell line (THP-1) and in cord blood–derived mononuclear cells, where production of the anti-inflammatory cytokine IL-10 was increased by retinoic acid in the same experiments (Wang, Allen, and Ballow 2007). Retinoic acid also inhibited production of TNF-α in rat peripheral blood monocytes and production of the prostaglandin-producing enzyme COX-2 in rat macrophages (Kim, Kang, and Lee 2004), consistent with a dampening effect of vitamin A on monocyte/macrophage-induced inflammatory activity. *Ex vivo* treatment of bone marrow–derived macrophages and a macrophage cell line with retinol, which is presumably converted to retinoic acid by these cells, decreases expression of several proinflammatory cytokines and chemokines (including TNF-α, IL-6, IL-12, IP-10, and CXCL9) (Kim et al. 2013).

While retinoic acid can decrease TNF-α production in macrophages, the role of specific RARs in this process is not clear. For example, production of TNF-α as well as IL-6 and IL-12 were all lower in macrophages from RARγ knockout mice, suggesting a role for retinoic acid and this receptor in enhancing the inflammatory activity of macrophages under some circumstances (Dzhagalov, Chambon, and He 2007). Retinoic acid receptors (both RARs and RXRs) act to directly regulate transcription by binding to retinoic-acid response elements (RARE) but work in murine splenic macrophages shows that RXR also interacts directly with the transcription factor NF-κB to decrease IL-12 production following LPS stimulation, indicating a second pathway for regulation of macrophage development (Na et al. 1999). Retinoic acid has also been shown to inhibit NF-κB activity in a human monocyte cell line and in vivo using NF-κB reporter mice (Austenaa et al. 2009). The ability of retinoic acid to decrease transcription of proinflammatory genes, such as IL-12 and TNF-α, may result in higher levels of inflammation in vitamin A–deficient animals during experimental infections, as discussed in an earlier review (Stephensen 2001).

The effect of retinoic acid on macrophage gene expression is not entirely anti-inflammatory. In *ex vivo* cultures of human alveolar macrophages, retinoic acid increased production of IL-1β and decreased IL-1 receptor antagonist (IL-1ra) production indicating that vitamin A can enhance the proinflammatory activity of this particular type of macrophage (Hashimoto et al. 1998). However, in a murine macrophage cell line (J774) retinoic acid decreased IL-1β production (Mathew and Sharma 2000). Retinoic acid also induces prostaglandin-E synthase in macrophages, resulting in increased PGE$_2$ synthesis. This process was seen in classically activated macrophages (induced from peripheral blood monocytes stimulated with M-CSF) but was much less pronounced in alternatively activated macrophages (induced with M-CSF plus IL-13) (Mamidi et al. 2012). While many studies on macrophage function in disease are carried out in model systems, a recent study in humans has shown that macrophages isolated from the intestinal tissue of patients with Crohn's disease produce retinoic acid that is associated with greater antigen-presenting ability and higher production of TNF-α, indicating that retinoic acid production in this inflammatory milieu is promoting, rather than dampening, inflammation (Sanders et al. 2014).

Recent work has shown that not all tissue macrophages are equal. Macrophages from different body sites develop distinct patterns of gene expression as a result of tissue-dependent factors affecting macrophage differentiation. For example, large peritoneal macrophages show a distinct pattern of gene expression that is dependent on the transcription factor GATA-6. The expression of GATA-6 itself is induced by retinoic acid apparently derived from omental fat-associated cells. Retinoic acid, along with other omental-derived factors, is thus a key regulator of the development of large peritoneal macrophages. One of the functions of these macrophages is to promote the development of IgA-producing B-1 cells in the peritoneal cavity via the production of TGF-β. These cells express the gut-homing receptors CCR9 and α4β7 integrin (the expression of which is induced by retinoic acid, as discussed below) and thus migrate to the intestinal lymphoid tissue where they secrete IgA, which is transported into the intestinal lumen where it provides important early responses to gut pathogens (Okabe and Medzhitov 2014).

While many *ex vivo* studies show that retinoic acid can dampen some aspects of macrophage function, *in vivo* studies may show different effects, perhaps as a result of the impact of physiologic factors (e.g., resulting from an ongoing infection in an animal model system) not completely reproduced in cell culture experiments. For example, high levels of vitamin A can increase the phagocytic and tumoricidal activities of rat alveolar macrophages (Tachibana et al. 1984). Peritoneal and splenic macrophages of rats treated with high levels of vitamin A had greater phagocytic activity (both percent of cells ingesting yeast particles and mean number of yeast ingested per cell) than did macrophages from control rats. The vitamin A–treated rats also had lower levels of *Salmonella* in both the liver and spleen after intraperitoneal infection (Hatchigian et al. 1989). In chickens, dietary vitamin A deficiency impaired the oxidative burst and phagocytosis of yeast particles by macrophages (Sijtsma et al. 1991). Thus, vitamin A deficiency *in vivo* tends to impair antimicrobial aspects of macrophage function, suggesting that impaired macrophage function may be one factor that can lead to impaired host resistance to infection during vitamin A deficiency.

11.3.4 VITAMIN A AND DENDRITIC CELL DEVELOPMENT AND FUNCTION

Dendritic cells of the innate immune system are also phagocytic cells. They take up microorganisms, particles, and soluble molecules by phagocytosis and pinocytosis. While dendritic cells kill ingested microorganisms, their more important role is transporting antigen from peripheral tissues, via the lymphatic circulation, to draining lymph nodes where they present antigen to lymphocytes to initiate the adaptive immune response. Dendritic cells are not the only cell type that can play the role of an antigen-presenting cell (APC), but they are particularly important in the development of naive T-cells into effector and memory T-cells. This role involves the presentation of antigen plus costimulation (e.g., from cell-surface molecules such as B7/CD86 on the APC, which interacts with CD28 on the surface of a naive T-cell) to ensure that the stimulated T-cells divide and survive. A third signal presented by APCs consists of cytokines, which stimulate T-cell differentiation. For example, IL-12 stimulates naive T-cells to develop into Th1 cells, IL-4 stimulates the development of Th2 cells, and IL-6 plus TGF-β stimulates the development of Th17 cells (Murphy et al. 2011). Some subsets of dendritic cells can also produce retinoic acid, which affects T-cell development in a variety of ways, as discussed below. CD103[+] dendritic cells in the gut, for example, typically produce retinoic acid which influences development of immune responses at that anatomical site (Guo et al. 2015).

The effects of vitamin A on dendritic cell development is often studied *ex vivo*, by stimulation of human peripheral blood monocytes with retinoic acid and, depending on the experiment, appropriate cytokines (e.g., granulocyte-macrophage colony-stimulating factor [GM-CSF] or IL-4). While results can vary with specific conditions, the effect of retinoic acid on dendritic cell development is often similar to what is described above for macrophages: expression of costimulatory molecules is decreased, reducing the ability of dendritic cells to stimulate T-cell proliferation and initiate adaptive immunity, and expression of cytokines is altered (Tao, Yang, and Wang 2006). In particular, expression of IL-12 is often reduced resulting in a decreased ability of these dendritic cells to stimulate development of Th1 cells (Wada et al. 2009), though this is not always the case (Mohty et al. 2003). While costimulatory ability and IL-12 production may be reduced by retinoic acid, other functions of dendritic cells may be enhanced, such as the expression of CD64, a cell-surface receptor that contributes to the uptake of soluble antigen for later presentation to T-cells, suggesting that lymphocyte responses to soluble antigens (including antibody responses) may be enhanced by retinoic acid (den Hartog et al. 2013). Studies of dendritic cell development with bone marrow precursors (rather than peripheral blood monocytes) from mice indicate that retinoic acid treatment increased the percentage of cells that develop a myeloid dendritic cell phenotype and also increased costimulatory molecule expression, but decreases expression of MHCII, which is required for antigen presentation (Hengesbach and Hoag 2004). Clearly specific conditions (e.g., presence of different cytokines) can modify the effect of retinoic acid on dendritic cell development.

While a complete picture of the overall effects of retinoic acid on dendritic cell development and function has not yet emerged, it does seem clear that retinoic acid may act to dampen development of inflammatory T-cell responses in some cases by decreasing antigen presentation by dendritic cells, as well as via other mechanisms (Beijer, Kraal, and den Haan 2014). On the other hand, the development of specific subsets of dendritic cells, such as CD11b$^+$ dendritic cells involved in antibacterial and antifungal responses, is impaired by vitamin A deficiency and may thus dampen certain protective responses (Bhatt et al. 2014). These apparently contradictory effects may be due to differences in timing, with retinoic acid acting during dendritic cell development affecting the type of dendritic cell that emerges, while retinoic acid present during the initial encounter of a dendritic cell with antigen and inflammatory signals during the initiation of an adaptive immune response may have a different, perhaps dampening, effect.

As the preceding paragraph indicates, the specific effects of retinoic acid on dendritic cell development can vary depending on experimental conditions. One consistent finding, however, is that gut-derived dendritic cells, which often express CD103 on their surface, produce retinoic acid in response to stimulation with appropriate cytokines or microbial stimuli (Manicassamy et al. 2009), as well as in response to retinoic acid itself (Iwata et al. 2004; Iwata and Yokota 2011; Ohoka et al. 2014). Dendritic cells in intestinal lymphoid compartment thus produce retinoic acid, which can act in a paracrine manner to affect other cells in the local environment, particularly the development of lymphocytes as will be discussed below. Other cells in the local environment of intestinal lymphoid tissue also produce retinoic acid (Vicente-Suarez et al. 2015). For these reasons, retinoic acid production is a relatively constant factor in this compartment of the immune system, while systemic lymphoid tissue does not typically produce retinoic acid, though specific conditions can induce its production as has been shown in the respiratory tract (Rudraraju et al. 2014).

11.3.5 Vitamin A and Innate Lymphoid Cell Development and Function

Natural killer (NK) cells are a type of innate lymphoid cell (Spits et al. 2013) that help protect against viral infections before the initiation of adaptive immunity. NK cells also play a role in cancer immunity by targeting some transformed cells (Murphy et al. 2011). As discussed in an earlier review (Stephensen 2001), vitamin A–deficient animals have lower numbers of NK cells with a decreased ability to kill damaged or virus-infected cells, and treatment with retinoic acid restores these NK functions. Thus, vitamin A deficiency impairs NK cell function and this deficit may result in a decreased ability to clear infections once they occur. However, recent work addressing NK cell function in the context of cancer therapy (Sanchez-Martinez et al. 2014), which at times involves retinoic acid therapy to individuals with adequate vitamin A status, found that retinoic acid treatment of NK cells *ex vivo* downregulates an activation step for cathepsin B, a molecule involved in cellular cytotoxicity of virally infected cells or cancer cells. Thus, retinoic acid therapy may have a role of dampening NK activity, a situation that is clearly different from the evaluation of the effects of vitamin A deficiency or adequacy on immune function.

Other innate lymphoid cells (ILC) play key roles in gut-barrier function (Spits and Di Santo 2011). These include ILCs that produce cytokines normally produced by adaptive immune cells. ILC1 cells (where NK cells can also be grouped) produce IFN-γ, as do Th1 cells, ILC2 cells

188

Nutrition, Immunity, and Infection

produce IL-4, -5, and -13, as do Th2 cells, and ILC3 cells produce IL-17A and IL-22, as do Th17 cells (Spits et al. 2013). Interestingly, vitamin A deficiency in mice decreases the presence of both ILC1 and ILC3 cells in the intestinal lymphoid tissue, but ILC2 numbers do not decrease and may increase (Spencer et al. 2014). This may result from the fact that homing of ILC1 and ILC3 cells to the intestine depends on retinoic acid–mediated induction of CCR9 and α4β7 integrin expression while expression of these homing factors in ILC2 cells is innate and does not require retinoic acid, and is thus not compromised by vitamin A deficiency (Kim, Taparowsky, and Kim 2015). Vitamin A deficiency, at least in this mouse model system, causes a relative enhancement of type 2 innate immunity in the gut while type 2 adaptive immunity in the gut is typically impaired by vitamin A deficiency, as discussed below.

11.4 VITAMIN A AND ADAPTIVE IMMUNE CELLS

11.4.1 Overview

The adaptive immune system is comprised primarily of lymphocytes, including T-cells and B-cells. Both cell types originate in the bone marrow from a common lymphoid progenitor and are then found in peripheral lymphoid tissue as well as blood. T-cell precursors undergo an additional maturation step in the thymus. Following stimulation in the peripheral tissue, antigenically naive CD4+ T-cells develop into either inflammatory helper T-cells (Th cells, including Th1, Th2, and Th17 cells) that are involved in clearing pathogenic organisms (or, in some cases, causing immune-mediated chronic diseases), follicular helper (Tfh) cells (which assist development of B cells), or into regulatory T-cells, including FOXP3-positive Treg cells or other subsets, including T-regulatory type 1 cells (Tr1 cells). Naive CD8+ T-cells develop into cytotoxic T-cells (Tc cells), while naive B-cells develop into memory B-cells and antibody-secreting plasma cells, as described in many basic immunology textbooks (Murphy et al. 2011). These cells provide immunologic memory to previous infections and are engaged following stimulation of the innate immune system by a vaccine, microorganisms, or other sources of antigen. These antigens, consisting primarily of short sequences of amino acids derived from antigenic proteins, are presented to lymphocytes by antigen-presenting cells such as dendritic cells. Dendritic cells provide the usual route of initiating a primary adaptive immune response. Dendritic cells, and other cells of the innate immune system, help steer the development of the adaptive immune response by producing cytokines, as described above, that promote T helper cell development along particular differentiation pathways toward Th1, Th2, Th17, Tfh, or Treg cells, for example, as was described above when discussing dendritic cells. As a result of antigen exposure over a lifetime, individuals have different levels of adaptive immunity depending on their exposure history. Such an adaptive immune response occurs more rapidly after the second exposure to an antigen than it does after the first exposure. Thus, the first encounter with a childhood pathogen (e.g., measles) can make a child quite ill, but subsequent infections will likely go unnoticed if an effective adaptive immune response has developed.

11.4.2 Vitamin A and Thymic Function

Vitamin A deficiency in rats causes a dramatic decrease in the size and cellularity of the thymus (Zile, Bunge, and DeLuca 1979). A similar effect is seen in mice (Ahmed, Jones, and Jackson 1990). Retinoic acid treatment of human thymocytes *ex vivo* increases cellular proliferation via the IL-2 pathway (Sidell and Ramsdell 1988), suggesting a role for this metabolite in thymocyte growth *in vivo*. However, retinoic acid, which can be produced in the thymus (Kiss et al. 2008), may have multiple effects on thymic development, as suggested by the observation that retinoic acid can also inhibit *ex vivo* maturation of a thymocyte cell line (Meco et al. 1994). Related work shows that retinoic acid can act via RARγ to induce apoptosis in mouse thymocytes (Szondy et al. 1997), though later work from the same group shows that retinoic acid may act via RARα to inhibit activation-induced apoptosis of thymocytes (Szondy et al. 1998). Both activities may participate in thymocyte maturation during different stages, and perhaps in physically different locations within the thymus during development. Apoptosis of self-reactive thymocytes is a normal function in thymocyte development, and one group suggests that interruption of this process by retinoic acid treatment in *ex vivo* thymic organ cultures increases the frequency of mature, self-reactive T-cells (Yagi et al. 1997). Later studies showed a similar role with a potential inhibition of negative selection (Szegezdi et al. 2003). *Ex vivo* treatment of human thymocytes with retinoic acid increased development of CD4$^+$ T-cells at the expense of CD8$^+$ T-cells (Zhou, Wang, and Yang 2008). Treatment with retinoic acid (Mulder, Manley, and Maggio-Price 1998) or a high dietary level of vitamin A (Mulder et al. 2000) during fetal development both have negative effects on thymic development in mice. One case report of treatment with 13-cis retinoic acid (all-trans is the principal *in vivo* metabolite) showed thymic hypoplasia in a human infant as well (Cohen et al. 1987). In summary, retinoic acid is produced in the thymus and appears to have multiple roles in both promoting thymocyte proliferation and survival, but a role in deletion of self-reactive thymocytes via induction of apoptosis is also evident. The net effect of severe dietary vitamin A deficiency is thymic atrophy, which will have negative impacts on adaptive immunity, though the effects of milder deficiency, or of supplementation, are not clearly described.

11.4.3 VITAMIN A AND T-CELL DEVELOPMENT AND FUNCTION

Following thymic development, retinoic acid is also required for normal proliferation and survival of T-cells in response to antigenic stimulation in the periphery (Engedal 2011). In addition, retinoic acid directly modulates development of T-cell differentiation following antigen exposure (Iwata 2009; Mucida, Park, and Cheroutre 2009). Naive CD4$^+$ T helper cells differentiate into many phenotypes based on the need to deal with different types of pathogens (Murphy et al. 2011). Th1 cells produce the effector cytokine IFN-γ that activates macrophages to kill intracellular pathogens (e.g., *Mycobacterium tuberculosis* and some *Salmonella* species) and promotes antiviral responses (e.g., development of CD8$^+$ Tc cells). Production of IL-12 by dendritic cells drives Th1 development (as well as production of IFN-γ itself by Th1 and other cell types). Th1 cell responses can be enhanced by vitamin A deficiency (Cantorna, Nashold, and Hayes 1994) perhaps primarily due to the ability of retinoic acid to decrease IFN-γ production, though this pattern is not unvarying and may depend on the patterns of cytokines produced in response to specific conditions (i.e., specific infections or types of vaccination). Th2 cells produce IL-4, IL-5, and IL-13 and promote "weep and sweep" responses in the gut and eosinophilic inflammation to expel metazoan parasites. Production of IL-4 by dendritic cells or other cell types drives Th2 development. Retinoic acid enhances Th2 development *ex vivo* in the presence of IL-4. Th17 cells produce the effector cytokines IL-17A and IL-22, which promote epithelial production of antibacterial peptides to kill extracellular bacteria and chemokines to attract neutrophils, which phagocytose and kill such bacteria. IL-17A also promotes neutrophil differentiation in the bone marrow. Th17 development is promoted by IL-6 from dendritic cells working together with TGF-β, which can be produced by many cell types, particularly in gut lymphoid tissue. Cytokines produced by Th17 cells, including IL-23, are also needed to sustain Th17 development. Treg cells also develop in the periphery after encountering antigen and act to inhibit rather than promote inflammation. This development of Treg cells is an inherent regulatory component of adaptive immunity to control inflammation in order to prevent excessive pathology. TGF-β in the absence of inflammatory cytokines drives Treg development but data also show that retinoic acid acts in concert with TGF-β to enhance Treg development. Both TGF-β and retinoic acid (Sun et al. 2007) are produced by immune cells in the gut and mesenteric lymph nodes, which are key sites of Treg development (Mucida, Park, and Cheroutre 2009). This role of retinoic acid in Treg/Th17 balance gives it an important action in development of tolerance to oral antigens and potentially beneficial bacteria (Hall et al. 2011). The effect of retinoic acid on T-cell development is complex and research has moved rapidly in recent years, though little research has been done on Tfh cells. There are many reviews that examine specific aspects of this topic in great detail (Hall et al. 2011; Raverdeau and Mills 2014; Ross 2012; Brown and Noelle 2015; Guo et al. 2015).

11.4.4   VITAMIN A, B-CELLS, AND ANTIBODY RESPONSES

Naive B-cells develop into antibody-producing plasma cells and memory B-cells following appropriate exposure to antigen. Thus B-cells are responsible for development of the humoral immune response (Murphy et al. 2011). Some antibody responses develop without T-cell help (e.g., bacterial polysaccharides), and these are not impaired by vitamin A deficiency but many humoral responses require such help. Vitamin A deficiency generally impairs T-cell–mediated antibody responses, particularly Th2-dependent antibody responses, such as IgE and IgG1 responses (Ertesvag, Naderi, and Blomhoff 2009; Ross, Chen, and Ma 2009). Antibody responses promoted by Th1 cells may not be affected or can be slightly increased by vitamin A deficiency in mice, as has been reviewed (Stephensen 2001).

IgA is secreted across mucosal surfaces to neutralize pathogens in the respiratory, urogenital, and intestinal tracts. It is a crucial part of the adaptive immune response protecting against mucosal pathogens (Murphy et al. 2011). Vitamin A deficiency impairs the serum and secretory IgA response in the gut and respiratory tracts, as has been reviewed (Stephensen 2001). This phenomenon is partially explained by diminished Th2 development and mucosal targeting of lymphocytes, but vitamin A also promotes IgA responses by enhancing class-switching to IgA by plasma cells (Watanabe et al. 2010). Thus, vitamin A deficiency impairs this crucial protective mechanism at mucosal surfaces.

11.4.5   VITAMIN A AND MUCOSAL TARGETING OF LYMPHOCYTES

Primary antigenic exposures at mucosal surfaces are likely to recur at the same mucosal sites. For example, exposure to enteric pathogens such as rotavirus is common, and to ensure a robust response at the site of exposure, an important component of memory responses, including T-cell responses, is the ability of lymphocytes first exposed to antigen at mucosal sites to return to mucosal sites as effector or memory cells (Murphy et al. 2011). Vitamin A plays a key role in targeting lymphocytes to mucosal surfaces. Retinoic acid produced by CD103+ dendritic cells in the gut facilitates such return by inducing the expression of CC-chemokine receptor 9 (CCR9) and the α4β7 integrin dimer on the surface of both T and B lymphocytes undergoing initial antigen exposure in the gut (Iwata and Yokota 2011). CCR9 responds to CC-chemokine ligand 25 (CCL25), which is constitutively expressed in the intestine, and α4β7 integrin binds to mucosal addressin cell adhesion molecule-1 (MAdCAM-1), which is expressed on the vascular endothelium associated with intestinal lymphoid tissue (Gorfu, Rivera-Nieves, and Ley 2009). CCR9 and α4β7 are induced by retinoic acid produced by intestinal dendritic cells (Iwata 2009). Dietary vitamin A deficiency decreases retinoic acid production by gut dendritic cells (Jaensson-Gyllenback et al. 2011; Molenaar et al. 2011).

11.5   CONCLUSIONS

Vitamin A deficiency impairs many aspects of innate and adaptive immunity, leading to an increased severity of infections and increased risk of death for infants and young children in areas of the world with a high burden of infection and a high risk of vitamin A deficiency. Vitamin A supplementation has been recommended in recent decades to decrease the risk of death from common infections, particularly enteric infections and measles. The role of vitamin A in enhancing mucosal immunity by affecting immune cell development and targeting to mucosal sites presumably accounts for some of this beneficial effect of vitamin A, and it might also be beneficial in diminishing chronic inflammation (e.g., inflammatory bowel disease) in the intestinal tract via enhancement of Treg development (Brown and Noelle 2015). In contrast, it is possible that treatment with vitamin A or other retinoids during active infections or other inflammatory conditions might enhance the activity of inflammatory T-cells that could cause immune pathology and perhaps increase the severity of some inflammatory conditions, perhaps including Th2-mediated responses (Schuster, Kenyon, and Stephensen 2008). Thus while prevention of vitamin A deficiency by use of supplements or fortification is reasonable in many areas of the world where vitamin A deficiency is a public health problem, caution is warranted in use of vitamin A supplements during active infections or inflammation.

REFERENCES

Ahmed, F., D. B. Jones, and A. A. Jackson. 1990. The interaction of vitamin A deficiency and rotavirus infection in the mouse. *Br J Nutr* 63 (2):363–73.

Austenaa, L. M., H. Carlsen, K. Hollung, H. K. Blomhoff, and R. Blomhoff. 2009. Retinoic acid dampens LPS-induced NF-kappaB activity: Results from human monoblasts and in vivo imaging of NF-kappaB reporter mice. *J Nutr Biochem* 20 (9):726–34.

Beijer, M. R., G. Kraal, and J. M. den Haan. 2014. Vitamin A and dendritic cell differentiation. *Immunology* 142 (1):39–45.

Benbrook, D. M., P. Chambon, C. Rochette-Egly, and M. A. Asson-Batres. 2014. History of retinoic acid receptors. *Subcell Biochem* 70:1–20.

Bhaskaram, P., R. Mathur, V. Rao, J. Madhusudan, K. V. Radhakrishna, N. Raghuramulu, and V. Reddy. 1986. Pathogenesis of corneal lesions in measles. *Hum Nutr Clin Nutr* 40 (3):197–204.

Bhatt, S., J. Qin, C. Bennett, S. Qian, J. J. Fung, T. A. Hamilton, and L. Lu. 2014. All-trans retinoic acid induces arginase-1 and inducible nitric oxide synthase-producing dendritic cells with T cell inhibitory function. *J Immunol* 192 (11):5098–108.

Biesalski, H. K. and D. Nohr. 2003. Importance of vitamin-A for lung function and development. *Mol Aspects Med* 24 (6):431–40.

Brown, C. C., and R. J. Noelle. 2015. Seeing through the dark: New insights into the immune regulatory functions of vitamin A. *Eur J Immunol* 45 (5):1287–95.

Cantorna, M. T., F. E. Nashold, and C. E. Hayes. 1994. In vitamin A deficiency multiple mechanisms establish a regulatory T helper cell imbalance with excess Th1 and insufficient Th2 function. *J Immunol* 152 (4):1515–22.

Chen, Q. and A. C. Ross. 2007. Retinoic acid regulates CD1d gene expression at the transcriptional level in human and rodent monocytic cells. *Exp Biol Med (Maywood)* 232 (4):488–94.

Cohen, M., A. Rubinstein, J. K. Li, and G. Nathenson. 1987. Thymic hypoplasia associated with isotretinoin embryopathy. *Am J Dis Child* 141 (3):263–6.

Denburg, J. A., R. Sehmi, and J. Upham. 2001. Regulation of IL-5 receptor on eosinophil progenitors in allergic inflammation: Role of retinoic acid. *Int Arch Allergy Immunol* 124 (1–3):246–8.

den Hartog, G., C. van Altena, H. F. Savelkoul, and R. J. van Neerven. 2013. The mucosal factors retinoic acid and TGF-beta1 induce phenotypically and functionally distinct dendritic cell types. *Int Arch Allergy Immunol* 162 (3):225–36.

Dzhagalov, I., P. Chambon, and Y. W. He. 2007. Regulation of CD8+ T lymphocyte effector function and macrophage inflammatory cytokine production by retinoic acid receptor gamma. *J Immunol* 178 (4):2113–21.

Edmond, K. M., S. Newton, C. Shannon, M. O'Leary, L. Hurt, G. Thomas, S. Amenga-Etego, C. Tawiah-Agyemang, L. Gram, C. N. Hurt et al. 2015. Effect of early neonatal vitamin A supplementation on mortality during infancy in Ghana (Neovita): A randomised, double-blind, placebo-controlled trial. *Lancet* 385 (9975):1315–23.

Eggersdorfer, M., D. Laudert, U. Letinois, T. McClymont, J. Medlock, T. Netscher, and W. Bonrath. 2012. One hundred years of vitamins-a success story of the natural sciences. *Angew Chem Int Ed Engl* 51 (52):12960–90.

Engedal, N. 2011. Immune regulator vitamin A and T cell death. *Vitam Horm* 86:153–78.

Ertesvag, A., S. Naderi, and H. K. Blomhoff. 2009. Regulation of B cell proliferation and differentiation by retinoic acid. *Semin Immunol* 21 (1):36–41.

Giguere, V., E. S. Ong, P. Segui, and R. M. Evans. 1987. Identification of a receptor for the morphogen retinoic acid. *Nature* 330 (6149):624–9.

Gorfu, G., J. Rivera-Nieves, and K. Ley. 2009. Role of beta7 integrins in intestinal lymphocyte homing and retention. *Curr Mol Med* 9 (7):836–50.

Green, H. N. and E. Mellanby. 1928. Vitamin A as an anti-infective agent. *Br Med J* 2 (3537):691–6.

Guimaraes, H., M. B. Guedes, G. Rocha, T. Tome, and A. Albino-Teixeira. 2012. Vitamin A in prevention of bronchopulmonary dysplasia. *Curr Pharm Des* 18 (21):3101–13.

Guo, Y., C. Brown, C. Ortiz, and R. J. Noelle. 2015. Leukocyte homing, fate, and function are controlled by retinoic acid. *Physiol Rev* 95 (1):125–48.

Haider, B. A. and Z. A. Bhutta. 2015. Neonatal vitamin A supplementation: Time to move on. *Lancet* 385 (9975):1268–71.

Hall, J. A., J. R. Grainger, S. P. Spencer, and Y. Belkaid. 2011. The role of retinoic acid in tolerance and immunity. *Immunity* 35 (1):13–22.

Hashimoto, S., S. Hayashi, S. Yoshida, K. Kujime, S. Maruoka, K. Matsumoto, Y. Gon, T. Koura, and T. Horie. 1998. Retinoic acid differentially regulates interleukin-1beta and interleukin-1 receptor antagonist production by human alveolar macrophages. *Leuk Res* 22 (11):1057–61.

Hatchigian, E. A., J. I. Santos, S. A. Broitman, and J. J. Vitale. 1989. Vitamin A supplementation improves macrophage function and bacterial clearance during experimental salmonella infection. *Proc Soc Exp Biol Med* 191 (1):47–54.

Hengesbach, L. M. and K. A. Hoag. 2004. Physiological concentrations of retinoic acid favor myeloid dendritic cell development over granulocyte development in cultures of bone marrow cells from mice. *J Nutr* 134 (10):2653–9.

Hubbard, B. A., J. G. Unger, and R. J. Rohrich. 2014. Reversal of skin aging with topical retinoids. *Plast Reconstr Surg* 133 (4):481e–90e.

Imdad, A., K. Herzer, E. Mayo-Wilson, M. Y. Yakoob, and Z. A. Bhutta. 2010. Vitamin A supplementation for preventing morbidity and mortality in children from 6 months to 5 years of age. *Cochrane Database Syst Rev* 8 (12):CD008524.

Iwata, M. 2009. Retinoic acid production by intestinal dendritic cells and its role in T-cell trafficking. *Semin Immunol* 21 (1):8–13.

Iwata, M., A. Hirakiyama, Y. Eshima, H. Kagechika, C. Kato, and S. Y. Song. 2004. Retinoic acid imprints gut-homing specificity on T cells. *Immunity* 21 (4):527–38.

Iwata, M., and A. Yokota. 2011. Retinoic acid production by intestinal dendritic cells. *Vitam Horm* 86:127–52.

Jaensson-Gyllenback, E., K. Kotarsky, F. Zapata, E. K. Persson, T. E. Gundersen, R. Blomhoff, and W. W. Agace. 2011. Bile retinoids imprint intestinal CD103(+) dendritic cells with the ability to generate gut-tropic T cells. *Mucosal Immunol* 4 (4):438–47.

Januszewicz, E. and I. A. Cooper. 1984. Inhibition of normal human macrophage progenitors by retinoic acid. *Br J Haematol* 58 (1):119–28.

Kastner, P. and S. Chan. 2001. Function of RARalpha during the maturation of neutrophils. *Oncogene* 20 (49):7178–85.

Kim, B. H., K. S. Kang, and Y. S. Lee. 2004. Effect of retinoids on LPS-induced COX-2 expression and COX-2 associated PGE(2) release from mouse peritoneal macrophages and TNF-alpha release from rat peripheral blood mononuclear cells. *Toxicol Lett* 150 (2):191–201.

Kim, S. Y., J. E. Koo, M. R. Song, and J. Y. Lee. 2013. Retinol suppresses the activation of Toll-like receptors in MyD88- and STAT1-independent manners. *Inflammation* 36 (2):426–33.

Kim, S. W., K. Y. Seo, T. Rhim, and E. K. Kim. 2012. Effect of retinoic acid on epithelial differentiation and mucin expression in primary human corneal limbal epithelial cells. *Curr Eye Res* 37 (1):33–42.

Kim, M. H., E. J. Taparowsky, and C. H. Kim. 2015. Retinoic acid differentially regulates the migration of innate lymphoid cell subsets to the gut. *Immunity* 43 (1):107–19.

Kinoshita, T., K. Koike, H. H. Mwamtemi, S. Ito, S. Ishida, Y. Nakazawa, Y. Kurokawa, K. Sakashita, T. Higuchi, K. Takeuchi et al. 2000. Retinoic acid is a negative regulator for the differentiation of cord blood-derived human mast cell progenitors. *Blood* 95 (9):2821–8.

Kiss, I., R. Ruhl, E. Szegezdi, B. Fritzsche, B. Toth, J. Pongracz, T. Perlmann, L. Fesus, and Z. Szondy. 2008. Retinoid receptor-activating ligands are produced within the mouse thymus during postnatal development. *Eur J Immunol* 38 (1):147–55.

Kozakova, H., L. A. Hanson, R. Stepankova, H. Kahu, U. I. Dahlgren, and U. Wiedermann. 2003. Vitamin A deficiency leads to severe functional disturbance of the intestinal epithelium enzymes associated with diarrhoea and increased bacterial translocation in gnotobiotic rats. *Microbes Infect* 5 (5):405–11.

Kreutz, M., J. Fritsche, U. Ackermann, S. W. Krause, and R. Andreesen. 1998. Retinoic acid inhibits monocyte to macrophage survival and differentiation. *Blood* 91 (12):4796–802.

Lawson, N. D. and N. Berliner. 1999. Neutrophil maturation and the role of retinoic acid. *Exp Hematol* 27 (9):1355–67.

Leber, B. F. and J. A. Denburg. 1997. Retinoic acid modulation of induced basophil differentiation. *Allergy* 52 (12):1201–6.

Mamidi, S., T. P. Hofer, R. Hoffmann, L. Ziegler-Heitbrock, and M. Frankenberger. 2012. All-trans retinoic acid up-regulates Prostaglandin-E Synthase expression in human macrophages. *Immunobiology* 217 (6):593–600.

Manicassamy, S., R. Ravindran, J. Deng, H. Oluoch, T. L. Denning, S. P. Kasturi, K. M. Rosenthal, B. D. Evavold, and B. Pulendran. 2009. Toll-like receptor 2-dependent induction of vitamin A-metabolizing enzymes in dendritic cells promotes T regulatory responses and inhibits autoimmunity. *Nat Med* 15:401–9.

Masanja, H., E. R. Smith, A. Muhihi, C. Briegleb, S. Mshamu, J. Ruben, R. A. Noor, P. Khudyakov, S. Yoshida, J. Martines et al. 2015. Effect of neonatal vitamin A supplementation on mortality in infants in Tanzania (Neovita): A randomised, double-blind, placebo-controlled trial. *Lancet* 385 (9975):1324–32.

Mathew, J. S. and R. P. Sharma. 2000. Effect of all-trans-retinoic acid on cytokine production in a murine macrophage cell line. *Int J Immunopharmacol* 22 (9):693–706.

Mazumder, S., S. Taneja, K. Bhatia, S. Yoshida, J. Kaur, B. Dube, G. S. Toteja, R. Bahl, O. Fontaine, J. Martines et al. 2015. Efficacy of early neonatal supplementation with vitamin A to reduce mortality in infancy in Haryana, India (Neovita): A randomised, double-blind, placebo-controlled trial. *Lancet* 385 (9975):1333–42.

McCullough, F. S., C. A. Northrop-Clewes, and D. I. Thurnham. 1999. The effect of vitamin A on epithelial integrity. *Proc Nutr Soc* 58 (2):289–93.

Meco, D., S. Scarpa, M. Napolitano, M. Maroder, D. Bellavia, R. De Maria, M. Ragano-Caracciolo, L. Frati, A. Modesti, A. Gulino et al. 1994. Modulation of fibronectin and thymic stromal cell-dependent thymocyte maturation by retinoic acid. *J Immunol* 153 (1):73–83.

Mehta, K., T. McQueen, S. Tucker, R. Pandita, and B. B. Aggarwal. 1994. Inhibition by all-trans-retinoic acid of tumor necrosis factor and nitric oxide production by peritoneal macrophages. *J Leukoc Biol* 55 (3):336–42.

Meunier, L., J. J. Voorhees, and K. D. Cooper. 1996. In vivo retinoic acid modulates expression of the class II major histocompatibility complex and function of antigen-presenting macrophages and keratinocytes in ultraviolet-exposed human skin. *J Invest Dermatol* 106 (5):1042–6.

Moens, E. and M. Veldhoen. 2012. Epithelial barrier biology: Good fences make good neighbours. *Immunology* 135 (1):1–8.

Mohty, M., S. Morbelli, D. Isnardon, D. Sainty, C. Arnoulet, B. Gaugler, and D. Olive. 2003. All-trans retinoic acid skews monocyte differentiation into interleukin-12-secreting dendritic-like cells. *Br J Haematol* 122 (5):829–36.

Molenaar, R., M. Knippenberg, G. Goverse, B. J. Olivier, A. F. de Vos, T. O'Toole, and R. E. Mebius. 2011. Expression of retinaldehyde dehydrogenase enzymes in mucosal dendritic cells and gut-draining lymph node stromal cells is controlled by dietary vitamin A. *J Immunol* 186 (4):1934–42.

Mucida, D., Y. Park, and H. Cheroutre. 2009. From the diet to the nucleus: Vitamin A and TGF-beta join efforts at the mucosal interface of the intestine. *Semin Immunol* 21 (1):14–21.

Mulder, G. B., N. Manley, J. Grant, K. Schmidt, W. Zeng, C. Eckhoff, and L. Maggio-Price. 2000. Effects of excess vitamin A on development of cranial neural crest-derived structures: A neonatal and embryologic study. *Teratology* 62 (4):214–26.

Mulder, G. B., N. Manley, and L. Maggio-Price. 1998. Retinoic acid-induced thymic abnormalities in the mouse are associated with altered pharyngeal morphology, thymocyte maturation defects, and altered expression of Hoxa3 and Pax1. *Teratology* 58 (6):263–75.

Murphy, K. P., P. Travers, M. Walport, and C. Janeway. 2011. *Janeway's Immunobiology*. New York, NY: Garland Science.

Na, S. Y., B. Y. Kang, S. W. Chung, S. J. Han, X. Ma, G. Trinchieri, S. Y. Im, J. W. Lee, and T. S. Kim. 1999. Retinoids inhibit interleukin-12 production in macrophages through physical associations of retinoid X receptor and NFkappaB. *J Biol Chem* 274 (12):7674–80.

Nauss, K. M., D. A. Mark, and R. M. Suskind. 1979. The effect of vitamin A deficiency on the in vitro cellular immune response of rats. *J Nutr* 109 (10):1815–23.

Ohoka, Y., A. Yokota-Nakatsuma, N. Maeda, H. Takeuchi, and M. Iwata. 2014. Retinoic acid and GM-CSF coordinately induce retinal dehydrogenase 2 (RALDH2) expression through cooperation between the RAR/RXR complex and Sp1 in dendritic cells. *PLOS ONE* 9 (5):e96512.

Okabe, Y. and R. Medzhitov. 2014. Tissue-specific signals control reversible program of localization and functional polarization of macrophages. *Cell* 157 (4):832–44.

Olson, J. A., D. B. Gunning, and R. A. Tilton. 1984. Liver concentrations of vitamin A and carotenoids, as a function of age and other parameters, of American children who died of various causes. *Am J Clin Nutr* 39 (6):903–10.

Olson, J. A., W. Rojanapo, and A. J. Lamb. 1981. The effect of vitamin A status on the differentiation and function of goblet cells in the rat intestine. *Ann N Y Acad Sci* 359:181–91.

Ongsakul, M., S. Sirisinha, and A. J. Lamb. 1985. Impaired blood clearance of bacteria and phagocytic activity in vitamin A-deficient rats. *Proc Soc Exp Biol Med* 178 (2):204–8.

Ozawa, K., N. Sato, A. Urabe, and F. Takaku. 1984. Modulation of normal myelopoiesis in vitro by retinoic acid. *Biochem Biophys Res Commun* 123 (1):128–32.

Paul, C. C., S. Mahrer, M. Tolbert, B. L. Elbert, I. Wong, S. J. Ackerman, and M. A. Baumann. 1995. Changing the differentiation program of hematopoietic cells: Retinoic acid-induced shift of eosinophil-committed cells to neutrophils. *Blood* 86 (10):3737–44.

Petkovich, M., N. J. Brand, A. Krust, and P. Chambon. 1987. A human retinoic acid receptor which belongs to the family of nuclear receptors. *Nature* 330 (6147):444–50.

Raverdeau, M. and K. H. Mills. 2014. Modulation of T cell and innate immune responses by retinoic Acid. *J Immunol* 192 (7):2953–8.

Rhodes, J. and S. Oliver. 1980. Retinoids as regulators of macrophage function. *Immunology* 40 (3):467–72.

Ross, A. C. 2012. Vitamin A and retinoic acid in T cell-related immunity. *Am J Clin Nutr* 96 (5):1166S–72S.

Ross, A. C., Q. Chen, and Y. Ma. 2009. Augmentation of antibody responses by retinoic acid and costimulatory molecules. *Semin Immunol* 21 (1):42–50.

Rudraraju, R., B. G. Jones, S. L. Surman, R. E. Sealy, P. G. Thomas, and J. L. Hurwitz. 2014. Respiratory tract epithelial cells express retinaldehyde dehydrogenase ALDH1A and enhance IgA production by stimulated B cells in the presence of vitamin A. *PLOS ONE* 9 (1):e86554.

Sanchez-Martinez, D., E. Krzywinska, M. G. Rathore, A. Saumet, A. Cornillon, N. Lopez-Royuela, L. Martinez-Lostao, A. Ramirez-Labrada, Z. Y. Lu, J. F. Rossi et al. 2014. All-trans retinoic acid (ATRA) induces miR-23a expression, decreases CTSC expression and granzyme B activity leading to impaired NK cell cytotoxicity. *Int J Biochem Cell Biol* 49:42–52.

Sanders, T. J., N. E. McCarthy, E. M. Giles, K. L. Davidson, M. L. Haltalli, S. Hazell, J. O. Lindsay, and A. J. Stagg. 2014. Increased production of retinoic acid by intestinal macrophages contributes to their inflammatory phenotype in patients with Crohn's disease. *Gastroenterology* 146 (5):1278–88. e1–2.

Schuster, G. U., N. J. Kenyon, and C. B. Stephensen. 2008. Vitamin A deficiency decreases and high dietary vitamin A increases disease severity in the mouse model of asthma. *J Immunol* 180 (3):1834–42.

Scrimshaw, N. S., C. E. Taylor, and J. E. Gordon. 1968. *Interactions of Nutrition and Infection, World Health Organization Monograph Series*. Geneva: World Health Organization.

Semba, R. D. 1999. Vitamin A as "anti-infective" therapy, 1920–1940. *J Nutr* 129 (4):783–91.

Semba, R. D. 2012a. Milk, butter, and early steps in human trials. *World Rev Nutr Diet* 104:106–31.

Semba, R. D. 2012b. On the 'discovery' of vitamin A. *Ann Nutr Metab* 61 (3):192–8.

Semba, R. D. 2012c. Rise of the 'anti-infective vitamin'. *World Rev Nutr Diet* 104:132–50.

Sidell, N. and F. Ramsdell. 1988. Retinoic acid upregulates interleukin-2 receptors on activated human thymocytes. *Cell Immunol* 115 (2):299–309.

Sijtsma, S. R., J. H. Rombout, M. J. Dohmen, C. E. West, and A. J. van der Zijpp. 1991. Effect of vitamin A deficiency on the activity of macrophages in Newcastle disease virus-infected chickens. *Vet Immunol Immunopathol* 28 (1):17–27.

Sommer, A. 1982. *Nutritional Blindness: Xerophthalmia and Keratomalacia*. New York, NY: Oxford University Press.

Sommer, A. 2014. Preventing blindness and saving lives: The centenary of vitamin A. *JAMA Ophthalmol* 132 (1):115–7.

Sommer, A., I. Tarwotjo, E. Djunaedi, K. P. West, Jr., A. A. Loeden, R. Tilden, and L. Mele. 1986. Impact of vitamin A supplementation on childhood mortality. A randomised controlled community trial. *Lancet* 1 (8491):1169–73.

Spencer, S. P., C. Wilhelm, Q. Yang, J. A. Hall, N. Bouladoux, A. Boyd, T. B. Nutman, J. F. Urban, Jr., J. Wang, T. R. Ramalingam et al. 2014. Adaptation of innate lymphoid cells to a micronutrient deficiency promotes type 2 barrier immunity. *Science* 343 (6169):432–7.

Spits, H., D. Artis, M. Colonna, A. Diefenbach, J. P. Di Santo, G. Eberl, S. Koyasu, R. M. Locksley, A. N. McKenzie, R. E. Mebius et al. 2013. Innate lymphoid cells—A proposal for uniform nomenclature. *Nat Rev Immunol* 13 (2):145–9.

Spits, H. and J. P. Di Santo. 2011. The expanding family of innate lymphoid cells: Regulators and effectors of immunity and tissue remodeling. *Nat Immunol* 12 (1):21–7.

Sporn, M. B., A. B. Roberts, and D. S. Goodman. 1994. *The Retinoids: Biology, Chemistry, and Medicine*, 2nd ed. New York, NY: Raven Press.

Stephensen, C. B. 2001. Vitamin A, infection, and immune function. *Annu Rev Nutr* 21:167–92.

Stephensen, C. B., S. R. Blount, T. R. Schoeb, and J. Y. Park. 1993. Vitamin A deficiency impairs some aspects of the host response to influenza A virus infection in BALB/c mice. *J Nutr* 123 (5):823–33.

Sun, C. M., J. A. Hall, R. B. Blank, N. Bouladoux, M. Oukka, J. R. Mora, and Y. Belkaid. 2007. Small intestine lamina propria dendritic cells promote de novo generation of Foxp3 T reg cells via retinoic acid. *J Exp Med* 204 (8):1775–85.

Szegezdi, E., I. Kiss, A. Simon, B. Blasko, U. Reichert, S. Michel, M. Sandor, L. Fesus, and Z. Szondy. 2003. Ligation of retinoic acid receptor alpha regulates negative selection of thymocytes by inhibiting both DNA binding of nur77 and synthesis of bim. *J Immunol* 170 (7):3577–84.

Szondy, Z., U. Reichert, J. M. Bernardon, S. Michel, R. Toth, P. Ancian, E. Ajzner, and L. Fesus. 1997. Induction of apoptosis by retinoids and retinoic acid receptor gamma-selective compounds in mouse thymocytes through a novel apoptosis pathway. *Mol Pharmacol* 51 (6):972–82.

Szondy, Z., U. Reichert, J. M. Bernardon, S. Michel, R. Toth, E. Karaszi, and L. Fesus. 1998. Inhibition of activation-induced apoptosis of thymocytes by all-trans- and 9-cis-retinoic acid is mediated via retinoic acid receptor alpha. *Biochem J* 331 (Pt 3):767–74.

Tachibana, K., S. Sone, E. Tsubura, and Y. Kishino. 1984. Stimulatory effect of vitamin A on tumoricidal activity of rat alveolar macrophages. *Br J Cancer* 49 (3):343–8.

Tao, Y., Y. Yang, and W. Wang. 2006. Effect of all-trans-retinoic acid on the differentiation, maturation and functions of dendritic cells derived from cord blood monocytes. *FEMS Immunol Med Microbiol* 47 (3):444–50.

Torii, A., M. Miyake, M. Morishita, K. Ito, S. Torii, and T. Sakamoto. 2004. Vitamin A reduces lung granulomatous inflammation with eosinophilic and neutrophilic infiltration in Sephadex-treated rats. *Eur J Pharmacol* 497 (3):335–42.

Twining, S. S. 1997. Vitamin A deficiency alters rat neutrophil function. *J Nutr* 127 (4):558–65.

Twining, S. S., D. P. Schulte, P. M. Wilson, B. L. Fish, and J. E. Moulder. 1996a. Retinol is sequestered in the bone marrow of vitamin A-deficient rats. *J Nutr* 126 (6):1618–26.

Twining, S. S., D. P. Schulte, P. M. Wilson, X. Zhou, B. L. Fish, and J. E. Moulder. 1996b. Neutrophil cathepsin G is specifically decreased under vitamin A deficiency. *Biochim Biophys Acta* 1317 (2):112–8.

Ueki, S., G. Mahemuti, H. Oyamada, H. Kato, J. Kihara, M. Tanabe, W. Ito, T. Chiba, M. Takeda, H. Kayaba et al. 2008. Retinoic acids are potent inhibitors of spontaneous human eosinophil apoptosis. *J Immunol* 181 (11):7689–98.

Ueki, S., J. Nishikawa, Y. Yamauchi, Y. Konno, M. Tamaki, M. Itoga, Y. Kobayashi, M. Takeda, Y. Moritoki, W. Ito et al. 2013. Retinoic acids up-regulate functional eosinophil-driving receptor CCR3. *Allergy* 68 (7):953–6.

Upham, J. W., R. Sehmi, L. M. Hayes, K. Howie, J. Lundahl, and J. A. Denburg. 2002. Retinoic acid modulates IL-5 receptor expression and selectively inhibits eosinophil-basophil differentiation of hemopoietic progenitor cells. *J Allergy Clin Immunol* 109 (2):307–13.

Vicente-Suarez, I., A. Larange, C. Reardon, M. Matho, S. Feau, G. Chodaczek, Y. Park, Y. Obata, R. Gold, Y. Wang-Zhu et al. 2015. Unique lamina propria stromal cells imprint the functional phenotype of mucosal dendritic cells. *Mucosal Immunol* 8 (1):141–51.

Wada, Y., T. Hisamatsu, N. Kamada, S. Okamoto, and T. Hibi. 2009. Retinoic acid contributes to the induction of IL-12-hypoproducing dendritic cells. *Inflamm Bowel Dis* 15 (10):1548–56.

Wang, X., C. Allen, and M. Ballow. 2007. Retinoic acid enhances the production of IL-10 while reducing the synthesis of IL-12 and TNF-alpha from LPS-stimulated monocytes/macrophages. *J Clin Immunol* 27 (2):193–200.

Watanabe, K., M. Sugai, Y. Nambu, M. Osato, T. Hayashi, M. Kawaguchi, T. Komori, Y. Ito, and A. Shimizu. 2010. Requirement for Runx proteins in IgA class switching acting downstream of TGF-beta 1 and retinoic acid signaling. *J Immunol* 184 (6):2785–92.

WHO. 2011a. *Guideline: Neonatal Vitamin A Supplementation*. Geneva: World Health Organization.

WHO. 2011b. *Guideline: Vitamin A Supplementation in Infants and Children 1–5 Months of Age*. Geneva: World Health Organization.

WHO. 2011c. *Guideline: Vitamin A Supplementation in Infants and Children 6–59 Months of Age*. Geneva: World Health Organization.

Wiedermann, U., X. J. Chen, L. Enerback, L. A. Hanson, H. Kahu, and U. I. Dahlgren. 1996a. Vitamin A deficiency increases inflammatory responses. *Scand J Immunol* 44 (6):578–84.

Wiedermann, U., A. Tarkowski, T. Bremell, L. A. Hanson, H. Kahu, and U. I. Dahlgren. 1996b. Vitamin A deficiency predisposes to Staphylococcus aureus infection. *Infect Immun* 64 (1):209–14.

Wolfson, M., E. S. Shinwell, M. Zvillich, and B. Rager-Zisman. 1988. Inhibitory effect of retinoic acid on the respiratory burst of adult and cord blood neutrophils and macrophages: Potential implication to broncho-pulmonary dysplasia. *Clin Exp Immunol* 72 (3):505–9.

Yagi, J., T. Uchida, K. Kuroda, and T. Uchiyama. 1997. Influence of retinoic acid on the differentiation pathway of T cells in the thymus. *Cell Immunol* 181 (2):153–62.

Zhao, Z. and A. C. Ross. 1995. Retinoic acid repletion restores the number of leukocytes and their subsets and stimulates natural cytotoxicity in vitamin A-deficient rats. *J Nutr* 125 (8):2064–73.

Zhou, X., W. Wang, and Y. Yang. 2008. The expression of retinoic acid receptors in thymus of young children and the effect of all-transretinoic acid on the development of T cells in thymus. *J Clin Immunol* 28 (1):85–91.

Zile, M. H., E. C. Bunge, and H. F. DeLuca. 1979. On the physiological basis of vitamin A-stimulated growth. *J Nutr* 109 (10):1787–96.

12 Vitamin E, Immunity, and Infection

Dayong Wu and Simin Nikbin Meydani

CONTENTS

12.1 Introduction..197
12.2 Vitamin E: Chemistry, Natural Source, and Intake 198
12.3 Vitamin E and Immune Function 199
    12.3.1 Vitamin E Deficiency and Immune Function...199
    12.3.2 Vitamin E Supplementation and Immune Function..200
    12.3.3 Mechanism of the Effect of Vitamin E on Immune Function............................201
12.4 Vitamin E and Infection 203
    12.4.1 Animal Models...203
    12.4.2 Human Studies...203
12.5 Non-α-Tocopherol Vitamin E 205
    12.5.1 Other Forms of Tocopherols 205
    12.5.2 Tocotrienols...206
12.6 Concluding Remarks..207
Acknowledgments...207
References...207

12.1 INTRODUCTION

A normally functioning immune system is critical for the body to fight against and eliminate invading environmental pathogens. The immune system also protects the body from internal risks such as neoplasia and autoimmune responses. It exerts its functions by orchestrating the activity and interaction of a variety of immune cells, as well as their soluble products, which together constitute the immune system (see Chapter 1). Increased risk of infection is the most noticeable consequence of compromised immune function, which is often related to multiple factors including genetic defects, environment, lifestyle, disease, drug side effects, aging, and diet.

Nutritional status can significantly impact immune function. Deficiency in macronutrients or micronutrients has long been known to cause impairment of immune function, which can be reversed by correcting the deficiency. Further, for some nutrients, additional intake above the currently recommended, adequate levels may optimize immune function and promote the body's defense against infection, particularly in individuals with compromised immune functions such as the elderly. A good example of this is vitamin E, a very effective chain-breaking, lipid-soluble antioxidant present in the membrane of all cells. Since vitamin E is particularly enriched in the membrane of immune cells, it can protect them from oxidative damage related to high metabolic activity and prevent lipid peroxidation of polyunsaturated fatty acids, which are high in content in these cells [1,2]. Vitamin E is considered one of the most effective nutrients known to enhance immune function. A number of animal and human studies have indicated that vitamin E deficiency impairs both humoral and cell-mediated immune functions [3]. Conversely, supplementation with vitamin E, especially in the elderly, has been shown to enhance the immune response, and in turn increase resistance against several pathogens [4–11]. This chapter provides an updated review of the research on the role of vitamin E in modulating immunity and resistance to infection.

12.2 VITAMIN E: CHEMISTRY, NATURAL SOURCE, AND INTAKE

Vitamin E is a collective term for a family of structurally related compounds (containing a common chromanol ring linked to a side chain) that possess the biological activity of α-tocopherol. There are eight naturally occurring forms of vitamin E, which are divided into two groups (i.e., tocopherols and tocotrienols) depending on whether they have a saturated or unsaturated (three double bonds) side chain, respectively. Both the tocopherol and tocotrienol groups each have four homologous types, designated as α, β, γ, and δ according to the number and position of substituent methyl groups on the chromanol ring (Figure 12.1). Tocopherols have three asymmetric carbon atoms at position 2, 4', and 8', which enable tocopherols to exist as one of eight stereoisomers. While the natural form of α-tocopherol is a single stereoisomer, RRR-α-tocopherol, chemical synthesis of α-tocopherol yields eight stereoisomers in equal proportions: RRR, RRS, RSR, RSS, SSS, SRR, SRS, SSR; thus, synthetic vitamin E is often designated as all racemic (or all rac) α-tocopherol. Vitamin E supplements are often made in an ester form (acetate, succinate, nicotinate) to prevent oxidation, which increases shelf life. These esters are hydrolyzed in the intestinal lumen and vitamin E is absorbed in the unesterified form. A great majority of studies use either all-rac-α-tocopherol (also expressed

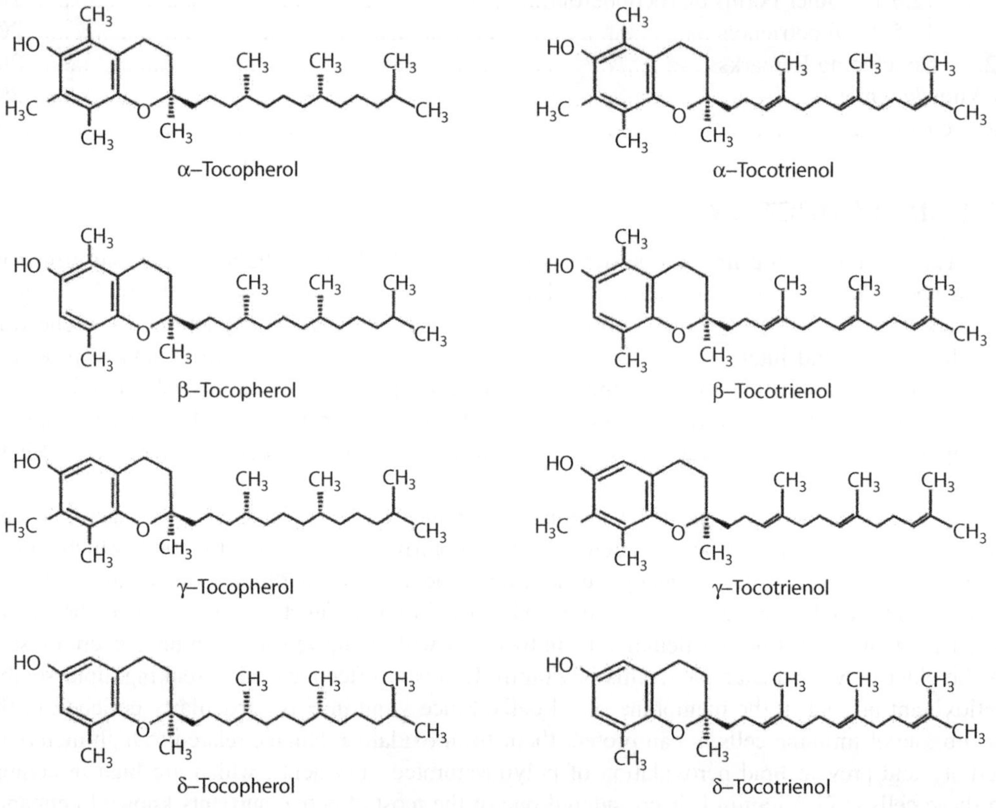

FIGURE 12.1 Chemical structure of vitamin E. All forms of vitamin E have the same chromanol ring. The phytyl tail is saturated in tocopherols and it contains three double bonds in tocotrienols. There are four homologues in both tocopherols and tocotrienols based on the difference in the number and position of methyl groups on the chromanol ring.

as dl-α-tocopherol) or RRR-α-tocopherol (also expressed as d-α-tocopherol); both are often used in the esterified forms. The quantity of vitamin E intake is expressed as either weight (mg) or international unit (IU), which reflects the relative biopotency of vitamin E based on prevention of fetal rat resorption. To help compare the results from the vitamin E studies in which different forms and doses of vitamin E are used but are sometimes referred to generically, it is necessary to provide the interconversion of common forms of vitamin E. One IU of vitamin E is defined as 1 mg of all-rac-α-tocopheryl acetate, 0.67 mg of RRR-α-tocopherol, or 0.74 mg of RRR-α-tocopheryl acetate; the IU equivalents of different forms of vitamin E are determined by the difference in biopotency among the eight stereoisomers (ranging from 100% for RRR to 21% for SSR) and by the adjustment for the difference in the molecular weights of esters. The biopotency ratio for natural vs. synthetic tocopherol is 1.36:1, initially determined by Harris and Ludwig [12], and later validated by several other investigators [13–15].

Different forms of vitamin E are present in foods with varying abundance and proportions. Synthesized by plants, the major dietary sources of vitamin E are edible vegetable oils, nuts, cereals, and vegetables [16]. While oils extracted from wheat germ, safflower, sunflower, grapeseed, and olive contain high amounts of α-tocopherol, the oils from soybean and corn are γ-tocopherol-dominant. In contrast, tocotrienols are mainly found in certain oils (palm oil, rice bran oil) and cereal grains (rye, barley, oat) [17]. α- and γ-tocopherols are the main forms of vitamin E in the common Western diet. α-tocopherol is the most bioavailable, and its plasma concentration is about tenfold higher than that of γ-tocopherol; all other forms of vitamin E are very low or even undetectable in the body. α-tocopherol is also recognized to be the most potent in a variety of biological activities, and is thus the most widely used form of vitamin E in supplements as well as in scientific research (representing roughly 90% of published vitamin E studies). Both synthetic and natural forms of α-tocopherol have been used in published studies, and no consistent evidence suggests a difference in the biological activities tested between these two forms of α-tocopherol.

Currently, the Dietary Reference Intake for vitamin E (DRI 2000) is 15 mg/day for teens and adults [18]. Although vitamin E deficiency rarely occurs, a large portion of the population does not consume the currently recommended daily intake of vitamin E. Primary deficiency is found in genetic defects in α-tocopherol-transfer protein and lipoprotein synthesis as well as in premature and low-birthweight infants; secondary causes are mainly fat malabsorption syndromes and some hematological disorders [19]. The main manifestations of vitamin E deficiency in humans include peripheral neuropathy, skeletal myopathy, reduced red blood cell half-life, and immunological impairments [3,20]. Since the current DRI is for the general population, it may not take into account the people who have specific conditions (aging, disease), which may require increased intake. Further, studies have provided evidence that vitamin E supplementation above currently recommended levels may provide additional health benefits in several bodily systems. The effect of vitamin E supplementation on immune function and resistance to infection is discussed in more detail below.

12.3 VITAMIN E AND IMMUNE FUNCTION

12.3.1 Vitamin E Deficiency and Immune Function

Since vitamin E is essential for maintaining the normal function of cells in almost all bodily systems, it is not surprising that its deficiency causes a variety of symptoms due to the corresponding pathological changes and impaired functionality. Immune cells are particularly enriched with vitamin E because these cells contain high levels of polyunsaturated fatty acids and have high metabolic activity, making them prone to oxidative damage [1,2]. Therefore, it is not difficult to understand the observed impairment in immune function reported in different species as a consequence of vitamin E deficiency. For example, mice fed a vitamin E–deficient diet had a lower humoral immune response (antibody production) than those fed an adequate diet [21]. Vitamin E–deficient rats, compared to their vitamin E–adequate counterparts, had a decrease in antigen presentation by macrophages [22], in phagocytic function of polymorphonuclear cells [23], and in lymphocyte proliferation [24]. Depressed lymphocyte response to T-cell mitogens was also found in vitamin E–deficient dogs [25], lambs [26], pigs [27], and chickens [28]. The observational studies on humans, though very limited, seem to draw the same conclusions. In one study, neutrophils from preterm infants with vitamin E deficiency showed impaired phagocytic and bactericidal activity [29]. In another study with healthy children (3 years old), those with low serum vitamin E levels (<10% percentile) were found to have lower lymphocyte proliferation and serum IgM compared to those with high vitamin E levels (>90% percentile). A case report showed that a 59-year-old woman who developed severe vitamin E deficiency due to intestinal malabsorption had impaired *in vivo* (delayed-type hypersensitivity skin test, DTH) and *in vitro* T-cell function (T-cell proliferation, IL-2 production), which was improved after vitamin E supplementation [3].

12.3.2 Vitamin E Supplementation and Immune Function

Although vitamin E deficiency causes impaired immune function (see previous section), vitamin E deficiency is not common in developed countries. Thus, the logical question is whether animals or humans without obvious vitamin E deficiency could still benefit from the additional intake of vitamin E in terms of an impact on their immune system. Studies over the past few decades have accumulated evidence to suggest that this might be the case. However, this is still a topic of ongoing debate due to some controversial results reported in the literature.

Studies on the immune-modulating effect of vitamin E supplementation started with the use of animal models in a variety of species. As early as the 1950s, vitamin E supplementation was shown to improve antibody production after vaccination in rabbits [30]. Results from later studies supported this initial finding. For examples, it has been reported that dietary supplementation with vitamin E enhances T-cell–mediated function including T-cell differentiation in rat thymus [31]; lymphocyte proliferation in mice [7,32,33], rats [34,35], and pigs [36]; helper T-cell activity and IL-2 production in mice [7,33]; and innate immune function such as natural killer cell activity and phagocytic ability of alveolar macrophages in rats [35]. Vitamin E was also shown in a tumor mouse model to reduce immunosuppression caused by myeloid-derived suppressor cells and to promote antigen-specific CD8+ T-cell activity leading to an enhanced antitumor effect [37]. A recent study showed that even in the Iberian green lizard, a species rarely used in studies of this kind, oral administration of vitamin E (synthetic α-tocopherol, 20 IU/d) could enhance the *in vivo* immune response as determined by T-cell mitogen phytohemagglutinin (PHA)-induced DTH skin response [38]. These results suggest that the immune-stimulating effect of vitamin E is more likely to be universal rather than species-specific.

Encouraged by the positive findings in animal studies, investigators advanced the research to clinical trials in humans. Baehner et al. [39] reported that administering 1,600 IU/d vitamin E (α-tocopherol) to unspecified volunteers for one week increased phagocytic rate but decreased bactericidal activity of polymorphonuclear leukocytes. The authors believed that this result was related to the free radical scavenging effect of vitamin E, which resulted in reduced H_2O_2 production. In another study by Prasad [40], decreased leukocyte bactericidal activity was also observed in young male subjects consuming 300 mg/d vitamin E (dl-α-tocopheryl acetate) for 3 weeks, but there were mixed results for cell-mediated immune function: reduced lymphocyte proliferation and unchanged DTH, both in response to the T-cell mitogen PHA. In a later double-blind, placebo-controlled trial, Meydani et al. [5] showed that healthy older adults (≥60 years old) who received vitamin E (dl-α-tocopheryl acetate) supplementation (800 mg/d) for 1 month had improved DTH response, *ex vivo* T-cell proliferation, IL-2 production, and a reduced production of prostaglandin (PG)E_2, a T-cell–suppressive eicosanoid. They also found a decrease in plasma lipid peroxide concentration compared to the study subjects' baseline values, while all these parameters remained unaltered in those receiving a placebo. To further determine the effect of long-term supplementation with lower doses of vitamin E in the older individuals, Meydani et al. conducted another randomized, double–blind, placebo-controlled trial (RCT) in which free-living elderly (≥65 years old) received 60, 200, or 800 mg/d of vitamin E (dl-α-tocopheryl acetate) or a placebo for 4.5 months [6]. In assessing the *in vivo* immune response with DTH, they found that all three vitamin E groups showed a significant increase in DTH response after supplementation compared to their respective baseline levels. However, the 200 mg/d group demonstrated a significantly greater increase compared to those receiving the placebo, and this group also showed a significant increase in antibody titers in response to hepatitis B and tetanus vaccines (T-cell–dependent antigens) [6]. These findings for the large part were confirmed by Pallast et al. [41], who showed that healthy older subjects (65–80 years old) administered 50 or 100 mg/d of vitamin E (dl-α-tocopheryl acetate) for 6 months had a significant increase in DTH (induration diameter and number of positive responses) compared with their own baseline values, and the change in the number of positive DTH responses tended to be greater in the 100 mg/d group than in the placebo group ($p = 0.06$). These marginal changes were reinforced by correlation analysis showing a significantly greater improvement in the cumulative DTH score and the number of positive DTH responses in a subgroup of subjects in the 100 mg vitamin E group who had lower levels of baseline DTH response. Further, evidence that is somewhat supportive came from a more recent study [42] showing that elderly participants receiving 200 mg/d vitamin E for 3 months had higher levels of PHA-stimulated lymphocyte proliferation, Con A–stimulated IL-2 production, natural killer cell activity, and neutrophil chemotaxis and phagocytosis but lower levels of neutrophil adherence and superoxide anion production. This study was not placebo-controlled; however, the potential bias due to this drawback is somewhat compensated by the observation that when the subjects were tested again 6 months after ending supplementation, the majority of improvements were reversed to baseline levels. Summarizing the results from several studies, Meydani et al. proposed that the net increase in plasma vitamin E levels up to 25 μmol/L are almost linearly associated with an increase in DTH response and that further increase in plasma vitamin E levels beyond this range does not seem to result in additional improvement in DTH [43]. Since it is estimated that a 25 μmol/L increase in plasma vitamin E can be achieved by consuming 200 mg/d of vitamin E [43], this provides a compelling argument to suggest 200 mg/d of vitamin E supplementation be recommended as an optimal dose for improving T-cell–mediated function in the elderly. Taken together, it appears that the evidence is strong to support a positive effect of vitamin E on the cell-mediated immune response. The information about its effect on innate immunity is limited and less clear, which calls for further research. Toward this end, it was recently reported that vitamin E attenuates dysregulated neutrophil function and enhances resistance to *Streptococcus pneumoniae* infection in a mouse model [11].

12.3.3 Mechanism of the Effect of Vitamin E on Immune Function

Unlike two other lipid-soluble vitamins (A and D), which act on their nuclear receptors to regulate the transcription of target genes, no receptor has yet been found for vitamin E. Although a fair amount of work has been accomplished contributing to our knowledge about the mechanisms underlying vitamin E's immunoenhancing effect, we still only partly understand the mode of its action. While the mechanistic investigation involves both human and animal studies, it is largely the results from animal studies combined with cell-based tests that have contributed to most of what we know today in this area.

Since vitamin E is a lipid-soluble antioxidant, a generally accepted mechanism is that vitamin E may exert its immunoenhancing effect by scavenging oxygen species to reduce oxidative stress. Indeed, vitamin E is a highly efficient antioxidant localized in lipid compartments, mainly the cell membranes, where it protects both membrane lipids and proteins from oxidative damage. The cell membrane plays a critical role in immune cell activity. Immune cells depend on proper membrane activity in carrying out a variety of important functions from early activation events to ultimate effector functions. Lipid peroxidation can damage cell membranes and membrane-associated functions. For example, lipid peroxidation can reduce membrane fluidity, which is implicated in a decreased ability of lymphocytes to respond to challenges [44]. It is therefore conceivable that vitamin E may help to maintain the integrity and functionality of immune cell membranes by preventing membrane lipid peroxidation. In addition, as a component residing around the membrane lipids, vitamin E may directly modulate certain properties of membranes, such as lipid raft mobility, which in turn may influence the lateral movement and activation condition of the signaling molecules [45].

More specifically, studies suggest that vitamin E may enhance T-cell–mediated function by influencing the process of signal transduction in T-cells or indirectly, by reducing production of suppressive factors such as PGE_2 by macrophages as summarized in the previous reviews [43,46,47]. The direct effect of vitamin E on T-cell response was established in mice using both *in vitro* and *in vivo* supplementation methods. *In vitro* supplementation with 46 μmol/L vitamin E (d-α-tocopherol) was shown to reverse the age-associated reduction in activation-induced T-cell division and IL-2 production in naive but not memory T-cells [48], which coincides with the reported higher susceptibility of naive T-cells to oxidative damage [49]. Studies also indicate that vitamin E may improve the early events in T-cell activation including formation of effective immune synapses, which have largely been shown to be impaired with aging in both animals and humans. For example, both *in vivo* (500 mg d-α-tocopherol/kg diet) and *in vitro* (46 μmol/L d-α-tocopherol in culture medium) vitamin E supplementation improved effective immune synapse formation and restored defective redistribution of signaling molecules Zap70, LAT, Vav, and PLCγ in the immune synapse formed between antigen-presenting cells and naive CD4+ T-cells from old mice [45]. Improved LAT distribution in immune synapse by vitamin E was later shown to be related to increased phosphorylation of LAT [50], a process required for recruitment of adaptor and effector proteins including Grb2, Gads, SLP76, Vav1, PLCγ1, and phosphoinositide 3-kinase [51,52].

In addition to its direct effect on T-cells, vitamin E can enhance T-cell function by reducing production of PGE_2, a product of arachidonic acid metabolism possessing potent proinflammatory and T-cell–suppressing activity. In the early 1970s, PGE_2 was first reported to suppress T-cell responses by activating adenylyl cyclase, thus increasing cAMP levels [53,54]. PGE_2 production was found to be elevated in animals after infection as well as in aged, but otherwise healthy, animals and humans. In both cases, elevated PGE_2 is believed to significantly contribute to the suppressed immune response. PGE_2 has a broad effect on different components of both the innate and adaptive immune systems [55–58]. Relevant to the topic under discussion here, PGE_2 inhibits T-cell proliferation, IL-2 production, and IL-2 receptor expression [56]. Both CD4+ and CD8+ T-cells are affected by PGE_2, but the effect is more pronounced in the former. Of note, the immune-enhancing effect of vitamin E is also more noticeable on CD4+ than CD8+ T-cells. Furthermore, the suppressive effect of PGE_2 on T-cell activity is related to the inhibition of several early signaling events that occur after T-cell activation [58]; importantly, some of these signaling processes are positively impacted by vitamin E. Studies have shown that macrophages and spleen cells from old mice and peripheral blood mononuclear cells from elderly human subjects produce more PGE_2 compared to those from their young counterparts [5,7,59,60], and this age-related increase in PGE_2 production contributes to impaired T-cell function [61,62]. Although it has long been known that vitamin E is effective in inhibiting prostaglandin synthesis in certain tissues, before the era of cyclooxygenase (COX) research, our understanding of the mode of action was limited to the speculation that vitamin E as an antioxidant might prevent arachidonic acid oxidation. This was later confirmed by Wu et al. [63], who reported that dietary supplementation with 500 mg/kg of vitamin E for 30 days reduced LPS-stimulated PGE_2 production by macrophages from old mice. They further showed that vitamin E exerted its effect by inhibiting the enzymatic activity of COX, a rate-limiting enzyme for prostaglandin synthesis, but without altering expression of either form of COX (COX-1 or COX-2) at either the protein or mRNA level [63]. These findings were later largely corroborated by other investigators [64,65]. While the mechanism of how vitamin E inhibits COX activity is not completely understood, the work of Beharka et al. suggests that, at least in old mice, this effect may be mediated through a reduced peroxynitrite production [66].

12.4   VITAMIN E AND INFECTION

A functional immune system is critical to the body's defense against infection. Existence of a strong association between impaired immune function and increased risk of infection is supported by numerous observational and experimental studies on a variety of pathogens. It is thus conceivable that vitamin E may help fight infection by modulating an appropriate, antipathogen immune response. Early demonstration of the protective effect of vitamin E on infection came from animal studies that used various infection models. Today, animal models are still a primary tool for investigating the role of vitamin E on infection. In contrast, due to ethical issues, the information for humans is from the studies conducted exclusively using the incidence of natural infections.

12.4.1   ANIMAL MODELS

Studies using various animal models have indicated that the immunostimulating effect of vitamin E may be associated with an improved host resistance to infections such as *Escherichia coli* in chicks [67] and pigs [68]; *Diplococcus pneumoniae* type I [69] and *Streptococcus pneumoniae* [11] in mice; *Listeria monocytogenes* in turkeys [70]; influenza infection in mice [8,9]; and also secondary *Staphylococcus aureus* infection after influenza infection in mice [10]. Since the incidence of, and mortality from, respiratory infection is profoundly higher in older adults and a compromised immune response is a significant contributing factor, using animal models of respiratory infection is preferred for vitamin E research. Thus, we will review a few such studies in more detail.

Hayek et al. [8] reported that compared to young mice, old mice had higher viral titers after being infected with influenza A/Port Chalmers/1/73 (H3N2); vitamin E supplementation (dl-α-tocopheryl acetate, 500 mg/kg diet) for 6 weeks reduced viral titers in both young and old mice but more so in the latter. This study also demonstrated that the age-related decline in natural killer cell activity was restored by vitamin E supplementation, suggesting involvement of the innate immune function in the protective effect of vitamin E. In another study of similar design, Han et al. [9] confirmed the protective effect of vitamin E in influenza infection. They further showed that the protective effect was also, in part, due to improved cell-mediated immune function: they found that old mice had more severe symptoms and delayed viral clearance, both of which were associated with lower IL-2 and higher PGE_2 production before infection, and in particular, with a lower IFN-γ production in response to viral infection. In a recent study using a bacterial infection model, Bou Ghanem et al. [11] showed that old mice compared to young mice had higher pulmonary bacterial burden, lethal septicemia, and lung inflammation (neutrophil infiltration) after being infected with *Streptococcus pneumoniae*. This age-related impairment in resistance to the infection was diminished by dietary vitamin E supplementation (d-α-tocopheryl acetate, 500 mg/kg diet) administered for 4 weeks. Their further mechanistic study showed that a key factor underlying vitamin E's protective effect is its reduction of neutrophil transepithelial migration (an adverse inflammatory process), which in turn may be attributed to altered expression of several epithelial and neutrophil adhesion molecules involved in neutrophil migration.

12.4.2   HUMAN STUDIES

Epidemiological evidence specifically linking vitamin E intake to infection is scarce. A retrospective study in healthy persons ($\geq$ 60 years old) found a negative relationship between plasma vitamin E levels and the number of infections over the past 3 years; however, there was no correlation found between vitamin E status and the indices of immune response including T-cell phenotype, PHA-induced lymphocyte proliferation, and DTH response to seven ubiquitous antigens [71]. Few clinical trials have directly examined how vitamin E supplementation impacts the host's resistance to infection. This type of study presents challenges since it depends on recording the natural occurrence of infection, but the incidence of a specific infection or even total infections is relatively low in many populations and thus would require a large sample size to detect significant differences. While the results generated from studies conducted thus far are promising, inconsistencies exist, necessitating more clinical trials to confirm the efficacy of vitamin E in reducing the risk or severity of infection. In the RCT mentioned above, which sought to determine (and indeed evidenced) the immune-enhancing effect of vitamin E [6], Meydani et al. also observed a nonsignificant ($p = 0.1$), 30% lower incidence of self-reported infections in all the vitamin E groups combined (60, 200, or 800 mg/d as dl-α-tocopheryl acetate) compared to the placebo group. Inspired by this, they later conducted an RCT in nursing home residents (>65 years old), a population that has a high incidence of infection, to specifically address whether vitamin E has a protective effect against respiratory infection. In this study, 617 participants received 200 mg/d vitamin E (dl-α-tocopheryl acetate) or placebo for one year, and their respiratory infections (RI) were objectively recorded during this time [72]. The authors found that significantly fewer participants acquired one or more RI or upper RI in the vitamin E–supplemented versus the placebo-treated subjects and that a lower incidence of common colds occurred in the vitamin E group. These studies support the notion that the immunostimulatory effect of vitamin E has clinical benefit in protecting against respiratory infections.

However, other studies in which infection was not the primary outcome have not produced consistent results. For example, Hemila et al., using data generated in the Alpha-Tocopherol Beta-Carotene Cancer Prevention (ATBC) study, showed a positive effect, no effect, or even a negative effect of vitamin E on pneumonia and the common cold depending on the age, smoking history, residence, exercise, and other subject characteristics [73–75]. This discrepancy may be attributed to a variety of confounding factors, especially the difference in the health conditions of participants and the intervention protocols. For instance, the ATBC study used a small dose (50 mg/d) of vitamin E in combination with 20 mg/d of β-carotene, which makes it difficult to compare this study's results with those reported by Meydani et al. In another RCT conducted in a Dutch elderly ($\geq$60 years old) cohort living in the community, the authors found no effect of 200 mg/d of vitamin E (200 mg dl-α-tocopheryl acetate) on the incidence of all RI [76]. Notably, since there are several differences in the study design and data analysis between the study by Graat et al., conducted with free-living participants, and the one conducted in managed nursing homes by Meydani et al. [72], these variations might have contributed to different outcomes of the two studies. One explanation could be that the immunoenhancing effect of vitamin E in the elderly might be associated with increased resistance to RI in nursing home residents, who, while frailer, might be under more controlled conditions. This may not be the case for those who are younger, healthier, living independently, and influenced by other lifestyle factors. Further studies are needed to answer these questions.

Finally, it is worth adding that the widely varied response to vitamin E supplementation observed among individuals, as well as from different studies, may be attributed to differences in baseline levels of immune response and genetic background of participants. For example, after analyzing the data generated from the study mentioned above [72], Belisle et al. conducted an analysis for interaction between the response to vitamin E treatment in cytokine production and the baseline levels of these cytokines, and concluded that the effect of vitamin E supplementation on cytokine production depended on presupplementation cytokine levels [77]. Further, they showed that single nucleotide polymorphisms also influenced whether and to what extent vitamin E treatment alters cytokine production [78]; common SNPs at cytokine genes may contribute to the individual risk of respiratory infection in the elderly, and both genetic factors and sex may have a significant bearing on the efficacy of vitamin E [79]. This should be considered when interpreting the inconsistent results of previous studies as well as when designing future studies to investigate effect of vitamin E on immune response and related disease.

12.5   NON-α-TOCOPHEROL VITAMIN E

12.5.1   OTHER FORMS OF TOCOPHEROLS

The amount of the four types of naturally occurring tocopherols from different food sources significantly varies as do their bioavailability and presence in the body. α-tocopherol and γ-tocopherol are the predominant forms of vitamin E in the human diet. Although the typical American diet contains even more γ- than α-tocopherol [80] due to the widespread use of corn and soybean oil [81], γ-tocopherol is only about one-tenth the amount of α-tocopherol in human plasma, which largely results from the preferential binding of α-tocopherol transfer protein to α-tocopherol over non-α-tocopherols. Likewise, less availability combined with low bioavailability makes β- and δ-tocopherols much lower or even undetectable in plasma. Accordingly, biological functions of non-α-tocopherols are less studied in general, and little is known about their effect on immune function in particular. Research on γ-tocopherol started much later relative to α-tocopherols; however, γ-tocopherol has received increasing attention in the past years and much progress has been made as demonstrated by the steadily growing findings about its anti-inflammatory properties and applications [82]. It is also worth noting that the recent positive findings related to anticancer activity of both γ- and δ-tocopherols in animal models have opened up a new area of research related to vitamin E's health benefits beyond the effects of α-tocopherol [83].

The research on non-α-tocopherols as mentioned above will not be discussed further, because this chapter is focused primarily on vitamin E's role in immunity and infection for which the information is very limited for non-α-tocopherols. An *in vitro* study showed that while all forms of tocopherols could enhance mitogen-induced T-cell lymphocyte proliferation, the dose required to reach maximal enhancement varied among the homologues in the order of α- > γ- > β- ≈ δ-tocopherol [84]. In addition, this study reported that these various forms of tocopherols had a differential effect on IL-2 and PGE_2 production. The difference in the nature and magnitude of the effect on immune cell function did not correspond to the relative antioxidant activity of these tocopherol homologues; thus, these results indicate unique biological activities related to the minor differences in their structure. More recently, Zingg et al. reported a study that determined the gene transcription profile of T-cells from old mice fed a diet supplemented with high amounts (500 mg/kg) of α- or γ-tocopherol (as RRR-tocopheryl acetate) relative to their respective control (adequate, 30 mg/kg) [85]. They found that expression of some genes was uniquely affected by either α-tocopherol (such as CD40 ligand, lymphotoxin A) or γ-tocopherol (such as poliovirus receptor-related-2). Overall, it appears that α-tocopherol activates gene clusters that promote lymphocyte proliferation and survival, whereas γ-tocopherol activates gene clusters that reduce lymphocyte proliferation and promote apoptosis and inflammation. These results further support the presence of biological functions unique to both α- and γ-tocopherols; however, given that α- and γ-tocopherols are known to compete for transport and metabolism (though α-tocopherol is more competitive), this leads to a reciprocal change in their tissue levels. Since vitamin E concentrations in T-cells or blood were not determined in this study, we do not know how much of the observed effects represent direct effects of each form of vitamin E or how much of the outcome was attributed to the altered tissue levels due to the competition in their incorporation into the target cells. Interestingly, although γ-tocopherol has been shown to possess anti-inflammatory properties unmatched by α-tocopherol both quantitatively and qualitatively, some studies found γ-tocopherol to be not only proinflammatory but also antagonistic to α-tocopherol's anti-inflammatory effect in animal models of inflammatory disorders. For example, γ-tocopherol administration (via subcutaneous injection) was reported to elevate its levels in plasma and lung resulting in increased inflammation in lung tissue of ovalbumin-induced allergic mice (asthma model), which was reversed by increasing α-tocopherol levels [86,87]. While it will require more research to resolve the discrepancies reported regarding the exact role of γ-tocopherol in inflammation, one possible explanation is that γ-tocopherol's effect may be dose-dependent. A proinflammatory effect was found in the above-mentioned studies after γ-tocopherol was administered via subcutaneous injection. Injections bypass liver metabolism resulting in more γ-tocopherol and fewer of its metabolites in blood and tissues; this is in contrast to oral administration, which was used by several other studies reporting an anti-inflammatory effect of γ-tocopherol. Although there has been steady progress in the study of γ-tocopherol, as well as recently elevated interest in other non-α-tocopherols, little information specific to the cell-mediated immune system is currently available. Nevertheless, the results reported thus far indicate that further research in this area might be fruitful.

12.5.2 TOCOTRIENOLS

In contrast to tocopherols, tocotrienols, the other half of the vitamin E family, are less well distributed in the food consumed by a great majority of people and are thus less studied. However, research on tocotrienols has accelerated and impressive progress has been made over the past decade. Growing evidence has suggested that tocotrienols may have multiple biological functions including potential anticancer [88,89], anti-angiogenic [90–92], blood cholesterol–lowering [93–95], anti-atherosclerotic [96–98], and neuroprotective effects [99–101]. A human study concluded that tocotrienols did not improve immune function in healthy individuals (20–50 years old). After daily supplementation with 200 mg of tocotrienol-rich fraction (TRF, composed of 70% tocotrienols including 113, 91, 36, and 10 mg/g α-, γ-, δ-, and β-tocotrienols, respectively, and 30% α-tocopherol) for 56 days, the authors found no effect on blood immune cell phenotype or production of cytokines IL-4 and IFN-γ compared to placebo or a 200 mg/d of α-tocopherol group [102]. Since these are the only parameters tested in defining an immune-modulating effect, a more comprehensive selection of markers may be required in future studies to confirm or refute this conclusion. Later, in an RCT conducted by the same group, results showed that young healthy individuals (18–25 years old) receiving 400 mg TRF/d for 2 months had higher antibody production in response to tetanus toxoid vaccine and higher IFN-γ and IL-4 production by their blood leukocytes after they were stimulated *in vitro* by tetanus toxoid antigen or Con A [103]. These authors also conducted an animal study of essentially the same design but added a group fed purified δ-tocotrienol. They were able to repeat their observations from the human study together with the new finding that δ-tocotrienol had a more pronounced effect than TRF and α-tocopherol in enhancing IFN-γ production [104]. In an animal study reported by Ren et al. [105], young (4 months old) and old (23 months old) C57BL/6 mice were fed 0.1% Tocomin® 50%, a mixture of natural tocotrienols (α-, β-, δ-, and γ-tocotrienols at 12.2%, 2%, 6.2%, and 20.1%, respectively) and α-tocopherol (10.7%), or a control diet containing an equal amount of α-tocopherol for 6 weeks. Lymphocyte proliferation was enhanced by feeding Tocomin® 50% relative to the control diet, but this effect was more pronounced in old than in young mice. Tocomin® 50% also increased IL-1β production and tended to increase IL-2 production by the splenocytes of old mice, and increased IL-1β production by macrophages of both young and old mice. *In vitro* supplementation with purified tocotrienols at all tested levels (0.01 to 5 μmol/L) enhanced lymphocyte proliferation with a potency order of α-> γ-> δ-tocotrienol with maximal enhancement reached at 0.15, 0.3, and 0.625 μmol/L, respectively. Similar to the findings in the *in vivo* study, this effect was more pronounced for cells from old compared to young mice.

Although tocotrienols are not present in significant amounts in a regular diet and they do not seem to be essential to life, studies have suggested their beneficial effects on several bodily systems. With the studies reviewed above, we are beginning to learn that tocotrienols may possess immune-modulating properties. This area of vitamin E research is still in its infancy; however, the preliminary results thus far suggest, with limited certainty, potential efficacy of tocotrienols in impacting the immune response. Future studies are needed to substantiate these assumptions.

12.6 CONCLUDING REMARKS

Vitamin E is a potent, lipid-soluble antioxidant. Its broad biological functions have been well-documented. Concerning the immune system, convincing evidence through descriptive studies suggests that vitamin E plays a key role in optimizing the immune response, particularly that involving T-cell–mediated function. A substantial body of work delineating the underlying mechanism of vitamin E's impact on the immune response supports the phenotypic observations. Furthermore, the clinical significance and potential applicability of this beneficial effect of vitamin E are supported by animal model studies and clinical trials using infection as an endpoint. Nevertheless, controversy still exists as not all investigators have observed the same positive results. This may be partly attributed to differences in study design, experimental protocols, and cohort characteristics including their genetic background. As with many other nutrients, a vitamin E deficiency state leads to impaired immune function, rendering an individual susceptible to infection. Although a large percentage of people do not consume the recommended dietary intake for vitamin E, cases of deficiency are rare in developed countries. Therefore, research on vitamin E and immune function has focused on determining the potential of vitamin E at higher than the recommended level (15 mg/day) for improving immune function in target populations such as older adults. Achieving this goal will provide an opportunity to expand the clinical applications of vitamin E in developing preventive and therapeutic strategies to combat age-related diseases, especially infection. α-tocopherol is the form of vitamin E used in a majority of human and animal studies. Emerging evidence however has revealed the uniqueness or higher efficacy of the non-α-tocopherol members of the vitamin E family on a variety of biological functions. These findings have been used to explain the reason for the failure of several intervention trials to support or even, in some cases, dispute, the health benefits of vitamin E intake suggested by the findings in epidemiologic studies. Based on preliminary observations, some investigators have suggested that increased intake of α-tocopherol may reduce the body's uptake of all the other forms of vitamin E, which otherwise might exert their unique or greater effect relative to α-tocopherol in promoting health. As we continue our efforts to better understand the actions of α-tocopherol, research should be expanded to include all members of the vitamin E family. Furthermore, studies which consider genetic background of study participants in terms of their responsiveness to vitamin E supplementation are needed to define target populations for vitamin E intervention. Advances in understanding the interactions of the different forms of vitamin E regarding uptake, metabolism, and biological function and its interaction with genetic background are needed in order to formulate accurate dietary guidance and supplementation strategies for optimizing immune and inflammatory responses and preventing related diseases.

ACKNOWLEDGMENTS

The authors are supported by the USDA/ARS under contract #58-1950-4-003. The authors thank Stephanie Marco for her help in the preparation of the manuscript.

REFERENCES

1. Coquette, A., B. Vray, and J. Vanderpas. 1986. Role of vitamin E in the protection of the resident macrophage membrane against oxidative damage. *Arch Int Physiol Biochim* 94: S29–S34.
2. Hatam, L. J. and H. J. Kayden. 1979. A high-performance liquid chromatographic method for the determination of tocopherol in plasma and cellular elements of the blood. *J Lipid Res* 20: 639–645.
3. Kowdley, K. V., J. B. Mason, S. N. Meydani, S. Cornwall, and R. J. Grand. 1992. Vitamin E deficiency and impaired cellular immunity related to intestinal fat malabsorption. *Gastroenterology* 102: 2139–2142.
4. Han, S. N. and S. N. Meydani. 1999. Vitamin E and infectious diseases in the aged. *Proc Nutr Soc* 58: 697–705.

5. Meydani, S. N., M. P. Barklund, S. Liu, M. Meydani, R. A. Miller, J. G. Cannon, F. D. Morrow, R. Rocklin, and J. B. Blumberg. 1990. Vitamin E supplementation enhances cell-mediated immunity in healthy elderly subjects. *Am J Clin Nutr* 52: 557–563.

6. Meydani, S. N., M. Meydani, J. B. Blumberg, L. S. Leka, G. Siber, R. Loszewski, C. Thompson, M. C. Pedrosa, R. D. Diamond, and B. D. Stollar. 1997. Vitamin E supplementation and in vivo immune response in healthy elderly subjects. A randomized controlled trial. *JAMA* 277: 1380–1386.

7. Meydani, S. N., M. Meydani, C. P. Verdon, A. A. Shapiro, J. B. Blumberg, and K. C. Hayes. 1986. Vitamin E supplementation suppresses prostaglandin E1(2) synthesis and enhances the immune response of aged mice. *Mech Ageing Dev* 34: 191–201.

8. Hayek, M. G., S. F. Taylor, B. S. Bender, S. N. Han, M. Meydani, D. E. Smith, S. Eghtesada, and S. N. Meydani. 1997. Vitamin E supplementation decreases lung virus titers in mice infected with influenza. *J Infect Dis* 176: 273–276.

9. Han, S. N., D. Wu, W. K. Ha, A. Beharka, D. E. Smith, B. S. Bender, and S. N. Meydani. 2000. Vitamin E supplementation increases T helper 1 cytokine production in old mice infected with influenza virus. *Immunology* 100: 487–493.

10. Gay, R., S. N. Han, M. Marko, S. Belisle, R. Bronson, and S. N. Meydani. 2004. The effect of vitamin E on secondary bacterial infection after influenza infection in young and old mice. *Ann N Y Acad Sci* 1031: 418–421.

11. Bou Ghanem, E. N., S. Clark, X. Du, D. Wu, A. Camilli, J. M. Leong, and S. N. Meydani. 2015. The alpha-tocopherol form of vitamin E reverses age-associated susceptibility to streptococcus pneumoniae lung infection by modulating pulmonary neutrophil recruitment. *J Immunol* 194: 1090–1099.

12. Harris, P. L. and M. I. Ludwig. 1949. Relative vitamin E potency of natural and of synthetic alpha-tocopherol. *J Biol Chem* 179: 1111–1115.

13. Leth, T. and H. Sondergaard. 1977. Biological activity of vitamin E compounds and natural materials by the resorption-gestation test, and chemical determination of the vitamin E activity in foods and feeds. *J Nutr* 107: 2236–2243.

14. Weiser, H., M. Vecchi, and M. Schlachter. 1985. Stereoisomers of alpha-tocopheryl acetate. III. Simultaneous determination of resorption-gestation and myopathy in rats as a means of evaluating bio-potency ratios of all-rac- and RRR-alpha-tocopheryl acetate. *Int J Vitam Nutr Res* 55: 149–158.

15. Weiser, H. and M. Vecchi. 1981. Stereoisomers of alpha-tocopheryl acetate--characterization of the samples by physico-chemical methods and determination of biological activities in the rat resorption-gestation test. *Int J Vitam Nutr Res* 51: 100–113.

16. Murphy, S. P., A. F. Subar, and G. Block. 1990. Vitamin E intakes and sources in the United States. *Am J Clin Nutr* 52: 361–367.

17. Aggarwal, B. B., C. Sundaram, S. Prasad, and R. Kannappan. 2010. Tocotrienols, the vitamin E of the 21st century: Its potential against cancer and other chronic diseases. *Biochem Pharmacol* 80: 1613–1631.

18. Food and Nutrition Board, Institute of Medicine. 2000. *Dietary Reference Intakes for Vitamin C, Vitamin E, Selenium, Carotenoids*. Washington, DC: National Academy Press.

19. Traber, M. G. 1999. *Vitamin E. In Modern Nutrition in Health and Disease*. M. E. Shils, J. A. Olson, M. Shike, and A. C. Ross, eds. Baltimore, MD: Williams & Wilkins. 347–362.

20. Traber, M. G., ed. 2012. *Vitamin E*. Washington, DC: ILSI Press.

21. Tengerdy, R. P., R. H. Henzerling, G. L. Brown, and M. M. Mathias. 1973. Enhancement of the humoral immune response by vitamin E. *Int Arch Allergy Appl Immunol* 44: 221–232.

22. Gebremichael, A., E. M. Levy, and L. M. Corwin. 1984. Adherent cell requirement for the effect of vitamin E on in vitro antibody synthesis. *J Nutr* 114: 1297–1305.

23. Harris, R. E., L. A. Boxer, and R. L. Baehner. 1980. Consequences of vitamin-E deficiency on the phagocytic and oxidative functions of the rat polymorphonuclear leukocyte. *Blood* 55: 338–343.

24. Eskew, M. L., R. W. Scholz, C. C. Reddy, D. A. Todhunter, and A. Zarkower. 1985. Effects of vitamin E and selenium deficiencies on rat immune function. *Immunology* 54: 173–180.

25. Langweiler, M., R. D. Schultz, and B. E. Sheffy. 1981. Effect of vitamin E deficiency on the proliferative response of canine lymphocytes. *Am J Vet Res* 42: 1681–1685.

26. Turner, R. J. and J. M. Finch. 1990. Immunological malfunctions associated with low selenium-vitamin E diets in lambs. *J Comp Pathol* 102: 99–109.

27. Jensen, M., C. Fossum, M. Ederoth, and R. V. Hakkarainen. 1988. The effect of vitamin E on the cell-mediated immune response in pigs. *Zentralbl Veterinarmed B* 35: 549–555.

28. Chang, W. P., J. S. Hom, R. R. Dietert, G. F. Combs, Jr., and J. A. Marsh. 1994. Effect of dietary vitamin E and selenium deficiency on chicken splenocyte proliferation and cell surface marker expression. *Immunopharmacol Immunotoxicol* 16: 203–223.

29. Miller, M. E. 1979. Phagocytic function in the same neonate: Selected aspects. *Pediatrics* 64: 5709–5712.
30. Segagni, E. 1955. Immunity phenomena and vitamin E; antityphus agglutinins and their behavior during treatment with vitamin E; experimental research. *Minerva Pediatr* 7: 985–988.
31. Moriguchi, S., H. Miwa, M. Okamura, K. Maekawa, Y. Kishino, and K. Maeda. 1993. Vitamin E is an important factor in T cell differentiation in thymus of F344 rats. *J Nutr Sci Vitaminol (Tokyo)* 39: 451–463.
32. Corwin, L. M. and J. Shloss. 1980. Influence of vitamin E on the mitogenic response of murine lymphoid cells. *J Nutr* 110: 916–923.
33. Wang, Y. and R. R. Watson. 1994. Vitamin E supplementation at various levels alters cytokine production by thymocytes during retrovirus infection causing murine AIDS. *Thymus* 22: 153–165.
34. Bendich, A., E. Gabriel, and L. J. Machlin. 1986. Dietary vitamin E requirement for optimum immune responses in the rat. *J Nutr* 116: 675–681.
35. Moriguchi, S., N. Kobayashi, and Y. Kishino. 1990. High dietary intakes of vitamin E and cellular immune functions in rats. *J Nutr* 120: 1096–1102.
36. Larsen, H. J. and S. Tollersrud. 1981. Effect of dietary vitamin E and selenium on the phytohaemagglutinin response of pig lymphocytes. *Res Vet Sci* 31: 301–305.
37. Kang, T. H., J. Knoff, W. H. Yeh, B. Yang, C. Wang, Y. S. Kim, T. W. Kim, T. C. Wu, and C. F. Hung. 2014. Treatment of tumors with vitamin E suppresses myeloid derived suppressor cells and enhances CD8+ T cell-mediated antitumor effects. *PLOS ONE* 9: e103562.
38. Kopena, R., P. Lopez, and J. Martin. 2014. What are carotenoids signaling? Immunostimulatory effects of dietary vitamin E, but not of carotenoids, in Iberian green lizards. *Naturwissenschaften* 101: 1107–1114.
39. Baehner, R. L., L. A. Boxer, J. M. Allen, and J. Davis. 1977. Autooxidation as a basis for altered function by polymorphonuclear leukocytes. *Blood* 50: 327–335.
40. Prasad, J. S. 1980. Effect of vitamin E supplementation on leukocyte function. *Am J Clin Nutr* 33: 606–608.
41. Pallast, E. G., E. G. Schouten, F. G. de Waart, H. C. Fonk, G. Doekes, B. M. von Blomberg, and F. J. Kok. 1999. Effect of 50- and 100-mg vitamin E supplements on cellular immune function in noninstitutionalized elderly persons. *Am J Clin Nutr* 69: 1273–1281.
42. De la Fuente, M., A. Hernanz, N. Guayerbas, V. M. Victor, and F. Arnalich. 2008. Vitamin E ingestion improves several immune functions in elderly men and women. *Free Radic Res* 42: 272–280.
43. Meydani, S. N., S. N. Han, and D. Wu. 2005. Vitamin E and immune response in the aged: Molecular mechanisms and clinical implications. *Immunol Rev* 205: 269–284.
44. Bendich, A., ed. 1990. *Antioxidant Vitamins and Their Functions in Immune Responses*. New York, NY: Plenum Press.
45. Marko, M. G., T. Ahmed, S. C. Bunnell, D. Wu, H. Chung, B. T. Huber, and S. N. Meydani. 2007. Age-associated decline in effective immune synapse formation of CD4(+) T cells is reversed by vitamin E supplementation. *J Immunol* 178: 1443–1449.
46. Wu, D. and S. N. Meydani. 2008. Age-associated changes in immune and inflammatory responses: Impact of vitamin E intervention. *J Leukoc Biol* 84: 900–914.
47. Wu, D. and S. N. Meydani. 2014. Age-associated changes in immune function: Impact of vitamin E intervention and the underlying mechanisms. *Endocr Metab Immune Disord Drug Targets* 14: 283–289.
48. Adolfsson, O., B. T. Huber, and S. N. Meydani. 2001. Vitamin E-enhanced IL-2 production in old mice: Naive but not memory T cells show increased cell division cycling and IL-2-producing capacity. *J Immunol* 167: 3809–3817.
49. Lohmiller, J. J., K. M. Roellich, A. Toledano, P. S. Rabinovitch, N. S. Wolf, and A. Grossmann. 1996. Aged murine T-lymphocytes are more resistant to oxidative damage due to the predominance of the cells possessing the memory phenotype. *J Gerontol A Biol Sci Med Sci* 51: B132–B140.
50. Marko, M. G., H. J. Pang, Z. Ren, A. Azzi, B. T. Huber, S. C. Bunnell, and S. N. Meydani. 2009. Vitamin E reverses impaired linker for activation of T cells activation in T cells from aged C57BL/6 mice. *J Nutr* 139: 1192–1197.
51. Paz, P. E., S. Wang, H. Clarke, X. Lu, D. Stokoe, and A. Abo. 2001. Mapping the Zap-70 phosphorylation sites on LAT (linker for activation of T cells) required for recruitment and activation of signalling proteins in T cells. *Biochem J* 356: 461–471.
52. Zhang, W., R. P. Trible, M. Zhu, S. K. Liu, C. J. McGlade, and L. E. Samelson. 2000. Association of Grb2, Gads, and phospholipase C-gamma 1 with phosphorylated LAT tyrosine residues. Effect of LAT tyrosine mutations on T cell angien receptor-mediated signaling. *J Biol Chem* 275: 23355–23361.
53. Smith, J. W., A. L. Steiner, W. M. Newberry, Jr., and C. W. Parker. 1971. Cyclic adenosine 3',5'-monophosphate in human lymphocytes. Alterations after phytohemagglutinin stimulation. *J Clin Invest* 50: 432–441.

54. Smith, J. W., A. L. Steiner, and C. W. Parker. 1971. Human lymphocytic metabolism. Effects of cyclic and noncyclic nucleotides on stimulation by phytohemagglutinin. *J Clin Invest* 50: 442–448.
55. Harris, S. G., J. Padilla, L. Koumas, D. Ray, and R. P. Phipps. 2002. Prostaglandins as modulators of immunity. *Trends Immunol* 23: 144–150.
56. Kalinski, P. 2012. Regulation of immune responses by prostaglandin E2. *J Immunol* 188: 21–28.
57. Rocca, B. and G. A. FitzGerald. 2002. Cyclooxygenases and prostaglandins: Shaping up the immune response. *Int Immunopharmacol* 2: 603–630.
58. Sreeramkumar, V., M. Fresno, and N. Cuesta. 2012. Prostaglandin E2 and T cells: Friends or foes? *Immunol Cell Biol* 90: 579–586.
59. Bartocci, A., F. M. Maggi, R. D. Welker, and F. Veronese. 1982. Age-related immunossuppresion: Putative role of prostaglandins. *In Prostaglandins and Cancer*. T. J. Powles, R. S. Backman, K. V. Honn, and P. Ramwell, eds. New York, NY: Alan R. Liss. 725–730.
60. Hayek, M. G., S. N. Meydani, M. Meydani, and J. B. Blumberg. 1994. Age differences in eicosanoid production of mouse splenocytes: Effects on mitogen-induced T-cell proliferation. *J Gerontol* 49: B197–B207.
61. Beharka, A. A., D. Wu, S. N. Han, and S. N. Meydani. 1997. Macrophage PGE₂ production contributes to the age-associated decrease in T cell function which is reversed by dietary antioxidants. *Mech Ageing Dev* 93: 59–77.
62. Franklin, R. A., S. Arkins, Y. M. Li, and K. W. Kelley. 1993. Macrophages suppress lectin-induced proliferation of lymphocytes from aged rats. *Mech Ageing Dev* 67: 33–46.
63. Wu, D., C. Mura, A. A. Beharka, S. N. Han, K. E. Paulson, D. Hwang, and S. N. Meydani. 1998. Age-associated increase in PGE2 synthesis and COX activity in murine macrophages is reversed by vitamin E. *Am J Physiol* 275: C661–C668.
64. Jiang, Q., I. Elson-Schwab, C. Courtemanche, and B. N. Ames. 2000. Gamma-tocopherol and its major metabolite, in contrast to alpha-tocopherol, inhibit cyclooxygenase activity in macrophages and epithelial cells. *Proc Natl Acad Sci U S A* 97: 11494–11499.
65. O'Leary, K. A., S. de Pascual-Tereasa, P. W. Needs, Y. P. Bao, N. M. O'Brien, and G. Williamson. 2004. Effect of flavonoids and vitamin E on cyclooxygenase-2 (COX-2) transcription. *Mutat Res* 551: 245–254.
66. Beharka, A. A., D. Wu, M. Serafini, and S. N. Meydani. 2002. Mechanism of vitamin E inhibition of cyclooxygenase activity in macrophages from old mice: Role of peroxynitrite. *Free Radic Boil Med* 32: 503–511.
67. Heinzerling, R. H., C. F. Nockels, C. L. Quarles, and R. P. Tengerdy. 1974. Protection of chicks against E. coli infection by dietary supplementation with vitamin E. *Proc Soc Exp Biol Med* 146: 279–283.
68. Ellis, R. P. and M. W. Vorhies. 1976. Effect of supplemental dietary vitamin E on the serologic response of swine to an Escherichia coli bacterin. *J Am Vet Med Assoc* 168: 231–232.
69. Heinzerling, R. H., R. P. Tengerdy, L. L. Wick, and D. C. Lueker. 1974. Vitamin E protects mice against Diplococcus pneumoniae type I infection. *Infect Immun* 10: 1292–1295.
70. Zhu, M., I. V. Wesley, R. Nannapaneni, M. Cox, A. Mendonca, M. G. Johnson, and D. U. Ahn. 2003. The role of dietary vitamin E in experimental Listeria monocytogenes infections in turkeys. *Poult Sci* 82: 1559–1564.
71. Chavance, M., B. Herbeth, C. Fournier, C. Janot, and G. Vernhes. 1989. Vitamin status, immunity and infections in an elderly population. *Eur J Clin Nutr* 43: 827–835.
72. Meydani, S. N., L. S. Leka, B. C. Fine, G. E. Dallal, G. T. Keusch, M. F. Singh, and D. H. Hamer. 2004. Vitamin E and respiratory tract infections in elderly nursing home residents: A randomized controlled trial. *JAMA* 292: 828–836.
73. Hemila, H. and J. Kaprio. 2011. Subgroup analysis of large trials can guide further research: A case study of vitamin E and pneumonia. *Clin Epidemiol* 3: 51–59.
74. Hemila, H., J. Virtamo, D. Albanes, and J. Kaprio. 2004. Vitamin E and beta-carotene supplementation and hospital-treated pneumonia incidence in male smokers. *Chest* 125: 557–565.
75. Hemila, H., J. Virtamo, D. Albanes, and J. Kaprio. 2006. The effect of vitamin E on common cold incidence is modified by age, smoking and residential neighborhood. *J Am Coll Nutr* 25: 332–339.
76. Graat, J. M., E. G. Schouten, and F. J. Kok. 2002. Effect of daily vitamin E and multivitamin-mineral supplementation on acute respiratory tract infections in elderly persons: A randomized controlled trial. *JAMA* 288: 715–721.
77. Belisle, S. E., L. S. Leka, G. E. Dallal, P. F. Jacques, J. Delgado-Lista, J. M. Ordovas, and S. N. Meydani. 2008. Cytokine response to vitamin E supplementation is dependent on pre-supplementation cytokine levels. *Biofactors* 33: 191–200.

78. Belisle, S. E., D. H. Hamer, L. S. Leka, G. E. Dallal, J. Delgado-Lista, B. C. Fine, P. F. Jacques, J. M. Ordovas, and S. N. Meydani. 2010. IL-2 and IL-10 gene polymorphisms are associated with respiratory tract infection and may modulate the effect of vitamin E on lower respiratory tract infections in elderly nursing home residents. *Am J Clin Nutr* 92: 106–114.

79. Belisle, S. E., L. S. Leka, J. Delgado-Lista, P. F. Jacques, J. M. Ordovas, and S. N. Meydani. 2009. Polymorphisms at cytokine genes may determine the effect of vitamin E on cytokine production in the elderly. *J Nutr* 139: 1855–1860.

80. Bieri, J. G. and R. P. Evarts. 1973. Tocopherols and fatty acids in American diets. The recommended allowance for vitamin E. *J Am Diet Assoc* 62: 147–151.

81. McLaughlin, P. J. and J. L. Weihrauch. 1979. Vitamin E content of foods. *J Am Diet Assoc* 75: 647–665.

82. Jiang, Q. 2014. Natural forms of vitamin E: Metabolism, antioxidant, and anti-inflammatory activities and their role in disease prevention and therapy. *Free Radic Biol Med* 72: 76–90.

83. Yang, C. S. and N. Suh. 2013. Cancer prevention by different forms of tocopherols. *Top Curr Chem* 329: 21–33.

84. Wu, D., M. Meydani, A. A. Beharka, M. Serafini, K. R. Martin, and S. N. Meydani. 2000. In vitro supplementation with different tocopherol homologues can affect the function of immune cells in old mice. *Free Radic Biol Med* 28: 643–651.

85. Zingg, J. M., S. N. Han, E. Pang, M. Meydani, S. N. Meydani, and A. Azzi. 2013. In vivo regulation of gene transcription by alpha- and gamma-tocopherol in murine T lymphocytes. *Arch Biochem Biophys* 538: 111–119.

86. Berdnikovs, S., H. Abdala-Valencia, C. McCary, M. Somand, R. Cole, A. Garcia, P. Bryce, and J. M. Cook-Mills. 2009. Isoforms of vitamin E have opposing immunoregulatory functions during inflammation by regulating leukocyte recruitment. *J Immunol* 182: 4395–4405.

87. McCary, C. A., H. Abdala-Valencia, S. Berdnikovs, and J. M. Cook-Mills. 2011. Supplemental and highly elevated tocopherol doses differentially regulate allergic inflammation: Reversibility of alpha-tocopherol and gamma-tocopherol's effects. *J Immunol* 186: 3674–3685.

88. Wada, S., Y. Satomi, T. Murakoshi, N. Noguchi, T. Yoshikawa, and H. Nishino. 2005. Tumor suppressive effects of tocotrienol in vivo and in vitro. *Cancer Lett* 229: 181–191.

89. Miyazawa, T., A. Shibata, P. Sookwong, Y. Kawakami, T. Eitsuka, A. Asai, S. Oikawa, and K. Nakagawa. 2009. Antiangiogenic and anticancer potential of unsaturated vitamin E (tocotrienol). *J Nutr Biochem* 20: 79–86.

90. Nakagawa, K., A. Shibata, S. Yamashita, T. Tsuzuki, J. Kariya, S. Oikawa, and T. Miyazawa. 2007. In vivo angiogenesis is suppressed by unsaturated vitamin E, tocotrienol. *J Nutr* 137: 1938–1943.

91. Inokuchi, H., H. Hirokane, T. Tsuzuki, K. Nakagawa, M. Igarashi, and T. Miyazawa. 2003. Anti-angiogenic activity of tocotrienol. *Biosci Biotechnol Biochem* 67: 1623–1627.

92. Miyazawa, T., A. Shibata, K. Nakagawa, and T. Tsuzuki. 2008. Anti-angiogenic function of tocotrienol. *Asia Pac J Clin Nutr* 17 (Suppl. 1): 253–256.

93. Baliarsingh, S., Z. H. Beg, and J. Ahmad. 2005. The therapeutic impacts of tocotrienols in type 2 diabetic patients with hyperlipidemia. *Atherosclerosis* 182: 367–374.

94. Black, T. M., P. Wang, N. Maeda, and R. A. Coleman. 2000. Palm tocotrienols protect ApoE +/- mice from diet-induced atheroma formation. *J Nutr* 130: 2420–2426.

95. Raederstorff, D., V. Elste, C. Aebischer, and P. Weber. 2002. Effect of either gamma-tocotrienol or a tocotrienol mixture on the plasma lipid profile in hamsters. *Ann Nutr Metab* 46: 17–23.

96. Naito, Y., M. Shimozawa, M. Kuroda, N. Nakabe, H. Manabe, K. Katada, S. Kokura, H. Ichikawa, N. Yoshida, N. Noguchi, and T. Yoshikawa. 2005. Tocotrienols reduce 25-hydroxycholesterol-induced monocyte-endothelial cell interaction by inhibiting the surface expression of adhesion molecules. *Atherosclerosis* 180: 19–25.

97. Qureshi, A. A., W. A. Salser, R. Parmar, and E. E. Emeson. 2001. Novel tocotrienols of rice bran inhibit atherosclerotic lesions in C57BL/6 ApoE-deficient mice. *J Nutr* 131: 2606–2618.

98. Theriault, A., J. T. Chao, and A. Gapor. 2002. Tocotrienol is the most effective vitamin E for reducing endothelial expression of adhesion molecules and adhesion to monocytes. *Atherosclerosis* 160: 21–30.

99. Khanna, S., S. Roy, A. Slivka, T. K. Craft, S. Chaki, C. Rink, M. A. Notestine, A. C. DeVries, N. L. Parinandi, and C. K. Sen. 2005. Neuroprotective properties of the natural vitamin E alpha-tocotrienol. *Stroke* 36: 2258–2264.

100. Osakada, F., A. Hashino, T. Kume, H. Katsuki, S. Kaneko, and A. Akaike. 2004. Alpha-tocotrienol provides the most potent neuroprotection among vitamin E analogs on cultured striatal neurons. *Neuropharmacology* 47: 904–915.

101. Sen, C. K., S. Khanna, and S. Roy. 2004. Tocotrienol: The natural vitamin E to defend the nervous system? *Ann N Y Acad Sci* 1031: 127–142.
102. Radhakrishnan, A. K., A. L. Lee, P. F. Wong, J. Kaur, H. Aung, and K. Nesaretnam. 2009. Daily supplementation of tocotrienol-rich fraction or alpha-tocopherol did not induce immunomodulatory changes in healthy human volunteers. *Br J Nutr* 101: 810–815.
103. Mahalingam, D., A. K. Radhakrishnan, Z. Amom, N. Ibrahim, and K. Nesaretnam. 2011. Effects of supplementation with tocotrienol-rich fraction on immune response to tetanus toxoid immunization in normal healthy volunteers. *Eur J Clin Nutr* 65: 63–69.
104. Radhakrishnan, A. K., D. Mahalingam, K. R. Selvaduray, and K. Nesaretnam. 2013. Supplementation with natural forms of vitamin E augments antigen-specific TH1-type immune response to tetanus toxoid. *Biomed Res Int* 2013: 782067.
105. Ren, Z., M. Pae, M. C. Dao, D. Smith, S. N. Meydani, and D. Wu. 2010. Dietary supplementation with tocotrienols enhances immune function in C57BL/6 mice. *J Nutr* 140: 1335–1341.

13 Iron, Immunity, and Infection

Hal Drakesmith

CONTENTS

13.1 Introduction: The Requirement for Iron...213
13.2 Iron Trafficking in Mammals 214
    13.2.1 Cellular Iron Homeostasis...214
    13.2.2 Systemic Iron Homeostasis 216
        13.2.2.1 Control of Hepcidin Synthesis 217
        13.2.2.2 Other Components of Systemic Iron Homeostasis 218
13.3 Regulation of Iron Handling by the Acute-Phase Response 218
13.4 How Important Is Iron Trafficking during Infections?...219
    13.4.1 Genetic Evidence 219
    13.4.2 Experimental Evidence 221
13.5 Effect of Iron Supplementation on Infections in Humans and Implications
    for Global Health 221
    13.5.1 Iron Supplementation and Infection—the Background 221
    13.5.2 The Iron–Malaria–Anemia Conundrum..222
    13.5.3 Other Effects of Iron Supplementation/Administration 223
13.6 Evidence That Iron Impacts Immune Cell Function 223
13.7 Summary and Perspectives 224
References...224

13.1 INTRODUCTION: THE REQUIREMENT FOR IRON

Iron is a highly abundant element and plays a critical role in basic physiological processes across almost all life-forms. The ability of iron to transition between its ferrous (Fe^{2+}) and ferric (Fe^{3+}) valency states, along with its capacity to form multiple chemical bonds in various orientations, imbues it with properties that are useful to catalyze biochemical reactions and transfer electrons. Iron plays a key role in generation of energy as the binder of oxygen in heme and as a component of the mitochondrial electron transport chain that generates ATP from oxygen by means of oxidative phosphorylation (Hatefi 1985). Furthermore, iron-dependent enzymes play many other important roles in cellular metabolism and macromolecular biogenesis, especially with respect to DNA (Zhang 2014), a key exemplar being ribonucleotide reductase, the enzyme responsible for the rate-limiting step in DNA synthesis (Jordan and Reichard 1998). Where iron is present in proteins, it is often as part of an iron-sulphur complex (Maio and Rouault 2015). Indeed, one explanation for the near-universal dependency of life-forms on iron is that the origins of life have an iron-sulphur–related basis. This "iron-sulphur world" hypothesis put forward by Günter Wächtershäuser posits that early life began autotrophically (Wächtershäuser 1992) in a volcanic hydrothermal flow at high pressure and temperature, such as in undersea hydrothermal vents, which can contain "micro-caverns" with walls of iron sulfide. Synthetic reactions involving hydrogen sulfide, water, and carbon monoxide in the presence of iron sulfide are believed to have generated early building blocks of biochemical molecules (Keller et al. 1994; Huber and Wachtershauser 1998; Cody et al. 2000). The theory holds that the Last Universal Common Ancestor may have emerged in hydrothermal vents—potentially explaining the near-universal presence of iron and iron-sulphur clusters in key physiological processes. However the ubiquity of iron came about, it is generally held that growth and proliferation of cellular life requires utilization of a source of iron. Two noteworthy exceptions to this general rule are the Lyme disease pathogen *Borrelia burgdorferi* and lactobacilli, a benevolent component of the human intestinal microbiota. Both of these otherwise distantly related organisms grow in the absence of iron, instead employing manganese to drive enzymatic biochemical processes (Imbert and Blondeau 1998; Posey and Gherardini 2000).

Since iron is required in general for growth, during infection, the pathogen must successfully acquire iron from its host to thrive, and so pathogenesis and virulence can be strongly influenced by iron (Payne and Finkelstein 1978). A key factor to be considered here is that iron, although abundant as an element, is not very bioavailable; in the presence of oxygen and at neutral pH, iron (Fe^{3+}) is poorly soluble in water, so that obtaining iron is often a rate-limiting step for microbial proliferation. Furthermore, the reactivity of iron, the basis of its usefulness, can be detrimental unless properly chaperoned because it can catalyze the generation of free radicals, in particular reactive oxygen species through the Fenton reaction. Excess host iron can therefore be dangerous for two reasons: because of the tissue damage that can be caused by free radicals and by providing a nutrient boost for infectious organisms. It follows that host iron homeostatic mechanisms must act to limit free iron and to be responsive to infectious stimuli to further deny access to this key nutrient (Ganz 2009; Weinberg 1984; Ganz and Nemeth 2015). This chapter will deal with these issues, beginning with a description of the normal processes of iron metabolism in mammals.

13.2   IRON TRAFFICKING IN MAMMALS

Total amount, distribution, and storage of iron are controlled by cellular homeostasis and systemic homeostasis, two distinct mechanisms (Hentze et al. 2010). Both are important to maintain viability, but will be considered separately in the main for ease of description, and evidence thus far indicates that regulation of systemic iron is more important for defense against infection. A list of important proteins regulating iron trafficking in humans appears in Table 13.1.

13.2.1   CELLULAR IRON HOMEOSTASIS

On a per-cell basis, enough iron must be available to serve metabolic functions, but it must be safely liganded to prevent formation of toxic reactants. Mammalian cells possess mechanisms to sense intracellular (cytoplasmic) levels of iron and to coordinately regulate iron uptake and storage systems appropriately to maintain equilibrium. This is achieved through the interaction of two sensing proteins, Iron Regulatory Proteins (IRP)-1 and -2, with Iron Response Elements (IREs) present in the untranslated regions of mRNAs encoding proteins that mediate iron trafficking and sequestration (Zhang, Ghosh, and Rouault 2014). IRP1 is an iron-sulphur cluster-containing enzyme with aconitase activity; however, during cellular iron deficiency, the iron-sulphur cluster is lost and the protein is then able to bind the stem-loop RNA structures that IREs form (Wilkinson and Pantopoulos 2014). IRP2 also binds IREs, but does not contain iron; instead, its stability is indirectly controlled by iron. Under conditions of cellular iron sufficiency, an E3 ubiquitin ligase complex containing a component, FBXL5, that requires iron and oxygen to function targets IRP2 for degradation (Vashisht et al. 2009; Salahudeen et al. 2009). Thus, when cellular iron is depleted, IRP1 and IRP2 bind to IRE mRNA structures. IREs are present in numerous genes, including transferrin receptor (TfR1), which mediates capture of transferrin-bound iron from the circulation, and ferritin, which safely encapsulates cytoplasmic iron in a protein shell. The 3' UTR of TfR1 mRNA contains multiple IRE sequences, and IRP binding stabilizes the mRNA-increasing transcript abundance and protein synthesis. Conversely, IRP binding to the IRE within the 5' UTR of ferritin decreases protein abundance by blocking the translation apparatus. Therefore, cellular iron

TABLE 13.1

Proteins Involved in Iron Trafficking and Iron Homeostasis

Protein	Major Sites of Expression	Function
IRP1/aconitase	Near-ubiquitous	} Regulation of expression of
		} genes containing Iron Response
IRP2	Near-ubiquitous	} Elements in their mRNA
FBXL5	Near-ubiquitous	Controls IRP2 stability
Transferrin	Secreted from liver to the circulation	Chaperoning and delivering iron to cells and tissues
Transferrin receptor 1	Near-ubiquitous	Internalization of transferrin
STEAP3	Erythroblasts	Reduces Fe^{3+} to Fe^{2+}
DMT1	Near-ubiquitous	Transmembrane Fe^{2+} importer
ZIP14	Hepatocytes	Transmembrane Fe^{2+} importer
NRAMP1	Macrophages	Metal (including iron) transporter
Ferritin	Present in cells and serum	Iron storage
Ferroportin	Macrophages, enterocytes, periportal hepatocytes	Only known cellular iron exporter
Ceruloplasmin	Soluble form in plasma	} Oxidizes Fe^{2+} released by
	GPI-anchored form on cells	} ferroportin to Fe^{3+}, enabling
Hephaestin	Duodenal enterocytes	} binding of iron to transferrin
FLVCR1	Erythroblasts, enterocytes	Export of heme
Hepcidin	Secreted from liver to the circulation	Master regulator of iron homeostasis: inhibits ferroportin
HFE	Hepatocytes, macrophages	Regulates hepcidin expression (+)
Transferrin receptor 2	Hepatocytes	Internalizes transferrin: regulates hepcidin expression (+)
Hemojuvelin	Hepatocytes, heart, muscle	Regulates hepcidin expression (+)
BMP6	Liver cell types	Regulates hepcidin expression (+)
Matriptase2 (TMPRSS6)	Hepatocytes	Regulates hepcidin expression (−)
Hemoglobin	Erythrocytes	Bind and deliver oxygen
Haptoglobin	Blood plasma	Sequester hemoglobin in plasma
Hemopexin	Blood plasma	Sequester free heme in plasma
Heme oxygenase-1	Macrophages, other cells	Liberates iron from heme; converts heme biliverdin, carbon monoxide, and Fe
Lipocalin-2	Blood plasma	Captures microbial siderophores to iron acquisition by pathogens

Abbreviations: IRP, iron response protein; FBXL5, F-box and leucine-rich repeat protein 5; STEAP3, Six-transmembrane epithelial antigen of the prostate 3; DMT1, divalent metal transporter 1; ZIP14, ZRT/IRT-like protein 14; NRAMP1, Natural resistance-associated macrophage protein 1; FLVCR1, feline leukemia virus subgroup C cellular receptor 1; BMP6, bone morphogenetic protein 6; TMPRSS6, transmembrane protease, serine 6.

deficiency increases the ability of a cell to obtain more iron through increased TfR1 and decreases storage of iron to ensure its utilization for metabolic processes. Other genes, including eALAS, which is involved in heme synthesis, and the iron transporter proteins DMT1 and ferroportin, also possess IREs in their mRNA. The importance of the IRE-IRP system, and of maintaining cellular iron homeostasis, is made apparent by the embryonic lethality of double IRP-1/IRP-2 knockout in mice (Smith et al. 2006). Mice lacking only one IRP are viable, although they display pathologies that are different depending upon which IRP is lacking; this demonstrates that the two have largely overlapping but also some specialized functions (LaVaute et al. 2001; Ghosh et al. 2013). However, it should be pointed out that regulation of iron genes occurs at transcriptional and posttranslational levels as well as by the IRE-IRP interaction. In the case of the iron-exporter protein ferroportin particularly, regulation is highly layered and complex (Drakesmith, Nemeth, and Ganz 2015).

The IRE-IRP system also plays a role in defense against *Salmonella* infection in macrophages. When both IRPs are lost from macrophages, ferritin levels increase, and this source of iron may facilitate the enhanced pathogen growth that is observed in mice lacking macrophage IRPs (Nairz et al. 2015). Further work is required to more fully investigate how the IRE-IRP system contributes to cell-specific immunity against intracellular pathogens in addition to its critical role in maintaining cellular iron homeostasis.

13.2.2 SYSTEMIC IRON HOMEOSTASIS

In broad terms, systemic iron trafficking can be thought of as an iron cycle—see Figure 13.1 (Ganz 2013; Silva and Faustino 2015). A small amount of iron is absorbed daily from the diet (around 1 mg) and enters the circulation where it is bound by a dedicated iron-chaperone protein, transferrin. Transferrin then delivers iron to cells and tissues expressing transferrin receptor—about 60% of total transferrin receptor is present in the bone marrow, where it functions to capture the circulating iron and deliver it intracellularly to developing erythrocytes for incorporation into the heme of hemoglobin. Most other tissues also express transferrin receptors and utilize or store iron, for example muscle (where heme iron is a component of myoglobin), and the liver, where iron is stored

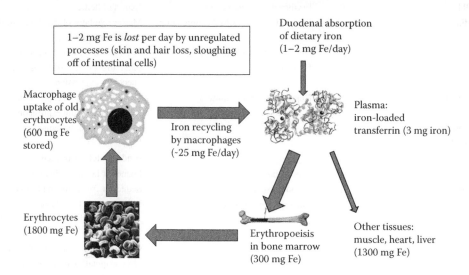

FIGURE 13.1   The iron cycle. Around 1–2 mg dietary iron (heme and/or non-heme associated) is absorbed per day through specialized transport mechanisms by duodenal enterocytes. Iron is exported from these cells into plasma, where it is chaperoned by transferrin. Each transferrin protein can bind up to two atoms of iron, and about 3 mg of iron is in the transferrin pool. Transferrin in the circulation delivers iron to cells and tissues that express transferrin receptors. 60% of all transferrin receptors are present in the bone marrow, where iron is captured and incorporated into heme in developing hematopoietic cells, especially erythrocytes (1800 mg iron). The life span of human erythrocytes averages 120 days, after which they are taken up by macrophages, and the iron is liberated from heme and recycled back into plasma (about 25 mg iron/day). Iron is also present in skeletal and cardiac muscle and liver (1300 mg iron in total), and stored in macrophages (600 mg iron) or the bone marrow (300 mg iron). Homeostatically controlled iron excretory mechanisms are not believed to exist, but iron is lost (about 1–2 mg iron/day) through unregulated processes; more iron is lost via menstruation. Note that iron deficiency, blood loss, hypoxia, or other causes of increased erythropoietic drive (for example thalassaemia) can enhance daily iron absorption to around 30 mg/day.

in hepatocytes. Red blood cells have a life span of about 120 days in humans, whereupon they are phagocytosed by macrophages in the red pulp of the spleen, which process the iron and return it to the circulation. Around 25 mg of iron per day is recycled in this way. Iron is lost from the cycle via mostly unregulated routes (skin, hair loss, sloughing off of intestinal cells) and menstruation in females. Absorption of iron from the diet is regulated to maintain homeostasis (McCance and Widdowson 1937), and this process is controlled by hepcidin (Ganz 2013; Andrews 2008).

The total amount of iron in mammals and its distribution within an organism is orchestrated by the hormone hepcidin (Ganz 2011). Produced primarily by the liver, circulating hepcidin is a 25-amino acid peptide containing 8 cysteine residues and 4 internal disulfide bonds. It is structurally and ancestrally related to antimicrobial peptides called beta-defensins, although hepcidin itself likely possesses only weak microbicidal properties. The receptor for hepcidin is the iron-exporter protein ferroportin (Nemeth et al. 2004b). Ferroportin is highly expressed by duodenal enterocytes, splenic red pulp macrophages, Kupffer cells, and to a lesser extent on periportally located hepatocytes (Drakesmith, Nemeth, and Ganz 2015). On enterocytes, ferroportin mediates the final step in transfer of dietary iron into the systemic circulation; on macrophages ferroportin returns iron derived from processing of senescent red blood cells to the plasma; and on hepatocytes, ferroportin releases stored iron. Hepcidin binds to ferroportin and causes the internalization and degradation of the transporter protein, thus inhibiting release of iron from cells (Nemeth et al. 2004b). Therefore, under conditions of high hepcidin, iron is not absorbed from the diet or released from macrophages, and serum iron levels fall. Persistently high hepcidin levels cause anemia by restricting the availability of iron for erythropoiesis (Du et al. 2008; Finberg et al. 2008; Prentice et al. 2012). Low hepcidin facilitates iron absorption from the diet, and allows release of iron from macrophage and hepatocyte stores. However, genetic disorders that lead to chronic low hepcidin result in iron overload (hereditary hemochromatosis and nontransfusion-dependent thalassemia) and associated toxicity in parenchymal organs where the iron excess is deposited, particularly the liver, pancreas, and heart (Ganz and Nemeth 2011; Pietrangelo 2010; Jones et al. 2015).

13.2.2.1   Control of Hepcidin Synthesis

Regulations of hepcidin is complex, and although many factors that alter expression of hepcidin are known, their molecular mechanistic modes of action are not in every case fully understood. Iron itself is a key regulator of hepcidin and appears to work in two ways (Corradini et al. 2011; Ramos et al. 2011). First, increases in the amount of iron in the blood (transferrin saturation) are sensed by hepatocyte surface proteins (including HFE, TfR2, and HJV) and this information is signaled to increase hepcidin synthesis (Corradini et al. 2011; Ramos et al. 2011). Secondly, intracellular accumulation of iron in the liver is also sensed and increases hepcidin synthesis. The bone morphogenetic protein (BMP) signaling pathway is involved in both these sensing mechanisms, and activation of this pathway increases hepcidin. Evidence in mice and humans strongly indicates that Bmp6 is the key member of the Bmp family that is induced by iron accumulation in the liver and exerts strong (but nevertheless partially redundant) control over hepcidin synthesis (Andriopoulos et al. 2009; Daher et al. 2015; Meynard et al. 2009). Genetic deficiency (naturally occurring or experimental) in components of liver BMP signaling results in aberrantly low hepcidin synthesis and hemochromatosis (Steinbicker et al. 2011); overactive BMP signaling leads to high hepcidin and severe iron deficiency anemia (Silvestri et al. 2008). Interestingly, the IRE-IRP system described above is not believed to play a major contributory role in the regulation of hepcidin by iron.

Two other important regulators of hepcidin have been characterized: inflammation and erythropoietic drive. In the case of inflammation, hepcidin transcription is induced by cytokines that signal through Jak-STAT pathways, and the promoter region of the hepcidin gene possesses Stat3 binding elements. Interleukin-6, interleukin-22, and type I interferon have been identified as mediators of hepcidin upregulation in the context of inflammation (Armitage et al. 2011; Nemeth et al. 2004a; Ryan et al. 2012; Smith et al. 2013; Wrighting and Andrews 2006). Because these mediators are released during acute-phase responses to infection, hepcidin increase and hypoferremia are observed during infections (Drakesmith and Prentice 2012). In murine models and/or in humans, hepcidin increases have been observed associated with malaria (Atkinson et al. 2014, 2015; de Mast et al. 2010; Portugal et al. 2011), HIV-1 (Armitage et al. 2014; Minchella et al. 2014; Minchella et al. 2015a), tuberculosis (Minchella et al. 2015b), influenza A virus (Armitage et al. 2011), *Candida albicans* (Armitage et al. 2011), *Vibrio vulnificus* (Arezes et al. 2015), and *Salmonella* infections (Darton et al. 2015). Two exceptions appear to be chronic hepatitis B and C viral infections that (more definitively in the latter) are linked to reduced hepcidin and hepatic iron accumulation that can exacerbate the liver pathology associated with the infection (Armitage et al. 2014; Fujita et al. 2007; Girelli et al. 2009). The significance of hepcidin and hepcidin-induced hypoferremia for the outcome of infections will be discussed in a later section.

Red blood cells constitute the major use of iron in the body, to carry oxygen to all tissues. Blood loss imparts a significant threat to viability and the capacity to replace lost erythrocytes as quickly as possible is important; as part of this process iron availability for erythropoiesis is increased (Finch 1994). This is achieved through the suppression of hepcidin expression as a consequence of increased erythroid drive; the mechanistic details of how this occurs are yet to be resolved, but a leading candidate to mediate hepcidin suppression is the erythroblast-secreted protein erythroferrone (Kautz et al. 2014). Increased erythropoiesis driven by erythropoietin in response to blood loss or hypoxia raises the level of erythroferrone, which is thought to travel in the circulation to the liver, where it acts to switch off hepcidin production. A lack of hepcidin then facilitates rapid release of iron from stores via ferroportin, raising transferrin saturation and enabling iron incorporation into developing red blood cells in the bone marrow. However, this suppression of hepcidin can be pathological in disorders of ineffective erythropoiesis, for example in nontransfusion-dependent thalassemia where globin gene mutations limit the life span of erythrocytes, and compensatory overactive erythropoiesis leads to persistently decreased hepcidin synthesis, in a partially erythroferrone-dependent manner (Kautz et al. 2014, 2015), leading to toxic iron accumulation in parenchymal organs.

13.2.2.2 Other Components of Systemic Iron Homeostasis

An additional source of systemic iron-related toxicity is from the release of heme and hemoglobin into circulation following tissue damage and/or hemolysis (rupture of red blood cells). However, two host proteins are deployed to counteract this effect: haptoglobin, which binds to free hemoglobin, and hemopexin, which binds to free heme. Haptoglobin-hemoglobin and hemopexin-heme complexes are taken up by receptors (CD163 and CD91 respectively) on hepatocytes and macrophages (Schaer et al. 2006; Hvidberg et al. 2005; Kristiansen et al. 2001). The heme-containing complexes are then safely processed by proteolysis and by heme-oxygenase-1, which converts heme-iron into free iron, carbon monoxide, and biliverdin; these latter two products also exert protective anti-inflammatory and antioxidant functions.

Having now described the basic mechanisms that exist to maintain cellular and systemic iron homeostasis, the chapter will move to consider how infections alter iron trafficking and the role of iron in immune responses.

13.3 REGULATION OF IRON HANDLING BY THE ACUTE-PHASE RESPONSE

The recognition of infection by innate immune sensors (toll-like receptors, NOD-like receptors, and other sensors of viral infections) leads to a rapid release of soluble mediators of inflammation including a range of cytokines. This rapid change in gene expression and secretion of powerful signaling factors is known as the acute-phase response. The cytokines involved bind to cellular receptors triggering expression of a battery of proteins that regulate multiple processes aimed at clearing infection and dealing with tissue damage associated with infection. Included within the genes that are regulated by inflammatory processes are several key components of the machinery that governs iron homeostasis (Ganz and Nemeth 2015). Notably hepcidin, ferritin, haptoglobin, hemopexin, and lipocalin-2 (see below) are all induced during the acute-phase response, while expression of ferroportin and transferrin is decreased. This combination maximizes the sequestration of iron away from invasive microbes (especially blood-borne bacteria) and severely decreases serum iron levels. Indeed, the "hypoferremia of infection" has been recognized since the 1940s (Cartwright et al. 1946a, b). The rapid increase in hepcidin—for example observed in humans experimentally challenged with typhoid infection (Darton et al. 2015)—coupled with the decrease in ferroportin expression—due to both the effect of hepcidin on ferroportin protein and the effect of inflammation suppressing transcription of the ferroportin gene (Drakesmith, Nemeth, and Ganz 2015; Liu et al. 2005; Guida et al. 2015)—results in a trapping of iron in macrophages. The continued consumption of iron by tissues, especially by the bone marrow, causes an acute scarcity of iron in the serum, so that transferrin saturation can fall below 5%. The concomitant increase of iron levels in macrophages may be, in part, why many types of pathogen target this cell type, and some are even obligate macrophage-tropic, for example *Mycobacterium tuberculosis*. As a result, macrophage-tropic pathogens in general are able to source iron from within this cell type even if the iron is sequestered within ferritin—for example *M. tuberculosis* has multiple iron-acquisition systems including heme uptake, transferrin binding, and siderophore utilization (Fang et al. 2015).

Siderophores are small molecules synthesized and secreted by bacteria that have very high affinity for iron and act to scavenge iron from the locale of the infection (Neilands 1995). Bacteria also encode mechanisms that export iron-free siderophores and capture siderophore-iron complexes that are then internalized and used as a source of iron. A well-studied example of a siderophore is enterobactin, which is made by several types of gram-negative bacteria including *E. coli* (Annamalai et al. 2004; Raymond, Dertz, and Kim 2003). However, enterobactin (and other siderophores such as carboxymycobactin) is rendered inactive by a component of human serum, lipocalin-2 (also known as 24p3, siderocalin, NGAL, or uterocalin), which binds to siderophore-iron complexes with a higher affinity than the bacterial siderophore receptor machinery (Goetz et al. 2002; Holmes et al. 2005). Expression of lipocalin-2 is induced by signaling downstream of toll-like receptor 4 binding of bacterial lipopolysaccharide, so that the presence of bacteria that use enterobactin is detected (because lipopolysaccharide is a component of gram-negative bacterial outer membranes), and the enterobactin-neutralizing activity of lipocalin-2 is mobilized (Flo et al. 2004). The importance of this defense mechanism is revealed by mice lacking the gene encoding lipocalin-2, which are susceptible to infection with enterocalin-utilizing strains of *E. coli*, while wild-type mice resist infection (Flo et al. 2004). Notably, some pathogens have responded to this defense mechanism by altering siderophore chemistry to resist binding by lipocalin-2. Salmochelins are siderophores used by *Salmonella* and are similar to enterobactin but modified by glucosylation, which enables escape from lipocalin-2 capture (Fischbach et al. 2006; Hantke et al. 2003; Muller, Valdebenito, and Hantke 2009). Other pathogens (for example *Bacillus*, *Mycobacteria* sp.) also use siderophores that are not sequestered by lipocalin-2 (Abergel et al. 2006; Fang et al. 2015). This specific strategy of evasion of host iron-restriction by lipocalin-2, along with other novel and emerging functions of siderophores, may be an important contributor to the pathogenicity and virulence of a bacterial infection (Holden and Bachman 2015).

13.4   HOW IMPORTANT IS IRON TRAFFICKING DURING INFECTIONS?

The information above describes how iron homeostasis is normally maintained and how iron trafficking is altered during the inflammatory response to infections. But what is the evidence that host control of iron is important for the outcome of infections in humans?

13.4.1   GENETIC EVIDENCE

If control of iron handling is important for defense against infection, one might expect (1) there is evidence for positive selection at the genomic level for alterations in genes that control iron transport, and (2) that genetic disorders of iron metabolism are associated with increased susceptibility to infections.

Evidence in support of both concepts is available. Host genes that are important for the immune response to infection can exhibit the hallmarks of positive selection. One manifestation of this is increased diversification; on the DNA level a proportional increase in nonsynonymous substitutions relative to neutral sites is detected. Sequence analysis can reveal specific regions or "hotspots" within proteins that have been selected by evolution and that may be critical for functionality during immunity (Daugherty and Malik 2012). The iron-binding protein transferrin was discovered in the 1940s, and was initially characterized by its ability to withhold iron from, and so inhibit the growth of, bacteria in culture broth (Schade and Caroline 1946). Recently the transferrin protein was shown to have been subjected to positive selection both across hominid genomes and within the standing human allele variants (Barber and Elde 2014). Transferrin binds iron with a high affinity so that "free" iron in serum is kept to an absolute minimum—the basis of the bacteriostatic effect noted by Schade and Caroline. However, *Neisseria* and *Haemophilus* bacteria encode their own transferrin-receptor protein complex (including the TbpA [transferrin-binding protein A] component) that scavenges iron from the host (Noinaj, Buchanan, and Cornelissen 2012). Transferrin gene orthologs from 21 hominid species, including humans, gorillas, chimpanzees, and Old and New World monkeys were sequenced, and 18 rapidly evolving sites were identified, 16 of which were located within the area of transferrin that binds to bacterial TbpA proteins. Using a solved-crystal structure of the TbpA:transferrin complex (Noinaj et al. 2012), it was apparent that 14 of these 16 sites localized to the interface between the bacterial and mammalian proteins, whereas only one site is in the area where transferrin contacts the mammalian transferrin receptor. Further analysis showed that alterations of amino acid residues at positions 589 and 591 of transferrin could completely control whether a bacterial TbpA could bind the transferrin or not (Barber and Elde 2014), with amino acid variation at position 591 being the most common alleles in humans. Reciprocal analysis of variation of bacterial TbpA genes showed that areas of rapid diversification mapped to the interface with mammalian transferrin (Barber and Elde 2014). Thus, a picture emerges of continual selection over recent evolutionary time of transferrin variants that evade capture by pathogenic bacteria, presumably conferring a survival advantage, with bacterial TbpA proteins undergoing counterselection to reacquire the iron source needed for growth and proliferation (Armitage and Drakesmith 2014).

The iron-overloading disorder hereditary hemochromatosis is caused by mutations in genes that control hepcidin synthesis (or very rarely in hepcidin itself). The most common mutations are in the HFE gene, and HFE mutants are common in Caucasian populations, although the penetrance of the mutations is variable and usually low, so that frank hemochromatosis is relatively infrequent (Pietrangelo 2010). Taken as a whole, patients with hemochromatosis are not markedly more predisposed to infections in general. However, there is likely an enhanced susceptibility to infections with "siderophilic" bacteria that thrive in high-iron environments, particularly *Vibrio vulnificus* (Barton and Acton 2009). Experimental analysis (described below) confirms a strong interaction of iron availability and pathogenicity of *V. vulnificus*. Other infections in hemochromatosis patients have been noted, a striking case being that of a fatal sepsis of a researcher using an "attenuated" strain of *Yersinia pestis*. This strain was thought to be relatively safe and unable to cause pathogenic infections in humans; the researcher using this bacteria was posthumously identified as harboring mutations in HFE and exhibited iron overload, and was presumed to have untreated hemochromatosis (Frank, Schneewind, and Shieh 2011). The attenuation of the *Y. pestis* strain was due to deletions in regions of the genome that encode high-affinity iron-uptake mechanisms (Carniel 1999; Parkhill et al. 2001); without these genes, the bacterial strain is unable to acquire iron from its host—however, this defect in the organism appears to have been complemented by the HFE mutations in the infected individual with fatal consequences. This singular case report (Frank, Schneewind, and Shieh 2011) highlights that iron availability can be critical in determining the outcome of infections.

13.4.2 EXPERIMENTAL EVIDENCE

The importance of host control of iron in response to infections has been further demonstrated by experimental analysis of *V. vulnificus* infections in mice (Arezes et al. 2015). In wild-type mice, *V. vulnificus* infection induces a rapid increase in hepcidin levels and a drop in serum iron. *V. vulnificus* requires high levels of serum iron in order to thrive; iron levels that oversaturate available binding sites on transferrin generate nontransferrin-bound iron (NTBI), and in the presence of NTBI, *V. vulnificus* proliferates exponentially with a doubling time of less than 15 minutes. The hypoferremic response in wild-type mice prevents acquisition of iron by *V. vulnificus*, and in general these mice survive and clear the infection. However, mice lacking the *Hamp1* gene that encodes hepcidin have very high serum iron including NTBI, fail to mount a strong hypoferremic response to *V. vulnificus*, and rapidly succumb to this infection within a few days or less (Arezes et al. 2015). This remarkable susceptibility to *V. vulnificus* of hepcidin-deficient mice can be almost entirely reversed by "minihepcidins," supraphysiological derivatives of hepcidin that induce hypoferremia (Preza et al. 2011), demonstrating that induction of hepcidin functionality during the acute response to *V. vulnificus* is necessary and sufficient for the containment of the infection (Arezes et al. 2015).

Further work must investigate the requirement for hepcidin in defense against other infections. The liver stage of *Plasmodium* infection is suppressed by increased levels of hepcidin, likely through decreasing hepatocyte iron levels (Portugal et al. 2011), but the effect on blood-stage malaria is not yet clear. There is conflicting evidence on the role and importance of hepcidin in murine models of *Salmonella* infection (Fang and Weiss 2014), with some investigations indicating that antagonism of hepcidin may be protective against infection, perhaps because iron levels will be lower in macrophages when hepcidin levels are low, so that growth of *Salmonella,* which targets this cell type, will be relatively inhibited (Kim et al. 2014; Nairz et al. 2007). However, in opposition to this idea, in mice entirely lacking *Hamp1* expression, susceptibility to *Salmonella* appears to be increased (Yuki et al. 2013); resolving the differences between the various studies of hepcidin–*Salmonella* interactions may not be straightforward. The effect of hepcidin deficiency or hepcidin overexpression *in vivo* on *M. tuberculosis*, another key macrophage-tropic pathogen, also needs further exploration, with mechanistic experiments investigating the effect of hepcidin/ferroportin activity in isolated infected *in vitro* cells (Olakanmi, Schlesinger, and Britigan 2007; Sow et al. 2007).

In sum, currently the importance of hepcidin induction and subsequent iron redistribution for protection against blood-dwelling siderophilic pathogens is clear, but the role of hepcidin in protection against other infections requires further investigation. Such ongoing mechanistic studies are warranted by longstanding and continuing observations in humans that changes in iron status can have profound effects on the frequency and severity of globally important infectious diseases.

13.5 EFFECT OF IRON SUPPLEMENTATION ON INFECTIONS IN HUMANS AND IMPLICATIONS FOR GLOBAL HEALTH

13.5.1 IRON SUPPLEMENTATION AND INFECTION—THE BACKGROUND

Iron deficiency and iron-deficiency anemia are held to be highly prevalent nutritional disorders worldwide, especially affecting infants and pregnant women (Lopez et al. 2015). The precise effects of iron deficiency on health at various ages are a matter of debate but fatigue, growth retardation, immune and cognitive impairment, and at a population level, poor socioeconomic performance, may be associated with low iron status and anemia (Lopez et al. 2015; Pasricha et al. 2013). To combat these effects, iron supplementation in various forms has been commonly used worldwide for many decades. Iron during pregnancy has been shown to improve maternal, neonatal, infant, and longer-term child outcomes. The benefits of iron supplementation to children are not so clear and require further definition (Pasricha et al. 2013).

One of the reasons that the desirability of iron supplementation is debated, particularly "universal" iron supplementation where iron is given to an entire age group in an area in which anemia is endemic, is because of many reported links between iron supplementation and infectious disease. This link is presumed to be because pathogen growth is stimulated by increased iron availability (Cassat and Skaar 2013; Cross et al. 2015). The first such associations were reported by Armand Trousseau more than 130 years ago, in which it appears that latent (or relatively inactive) tuberculosis was reactivated in two young women given iron-containing solutions ("ferruginous remedies") with fatal consequences (Trousseau 1872). In the 1970s, a study amongst Somali nomads suggested that oral iron could exacerbate malaria, and an increase in fevers and in excretion of *Schistosoma* eggs were also observed (Murray et al. 1978). Up until the early 2000s, many other studies had been conducted in which infectious disease incidence or severity was examined in the context of iron supplementation. But variations in age group studied, form of iron given, time scale of the study, location of the study (e.g., in malarious or nonmalarious areas), and nature of the study and of controls meant that drawing clear, generalizable conclusions was extremely difficult (Oppenheimer 2001). Nevertheless, even at this time there was already an indication that for malaria, iron deficiency may be mildly protective and that iron supplementation carried some risks (Oppenheimer 2001). These two propositions have been more closely examined in recent years.

13.5.2 THE Iron–Malaria–Anemia CONUNDRUM

A large randomized trial of iron supplements conducted on 24,000 infants on the malaria-endemic Tanzanian island of Pemba had to be prematurely stopped because of a statistically significant increase in the number of cases of malaria and mortality in the children receiving iron and folic acid (Sazawal et al. 2006). The results from this one trial, which had an enormous sample size and analytical power compared to previous studies relating iron to infection, have had important consequences for global health (Schumann and Solomons 2013). As stated previously, anemia is a major global health concern, and decreasing the prevalence of anemia worldwide has proved to be very challenging (Kassebaum et al. 2014). Iron is a cheap nutrient in that its abundance enables relatively cheap manufacture, and this has perhaps been an encouragement for deploying iron-containing supplements at high doses (up to 200 mg per day as an oral dose, when the limit for intestinal absorption is usually in the low tens of milligrams per day) to large swathes of populations worldwide. The results of the Pemba trial have necessitated rethinking of global iron supplementation policies that has yet to be adequately resolved (Raiten 2015). Subsequent trials have in part confirmed, but some have refuted, the effect of iron supplementation on exacerbation of malaria (Mwangi et al. 2015; Prentice, Verhoef, and Cerami 2013; Zlotkin et al. 2013). Consequently, the overall picture remains complex, particularly with respect to the variation of risk-benefit balance for providing iron to children or pregnant women with mild versus severe iron deficiency in areas of high or low malaria burden. Moreover, evidence has accumulated indicating that iron deficiency is likely mildly protective against malaria in children and perhaps also in pregnant women (Spottiswoode, Duffy, and Drakesmith 2014; Gwamaka et al. 2012; Kabyemela et al. 2008). Iron-deficient erythrocytes appear to be relatively resistant to *Plasmodium falciparum* infection, but this effect is reversed by iron supplementation at least in part because iron-stimulated erythropoiesis increases the number of immature erythrocytes that are the preferential target for *P. falciparum* merozoites (Clark et al. 2014). Therefore, a conundrum exists whereby iron deficiency is common and undesirable but may protect against malaria, whereas treating iron deficiency has hematological benefit but confers susceptibility to infection. Solutions to this problem may lie in focusing more on antimalarial provision (especially as malaria is itself a major cause of anemia and can coexist with iron deficiency) than on blanket iron supplementation policies, and in targeting iron more effectively to individuals and populations who are most likely to benefit from it (Spottiswoode, Duffy, and Drakesmith 2014). Targeting could be via providing iron during the dry season when malaria infection is less likely (Atkinson et al. 2014), or a screen-and-treat approach in which a "need iron" serum marker is rapidly assessed and used to guide supplementation—hepcidin is just such a candidate serum marker currently under investigation (Pasricha et al. 2014).

13.5.3 OTHER EFFECTS OF IRON SUPPLEMENTATION/ADMINISTRATION

It must be noted also that deleterious effects of iron supplementation are not limited to exacerbating malaria. Other infections have been shown to be associated with increased iron, for example respiratory infections as found in a large trial of iron-containing multiple micronutrient powders in a nonmalarious area of Pakistan (Soofi et al. 2013). Gastrointestinal disorders are also often recorded as being increased in the context of oral iron. This has been observed especially in populations in which pathogenic microflora are already present in the intestine; such bacteria then appear to outgrow barrier protective microbiota leading to intestinal inflammation and bloody diarrhea (Zimmermann et al. 2010; Jaeggi et al. 2015). The barrier bacteria include lactobacilli, which do not require iron to grow, utilizing manganese instead for critical cellular processes; this may be part of the reason why their protective function can be relatively compromised by high iron doses that preferentially favor the growth of iron-requiring pathogenic microflora (Kortman et al. 2012). Therefore, factored into a risk-benefit analysis of iron supplementation must also be potential side effects of altered microbiota profile, which could be directly pathogenic and is increasingly understood to also affect many other physiological processes beyond the intestine itself.

13.6 EVIDENCE THAT IRON IMPACTS IMMUNE CELL FUNCTION

Iron impacts the host immune system as well as infectious organisms and the intestinal microbiota. Individual components of immunity are influenced by iron availability. For example, the neutrophil oxidative burst that is an important component of antibacterial activity is depressed by dietary iron deficiency at least in rodent models (Murakawa et al. 1987). Increased iron retention by macrophages impairs interferon-gamma signaling (Weiss et al. 1992). One aspect of the macrophage response to infection with intracellular bacteria such as *Salmonella typhimurium* is to increase ferroportin transcription so enhancing the microbicidal functions of interferon-gamma at the same time as lowering availability of iron for the resident pathogen (Fang and Weiss 2014). In general, it appears that cell-mediated immunity is more influenced by fluctuations in iron levels than humoral immunity, although this concept requires a great deal of further work, especially in human contexts. In particular, mechanistic analysis of how iron can influence the development, polarization, and resolution of immune responses to human pathogens is mostly lacking.

Nevertheless, recent genetic evidence points to a critical role for cellular iron acquisition in modulating the adaptive immune response in humans. A study found that members of two families with a severe combined immunodeficiency all harbored the same mutation in the gene encoding transferrin receptor 1, causing an amino acid substitution in the cytoplasmic tail of the protein (Jabara et al. 2016). The specific amino acid altered (Tyr20 [in humans] changed to a histidine in patients) is conserved across dozens of vertebrate species and is a critical part of a motif that governs protein recycling between the cell surface (where the transferrin receptor captures transferrin-iron) and the endosomal compartments (where iron is liberated and is transported into the cytoplasm). Lymphocytes from patients accumulated more transferrin receptor on the cell surface but were defective at internalizing the protein (Jabara et al. 2016). Intriguingly, the patients were not anemic or had only mildly reduced hemoglobin levels, suggesting that erythrocytic acquisition of iron is not markedly abrogated by the substitution of Tyr20. Instead, patients in the families were highly susceptible to infections despite normal lymphocyte numbers (although there was a reduced number of memory B-cells and occasional neutropenia) (Jabara et al. 2016). T lymphocytes from the patients displayed a suppressed response to mitogens, and B lymphocytes showed both reduced proliferative activity and defective class-switching *in vitro*. Therefore, the defect in transferrin receptor activity likely acts on adaptive immune cell function in response to infection, rather than at the stage of lymphocyte development and maturation; however, further characterization of the effect of mutated transferrin receptor on immune function is required. The generation of $Tfrc^{Y20H/Y20H}$ knock-in mice, which appear to mostly recapitulate the patients' phenotype (Jabara et al. 2016), should help with this objective.

13.7 SUMMARY AND PERSPECTIVES

The importance of iron as a key nutrient in the context of immunity and infection has become more apparent over time. The recent discoveries of positive selection of transferrin during evolutionary timescales to generate variants capable of escaping bacterial capture (Barber and Elde 2014), and of severe immunodeficiency caused by a mutation in transferrin receptor (Jabara et al. 2016), show how genetic investigations have confirmed longstanding clinical and experimental observations of the impact of iron on infectious disease. The mechanistic dissection of iron homeostasis over the past 10 years, especially the identification of hepcidin as the master regulator of iron homeostasis, have enabled more precise molecular studies of how hosts regulate iron traffic during infections. The challenge is to use the basic knowledge gained to generate new strategies to combat disease. In the era of increasing antibiotic resistance, manipulating iron transport to decrease iron availability to iron-sensitive pathogens is an attractive idea. Newly available tools such as minihepcidins and hepcidin antagonists that alter whole-organism homeostasis may be of use in certain circumstances (Arezes et al. 2015; Schwoebel et al. 2013; van Eijk et al. 2014); further iterations that more specifically target iron trafficking by cell-types (hepatocytes, macrophage subsets, and lymphocytes), which harbor specific pathogen types, may be worth investigating.

Many areas of how iron availability influences the generation and polarization of immune responses are unexplored, but given that progression of T-cell responses is characterized by striking metabolic reprogramming and sensitivity to nutrients (Blagih et al. 2015; Slack, Wang, and Wang 2015), it is at least possible that variations in iron availability could influence the efficacy of adaptive immunity; such effects may underlie the severe phenotype of the transferrin receptor mutant patients described above (Jabara et al. 2016). Should iron influence generation of immune responses in a clear and well-understood manner, vaccination strategies might benefit from appurtenant manipulation of iron availability.

Lastly, the global health problems of iron deficiency and anemia remain challenging in the extreme, but here again there may be opportunities to use the information gleaned from studying hepcidin, iron transport, and infection to design new approaches of diagnosing and redefining individuals and populations not as "iron-deficient" but as "in need of and able to utilize iron." This distinction may be critically important if the exacerbation of infection and gastrointestinal adverse effects that can be caused by iron are to be avoided, while ensuring that deficits in iron are effectively treated.

REFERENCES

Abergel, R. J., M. K. Wilson, J. E. Arceneaux, T. M. Hoette, R. K. Strong, B. R. Byers, and K. N. Raymond. 2006. Anthrax pathogen evades the mammalian immune system through stealth siderophore production. *Proc Natl Acad Sci U S A* 103 (49):18499–503. doi: 10.1073/pnas.0607055103.

Andrews, N. C. 2008. Forging a field: The golden age of iron biology. *Blood* 112 (2):219–30.

Andriopoulos, B., Jr., E. Corradini, Y. Xia, S. A. Faasse, S. Chen, L. Grgurevic, M. D. Knutson, A. Pietrangelo, S. Vukicevic, H. Y. Lin, and J. L. Babitt. 2009. BMP6 is a key endogenous regulator of hepcidin expression and iron metabolism. *Nat Genet* 41 (4):482–7.

Annamalai, R., B. Jin, Z. Cao, S. M. Newton, and P. E. Klebba. 2004. Recognition of ferric catecholates by FepA. *J Bacteriol* 186 (11):3578–89. doi: 10.1128/JB.186.11.3578–3589.2004.

Arezes, J., G. Jung, V. Gabayan, E. Valore, P. Ruchala, P. A. Gulig, T. Ganz, E. Nemeth, and Y. Bulut. 2015. Hepcidin-induced hypoferremia is a critical host defense mechanism against the siderophilic bacterium Vibrio vulnificus. *Cell Host Microbe* 17 (1):47–57. doi: 10.1016/j.chom.2014.12.001.

Armitage, A. E. and H. Drakesmith. 2014. Genetics. The battle for iron. *Science* 346 (6215):1299–300. doi: 10.1126/science.aaa2468.

Armitage, A. E., L. A. Eddowes, U. Gileadi, S. Cole, N. Spottiswoode, T. A. Selvakumar, L. P. Ho, A. R. Townsend, and H. Drakesmith. 2011. Hepcidin regulation by innate immune and infectious stimuli. *Blood* 118:4129–39. doi: 10.1182/blood-2011-04-351957.

Armitage, A. E., A. R. Stacey, E. Giannoulatou, E. Marshall, P. Sturges, K. Chatha, N. M. Smith, X. Huang, X. Xu, S. R. Pasricha, N. Li, H. Wu, C. Webster, A. M. Prentice, P. Pellegrino, I. Williams, P. J. Norris, H. Drakesmith, and P. Borrow. 2014. Distinct patterns of hepcidin and iron regulation during HIV-1, HBV, and HCV infections. *Proc Natl Acad Sci U S A* 111 (33):12187–92. doi: 10.1073/pnas.1402351111.

Atkinson, S. H., A. E. Armitage, S. Khandwala, T. W. Mwangi, S. Uyoga, P. A. Bejon, T. N. Williams, A. M. Prentice, and H. Drakesmith. 2014. Combinatorial effects of malaria season, iron deficiency, and inflammation determine plasma hepcidin concentration in African children. *Blood* 123 (21):3221–9. doi: 10.1182/blood-2013-10-533000.

Atkinson, S. H., S. M. Uyoga, A. E. Armitage, S. Khandwala, C. K. Mugyenyi, P. Bejon, K. Marsh, J. G. Beeson, A. M. Prentice, H. Drakesmith, and T. N. Williams. 2015. Malaria and age variably but critically control hepcidin throughout childhood in Kenya. *EBioMedicine* 2 (10):1478–86. doi: 10.1016/j.ebiom.2015.08.016.

Barber, M. F. and N. C. Elde. 2014. Nutritional immunity. Escape from bacterial iron piracy through rapid evolution of transferrin. *Science* 346 (6215):1362–6. doi: 10.1126/science.1259329.

Barton, J. C. and R. T. Acton. 2009. Hemochromatosis and Vibrio vulnificus wound infections. *J Clin Gastroenterol* 43 (9):890–3. doi: 10.1097/MCG.0b013e31819069c1.

Blagih, J., F. Coulombe, E. E. Vincent, F. Dupuy, G. Galicia-Vazquez, E. Yurchenko, T. C. Raissi, G. J. van der Windt, B. Viollet, E. L. Pearce, J. Pelletier, C. A. Piccirillo, C. M. Krawczyk, M. Divangahi, and R. G. Jones. 2015. The energy sensor AMPK regulates T cell metabolic adaptation and effector responses in vivo. *Immunity* 42 (1):41–54. doi: 10.1016/j.immuni.2014.12.030.

Carniel, E. 1999. The Yersinia high-pathogenicity island. *Int Microbiol* 2 (3):161–7.

Cartwright, G. E., M. A. Lauritsen, S. Humphreys, P. J. Jones, I. M. Merrill, and M. M. Wintrobe. 1946a. The anemia of infection. II. The experimental production of hypoferremia and anemia in dogs. *J Clin Invest* 25 (1):81–6. doi: 10.1172/JCI101691.

Cartwright, G. E., M. A. Lauritsen, P. J. Jones, I. M. Merrill, and M. M. Wintrobe. 1946b. The anemia of infection. I. Hypoferremia, hypercupremia, and alterations in porphyrin metabolism in patients. *J Clin Invest* 25 (1):65–80. doi: 10.1172/JCI101690.

Cassat, J. E. and E. P. Skaar. 2013. Iron in infection and immunity. *Cell Host Microbe* 13 (5):509–19. doi: 10.1016/j.chom.2013.04.010.

Clark, M. A., M. M. Goheen, A. Fulford, A. M. Prentice, M. A. Elnagheeb, J. Patel, N. Fisher, S. M. Taylor, R. S. Kasthuri, and C. Cerami. 2014. Host iron status and iron supplementation mediate susceptibility to erythrocytic stage Plasmodium falciparum. *Nat Commun* 5:4446. doi: 10.1038/ncomms5446.

Cody, G. D., N. Z. Boctor, T. R. Filley, R. M. Hazen, J. H. Scott, A. Sharma, and H. S. Yoder, Jr. 2000. Primordial carbonylated iron-sulfur compounds and the synthesis of pyruvate. *Science* 289 (5483):1337–40.

Corradini, E., D. Meynard, Q. Wu, S. Chen, P. Ventura, A. Pietrangelo, and J. L. Babitt. 2011. Serum and liver iron differently regulate the bone morphogenetic protein 6 (BMP6)-SMAD signaling pathway in mice. *Hepatology* 54 (1):273–84. doi: 10.1002/hep.24359.

Cross, J. H., R. S. Bradbury, A. J. Fulford, A. T. Jallow, R. Wegmuller, A. M. Prentice, and C. Cerami. 2015. Oral iron acutely elevates bacterial growth in human serum. *Sci Rep* 5:16670. doi: 10.1038/srep16670.

Daher, R., C. Kannengiesser, D. Houamel, T. Lefebvre, E. Bardou-Jacquet, N. Ducrot, C. de Kerguenec, A. M. Jouanolle, A. M. Robreau, C. Oudin, G. Le Gac, B. Moulouel, V. Loustaud-Ratti, P. Bedossa, D. Valla, L. Gouya, C. Beaumont, P. Brissot, H. Puy, Z. Karim, and D. Tchernitchko. 2015. Heterozygous mutations in BMP6 pro-peptide lead to inappropriate hepcidin synthesis and moderate iron overload in humans. *Gastroenterology* 150:672–83. doi: 10.1053/j.gastro.2015.10.049.

Darton, T. C., C. J. Blohmke, E. Giannoulatou, C. S. Waddington, C. Jones, P. Sturges, C. Webster, H. Drakesmith, A. J. Pollard, and A. E. Armitage. 2015. Rapidly escalating hepcidin and associated serum iron starvation are features of the acute response to typhoid infection in humans. *PLOS Negl Trop Dis* 9 (9):e0004029. doi: 10.1371/journal.pntd.0004029.

Daugherty, M. D. and H. S. Malik. 2012. Rules of engagement: Molecular insights from host-virus arms races. *Annu Rev Genet* 46:677–700. doi: 10.1146/annurev-genet-110711-155522.

de Mast, Q., D. Syafruddin, S. Keijmel, T. Olde Riekerink, O. Deky, P. B. Asih, D. W. Swinkels, and A. J. van der Ven. 2010. Increased serum hepcidin and alterations in blood iron parameters associated with asymptomatic P. falciparum and P. vivax malaria. *Haematologica* 95:1068–74.

Drakesmith, H., E. Nemeth, and T. Ganz. 2015. Ironing out ferroportin. *Cell Metab* 22 (5):777–87. doi: 10.1016/j.cmet.2015.09.006.

Drakesmith, H. and A. M. Prentice. 2012. Hepcidin and the iron-infection axis. *Science* 338 (6108):768–72. doi: 10.1126/science.1224577.

Du, X., E. She, T. Gelbart, J. Truksa, P. Lee, Y. Xia, K. Khovananth, S. Mudd, N. Mann, E. M. Moresco, E. Beutler, and B. Beutler. 2008. The serine protease TMPRSS6 is required to sense iron deficiency. *Science* 320 (5879):1088–92.

Fang, Z., S. L. Sampson, R. M. Warren, N. C. Gey van Pittius, and M. Newton-Foot. 2015. Iron acquisition strategies in mycobacteria. *Tuberculosis (Edinb)* 95 (2):123–30. doi: 10.1016/j.tube.2015.01.004.

Fang, F. C. and G. Weiss. 2014. Iron ERRs with Salmonella. *Cell Host Microbe* 15 (5):515–6. doi: 10.1016/j.chom.2014.04.012.

Finberg, K. E., M. M. Heeney, D. R. Campagna, Y. Aydinok, H. A. Pearson, K. R. Hartman, M. M. Mayo, S. M. Samuel, J. J. Strouse, K. Markianos, N. C. Andrews, and M. D. Fleming. 2008. Mutations in TMPRSS6 cause iron-refractory iron deficiency anemia (IRIDA). *Nat Genet* 40 (5):569–71.

Finch, C. 1994. Regulators of iron balance in humans. *Blood* 84 (6):1697–702.

Fischbach, M. A., H. Lin, L. Zhou, Y. Yu, R. J. Abergel, D. R. Liu, K. N. Raymond, B. L. Wanner, R. K. Strong, C. T. Walsh, A. Aderem, and K. D. Smith. 2006. The pathogen-associated iroA gene cluster mediates bacterial evasion of lipocalin 2. *Proc Natl Acad Sci U S A* 103 (44):16502–7. doi: 10.1073/pnas.0604636103.

Flo, T. H., K. D. Smith, S. Sato, D. J. Rodriguez, M. A. Holmes, R. K. Strong, S. Akira, and A. Aderem. 2004. Lipocalin 2 mediates an innate immune response to bacterial infection by sequestrating iron. *Nature* 432 (7019):917–21. doi: 10.1038/nature03104.

Frank, K. M., O. Schneewind, and W. J. Shieh. 2011. Investigation of a researcher's death due to septicemic plague. *N Engl J Med* 364 (26):2563–4. doi: 10.1056/NEJMc1010939.

Fujita, N., R. Sugimoto, M. Takeo, N. Urawa, R. Mifuji, H. Tanaka, Y. Kobayashi, M. Iwasa, S. Watanabe, Y. Adachi, and M. Kaito. 2007. Hepcidin expression in the liver: Relatively low level in patients with chronic hepatitis C. *Mol Med* 13 (1–2):97–104.

Ganz, T. 2009. Iron in innate immunity: Starve the invaders. *Curr Opin Immunol* 21 (1):63–7. doi: 10.1016/j.coi.2009.01.011.

Ganz, T. 2011. Hepcidin and iron regulation, 10 years later. *Blood* 117 (17):4425–33. doi: 10.1182/blood-2011-01-258467.

Ganz, T. 2013. Systemic iron homeostasis. *Physiol Rev* 93 (4):1721–41. doi: 10.1152/physrev.00008.2013.

Ganz, T. and E. Nemeth. 2011. Hepcidin and disorders of iron metabolism. *Annu Rev Med* 62:347–60. doi: 10.1146/annurev-med-050109-142444.

Ganz, T. and E. Nemeth. 2015. Iron homeostasis in host defence and inflammation. *Nat Rev Immunol* 15 (8):500–10. doi: 10.1038/nri3863.

Ghosh, M. C., D. L. Zhang, S. Y. Jeong, G. Kovtunovych, H. Ollivierre-Wilson, A. Noguchi, T. Tu, T. Senecal, G. Robinson, D. R. Crooks, W. H. Tong, K. Ramaswamy, A. Singh, B. B. Graham, R. M. Tuder, Z. X. Yu, M. Eckhaus, J. Lee, D. A. Springer, and T. A. Rouault. 2013. Deletion of iron regulatory protein 1 causes polycythemia and pulmonary hypertension in mice through translational derepression of HIF2alpha. *Cell Metab* 17 (2):271–81. doi: 10.1016/j.cmet.2012.12.016.

Girelli, D., M. Pasino, J. B. Goodnough, E. Nemeth, M. Guido, A. Castagna, F. Busti, N. Campostrini, N. Martinelli, I. Vantini, R. Corrocher, T. Ganz, and G. Fattovich. 2009. Reduced serum hepcidin levels in patients with chronic hepatitis C. *J Hepatol* 51 (5):845–52.

Goetz, D. H., M. A. Holmes, N. Borregaard, M. E. Bluhm, K. N. Raymond, and R. K. Strong. 2002. The neutrophil lipocalin NGAL is a bacteriostatic agent that interferes with siderophore-mediated iron acquisition. *Mol Cell* 10 (5):1033–43.

Guida, C., S. Altamura, F. A. Klein, B. Galy, M. Boutros, A. J. Ulmer, M. W. Hentze, and M. U. Muckenthaler. 2015. A novel inflammatory pathway mediating rapid hepcidin-independent hypoferremia. *Blood* 125 (14):2265–75. doi: 10.1182/blood-2014-08-595256.

Gwamaka, M., J. D. Kurtis, B. E. Sorensen, S. Holte, R. Morrison, T. K. Mutabingwa, M. Fried, and P. E. Duffy. 2012. Iron deficiency protects against severe Plasmodium falciparum malaria and death in young children. *Clin Infect Dis* 54:1137–44. doi: 10.1093/cid/cis010.

Hantke, K., G. Nicholson, W. Rabsch, and G. Winkelmann. 2003. Salmochelins, siderophores of Salmonella enterica and uropathogenic Escherichia coli strains, are recognized by the outer membrane receptor IroN. *Proc Natl Acad Sci U S A* 100 (7):3677–82. doi: 10.1073/pnas.0737682100.

Hatefi, Y. 1985. The mitochondrial electron transport and oxidative phosphorylation system. *Annu Rev Biochem* 54:1015–69. doi: 10.1146/annurev.bi.54.070185.005055.

Hentze, M. W., M. U. Muckenthaler, B. Galy, and C. Camaschella. 2010. Two to tango: Regulation of Mammalian iron metabolism. *Cell* 142 (1):24–38.

Holden, V. I. and M. A. Bachman. 2015. Diverging roles of bacterial siderophores during infection. *Metallomics* 7 (6):986–95. doi: 10.1039/c4mt00333k.

Holmes, M. A., W. Paulsene, X. Jide, C. Ratledge, and R. K. Strong. 2005. Siderocalin (Lcn 2) also binds carboxymycobactins, potentially defending against mycobacterial infections through iron sequestration. *Structure* 13 (1):29–41. doi: 10.1016/j.str.2004.10.009.

Huber, C. and G. Wachtershauser. 1998. Peptides by activation of amino acids with CO on (Ni,Fe)S surfaces: Implications for the origin of life. *Science* 281 (5377):670–2.

Hvidberg, V., M. B. Maniecki, C. Jacobsen, P. Hojrup, H. J. Moller, and S. K. Moestrup. 2005. Identification of the receptor scavenging hemopexin-heme complexes. *Blood* 106 (7):2572–9.

Imbert, M. and R. Blondeau. 1998. On the iron requirement of lactobacilli grown in chemically defined medium. *Curr Microbiol* 37 (1):64–6.

Jabara, H. H., S. E. Boyden, J. Chou, N. Ramesh, M. J. Massaad, H. Benson, W. Bainter, D. Fraulino, F. Rahimov, C. Sieff, Z. J. Liu, S. H. Alshemmari, B. K. Al-Ramadi, H. Al-Dhekri, R. Arnaout, M. Abu-Shukair, A. Vatsayan, E. Silver, S. Ahuja, E. G. Davies, M. Sola-Visner, T. K. Ohsumi, N. C. Andrews, L. D. Notarangelo, M. D. Fleming, W. Al-Herz, L. M. Kunkel, and R. S. Geha. 2016. A missense mutation in TFRC, encoding transferrin receptor 1, causes combined immunodeficiency. *Nat Genet* 48 (1):74–8. doi: 10.1038/ng.3465.

Jaeggi, T., G. A. Kortman, D. Moretti, C. Chassard, P. Holding, A. Dostal, J. Boekhorst, H. M. Timmerman, D. W. Swinkels, H. Tjalsma, A. Njenga, A. Mwangi, J. Kvalsvig, C. Lacroix, and M. B. Zimmermann. 2015. Iron fortification adversely affects the gut microbiome, increases pathogen abundance and induces intestinal inflammation in Kenyan infants. *Gut* 64 (5):731–42. doi: 10.1136/gutjnl-2014-307720.

Jones, E., S. R. Pasricha, A. Allen, P. Evans, C. A. Fisher, K. Wray, A. Premawardhena, D. Bandara, A. Perera, C. Webster, P. Sturges, N. F. Olivieri, T. St Pierre, A. E. Armitage, J. B. Porter, D. J. Weatherall, and H. Drakesmith. 2015. Hepcidin is suppressed by erythropoiesis in hemoglobin E beta-thalassemia and beta-thalassemia trait. *Blood* 125 (5):873–80. doi: 10.1182/blood-2014-10-606491.

Jordan, A. and P. Reichard. 1998. Ribonucleotide reductases. *Annu Rev Biochem* 67:71–98. doi: 10.1146/annurev.biochem.67.1.71.

Kabyemela, E. R., M. Fried, J. D. Kurtis, T. K. Mutabingwa, and P. E. Duffy. 2008. Decreased susceptibility to Plasmodium falciparum infection in pregnant women with iron deficiency. *J Infect Dis* 198 (2):163–6. doi: 10.1086/589512.

Kassebaum, N. J., R. Jasrasaria, M. Naghavi, S. K. Wulf, N. Johns, R. Lozano, M. Regan, D. Weatherall, D. P. Chou, T. P. Eisele, S. R. Flaxman, R. L. Pullan, S. J. Brooker, and C. J. Murray. 2014. A systematic analysis of global anemia burden from 1990 to 2010. *Blood* 123 (5):615–24. doi: 10.1182/blood-2013-06-508325.

Kautz, L., G. Jung, X. Du, V. Gabayan, J. Chapman, M. Nasoff, E. Nemeth, and T. Ganz. 2015. Erythroferrone contributes to hepcidin suppression and iron overload in a mouse model of beta-thalassemia. *Blood* 126 (17):2031–7. doi: 10.1182/blood-2015-07-658419.

Kautz, L., G. Jung, E. V. Valore, S. Rivella, E. Nemeth, and T. Ganz. 2014. Identification of erythroferrone as an erythroid regulator of iron metabolism. *Nat Genet* 46 (7):678–84. doi: 10.1038/ng.2996.

Keller, M., E. Blochl, G. Wachtershauser, and K. O. Stetter. 1994. Formation of amide bonds without a condensation agent and implications for origin of life. *Nature* 368 (6474):836–8. doi: 10.1038/368836a0.

Kim, D. K., J. H. Jeong, J. M. Lee, K. S. Kim, S. H. Park, Y. D. Kim, M. Koh, M. Shin, Y. S. Jung, H. S. Kim, T. H. Lee, B. C. Oh, J. I. Kim, H. T. Park, W. I. Jeong, C. H. Lee, S. B. Park, J. J. Min, S. I. Jung, S. Y. Choi, H. E. Choy, and H. S. Choi. 2014. Inverse agonist of estrogen-related receptor gamma controls Salmonella typhimurium infection by modulating host iron homeostasis. *Nat Med* 20 (4):419–24. doi: 10.1038/nm.3483.

Kortman, G. A., A. Boleij, D. W. Swinkels, and H. Tjalsma. 2012. Iron availability increases the pathogenic potential of Salmonella typhimurium and other enteric pathogens at the intestinal epithelial interface. *PLOS ONE* 7 (1):e29968. doi: 10.1371/journal.pone.0029968.

Kristiansen, M., J. H. Graversen, C. Jacobsen, O. Sonne, H. J. Hoffman, S. K. Law, and S. K. Moestrup. 2001. Identification of the haemoglobin scavenger receptor. *Nature* 409 (6817):198–201.

LaVaute, T., S. Smith, S. Cooperman, K. Iwai, W. Land, E. Meyron-Holtz, S. K. Drake, G. Miller, M. Abu-Asab, M. Tsokos, R. Switzer, 3rd, A. Grinberg, P. Love, N. Tresser, and T. A. Rouault. 2001. Targeted deletion of the gene encoding iron regulatory protein-2 causes misregulation of iron metabolism and neurodegenerative disease in mice. *Nat Genet* 27 (2):209–14. doi: 10.1038/84859.

Liu, X. B., N. B. Nguyen, K. D. Marquess, F. Yang, and D. J. Haile. 2005. Regulation of hepcidin and ferroportin expression by lipopolysaccharide in splenic macrophages. *Blood Cells Mol Dis* 35 (1):47–56.

Lopez, A., P. Cacoub, I. C. Macdougall, and L. Peyrin-Biroulet. 2015. Iron deficiency anaemia. *Lancet* 387:907–16. doi: 10.1016/S0140-6736(15)60865-0.

Maio, N. and T. A. Rouault. 2015. Iron-sulfur cluster biogenesis in mammalian cells: New insights into the molecular mechanisms of cluster delivery. *Biochim Biophys Acta* 1853 (6):1493–512. doi: 10.1016/j.bbamcr.2014.09.009.

McCance, R. A. and E. M. Widdowson. 1937. Absorption and excretion of iron. *Lancet* 2:680.

Meynard, D., L. Kautz, V. Darnaud, F. Canonne-Hergaux, H. Coppin, and M. P. Roth. 2009. Lack of the bone morphogenetic protein BMP6 induces massive iron overload. *Nat Genet* 41 (4):478–81.

Minchella, P. A., A. E. Armitage, B. Darboe, M. W. Jallow, H. Drakesmith, A. Jaye, A. M. Prentice, and J. M. McDermid. 2014. Elevated hepcidin at HIV diagnosis is associated with incident tuberculosis in a retrospective cohort study. *Int J Tuberc Lung Dis* 18 (11):1337–9. doi: 10.5588/ijtld.14.0143.

Minchella, P. A., A. E. Armitage, B. Darboe, M. W. Jallow, H. Drakesmith, A. Jaye, A. M. Prentice, and J. M. McDermid. 2015a. Elevated hepcidin is part of a complex relation that links mortality with iron homeostasis and anemia in men and women with HIV infection. *J Nutr* 145 (6):1194–201. doi: 10.3945/jn.114.203158.

Minchella, P. A., S. Donkor, O. Owolabi, J. S. Sutherland, and J. M. McDermid. 2015b. Complex anemia in tuberculosis: The need to consider causes and timing when designing interventions. *Clin Infect Dis* 60 (5):764–72. doi: 10.1093/cid/ciu945.

Muller, S. I., M. Valdebenito, and K. Hantke. 2009. Salmochelin, the long-overlooked catecholate siderophore of Salmonella. *Biometals* 22 (4):691–5. doi: 10.1007/s10534-009-9217-4.

Murakawa, H., C. E. Bland, W. T. Willis, and P. R. Dallman. 1987. Iron deficiency and neutrophil function: Different rates of correction of the depressions in oxidative burst and myeloperoxidase activity after iron treatment. *Blood* 69 (5):1464–8.

Murray, M. J., A. B. Murray, M. B. Murray, and C. J. Murray. 1978. The adverse effect of iron repletion on the course of certain infections. *Br Med J* 2 (6145):1113–5.

Mwangi, M. N., J. M. Roth, M. R. Smit, L. Trijsburg, A. M. Mwangi, A. Y. Demir, J. P. Wielders, P. F. Mens, J. J. Verweij, S. E. Cox, A. M. Prentice, I. D. Brouwer, H. F. Savelkoul, P. E. Andang'o, and H. Verhoef. 2015. Effect of daily antenatal iron supplementation on plasmodium infection in kenyan women: A randomized clinical trial. *JAMA* 314 (10):1009–20. doi: 10.1001/jama.2015.9496.

Nairz, M., D. Ferring-Appel, D. Casarrubea, T. Sonnweber, L. Viatte, A. Schroll, D. Haschka, F. C. Fang, M. W. Hentze, G. Weiss, and B. Galy. 2015. Iron regulatory proteins mediate host resistance to Salmonella infection. *Cell Host Microbe* 18 (2):254–61. doi: 10.1016/j.chom.2015.06.017.

Nairz, M., I. Theurl, S. Ludwiczek, M. Theurl, S. M. Mair, G. Fritsche, and G. Weiss. 2007. The co-ordinated regulation of iron homeostasis in murine macrophages limits the availability of iron for intracellular Salmonella typhimurium. *Cell Microbiol* 9 (9):2126–40.

Neilands, J. B. 1995. Siderophores: Structure and function of microbial iron transport compounds. *J Biol Chem* 270 (45):26723–6.

Nemeth, E., S. Rivera, V. Gabayan, C. Keller, S. Taudorf, B. K. Pedersen, and T. Ganz. 2004a. IL-6 mediates hypoferremia of inflammation by inducing the synthesis of the iron regulatory hormone hepcidin. *J Clin Invest* 113 (9):1271–6.

Nemeth, E., M. S. Tuttle, J. Powelson, M. B. Vaughn, A. Donovan, D. M. Ward, T. Ganz, and J. Kaplan. 2004b. Hepcidin regulates cellular iron efflux by binding to ferroportin and inducing its internalization. *Science* 306 (5704):2090–3.

Noinaj, N., S. K. Buchanan, and C. N. Cornelissen. 2012. The transferrin-iron import system from pathogenic Neisseria species. *Mol Microbiol* 86 (2):246–57. doi: 10.1111/mmi.12002.

Noinaj, N., N. C. Easley, M. Oke, N. Mizuno, J. Gumbart, E. Boura, A. N. Steere, O. Zak, P. Aisen, E. Tajkhorshid, R. W. Evans, A. R. Gorringe, A. B. Mason, A. C. Steven, and S. K. Buchanan. 2012. Structural basis for iron piracy by pathogenic Neisseria. *Nature* 483 (7387):53–8. doi: 10.1038/nature10823.

Olakanmi, O., L. S. Schlesinger, and B. E. Britigan. 2007. Hereditary hemochromatosis results in decreased iron acquisition and growth by Mycobacterium tuberculosis within human macrophages. *J Leukoc Biol* 81 (1):195–204.

Oppenheimer, S. J. 2001. Iron and its relation to immunity and infectious disease. *J Nutr* 131 (2S–2):616S–633S; discussion 633S–635S.

Parkhill, J., B. W. Wren, N. R. Thomson, R. W. Titball, M. T. Holden, M. B. Prentice, M. Sebaihia, K. D. James, C. Churcher, K. L. Mungall, S. Baker, D. Basham, S. D. Bentley, K. Brooks, A. M. Cerdeno-Tarraga, T. Chillingworth, A. Cronin, R. M. Davies, P. Davis, G. Dougan, T. Feltwell, N. Hamlin, S. Holroyd, K. Jagels, A. V. Karlyshev, S. Leather, S. Moule, P. C. Oyston, M. Quail,

K. Rutherford, M. Simmonds, J. Skelton, K. Stevens, S. Whitehead, and B. G. Barrell. 2001. Genome sequence of Yersinia pestis, the causative agent of plague. *Nature* 413 (6855):523–7. doi: 10.1038/35097083.

Pasricha, S. R., S. H. Atkinson, A. E. Armitage, S. Khandwala, J. Veenemans, S. E. Cox, L. A. Eddowes, T. Hayes, C. P. Doherty, A. Y. Demir, E. Tijhaar, H. Verhoef, A. M. Prentice, and H. Drakesmith. 2014. Expression of the iron hormone hepcidin distinguishes different types of anemia in African children. *Sci Transl Med* 6 (235):235re3. doi: 10.1126/scitranslmed.3008249.

Pasricha, S. R., H. Drakesmith, J. Black, D. Hipgrave, and B. A. Biggs. 2013. Control of iron deficiency anemia in low- and middle-income countries. *Blood* 121 (14):2607–17. doi: 10.1182/blood-2012-09-453522.

Payne, S. M. and R. A. Finkelstein. 1978. The critical role of iron in host-bacterial interactions. *J Clin Invest* 61 (6):1428–40.

Pietrangelo, A. 2010. Hereditary hemochromatosis: Pathogenesis, diagnosis, and treatment. *Gastroenterology* 139 (2):393–408, 408. e1–2.

Portugal, S., C. Carret, M. Recker, A. E. Armitage, L. A. Goncalves, S. Epiphanio, D. Sullivan, C. Roy, C. I. Newbold, H. Drakesmith, and M. M. Mota. 2011. Host-mediated regulation of superinfection in malaria. *Nat Med* 17 (6):732–7. doi: 10.1038/nm.2368.

Posey, J. E. and F. C. Gherardini. 2000. Lack of a role for iron in the Lyme disease pathogen. *Science* 288 (5471):1651–3.

Prentice, A. M., C. P. Doherty, S. A. Abrams, S. E. Cox, S. H. Atkinson, H. Verhoef, A. E. Armitage, and H. Drakesmith. 2012. Hepcidin is the major predictor of erythrocyte iron incorporation in anemic African children. *Blood* 119 (8):1922–8. doi: 10.1182/blood-2011-11-391219.

Prentice, A. M., H. Verhoef, and C. Cerami. 2013. Iron fortification and malaria risk in children. *JAMA* 310 (9):914–5. doi: 10.1001/jama.2013.6771.

Preza, G. C., P. Ruchala, R. Pinon, E. Ramos, B. Qiao, M. A. Peralta, S. Sharma, A. Waring, T. Ganz, and E. Nemeth. 2011. Minihepcidins are rationally designed small peptides that mimic hepcidin activity in mice and may be useful for the treatment of iron overload. *J Clin Invest* 121 (12):4880–8. doi: 10.1172/JCI57693.

Raiten, D. J. 2015. Iron: Current landscape and efforts to address a complex issue in a complex world. *J Pediatr* 167 (4 Suppl):S3–7. doi: 10.1016/j.jpeds.2015.07.013.

Ramos, E., L. Kautz, R. Rodriguez, M. Hansen, V. Gabayan, Y. Ginzburg, M. P. Roth, E. Nemeth, and T. Ganz. 2011. Evidence for distinct pathways of hepcidin regulation by acute and chronic iron loading in mice. *Hepatology* 53 (4):1333–41. doi: 10.1002/hep.24178.

Raymond, K. N., E. A. Dertz, and S. S. Kim. 2003. Enterobactin: An archetype for microbial iron transport. *Proc Natl Acad Sci U S A* 100 (7):3584–8. doi: 10.1073/pnas.0630018100.

Ryan, J. D., S. Altamura, E. Devitt, S. Mullins, M. W. Lawless, M. U. Muckenthaler, and J. Crowe. 2012. Pegylated interferon-alpha induced hypoferremia is associated with the immediate response to treatment in hepatitis C. *Hepatology* 56:492–500. doi: 10.1002/hep.25666.

Salahudeen, A. A., J. W. Thompson, J. C. Ruiz, H. W. Ma, L. N. Kinch, Q. Li, N. V. Grishin, and R. K. Bruick. 2009. An E3 ligase possessing an iron-responsive hemerythrin domain is a regulator of iron homeostasis. *Science* 326 (5953):722–6.

Sazawal, S., R. E. Black, M. Ramsan, H. M. Chwaya, R. J. Stoltzfus, A. Dutta, U. Dhingra, I. Kabole, S. Deb, M. K. Othman, and F. M. Kabole. 2006. Effects of routine prophylactic supplementation with iron and folic acid on admission to hospital and mortality in preschool children in a high malaria transmission setting: Community-based, randomised, placebo-controlled trial. *Lancet* 367 (9505):133–43.

Schade, A. L. and L. Caroline. 1946. An Iron-binding component in human blood plasma. *Science* 104 (2702):340–1.

Schaer, D. J., C. A. Schaer, P. W. Buehler, R. A. Boykins, G. Schoedon, A. I. Alayash, and A. Schaffner. 2006. CD163 is the macrophage scavenger receptor for native and chemically modified hemoglobins in the absence of haptoglobin. *Blood* 107 (1):373–80.

Schumann, K. and N. W. Solomons. 2013. Can iron supplementation be reconciled with benefits and risks in areas hyperendemic for malaria? *Food Nutr Bull* 34 (3):349–56.

Schwoebel, F., L. T. van Eijk, D. Zboralski, S. Sell, K. Buchner, C. Maasch, W. G. Purschke, M. Humphrey, S. Zollner, D. Eulberg, F. Morich, P. Pickkers, and S. Klussmann. 2013. The effects of the anti-hepcidin Spiegelmer NOX-H94 on inflammation-induced anemia in cynomolgus monkeys. *Blood* 121 (12):2311–5. doi: 10.1182/blood-2012-09-456756.

Silva, B. and P. Faustino. 2015. An overview of molecular basis of iron metabolism regulation and the associated pathologies. *Biochimica et biophysica acta* 1852 (7):1347–59. doi: 10.1016/j.bbadis.2015.03.011.

Silvestri, L., A. Pagani, A. Nai, I. De Domenico, J. Kaplan, and C. Camaschella. 2008. The serine protease matriptase-2 (TMPRSS6) inhibits hepcidin activation by cleaving membrane hemojuvelin. *Cell Metab* 8 (6):502–11.

Slack, M., T. Wang, and R. Wang. 2015. T cell metabolic reprogramming and plasticity. *Mol Immunol* 68 (2 Pt C):507–12. doi: 10.1016/j.molimm.2015.07.036.

Smith, C. L., T. L. Arvedson, K. S. Cooke, L. J. Dickmann, C. Forte, H. Li, K. L. Merriam, V. K. Perry, L. Tran, J. B. Rottman, and J. R. Maxwell. 2013. IL-22 regulates iron availability in vivo through the induction of hepcidin. *J Immunol* 191 (4):1845–55. doi: 10.4049/jimmunol.1202716.

Smith, S. R., M. C. Ghosh, H. Ollivierre-Wilson, W. Hang Tong, and T. A. Rouault. 2006. Complete loss of iron regulatory proteins 1 and 2 prevents viability of murine zygotes beyond the blastocyst stage of embryonic development. *Blood Cells Mol Dis* 36 (2):283–7. doi: 10.1016/j.bcmd.2005.12.006.

Soofi, S., S. Cousens, S. P. Iqbal, T. Akhund, J. Khan, I. Ahmed, A. K. Zaidi, and Z. A. Bhutta. 2013. Effect of provision of daily zinc and iron with several micronutrients on growth and morbidity among young children in Pakistan: A cluster-randomised trial. *Lancet* 382:29–40. doi: 10.1016/S0140-6736(13)60437-7.

Sow, F. B., W. C. Florence, A. R. Satoskar, L. S. Schlesinger, B. S. Zwilling, and W. P. Lafuse. 2007. Expression and localization of hepcidin in macrophages: A role in host defense against tuberculosis. *J Leukoc Biol* 82 (4):934–45. doi: 10.1189/jlb.0407216.

Spottiswoode, N., P. E. Duffy, and H. Drakesmith. 2014. Iron, anemia and hepcidin in malaria. *Front Pharmacol* 5:125. doi: 10.3389/fphar.2014.00125.

Steinbicker, A. U., T. B. Bartnikas, L. K. Lohmeyer, P. Leyton, C. Mayeur, S. M. Kao, A. E. Pappas, R. T. Peterson, D. B. Bloch, P. B. Yu, M. D. Fleming, and K. D. Bloch. 2011. Perturbation of hepcidin expression by BMP type I receptor deletion induces iron overload in mice. *Blood* 118 (15):4224–30. doi: 10.1182/blood-2011-03-339952.

Trousseau, A. 1872. True and false chlorosis. *In Lectures on Clinical Medicine* Bazire, V. (ed.), 95–117. Philadelphia, PA: Lindsay & Blakiston.

van Eijk, L. T., A. S. John, F. Schwoebel, L. Summo, S. Vauleon, S. Zollner, C. M. Laarakkers, M. Kox, J. G. van der Hoeven, D. W. Swinkels, K. Riecke, and P. Pickkers. 2014. Effect of the antihepcidin Spiegelmer lexaptepid on inflammation-induced decrease in serum iron in humans. *Blood* 124 (17):2643–6. doi: 10.1182/blood-2014-03-559484.

Vashisht, A. A., K. B. Zumbrennen, X. Huang, D. N. Powers, A. Durazo, D. Sun, N. Bhaskaran, A. Persson, M. Uhlen, O. Sangfelt, C. Spruck, E. A. Leibold, and J. A. Wohlschlegel. 2009. Control of iron homeostasis by an iron-regulated ubiquitin ligase. *Science* 326 (5953):718–21.

Wachtershauser, G. 1992. Groundworks for an evolutionary biochemistry: The iron-sulphur world. *Prog Biophys Mol Biol* 58 (2):85–201.

Weinberg, E. D. 1984. Iron withholding: A defense against infection and neoplasia. *Physiol Rev* 64 (1):65–102.

Weiss, G., D. Fuchs, A. Hausen, G. Reibnegger, E. R. Werner, G. Werner-Felmayer, and H. Wachter. 1992. Iron modulates interferon-gamma effects in the human myelomonocytic cell line THP-1. *Exp Hematol* 20 (5):605–10.

Wilkinson, N. and K. Pantopoulos. 2014. The IRP/IRE system in vivo: Insights from mouse models. *Front Pharmacol* 5:176. doi: 10.3389/fphar.2014.00176.

Wrighting, D. M. and N. C. Andrews. 2006. Interleukin-6 induces hepcidin expression through STAT3. *Blood* 108 (9):3204–9.

Yuki, K. E., M. M. Eva, E. Richer, D. Chung, M. Paquet, M. Cellier, F. Canonne-Hergaux, S. Vaulont, S. M. Vidal, and D. Malo. 2013. Suppression of hepcidin expression and iron overload mediate Salmonella susceptibility in ankyrin 1 ENU-induced mutant. *PLOS ONE* 8 (2):e55331. doi: 10.1371/journal.pone.0055331.

Zhang, C. 2014. Essential functions of iron-requiring proteins in DNA replication, repair and cell cycle control. *Protein Cell* 5 (10):750–60. doi: 10.1007/s13238-014-0083-7.

Zhang, D. L., M. C. Ghosh, and T. A. Rouault. 2014. The physiological functions of iron regulatory proteins in iron homeostasis - an update. *Front Pharmacol* 5:124. doi: 10.3389/fphar.2014.00124.

Zimmermann, M. B., C. Chassard, F. Rohner, E. K. N'Goran, C. Nindjin, A. Dostal, J. Utzinger, H. Ghattas, C. Lacroix, and R. F. Hurrell. 2010. The effects of iron fortification on the gut microbiota in African children: A randomized controlled trial in Cote d'Ivoire. *Am J Clin Nutr* 92 (6):1406–15. doi: 10.3945/ajcn.110.004564.

Zlotkin, S., S. Newton, A. M. Aimone, I. Azindow, S. Amenga-Etego, K. Tchum, E. Mahama, K. E. Thorpe, and S. Owusu-Agyei. 2013. Effect of iron fortification on malaria incidence in infants and young children in Ghana: A randomized trial. *JAMA* 310 (9):938–47. doi: 10.1001/jama.2013.277129.

14 Selenium as a Regulator of Inflammation and Immunity

Aaron H. Rose and Peter R. Hoffmann

CONTENTS

14.1 Introduction 231
14.2 Dietary Sources of Selenium and its Metabolism 232
14.3 The Family of Selenoproteins...233
14.4 Selenium Status and Biomarkers...233
14.5 Effects of Selenium on Different Immune Cells 235
14.6 Selenium, Immunity, and Cancer 238
14.7 Selenium and Viral Infections 238
14.8 Selenium and Bacterial and Parasitic Infections 239
14.9 Selenium and Inflammatory Bowel Diseases 239
14.10 Selenium and Asthma..240
14.11 Conclusions 240
References...240

14.1 INTRODUCTION

The element selenium was discovered in 1817 by the Swedish chemist, Jöns Jakob Berzelius. The first descriptions of this element in relation to human health involved its role as a toxin that caused neurological defects at high doses (Oldfield 2006). The beneficial effects of selenium were not described until the latter half of the twentieth century, when it became evident that selenium was essential for the health of laboratory animals and livestock (Schwarz and Foltz 1957; Patterson, Milstrey, and Stokstad 1957; Muth et al. 1958). These findings were extended to human health as selenium was subsequently recognized to be important for preventing diseases including Keshan disease (Ge et al. 1983), Keshan-Beck disease (Yao, Pei, and Kang 2011), and myxedematous endemic cretinism (Contempre, Vanderpas, and Dumont 1991). Over the past several decades, there have been a multitude of studies of animals and humans showing both beneficial and detrimental effects of altering selenium intake in humans. The effects of dietary selenium on inflammation and immunity have mostly been studied in cell culture systems and animal studies, although there have been some limited investigations in humans as well (Huang, Rose, and Hoffmann 2012). The benefits of increasing levels of selenium intake mainly apply to individuals with low baseline selenium status, while supplementation of diets to pharmacological levels of selenium has not demonstrated much increase in immune system function (Hoffmann and Berry 2008). These varying results highlight the multiple ways in which inflammation and immunity may be impacted by selenium status. Determining specific mechanisms by which selenium intake regulates inflammation and immunity has been a major challenge due to the wide variety of effects exerted by this micronutrient. In this chapter, the current understanding of the effects of selenium on immunity will be discussed as well as mechanisms through which selenium exerts its biological effects on the immune system and tissues that drive inflammation.

14.2   DIETARY SOURCES OF SELENIUM AND ITS METABOLISM

Humans acquire selenium exclusively through diet, and a wide variety of foods can serve as sources of selenium. These include foods from plants and animals, and they can all differ in selenium content as the soils and waters in different geographical regions may differ in selenium content. Thus, selenium enters the body through the consumption of grains, vegetables, legumes, nuts, meats, seafoods, and other foods (National Institutes of Health 2013). The main selenocompound in plants is selenomethionine, but also present are selenate, selenite, selenocysteine, dimethyl diselenide, and others. Animal tissues mainly contain selenocysteine, selenomethionine, selenotrisulfides of cystine, selenate and selenite (Navarro-Alarcon and Cabrera-Vique 2008). The major form of selenium ingested by humans is selenomethionine. Absorption of Se into duodenum capillaries is efficient and is not regulated. More than 90% of selenomethionine is absorbed by the same mechanism as methionine itself (Navarro-Alarcon and Cabrera-Vique 2008). Although less is known about selenocysteine absorption, it appears to be absorbed very well. Selenate is absorbed almost completely, but a significant fraction of it is lost in the urine before it can be incorporated into tissues. Excretion of excess selenium in urine is also a mechanism by which selenium levels are regulated in the body (Navarro-Alarcon and Cabrera-Vique 2008). Interestingly, organic and inorganic selenium compounds are metabolized and eliminated in human urine differently (Jager, Drexler, and Goen 2016). The kidneys play a key role in maintaining proper selenium homeostasis by scavenging selenium in glomerular filtrate via megalin receptor–mediated uptake of the key selenium

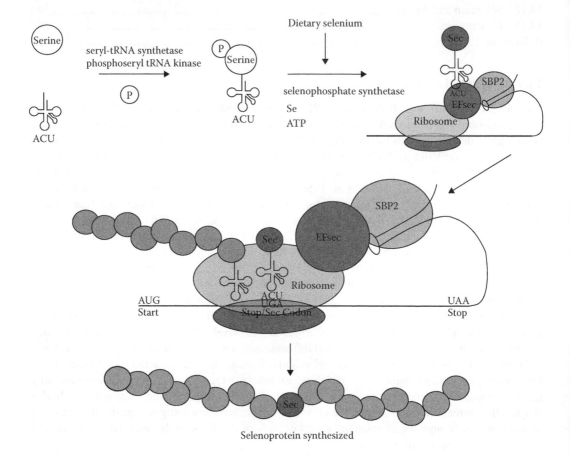

FIGURE 14.1   Selenoprotein synthesis involves assembly of Sec-tRNA and insertion of selenium into polypeptide by SECIS/SBP2/EFsec coded by UGA on the mRNA.

transporter, selenoprotein P. The major urinary selenium metabolites are selenosugars (Francesconi and Pannier 2004).

Within cells, various forms of selenium are ultimately shunted into the pathway shown in Figure 14.1 that leads to synthesis of a very special amino acid, selenocysteine. Selenocysteine has a structure similar to cysteine, hence the name. However, the precursor to selenocysteine in the synthesis pathway is the amino acid serine provided by seryl-tRNA synthetase. The details of selenocysteine synthesis and its incorporation into newly formed selenoproteins are covered in detail in several excellent reviews (Labunskyy, Hatfield, and Gladyshev 2014; Gonzalez-Flores et al. 2013; Squires and Berry 2008). Selenocysteine is unique among the amino acids in that for its incorporation into proteins during translation, it requires its own dedicated machinery and it uses a stop codon, UGA, as its insertion codon. The ribosomes are the same as those used for other proteins, but the dedicated translational machinery includes a special tRNA called Sec tRNA[Ser]Sec, SBP2, and a selenium-specific eukaryotic elongation factor called eEFSec. This machinery associates with the mRNA for an individual selenoprotein and facilitates the recoding of the UGA stop codon to a selenium insertion codon, thereby allowing uninterrupted polypeptide synthesis to occur on the ribosome.

14.3 THE FAMILY OF SELENOPROTEINS

The complete list of human selenoproteins was revealed with the hallmark paper published by the Gladyshev laboratory in which bioinformatic analyses of the human genome were successfully employed to identify all family members of the selenoproteome (Kryukov et al. 2003). As shown in Table 14.1, this family consists of 25 selenoproteins that all contain the selenium residue as part of their amino acid sequence, and they exhibit a wide range of tissue distribution and functions (Reeves and Hoffmann 2009). Many of the selenoproteins are enzymes such as the glutathione peroxidases, thioredoxin reductases, deiodinases, and methionine sulfoxide reductase. Other selenoproteins may or may not function as enzymes, and investigations are ongoing to determine exact physiological roles for all of the family members. Cells of the immune system express many of the selenoproteins and the antioxidant- or redox-regulating roles they play seem to be similar to those roles played in nonimmune cells. It must be noted that in addition to the selenoproteins, small-molecule selenocompounds also are found in immune cells, and these affect cell functions such as DNA repair and other less-known processes.

14.4 SELENIUM STATUS AND BIOMARKERS

Like many other nutrients, the health benefits of increasing selenium intake follow a U-shaped curve (Figure 14.2). An absence of dietary selenium and/or selenoproteins during development is lethal (Bosl et al. 1997). Raising levels of selenium intake from 0 µg/day increases the health status of an individual, but low selenium status may still impact several physiological processes. At the other end of the spectrum is the effects of extremely high selenium intake (300–800 µg/day) that can lead to a variety of negative health outcomes, and reducing intake to safe levels will reduce those effects (Vinceti et al. 2001). The optimal part of the U-shaped curve is not defined, particularly for immune responses. The data available suggest that individuals with marginally low selenium status will have relatively low selenoprotein expression and this can lead to suboptimal immune responses (Huang, Rose, and Hoffmann 2012).

To determine selenium status of an individual, one can collect different types of samples including toenails, hair, tissue, blood, or urine. Toenail selenium level is recognized as a reliable biomarker reflecting long-term selenium status (Hunter et al. 1990), and is often used for population-based studies. For individuals, most commonly the plasma is sampled and can be analyzed for total selenium by mass spectrophotometry, for individual selenoprotein levels, or selenoenzyme activity (Combs 2015). The recommended daily intakes for each country are based on the amount needed to maximize activity of the selenoprotein plasma glutathione peroxidase. However, there is

TABLE 14.1

Selenoproteins with Their Abbreviations and Functions

Selenoprotein	Abbreviation	Function
Cytosolic glutathione peroxidase	GPX1	Reduces cellular H_2O_2. GPX1 knockout is more susceptible to oxidative challenge. Overexpression of GPX1 increases risk of diabetes. KO of GPx1 and 2 leads to spontaneous colitis.
Gastrointestinal glutathione peroxidase	GPX2	Reduces peroxide in gut. GPX1/GPX2 double knockout mice develop intestinal cancer, one allele of GPX2 added back confers protection. KO of GPx1 and 2 leads to spontaneous colitis.
Plasma glutathione peroxidase	GPX3	Reduces peroxide in blood. Important for cardiovascular protection, perhaps through modulation of nitrous oxide levels.
Phosholipid hydroperoxide glutathione peroxidase	GPX4	Reduces phospholipid peroxide. Genetic deletion is embryonic lethal; GPX4 acts as crucial antioxidant, and sensor of oxidative stress and proapoptotic signals.
Olfactory glutathione peroxidase	GPX6	Age-related expression. Modulates toxicity in Huntington's disease.
Thioredoxin reductase Type I	TrxR1, Trxrd1, TR1	Localized to cytoplasm and nucleus. Genetic deletion is embryonic lethal. Regenerates reduced thioredoxin; controls glucose-derived H_2O_2.
Thioredoxin reductase Type II	TrxR2, Trxrd2, TR2	Localized to mitochondria. Genetic deletion in mice is embryonic lethal, but TXNRD2-deficiency in humans leads to glucocorticoid deficiency.
Thioredoxin reductase Type III	TRxR3, Trxrd3, TR3, TGR	Testes-specific expression.
Deiodinase Type I	D1, DI01	Important for systemic active thyroid hormone levels.
Deiodinase Type II	D2, DI02	Important for local active thyroid hormone levels.
Deiodinase Type III	D3, DI03	Inactivates thyroid hormone.
Selenoprotein H	Sel H	Nuclear localization, involved in transcription. Essential for viability and antioxidant defense in Drosophila.
Selenoprotein I	Sel 1, hEPT1	Transmembrane protein involved in phosphatidylethanolamine biosynthesis.
Selenoprotein K	Sel K	Transmembrane protein localized in ER and involved in calcium flux in immune cells. Also associated with ER associated degradation.

(Continued)

TABLE 14.1 (*Continued*)
Selenoproteins with Their Abbreviations and Functions

Selenoprotein	Abbreviation	Function
Selenoprotein M	Sel M	Thioredoxin-like ER-resident protein that may be involved in regulation of body weight and energy metabolism.
Selenoprotein 15	Sep 15	Thiol-disulfide oxidoreductase involved in protein folding in the ER. Possibly a procancer selenoprotein and knockout mice are protected from chemically induced colon carcinogenesis.
Selenoprotein N	Sel N, SEPN 1, SepN	Potential role in early muscle formation; mutations lead to multiminicore disease and other myopathies. Knockout affects muscle function and also impairs lung function independent of respiratory muscles.
Selenoprotein O	Sel O	Contains a Cys-X-X-Sec motif suggestive of redox function, but importance remains unknown. Localized to mitochondria across mouse tissues.
Selenoprotein P	Sel P, SepP	Selenium transport to brain and tests – Sel P knockout leads to neurological problems and male sterility. Sel P also functions an intracellular antioxidant in phagocytes. Helps regulate oxidative stress and epithelial stem cell functions during IBD.
Selenoprotein R	Sel R, MsrB1	Functions as a methionine sulfoxide reductase and Sel R knockouts show mild damage to oxidative insult and impaired actin dynamics.
Selenoprotein S	Sel S, SEPS1, SELENOS, VIMP	Transmembrane protein found in ER. Complexes with many proteins and may be involved in ER associated degradation.

growing debate over the use of plasma glutathione peroxidase activity as a basis for setting selenium requirements, and other biomarkers like plasma selenoprotein P have been suggested as superior biomarkers. Selenoprotein P has been shown to exhibit a better response to different dietary forms of selenium and a higher plateau with increasing selenium intake (Hurst et al. 2010; Xia et al. 2010).

14.5 EFFECTS OF SELENIUM ON DIFFERENT IMMUNE CELLS

There are many effects of selenium on immune cells (Figure 14.3). As this figure shows, cell lineages throughout the hematopoietic system rely on selenium for proper functioning.

Macrophages are one type of immune cell for which the effects of selenium have been well studied. Selenium metabolites, as well as the different selenoproteins, can have significant effects on macrophage activation, differentiation, and effector functions. Low selenium status can reduce phagocytic capacity, superoxide production, and cytokine secretion by macrophages

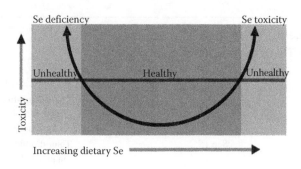

Se deficiency
(associated disease outcomes)

Keshan disease

Male infertility

Potential of increased risk of
infection with:
  HIV, Hep C, polio,
  West Nile virus, Tuberculosis
  L. monocytogenes, H. bakeri
Inflammatory Bowel Disease

Se toxicity
(associated disease outcomes)

Increased cancer growth

Se toxicity

FIGURE 14.2 The relationship between selenium intake and health outcomes.

The Effect of Dietary Selenium Status on Specific Immune Cells

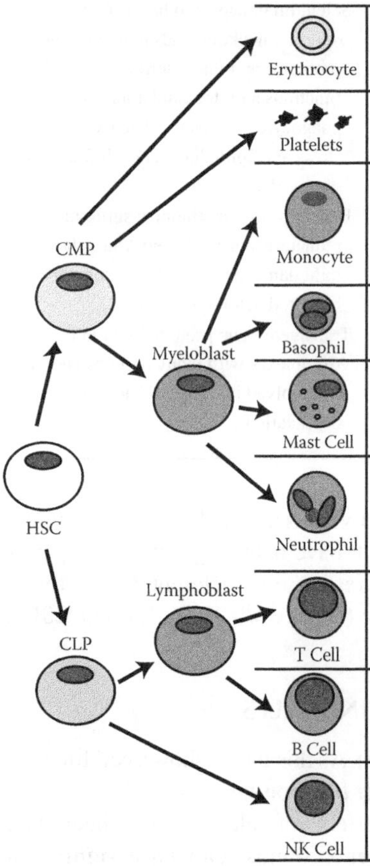

Erythrocyte	More than 95% of blood Se is contained in red blood cells and therefore red blood cell GPx activity has been considered as a potentially valuable intermediate time frame (cell lifespan of around 150 days) assessment tool of overall Se status.
Platelets	Similarly to red blood cells, platelet GPx activity may be useful as an assessment tool of overall Se status but for a much shorter timeframe (5–9 days).
Monocyte	Se status has significant effects on macrophage activation, differentiation, and function. Some studies have shown that insufficient Se leads to greater inflammatory activation and nitric oxide production through NFkB signaling,while higher levels of selenium shifts macrophages to an M2 inflammation resolving phenoype through PPARy sigaling
Basophil	Se status and the function of basophils has not been investigated in depth and is an important cell popultation for future studies.
Mast Cell	Mast cell mediators, which are intimately involved in allergy and asthma, may be decreased in cells supplemented with Se and this may help to account for some of the observed relationship between selenium status and asthma.
Neutrophil	Neutrophils, in Se deficient rat studies, have been shown to produce less oxidative burst. However, the opposite results have been found in chickens. In human studies Se deficiency has been correlated with greater oxidative stress, due in part to neutrophil ROS production.
T Cell	Se can effect the differentitation of T-cells to Th1 or Th2 phenotypes. Higher Se shifts toward TH1 while lower Se shifts toward Th2. In mice, high levels of dietary Se increased T-cell function and proliferation.
B Cell	Both low and high dietary Se levels have been shown to decrease B-cells in mice, while in humans increased Se has produced greater numbers of circulating B-cells.
NK Cell	NK cells are involved in clearing cancerous cells. Multiple studies have demonstrated that selenium in various forms can alter the expression of surface proteins on cancer cells that control the response of NK cells. Generally higher levels of selenium have been shown to enhance NK cell detection of cancer.

CMP

Myeloblast

HSC

CLP

Lymphoblast

FIGURE 14.3 The development of different cells of the immune system and the effects of selenium (Se) on their functions.

(Safir et al. 2003). At the level of DNA, selenium status can also affect macrophage biology. An interesting study by the Prabhu laboratory showed that selenium controls epigenetic modulation of proinflammatory genes in macrophages (Narayan et al. 2015). Selenium can also affect how arachidonic acid is metabolized into lipid mediators in macrophages, affecting both the macrophages themselves and other target cells (Gandhi et al. 2011). Upon activation, macrophages differentiate into different phenotypes that include inflammatory (M1) and anti-inflammatory (M2) types. Studies with mouse macrophages suggest that selenium supplementation leads to endogenous activation of the PPARγ-dependent switch from M1 to M2 phenotype in the presence of IL-4, possibly affecting pathways of wound healing and inflammation resolution (Nelson, Lei, and Prabhu 2011). Related to this, low selenium status can affect nitric oxide production through the enzyme iNOS (Prabhu et al. 2002). Finally, macrophages deficient in selenoprotein synthesis did not show the same defects as selenium-deficient macrophages, but were impaired in regulating extracellular matrix–related gene expression related to their ability to navigate through tissues (Carlson et al. 2010). Thus, the small molecular selenocompounds that are still present in the selenoprotein-deficient macrophages may be important for many macrophage functions.

Other innate immune cells rely on adequate selenium supply for carrying out functions during immune responses. For example, neutrophils from selenium-deficient rats exhibited reduced oxidative burst compared to neutrophils from controls (Baker and Cohen 1983). However, other functions may be more resistant to changes in selenium, such as phagocytosis or degranulation (Baker and Cohen 1984). In humans, there is some evidence to suggest that subjects with a lower serum selenium concentration may be exposed to a greater chronic oxidative stress due to neutrophil ROS production (Lee et al. 2011). Mechanistic studies have shown that increased selenium appears to provide a protective effect in neutrophils from patients with polycystic ovary syndrome against oxidative stress and calcium entry through modulation of TRPV1 calcium channels (Lee et al. 2011). Dendritic cells are also affected by redox status and selenium almost certainly affects their function, but limited data are available regarding these effects. One study showed that a selenium-containing compound, ebselen, reduced activation capacity of dendritic cells when T-cells were present (Matsue et al. 2003). Mast cell mediator release was decreased with supplementation of selenium in the culture medium, although the physiological relationship to doses used was not fully illustrated (Safaralizadeh et al. 2013).

T-cells are a crucial member of the adaptive immune system, and selenium levels as well as expression levels of individual selenoproteins can impact the ability of these cells to properly function. Selenium had a protective effect on T-cells when mice were challenged with a potent mytotoxin compared to other nutrients like vitamin E (Salimian et al. 2014). The differentiation of CD4+ T helper cells into effectors like T helper 1 or 2 (Th1 or Th2) cells may be impacted by levels of selenium intake, and this can affect how the immune system is directed toward fighting certain infections or give rise to allergic reactions. In mice, higher selenium intake biased the differentiation of naive T helper cells into Th1 cells and away from Th2 cells (Hoffmann et al. 2010). Several aspects of activation of naive CD4+ T-cells were enhanced by increasing dietary selenium in mice, including calcium mobilization, oxidative burst, translocation of nuclear factor of activated T-cells, and proliferation. This is consistent with studies in mice deficient for selenoprotein expression in T-cells, where T-cell proliferation and T-cell–dependent antibody responses were reduced (Shrimali et al. 2008). B-cells appear to be affected differently from T-cells in relation to selenium status (Cheng et al. 2012): while T-cell function was enhanced, the total numbers of peripheral B-cells decreased in both the selenium supplemented and the selenium-deficient mice. These results are not in line with data from a study showing that in human males, selenium supplementation produced greater numbers of circulating B-cells (Hawkes, Kelley, and Taylor 2001). The exact role of selenium status in B-cell function remains to be determined.

14.6 SELENIUM, IMMUNITY, AND CANCER

Early animal studies showed very promising results for selenium supplementation in exerting antitumor effects (Yan et al. 1999; Ankerst and Sjogren 1982). These were followed by positive findings in humans receiving selenium supplementation leading to reduced cancer (Clark et al. 1996; Comstock, Bush, and Helzlsouer 1992). However, other studies have not supported a beneficial role of selenium supplementation in preventing different types of cancer (Rose et al. 2014; Lippman et al. 2009; Klein et al. 2011). A potential reason for these different findings may by that selenium has different effects on different stages of cancer. For example, higher levels of selenium within tissues and cells may benefit the DNA-repair process and help prevent carcinogenic processes. However, once tumorigenesis has occurred, higher levels of selenium may increase the rate of progression of tumors (Bera et al. 2013). Interestingly, the different forms of selenium that are ingested or are metabolized after ingestion can have different effects on cancer (Ip 1998; Chen et al. 2013). Compounds such as methylseleninic acid show greater uptake and metabolic activity for the production of methylselenol (CH3SeH), a major anticancer selenium metabolite, but are unstable; therefore these advantages may be countered by their instability *in vivo* (Ip et al. 2000; Suzuki et al. 2008).

Of course, the effects of dietary selenium or selenium supplementation on tumors themselves may be quite different from the immune cells responsible for eradicating those tumors. Like many other types of immune responses, anticancer immunity may be jeopardized with a low selenium diet. One mechanism by which selenium may prevent tumor development was described in a study showing that methylselenol was not only acting directly on cancer cell metabolism but also effective in increasing cell surface expression of NKG2D ligands (Hagemann-Jensen et al. 2014). This is important since expression of NKG2D ligands is induced by stress-associated pathways that occur early during malignant transformation, and this enables the recognition and elimination of tumors by activating the lymphocyte receptor NKG2D. Another study determined that selenium in the form of selenite induces a posttranscriptional blockade of HLA-E expression on cancer cells (Enqvist et al. 2011). This surface protein normally inhibits the killing function of NK cells by binding to CD94/NKG2A receptors. Some studies have combined selenium with other cancer therapeutics with positive results. Selenium enriched *Bifidobacterium longum* was able to enhance anticancer activity of T-cells and NK cells in H22 tumor–bearing mice (Yin et al. 2014). In another study, mice bearing H22 tumors were treated with polysaccharides from roots of *Astraguls membranaceus* with or without selenium, and the selenium improved the phagocytotic function of intra-abdominal macrophages and suppressed M2-like polarization of tumor-associated macrophages (Li et al. 2014). In a small study in human subjects (N = 33), selenium supplementation increased cytotoxic T-cell–driven tumor lysis (Kiremidjian-Schumacher and Roy 2001). However, there is not currently enough evidence to support a therapeutic role for selenium supplementation in all cancer patients.

14.7 SELENIUM AND VIRAL INFECTIONS

Effective antiviral immunity requires effective cell-mediated immunity and in many cases strong neutralizing antibodies produced through the humoral immune response. Selenium status may affect antiviral immune responses, and one study in the United Kingdom involving a small group of human subjects (N = 22) showed that individuals with a low baseline selenium status benefited from supplementation with up to 100 µg/day sodium selenite reflected by increased T-cell responses to poliovirus and by improved poliovirus clearance (Broome et al. 2004). Humoral responses did not seem to improve with supplementation. In selenium deficiency, benign strains of Coxsackievirus and influenza virus can mutate to highly pathogenic strains. Perhaps the best example of this is the altered virulance of Coxsackievirus B3 under conditions of low selenium and its role in Keshan disease (Beck 1997). Keshan disease in parts of China has been shown to be fully preventable with selenium supplementation. Selenium status or deficiencies in specific selenoproteins may affect many other viral infections including influenza, HIV, IAV, hepatitis C virus, poliovirus, and West

Nile virus (Steinbrenner et al. 2015). HIV infection is particularly interesting in that selenium status can influence the course of infection, and the infection can affect the selenium status of the individual. For example, there is a direct correlation between a low dietary selenium intake and a 20-fold increase in the risk of developing AIDS in HIV-infected individuals (Baum et al. 1997). Studies have also shown that plasma selenium levels tend to be low in infected individuals and to rise again in populations that are undergoing antiretroviral therapy (ART) with a concurrent suppression of viral titers (de Menezes Barbosa et al. 2015). In a study conducted to examine the correlation between plasma selenium levels and treatment in HIV-positive patients undergoing ART it was shown that there was a positive correlation between plasma selenium concentration, CD8$^+$ T-cell activation, and lower body mass (Hileman et al. 2015). The notion that there may be a beneficial role of selenium for HIV-infected individuals is further supported by evidence showing decreased levels of major selenoproteins in Jurkat T-cells during HIV infection accompanied by an increase in low molecular mass selenium compounds (Gladyshev et al. 1999). However, it remains unclear whether selenium supplementation benefits HIV-infected individuals (Nunnari et al. 2012). Perhaps targeting selenium therapy to individuals who are more likely to be selenium deficient during infection is a more viable approach. In fact, this is being done in places like Rwanda and results from these studies will be informative (Kamwesiga et al. 2011).

14.8   SELENIUM AND BACTERIAL AND PARASITIC INFECTIONS

Selenium deficiency is very likely to have a negative impact on the ability of an individual to fight bacterial or parasitic infections. This is supported by animal studies, such as those showing that low selenium diets led to impaired host innate immune responses against *Listeria monocytogenes* (Wang et al. 2009). Selenium deficiency in mice led to more severe infection with the nematode *Heligmosomoides bakeri* (Smith et al. 2013). Lower selenium status was associated with reduced Th2 responses and lower anti-*H. bakeri* IgG1 production, which both are protective in this infection. Like HIV, tuberculosis infection has been associated with lower selenium status (Kassu et al. 2006). This has led to small intervention studies where micronutrients like selenium have shown potential for supportive therapy in tuberculosis patients (Villamor et al. 2008). This may be due in part to proimmune effects, although attempts to apply micronutrient supplementation that included selenium to tuberculosis infection in Tanzania did not show significant improvements in T-cell mediated responses (Kawai et al. 2014). The boost in selenium may alternatively increase antioxidant selenoenzyme activity that provides beneficial effects for these patients.

Other bacterial infections studied in mice show some promising results. One study involving selenium-enriched probiotics for reducing pathogenic *Escherichia coli* infections showed that antioxidant status improved, immunity was enhanced, and the internal environment of the intestinal tract was modified (Yang et al. 2009). Genetic models in mice have provided some insight into the roles of certain selenoproteins in susceptibility to bacterial infections. For example, mice deficient for both glutathione peroxidase 1 and 2 on some genetic backgrounds (e.g. 129S1/SvImJ) develop spontaneous colitis (Broome et al. 2004). These studies provide evidence to demonstrate the function of GPx1 and GPx2 against *Salmonella typhimmurium* colonization and infection, but whether this is due to defects in immune-system surveillance or gut epithelial homeostasis is unclear. However, there is an adverse effect from enhanced inflammation in GPx2 deficiency with the development of tumors (Krehl et al. 2012).

14.9   SELENIUM AND INFLAMMATORY BOWEL DISEASES

The human inflammatory bowel diseases (IBDs) include Crohn's disease and ulcerative colitis, which both involve chronic inflammation. Human studies have suggested that IBDs are often accompanied by lower serum selenium concentrations, along with reduced antioxidant and increased pro-inflammatory activities (Nagy, Fulesdi, and Hallay 2013). Encouraging results from animal studies support the notion that higher selenium intake can lower intestinal damage during IBD and chronic inflammation–induced colon cancer (Kaushal et al. 2014; Barrett et al. 2013). Some of these effects may be attributed to the role that selenoproteins play in regulating macrophage activation and differentiation. In particular, IBD can involve changes in cellular oxidative state coupled with altered expression of selenoproteins in macrophages that drive the switch from a proinflammatory pheno-type to an anti-inflammatory phenotype to efficiently resolve inflammation in the gut and restore epithelial barrier integrity (Kudva, Shay, and Prabhu 2015). In addition, selenoprotein P plays a role in regulating oxidative stress and epithelial stem cell functions during IBD (Barrett et al. 2015).

14.10   SELENIUM AND ASTHMA

There has been a long-standing interest in the role of dietary selenium in the development of asthma based on the simplified notion that this multifactorial disease involves increased oxida-tive stress in the lungs, and selenium may function as a protective antioxidant. In support of this idea, some studies have found asthmatics had lower concentrations of selenium compared with healthy subjects (Guo et al. 2011). Some small intervention studies with antioxidants that included selenium showed improved outcomes for those suffering from asthma. (Guo et al. 2012). However, other studies have not provided supportive data and there appear to be confounding effects of increased selenium on the development or severity of this very complex disease (Norton and Hoffmann 2012; Hoffmann 2012). There have been several promising results in mouse models of asthma suggesting that selenium supplementation may be beneficial for limiting the morbid-ity caused by this disease (Hoffmann et al. 2007). In another study using cockroach extract as an allergen, a combination of choline chloride, vitamin C, and selenium via the intranasal route reduced airway hyperresponsiveness, inflammation, and oxidative stress (Bansal et al. 2014). This seemed to involve IL-10 production by FoxP3$^+$ cells, and offers one possible therapeutic approach against allergic airway disease.

14.11   CONCLUSIONS

There is an abundance of evidence in animal models and immune cell culture systems to suggest that marginally low selenium status leads to impaired immune responses. There are limited stud-ies involving human subjects, but this notion is generally in agreement where data are available. The benefits of supplementing individuals with selenium to boost immunity may apply mostly to those who have a low baseline selenium status, or in some cases of ongoing HIV-1 infection. The mechanisms by which selenium affects immunity lie in the metabolism of this micronutrient into small compounds and incorporation into selenoproteins. Much more information is needed for a better understanding of these mechanisms in order to selectively and more effectively utilize the therapeutic potential of dietary selenium.

REFERENCES

Ankerst, J. and H. O. Sjogren. 1982. Effect of selenium on the induction of breast fibroadenomas by adenovirus type 9 and 1,2-dimethylhydrazine-induced bowel carcinogenesis in rats. *Int J Cancer* 29 (6):707–10.
Baker, S. S. and H. J. Cohen. 1983. Altered oxidative metabolism in selenium-deficient rat granulocytes. *J Immunol* 130 (6):2856–60.
Baker, S. S. and H. J. Cohen. 1984. Increased sensitivity to H2O2 in glutathione peroxidase-deficient rat granu-locytes. *J Nutr* 114 (11):2003–9.
Bansal, P., S. Saw, D. Govindaraj, et al. 2014. Intranasal administration of a combination of choline chloride, vitamin C, and selenium attenuates the allergic effect in a mouse model of airway disease. *Free Radic Biol Med* 73:358–65.
Barrett, C. W., V. K. Reddy, S. P. Short, et al. 2015. Selenoprotein P influences colitis-induced tumorigenesis by mediating stemness and oxidative damage. *J Clin Invest* 125 (7):2646–60.

Barrett, C. W., K. Singh, A. K. Motley, et al. 2013. Dietary selenium deficiency exacerbates DSS-induced epithelial injury and AOM/DSS-induced tumorigenesis. *PLOS ONE* 8 (7):e67845.

Baum, M. K., G. Shor-Posner, S. Lai, et al. 1997. High risk of HIV-related mortality is associated with selenium deficiency. *J Acquir Immune Defic Syndr Hum Retrovirol* 15 (5):370–4.

Beck, M. A. 1997. Rapid genomic evolution of a non-virulent coxsackievirus B3 in selenium-deficient mice. *Biomed Environ Sci* 10 (2–3):307–15.

Bera, S., V. De Rosa, W. Rachidi, et al. 2013. Does a role for selenium in DNA damage repair explain apparent controversies in its use in chemoprevention? *Mutagenesis* 28 (2):127–34.

Bosl, M. R., K. Takaku, M. Oshima, et al. 1997. Early embryonic lethality caused by targeted disruption of the mouse selenocysteine tRNA gene (Trsp). *Proc Natl Acad Sci U S A* 94 (11):5531–4.

Broome, C. S., F. McArdle, J. A. Kyle, et al. 2004. An increase in selenium intake improves immune function and poliovirus handling in adults with marginal selenium status. *Am J Clin Nutr* 80 (1):154–62.

Carlson, B. A., M. H. Yoo, R. K. Shrimali, et al. 2010. Role of selenium-containing proteins in T-cell and macrophage function. *Proc Nutr Soc* 69 (3):300–10.

Chen, Y. C., K. S. Prabhu, A. Das, et al. 2013. Dietary selenium supplementation modifies breast tumor growth and metastasis. *Int J Cancer* 133 (9):2054–64.

Cheng, W. H., A. Holmstrom, X. Li, et al. 2012. Effect of dietary selenium and cancer cell xenograft on peripheral T and B lymphocytes in adult nude mice. *Biol Trace Elem Res* 146 (2):230–5.

Clark, L. C., G. F. Combs, Jr., B. W. Turnbull, et al. 1996. Effects of selenium supplementation for cancer prevention in patients with carcinoma of the skin. A randomized controlled trial. Nutritional Prevention of Cancer Study Group. *JAMA* 276 (24):1957–63.

Combs, G. F., Jr. 2015. Biomarkers of selenium status. *Nutrients* 7 (4):2209–36.

Comstock, G. W., T. L. Bush, and K. Helzlsouer. 1992. Serum retinol, beta-carotene, vitamin E, and selenium as related to subsequent cancer of specific sites. *Am J Epidemiol* 135 (2):115–21.

Contempre, B., J. Vanderpas, and J. E. Dumont. 1991. Cretinism, thyroid hormones and selenium. *Mol Cell Endocrinol* 81 (1–3):C193–5.

de Menezes Barbosa, E. G., F. B. Junior, A. A. Machado, et al. 2015. A longer time of exposure to antiretroviral therapy improves selenium levels. *Clin Nutr* 34 (2):248–51.

Enqvist, M., G. Nilsonne, O. Hammarfjord, et al. 2011. Selenite induces posttranscriptional blockade of HLA-E expression and sensitizes tumor cells to CD94/NKG2A-positive NK cells. *J Immunol* 187 (7):3546–54.

Francesconi, K. A. and F. Pannier. 2004. Selenium metabolites in urine: A critical overview of past work and current status. *Clin Chem* 50 (12):2240–53.

Gandhi, U. H., N. Kaushal, K. C. Ravindra, et al. 2011. Selenoprotein-dependent up-regulation of hematopoietic prostaglandin D2 synthase in macrophages is mediated through the activation of peroxisome proliferator-activated receptor (PPAR) gamma. *J Biol Chem* 286 (31):27471–82.

Ge, K., A. Xue, J. Bai, et al. 1983. Keshan disease-an endemic cardiomyopathy in China. *Virchows Arch A Pathol Anat Histopathol* 401 (1):1–15.

Gladyshev, V. N., T. C. Stadtman, D. L. Hatfield, et al. 1999. Levels of major selenoproteins in T cells decrease during HIV infection and low molecular mass selenium compounds increase. *Proc Natl Acad Sci U S A* 96 (3):835–9.

Gonzalez-Flores, J. N., S. P. Shetty, A. Dubey, et al. 2013. The molecular biology of selenocysteine. *Biomol Concepts* 4 (4):349–65.

Guo, C. H., P. J. Liu, S. Hsia, et al. 2011. Role of certain trace minerals in oxidative stress, inflammation, CD4/CD8 lymphocyte ratios and lung function in asthmatic patients. *Ann Clin Biochem* 48 (Pt 4):344–51.

Guo, C. H., P. J. Liu, K. P. Lin, et al. 2012. Nutritional supplement therapy improves oxidative stress, immune response, pulmonary function, and quality of life in allergic asthma patients: An open-label pilot study. *Altern Med Rev* 17 (1):42–56.

Hagemann-Jensen, M., F. Uhlenbrock, S. Kehlet, et al. 2014. The selenium metabolite methylselenol regulates the expression of ligands that trigger immune activation through the lymphocyte receptor NKG2D. *J Biol Chem* 289 (45):31576–90.

Hawkes, W. C., D. S. Kelley, and P. C. Taylor. 2001. The effects of dietary selenium on the immune system in healthy men. *Biol Trace Elem Res* 81 (3):189–213.

Hileman, C. O., S. Dirajlal-Fargo, S. K. Lam, et al. 2015. Plasma selenium concentrations are sufficient and associated with protease inhibitor use in treated HIV-infected adults. *J Nutr* 145:2293–9.

Hoffmann, P. R. 2012. Asthma in children and nutritional selenium get another look. *Clin Exp Allergy* 42 (4):488–9.

Hoffmann, P. R. and M. J. Berry. 2008. The influence of selenium on immune responses. *Mol Nutr Food Res* 52 (11):1273–80.

Hoffmann, F. W., A. C. Hashimoto, L. A. Shafer, et al. 2010. Dietary selenium modulates activation and differentiation of CD4+ T cells in mice through a mechanism involving cellular free thiols. *J Nutr* 140 (6):1155–61.

Hoffmann, P. R., C. Jourdan-Le Saux, F. W. Hoffmann, et al. 2007. A role for dietary selenium and selenoproteins in allergic airway inflammation. *J Immunol* 179 (5):3258–67.

Huang, Z., A. H. Rose, and P. R. Hoffmann. 2012. The role of selenium in inflammation and immunity: From molecular mechanisms to therapeutic opportunities. *Antioxid Redox Signal* 16 (7):705–43.

Hunter, D. J., J. S. Morris, C. G. Chute, et al. 1990. Predictors of selenium concentration in human toenails. *Am J Epidemiol* 132 (1):114–22.

Hurst, R., C. N. Armah, J. R. Dainty, et al. 2010. Establishing optimal selenium status: Results of a randomized, double-blind, placebo-controlled trial. *Am J Clin Nutr* 91 (4):923–31.

Ip, C. 1998. Lessons from basic research in selenium and cancer prevention. *J Nutr* 128 (11):1845–54.

Ip, C., H. J. Thompson, Z. Zhu, and H. E. Ganther. 2000. In vitro and in vivo studies of methylseleninic acid: Evidence that a monomethylated selenium metabolite is critical for cancer chemoprevention. *Cancer Res* 60 (11):2882–6.

Jager, T., H. Drexler, and T. Goen. 2016. Human metabolism and renal excretion of selenium compounds after oral ingestion of sodium selenite and selenized yeast dependent on the trimethylselenium ion (TMSe) status. *Arch Toxicol* 90:1069.

Kamwesiga, J., V. Mutabazi, J. Kayumba, et al. 2011. Effect of selenium supplementation on CD4 T-cell recovery, viral suppression, morbidity and quality of life of HIV-infected patients in Rwanda: Study protocol for a randomized controlled trial. *Trials* 12:192.

Kassu, A., T. Yabutani, Z. H. Mahmud, et al. 2006. Alterations in serum levels of trace elements in tuberculosis and HIV infections. *Eur J Clin Nutr* 60 (5):580–6.

Kaushal, N., A. K. Kudva, A. D. Patterson, et al. 2014. Crucial role of macrophage selenoproteins in experimental colitis. *J Immunol* 193 (7):3683–92.

Kawai, K., S. N. Meydani, W. Urassa, et al. 2014. Micronutrient supplementation and T cell-mediated immune responses in patients with tuberculosis in Tanzania. *Epidemiol Infect* 142 (7):1505–9.

Kiremidjian-Schumacher, L. and M. Roy. 2001. Effect of selenium on the immunocompetence of patients with head and neck cancer and on adoptive immunotherapy of early and established lesions. *Biofactors* 14 (1–4):161–8.

Klein, E. A., I. M. Thompson, Jr., C. M. Tangen, et al. 2011. Vitamin E and the risk of prostate cancer: The Selenium and Vitamin E Cancer Prevention Trial (SELECT). *JAMA* 306 (14):1549–56.

Krehl, S., M. Loewinger, S. Florian, et al. 2012. Glutathione peroxidase-2 and selenium decreased inflammation and tumors in a mouse model of inflammation-associated carcinogenesis whereas sulforaphane effects differed with selenium supply. *Carcinogenesis* 33 (3):620–8.

Kryukov, G. V., S. Castellano, S. V. Novoselov, et al. 2003. Characterization of mammalian selenoproteomes. *Science* 300 (5624):1439–43.

Kudva, A. K., A. E. Shay, and K. S. Prabhu. 2015. Selenium and inflammatory bowel disease. *Am J Physiol Gastrointest Liver Physiol* 309 (2):G71–7.

Labunskyy, V. M., D. L. Hatfield, and V. N. Gladyshev. 2014. Selenoproteins: Molecular pathways and physiological roles. *Physiol Rev* 94 (3):739–77.

Lee, S., I. Takahashi, M. Matsuzaka, et al. 2011. The relationship between serum selenium concentration and neutrophil function in peripheral blood. *Biol Trace Elem Res* 144 (1–3):396–406.

Li, S., F. Bian, L. Yue, et al. 2014. Selenium-dependent antitumor immunomodulating activity of polysaccharides from roots of A. membranaceus. *Int J Biol Macromol* 69:64–72.

Lippman, S. M., E. A. Klein, P. J. Goodman, et al. 2009. Effect of selenium and vitamin E on risk of prostate cancer and other cancers: The Selenium and Vitamin E Cancer Prevention Trial (SELECT). *JAMA* 301 (1):39–51.

Matsue, H., D. Edelbaum, D. Shalhevet, et al. 2003. Generation and function of reactive oxygen species in dendritic cells during antigen presentation. *J Immunol* 171 (6):3010–8.

Muth, O. H., J. E. Oldfield, L. F. Remmert, et al. 1958. Effects of selenium and vitamin E on white muscle disease. *Science* 128 (3331):1090.

Nagy, D. T., B. Fulesdi, and J. Hallay. 2013. The relationship between selenium and gastrointestinal inflammatory diseases. *Orv Hetil* 154 (41):1636–40.

Narayan, V., K. C. Ravindra, C. Liao et al. 2015. Epigenetic regulation of inflammatory gene expression in macrophages by selenium. *J Nutr Biochem* 26 (2):138–45.

National Institutes of Health. *Selenium, Dietary Supplement Fact Sheet.* Office of Dietary Supplements 2013. Available from https://ods.od.nih.gov/factsheets/Selenium-HealthProfessional/#h3.

Navarro-Alarcon, M. and C. Cabrera-Vique. 2008. Selenium in food and the human body: A review. *Sci Total Environ* 400 (1–3):115–41.

Nelson, S. M., X. Lei, and K. S. Prabhu. 2011. Selenium levels affect the IL-4-induced expression of alternative activation markers in murine macrophages. *J Nutr* 141 (9):1754–61.

Norton, R. L. and P. R. Hoffmann. 2012. Selenium and asthma. *Mol Aspects Med* 33 (1):98–106.

Nunnari, G., C. Coco, M. R. Pinzone, et al. 2012. The role of micronutrients in the diet of HIV-1-infected individuals. *Front Biosci (Elite Ed)* 4:2442–56.

Oldfield, J.E. 2006. Selenium: A historical perspective. In *Selenium: Its Molecular Biology and Role in Human Health*, edited by D. L. Hatfield, M. J. Berry, and V. N. Gladyshev. New York, NY: Springer Science+Business Media.

Patterson, E. L., R. Milstrey, and E. L. Stokstad. 1957. Effect of selenium in preventing exudative diathesis in chicks. *Proc Soc Exp Biol Med* 95 (4):617–20.

Prabhu, K. S., F. Zamamiri-Davis, J. B. Stewart, et al. 2002. Selenium deficiency increases the expression of inducible nitric oxide synthase in RAW 264.7 macrophages: Role of nuclear factor-kappaB in up-regulation. *Biochem J* 366 (Pt 1):203–9.

Reeves, M. A. and P. R. Hoffmann. 2009. The human selenoproteome: Recent insights into functions and regulation. *Cell Mol Life Sci* 66 (15):2457–78.

Rose, A. H., P. Bertino, F. W. Hoffmann, et al. 2014. Increasing dietary selenium elevates reducing capacity and ERK activation associated with accelerated progression of select mesothelioma tumors. *Am J Pathol* 184 (4):1041–9.

Safaralizadeh, R., M. Nourizadeh, A. Zare, et al. 2013. Influence of selenium on mast cell mediator release. *Biol Trace Elem Res* 154 (2):299–303.

Safir, N., A. Wendel, R. Saile, et al. 2003. The effect of selenium on immune functions of J774.1 cells. *Clin Chem Lab Med* 41 (8):1005–11.

Salimian, J., M. A. Arefpour, M. Riazipour, et al. 2014. Immunomodulatory effects of selenium and vitamin E on alterations in T lymphocyte subsets induced by T-2 toxin. *Immunopharmacol Immunotoxicol* 36 (4):275–81.

Schwarz, K. and C.M. Foltz. 1957. Selenium as an integral part of factor 3 against dietary necrotic liver degeneration. *J Am Chem Soc* 78:3292–3293.

Shrimali, R. K., R. D. Irons, B. A. Carlson, et al. 2008. Selenoproteins mediate T cell immunity through an antioxidant mechanism. *J Biol Chem* 283 (29):20181–5.

Smith, A. D., L. Cheung, E. Beshah, et al. 2013. Selenium status alters the immune response and expulsion of adult Heligmosomoides bakeri worms in mice. *Infect Immun* 81 (7):2546–53.

Squires, J. E. and M. J. Berry. 2008. Eukaryotic selenoprotein synthesis: Mechanistic insight incorporating new factors and new functions for old factors. *IUBMB Life* 60 (4):232–5.

Steinbrenner, H., S. Al-Quraishy, M. A. Dkhil, et al. 2015. Dietary selenium in adjuvant therapy of viral and bacterial infections. *Adv Nutr* 6 (1):73–82.

Suzuki, K. T., Y. Tsuji, Y. Ohta, et al. 2008. Preferential organ distribution of methylselenol source Se-methylselenocysteine relative to methylseleninic acid. *Toxicol Appl Pharmacol* 227 (1):76–83.

Villamor, E., F. Mugusi, W. Urassa, et al. 2008. A trial of the effect of micronutrient supplementation on treatment outcome, T cell counts, morbidity, and mortality in adults with pulmonary tuberculosis. *J Infect Dis* 197 (11):1499–505.

Vinceti, M., E. T. Wei, C. Malagoli, et al. 2001. Adverse health effects of selenium in humans. *Rev Environ Health* 16 (4):233–51.

Wang, C., H. Wang, J. Luo, et al. 2009. Selenium deficiency impairs host innate immune response and induces susceptibility to Listeria monocytogenes infection. *BMC Immunol* 10:55.

Xia, Y., K. E. Hill, P. Li, et al. 2010. Optimization of selenoprotein P and other plasma selenium biomarkers for the assessment of the selenium nutritional requirement: A placebo-controlled, double-blind study of selenomethionine supplementation in selenium-deficient Chinese subjects. *Am J Clin Nutr* 92 (3):525–31.

Yan, L., J. A. Yee, D. Li, et al. 1999. Dietary supplementation of selenomethionine reduces metastasis of melanoma cells in mice. *Anticancer Res* 19 (2A):1337–42.

Yang, J., K. Huang, S. Qin, et al. 2009. Antibacterial action of selenium-enriched probiotics against pathogenic Escherichia coli. *Dig Dis Sci* 54 (2):246–54.

Yao, Y., F. Pei, and P. Kang. 2011. Selenium, iodine, and the relation with Kashin-Beck disease. *Nutrition* 27 (11–12):1095–100.

Yin, Y., R. R. Wang, Y. Wang, et al. 2014. Preparation of selenium-enriched Bifidobacterium longum and its effect on tumor growth and immune function of tumor-bearing mice. *Asian Pac J Cancer Prev* 15 (8):3681–6.

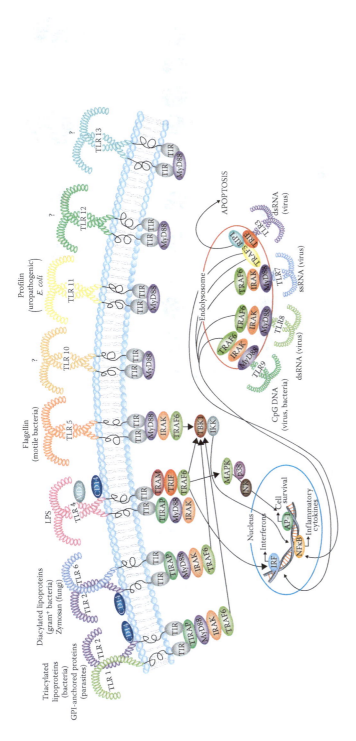

FIGURE 1.1 Toll-like receptor (TLR) signaling. Individual TLRs initiate overlapping and distinct signaling pathways in various cell types such as macrophages, dendritic cells, and inflammatory monocytes. Engagement of TLRs with their ligands induces conformational changes of TLRs that lead to recruitment of adaptor proteins such as MyD88, TIRAP, TRIF, TRAF, and TRAM. TLR4, TLR5, TLR10, TLR11, TLR12, and TR13 exist as surface-bound homodimers, while TLR2 can form surface-bound heterodimers with TLR1 or TLR6. TLR3, TLR7, TLR8, and TLR9 are homodimers bound to the endolysosome membrane. All TLRs are capable of activating nuclear factor kappa B (NFκB) and inducing inflammatory cytokine production. Some TLRs also signal to promote production of type-1 interferon (interferon-α). Reproduced with permission from Cayman Chemical Company.

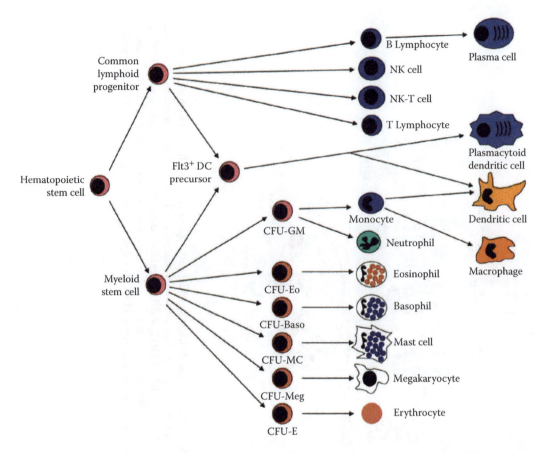

FIGURE 1.2 Hematopoietic stem cell-derived lineages. Pluripotent hematopoietic stem cells differentiate in bone marrow into common lymphoid progenitor cells or myeloid stem cells. Lymphoid stem cells give rise to B-cell, T-cell, and natural killer (NK) cell lineages. Myeloid stem cells give rise to a second level of lineage-specific colony-forming unit (CFU) cells that go on to produce neutrophils and monocytes (granulocyte macrophage [GM]), eosinophils (Eo), basophils (Baso), mast cells (MC), megakaryocytes (Meg), and erythrocytes (E). Monocytes differentiate further into macrophages in peripheral tissue compartments. Dendritic cells (DC) appear to develop primarily from a dendritic cell precursor that is distinguished by its expression of the Fms-like tyrosine kinase 3 (Flt3) receptor. This precursor can derive from either lymphoid or myeloid stem cells, and gives rise to both classical and plasmacytoid dendritic cells. Classical dendritic cells can also derive from differentiation of monocytoid precursor cells. (Reprinted from *J. Allergy Clin. Immunol.*, 125, Chaplin, D. D. (2010) Overview of the immune response, S3–S23, with permission from Elsevier.)

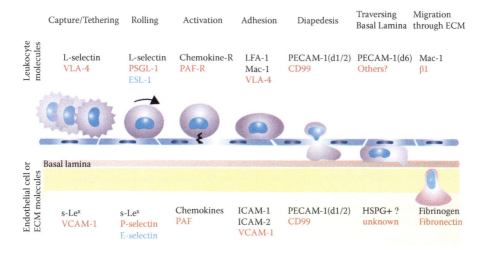

FIGURE 1.3   Leukocyte–endothelial cell interactions. Leukocyte recruitment is a multistep process involving initial attachment and rolling, tight binding, and transmigration across the vascular endothelium. Steps in leukocyte emigration are controlled by specific adhesion molecules on leukocytes and endothelial cells (see Table 1.3). The various steps of leukocyte emigration are depicted schematically here; interacting pairs of molecules are shown in the same color. The activated endothelium expresses selectins, which when binding to leukocytes initiate a rolling adhesion of leukocytes to the vessel's luminal wall. Integrins become activated by chemokines and bind to endothelial intercellular adhesion molecules (ICAMs) and vascular cell adhesion molecules (VCAMs), permitting a firmer adhesion. Transmigration across the vascular endothelium may be guided by further adhesive interactions, perhaps involving molecules such as platelet-endothelial cell adhesion molecule (PECAM)-1, which endothelial cells express at intercellular junctions. ESL, E-selectin ligand; HSPG, heparin sulfate proteoglycan; LFA, leukocyte function-associated antigen; PAF, platelet activating factor; PECAM-1 (d1/2), interaction involves immunoglobulin domains 1 and/or 2 of PECAM-1; PECAM-1 (d6), interaction involves immunoglobulin domain 6 of PECAM-1; PSGL, P-selectin glycoprotein ligand; s-Lex, sialyl-Lewisx carbohydrate antigen; VLA, very late (activation) antigen. (Reprinted with permission from Macmillan Publishers Ltd: Laboratory Investigation Muller, W. A. (2002) Leukocyte-endothelial cell interactions in the inflammatory response, 82, 521–533.)

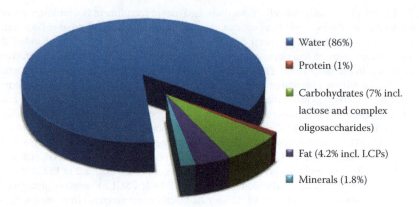

FIGURE 9.1 Summary of the composition of human milk.

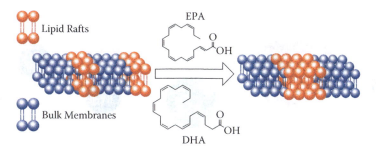

FIGURE 17.2 Phospholipid-membrane effects of n-3 PUFA. When highly unsaturated EPA and DHA incorporate into plasma membrane phospholipids, they modify the lateral organization of the lipid bilayer. This results in an alteration in the size/stability of lipid rafts in the plasma membrane, perturbing membrane-regulated signal transduction.

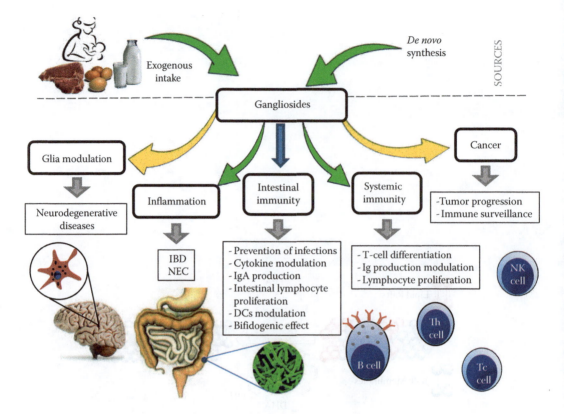

FIGURE 24.1 Summary of the roles of gangliosides related to immune function and inflammation. Gangliosides can derive from *de novo* synthesis or exogenous intake from the diet. Gangliosides are important components of lipid rafts, which account for a wide range of biological functions; they are involved in glia modulation, inflammation, intestinal immunity, microbiota regulation, systemic immunity, and cancer.

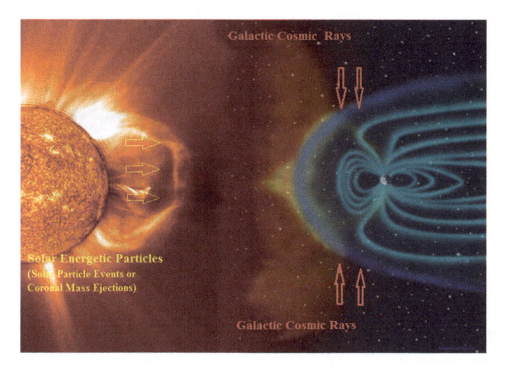

FIGURE 26.1 The interplanetary space environment showing the toxic combination of galactic cosmic radiation (GCR) and (largely) proton radiation due to solar particle events (SPEs). Figure courtesy of NASA/JPL-Caltech.

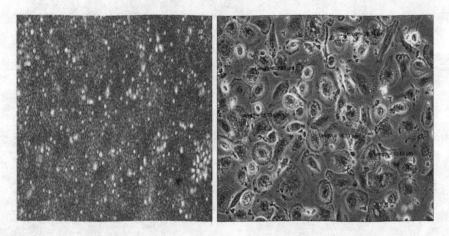

FIGURE 26.2 Representative image of AHCC-treated lymphocytes. Cells were treated with 50 μg/mL AHCC and are shown at 20 × magnification. Note the morphological changes of lymphocytes from 96 hours to 360 hours posttreatment with AHCC. Cells become adherent and phenotypic changes were observed.

15 Zinc Regulation of the Immune Response

Veronika Kloubert and Lothar Rink

CONTENTS

15.1 Introduction...245
15.2 Zinc Homeostasis..246
    15.2.1 Overview of Zinc Homeostasis...246
    15.2.2 Zinc Regulation by Transporters and Intracellular Proteins 247
15.3 Zinc Deficiency...253
15.4 Nutritional Aspects of Zinc..254
    15.4.1 General Considerations 254
    15.4.2 Assessment of Zinc Status...255
    15.4.3 Investigation of Intracellular Zinc Pools 255
15.5 Effects of Zinc on Immune Function 255
    15.5.1 Zinc and Innate Immunity...255
        15.5.1.1 Granulocytes..255
        15.5.1.2 Monocytes/Macrophages...256
        15.5.1.3 Dendritic Cells..259
        15.5.1.4 Natural Killer Cells...259
    15.5.2 Zinc and Adaptive Immunity...260
        15.5.2.1 B-Cells..260
        15.5.2.2 T-Cells...260
15.6 Zinc and Allergy, Autoimmunity, Infections, and Neoplasia.........................265
    15.6.1 Zinc and Allergies 265
    15.6.2 Zinc and Autoimmune Diseases 265
    15.6.3 Zinc and Infectious Disease...267
        15.6.3.1 Zinc and Diarrhea...267
        15.6.3.2 Zinc and HIV Infection 267
        15.6.3.3 Zinc and Malaria...267
        15.6.3.4 Zinc and the Common Cold 268
    15.6.4 Zinc and Neoplasia 268
        15.6.4.1 Zinc and Breast Cancer 268
        15.6.4.2 Zinc and Prostate Cancer..269
        15.6.4.3 Zinc and p53 269
References..269

15.1 INTRODUCTION

In 1869 Raulin was the first to describe the need of zinc in biological systems, namely in studying the growth of *Aspergillus niger* (Raulin 1869). The essentiality of zinc for animals was described for the first time several decades later in 1934 by Todd and his group (Todd, Evelym, and Hart 1934). It was not until the 1960s that zinc deficiency was observed in humans by Ananda Prasad. He described a zinc deficiency syndrome in Iranian and Egyptian subjects who were extremely susceptible to bacterial, fungal, and parasitic infections. More precisely, they suffered from anemia, skin alterations, hypogonadism, hepatosplenomegaly, and mental retardation (Prasad et al. 1963; Prasad 1991). It was possible to completely reverse all symptoms by supplementation with high doses of zinc, leading to the assumption that the symptoms were a result of zinc deficiency. Only anemia was shown to be due to iron deficiency and reversed by iron supplementation (Prasad 1991). Impaired zinc absorption due to phytates, which are present in cereal grains, was observed by O'Dell and Savage (1960). This may be relevant to the apparent zinc deficiency in the Iranian and Egyptian subjects studied by Prasad, since their diet comprised largely plant-based foods without any meat (O'Dell and Savage 1960). Another cause promoting zinc deficiency was the practice of geophagia, driven by a lack of food (Prasad et al. 1963).

One inherited disease related to malabsorption of zinc is called acrodermatitis enteropathica (AE), which is mostly based on a mutation in the gene encoding for the zinc transporter Zip4. AE is a rare, autosomal recessively inherited disease. Affected patients suffer from symptoms of zinc deficiency, including severe dermatitis, immune dysfunction, diarrhea, growth retardation, alopecia, and, occasionally, mental retardation (Wang et al. 2002).

Reversion of AE symptoms in infants is achieved after high-dose zinc supplementation. Thus, other transporters than Zip4 seem to be present, and these allow zinc uptake by enterocytes (Eide 2006).

Zinc is essential for the growth and development of all organisms; it is important for the function of more than 300 enzymes, covering all enzyme classes. Apart from this, zinc is involved in essential cellular functions, comprising DNA and RNA synthesis, proliferation, and apoptosis. Since the immune system has one of the highest requirements for proliferation in the human body and also has a high capacity for biosynthesis, zinc deficiency is readily seen to cause impaired immune functions, leading to suppressed cell proliferation and differentiation (Rink and Gabriel 2000) and increased susceptibility to infection. However, zinc also has specific effects on the immune function besides those general effects on cell physiology, which will be discussed in detail below.

15.2   ZINC HOMEOSTASIS

15.2.1   OVERVIEW OF ZINC HOMEOSTASIS

The essentiality of zinc for the function of more than 300 enzymes emphasizes the importance of this trace element in signaling cascades. Moreover, it is essential for different basic cellular functions (e.g. participation in cell division, DNA and RNA synthesis, and apoptosis) (Vallee and Falchuk 1993). Thus, the importance of zinc for highly proliferating organ systems, such as the already mentioned immune system, can be readily assumed.

Zinc is widespread throughout the body, but the highest amounts, in terms of the percentage of whole body zinc, are in the liver, skin, skeletal muscle, and bones (Favier and Favier 1990; Mills 1989). The total amount of zinc in the human body is 2–4 g and the plasma or serum concentration is 12–16 µM (Rink and Gabriel 2000). The serum zinc pool is small but mobile and thus important for the distribution of zinc in the body. Within the serum, zinc is predominantly bound with a low affinity to albumin (60%), and with a high affinity to α_2-macroglobulin (30%) and to transferrin (10%) (Scott and Bradwell 1983). Since there is no existing storage system for zinc in the human body, as for example for iron, a steady state of zinc intake and excretion is necessary. The recommendations for daily zinc intake vary between different countries. The recommended zinc intake given by the German Society of Nutrition is 10 mg/d for adult males and 7 mg/d for adult females (Deutsche Gesellschaft für Ernährung [DGE] 2015). However, the recommended zinc intake given by the U.S. Food and Nutrition Board varies slightly from that of the DGE; it is 11 mg/d for adult males and 8 mg/d for adult females (Food and Nutrition Board 2001).

Different sites of homeostatic regulation of zinc were identified by examining the effects of oral zinc intake. Namely, homeostatic regulation was detected in gastrointestinal absorption and secretion, renal excretion, release from muscles, and exchange with erythrocytes (Hotz et al. 2003).

15.2.2 ZINC REGULATION BY TRANSPORTERS AND INTRACELLULAR PROTEINS

To maintain zinc homeostasis and to prevent cellular overaccumulation of zinc accompanied by toxic effects, regulatory mechanisms are of high importance (Eide 2006). Neurons, prostate cells, and cells of the eye, especially choroid and retina cells, accumulate higher levels of zinc than cells of other tissues, suggesting specialized functions of zinc within different cell types (Frederickson et al. 2000; Costello and Franklin 1998; Karcioglu 1982). Another example of zinc regulation is the transport of zinc into enterocytes of the mammalian intestine. Here, zinc transporters are responsible for the uptake of zinc from the intestinal lumen and the following efflux across the basolateral membrane into the portal blood, emphasizing again the need of tight regulatory mechanisms in the distribution of zinc (Gaither and Eide 2001a).

Because zinc is a charged divalent cation, passive diffusion across membranes is not possible. Thus, special transport mechanisms are required for zinc transport into and out of the cytosol ensuring tight control of zinc levels. Two families of zinc transporters are identified in mammals, comprising the Zip- (Zrt-, Irt-like protein)/SLC39A- (solute carrier family 39) family and the ZnT- (zinc transporter)/SLC30A-family (Figure 15.1). The latter is also described as a cation diffusion facilitator (CDF). Both families of zinc transporter are found at all phylogenetic levels, comprising bacteria, fungi, plants, and mammals (Nies and Silver 1995; Gaither and Eide 2001a). Zip transporters perform zinc transport out from organelles and the extracellular space into the cytosol, whereas the ZnT transporters are responsible for zinc transport from the cytosol into the extracellular space or into the lumen of intracellular organelles (Eide 2006). So far, 14 Zip transporters and 10 ZnT transporters encoded by the human genome have been identified (Jeong and Eide 2013; Lichten and Cousins 2009). An overview of ZnT and Zip transporter functions and localization is presented in Tables 15.1 and 15.2, respectively.

One example of a Zip transporter is Zip1, which is expressed ubiquitously in human tissues and localized to the plasma membrane in some cell types (Gaither and Eide 2001b). Interestingly, in zinc-deficient murine cells, Zip1 and Zip3 were found to migrate to the plasma membrane, whereas they associated within the membrane of intracellular compartments in zinc-repleted cells. Thus, posttranslational control of zinc transporters seems to be important in zinc homeostasis, as, for example, phosphorylation of the Zip7 transporter by protein kinase casein kinase (CK)2 leading to opening of the channel or homodimerization of ZnT8, which requires biological membranes for proper assembly (Wang et al. 2004; Taylor et al. 2012; Murgia et al. 2009).

Zip transporters are involved in immunologic functions. For example, Zip14 is involved in the uptake of zinc by hepatocytes during the acute-phase response, leading to the suggestion that Zip14 induction is a cause of serum hypozincemia linked to infection (Liuzzi et al. 2005).

The exact transport mechanism of eukaryotic Zip proteins remains to be solved. So far, it is known that zinc transporters are energy independent (i.e., they act without adenosine triphosphate [ATP] as a source of energy). In contrast, the yeast zinc transporters Zrt1 and Zrt2 seem to be energy dependent. It was shown that energy-independent zinc uptake by the human Zip2 transporter is possibly conducted by a Zn^{2+}-HCO_3- cotransport (Gaither and Eide 2000; Zhao and Eide 1996). Since concentrations of the intracellular labile zinc pool are in the nanomolar range, another possibility may be the transport is simply due to a concentration gradient (Gaither and Eide 2001a).

Concerning the ZnT transport mechanism, studies were first carried out with the prokaryotic homologue YiiP in *Eschericia coli*, catalyzing Zn^{2+}/H^+ antiport across the membrane (Lu and Fu 2007; Grass et al. 2005). Four amino acid residues were found to serve as potential zinc-binding sites in the mammalian zinc transporter ZnT5, based on x-ray structure analysis of YiiP. Indeed,

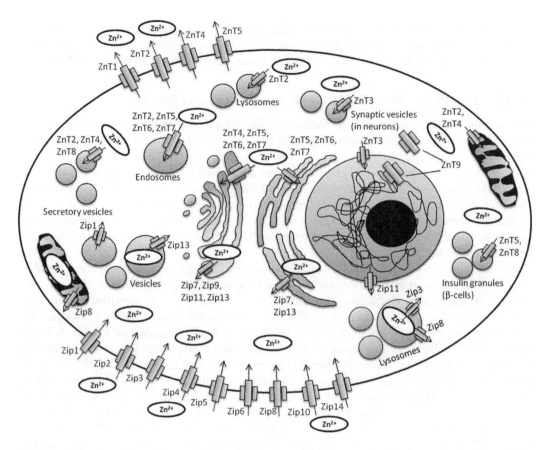

FIGURE 15.1 Overview of intracellular zinc transporter. In the upper half of the cell, the intracellular localization of a ZnT transporter is represented leading to reduction of cytosolic zinc. ZnT1 is ubiquitously expressed within the plasma membrane of mammalian cells, conducting zinc transport from the cytoplasm into the extracellular space. Apart from that, ZnT4 and isoforms of ZnT2 and ZnT5 are found within the plasma membrane. The majority of the ZnT transporter (ZnT2–ZnT8) is localized within membranes of different intracellular organelles, (i.e., in the membranes of endosomes, secretory vesicles, lysosomes, endoplasmic reticulum, mitochondria, and Golgi apparatus). ZnT9 is predominantly found in an unbound form within the cytoplasm and nucleus. The expression of ZnT3 was found in high amounts especially on mRNA levels in the brain. The indicated localization of ZnT4 within the membrane of mitochondria was only analyzed in rats so far. The lower half of the cell shows the intracellular localization of a Zip transporter resulting in increased cytosolic zinc. The majority of the Zip transporter (Zip1–6, Zip8, Zip10, Zip14) is localized within the plasma membrane, conducting zinc transport from the extracellular space into the cytoplasm. Apart from that, some Zip transporters manage zinc import out from intracellular organelles into the cytoplasm, such as Zip7 localized within the membrane of the endoplasmic reticulum and the Golgi apparatus. The indicated localization of Zip11 within the membrane of the nucleus was so far only investigated within mice and expression of Zip13 within the endoplasmic reticulum was found in rats so far.

replacement of the identified amino acid residues successfully blocked zinc transport. In conclusion, those results indicate a Zn^{2+}/H^+ antiport action of mammalian ZnT transporters, similar to the zinc transport system of the prokaryotic homologues (Ohana et al. 2009).

In addition to zinc transporters, other mechanisms exist to bind zinc and thus regulate over-accumulation of intracellular zinc. The metal regulatory transcription factor-1 (MTF-1) is a zinc finger protein, conserved from insects to mammals (Radtke et al. 1993). Increased cellular zinc concentrations can be sensed by MTF-1 followed by zinc-dependent gene induction, as, for example,

TABLE 15.1
Tissue Distribution, Subcellular Localization, and Characteristics of the ZnT Family of Zinc Exporters

Transporter	Tissue Distribution	Subcellular Localization	Characteristics	References
ZnT1	Ubiquitous, especially found in leukocytes	Plasma membrane	Zinc export into extracellular space; significantly increased in the brain of patients with Alzheimer's disease	Kolaj-Robin et al. (2015), Huang and Tepaamorndech (2013), Overbeck et al. (2008)
ZnT2	Mammary gland, pancreas, prostate, small intestine, and elsewhere	Endosomal/lysosomal/secretory vesicles, mitochondria, isoform found in plasma membrane	Enrichment of vesicular zinc; mutation in breast epithelial cells causes decreased zinc transport into breast milk of nursing women	Huang and Tepaamorndech (2013), Overbeck et al. (2008), Chowanadisai, Lonnerdal, and Kelleher (2006), Lee et al. (2015a)
ZnT3	Brain, leukocytes, pancreas, testis	Synaptic vesicles, nucleus of neurons (in mice and rats)	Zinc transport into synaptic vesicles of nerve cells; high amounts of mRNA found within mouse brain	Kolaj-Robin et al. (2015), Huang and Tepaamorndech (2013), Shen et al. (2007), Kodirov et al. (2006), Overbeck et al. (2008)
ZnT4	Brain, intestine, kidney, leukocytes, mammary gland	Mitochondria, plasma membrane, secretory vesicles, trans-Golgi network	Regulates milk zinc concentration in breast epithelium; *SLC30A4* mutation causes lethal milk in mice	Kolaj-Robin et al. (2015), Overbeck et al. (2008), Huang and Gitschier (1997), Sun et al. (2015)
ZnT5	Ubiquitous, especially found in leukocytes	Endoplasmic reticulum, Golgi apparatus, isoform found in plasma membrane, secretory granules of pancreatic β-cells	Involved in formation of zinc/insulin crystals; in the human colorectal adenocarcinoma cell line Caco-2 high zinc levels inhibit *SLC30A5* transcription and translation *in vitro*, whereas stability of *SLC30A5* mRNA is increased	Huang and Tepaamorndech (2013), Overbeck et al. (2008), Petkovic, Miletta, and Mullis (2012)
ZnT6	Brain, intestine, kidney, leukocytes, liver, lung	Endoplasmic reticulum, Golgi apparatus, vesicles	Elevated expression in Alzheimer's disease; RNA expression detected in the brain, intestine, kidney, and liver; protein expression in brain and lung	Overbeck et al. (2008), Petkovic, Miletta, and Mullis (2012), Dubben et al. (2010)
ZnT7	Intestine, leukocytes, pancreas, prostate, retina, testis, and elsewhere	Endoplasmic reticulum, Golgi apparatus, vesicles	Insulin gene expression up-regulated via transcription factor MTF-1 in mice	Huang and Tepaamorndech (2013), Overbeck et al. (2008)

(Continued)

TABLE 15.1 (*Continued*)

Tissue Distribution, Subcellular Localization, and Characteristics of the ZnT Family of Zinc Exporters

Transporter	Tissue Distribution	Subcellular Localization	Characteristics	References
ZnT8	Adrenal gland, leukocytes, liver, pancreas, pancreatic β-cells, testis, thyroid	Secretory vesicles	Involved in formation of zinc/insulin crystals; important for maturation and storage of insulin; major autoantigen in the development of autoimmunity in type I diabetes	Kolaj-Robin et al. (2015), Huang and Tepaamorndech (2013), Overbeck et al. (2008)
ZnT9	Kidney, leukocytes, pancreas, thymus, and elsewhere	Cytoplasm, nucleus	Functions as a transcriptional coactivator of nuclear receptors	Huang and Tepaamorndech (2013), Sim and Chow (1999), Overbeck et al. (2008)
ZnT10	Brain, liver, retina	Not described	No expression in PBMCs; ZnT10 expression at mRNA and protein levels is down-regulated after zinc supplementation; potentially higher affinity to manganese than to zinc; might be involved in Alzheimer's disease	Huang and Tepaamorndech (2013), Wex et al. (2014), Bosomworth et al. (2013)

TABLE 15.2

Tissue Distribution, Subcellular Localization, and Characteristics of the Zip Family of Zinc Importers

Transporter	Tissue Distribution	Subcellular Localization	Characteristics	References
Zip1	Ubiquitous, especially found in leukocytes	Plasma membrane, vesicles	Main zinc uptake transporter in K562 erythroleukemia and prostate cells; localized within membranes of intracellular organelles when cells are cultured in zinc-repleted media; translocated to cell surface when zinc is limited; probable key role in pregnancy; suppressed expression associated with prostate cancer	Jeong and Eide (2013), Kelleher et al. (2011), Haase et al. (2007), Andree et al. (2004)
Zip2	Cervix, epidermis, optic nerve, prostate, uterus	Plasma membrane	Suppressed expression associated with prostate cancer; potential key role during pregnancy; knockdown causes decreased intracellular zinc levels within keratinocytes, leading to inhibited differentiation	Jeong and Eide (2013), Kelleher et al. (2011), Inoue et al. (2014), Lichten and Cousins (2009)

(Continued)

TABLE 15.2 (*Continued*)

Tissue Distribution, Subcellular Localization, and Characteristics of the Zip Family of Zinc Importers

Transporter	Tissue Distribution	Subcellular Localization	Characteristics	References
Zip3	Leukocytes, mammary gland, prostate, testis	Lysosomes, plasma membrane	Probable key role during pregnancy; suppressed expression associated with prostate cancer	Jeong and Eide (2013), Kelleher et al. (2011), Lichten and Cousins (2009), Andree et al. (2004), Aydemir, Blanchard, and Cousins (2006)
Zip4	Colon, kidney, pancreatic β-cells, small intestine	Plasma membrane	Defect causes *acrodermatitis enteropathica*; zinc uptake from gut lumen; expression regulated by Klf-4; localized to apical membranes of enterocytes during zinc deficiency; zinc repletion causes mRNA degradation and rapid Zip4 endocytosis	Jeong and Eide (2013), Kelleher et al. (2011), Lichten and Cousins (2009)
Zip5	Colon, kidney, liver, pancreas, small intestine	Plasma membrane	Possibly unique role in polarized cells, sensing body zinc status by serosal-to-mucosal zinc transport; causes increased accumulation of endogenous zinc in enterocytes during high-zinc conditions, leading to clearance of excess systemic zinc through the intestine and intestinal lumen	Jeong and Eide (2013), Kelleher et al. (2011), Guthrie et al. (2015)
Zip6	Mammary gland, placenta, prostate, T-cells	Plasma membrane	Decreased expression in dendritic cells upon LPS stimulation, accompanied by reduced intracellular zinc levels; increased expression in breast cancer; reliable marker of oestrogen-receptor-positive cancers	Jeong and Eide (2013), Lichten and Cousins (2009), Taylor, Gee, and Kille (2011), Yu et al. (2011)
Zip7	Ubiquitous, especially in mammary gland	Endoplasmic reticulum, Golgi apparatus	Increased expression in breast cancer; increases intracellular zinc levels, resulting in growth and invasion which is a hallmark of the aggressive phenotype of tamoxifen resistant cells	Petkovic, Miletta, and Mullis (2012), Taylor et al. (2007)

(Continued)

TABLE 15.2 (*continued*)
Tissue Distribution, Subcellular Localization, and Characteristics of the Zip Family of Zinc Importers

Transporter	Tissue Distribution	Subcellular Localization	Characteristics	References
Zip8	Brain, kidney, leukocytes, liver, lung, mammary gland, small intestine, testis	Lysosomes, mitochondria, plasma membrane	Knockdown causes reduced IFN-γ and perforin secretion; transient overexpression leads to enhanced T-cell activation; decreases lysosomal labile zinc upon T-cell activation	Lichten and Cousins (2009), Aydemir et al. (2009), Besecker et al. (2008), Aydemir, Blanchard, and Cousins (2006)
Zip9	Breast cancer cells, prostate cancer cells	Golgi apparatus	Up-regulated in malignant breast and prostate cancers; functions as a membrane androgen receptor; mediates testosterone-induced apoptosis	Jeong and Eide (2013), Pascal and Wang (2014), Berg et al. (2014)
Zip10	Brain, liver, leukocytes (human B-cells and murine T-cells), mammary gland, pancreatic α-cells	Plasma membrane	Expression is suppressed by MTF-1; potential role in metastatic breast cancer progression; necessary for proper antibody responses upon BCR activation; important for mature B-cell maintenance and humoral immune responses	Jeong and Eide (2013), Kelleher et al. (2011), Lichten and Cousins (2009), Hojyo et al. (2014), Ryu et al. (2012), Daaboul et al. (2012)
Zip11	Lactating mammary gland	Golgi apparatus, nucleus of mice	Potential role in the transfer of zinc into milk	Kelleher et al. (2012), Martin et al. (2013)
Zip12	Brain, murine T-cells	Not described	Required for the development of the nervous system; possible participation in embryogenesis; mutation in the underlying gene might be related to schizophrenia development	Lichten and Cousins (2009), Chowanadisai (2014), Daaboul et al. (2012)
Zip13	Chondrocytes, fibroblasts, odontoblasts, osteoblasts	Endoplasmic reticulum of rats, Golgi apparatus, intracellular vesicles	Important for connective tissue development; mutation of *SLC39A13* causes spondylocheiro dysplastic Ehlers-Danlos syndrome (SCD-EDS)	Sun et al. (2015), Jeong and Eide (2013), Hirose et al. (2015)
Zip14	Liver, pancreatic α-cells	Plasma membrane	Increased expression in the liver after interleukin (IL)-6 stimulation; possibly related to hypozincemia in serum during acute-phase reaction, accompanied by elevated zinc levels within hepatocytes; potential role in maintaining intestinal barrier function for the gastrointestinal tract via stabilization of a tight junction protein	Kelleher et al. (2011), Guthrie et al. (2015), Liuzzi et al. (2005)

transcription of the metallothionein (MT) encoding gene (Gunther, Lindert, and Schaffner 2012). Zinc can be bound by cytoplasmic macromolecules (e.g., by MT or proteins of the S100 family, such as S100A8, S100A9, or S100A12, acting as zinc buffers) (Hamer 1986; Goyette and Geczy 2011). Characteristics of MTs comprise the low molecular weight of 6–7 kDa, the ability to complex metal ions, the high content of cysteine residues, and the involvement in a variety of cellular processes, such as metal detoxification and metal homeostasis. Up to seven zinc ions can be bound by MT, which are presented in the form of two clusters (Vallee and Falchuk 1993). Interestingly, the binding constants of MT vary among the bound zinc ions. Total zinc concentration in the cytoplasm of eukaryotic cells is relatively high, comprising a few hundred micromolar. However, the percentage in the "free" form finally depends on the zinc buffering capacity (Maret and Krezel 2007).

Circumstances such as oxidative stress or the presence of reactive compounds, such as electrophiles, are responsible for oxidizing or at least modifying the cysteine sulfur groups of MTs. This is essential for zinc ion release from MT and zinc buffering, leading to increased free zinc concentrations. The increased free zinc concentration thus leads to modified intracellular signaling at only picomolar concentrations (Maret and Krezel 2007). Therefore, MTs are redox-active proteins, whereas zinc itself is redox inert. Zinc ions are released when oxidants react with MT and the oxidized protein is formed.

The metal-free protein thionein is supposed to be the biologically active form of MT. A variety of signals induce thionein synthesis *in vivo*, including cytokines and phorbol esters. MT-bound zinc ions are not trapped in an inflexible conformation. In fact, metal transfer exists due to metal exchange within each MT cluster. Moreover, cluster-bound metals can exchange with metals in solution or with metals in different MT proteins. For instance, the transport of metals from MT to thymulin or glutathione has been described (Vallee and Falchuk 1993). To sum up, MT proteins are able to bind or release zinc into the cytoplasm depending on their redox status.

15.3 ZINC DEFICIENCY

Different forms of zinc deficiency have to be distinguished (i.e., marginal zinc deficiency and severe zinc deficiency). Subjects with marginal zinc deficiency show impaired memory, smell, and taste; depressed immunity; onset of night blindness; and, in males, reduced spermatogenesis (Shankar and Prasad 1998). Zinc deficiency has a higher prevalence in areas with low animal food intake, but high cereal consumption. The reason for this is not necessarily a low zinc content of food, but the reduced bioavailability, particularly due to phytates. Especially prone to zinc deficiencies are individuals in the growth phase (i.e., infants, children, and adolescents), as well as pregnant and lactating women (Roohani et al. 2013). Not all causes of zinc deficiency are due to malnutrition. Some rare forms are based on inherited disorders. Probably the most studied one is the already mentioned *Acrodermatitis enteropathica* with an incidence of 1 per 500,000 children (Maverakis et al. 2007). In Friesian calves, hereditary zinc deficiency (lethal trait A 46) was observed, caused by the failure to absorb zinc from the gastrointestinal tract. If these calves do not receive zinc supplements, it is likely that they will die due to increased infections (Bosma et al. 1988). In addition, a mutation affecting the zinc transporter ZnT2 was found, which in lactating women results in transient neonatal zinc deficiency (Chowanadisai, Lonnerdal, and Kelleher 2006). This mutation causes reduced zinc concentration in the breast milk and cannot be corrected in the mother. However, the mother herself does not suffer any symptoms, although she presents the genotype and with the phenotype of low milk zinc concentration. Symptoms are only seen in the breast-fed infant: growth retardation, skin alterations, and impaired immune function, which can be reversed by zinc supplements during the suckling period. Apart from that, a genetic defect was found in lethal milk mice to be due to disturbed zinc metabolism. A mutation in the *SLC30A4* gene causes premature translational termination and truncation of the ZnT4 transporter. This is accompanied by reduced zinc concentrations within the milk, resulting in neonatal zinc deficiency in pups nursed from affected mice. In contrast to transient neonatal zinc deficiency in humans where only the breastfed infant is affected, the lethal milk mice develop zinc deficiency with proceeding age (Chowanadisai, Lonnerdal, and Kelleher 2006).

Zinc deficiency is not only a major problem in the developing world, but also in the industrialized world, especially in the elderly: 60% of the elderly among the U.S. population were shown to be zinc deficient (Prasad et al. 1993; Briefel et al. 2000). Related to this zinc deficiency, an association to low-grade inflammation is observed in aging, and moderate zinc supplementation leads to a significant reduction of basal interleukin (IL)-6 release (Kahmann et al. 2008). Zinc deficiency was related to decreased IL-6 promotor methylation, causing an increase in IL-6 production, leading to enhanced inflammation which was observed in the context of aging in an animal and cell model (Wong, Rinaldi, and Ho 2015). An ongoing zinc supplementation study in elderly residents in nursing homes revealed an association between increased serum zinc concentration and an enhancement of T-cell function, mainly due to an increase in the number of T-cells (Barnett et al. 2016).

Apoptosis of cells is increased under conditions of zinc deficiency and conversely prevented by zinc treatment (Treves et al. 1994; Zalewski, Forbes, and Betts 1993). In particular, inhibition of apoptosis by zinc is achieved by inhibiting the activity of caspases (Stennicke and Salvesen 1997; Kown et al. 2000). Caspase-3 was shown to be directly inhibited by zinc binding (Maret et al. 1999). A short delay upon induction of zinc deficiency using N,N,N',N'-Tetrakis-(2-pyridyl-methyl)-ethylenediamine (TPEN) and an increase of caspase-3 activity was observed. The decline in zinc concentrations might favor formation of the active form of caspase-3 from procaspase-3 by removing the inhibitory acting zinc or alternatively by inactivating a zinc-dependent inhibitor. Apart from caspase-3, zinc was shown to inhibit caspase-6 and caspase-9 (Zalewski 2011; Truong-Tran et al. 2000). In a Mongolian gerbil model zinc supplements prevented cell death caused by an ischemic insult, probably due to an antiendonuclease activity of zinc (Matsushita et al. 1996).

15.4 NUTRITIONAL ASPECTS OF ZINC

15.4.1 GENERAL CONSIDERATIONS

Zinc absorption is generally based on the zinc content of the food and its bioavailability. The content of zinc within foods varies at least one order of magnitude. Overviews of the zinc content of different foods can be found elsewhere (U.S. Department of Agriculture 2011; Kloubert and Rink 2015). Worldwide, the major sources of zinc for most people are cereals and legumes (Maret and Sandstead 2006; Gibson 1994). In contrast, one of the richest sources of readily bioavailable zinc is meat, including red meat. Thus, unavailability or avoidance of certain foods increases the risk of zinc deficiency, as for example for people living in the developing world or for vegetarians. Moreover, the bioavailability of zinc is markedly influenced by other food constituents, such as phytates (Solomons et al. 1979). However, not all kinds of legumes seem to negatively influence zinc uptake. The soybean extract soyasaponin Bb was shown to increase the expression of the zinc importer Zip4, followed by increased intracellular zinc levels (Hashimoto et al. 2015). Besides phytates, calcium is able to inhibit zinc absorption and in the presence of phytates even augments inhibition of zinc absorption (Maret and Sandstead 2006). Another nutritional cause of decreased zinc absorption is use of high-dose iron supplements (Solomons 1986). The influence of iron on zinc absorption is discussed elsewhere (Fischer Walker et al. 2005; Lim et al. 2013). The form of zinc consumed is also important, especially from supplements. The highest absorption is achieved by amino acid–bound zinc, in particular zinc bound to aspartate, cysteine, histidine, and methionine. In contrast, bioavailability of zinc oxide is very low (Brieger and Rink 2010).

15.4.2   Assessment of Zinc Status

Correct assessment of zinc status to evaluate zinc deficiency is difficult since there is no exist-ing zinc storage system or an established biomarker. Zinc measurements lack both sensitivity and specificity since serum zinc levels are maintained at a stable and physiological level for some time, even with insufficient zinc intake. Thus, the search for a reliable indicator of zinc status represents an important issue. The quality of different zinc biomarkers was analyzed and discussed previously (Lowe, Fekete, and Decsi 2009). Although serum or plasma zinc concentration has limitations, as just described, it seems to be the most reliable biomarker for measuring zinc status at the moment. Besides serum/plasma zinc, urinary zinc excretion and hair zinc seem to be responsive to zinc supplementation. However, data are missing to evaluate responsiveness of those biomarkers to zinc depletion (Lowe, Fekete, and Decsi 2009).

A possibility to assess dietary zinc intake might be the use of a questionnaire as during the ZINCAGE study (Kanoni et al. 2010). A zinc score was calculated for every participant based on a food question-naire, taking the zinc content of the food, the quantity of the consumed food, and the frequency of food consumption into consideration. Interestingly, plasma zinc levels and zinc score were found to be posi-tively associated among the studied elderly individuals. This zinc score might serve as a suitable tool in the analysis of gene-nutrient and biochemical-nutrient interactions (Kanoni et al. 2010).

15.4.3   Investigation of Intracellular Zinc Pools

Zinc-responsive fluorophores (e.g., FluoZin-3 AM and Zinquin) were used in several studies to examine the distribution of intracellular labile zinc (Coyle et al. 1994; Gee et al. 2002). Thereby, it was shown that free zinc can be detected within vesicles in a variety of mammalian cell types. Those vesicles seem to serve as zinc storage vesicles, providing zinc to the cell under conditions of zinc deficiency, and were named "zincosomes" (Beyersmann and Haase 2001; Eide 2006). Another function of those zincosomes could be as a buffer system, thereby preventing toxicity due to excess zinc and releasing zinc after an appropriate stimulus, which induces zinc signals (Palmiter, Cole, and Findley 1996; Brieger, Rink, and Haase 2013).

15.5   EFFECTS OF ZINC ON IMMUNE FUNCTION

The immune system has a high proliferation rate, and, thus, impaired immune functions during zinc deficiency are readily seen, causing suppressed cell proliferation and differentiation (Rink and Gabriel 2000). The effects of zinc on immune functions are diverse and manifold. Zinc signals have been observed in different cell types of the innate immune system, comprising dendritic cells (DCs), mast cells, monocytes/macrophages, natural killer (NK) cells, as well as in the adaptive immune system, comprising T-cells and B-cells (Haase and Rink 2009; Kaltenberg et al. 2010). During the last years, a variety of studies carried out in humans and animals indicate suppressed immune responses as a result of zinc deficiency, accompanied by increased susceptibility to a mul-titude of infectious agents (Shankar and Prasad 1998).

15.5.1   Zinc and Innate Immunity

15.5.1.1   Granulocytes

Neutrophils are usually the first immune cells actively entering the site of infection; they do this by following a chemotactic gradient. Very high zinc concentrations of around 500 μM promote neutro-phil chemotaxis, whereas zinc deficiency reduces chemotaxis, resulting in fewer neutrophils at the site of infection (Ibs and Rink 2003; Hujanen, Seppa, and Virtanen 1995). Among the granulocytes, neu-trophils are phagocytically the most efficient (Cadman and Lawrence 2010). Neutrophil phagocytosis

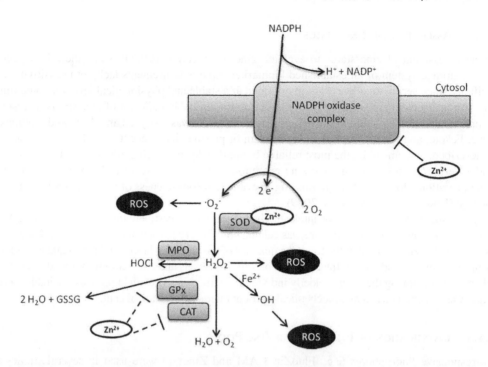

FIGURE 15.2 Zinc-affected ROS production. NADPH oxidase is localized within the membrane of pathogen engulfing vesicles in phagocytes. ROS comprise superoxide radicals (·O_2^-), hydroxyl radicals (·OH), and hydrogen peroxide (H_2O_2). Zinc is able to inhibit NADPH oxidase, which normally generates ·O_2^- from oxygen (O_2) and cytosolic NADPH. During the following downstream events ·O_2^- is dismutated by superoxide dismutase (SOD), using zinc as a cofactor which leads to H_2O_2 formation. In the presence of iron (Fe^{2+}), H_2O_2 is transformed into OH, into water and oxygen molecules by catalase (CAT), into hypochlorous acid (HOCl) by myeloperoxidase (MPO), or into water and glutathione disulfide (GSSG) by glutathione peroxidase (GPx), which can further react to glutathione. Zinc might cause decreased CAT and GPx activity. (Modified from Kloubert, V. and L. Rink, *Food Funct.*, 6, 3195–3204, 2015.)

uses so-called neutrophil extracellular traps (NETs). During NET formation, neutrophils release a matrix composed of DNA, chromatin, and granule molecules to capture extracellular pathogens prior to phagocytosing them. It was shown that phorbol-12-myristate-13-acetate (PMA) stimulation causes a zinc signal via protein kinase C (PKC) activation, resulting in NET formation. Consistent with a role for zinc in NET formation, zinc chelation inhibited NETosis. It is likely that NET formation is dependent on the production of reactive oxygen species (ROS) and zinc signals seem to be required for ROS-dependent signal transduction, finally leading to NET formation (Hasan, Rink, and Haase 2013). The heterodimeric antimicrobial peptide calprotectin is found in NETs and is assumed to exert its effect once being released from neutrophils (Djoko et al. 2015). Calprotectin can bind extracellular zinc and manganese, limiting their availability to microbes and so contributing positively to the battle between host and microbe (Crawford and Wilson 2015). Phagocytosed pathogens are killed by neutrophils due to production of ROS, such as the superoxide anion. The superoxide anion is produced by NADPH oxidase, which in turn can be inhibited by zinc (Figure 15.2) (Prasad 2014). The effect of this on bacterial killing is not clear. On balance, it appears that zinc is required for optimal neutrophil function and that zinc deficiency impairs neutrophil responses (Hasegawa et al. 2000).

15.5.1.2 Monocytes/Macrophages

Monocytes circulate within the blood, and migrate into tissues where they mature into different types of tissue-resident macrophages. Adherence to endothelial cells is the first step in this chemotactic process and zinc was shown to augment monocyte adhesion *in vitro*. Stimulation of monocytes with PMA or monocyte chemoattractant protein-1 (MCP-1) leads to the induction of intracellular zinc signals and thus promotes adhesion to endothelial cells (Kojima et al. 2007). In contrast, reduced extracellular zinc levels might serve as a signal to induce monocyte differentiation (Dubben et al. 2010). Elimination of bacterial pathogens by phagocytosis and oxidative burst was increased under conditions of zinc deficiency, whereas production of IL-6 and tumor necrosis factor (TNF)-α was decreased, suggesting a shift from intercellular communication to basic innate defensive functions (Mayer et al. 2014). The reduction in cytokine expression might be a result of short-term zinc deficiency, since under conditions of long-term zinc deficiency, cytokine expression is increased due to constitutive promoter activity regulated by redox and epigenetic mechanisms (Wessels et al. 2013). Nevertheless, intracellular zinc signals are needed to induce the synthesis of proinflammatory cytokines, such as IL-1β, IL-6, and TNF-α. Those cytokines are probably well induced in the presence of high extracellular zinc concentrations (Wellinghausen and Rink 1998; Wellinghausen, Kirchner, and Rink 1997). Influenced by the local cytokine and growth factor microenvironment, monocytes terminally differentiate to M1 or M2 macrophages after localization into the tissue. Individual structural contributions of different zinc-fingers to DNA-binding is linked to the function of regulatory proteins related to terminal monocyte differentiation. As an example, the mutant of the zinc-finger domain of Krüppel-like factor 4 (Klf-4), which lacks the DNA-binding domain, was able to induce cellular self-renewal and to inhibit maturation (Schuetz et al. 2011). Thus, zinc seems to play a role in monocyte differentiation.

Macrophages play an important role in regulating trace element availability to pathogens during infection (Haase and Rink 2014a). They are able to sequester certain trace elements causing "metal starvation" of pathogens; on the other hand, they can cause metal intoxication as a tool in host defense. One example is the infection of a host with the fungal pathogen *Histoplasma capsulatum*. Zinc was shown to be essential for the survival of the pathogen within granulocyte macrophage colony-stimulating factor (GM-CSF)-stimulated macrophages, whereas chelation of zinc-caused retardation of fungal growth. Different mechanisms within macrophages help to sequester zinc, thus making it inaccessible to the pathogen. Those mechanisms comprise the upregulation of the zinc exporters ZnT4 and ZnT7, shifting zinc ions into the Golgi apparatus, and MT upregulation, resulting in the protein binding of more intracellular zinc. In particular, it seems likely that GM-CSF–activated macrophages sequester free zinc accompanied by increased ROS production, which in turn causes pathogen clearance (Subramanian Vignesh et al. 2013).

Apart from that, zinc seems to affect the toll-like receptor (TLR) 4–induced cytokine secretion in monocytes (Figure 15.3). Monocytes, macrophages, and DCs carry TLR4, which can be activated by lipopolysaccharide (LPS). These cell populations are able to present antigens to T-cells after activation, thereby coordinating the immune response and linking innate and adaptive immunity. In particular, TLR4 signaling leads to production and secretion of proinflammatory cytokines (Haase and Rink 2009). Moderate zinc increase seems to be involved in TLR4 signal transduction at the level of downstream mitogen-activated protein kinases (MAPKs), whereas high concentrations of zinc are inhibitory (Haase et al. 2008). The inhibitory effect of elevated free zinc on TLR4 signaling is based on the modulation of cyclic nucleotide signals (Haase and Rink 2009). Cyclic adenosine monophosphate (cAMP) and cyclic guanosine monophosphate (cGMP) are synthesized by the adenylate cyclase (AC) or the guanylate cyclase (GC), respectively. Degradation of cAMP and cGMP is carried out by cyclic nucleotide phosphodiesterases (PDEs). Whereas low zinc concentrations are able to activate some PDE isoforms, high zinc concentrations inhibit PDEs, leading to reduced cyclic nucleotide degradation, therefore causing prolonged signaling (Francis et al. 1994). The anti-inflammatory effect of zinc can be explained by cross-activation of protein kinase A (PKA) as a result of elevated cAMP, which in turn is caused by zinc-induced inhibition of PDE. This is followed by phosphorylation of the inhibitory serine residue 259 of the Raf kinase, leading to Raf inactivation. Inhibition of the PKA/Raf pathway causes suppressed "nuclear factor 'kappa-light-chain-enhancer' of activated B-cells" (NF-κB) formation, accompanied by suppressed proinflammatory cytokine

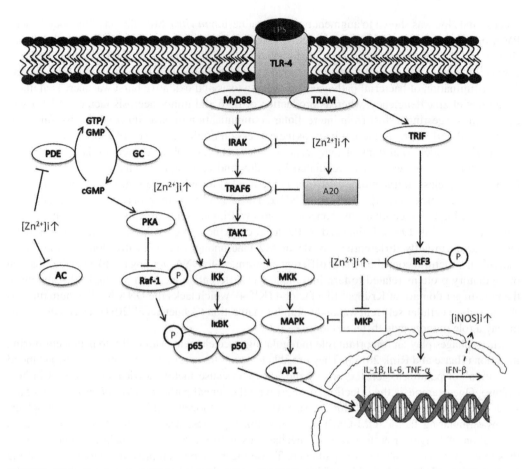

FIGURE 15.3 Involvement of zinc in LPS-induced TLR-4 signaling. Lipopolysaccharide (LPS)-induced toll-like receptor (TLR)-4 signaling initiates a cascade of signaling molecules, which are affected by zinc on different levels. High concentrations of zinc inhibit interleukin-1 receptor-associated kinase (IRAK), and zinc induces A20 upregulation thereby negatively affecting tumor necrosis factor receptor–associated factor 6 (TRAF6). Inhibition of phosphodiesterase (PDE) by zinc causes elevated cGMP levels accompanied by protein kinase A (PKA) cross-activation, which in turn inhibits Raf and subsequently nuclear factor kappa B (NF-κB) activation, represented in its subunits p65 and p50. In contrast, zinc signals are essential for mitogen-activated protein kinases (MAPK), which are not dephosphorylated due to inhibition of MAPK phosphatases (MKP) by zinc. This is followed by induction of proinflammatory cytokine expression. Another zinc affected pathway is the Toll/IL-1R domain-containing adaptor inducing IFN-β (TRIF) pathway where zinc inhibits IFN regulatory factor 3 (IRF3) dephosphorylation. Thereby expression of IFN-β is increased, which in turn is able to induce inducible nitric monoxide synthase (iNOS) via type I IFNR activation. (Modified from Haase, H. and L. Rink, *Annu Rev Nutr.*, 29, 133–152, 2009.) AC, adenylate cyclase; AP1, activator protein 1; GC, guanylate cyclase; cGMP, cyclic guanosine monophosphate; GTP, guanosine trisphosphate; IKK, I kappa B kinase; TAK1, transforming growth factor beta-activated kinase 1.

production (von Bulow et al. 2007). Apart from zinc induced PDE inhibition, AC is also negatively affected by zinc. The conformation of AC seems to be sensitive to zinc and this might change its enzymatic activity (Haase and Rink 2009).

MAPKs are responsible for the transduction of extracellular signals from cytokines, growth factors, hormones, and environmental stress, thereby regulating a variety of cellular responses including differentiation, proliferation, and apoptosis (Junttila, Li, and Westermarck 2008). The activation of MAPKs, such as the extracellular signal-related kinase (ERK), p38, MEK1/2, and Jun N-terminal kinase (JNK), by zinc is a common event in several cell types (Haase and Rink 2009). Moreover, regulation of kinase activation by zinc seems to be concentration-dependent, as for the kinase ERK. Dephosphorylation of ERK was shown to be inhibited by zinc in monocytes (Haase et al. 2008). However, MAPKs seem not always to serve as direct zinc targets, but rather might be activated indirectly by MAP-kinase phosphatases (MKPs). MKPs are responsible for dephosphorylation of threonine and tyrosine residues in activated MAPKs. Inhibition of MKPs by zinc was shown to be involved in ERK activation during oxidative stress in neurons (Ho et al. 2008).

However, not all effects on MAPK phosphorylation can be explained by zinc inhibition of MKP. Zinc is also able to affect targets upstream of MAPKs, shown by MAPK activation in airway epithelial cells, where zinc affects tyrosine phosphorylation upstream of ERK (Wu et al. 2002). Another zinc-affected pathway downstream of LPS-induced TLR4 signaling comprises the Toll/IL-1R domain–containing adaptor inducing interferon (IFN)-β (TRIF) pathway (Figure 15.3). Zinc is able to inhibit downstream IFN regulatory factor 3 (IRF3) dephosphorylation, resulting in IFN-β expression. IFN-β in turn activates type I IFNR, causing induction of the inducible nitric monoxide synthase (iNOS) (Brieger, Rink, and Haase 2013).

15.5.1.3 Dendritic Cells

Acting via pattern recognition receptors (PRRs), activated DCs are important in innate and adaptive immunity, promoting the activation of antigen-specific T-cells and thereby functioning as mediators between the two parts of the immune system (Pearce and Everts 2015).

DC activation upon LPS stimulation, which activates TLR4, caused reduced Zip6 expression. This phenomenon was accompanied by reduced free zinc, which in turn is required for cell maturation. Interestingly, zinc deficiency induced by the addition of a zinc chelator led to increased surface expression of major histocompatibility complex (MHC) class II molecules and costimulatory molecules on DCs, mimicking the LPS effects. In contrast, zinc supplementation or Zip6 overexpression inhibited those effects. Zinc homeostasis is at least partly involved in DC maturation and thus may affect the magnitude of adaptive immune responses (Kitamura et al. 2006). The exact underlying molecular mechanisms are described in the monocyte/macrophage section (Section 15.5.1.2).

The zinc-finger transcription factor CTCF, belonging to the C_2H_2 group of transcription factors, was identified as a regulator of DC differentiation. This transcription factor is expressed in human as well as in murine DCs. During differentiation of human monocyte-derived DCs, CTCF is downregulated. Moreover, increased CTCF expression in mice during the differentiation of bone marrow–derived DCs caused increased apoptosis and decreased proliferation. This results in a decreased number of CTCF transduced DCs accompanied by a more immature phenotype, revealing maturation defects upon stimulation (Koesters et al. 2007).

15.5.1.4 Natural Killer Cells

Another zinc-affected cell population comprises NK cells. NK cells are able to recognize and eliminate virus-infected cells and tumor cells by detecting the "missing self" (i.e., the absence of MHC class I molecules on the cell surface). Another defense mechanism of NK cells is antibody-dependent cellular cytotoxicity (ADCC), by which target cell surface bound antibodies are recognized. Finally, NK cells are able to kill target cells due to the release of cytotoxic granules (Haase and Rink 2014b). Zinc deficiency decreases lytic activity of NK cells, which might be related to decreased IL-2 production of T-cells (Prasad 2000). The killer cell–inhibitory receptor (KIR) family expressed by NK cells harbors a zinc-binding site and recognizes MHC class I molecules presented on target cells, causing suppressed target cell killing. Deletion of the KIR-zinc–binding site led to impaired inhibitory functions on the activity of NK cells (Rajagopalan and Long 1998).

15.5.2 ZINC AND ADAPTIVE IMMUNITY

15.5.2.1 B-Cells

Zinc deficiency causes lymphopenia and attenuation of cellular and humoral immunity, leading to increased susceptibility to pathogens (Shankar and Prasad 1998). B-cell development and function is not impaired to the same extent by zinc deficiency as seen in T-cells. However, zinc deficiency is known to cause decreased antibody production and loss of premature and immature B-cells (Haase and Rink 2014b). Moreover, zinc deficiency blocks the development of B-cells in the bone marrow, resulting in reduced numbers of B-cells within the spleen (Shankar and Prasad 1998).

The impact of zinc supplementation on vaccination in zinc-deficient subjects has been investigated, revealing contradictory results depending upon the study design. Extremely high amounts of supplemental zinc combined with the vaccine led to either no or contrary effects (Overbeck, Rink, and Haase 2008). Thus, giving zinc at the same time as the vaccination seems not to be useful. So far, only one study revealed beneficial effects of zinc supplementation on vaccination. In contrast to the other studies, patients started zinc supplementation one month prior to vaccination and stopped the intake during the vaccination procedure. Zinc-supplemented subjects, who were older than 70 years, showed increases in the antibody titer, increased circulating T-cells, and improved delayed-type hypersensitivity reaction toward several antigens (Duchateau et al. 1981). This study suggests that zinc supplementation before vaccination might be beneficial in the elderly.

Zinc importer Zip10 was shown to be required for proper antibody responses after B-cell receptor (BCR) activation. Deficiencies in Zip10 are followed by hyperactivated BCR signaling, which in turn causes reduced cell proliferation (Hojyo et al. 2014). In particular, Zip10 is involved in the early B-cell developmental process. Inducible deletion of Zip10 in pro-B-cells caused increased caspase activity going along with decreased intracellular zinc levels. Concordantly, intracellular zinc depletion led to spontaneous caspase activity, resulting in B-cell apoptosis. Thus, Zip10-mediated zinc homeostasis might be crucial for survival of early B-cells. Apart from that, Zip10 expression was found to be regulated in a Janus kinase (JAK)-signal transducer and activator of transcription (STAT)-dependent manner. Its expression is correlated with STAT activation in human B-cell lymphoma, indicating any influence on B-cell homeostasis by a possible JAK-STAT-Zip10-zinc signaling axis (Miyai et al. 2014).

15.5.2.2 T-Cells

In adaptive immunity zinc is especially important for T-cell development and subsequent peripheral functions. A variety of different studies tried to elucidate the importance of zinc for T-cells, revealing impaired T-cell development and function upon zinc deficiency. The maturation of T-cell progenitors takes place in the thymus. However, zinc deficiency causes thymic atrophy and T-cell lymphopenia (Haase and Rink 2014b). Moreover, the peptide hormone thymulin is dependent on zinc ions, which act as a cofactor. Zinc deficiency decreases the biological activity of thymulin, thereby negatively affecting T-cell functions and differentiation (Prasad et al. 1988).

Apart from that, zinc deficiency alters the T helper cell balance of Th1 and Th2, this imbalance being restored after zinc supplementation (Figure 15.4). T helper cells promote functions of other cells (e.g., by activating infected macrophages to kill phagocytosed pathogens, namely by Th1 cells, or by supporting antibody production in B-cells, namely by Th2 cells). Long-term zinc deficiency decreases the production of the Th1 cytokines IFN-γ, IL-2, and TNF-α, whereas production of the Th2 cytokines IL-4, IL-6, and IL-10 is not affected. Thus, the imbalance of secreted cytokines favors the production of Th2 cytokines in contrast to Th1 cytokines (Cakman et al. 1996; Beck et al. 1997). This could result in impairment of defense against bacteria and viruses in particular.

Considering the involved signaling pathways, zinc seems to be required for p38 activation within Th1 cells whereas it inhibits the activity of ERK in Th2 cells. The activity of the phosphatase calcineurin was shown to be inhibited by zinc; this enzyme normally inactivates cAMP response element-binding protein (CREB) by dephosphorylation. The influence of zinc on calcineurin causes

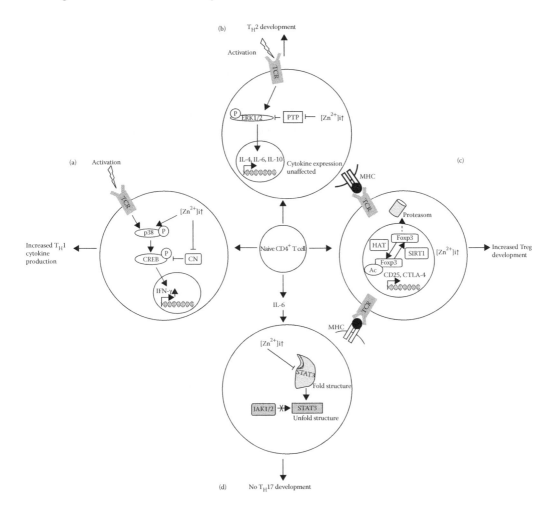

FIGURE 15.4 Overview of zinc effects on development of naive CD4+ T-cells. Zinc differentially influences the fate of the development of naive CD4+ T cells. (a) T_H1 cytokine production is increased upon zinc supplementation, causing a shift towards T_H1 cells within the T_H1/T_H2 cell balance. Zinc positively affects p38, whereas it inhibits the activity of calcineurin (CN), which is not able to dephosphorylate cAMP response element-binding protein (CREB) anymore. (b) The cytokine expression of T_H2 remains unaffected by zinc. (c) Differentiation into the Treg phenotype is increased upon zinc supplementation. Zinc inhibits the histondeacetlyase SIRT1, causing increased Foxp3 acetylation by histonacetylases (HAT). (d) Zinc supplementation causes decreased differentiation of naive CD4+ T cells into pathogenic T_H17 cells, resulting in autoimmunity. IL-6-stimulated CD4+ T-cells show inhibition of signal transducer and activator of transcription 3 (STAT3). STAT3 is inhibited by zinc binding, promoting the unfold structure of STAT3. Consequently, the Janus kinase (JAK) is not able to phosphorylate STAT3, thereby inhibiting T_H17 development.

increased CREB phosphorylation, which in turn results in increased expression of the Th1 cytokine IFN-γ. The activating phosphorylation of CREB is dependent on p38 activity, which is associated with participation of zinc, indicating once again a role of zinc in the regulation of the Th1/Th2 balance by inducing IFN-γ (Honscheid et al. 2012; Aydemir et al. 2009).

T-cell functions are susceptible to zinc deprivation and zinc signals seem likely to activate PKC within T-cells. This indicates involvement of zinc in the "cross-talk" of second messengers involved in T-cell signal transduction (Csermely and Somogyi 1989). Further involvement of zinc was assumed in the activation of the lymphocyte-specific protein tyrosine kinase (Lck) by the T-cell receptor (TCR), which belongs to the Src family of kinases (Figure 15.5). Zinc ions are required

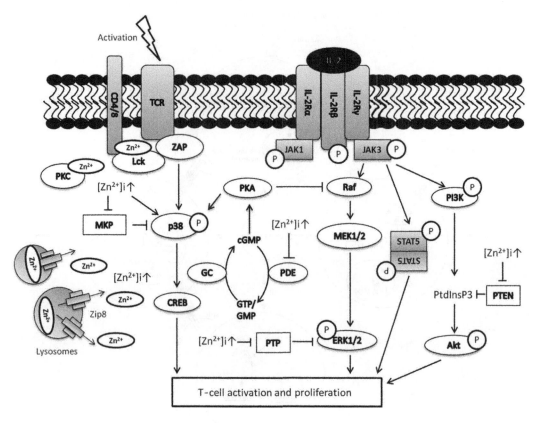

FIGURE 15.5 Involvement of zinc in T-cell signaling. Upon IL-2-induced T-cell activation lysosomal zinc is transported via Zip8 into the cytoplasm, revealing activating and inhibiting functions. Due to inhibition of MKP and protein tyrosine phosphatases (PTP) dephosphorylation of p38 and extracellular signal-related kinase (ERK1/2) is inhibited by zinc, respectively, causing prolonged T-cell activation and proliferation. Apart from that protein kinase C (PKC) is activated by zinc, which is involved in various intracellular signaling cascades. As in the signaling cascade of the TLR-4, zinc inhibits PDE causing cross-activation of PKA, which in turn promotes p38, whereas Raf is inhibited. Another zinc-affected pathway is the phosphoinositide 3-kinase (PI3K)/Akt pathway, where zinc inhibits phosphatase and tensin homologue deleted on chromosome 10 (PTEN). PTEN in turn is responsible for degradation of phosphatidylinositol (3,4,5)-trisphosphate (PtdIns (3,4,5)P3). Due to PTEN inhibition by zinc, Akt signaling is sustained, causing increased T-cell activation. Besides, zinc ions are required for stabilizing the interaction between lymphocyte-specific protein tyrosine kinase (Lck) and CD4/CD8 by recruiting Lck to the T-cell receptor (TCR) after activation. Subsequent phosphorylation of p38 is increased by zinc, causing increased CREB function, which in turn results in increased T-cell activation and proliferation. Apart from that, p38 affecting MKP is inhibited by zinc leading as well to increased p38 function. The STAT5 pathway within T-cells is not affected by zinc.

to stabilize the interaction between Lck and CD4/CD8 by recruiting the kinase to the TCR (Lin et al. 1998). Moreover, zinc ions are required for stabilizing the homodimerization of Lck, which promotes the activating transphosphorylation between two Lck molecules (Romir et al. 2007).

The zinc transporter Zip8 is highly expressed in human T-cells. Zip8 localization is predominantly found within the membranes of lysosomes, being upregulated after stimulation. Upon TCR-mediated T-cell activation, cytoplasmic zinc is increased due to zinc release from the lysosomal compartments via Zip8. Intracellular zinc accumulation might be an important event in response to TCR-mediated activation (Aydemir et al. 2009). Apart from that, zinc ions seem to play a crucial role in T-cell activation induced by IL-2 (Figure 15.5) (Kaltenberg et al. 2010; Tanaka et al. 1990). Stimulation of the IL-2 receptor (IL-2R) results in ERK dephosphorylation and IL-2-induced T-cell proliferation due to elevated intracellular zinc signals. Additionally, translocation of zinc ions from lysosomes into the cytosol was shown as a result of IL-2 induction (Kaltenberg et al. 2010). Phosphorylation of a specific tyrosine residue in the IL-2R β-chain promotes the assembly of adaptor proteins, triggering a MAPK cascade comprising the dual-specific kinases MEK and Raf. MEK and Raf in turn activate ERK via phosphorylation of conserved threonine and tyrosine residues in its catalytic domain (Gaffen 2001). ERK activation is followed by phosphorylation of further kinases and transcription factors (Cahill, Janknecht, and Nordheim 1996). In contrast, negative regulation of the ERK pathway is mediated by different phosphatases, which in turn can be inhibited by zinc (Ho et al. 2008).

The phosphatase and tensin homolog deleted on chromosome 10 (PTEN) is another enzyme affected by zinc in the downstream signaling cascade of IL-2 (Figure 15.5). PTEN seems to be inactivated by zinc binding, resulting in Akt activation and thus cell survival. In detail, the second messenger phosphatidylinositol (3,4,5)-trisphosphate (PtdIns(3,4,5)P3) is produced by phosphoinositide 3-kinase (PI3K) leading to Akt activation. Conversely, PTEN is responsible for PtdIns(3,4,5)P3 degradation. Zinc signals affect the IL-2-dependent PI3K/Akt pathway by inhibiting the negative regulator PTEN via binding to its catalytic cysteine residues. Binding of zinc to the catalytic cysteine residues protects PTEN from oxidation by H_2O_2 (Plum et al. 2014).

IL-1β-induced IL-2 production in humans is negatively affected by mild zinc deficiency (Figure 15.6). Zinc concentrations within T-cells are slightly below the optimal concentration for T-cell functions. Thus, further reduction of intracellular zinc leads to T-cell dysfunction and autoreactivity, whereas high zinc concentrations inhibit the activation of IL-1-induced IL-1 receptor kinase (IRAK). It seems likely that zinc represses the Th17 responses in humans by increasing intracellular zinc within T-cells and thereby inhibiting the IL-1β-signaling via inhibition of IRAK4 phosphorylation (Lee et al. 2015b).

Zinc supplementation was able to increase the intracellular zinc levels of zinc-deficient T-cells. In a murine T-cell line this increase was shown to be essential for the phosphorylation of p38 and for the phosphorylation of the subunit p65 of NF-κB, followed by IL-1β-induced IL-2 production. Intracellular zinc signals in T-cells were induced by IL-1β due to increased zinc transporter expression within the plasma membrane, namely Zip10 and Zip12. Specific inhibition of the MAPK p38 was shown to decrease IL-2 production. However, IL-2 synthesis could not be completely inhibited, assuming the participation of other molecules in this mechanism (Daaboul et al. 2012).

Zinc is described to suppress Th17 cell development by inhibiting the IL-6-induced STAT3 activation (Figure 15.4). In detail, zinc binds to STAT3 resulting in changes of its conformation, thereby causing the inability of STAT3 to interact with the appropriate Janus kinase (Kitabayashi et al. 2010). Zinc supplementation decreases the number of Th17 cells whereas it increases the number of T regulatory cells (Tregs). Namely, zinc supplementation was shown to induce and to elevate the number of CD4+CD25+Foxp3+ Tregs *in vitro* and *in vivo* (Figure 15.4). This was accompanied by decreased reactivity of Th1 and Th2 cells as well as decreased Th17-mediated experimental autoimmune encephalomyelitis (EAE). It seems that high zinc concentrations induce Tregs, which are normally responsible for the suppression of allo- or autoreactive effector cells (Rosenkranz et al. 2016a). Thus, zinc could play a role in decreasing risk of autoimmunity.

Another zinc-affected system is the mixed lymphocyte culture (MLC), serving as an *in vitro* model for allogeneic reactions and transplantation to determine the compatibility between the host and donor. Therein, the proliferation of T-cells seems to be a good indicator to assess the success of the transplantation. However, cytokines, such as IFN-γ, seem to be more reliable in assessing graft rejection. IFN-γ is able to induce cytotoxic T-cells by enhancing MHC I and MHC II expression, thereby representing reactivity between two individuals. Since immunosuppressive substances reveal toxicity *in vivo*, it is important to find new substances with less toxicity, as for example zinc. Zinc supplementation was shown to inhibit alloreactivity in the MLC. In contrast, T-cell proliferation *in vitro* was not decreased and no immunosuppressive effects were seen *in vivo*. Stimulation of T-cells by an HLA-different cell population might be blocked by zinc via specific inhibition of phosphorylation processes, causing reduced signal transduction. This in turn leads to reduced cytokine

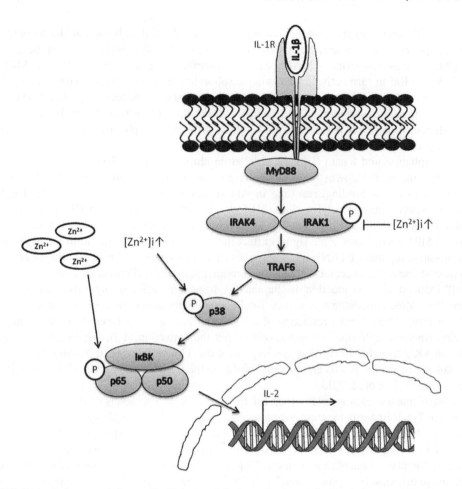

FIGURE 15.6 Influence of zinc on IL-1β-induced IL-2 production. After IL-1 receptor (IL-1R) activation, p38 gets phosphorylated via different upstream signaling events. p38 phosphorylation is increased after zinc supplementation due to elevated Zip transporter expression within the T cell membrane. Increases in p38 phosphorylation in turn cause increased NF-κB activity, represented in its subunits p65 and p50, followed by increased IL-2 production. Moreover, zinc is able to enhance p65 phosphorylation thereby enhancing NF-κB activity with subsequent increased IL-2 production.

secretion, which is related related to reduced graft rejection *in vivo*. Therefore, the infection rate will be reduced by the use of zinc compared to current immunosuppressive drugs (Campo et al. 2001). Zinc maintains the antigenic potency of the host *in vitro* since antigen recognition is not influenced by zinc, whereas allogeneic responses are suppressed. Oral zinc supplementation of different individuals for one week induced the same effect, showing suppression of the MLC. Increased inhibition of the MLC was observed *ex vivo* in cases where higher IFN-γ release occurred prior to zinc intake (Faber et al. 2004). New data indicate that the induction and stabilization of Treg cells is also involved in the MLC (Rosenkranz et al. 2015, Rosenkranz et al. 2016b). Zinc supplementation of the MLC results in decreased synthesis of IFN-γ, which is possibly related to the inhibition of the histone deacetylase Sirtuin-1. This inhibition stabilizes Foxp3, favoring Treg cell differentiation, which in turn might be beneficial during transplantation (Rosenkranz et al. 2016b).

Furthermore, Treg cell induction and stabilization in the MLC after zinc supplementation might be explained with zinc-induced upregulation of Foxp3 and Krüppel-like factor 10 (Klf-10) on the one hand and downregulation of interferon regulatory factor (IRF)-1 on the other hand. Klf-10 is an essential transcription factor for proper Treg cell function, whereas IRF-1 is a negative Foxp3 regulator, repressing its transcriptional activity. Thereby, zinc might be able to downregulate allogeneic immune reactions due to stabilization of induced Treg cells (Maywald and Rink 2016).

The treatment of peripheral blood mononuclear cells (PBMCs) and the MLC with a combination of zinc and transforming growth factor (TGF)-β1 revealed synergistic effects on Foxp3 expression. TGF-β1 mediates an increase of intracellular free zinc in T helper cells and in combination with zinc elevates phosphorylation of the signal transduction molecules Smad2/3, which is important for Foxp3 expression. Apart from that, zinc and TGF-β1 are able to significantly reduce the IFN-γ secretion in the MLC. Taken together, a combined treatment of zinc and TGF-β1 induces Treg cells and causes an increase of Smad2/3 activation, accompanied by increased Foxp3 expression, which suggests a possible beneficial use of zinc during transplantation (Maywald et al. unpublished data).

15.6 ZINC AND ALLERGY, AUTOIMMUNITY, INFECTIONS, AND NEOPLASIA

15.6.1 Zinc and Allergies

Allergic reactions (e.g., atopic dermatitis, allergic asthma, and anaphylaxis) are caused by basophils, eosinophils, and mast cells. After activation, mast cells are able to secrete chemokines and cytokines, which are important in the inflammatory reactions observed in allergic patients (Galli, Tsai, and Piliponsky 2008). Use of the zinc probe Zinquin revealed highly fluorescent granules within mast cells, indicating elevated zinc concentrations. Zinc was also detected by Zinquin staining within respiratory epithelial cells. However, human asthma is related to hypozincemia and epithelial damage (Truong-Tran, Ruffin, and Zalewski 2000; Zalewski et al. 2005). Concerning allergic eosinophilic inflammation, zinc deficiency led to increased inflammation, which is reversed by zinc supplementation. Moreover, zinc deficiency seems likely to induce a relative decrease in the Th1 immune response and therefore promotes the Th2 response, which is a key feature of asthma immunopathology. To test the hypothesis that zinc deficiency causes an imbalance in the Th1/Th2 ratio, a murine mouse model was used, showing increased eosinophilic inflammation with zinc deficiency (Richter et al. 2003). Thus, zinc deficiency might be a risk factor for developing asthma. However, results of different studies are controversial. Although some results reveal significantly reduced zinc levels in healthy individuals compared to patients with asthma, other studies could not show any significant differences in zinc plasma concentrations. Apart from that, there are also existing studies which show increased zinc plasma concentrations, being proportionally related to the severity degree of asthma (Riccioni and D'Orazio 2005). However, results of different human studies are inconsistent. Furthermore, zinc deficiency is associated with inhibited FcεRI-induced degranulation and cytokine production in mast cells. The PKC/NF-κB signaling pathway seems to be modulated by zinc transporters, which in turn regulate chemokine and cytokine gene expression. This might be an important aspect in the development of new antiallergic treatments, whereby the control of zinc concentration within mast cells might be a promising strategy (Kabu et al. 2006). Furthermore, zinc is able to induce Treg cells in *in vitro* allergic models, indicating a possible use of zinc in the therapy of allergies (Rosenkranz et al. 2015).

15.6.2 Zinc and Autoimmune Diseases

Autoimmune diseases include diabetes mellitus type I, rheumatoid arthritis (RA), systemic lupus erythematosus (SLE), multiple sclerosis (MS), and many others. The autoimmune destruction of insulin producing β-cells by the cellular und humoral immune response in the pancreatic islets of Langerhans is characteristic for diabetes mellitus type I, consequently causing insulin deficiency. The onset of this type of diabetes mostly occurs before 20 years of age, but disease manifestation is also observed in older adults. However, the maintenance of glucose homeostasis by administration of insulin is necessary to prevent subsequent diabetic complications (Daneman 2006). Zinc was

shown to be part of the insulin complex, suggesting a possible link between zinc status and development of type I diabetes (Scott 1934). Indeed, patients suffering from type I diabetes show higher
elimination rates of zinc via the urine, accompanied by significantly reduced plasma zinc levels
compared to healthy individuals (McNair et al. 1981). Blood glucose levels in animal models were
reduced after zinc supplementation, indicating insulinomimetic properties of zinc (Jansen, Karges,
and Rink 2009). However, whether the immunologic effects of zinc play a role in development, rate
of progression, or severity of type I diabetes is not clear.

Another possibly zinc-affected autoimmune disease is RA, a disease characterized by high concentrations of proinflammatory cytokines, especially of IL-1β, IL-6, and TNF-α, accompanied by
synovial inflammation and destruction of bone and cartilage (Koenders and van den Berg 2015;
Choy and Panayi 2001). Free radical oxidation products were identified in the synovial fluid of
patients suffering from RA, probably produced by phagocytes. Because ROS production seems
to be involved in RA development, the intake of antioxidant micronutrients, such as zinc, could
have protective effects (Cerhan et al. 2003). Additionally, the zinc-containing enzyme superoxide
dismutase (SOD) acts as a scavenger for toxic oxygen in tissues and might thus act as a preventing
factor in the onset of RA by reducing the free radical burden (Aaseth, Haugen, and Forre 1998).
Measurements within the serum/blood, scalp hair, and urine revealed low zinc concentrations in
RA patients (Niedermeier and Griggs 1971; Afridi et al. 2013). Moreover, reduced zinc levels within
the serum seem to be associated with increased levels of IL-1β and TNF-α (Zoli et al. 1998). Zinc
supplementation studies in RA patients showed beneficial effects. Joint swelling, walking time, and
morning stiffness were at least partly improved, suggesting a protective role of zinc (Simkin 1976;
Cerhan et al. 2003). However, other studies could not show a beneficial effect of zinc supplementation (Peretz et al. 1993; Mattingly and Mowat 1982; Rasker and Kardaun 1982). Nevertheless, it
seems evident that antioxidants, such as zinc, might at least positively influence the disease state in
patients with RA or might even slow progression of RA. However, a recent study showed that IL-17-
and TNF-α-mediated inflammation enhanced zinc uptake by synoviocytes and this in turn further
increased inflammation (Bonaventura et al. 2016).

MS is another autoimmune disease possibly affected by zinc. MS is a neurodegenerative auto-
immune-mediated disorder of the central nervous system (Ramsaransing, Mellema, and De Keyser
2009). The animal model for MS is the experimental autoimmune encephalomyelitis (EAE). Using
this model, zinc supplementation was shown to reduce symptoms, suggesting possible beneficial
effects of zinc supplementation in MS (Schubert et al. 2014; Stoye et al. 2012). Metal concentrations
within the cerebrospinal fluid (CSF) were shown to be lower in patients with MS than in controls
and to be held at constant levels compared to levels within the blood due to carefully controlled
metal permeability of the blood-brain barrier. Hence, the metal composition of the CSF may reflect
metabolic processes in the brain more reliably than the metal composition in the blood. However,
no significant differences were observed in the CSF of MS patients with regard to the zinc status nor
was a significant difference observed in the serum zinc levels of MS patients compared to a control
group (Sedighi et al. 2013; Melo et al. 2003).

At the molecular level, deficiency of the Th17 secreted proinflammatory cytokine IL-17A results
in resistance to EAE and to collagen-induced arthritis (CIA) in mice (Nishida et al. 2011). The
development of pathogenic Th17 cells from naive CD4+ T-cells was shown to be inhibited by zinc.
In contrast, zinc was not able to alter cytokine expression of T-cells, which had already developed
into a pathogenic state. Zinc supplementation led to a decrease in the number of Th17 cells in
regional lymph nodes accompanied by decreased IL-17A within the serum. Inhibition of STAT3
activation in CD4+ T-cells stimulated *in vivo* with IL-6 was induced by zinc supplementation. Zinc
binding alters STAT3, subsequently resulting in an unfolded structure. This in turn leads to the
inhibition of STAT3 phosphorylation by JAK kinases. All in all, it might be possible that zinc
suppresses the development of autoimmune diseases by inhibiting Th17 cell development via the
IL-6-STAT3 signaling axis in naive CD4+ T-cells and inducing Treg (Figure 15.4) (Rosenkranz
et al. 2016a; Nishida et al. 2011).

15.6.3 ZINC AND INFECTIOUS DISEASE

Infectious diseases, such as pneumonia, diarrhea, and malaria, remain a leading cause of morbidity and mortality, especially among children younger than 5 years of age (Black et al. 2010). A variety of observational studies linked susceptibility of increased infection rates to zinc status (Fischer Walker et al. 2011). Interestingly, zinc supplementation has been shown to be beneficial regarding the incidence of pneumonia and diarrhea, and might lead to reduced incidence of malaria. Zinc might have an important role, especially in infant and childhood infectious disease (Fischer Walker and Black 2004).

15.6.3.1 Zinc and Diarrhea

Zinc-deficient children seem to be more susceptible to diarrheal pathogens than children with normal zinc levels, suggesting an association between low zinc and risk of diarrhea (Fischer Walker et al. 2011). In addition, increased zinc loss was seen during acute diarrhea in hospitalized infants (Castillo-Duran, Vial, and Uauy 1988). Zinc supplementation reduced diarrheal morbidity, and nowadays the treatment of diarrhea in children with zinc is recommended by the World Health Organization (WHO) (Brown et al. 2009; WHO/UNICEF 2004).

15.6.3.2 Zinc and HIV Infection

Involvement of zinc is assumed in human immunodeficiency virus (HIV) disease where a significant association between low zinc and progression to acquired immunodeficiency syndrome (AIDS) was described (Coodley and Girard 1991; Beach et al. 1992), although results are inconsistent. Zinc utilization by the HIV for gene expression, multimerization, and integration characterizes HIV as a zinc-dependent virus, which may at least in part explain the low plasma zinc levels frequently observed in HIV-infected patients (Mocchegiani et al. 1995; Baum, Shor-Posner, and Campa 2000). Futhermore, patients with AIDS show clinical symptoms similar to symptoms associated with zinc deficiency (Baum, Shor-Posner, and Campa 2000). However, increased intake of micronutrients, including zinc, was shown to be associated with a more rapid disease progression to AIDS (Tang et al. 1993).

It is of special interest to elucidate the effect of zinc supplementation in children and pregnant women. It was seen that, apart from reduced opportunistic infections due to zinc supplementation, zinc levels and CD4 counts were increased in HIV-infected adults given zinc. However, no beneficial differences were seen after zinc supplementation with regard to viral load, mortality, and mother-to-child transmission of the virus (Zeng and Zhang 2011). The increase of CD4+ cells is in agreement with another study showing an increase in CD4+ cells in HIV-infected patients after zinc supplementation, accompanied by increased levels of active zinc-bound thymulin (Mocchegiani et al. 1995).

During progression of HIV infection to AIDS, the zinc-bound form of thymulin is strongly reduced, accompanied by decreased CD4 cell counts and decreased zinc levels within the blood. *In vitro* addition of zinc to plasma samples was shown to induce recovery of the active thymulin form, suggesting low zinc bioavailability as a cause of impaired thymic functions. Administration of the widely used antiretroviral agent zidovudine (AZT) combined with zinc supplements in patients with AIDS restored active zinc-bound thymulin, zinc levels within the blood, and CD4 T-cells accompanied by reduced opportunistic infections compared with the group of solely AZT-treated individuals (Mocchegiani and Muzzioli 2000). To sum up, while HIV-infected individuals seem to be especially susceptible to zinc deficiency, excessive zinc may stimulate HIV progression to AIDS.

15.6.3.3 Zinc and Malaria

Morbidity and mortality caused by malaria is especially high in areas with predominant malnutrition and exposure to the malaria parasite. Plasma zinc concentrations in children showing acute malaria infection are low and inversely correlated with the C-reactive protein (CRP) and the density of parasites within the blood. The children are likely to be at risk of zinc deficiency and zinc redistribution into the liver as part of the acute-phase reaction might not be the only cause for the observed deficiency. Zinc supplementation increased the plasma zinc levels in those patients (Duggan et al. 2005). There are few studies of zinc supplementation and malaria and the existing studies show inconsistent results. On the one hand, beneficial outcomes of zinc intake on malaria were shown, whereas on the other hand no differences between zinc supplemented individuals and a control group were observed (Caulfield, Richard, and Black 2004).

15.6.3.4 Zinc and the Common Cold

Interestingly, the duration of the common cold was shown to be decreased after zinc gluconate supplementation (Mossad et al. 1996). Another study analyzing a possible relation between the common cold and zinc supplements revealed reduced disease duration when zinc was administered immediately after the appearance of the first disease symptoms. Although duration of the common cold was reduced, severity was not (Das and Singh 2014). A Cochrane analysis revealed that zinc supplementation within 24 hours of the onset of common cold symptoms reduced the severity and duration in otherwise healthy people. Moreover, zinc supplementation for at least 5 months showed beneficial effects in terms of reduced cold incidence, less school absence, and lower intake of antibiotics (Singh and Das 2011). Nevertheless, a distinction between children and adults needs to be made, since one study could show reduced incidence of the common cold due to prophylactic zinc intake by children and in contrast, prophylactic zinc intake by adults was not studied (Das and Singh 2014).

15.6.4 ZINC AND NEOPLASIA

Studies analyzing zinc levels in tumors are inconsistent and reveal both increase of zinc as an indicator of unfavorable outcome as well as decrease of zinc associated with a poor outlook depending on the tumor (Taylor, Gee, and Kille 2011). Although in patients with several tumor types, including breast cancer, cervical cancer, lung cancer, and neck cancer, the levels of serum and plasma zinc were shown to be decreased, other studies did not show an association between zinc deficiency and the risk to develop cancer (Navarro Silvera and Rohan 2007; Taylor, Gee, and Kille 2011).

15.6.4.1 Zinc and Breast Cancer

Many studies have examined the relationship between breast cancer and serum or plasma zinc levels, revealing inconsistent results. Due to the uncontrolled cell growth during tumor progression, cells might require higher amounts of zinc and therefore replenish zinc from the plasma, which in turn reduces serum/plasma zinc levels (Taylor, Gee, and Kille 2011). One important zinc transporter involved in breast cancer is Zip6. Zip6 was shown to be estrogen-regulated and its presence in estrogen-receptor positive breast cancers is increased. Moreover, the association of Zip6 with estrogen-receptor positive breast cancers serves as a reliable marker for those cancer types, and it is one of the genes used routinely for determination. STAT3 is activated by growth factors or other agents and induces Zip6 transcription, which in turn manages the zinc influx into the cells, causing cell activation. This mechanism may explain the previously observed increased expression of Zip6 in breast cancers that have metastasized to lymph nodes (Taylor, Gee, and Kille 2011). Another zinc transporter involved is Zip7, which is primarily found in the membrane of the endoplasmic reticulum (ER), and is responsible for zinc release out of the ER into the cytosol. Expression of Zip7 was shown to be increased in clinical breast cancer samples where it is in the top 10% of genes overexpressed in poor prognostic breast cancer states (Taylor, Gee, and Kille 2011). Intracellular released zinc is able to inhibit various phosphatases, and this might explain how the presence of abnormally high zinc levels within the cells is thereby able to keep different tyrosine kinase signaling pathways activated. This might lead to increased invasion and growth accompanied by a more aggressive phenotype, as especially seen in tamoxifen-resistant cells (Taylor et al. 2008). Especially in breast cancer aberrant growth factor signaling supports rapid tumor cell proliferation and loss of therapeutic response to antihormonal drugs. A model of tamoxifen-resistant breast cancer revealed increased intracellular zinc levels compared to hormone-responsive counterparts. Increased expression of Zip7 in breast cancer might provide a novel target for blocking multiple antihormone-resistant signaling pathways (Taylor et al. 2008). However, targeting signaling pathways in the clinic to prevent tumor growth loses its effect when cells use new signaling pathways, potentially resulting in a more aggressive tumor growth. The benefit to targeting zinc might be to turn off its ability to inhibit phosphatases, thereby blocking various signaling pathways at the same time instead of blocking one specific pathway (Taylor, Gee, and Kille 2011).

15.6.4.2   Zinc and Prostate Cancer

Patients suffering from prostate cancer show reduced plasma zinc levels compared to patients affected by noncancer-related prostate diseases, normally presenting an organ with higher zinc content. The malignant prostate cells lose their ability to accumulate zinc, especially due to a decrease of the Zip1 importer (Taylor, Gee, and Kille 2011). The observed changes of intracellular zinc in the prostate during prostate cancer appear to be the direct opposite of what has been observed in breast cancer. Under normal conditions, the accumulation of high cellular zinc in prostate epithelial cells is necessary to carry out the major physiological functions of citrate production and secretion, which is important for reproduction. Prostate cancer is accompanied by the inability to accumulate zinc and citrate. This might be associated with decreased zinc transporter expression (Franklin et al. 2005; Franz et al. 2013). Zinc accumulation within the prostate is mainly by Zip1, with Zip2 and Zip3 being responsible for zinc maintenance within the cells. However, the ability to accumulate zinc is lost in prostate cancer cells (Desouki et al. 2007). Most studies revealed no significant effect of zinc supplementation on advanced prostate cancer (Gathirua-Mwangi and Zhang 2014).

15.6.4.3   Zinc and p53

An association between zinc and the tumor suppressor p53 is proposed, which is another interesting aspect to consider in the development of neoplasia. Intracellular free zinc seems to modulate p53 activity and stability. Excess zinc alters p53 protein structure and leads to decreased binding of p53 to the DNA. Copper is able to displace zinc from its binding site at p53, leading to wrong protein folding and disruption of p53 function. Moreover, p53 plays an important role in the transcriptional regulation of MT, indicating a novel regulatory role for p53 (Formigari, Gregianin, and Irato 2013).

REFERENCES

Aaseth, J., M. Haugen, and O. Forre. 1998. Rheumatoid arthritis and metal compounds--perspectives on the role of oxygen radical detoxification. *Analyst* 123 (1):3–6.

Afridi, H. I., T. G. Kazi, N. Kazi, F. N. Talpur, F. Shah, K. Naeemullah, S. S. Arain, and K. D. Brahman. 2013. Evaluation of status of arsenic, cadmium, lead and zinc levels in biological samples of normal and arthritis patients of age groups (46–60) and (61–75) years. *Clin Lab* 59 (1–2):143–53.

Andree, K. B., J. Kim, C. P. Kirschke, J. P. Gregg, H. Paik, H. Joung, L. Woodhouse, J. C. King, and L. Huang. 2004. Investigation of lymphocyte gene expression for use as biomarkers for zinc status in humans. *J Nutr* 134 (7):1716–23.

Aydemir, T. B., R. K. Blanchard, and R. J. Cousins. 2006. Zinc supplementation of young men alters metallothionein, zinc transporter, and cytokine gene expression in leukocyte populations. *Proc Natl Acad Sci U S A* 103 (6):1699–704. doi: 10.1073/pnas.0510407103.

Aydemir, T. B., J. P. Liuzzi, S. McClellan, and R. J. Cousins. 2009. Zinc transporter ZIP8 (SLC39A8) and zinc influence IFN-gamma expression in activated human T cells. *J Leukoc Biol* 86 (2):337–48. doi: 10.1189/jlb.1208759.

Barnett, J. B., M. C. Dao, D. H. Hamer, R. Kandel, G. Brandeis, D. Wu, G. E. Dallal, P. F. Jacques, R. Schreiber, E. Kong, and S. N. Meydani. 2016. Effect of zinc supplementation on serum zinc concentration and T cell proliferation in nursing home elderly: A randomized, double-blind, placebo-controlled trial. *Am J Clin Nutr* 103 (3):942–51. doi: 10.3945/ajcn.115.115188.

Baum, M. K., G. Shor-Posner, and A. Campa. 2000. Zinc status in human immunodeficiency virus infection. *J Nutr* 130 (5S Suppl):1421S–3S.

Beach, R. S., E. Mantero-Atienza, G. Shor-Posner, J. J. Javier, J. Szapocznik, R. Morgan, H. E. Sauberlich, P. E. Cornwell, C. Eisdorfer, and M. K. Baum. 1992. Specific nutrient abnormalities in asymptomatic HIV-1 infection. *AIDS* 6 (7):701–8.

Beck, F. W., A. S. Prasad, J. Kaplan, J. T. Fitzgerald, and G. J. Brewer. 1997. Changes in cytokine production and T cell subpopulations in experimentally induced zinc-deficient humans. *Am J Physiol* 272 (6 Pt 1):E1002–7.

Berg, A. H., C. D. Rice, M. S. Rahman, J. Dong, and P. Thomas. 2014. Identification and characterization of membrane androgen receptors in the ZIP9 zinc transporter subfamily: I. Discovery in female atlantic croaker and evidence ZIP9 mediates testosterone-induced apoptosis of ovarian follicle cells. *Endocrinology* 155 (11):4237–49. doi: 10.1210/en.2014-1198.

Besecker, B., S. Bao, B. Bohacova, A. Papp, W. Sadee, and D. L. Knoell. 2008. The human zinc transporter SLC39A8 (Zip8) is critical in zinc-mediated cytoprotection in lung epithelia. *Am J Physiol Lung Cell Mol Physiol* 294 (6):L1127–36. doi: 10.1152/ajplung.00057.2008.

Beyersmann, D. and H. Haase. 2001. Functions of zinc in signaling, proliferation and differentiation of mammalian cells. *Biometals* 14 (3–4):331–41.

Black, R. E., S. Cousens, H. L. Johnson, J. E. Lawn, I. Rudan, D. G. Bassani, P. Jha, H. Campbell, C. F. Walker, R. Cibulskis, T. Eisele, L. Liu, and C. Mathers. 2010. Global, regional, and national causes of child mortality in 2008: A systematic analysis. *Lancet* 375 (9730):1969–87. doi: 10.1016/s0140-6736(10)60549-1.

Bonaventura, P., A. Lamboux, F. Albarede, and P. Miossec. 2016. A feedback loop between inflammation and Zn uptake. *PLOS ONE* 11 (2):e0147146. doi: 10.1371/journal.pone.0147146.

Bosma, A. A., B. M. Mannaerts, N. A. de Haan, and J. Kroneman. 1988. Sister chromatid exchanges in calves with hereditary zinc deficiency (lethal trait A 46). *Vet Q* 10 (4):230–3. doi: 10.1080/01652176.1988.9694177.

Bosomworth, H. J., P. A. Adlard, D. Ford, and R. A. Valentine. 2013. Altered expression of ZnT10 in Alzheimer's disease brain. *PLOS ONE* 8 (5):e65475. doi: 10.1371/journal.pone.0065475.

Briefel, R. R., K. Bialostosky, J. Kennedy-Stephenson, M. A. McDowell, R. B. Ervin, and J. D. Wright. 2000. Zinc intake of the U.S. population: Findings from the third National Health and Nutrition Examination Survey, 1988–1994. *J Nutr* 130 (5S Suppl):1367S–73S.

Brieger, A. and L. Rink. 2010. Zink und Immunfunktion. *Ernährung & Medizin* 24 (4):156–160.

Brieger, A., L. Rink, and H. Haase. 2013. Differential regulation of TLR-dependent MyD88 and TRIF signaling pathways by free zinc ions. *J Immunol* 191 (4):1808–17. doi: 10.4049/jimmunol.1301261.

Brown, K. H., J. M. Peerson, S. K. Baker, and S. Y. Hess. 2009. Preventive zinc supplementation among infants, preschoolers, and older prepubertal children. *Food Nutr Bull* 30 (1 Suppl):S12–40.

Cadman, E. T. and R. A. Lawrence. 2010. Granulocytes: Effector cells or immunomodulators in the immune response to helminth infection? *Parasite Immunol* 32 (1):1–19. doi: 10.1111/j.1365-3024.2009.01147.x.

Cahill, M. A., R. Janknecht, and A. Nordheim. 1996. Signalling pathways: Jack of all cascades. *Curr Biol* 6 (1):16–9.

Cakman, I., J. Rohwer, R. M. Schutz, H. Kirchner, and L. Rink. 1996. Dysregulation between TH1 and TH2 T cell subpopulations in the elderly. *Mech Ageing Dev* 87 (3):197–209.

Campo, C. A., N. Wellinghausen, C. Faber, A. Fischer, and L. Rink. 2001. Zinc inhibits the mixed lymphocyte culture. *Biol Trace Elem Res* 79 (1):15–22. doi: 10.1385/bter:79:1:15.

Castillo-Duran, C., P. Vial, and R. Uauy. 1988. Trace mineral balance during acute diarrhea in infants. *J Pediatr* 113 (3):452–7.

Caulfield, L. E., S. A. Richard, and R. E. Black. 2004. Undernutrition as an underlying cause of malaria morbidity and mortality in children less than five years old. *Am J Trop Med Hyg* 71 (2 Suppl):55–63.

Cerhan, J. R., K. G. Saag, L. A. Merlino, T. R. Mikuls, and L. A. Criswell. 2003. Antioxidant micronutrients and risk of rheumatoid arthritis in a cohort of older women. *Am J Epidemiol* 157 (4):345–54.

Chowanadisai, W. 2014. Comparative genomic analysis of slc39a12/ZIP12: Insight into a zinc transporter required for vertebrate nervous system development. *PLOS ONE* 9 (11):e111535. doi: 10.1371/journal.pone.0111535.

Chowanadisai, W., B. Lonnerdal, and S. L. Kelleher. 2006. Identification of a mutation in SLC30A2 (ZnT-2) in women with low milk zinc concentration that results in transient neonatal zinc deficiency. *J Biol Chem* 281 (51):39699–707. doi: 10.1074/jbc.M605821200.

Choy, E. H. and G. S. Panayi. 2001. Cytokine pathways and joint inflammation in rheumatoid arthritis. *N Engl J Med* 344 (12):907–16. doi: 10.1056/nejm200103223441207.

Coodley, G. and D. E. Girard. 1991. Vitamins and minerals in HIV infection. *J Gen Intern Med* 6 (5):472–9.

Costello, L. C. and R. B. Franklin. 1998. Novel role of zinc in the regulation of prostate citrate metabolism and its implications in prostate cancer. *Prostate* 35 (4):285–96.

Coyle, P., P. D. Zalewski, J. C. Philcox, I. J. Forbes, A. D. Ward, S. F. Lincoln, I. Mahadevan, and A. M. Rofe. 1994. Measurement of zinc in hepatocytes by using a fluorescent probe, zinquin: Relationship to metallothionein and intracellular zinc. *Biochem J* 303 (Pt 3):781–6.

Crawford, A. and D. Wilson. 2015. Essential metals at the host-pathogen interface: Nutritional immunity and micronutrient assimilation by human fungal pathogens. *FEMS Yeast Res* 15 (7). doi: 10.1093/femsyr/fov071.

Csermely, P. and J. Somogyi. 1989. Zinc as a possible mediator of signal transduction in T lymphocytes. *Acta Physiol Hung* 74 (2):195–9.

Daaboul, D., E. Rosenkranz, P. Uciechowski, and L. Rink. 2012. Repletion of zinc in zinc-deficient cells strongly up-regulates IL-1beta-induced IL-2 production in T-cells. *Metallomics* 4 (10):1088–97. doi: 10.1039/c2mt20118f.

Daneman, D. 2006. Type 1 diabetes. *Lancet* 367 (9513):847–58. doi: 10.1016/s0140-6736(06)68341-4.

Das, R. R. and M. Singh. 2014. Oral zinc for the common cold. *JAMA* 311 (14):1440–1. doi: 10.1001/jama.2014.1404.

Desouki, M. M., J. Geradts, B. Milon, R. B. Franklin, and L. C. Costello. 2007. hZip2 and hZip3 zinc transporters are down regulated in human prostate adenocarcinomatous glands. *Mol Cancer* 6:37. doi: 10.1186/1476-4598-6-37.

Deutsche Gesellschaft für Ernährung (DGE), Österreichische Gesellschaft für Ernährung (ÖGE), Schweizerische Gesellschaft für Ernährung (SGE). 2015. *Referenzwerte für die Nährstoffzufuhr*. 2nd ed. Bonn, Germany.

Djoko, K. Y., C. L. Ong, M. J. Walker, and A. G. McEwan. 2015. The role of copper and zinc toxicity in innate immune defense against bacterial pathogens. *J Biol Chem* 290 (31):18954–61. doi: 10.1074/jbc.R115.647099.

Dubben, S., A. Honscheid, K. Winkler, L. Rink, and H. Haase. 2010. Cellular zinc homeostasis is a regulator in monocyte differentiation of HL-60 cells by 1 alpha,25-dihydroxyvitamin D3. *J Leukoc Biol* 87 (5):833–44. doi: 10.1189/jlb.0409241.

Duchateau, J., G. Delepesse, R. Vrijens, and H. Collet. 1981. Beneficial effects of oral zinc supplementation on the immune response of old people. *Am J Med* 70 (5):1001–4.

Duggan, C., W. B. MacLeod, N. F. Krebs, J. L. Westcott, W. W. Fawzi, Z. G. Premji, V. Mwanakasale, J. L. Simon, K. Yeboah-Antwi, and D. H. Hamer. 2005. Plasma zinc concentrations are depressed during the acute phase response in children with falciparum malaria. *J Nutr* 135 (4):802–7.

Eide, D. J. 2006. Zinc transporters and the cellular trafficking of zinc. *Biochim Biophys Acta* 1763 (7):711–22. doi: 10.1016/j.bbamcr.2006.03.005.

Faber, C., P. Gabriel, K. H. Ibs, and L. Rink. 2004. Zinc in pharmacological doses suppresses allogeneic reaction without affecting the antigenic response. *Bone Marrow Transplant* 33 (12):1241–6. doi: 10.1038/sj.bmt.1704509.

Favier, A. and M. Favier. 1990. Effects of zinc deficiency in pregnancy on the mother and the newborn infant. *Rev Fr Gynecol Obstet* 85 (1):13–27.

Fischer Walker, C. and R. E. Black. 2004. Zinc and the risk for infectious disease. *Annu Rev Nutr* 24:255–75. doi: 10.1146/annurev.nutr.23.011702.073054.

Fischer Walker, C., K. Kordas, R. J. Stoltzfus, and R. E. Black. 2005. Interactive effects of iron and zinc on biochemical and functional outcomes in supplementation trials. *Am J Clin Nutr* 82 (1):5–12.

Fischer Walker, C., L. Lamberti, D. Roth, and R. E. Black. 2011. Zinc and infectious diseases. In *Zinc in Human Health*, edited by L. Rink, 234–253. Netherlands: IOS Press BV.

Food and Nutrition Board, Institute of Medicine. 2001. *Dietary Reference Intakes for Vitamin A, Vitamin K, Arsenic, Boron, Chromium, Copper, Iodine, Iron, Manganese, Molybdenum, Nickel, Silicon, Vanadium, and Zinc*. Washington, DC: The National Academies Press.

Formigari, A., E. Gregianin, and P. Irato. 2013. The effect of zinc and the role of p53 in copper-induced cellular stress responses. *J Appl Toxicol* 33 (7):527–36. doi: 10.1002/jat.2854.

Francis, S. H., J. L. Colbran, L. M. McAllister-Lucas, and J. D. Corbin. 1994. Zinc interactions and conserved motifs of the cGMP-binding cGMP-specific phosphodiesterase suggest that it is a zinc hydrolase. *J Biol Chem* 269 (36):22477–80.

Franklin, R. B., B. Milon, P. Feng, and L. C. Costello. 2005. Zinc and zinc transporters in normal prostate and the pathogenesis of prostate cancer. *Front Biosci* 10:2230–9.

Franz, M. C., P. Anderle, M. Burzle, Y. Suzuki, M. R. Freeman, M. A. Hediger, and G. Kovacs. 2013. Zinc transporters in prostate cancer. *Mol Aspects Med* 34 (2–3):735–41. doi: 10.1016/j.mam.2012.11.007.

Frederickson, C. J., S. W. Suh, D. Silva, C. J. Frederickson, and R. B. Thompson. 2000. Importance of zinc in the central nervous system: The zinc-containing neuron. *J Nutr* 130 (5S Suppl):1471S–83.

Gaffen, S. L. 2001. Signaling domains of the interleukin 2 receptor. *Cytokine* 14 (2):63–77. doi: 10.1006/cyto.2001.0862.

Gaither, L. A. and D. J. Eide. 2000. Functional expression of the human hZIP2 zinc transporter. *J Biol Chem* 275 (8):5560–4.

Gaither, L. A. and D. J. Eide. 2001a. Eukaryotic zinc transporters and their regulation. *Biometals* 14 (3–4):251–70.

Gaither, L. A. and D. J. Eide. 2001b. The human ZIP1 transporter mediates zinc uptake in human K562 erythroleukemia cells. *J Biol Chem* 276 (25):22258–64. doi: 10.1074/jbc.M101772200.

Galli, S. J., M. Tsai, and A. M. Piliponsky. 2008. The development of allergic inflammation. *Nature* 454 (7203):445–54. doi: 10.1038/nature07204.

Gathirua-Mwangi, W. G. and J. Zhang. 2014. Dietary factors and risk for advanced prostate cancer. *Eur J Cancer Prev* 23 (2):96–109. doi: 10.1097/CEJ.0b013e3283647394.

Gee, K. R., Z. L. Zhou, D. Ton-That, S. L. Sensi, and J. H. Weiss. 2002. Measuring zinc in living cells. A new generation of sensitive and selective fluorescent probes. *Cell Calcium* 31 (5):245–51. doi: 10.1016/s0143-4160(02)00053-2.

Gibson, R. S. 1994. Zinc nutrition in developing countries. *Nutr Res Rev* 7 (1):151–73. doi: 10.1079/nrr19940010.

Goyette, J. and C. L. Geczy. 2011. Inflammation-associated S100 proteins: New mechanisms that regulate function. *Amino Acids* 41 (4):821–42. doi: 10.1007/s00726-010-0528-0.

Grass, G., M. Otto, B. Fricke, C. J. Haney, C. Rensing, D. H. Nies, and D. Munkelt. 2005. FieF (YiiP) from Escherichia coli mediates decreased cellular accumulation of iron and relieves iron stress. *Arch Microbiol* 183 (1):9–18. doi: 10.1007/s00203-004-0739-4.

Gunther, V., U. Lindert, and W. Schaffner. 2012. The taste of heavy metals: Gene regulation by MTF-1. *Biochim Biophys Acta* 1823 (9):1416–25. doi: 10.1016/j.bbamcr.2012.01.005.

Guthrie, G. J., T. B. Aydemir, C. Troche, A. B. Martin, S. M. Chang, and R. J. Cousins. 2015. Influence of ZIP14 (slc39A14) on intestinal zinc processing and barrier function. *Am J Physiol Gastrointest Liver Physiol* 308 (3):G171–8. doi: 10.1152/ajpgi.00021.2014.

Haase, H., D. J. Mazzatti, A. White, K. H. Ibs, G. Engelhardt, S. Hebel, J. R. Powell, and L. Rink. 2007. Differential gene expression after zinc supplementation and deprivation in human leukocyte subsets. *Mol Med* 13 (7–8):362–70. doi: 10.2119/2007-00049.Haase.

Haase, H., J. L. Ober-Blobaum, G. Engelhardt, S. Hebel, A. Heit, H. Heine, and L. Rink. 2008. Zinc signals are essential for lipopolysaccharide-induced signal transduction in monocytes. *J Immunol* 181 (9):6491–502.

Haase, H. and L. Rink. 2009. Functional significance of zinc-related signaling pathways in immune cells. *Annu Rev Nutr* 29:133–52. doi: 10.1146/annurev-nutr-080508-141119.

Haase, H. and L. Rink. 2014a. Multiple impacts of zinc on immune function. *Metallomics* 6 (7):1175–80. doi: 10.1039/c3mt00353a.

Haase, H. and L. Rink. 2014b. Zinc signals and immune function. *Biofactors* 40 (1):27–40. doi: 10.1002/biof.1114.

Hamer, D. H. 1986. Metallothionein. *Annu Rev Biochem* 55:913–51. doi: 10.1146/annurev.bi.55.070186.004405.

Hasan, R., L. Rink, and H. Haase. 2013. Zinc signals in neutrophil granulocytes are required for the formation of neutrophil extracellular traps. *Innate Immun* 19 (3):253–64. doi: 10.1177/1753425912458815.

Hasegawa, H., K. Suzuki, K. Suzuki, S. Nakaji, and K. Sugawara. 2000. Effects of zinc on the reactive oxygen species generating capacity of human neutrophils and on the serum opsonic activity in vitro. *Luminescence* 15 (5):321–7. doi: 10.1002/1522-7243(200009/10)15:5<321::aid-bio605>3.0.co;2-o.

Hashimoto, A., K. Ohkura, M. Takahashi, K. Kizu, H. Narita, S. Enomoto, Y. Miyamae, S. Masuda, M. Nagao, K. Irie, H. Ohigashi, G. K. Andrews, and T. Kambe. 2015. Soybean extracts increase cell surface ZIP4 abundance and cellular zinc levels: A potential novel strategy to enhance zinc absorption by ZIP4 targeting. *Biochem J* 472 (2):183–93. doi: 10.1042/bj20150862.

Hirose, T., T. Ogura, K. Tanaka, J. Minaguchi, T. Yamauchi, T. Fukada, Y. I. Koyama, and K. Takehana. 2015. Comparative study of dermal components and plasma TGF-beta1 levels in Slc39a13/Zip13-KO mice. *J Vet Med Sci.* 77:1385–9. doi: 10.1292/jvms.15-0015.

Ho, Y., R. Samarasinghe, M. E. Knoch, M. Lewis, E. Aizenman, and D. B. DeFranco. 2008. Selective inhibition of mitogen-activated protein kinase phosphatases by zinc accounts for extracellular signal-regulated kinase 1/2-dependent oxidative neuronal cell death. *Mol Pharmacol* 74 (4):1141–51. doi: 10.1124/mol.108.049064.

Hojyo, S., T. Miyai, H. Fujishiro, M. Kawamura, T. Yasuda, A. Hijikata, B. H. Bin, T. Irie, J. Tanaka, T. Atsumi, M. Murakami, M. Nakayama, O. Ohara, S. Himeno, H. Yoshida, H. Koseki, T. Ikawa, K. Mishima, and T. Fukada. 2014. Zinc transporter SLC39A10/ZIP10 controls humoral immunity by modulating B-cell receptor signal strength. *Proc Natl Acad Sci U S A* 111 (32):11786–91. doi: 10.1073/pnas.1323557111.

Honscheid, A., S. Dubben, L. Rink, and H. Haase. 2012. Zinc differentially regulates mitogen-activated protein kinases in human T cells. *J Nutr Biochem* 23 (1):18–26. doi: 10.1016/j.jnutbio.2010.10.007.

Hotz, C., N. M. Lowe, M. Araya, and K. H. Brown. 2003. Assessment of the trace element status of individuals and populations: The example of zinc and copper. *J Nutr* 133 (5 Suppl 1):1563S–8S.

Huang, L. and J. Gitschier. 1997. A novel gene involved in zinc transport is deficient in the lethal milk mouse. *Nat Genet* 17 (3):292–7. doi: 10.1038/ng1197-292.

Huang, L. and S. Tepaamorndech. 2013. The SLC30 family of zinc transporters – a review of current understanding of their biological and pathophysiological roles. *Mol Aspects Med* 34 (2–3):548–60. doi: 10.1016/j.mam.2012.05.008.

Hujanen, E. S., S. T. Seppa, and K. Virtanen. 1995. Polymorphonuclear leukocyte chemotaxis induced by zinc, copper and nickel in vitro. *Biochim Biophys Acta* 1245 (2):145–52.

Ibs, K. H. and L. Rink. 2003. Zinc-altered immune function. *J Nutr* 133 (5 Suppl 1):1452S–6S.

Inoue, Y., S. Hasegawa, S. Ban, T. Yamada, Y. Date, H. Mizutani, S. Nakata, M. Tanaka, and N. Hirashima. 2014. ZIP2 protein, a zinc transporter, is associated with keratinocyte differentiation. *J Biol Chem* 289 (31):21451–62. doi: 10.1074/jbc.M114.560821.

Jansen, J., W. Karges, and L. Rink. 2009. Zinc and diabetes–clinical links and molecular mechanisms. *J Nutr Biochem* 20 (6):399–417. doi: 10.1016/j.jnutbio.2009.01.009.

Jeong, J. and D. J. Eide. 2013. The SLC39 family of zinc transporters. *Mol Aspects Med* 34 (2–3):612–9. doi: 10.1016/j.mam.2012.05.011.

Junttila, M. R., S. P. Li, and J. Westermarck. 2008. Phosphatase-mediated crosstalk between MAPK signaling pathways in the regulation of cell survival. *FASEB J* 22 (4):954–65. doi: 10.1096/fj.06-7859rev.

Kabu, K., S. Yamasaki, D. Kamimura, Y. Ito, A. Hasegawa, E. Sato, H. Kitamura, K. Nishida, and T. Hirano. 2006. Zinc is required for Fc epsilon RI-mediated mast cell activation. *J Immunol* 177 (2):1296–305.

Kahmann, L., P. Uciechowski, S. Warmuth, B. Plumakers, A. M. Gressner, M. Malavolta, E. Mocchegiani, and L. Rink. 2008. Zinc supplementation in the elderly reduces spontaneous inflammatory cytokine release and restores T cell functions. *Rejuvenation Res* 11 (1):227–37. doi: 10.1089/rej.2007.0613.

Kaltenberg, J., L. M. Plum, J. L. Ober-Blobaum, A. Honscheid, L. Rink, and H. Haase. 2010. Zinc signals promote IL-2-dependent proliferation of T cells. *Eur J Immunol* 40 (5):1496–503. doi: 10.1002/eji.200939574.

Kanoni, S., G. V. Dedoussis, G. Herbein, T. Fulop, A. Varin, J. Jajte, L. Rink, D. Monti, E. Mariani, M. Malavolta, R. Giacconi, F. Marcellini, and E. Mocchegiani. 2010. Assessment of gene-nutrient interactions on inflammatory status of the elderly with the use of a zinc diet score--ZINCAGE study. *J Nutr Biochem* 21 (6):526–31. doi: 10.1016/j.jnutbio.2009.02.011.

Karcioglu, Z. A. 1982. Zinc in the eye. *Surv Ophthalmol* 27 (2):114–22.

Kelleher, S. L., N. H. McCormick, V. Velasquez, and V. Lopez. 2011. Zinc in specialized secretory tissues: Roles in the pancreas, prostate, and mammary gland. *Adv Nutr* 2 (2):101–11. doi: 10.3945/an.110.000232.

Kelleher, S. L., V. Velasquez, T. P. Croxford, N. H. McCormick, V. Lopez, and J. MacDavid. 2012. Mapping the zinc-transporting system in mammary cells: Molecular analysis reveals a phenotype-dependent zinc-transporting network during lactation. *J Cell Physiol* 227 (4):1761–70. doi: 10.1002/jcp.22900.

Kitabayashi, C., T. Fukada, M. Kanamoto, W. Ohashi, S. Hojyo, T. Atsumi, N. Ueda, I. Azuma, H. Hirota, M. Murakami, and T. Hirano. 2010. Zinc suppresses Th17 development via inhibition of STAT3 activation. *Int Immunol* 22 (5):375–86. doi: 10.1093/intimm/dxq017.

Kitamura, H., H. Morikawa, H. Kamon, M. Iguchi, S. Hojyo, T. Fukada, S. Yamashita, T. Kaisho, S. Akira, M. Murakami, and T. Hirano. 2006. Toll-like receptor-mediated regulation of zinc homeostasis influences dendritic cell function. *Nat Immunol* 7 (9):971–7. doi: 10.1038/ni1373.

Kloubert, V. and L. Rink. 2015. Zinc as a micronutrient and its preventive role of oxidative damage in cells. *Food Funct* 6 (10):3195–204. doi: 10.1039/c5fo00630a.

Kodirov, S. A., S. Takizawa, J. Joseph, E. R. Kandel, G. P. Shumyatsky, and V. Y. Bolshakov. 2006. Synaptically released zinc gates long-term potentiation in fear conditioning pathways. *Proc Natl Acad Sci U S A* 103 (41):15218–23. doi: 10.1073/pnas.0607131103.

Koenders, M. I. and W. B. van den Berg. 2015. Novel therapeutic targets in rheumatoid arthritis. *Trends Pharmacol Sci* 36 (4):189–95. doi: 10.1016/j.tips.2015.02.001.

Koesters, C., B. Unger, I. Bilic, U. Schmidt, S. Bluml, B. Lichtenberger, M. Schreiber, J. Stockl, and W. Ellmeier. 2007. Regulation of dendritic cell differentiation and subset distribution by the zinc finger protein CTCF. *Immunol Lett* 109 (2):165–74. doi: 10.1016/j.imlet.2007.02.006.

Kojima, C., A. Kawakami, T. Takei, K. Nitta, and M. Yoshida. 2007. Angiotensin-converting enzyme inhibitor attenuates monocyte adhesion to vascular endothelium through modulation of intracellular zinc. *J Pharmacol Exp Ther* 323 (3):855–60. doi: 10.1124/jpet.107.127944.

Kolaj-Robin, O., D. Russell, K. A. Hayes, J. T. Pembroke, and T. Soulimane. 2015. Cation diffusion facilitator family: Structure and function. *FEBS Lett* 589 (12):1283–1295. doi: 10.1016/j.febslet.2015.04.007.

Kown, M. H., T. Van der Steenhoven, F. G. Blankenberg, G. Hoyt, G. J. Berry, J. F. Tait, H. W. Strauss, and R. C. Robbins. 2000. Zinc-mediated reduction of apoptosis in cardiac allografts. *Circulation* 102 (19 Suppl 3):III228–32.

Lee, S., S. R. Hennigar, S. Alam, K. Nishida, and S. L. Kelleher. 2015a. Essential role for zinc transporter 2 (ZnT2)-mediated zinc transport in mammary gland development and function during lactation. *J Biol Chem* 290 (21):13064–78. doi: 10.1074/jbc.M115.637439.

Lee, H., B. Kim, Y. H. Choi, Y. Hwang, D. H. Kim, S. Cho, S. J. Hong, and W. W. Lee. 2015b. Inhibition of interleukin-1beta-mediated interleukin-1 receptor-associated kinase 4 phosphorylation by zinc leads to repression of memory T helper type 17 response in humans. *Immunology* 146 (4):645–56. doi: 10.1111/imm.12536.

Lichten, L. A. and R. J. Cousins. 2009. Mammalian zinc transporters: Nutritional and physiologic regulation. *Annu Rev Nutr* 29:153–76. doi: 10.1146/annurev-nutr-033009-083312.

Lim, K. H., L. J. Riddell, C. A. Nowson, A. O. Booth, and E. A. Szymlek-Gay. 2013. Iron and zinc nutrition in the economically-developed world: A review. *Nutrients* 5 (8):3184–211. doi: 10.3390/nu5083184.

Lin, R. S., C. Rodriguez, A. Veillette, and H. F. Lodish. 1998. Zinc is essential for binding of p56(lck) to CD4 and CD8alpha. *J Biol Chem* 273 (49):32878–82.

Liuzzi, J. P., L. A. Lichten, S. Rivera, R. K. Blanchard, T. B. Aydemir, M. D. Knutson, T. Ganz, and R. J. Cousins. 2005. Interleukin-6 regulates the zinc transporter Zip14 in liver and contributes to the hypozincemia of the acute-phase response. *Proc Natl Acad Sci U S A* 102 (19):6843–8. doi: 10.1073/pnas.0502257102.

Lowe, N. M., K. Fekete, and T. Decsi. 2009. Methods of assessment of zinc status in humans: A systematic review. *Am J Clin Nutr* 89 (6):2040S–51. doi: 10.3945/ajcn.2009.27230G.

Lu, M. and D. Fu. 2007. Structure of the zinc transporter YiiP. *Science* 317 (5845):1746–8. doi: 10.1126/science.1143748.

Maret, W., C. Jacob, B. L. Vallee, and E. H. Fischer. 1999. Inhibitory sites in enzymes: Zinc removal and reactivation by thionein. *Proc Natl Acad Sci U S A* 96 (5):1936–40.

Maret, W. and A. Krezel. 2007. Cellular zinc and redox buffering capacity of metallothionein/thionein in health and disease. *Mol Med* 13 (7–8):371–5. doi: 10.2119/2007–00036.Maret.

Maret, W. and H. H. Sandstead. 2006. Zinc requirements and the risks and benefits of zinc supplementation. *J Trace Elem Med Biol* 20 (1):3–18. doi: 10.1016/j.jtemb.2006.01.006.

Martin, A. B., T. B. Aydemir, G. J. Guthrie, D. A. Samuelson, S. M. Chang, and R. J. Cousins. 2013. Gastric and colonic zinc transporter ZIP11 (Slc39a11) in mice responds to dietary zinc and exhibits nuclear localization. *J Nutr* 143 (12):1882–8. doi: 10.3945/jn.113.184457.

Matsushita, K., K. Kitagawa, T. Matsuyama, T. Ohtsuki, A. Taguchi, K. Mandai, T. Mabuchi, Y. Yagita, T. Yanagihara, and M. Matsumoto. 1996. Effect of systemic zinc administration on delayed neuronal death in the gerbil hippocampus. *Brain Res* 743 (1–2):362–5.

Mattingly, P. C. and A. G. Mowat. 1982. Zinc sulphate in rheumatoid arthritis. *Ann Rheum Dis* 41 (5):456–7.

Maverakis, E., M. A. Fung, P. J. Lynch, M. Draznin, D. J. Michael, B. Ruben, and N. Fazel. 2007. Acrodermatitis enteropathica and an overview of zinc metabolism. *J Am Acad Dermatol* 56 (1):116–24. doi: 10.1016/j.jaad.2006.08.015.

Mayer, L. S., P. Uciechowski, S. Meyer, T. Schwerdtle, L. Rink, and H. Haase. 2014. Differential impact of zinc deficiency on phagocytosis, oxidative burst, and production of pro-inflammatory cytokines by human monocytes. *Metallomics* 6 (7):1288–95. doi: 10.1039/c4mt00051j.

Maywald, M. and L. Rink. 2016. Zinc supplementation induces CD4+CD25+Foxp3+ antigen-specific regulatory T cells and suppresses IFN-g production by upregulation of Foxp3 and KLF-10 and downregulation of IRF-1. *Eur J Nutr*. doi: 10.1007/s00394-016-1228-7.

McNair, P., S. Kiilerich, C. Christiansen, M. S. Christensen, S. Madsbad, and I. Transbol. 1981. Hyperzincuria in insulin treated diabetes mellitus--its relation to glucose homeostasis and insulin administration. *Clin Chim Acta* 112 (3):343–8.

Melo, T. M., C. Larsen, L. R. White, J. Aasly, T. E. Sjobakk, T. P. Flaten, U. Sonnewald, and T. Syversen. 2003. Manganese, copper, and zinc in cerebrospinal fluid from patients with multiple sclerosis. *Biol Trace Elem Res* 93 (1–3):1–8. doi: 10.1385/bter:93:1-3:1.

Mills, C.F. 1989. *Zinc in Human Biology*. New York, NY: Springer.

Miyai, T., S. Hojyo, T. Ikawa, M. Kawamura, T. Irie, H. Ogura, A. Hijikata, B. H. Bin, T. Yasuda, H. Kitamura, M. Nakayama, O. Ohara, H. Yoshida, H. Koseki, K. Mishima, and T. Fukada. 2014. Zinc transporter SLC39A10/ZIP10 facilitates antiapoptotic signaling during early B-cell development. *Proc Natl Acad Sci U S A* 111 (32):11780–5. doi: 10.1073/pnas.1323549111.

Mocchegiani, E. and M. Muzzioli. 2000. Therapeutic application of zinc in human immunodeficiency virus against opportunistic infections. *J Nutr* 130 (5S Suppl):1424S–31S.

Mocchegiani, E., S. Veccia, F. Ancarani, G. Scalise, and N. Fabris. 1995. Benefit of oral zinc supplementation as an adjunct to zidovudine (AZT) therapy against opportunistic infections in AIDS. *Int J Immunopharmacol* 17 (9):719–27.

Mossad, S. B., M. L. Macknin, S. V. Medendorp, and P. Mason. 1996. Zinc gluconate lozenges for treating the common cold. A randomized, double-blind, placebo-controlled study. *Ann Intern Med* 125 (2):81–8.

Murgia, C., C. Devirgiliis, E. Mancini, G. Donadel, P. Zalewski, and G. Perozzi. 2009. Diabetes-linked zinc transporter ZnT8 is a homodimeric protein expressed by distinct rodent endocrine cell types in the pancreas and other glands. *Nutr Metab Cardiovasc Dis* 19 (6):431–9. doi: 10.1016/j.numecd.2008.09.004.

Navarro Silvera, S. A. and T. E. Rohan. 2007. Trace elements and cancer risk: A review of the epidemiologic evidence. *Cancer Causes Control* 18 (1):7–27. doi: 10.1007/s10552-006-0057-z.

Niedermeier, W. and J. H. Griggs. 1971. Trace metal composition of synovial fluid and blood serum of patients with rheumatoid arthritis. *J Chronic Dis* 23 (8):527–36.

Nies, D. H. and S. Silver. 1995. Ion efflux systems involved in bacterial metal resistances. *J Ind Microbiol* 14 (2):186–99.

Nishida, K., T. Fukada, S. Yamasaki, M. Murakami, and T. Hirano. 2011. Zinc in allergy, autoimmune, and hard and connective tissue diseases. In *Zinc in Human Health*, edited by L. Rink, 268–282. Netherlands: IOS Press BV.

O'Dell, B. L. and J. E. Savage. 1960. Effect of phytic acid on zinc availability. *Proc Soc Exp Biol Med* 103:304–6.

Ohana, E., E. Hoch, C. Keasar, T. Kambe, O. Yifrach, M. Hershfinkel, and I. Sekler. 2009. Identification of the Zn2+ binding site and mode of operation of a mammalian Zn2+ transporter. *J Biol Chem* 284 (26):17677–86. doi: 10.1074/jbc.M109.007203.

Overbeck, S., L. Rink, and H. Haase. 2008. Modulating the immune response by oral zinc supplementation: A single approach for multiple diseases. *Arch Immunol Ther Exp (Warsz)* 56 (1):15–30. doi: 10.1007/s00005-008-0003-8.

Overbeck, S., P. Uciechowski, M. L. Ackland, D. Ford, and L. Rink. 2008. Intracellular zinc homeostasis in leukocyte subsets is regulated by different expression of zinc exporters ZnT-1 to ZnT-9. *J Leukoc Biol* 83 (2):368–80. doi: 10.1189/jlb.0307148.

Palmiter, R. D., T. B. Cole, and S. D. Findley. 1996. ZnT-2, a mammalian protein that confers resistance to zinc by facilitating vesicular sequestration. *EMBO J* 15 (8):1784–91.

Pascal, L. E. and Z. Wang. 2014. Unzipping androgen action through ZIP9: A novel membrane androgen receptor. *Endocrinology* 155 (11):4120–3. doi: 10.1210/en.2014-1749.

Pearce, E. J. and B. Everts. 2015. Dendritic cell metabolism. *Nat Rev Immunol* 15 (1):18–29. doi: 10.1038/nri3771.

Peretz, A., J. Neve, O. Jeghers, and F. Pelen. 1993. Zinc distribution in blood components, inflammatory status, and clinical indexes of disease activity during zinc supplementation in inflammatory rheumatic diseases. *Am J Clin Nutr* 57 (5):690–4.

Petkovic, V., M. C. Miletta, and P. E. Mullis. 2012. From endoplasmic reticulum to secretory granules: Role of zinc in the secretory pathway of growth hormone. *Endocr Dev* 23:96–108. doi: 10.1159/000341763.

Plum, L. M., A. Brieger, G. Engelhardt, S. Hebel, A. Nessel, M. Arlt, J. Kaltenberg, U. Schwaneberg, M. Huber, L. Rink, and H. Haase. 2014. PTEN-inhibition by zinc ions augments interleukin-2-mediated Akt phosphorylation. *Metallomics* 6 (7):1277–87. doi: 10.1039/c3mt00197k.

Prasad, A. S. 1991. Discovery of human zinc deficiency and studies in an experimental human model. *Am J Clin Nutr* 53 (2):403–12.

Prasad, A. S. 2000. Effects of zinc deficiency on Th1 and Th2 cytokine shifts. *J Infect Dis* 182 Suppl 1:S62–8. doi: 10.1086/315916.

Prasad, A. S. 2014. Zinc: An antioxidant and anti-inflammatory agent: Role of zinc in degenerative disorders of aging. *J Trace Elem Med Biol* 28 (4):364–71. doi: 10.1016/j.jtemb.2014.07.019.

Prasad, A. S., J. T. Fitzgerald, J. W. Hess, J. Kaplan, F. Pelen, and M. Dardenne. 1993. Zinc deficiency in elderly patients. *Nutrition* 9 (3):218–24.

Prasad, A. S., S. Meftah, J. Abdallah, J. Kaplan, G. J. Brewer, J. F. Bach, and M. Dardenne. 1988. Serum thymulin in human zinc deficiency. *J Clin Invest* 82 (4):1202–10. doi: 10.1172/jci113717.

Prasad, A. S., A. Miale, Jr., Z. Farid, H. H. Sandstead, and A. R. Schulert. 1963. Zinc metabolism in patients with the syndrome of iron deficiency anemia, hepatosplenomegaly, dwarfism, and hypognadism. *J Lab Clin Med* 61:537–49.

Radtke, F., R. Heuchel, O. Georgiev, M. Hergersberg, M. Gariglio, Z. Dembic, and W. Schaffner. 1993. Cloned transcription factor MTF-1 activates the mouse metallothionein I promoter. *EMBO J* 12 (4):1355–62.

Rajagopalan, S. and E. O. Long. 1998. Zinc bound to the killer cell-inhibitory receptor modulates the negative signal in human NK cells. *J Immunol* 161 (3):1299–305.

Ramsaransing, G. S., S. A. Mellema, and J. De Keyser. 2009. Dietary patterns in clinical subtypes of multiple sclerosis: An exploratory study. *Nutr J* 8:36. doi: 10.1186/1475-2891-8-36.

Rasker, J. J. and S. H. Kardaun. 1982. Lack of beneficial effect of zinc sulphate in rheumatoid arthritis. *Scand J Rheumatol* 11 (3):168–70.

Raulin, J. 1869. Études Chimique sur la Végétation. *Annales des Sciences Naturelles Botanique et Biologie Végétale* 11:293–299.

Riccioni, G. and N. D'Orazio. 2005. The role of selenium, zinc and antioxidant vitamin supplementation in the treatment of bronchial asthma: Adjuvant therapy or not? *Expert Opin Investig Drugs* 14 (9):1145–55. doi: 10.1517/13543784.14.9.1145.

Richter, M., R. Bonneau, M. A. Girard, C. Beaulieu, and P. Larivee. 2003. Zinc status modulates bronchopulmonary eosinophil infiltration in a murine model of allergic inflammation. *Chest* 123 (3 Suppl):446S.

Rink, L. and P. Gabriel. 2000. Zinc and the immune system. *Proc Nutr Soc* 59 (4):541–52.

Romir, J., H. Lilie, C. Egerer-Sieber, F. Bauer, H. Sticht, and Y. A. Muller. 2007. Crystal structure analysis and solution studies of human Lck-SH3; zinc-induced homodimerization competes with the binding of proline-rich motifs. *J Mol Biol* 365 (5):1417–28. doi: 10.1016/j.jmb.2006.10.058.

Roohani, N., R. Hurrell, R. Kelishadi, and R. Schulin. 2013. Zinc and its importance for human health: An integrative review. *J Res Med Sci* 18 (2):144–57.

Rosenkranz, E., R. D. Hilgers, P. Uciechowski, A. Petersen, B. Plumakers, and L. Rink. 2015. Zinc enhances the number of regulatory T cells in allergen-stimulated cells from atopic subjects. *Eur J Nutr.* doi: 10.1007/s00394-015-1100-1.

Rosenkranz, E., M. Maywald, R. D. Hilgers, A. Brieger, T. Clarner, M. Kipp, B. Plumakers, S. Meyer, T. Schwerdtle, and L. Rink. 2016a. Induction of regulatory T cells in Th1-/Th17-driven experimental autoimmune encephalomyelitis by zinc administration. *J Nutr Biochem* 29:116–23. doi: 10.1016/j.jnutbio.2015.11.010.

Rosenkranz, E., C. H. Metz, M. Maywald, R. D. Hilgers, I. Wessels, T. Senff, H. Haase, M. Jager, M. Ott, R. Aspinall, B. Plumakers, and L. Rink. 2016b. Zinc supplementation induces regulatory T cells by inhibition of Sirt-1 deacetylase in mixed lymphocyte cultures. *Mol Nutr Food Res* 60 (3):661–71. doi: 10.1002/mnfr.201500524.

Ryu, M. S., G. J. Guthrie, A. B. Maki, T. B. Aydemir, and R. J. Cousins. 2012. Proteomic analysis shows the upregulation of erythrocyte dematin in zinc-restricted human subjects. *Am J Clin Nutr* 95 (5):1096–102. doi: 10.3945/ajcn.111.032862.

Schubert, C., K. Guttek, K. Grungreiff, A. Thielitz, F. Buhling, A. Reinhold, S. Brocke, and D. Reinhold. 2014. Oral zinc aspartate treats experimental autoimmune encephalomyelitis. *Biometals* 27 (6):1249–62. doi: 10.1007/s10534-014-9786-8.

Schuetz, A., D. Nana, C. Rose, G. Zocher, M. Milanovic, J. Koenigsmann, R. Blasig, U. Heinemann, and D. Carstanjen. 2011. The structure of the Klf4 DNA-binding domain links to self-renewal and macrophage differentiation. *Cell Mol Life Sci* 68 (18):3121–31. doi: 10.1007/s00018-010-0618-x.

Scott, D. A. 1934. Crystalline insulin. *Biochem J* 28 (4):1592–1602.1.

Scott, B. J. and A. R. Bradwell. 1983. Identification of the serum binding proteins for iron, zinc, cadmium, nickel, and calcium. *Clin Chem* 29 (4):629–33.

Sedighi, B., H. A. Ebrahimi, A. A. Haghdoost, and M. Abotorabi. 2013. Comparison of serum levels of copper and zinc among multiple sclerosis patients and control group. *Iran J Neurol* 12 (4):125–8.

Shankar, A. H. and A. S. Prasad. 1998. Zinc and immune function: The biological basis of altered resistance to infection. *Am J Clin Nutr* 68 (2 Suppl):447S–63.

Shen, H., Y. Zhang, J. Xu, J. Long, H. Qin, F. Liu, and J. Guo. 2007. Zinc distribution and expression pattern of ZnT3 in mouse brain. *Biol Trace Elem Res* 119 (2):166–74. doi: 10.1007/s12011-007-0056-2.

Sim, D. L. and V. T. Chow. 1999. The novel human HUEL (C4orf1) gene maps to chromosome 4p12-p13 and encodes a nuclear protein containing the nuclear receptor interaction motif. *Genomics* 59 (2):224–33. doi: 10.1006/geno.1999.5856.

Simkin, P. A. 1976. Oral zinc sulphate in rheumatoid arthritis. *Lancet* 2 (7985):539–42.

Singh, M. and R. R. Das. 2011. Zinc for the common cold. *Cochrane Database Syst Rev* (2):Cd001364. doi: 10.1002/14651858.CD001364.pub3.

Solomons, N. W. 1986. Competitive interaction of iron and zinc in the diet: Consequences for human nutrition. *J Nutr* 116 (6):927–35.

Solomons, N. W., R. A. Jacob, O. Pineda, and F. Viteri. 1979. Studies on the bioavailability of zinc in man. II. Absorption of zinc from organic and inorganic sources. *J Lab Clin Med* 94 (2):335–43.

Stennicke, H. R. and G. S. Salvesen. 1997. Biochemical characteristics of caspases-3, -6, -7, and -8. *J Biol Chem* 272 (41):25719–23.

Stoye, D., C. Schubert, A. Goihl, K. Guttek, A. Reinhold, S. Brocke, K. Grungreiff, and D. Reinhold. 2012. Zinc aspartate suppresses T cell activation in vitro and relapsing experimental autoimmune encephalomyelitis in SJL/J mice. *Biometals* 25 (3):529–39. doi: 10.1007/s10534-012-9532-z.

Subramanian Vignesh, K., J. A. Landero Figueroa, A. Porollo, J. A. Caruso, and G. S. Deepe, Jr. 2013. Granulocyte macrophage-colony stimulating factor induced Zn sequestration enhances macrophage superoxide and limits intracellular pathogen survival. *Immunity* 39 (4):697–710. doi: 10.1016/j.immuni.2013.09.006.

Sun, Q., W. Zhong, W. Zhang, Q. Li, X. Sun, X. Tan, X. Sun, D. Dong, and Z. Zhou. 2015. Zinc deficiency mediates alcohol-induced apoptotic cell death in the liver of rats through activating ER and mitochondrial cell death pathways. *Am J Physiol Gastrointest Liver Physiol* 308 (9):G757–66. doi: 10.1152/ajpgi.00442.2014.

Tanaka, Y., S. Shiozawa, I. Morimoto, and T. Fujita. 1990. Role of zinc in interleukin 2 (IL-2)-mediated T-cell activation. *Scand J Immunol* 31 (5):547–52.

Tang, A. M., N. M. Graham, A. J. Kirby, L. D. McCall, W. C. Willett, and A. J. Saah. 1993. Dietary micronutrient intake and risk of progression to acquired immunodeficiency syndrome (AIDS) in human immunodeficiency virus type 1 (HIV-1)-infected homosexual men. *Am J Epidemiol* 138 (11):937–51.

Taylor, K., J. Gee, and P. Kille. 2011. Zinc and cancer. In *Zinc in Human Health*, edited by L. Rink, 283–304. Netherlands: IOS Press BV.

Taylor, K. M., S. Hiscox, R. I. Nicholson, C. Hogstrand, and P. Kille. 2012. Protein kinase CK2 triggers cytosolic zinc signaling pathways by phosphorylation of zinc channel ZIP7. *Sci Signal* 5 (210):ra11. doi: 10.1126/scisignal.2002585.

Taylor, K. M., H. E. Morgan, K. Smart, N. M. Zahari, S. Pumford, I. O. Ellis, J. F. Robertson, and R. I. Nicholson. 2007. The emerging role of the LIV-1 subfamily of zinc transporters in breast cancer. *Mol Med* 13 (7–8):396–406. doi: 10.2119/2007-00040.Taylor.

Taylor, K. M., P. Vichova, N. Jordan, S. Hiscox, R. Hendley, and R. I. Nicholson. 2008. ZIP7-mediated intracellular zinc transport contributes to aberrant growth factor signaling in antihormone-resistant breast cancer Cells. *Endocrinology* 149 (10):4912–20. doi: 10.1210/en.2008-0351.

Todd, W.K., A. Evelym, and E.B. Hart. 1934. Zinc in the nutrition of the rat. *Am J Physiol* 107:146–56.

Treves, S., P. L. Trentini, M. Ascanelli, G. Bucci, and F. Di Virgilio. 1994. Apoptosis is dependent on intracellular zinc and independent of intracellular calcium in lymphocytes. *Exp Cell Res* 211 (2):339–43. doi: 10.1006/excr.1994.1096.

Truong-Tran, A. Q., L. H. Ho, F. Chai, and P. D. Zalewski. 2000. Cellular zinc fluxes and the regulation of apoptosis/gene-directed cell death. *J Nutr* 130 (5S Suppl):1459S–66.

Truong-Tran, A. Q., R. E. Ruffin, and P. D. Zalewski. 2000. Visualization of labile zinc and its role in apoptosis of primary airway epithelial cells and cell lines. *Am J Physiol Lung Cell Mol Physiol* 279 (6):L1172–83.

U.S. Department of Agriculture, Agricultural Research Service. 2011. USDA National Nutrient Database for Standard References, Release 24. Nutrient Data Labratory Home Page, http://www.ars.usda.gov/ba/bhnrc/ndl.

Vallee, B. L. and K. H. Falchuk. 1993. The biochemical basis of zinc physiology. *Physiol Rev* 73 (1):79–118.

von Bulow, V., S. Dubben, G. Engelhardt, S. Hebel, B. Plumakers, H. Heine, L. Rink, and H. Haase. 2007. Zinc-dependent suppression of TNF-alpha production is mediated by protein kinase A-induced inhibition of Raf-1, I kappa B kinase beta, and NF-kappa B. *J Immunol* 179 (6):4180–6.

Wang, F., J. Dufner-Beattie, B. E. Kim, M. J. Petris, G. Andrews, and D. J. Eide. 2004. Zinc-stimulated endocytosis controls activity of the mouse ZIP1 and ZIP3 zinc uptake transporters. *J Biol Chem* 279 (23):24631–9. doi: 10.1074/jbc.M400680200.

Wang, K., B. Zhou, Y. M. Kuo, J. Zemansky, and J. Gitschier. 2002. A novel member of a zinc transporter family is defective in acrodermatitis enteropathica. *Am J Hum Genet* 71 (1):66–73. doi: 10.1086/341125.

Wellinghausen, N., H. Kirchner, and L. Rink. 1997. The immunobiology of zinc. *Immunol Today* 18 (11):519–21.

Wellinghausen, N. and L. Rink. 1998. The significance of zinc for leukocyte biology. *J Leukoc Biol* 64 (5):571–7.

Wessels, I., H. Haase, G. Engelhardt, L. Rink, and P. Uciechowski. 2013. Zinc deficiency induces production of the proinflammatory cytokines IL-1beta and TNFalpha in promyeloid cells via epigenetic and redox-dependent mechanisms. *J Nutr Biochem* 24 (1):289–97. doi: 10.1016/j.jnutbio.2012.06.007.

Wex, T., K. Grungreiff, K. Schutte, M. Stengritt, and D. Reinhold. 2014. Expression analysis of zinc transporters in resting and stimulated human peripheral blood mononuclear cells. *Biomed Rep* 2 (2):217–222. doi: 10.3892/br.2014.219.

WHO/UNICEF. 2004. *Joint Statement—Clinical Management of Acute Diarrhoea*. New York, NY/Geneva: The United Nations Children's Fund/World Health Organization.

Wong, C. P., N. A. Rinaldi, and E. Ho. 2015. Zinc deficiency enhanced inflammatory response by increasing immune cell activation and inducing IL6 promoter demethylation. *Mol Nutr Food Res* 59 (5):991–9. doi: 10.1002/mnfr.201400761.

Wu, W., I. Jaspers, W. Zhang, L. M. Graves, and J. M. Samet. 2002. Role of Ras in metal-induced EGF receptor signaling and NF-kappaB activation in human airway epithelial cells. *Am J Physiol Lung Cell Mol Physiol* 282 (5):L1040–8. doi: 10.1152/ajplung.00390.2001.

Yu, M., W. W. Lee, D. Tomar, S. Pryshchep, M. Czesnikiewicz-Guzik, D. L. Lamar, G. Li, K. Singh, L. Tian, C. M. Weyand, and J. J. Goronzy. 2011. Regulation of T cell receptor signaling by activation-induced zinc influx. *J Exp Med* 208 (4):775–85. doi: 10.1084/jem.20100031.

Zalewski, P. 2011. Zinc in mammalian cell cycle and cell death. In *Zinc in Human Health*, edited by L. Rink, 63–93. Netherlands: IOS Press BV.

Zalewski, P. D., I. J. Forbes, and W. H. Betts. 1993. Correlation of apoptosis with change in intracellular labile Zn(II) using zinquin [(2-methyl-8-p-toluenesulphonamido-6-quinolyloxy)acetic acid], a new specific fluorescent probe for Zn(II). *Biochem J* 296 (Pt 2):403–8.

Zalewski, P. D., A. Q. Truong-Tran, D. Grosser, L. Jayaram, C. Murgia, and R. E. Ruffin. 2005. Zinc metabolism in airway epithelium and airway inflammation: Basic mechanisms and clinical targets. A review. *Pharmacol Ther* 105 (2):127–49. doi: 10.1016/j.pharmthera.2004.09.004.

Zeng, L. and L. Zhang. 2011. Efficacy and safety of zinc supplementation for adults, children and pregnant women with HIV infection: Systematic review. *Trop Med Int Health* 16 (12):1474–82. doi: 10.1111/j.1365-3156.2011.02871.x.

Zhao, H. and D. Eide. 1996. The yeast ZRT1 gene encodes the zinc transporter protein of a high-affinity uptake system induced by zinc limitation. *Proc Natl Acad Sci U S A* 93 (6):2454–8.

Zoli, A., L. Altomonte, R. Caricchio, A. Galossi, L. Mirone, M. P. Ruffini, and M. Magaro. 1998. Serum zinc and copper in active rheumatoid arthritis: Correlation with interleukin 1 beta and tumour necrosis factor alpha. *Clin Rheumatol* 17 (5):378–82.

16 Short-Chain Fatty Acids, G Protein-Coupled Receptors, and Immune Cells

José Luís Fachi, Renan O. Corrêa, Fabio T. Sato, Angélica T. Vieira, Hosana G. Rodrigues, and Marco Aurélio R. Vinolo

CONTENTS

16.1 Introduction 279
16.2 G Protein-Coupled Receptors 281
16.3 Effect of SCFAs In Epithelial Cells and Leukocytes 282
16.4 Regulation of Inflammation by SCFAs 285
16.5 SCFAs and Infection 286
References 288

16.1 INTRODUCTION

Short-chain fatty acids (SCFAs) are a group of fatty acids that comprises small carboxylic acids (from 1 to 6 carbons in their structure) produced mainly, but not exclusively, by anaerobic bacteria as end products of fermentation. The main components of this class of molecules are acetic, propionic, and butyric acids, which are usually found in the deprotonated forms (salts) as acetate, propionate, and butyrate (Figure 16.1a). As expected, SCFA concentrations are high in the gastrointestinal tract (GI tract), where they are released by bacteria of the microbiota after fermentation of fiber and resistant starches. In the proximal colon, their concentrations range from 70 to 140 mM, while in the distal colon lower concentrations have been described (20–70 mM) (Wong et al. 2006). Additionally, these bacterial metabolites are also present in high concentrations in the oral cavity and female genital tract, where, as described later in the chapter, they may play a role in tissue homeostasis, particularly in the immune interactions with bacteria and other microorganisms.

Different metabolic pathways are involved in the production of SCFAs. Depending on the bacterial species involved and on environmental factors, including type and availability of substrate, pH, and oxygen tension, the flow through the metabolic pathways may be different, affecting the amount and proportions of SCFAs produced (Louis, Hold, and Flint 2014). In general, the major metabolic pathways involved in the production of SCFAs are the Embden–Meyerhof–Parnas (glycolysis) and the pentose pathways (Tan et al. 2014; Miller and Wolin 1996) as summarized in Figure 16.1b. Pyruvate produced in these pathways is in part converted to acetyl-CoA, which can be hydrolyzed, generating acetate. Additionally, acetate can be produced in the Wood-Ljungdahl pathway from CO_2 and hydrogen or from formate (Figure 16.1b).

Propionate is mainly produced in the succinate pathway, but other pathways, which use lactate or deoxyhexose sugars as substrate (propanediol and acrylate pathways), also contribute to the generation of propionate. Butyrate is produced from two molecules of acetyl-CoA, which are converted to

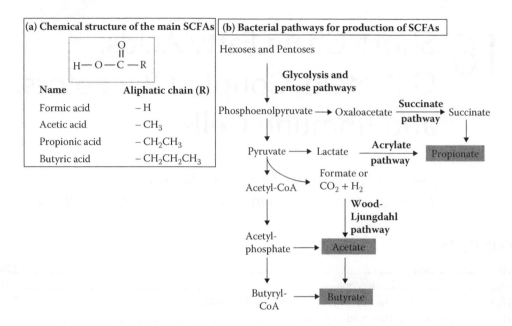

FIGURE 16.1 (a) Chemical structure and (b) bacterial pathways for the production of short-chain fatty acids (SCFAs).

butyryl CoA. This latter molecule is converted by butyrate kinase or via butyryl CoA:acetate CoA transferase to butyrate (Pryde et al. 2002; Louis, Hold, and Flint 2014) (Figure 16.1b).

It is important to highlight that there is a complex metabolic interaction between different species of bacteria, which is important for their survival and colonization. The cooperation between *Aggregatibacter actinomycetemcomitans*, an oral pathogen, and *Streptococcus gordonii*, a common component of oral microbiota (Ramsey, Rumbaugh, and Whiteley 2011), is an example of this. Briefly, the ability of *A. actinomycetemcomitans* to cause infection is enhanced in the presence of the commensal bacteria *S. gordonii*. The mechanism behind this effect involves lactate, the main metabolite of *S. gordonii*, which is an important substrate catabolized by *A. actinomycetemcomitans* (Ramsey, Rumbaugh, and Whiteley 2011). In other tissues, a similar metabolic cooperation between bacteria is observed, as in the intestine, where a close relation between, for example, acetate-producing bacteria and butyrate-producers (these latter bacteria can use acetate as substrate) has been demonstrated (Barcenilla et al. 2000; Duncan et al. 2004).

In addition to their uptake and use by other bacteria, SCFAs released in the intestine cross the epithelial cells through passive (nonionized form) or active (ionized form that is transported by receptors such as monocarboxylate transporter 1 [MCT-1] and sodium-coupled monocarboxylate transporter 1 [SMCT-1]) mechanisms and reach the blood circulation. A small fraction of the SCFAs absorbed in the intestine enters the systemic circulation, since they are metabolized by epithelial cells and in the liver. Indeed, the serum/plasma concentrations of these bacterial metabolites are much lower than their intestinal concentrations: serum concentration of acetate has been reported to be between 60 and 150 µM, while propionate and butyrate are found in even lower concentrations, respectively, 3–7 µM and 1–4 µM (Vogt, Pencharz, and Wolever 2004; Wolever et al. 1997, 2002).

In this chapter, we summarize the cellular responses induced/modulated by SCFAs focusing on their G protein–coupled receptor–dependent effects on cells involved in the immune response and protection of the host (i.e., leukocytes and epithelial cells). We also discuss some recent studies that implicate SCFAs in the regulation of inflammation and the response to infectious agents.

16.2   G PROTEIN-COUPLED RECEPTORS

SCFAs activate different biological responses depending mainly on their concentrations, the target tissue and the receptor/mechanism activated. There are at least two major molecular mechanisms that account for the cellular effects of SCFAs (reviewed by Vinolo et al. 2011c; Tan et al. 2014). The first involves activation of membrane receptors coupled to G proteins (GPCRs), which will be discussed in more detail below. The second is through inhibition of a class of enzymes called histone deacetylases (HDACs). These latter enzymes are divided into four classes: class I (HDACs 1, 2, 3, and 8), class IIa (HDACs 4, 5, 7, and 9) and IIb (HDACs 6 and 10), class III (SIRT 1, 2, and 3) and class IV (HDAC 11). The HDACs, which remove acetyl groups from lysine residues of proteins, together with the histone acetyltransferases, enzymes that add acetyl groups to the lysine residues of proteins, control the acetylation status of histones and nonhistone proteins. SCFAs inhibit HDACs (isoforms of class I and II HDACs, in this order of potency: butyrate>propionate>acetate) and, by doing that, they modulate the expression of several genes. Within the effects that seem to be mediated by inhibition of HDACs are their actions on dendritic cell differentiation and activation, regulation of the production of inflammatory mediators by neutrophils and macrophages, and stimulation of regulatory T cell generation (Vinolo et al. 2011c; Smith et al. 2013; Wong et al. 2006).

GPCRs constitute a family of membrane proteins characterized by a common motif, the seven-transmembrane domain. These receptors are activated by numerous ligands including photons, ions (e.g., calcium-sensing receptor [CaSR]), nucleoside phosphates (e.g., receptors P2Y whose ligands include ATP, ADP, and UDP), fatty acids and other lipids (e.g., free fatty acid receptors [FFAR 1, 2, 3 and 4]), and prostanoids (e.g., receptors such as the prostaglandin D receptors DP-1 and 2, and the prostaglandin E receptors EP1, 2, 3, and 4) (http://www.guidetopharmacology.org/GRAC). The GPCRs and their ligands present a crucial role in different physiological and pathological conditions and are important targets of drugs.

Regarding the immune system, the chemoattractant receptors, which are GPCRs activated by chemokines, lipid mediators including platelet-activating factor (PAF) and leukotriene B_4 (LTB_4), complement fragments C3a and C5a, and other molecules including microbe ligands, such as the formylated peptides, are essential for normal function. The binding of ligands to these receptors leads to conformational changes and activation of heterotrimeric G proteins. These latter proteins are formed by three components, α, β, and γ, that are released (α and $\beta\gamma$ subunits) after receptor activation. Through interaction with intracellular proteins, these subunits can increase or decrease the activity of effector proteins such as adenylyl and guanylyl cyclases, ion channels, phospholipases (PLA_2 and C), and phosphatidylinositol 3-kinases (PI3Ks), leading to distinct downstream signaling pathways (further details in Katritch, Cherezov, and Stevens 2013).

As already mentioned, some of the biological responses to SCFAs are secondary to the activation of GPCRs. At least three GPCRs are activated by SCFAs: GPR41, also known as free fatty acid receptor-3 (FFAR3), GPR43 (FFAR2), and GPR109A, also known as Niacin receptor-1 or hydroxycarboxylic acid receptor-2 (HCA2) (Table 16.1). FFAR2 and FFAR3 are activated by acetate, propionate, and butyrate, but these ligands present a different order of potency depending on the receptor: for FFAR2, the potency is acetate=propionate>butyrate>other SCFAs and for FFAR3 propionate and butyrate are more potent than acetate (Brown et al. 2003). These receptors also show some differences in their tissue distribution and biological functions, as reviewed by us and others (Vinolo, Hirabara, and Curi 2012; Tan et al. 2014; Hara et al. 2014) (Table 16.1). In the context of the immune response, it is important to highlight that FFAR2 is highly expressed in myeloid cells, especially in neutrophils, and that both FFAR2 and FFAR3 are expressed by intestinal epithelial cells (Kim et al. 2013; Park et al. 2015). As described later in this chapter, the activation of the latter cells leads to the production of important inflammatory mediators including cytokines and chemokines (Kim et al. 2013). Additionally, high expression of FFAR2 has been observed in colonic regulatory T cells in which this receptor seems to play a role in the differentiation process (Smith et al. 2013).

TABLE 16.1
Overview of the Receptors Activated by SCFAs

Nomenclature	FFAR3 (GPR41)	FFAR2 (GPR43)	GPR109A (HCA2)
SCFA agonists	Propionate = butyrate > acetate	Acetate = propionate > butyrate	Butyrate
Other agonists	Synthetic agonists	Phenilacetamides	Nicotinic acid, (D)-beta-hydroxybutyrate, MK-0354, and others
Tissue expression	Adipose tissue, GI tract, liver, spleen, bone marrow, brain, pancreas, leukocytes, and others	Leukocytes, pancreas, adipose tissue, and GI tract	Adipose tissue, pancreas, leukocytes, and GI tract
Main biological effects in the immune system	Modulation of cytokine production; production of antimicrobial peptides	Modulation of cytokine production; production of antimicrobial peptides; neutrophil chemotaxis; regulatory T cell homeostasis; inflammasome activation; apoptosis	Anti-inflammatory; apoptosis; regulatory T cell homeostasis; inflammasome activation

GPR109A was first described as a receptor for nicotinic acid and it was associated with the antilipolytic effect of nicotinic acid (Soga et al. 2003; Brown et al. 2003; Tunaru et al. 2003). A subsequent study demonstrated that, in addition to nicotinic acid, (D)-beta-hydroxybutyrate, butyrate, and other molecules act as ligands (Taggart et al. 2005). GPR109A is expressed by several cell types (e.g., macrophages, dendritic cells, epithelial cells, adipocytes, neutrophils, and lymphocytes) and different biological responses including modulation of the production of anti-inflammatory cytokines and apoptosis have been associated with its activation by butyrate and its other ligands (Taggart et al. 2005; Zimmerman et al. 2012; Singh et al. 2014).

16.3   EFFECT OF SCFAs IN EPITHELIAL CELLS AND LEUKOCYTES

Epithelial cells of the skin, gastrointestinal, respiratory, and genitourinary tracts act as a physical and chemical barrier to the entrance of microorganisms. These cells are especially important in the detection of microorganisms and harmful substances outside the body and not only protect the host organism passively through their physical barrier function, but also actively by secreting substances such as mucus and antimicrobial molecules (e.g., lysozyme, defensins, and cathelicidins). Additionally, through the production of cytokines and chemokines, they regulate immune processes (Shaykhiev and Bals 2007).

The role of SCFAs as an energetic substrate for colonic epithelial cells is well established in the literature (Roediger 1982). Indeed, reductions in their concentrations in the colon may lead to mucosal atrophy, diminished absorption, and colitis. Soon after their production in the colon by the microbiota, butyrate is rapidly metabolized by colonocytes, being their major energy source, while acetate and propionate are directed to the liver by the portal vein. A large amount of propionate is utilized by the hepatocytes, while acetate enters the systemic circulation and is metabolized by peripheral tissues (Pomare, Branch, and Cummings 1985). Moreover, SCFAs drive many other roles in colonic physiology including regulation of colonocyte proliferation and differentiation, gut mobility, and immune responses/inflammation.

In the 1950s, Nieman (1954) described the direct antimicrobial activities of free fatty acids, acting probably by disrupting the membrane structure, electron transport, proton gradient, or even the membrane potential of the microorganisms. More recently, it has been suggested that SCFAs modulate the expression of host defense peptides (HDPs) in colonocytes or even in some immune/inflammatory cells (Raqib et al. 2006). HDPs, also known as antimicrobial peptides, constitute a defense mechanism of the innate immune system and are found in nearly all forms of life. HDPs are able to kill a broad range of microorganisms through physical interaction and disruption of the membrane (Hancock 2006; Zasloff 2002). Among the SCFAs, butyrate was the most potent enhancer of multiple (porcine) β-defensin and cathelicidin genes (Zeng et al. 2013). Butyrate increased cathelicidin LL-37 mRNA and protein expression in both rabbits and humans (Raqib et al. 2006, 2012). Butyrate acts mainly due to inhibition of HDACs, which results in a less-compact chromatin, modulating the transcription of different genes (Sunkara, Jiang, and Zhang 2012).

In addition to their effect on the production of antimicrobial peptides, SCFAs also modulate the production of cytokines and chemokines by epithelial cells. Kim et al. (2013) suggested that mice enteroendocrine cells and colonic enterocytes play an important role in the inflammatory response dependent on SCFAs. They found high expression of FFAR2 and FFAR3 in these cells and demonstrated that SCFAs, through these receptors, regulate the production of proinflammatory cytokines and chemokines in response to bacterial products. After *in vitro* activation of epithelial cells with bacterial products for 24 hours, there was an increase in the expression of the *Il6*, *Cxcl1*, and *Cxcl10* genes in the presence of acetate and propionate. Additionally, the expression of *Il6* was slightly increased in cells incubated with acetate and propionate in the absence of bacterial products. These responses were abrogated when cells were pretreated with pertussis toxin (an inhibitor of GPCRs) or when using cells from FFAR2$^{-/-}$ or FFAR3$^{-/-}$ mice, indicating the participation of these receptors in this effect of SCFAs. This study also suggested that phosphorylation of extracellular signal-regulated kinase (ERK) through FFAR2 and FFAR3 by acetate and propionate is involved in the effect on colonic epithelial cells.

Other studies have explored the effect of SCFAs on various types of leukocyte. *In vivo* and *in vitro* evidence suggests that, in the absence of inflammation, SCFAs act as neutrophil chemoattractants through activation of FFAR2 (Le Poul et al. 2003; Vinolo et al. 2009b, 2011a; Sina et al. 2009; Maslowski et al. 2009). However, in the presence of other chemoattractants or during inflammation, the effect of SCFAs on neutrophil recruitment is less clear, as discussed in a recent review (Rodrigues et al. 2015). Other functional aspects of neutrophils modulated by SCFAs include the production of reactive oxygen species (ROS), degranulation, and their ability to phagocytose microorganisms and particles. Regarding ROS production and phagocytosis of microorganisms and particles by neutrophils, both increases and decreases have been described in the literature. Murine bone marrow isolated neutrophils showed increased production of ROS and enhanced phagocytosis when incubated with acetate, an effect not observed in cells from FFAR2$^{-/-}$ mice (Maslowski et al. 2009). Human neutrophils incubated with butyrate or acetate also show increased ROS production, as shown by Mirmonsef et al. (2012). However, other studies performed with neutrophils found that SCFAs do not affect, or even inhibit, ROS production and phagocytosis (Mills, Montgomery, and Morck 2006; Sandoval et al. 2007; Vinolo et al. 2009a; Liu et al. 2001). It is not clear why these findings are inconsistent.

Neutrophils are an important source of signaling molecules including cytokines (i.e., tumor necrosis factor-α [TNF-α], interleukin-1β, and interleukin-6), chemokines (i.e., CXCL1, CXCL2, CXCL3, CCL2, CCL3, and CXCL8), and lipid mediators (i.e., lipoxins, leukotrienes, prostaglandins, hydroxyeicosotetraenoic acids, and resolvins) (Dalli and Serhan 2012; Mantovani et al. 2011; Tecchio and Cassatella 2014). In this context, it has been shown that SCFAs decrease the production of TNF-α by neutrophils (Tedelind et al. 2007; Vinolo et al. 2011b), and that butyrate and propionate decrease the production of CXCL3/CINC-2 by rat neutrophils (Vinolo et al. 2011b).

Some studies also indicate that SCFAs can induce apoptosis in neutrophils (Aoyama, Kotani, and Usami 2010; Maslowski et al. 2009). Aoyama, Kotani, and Usami (2010) found that propionate and butyrate, through a GPCR-independent mechanism, activate caspases leading to apoptosis. Maslowski et al. (2009) also demonstrated that SCFA activate apoptotic pathways, but in this case an association with FFAR2 activation was found.

The function of dendritic cells (DCs) and macrophages, two other important components of the innate immune system, is also modified by SCFAs. Millard et al. (2002) reported that butyrate reduced the phagocytic activity of macrophages by inhibiting their differentiation and maturation. However, the mechanisms for this action are not clear. Park et al. (2007) found a reduction in the interferon (IFN)-γ-induced expression of iNOS, TNF-α, and IL-6 in RAW264.7 macrophage-like cells incubated with butyrate. Moreover, an increase in the production of the anti-inflammatory cytokine IL-10 was also observed in these cells incubated with butyrate. A similar pattern of cytokine production was seen by Liu et al. (2012a). In this latter study, the authors also demonstrated that SCFAs, especially propionate, reduce NO production in a concentration-dependent manner. Moreover, LPS-induced translocation of p65 to the nucleus and NF-kB activity have been shown to be attenuated by SCFAs, suggesting that SCFAs reduce the production of these inflammatory mediators by interfering with the NF-kB pathway, an effect also observed in neutrophils (Vinolo et al. 2011b; Liu et al. 2012b). More recently, Chang et al. (2013) found that butyrate decreases the expression of some proinflammatory genes including *Nos2*, *Il6*, and *Il12*, while it did not affect the expression of others, including *Tnfa* and *Ccl2*. This study, conducted using murine bone marrow–derived macrophages (BMDMs), indicated that the effects on gene expression are due to the ability of butyrate to inhibit HDACs. Additionally, Singh et al. (2014) described a macrophage-dependent anti-inflammatory profile of colonic CD4+ cells, through activation of GPR109A by butyrate, in which macrophages (and DCs) were able to induce differentiation of naive T cells into regulatory T cells (Tregs). This study showed that *Niacr1−/−* mice (mice lacking GPR109A) have a reduced number of colonic Foxp3+ (Treg) cells/IL-10-producing T cells and an enhanced number of proinflammatory IL-17-producing CD4+ T cells when compared to wild-type animals. However, since T cells (as well as B-cells and NK cells) do not express GPR109A, these effects could not be explained by a direct action on them. On the other hand, macrophages and DCs do express this receptor, and the authors demonstrated that these cells, when taken from *Niacr1−/−* mice, lack the ability to induce differentiation of Tregs/IL-10-producing T cells. In addition, by incubating wild-type macrophages and DCs with butyrate, there was an increase in the expression of anti-inflammatory genes as *Il10* and *Aldh1a1*, which are important mediators toward Treg differentiation.

An effect of SCFAs on differentiation and maturation of DCs from human monocytes was proposed by Millard et al. (2002). Butyrate treatment partially inhibited the differentiation of DCs into mature cells (probably by modulating NF-kB/Rel transcription factor family activation), since there was a maintenance of CD14 and a decrease of CD54, CD86, and HLA class II in the cells treated with butyrate. In addition, these cells had high phagocytic capacity and an altered capacity to produce IL-10 and IL-12, revealing their immature profile. Berndt et al. (2012) demonstrated that butyrate inhibited maturation of LPS-stimulated murine bone marrow-derived DCs. Furthermore, Liu et al. (2012a) showed that butyrate was able to inhibit dendrite formation (a distinctive morphology of mature DCs) of human monocyte-derived DCs *in vitro* when compared to LPS-induced DCs; furthermore, butyrate also led to formation of clusters and an increase in the cell volume (immature DC morphology). More importantly, the authors showed that butyrate downregulates HLA molecules, costimulatory molecules (CD80), CD1a, and specific maturation molecules (CD83), which are related to optimal T cell stimulatory capacity.

DCs are the bridge between innate and adaptive immunity, playing an important role in T cell activation, so alterations in DC effector mechanisms certainly lead to changes in T cell responses. Trompette et al. (2014), by studying allergic airway disease in mice, demonstrated that SCFAs produced in the intestine not only alter the gut microbiota but also impair Th2 differentiation. This latter effect was associated with the capacity of propionate (through FFAR3) to enhance hematopoiesis and the recruitment of DC precursors expressing lower levels of MHCII and CD40 to the lung, which showed a lower ability to activate effector Th2 cells. Another study showed how SCFAs interfere with DCs and generation of Tregs (Arpaia et al. 2013). The authors demonstrated that butyrate leads to an *in vitro* extrathymic Treg Foxp3+ differentiation, which is TGF-β-dependent. *In vivo*, there was a robust increase in the number of the peripheral Treg cells in microbiota-deficient mice (treated with broad-spectrum antibiotics [AVNM]) that received butyrate supplementation in their drinking water (pattern not seen for the thymic or colonic Treg cells). Similar experiments with CNS1$^{-/-}$ mice (CNS1 being an intronic *Foxp3* enhancer: animals have intact thymic differentiation, but they lack extrathymic Treg differentiation) revealed that this increase was not due to altered thymic output, but was due to increased extrathymic generation of this cell type. However, local provision of butyrate (and also acetate and propionate) was able to promote CNS1-dependent extrathymic generation of Tregs in the colonic epithelium. Furthermore, even though butyrate acts directly in the T cell promoting Treg differentiation, this SCFA has a bigger effect in the DCs, through HDAC inhibition, facilitating the generation of the Foxp3+ cells. Altogether, these pieces of information highlight the ability of SCFAs to modulate DCs and T cells toward a tolerogenic profile.

Zimmerman et al. (2012) demonstrated that butyrate was able to inhibit T cell proliferation (both CD4+ and CD8+ cells) in a dose-dependent manner. This inhibition was due to an increase of T cell death by Fas-dependent apoptosis. A low concentration of butyrate was able to increase the expression of Fas in T cells (both CD4+ and CD8+) by inhibiting HDACI enzymatic activity, which led to hyperacetylation of the Fas promoter. In humans, this T cell inhibition contributes to the anti-inflammatory effect of butyrate, since it acts together with a partial suppression of colonic inflammation by decreasing production of iNOS in colonic epithelial cells.

Park et al. (2015) reported that acetate, propionate, and butyrate support polarization of naive T cells into Th1, Th17, and Treg effector cells, this effect occurring through direct HDAC inhibition and independent of FFAR3/FFAR2. By incubating naive T cells *in vitro* with the SCFAs, the authors demonstrated that acetate (5–20 mM), propionate (0.5–1 mM), and butyrate (0.5 mM) increased polarization into Th17 cells, and when incubated with IL-12, also increased polarization into Th1 cells. However, even with higher expression of effector cytokines, the acetate-treated Th1 or Th17 cells did not show a high inflammatory profile *in vivo*. This is mainly explained by the fact that these cells produce high levels of IL-10 (a cytokine with regulatory activities on T cell responses) since SCFAs enhanced activation of STAT3, which coordinates the expression of cytokines, such as IL-10, IFN-γ, and IL-17. Moreover, administration of acetate in drinking water of mice did not change Th1 and Th17 balance in the absence of infection, but it changed this balance during infection with *C. rodentium*, while the infection itself decreased the number of IL-10-producing CD4+ T cells. As pointed out earlier, this effect of the SCFAs on T cells is associated with HDAC inhibition, which is independent of the FFAR3/FFAR2 receptors, since according to this study, T cells do not express FFAR3 and FFAR2 at functional levels.

16.4 REGULATION OF INFLAMMATION BY SCFAs

It has been shown that SCFAs induce significant anti-inflammatory effects and may have beneficial effects in chronic diseases such as inflammatory bowel disease, arthritis, asthma, and gout (Maslowski et al. 2009; Smith et al. 2013; Trompette et al. 2014). Administration of SCFAs to mice and humans alleviates certain inflammatory conditions (Harig et al. 1989; Maslowski et al. 2009; Chervonsky 2010). Therapeutic effects of SCFAs have been explored in patients with inflammatory bowel disease, especially with Crohn's disease. Daily enteric administration of butyrate-induced clinical improvement and remission of disease and also decreased mucosal levels of NF-kB and IL-1β (Di Sabatino et al. 2005). In experimental murine models of colitis, treatment with butyrate reduced inflammation in the colon and attenuated neutrophilic infiltration and proinflammatory cytokine release in the colonic mucosa, an effect that was also demonstrated with acetate treatment (Maslowski et al. 2009). Moreover, inflammatory responses are exacerbated in mice that lack the *Ffar2* gene, and these mice show poor ability to resolve inflammation. This receptor, which is highly expressed by polymorphonuclear cells (neutrophils and eosinophils) and macrophages, seems to participate in the beneficial effects of SCFAs on colitis.

Most of the anti-inflammatory functions of SCFAs are associated with their ability to modulate inflammatory cell migration, ROS release, and cytokine production, as previously described. Recently, new mechanisms, including induction of apoptosis of inflammatory leukocytes and on activation of the inflammasome, have been demonstrated. Apoptosis is essential for the safe clearance of inflammatory cells, including neutrophils. This process is part of a series of cellular/tissue changes associated with the regulation/resolution of inflammation and minimization of tissue damage (Savill and Haslett 1995; Serhan et al. 2007). Efficient resolution of inflammation requires the shutting down of the production of proinflammatory factors (Perez et al. 2014; Serhan, Chiang, and Van Dyke 2008; Buckley et al. 2013). Apoptotic leukocytes sequester cytokines thereby limiting the release of proinflammatory signals that perpetuate an inflammatory response. In this context, it is important to highlight that butyrate (and also propionate) induce apoptosis of nonactivated and LPS- or TNF-α-activated neutrophils by caspase-8 and caspase-9 pathways (Aoyama, Kotani, and Usami 2010), an effect that may be relevant for the resolution of inflammation.

Inflammasome activation has been reported to be important for maintenance of gut epithelial integrity by ensuring repair and cell survival under stress conditions (Zaki et al. 2010a, b; Dupaul-Chicoine et al. 2010; Elinav et al. 2011; Hirota et al. 2011). Indeed, factors that trigger activation of the inflammasome in nonhematopoietic cells in the gut are essential for repair and intestinal homeostasis, especially through IL-18 production (Zaki et al. 2010b; Elinav et al. 2011). More recently, the molecular pathways by which SCFAs may promote protection to the gut epithelium in colitis were clarified (Macia et al. 2015). Acetate was found to activate the inflammasome in colonic epithelial cells thought mechanisms that involve mobilization of intracellular Ca^{2+}, membrane hyperpolarization, and K^+ efflux (Macia et al. 2015). The mechanisms behind these effects involve the activation of FFAR2 and GPR109A in colonic cells, which leads to NLRP3 activation and release of IL-18, a cytokine that promotes epithelial repair and protection from colitis development.

16.5 SCFAs AND INFECTION

The microorganisms that colonize mucosal surfaces, which constitute the microbiota, contribute through several mechanisms toward the resistance against infections, including stimulation of the production of mucin and antimicrobial peptides by epithelial cells and immune system development and activation. Additionally, they limit the capacity of pathogens to colonize the tissue through, for example, generation of toxic metabolites derived from bile acid; physical and nutrient/metabolic competition; and production of antimicrobial molecules including bacteriocins (Stecher and Hardt 2008). Considering that, it is not a surprise that quali- or quantitative changes in the microbiota have been associated with modifications in the resistance or susceptibility to certain pathogens. In this context, SCFAs, which, as highlighted before, are bacterial metabolites that present several effects on cells involved in the immune defense, may be a key link between microbiota and host resistance to pathogens. Additionally, pathogenic bacteria can also produce and release SCFAs, which under certain circumstances may act as a virulence factor. Some studies described changes in SCFA concentrations in infectious conditions including periodontitis, vaginosis, and intestinal infections, as described below.

Periodontitis, a chronic inflammatory disease induced by bacteria, is characterized by a weakening of the structure that gives support to the teeth, which may lead to tooth loss (Darveau 2010). There is some evidence in the literature that supports a role of the SCFAs in this condition. First, anaerobic periodontopathic bacteria including *Aggregatibacter actinomycetemcomitans*, *Fusobacterium nucleatum*, and *Porphyromonas gingivalis* produce high amounts of SCFAs (Abe 2012). Secondly, higher concentrations of SCFAs were described in the gingival crevicular fluid of individuals with periodontitis in comparison to individuals without periodontitis (Lu et al.

2014; Qiqiang, Huanxin, and Xuejun 2012). Additionally, a reduction in their concentrations was observed after periodontitis treatment. Thirdly, direct application of SCFAs in the gingiva of healthy individuals causes a local inflammation, which may be relevant for the initiation of the infection (Niederman, Zhang, and Kashket 1997). Finally, in addition to their effects on leukocytes and epithelial cells, *in vitro* studies indicate that SCFAs modify the growth and function of gingival fibroblasts, an effect that may be relevant for the periodontal tissue healing (Chang, Huang, and Liou 2012).

An increase in the concentrations of SCFAs has also been found in other types of infections including anaerobic bacteria abscesses (Gorbach et al. 1976) and bacterial vaginosis (Al-Mushrif, Eley, and Jones 2000). This latter condition is defined as a dysbiosis of the vaginal microbiota and is characterized by local discomfort, elevation in vaginal pH, and unpleasant odor (Niederman, Zhang, and Kashket 1997; Spiegel, Amsel, and Holmes 1983). Bacterial vaginosis is accompanied by a reduction in lactobacilli (the dominant component of vaginal microbiota) and an increase of several other bacteria including *Gardnerella*, *Prevotella*, *Bacteroides*, and *Mobiluncus* spp., as recently reviewed (Aldunate et al. 2015). Concomitant with these changes, a shift in the pattern and amount of bacterial metabolites present in the vagina is observed. Specifically, a reduction in lactic acid and an increase in the concentrations of SCFAs, mainly acetate, but also propionate and butyrate, is observed (Al-Mushrif, Eley, and Jones 2000; Mirmonsef et al. 2011; Chaudry et al. 2004). In this context, Chaudry et al. (2004) showed that the vaginal concentration of acetic acid is high in infected women and drops markedly after treatment. A role of these SCFAs in this condition has been suggested and SCFAs found in the genital tract of women with bacterial vaginosis inhibit monocyte chemotaxis *in vitro*, an effect that suggests that the SCFAs are an important factor in the early stages of the disease (Al-Mushrif, Eley, and Jones 2000).

The studies on periodontitis, anaerobic abscess, and bacterial vaginosis, despite being preliminary, indicate that a local increase in SCFA concentration is associated with an impaired function of immune cells. In this context, SCFAs can be seen as virulence factors produced directly by pathogenic bacteria or indirectly as a result of dysbiosis. However, an increase in SCFAs is not always associated with a worsening of the immune response. In some cases, as described below for some intestinal infections, an increase in SCFA concentrations seems to be beneficial for the host.

Fukuda et al. (2012) described that administration of certain strains of bifidobacteria protect mice against intestinal infection caused by enterohemorrhagic *E. coli* O157:H7. This effect was attributed to the production and release of acetate by bifidobacteria. Other SCFAs, such as butyrate, do not seem to have the beneficial effect of acetate, since in another study conducted with *E. coli* infection, an inverse relation between butyrate concentrations and resistance to infection was described (Zumbrun et al. 2013).

Pseudomembranous colitis is a disease associated with the intensive use of antibiotics and is caused primarily by *Clostridium difficile* toxins. The Gram-negative bacillus spore-forming *C. difficile*, which is resistant to various antimicrobial agents such as clindamycin, ampicillin, and third-generation cephalosporins, is normally found in the intestinal microbiota, but its numbers increase after depletion of other bacteria by antibiotic therapy (Chen et al. 2008). van Nood et al. (2013) showed that the infusion of stools from healthy donors to patients with recurrent *C. difficile* infection was significantly more effective for treatment (94%) than the use of vancomycin (31%) or vancomycin followed by intestinal washings (23%). In this context, the analysis of microbial diversity in the treated patients showed an increase in quantity of commensal bacteria after fecal infusion and resolution of the disease. It has been demonstrated that the depletion of microbiota components is associated with a drastic reduction in the intestinal concentrations of SCFAs, a fact that possibly contributes to the *C. difficile* infection, since SCFAs increase the production and release of antimicrobial peptides by epithelial cells, which inhibit *C. difficile* (Antharam et al. 2013; Schauber et al. 2003; Theriot et al. 2014).

Using a murine model of intestinal inflammation caused by *C. rodentium*, Kim et al. (2013) demonstrated that the SCFAs activate GPCRs, resulting in the rapid production of inflammatory mediators and that knockout mice for FFAR2 resulted in lower production of these mediators and less activation of neutrophils and CD4+ T cells, which was associated with an increased loss of body mass and persistent infection.

Hung et al. (2013) showed that propionate directly reduces the expression of genes involved with *Salmonella* invasion of cells and inhibit the invasion of intestinal epithelial cells by this bacterium. Others showed that supplementation of drinking water of chickens with butyrate reduced cecum colonization with *Salmonella enteritidis*, an effect associated with enhancement in antimicrobial perptide production (Sunkara, Jiang, and Zhang 2012).

In addition to bacterial infections, it is possible that SCFAs affect susceptibility to viral infections. Graham et al. (2013) studied how SCFAs impact HIV expression in macrophages, which are known for being the first cell to be infected by HIV, and also for being an important reservoir for maintaining latent forms of the virus (Sharova et al. 2005), and found that butyrate (but not acetate or propionate) reduces the expression of HIV, while succinic acid had the opposite effect. Other studies indicate that some SCFAs induce epigenetic changes in cells that participate in the process of latent virus reactivation. Das et al. (2015) demonstrated that SCFAs (excluding acetic acid) stimulate transactivation and transcription of latent HIV-1 in T cells. Yu et al. (2014) showed that changes in gene expression caused by SCFAs during periodontitis infection also stimulate replication of the herpes virus associated with Kaposi's sarcoma in the oral cavity. In other study, reactivation of Epstein-Barr virus by butyrate was demonstrated. This latter effect was attributed to modifications of chromatin acetylation state, which are secondary to the inhibition of HDAC activity by butyrate (Daigle et al. 2010).

Taken together, the studies described above indicate that changes in SCFA concentrations may play an important role in the development of infectious conditions. However, the overall picture that emerges is inconsistent. In some studies, SCFAs act to increase resistance to infection, while in other studies, they show effects that increase susceptibility. Clearly, the nature of the infectious agent might be important in determining the observed effects. Other important factors might be the differences among experimental settings (host organism, *in vivo* versus *in vitro* model, used concentration of SCFAs and mode of delivery, site of infection, etc). Additionally in the defense against a specific pathogenic organism and which precise effects of SCFAs are connected to those mechanisms; SCFAs can enhance immune mechanisms that act against certain pathogens but suppress mechanisms that act against others. More studies are necessary in order to better identify the cellular mechanisms behind the effects of SCFAs on host defense and to better clarify how different SCFAs act towards infectious challenges in experimental animal systems and in humans.

REFERENCES

Abe, K. 2012. Butyric acid induces apoptosis in both human monocytes and lymphocytes equivalently. *Journal of Oral Science* 54 (1):7–14.

Aldunate, M., D. Srbinovski, A. C. Hearps, C. F. Latham, P. A. Ramsland, R. Gugasyan, R. A. Cone, and G. Tachedjian. 2015. Antimicrobial and immune modulatory effects of lactic acid and short chain fatty acids produced by vaginal microbiota associated with eubiosis and bacterial vaginosis. *Frontier in Physiology* 6:164.

Al-Mushrif, S., A. Eley, and B. M. Jones. 2000. Inhibition of chemotaxis by organic acids from anaerobes may prevent a purulent response in bacterial vaginosis. *Journal of Medical Microbiology* 49 (11):1023–30.

Antharam, V. C., E. C. Li, A. Ishmael, A. Sharma, V. Mai, K. H. Rand, and G. P. Wang. 2013. Intestinal dysbiosis and depletion of butyrogenic bacteria in Clostridium difficile infection and nosocomial diarrhea. *Journal of Clinical Microbiology* 51 (9):2884–92. doi: 10.1128/JCM.00845-13.

Aoyama, M., J. Kotani, and M. Usami. 2010. Butyrate and propionate induced activated or non-activated neutrophil apoptosis via HDAC inhibitor activity but without activating GPR-41/GPR-43 pathways. *Nutrition* 26 (6):653–61. doi: 10.1016/j.nut.2009.07.006.

Arpaia, N., C. Campbell, X. Fan, S. Dikiy, J. van der Veeken, P. deRoos, H. Liu, J. R. Cross, K. Pfeffer, P. J. Coffer, and A. Y. Rudensky. 2013. Metabolites produced by commensal bacteria promote peripheral regulatory T-cell generation. *Nature* 504 (7480):451–5. doi: 10.1038/nature12726.

Barcenilla, A., S. E. Pryde, J. C. Martin, S. H. Duncan, C. S. Stewart, C. Henderson, and H. J. Flint. 2000. Phylogenetic relationships of butyrate-producing bacteria from the human gut. *Applied and Environmental Microbiology* 66 (4):1654–61.

Berndt, B. E., M. Zhang, S. Y. Owyang, T. S. Cole, T. W. Wang, J. Luther, N. A. Veniaminova, J. L. Merchant, C. C. Chen, G. B. Huffnagle, and J. Y. Kao. 2012. Butyrate increases IL-23 production by stimulated dendritic cells. *American Journal of Physiology. Gastrointestinal and Liver Physiology* 303 (12):G1384–92. doi: 10.1152/ajpgi.00540.2011.

Brown, A. J., S. M. Goldsworthy, A. A. Barnes, M. M. Eilert, L. Tcheang, D. Daniels, A. I. Muir, M. J. Wigglesworth, I. Kinghorn, N. J. Fraser, N. B. Pike, J. C. Strum, K. M. Steplewski, P. R. Murdock, J. C. Holder, F. H. Marshall, P. G. Szekeres, S. Wilson, D. M. Ignar, S. M. Foord, A. Wise, and S. J. Dowell. 2003. The Orphan G protein-coupled receptors GPR41 and GPR43 are activated by propionate and other short chain carboxylic acids. *Journal of Biological Chemistry* 278 (13):11312–9.

Buckley, C. D., D. W. Gilroy, C. N. Serhan, B. Stockinger, and P. P. Tak. 2013. The resolution of inflammation. *Nature Reviews. Immunology* 13 (1):59–66. doi: 10.1038/nri3362.

Chang, W. T., W. C. Huang, and C. J. Liou. 2012. Evaluation of the anti-inflammatory effects of phloretin and phlorizin in lipopolysaccharide-stimulated mouse macrophages. *Food Chemistry* 134 (2):972–9. doi: 10.1016/j.foodchem.2012.03.002.

Chang, Y., X. Huang, Z. Liu, G. Han, L. Huang, Y. C. Xiong, and Z. Wang. 2013. Dexmedetomidine inhibits the secretion of high mobility group box 1 from lipopolysaccharide-activated macrophages in vitro. *Journal of Surgical Research* 181 (2):308–14. doi: 10.1016/j.jss.2012.07.017.

Chaudry, A. N., P. J. Travers, J. Yuenger, L. Colletta, P. Evans, J. M. Zenilman, and A. Tummon. 2004. Analysis of vaginal acetic acid in patients undergoing treatment for bacterial vaginosis. *Journal of Clinical Microbiology* 42 (11):5170–5. doi: 10.1128/JCM.42.11.5170-5175.2004.

Chen, X., K. Katchar, J. D. Goldsmith, N. Nanthakumar, A. Cheknis, D. N. Gerding, and C. P. Kelly. 2008. A mouse model of Clostridium difficile-associated disease. *Gastroenterology* 135 (6):1984–92. doi: 10.1053/j.gastro.2008.09.002.

Chervonsky, A. V. 2010. Influence of microbial environment on autoimmunity. *Nature Immunology* 11 (1):28–35. doi: 10.1038/ni.1801.

Daigle, D., C. Megyola, A. El-Guindy, L. Gradoville, D. Tuck, G. Miller, and S. Bhaduri-McIntosh. 2010. Upregulation of STAT3 marks Burkitt lymphoma cells refractory to Epstein-Barr virus lytic cycle induction by HDAC inhibitors. *Journal of Virology* 84 (2):993–1004. doi: 10.1128/JVI.01745-09.

Dalli, J. and C. N. Serhan. 2012. Specific lipid mediator signatures of human phagocytes: Microparticles stimulate macrophage efferocytosis and pro-resolving mediators. *Blood* 120 (15):e60–72. doi: 10.1182/blood-2012-04-423525.

Darveau, R. P. 2010. Periodontitis: A polymicrobial disruption of host homeostasis. *Nature Reviews. Microbiology* 8 (7):481–90. doi: 10.1038/nrmicro2337.

Das, B., C. Dobrowolski, A. M. Shahir, Z. Feng, X. Yu, J. Sha, N. F. Bissada, A. Weinberg, J. Karn, and F. Ye. 2015. Short chain fatty acids potently induce latent HIV-1 in T-cells by activating P-TEFb and multiple histone modifications. *Virology* 474:65–81. doi: 10.1016/j.virol.2014.10.033.

Di Sabatino, A., R. Morera, R. Ciccocioppo, P. Cazzola, S. Gotti, F. P. Tinozzi, S. Tinozzi, and G. R. Corazza. 2005. Oral butyrate for mildly to moderately active Crohn's disease. *Alimentary Pharmacology & Therapeutics* 22 (9):789–94. doi: 10.1111/j.1365-2036.2005.02639.x.

Duncan, S. H., G. Holtrop, G. E. Lobley, A. G. Calder, C. S. Stewart, and H. J. Flint. 2004. Contribution of acetate to butyrate formation by human faecal bacteria. *British Journal of Nutrition* 91 (6):915–23. doi: 10.1079/BJN20041150.

Dupaul-Chicoine, J., G. Yeretssian, K. Doiron, K. S. Bergstrom, C. R. McIntire, P. M. LeBlanc, C. Meunier, C. Turbide, P. Gros, N. Beauchemin, B. A. Vallance, and M. Saleh. 2010. Control of intestinal homeostasis, colitis, and colitis-associated colorectal cancer by the inflammatory caspases. *Immunity* 32 (3):367–78. doi: 10.1016/j.immuni.2010.02.012; S1074-7613(10)00082-8 [pii].

Elinav, E., T. Strowig, A. L. Kau, J. Henao-Mejia, C. A. Thaiss, C. J. Booth, D. R. Peaper, J. Bertin, S. C. Eisenbarth, J. I. Gordon, and R. A. Flavell. 2011. NLRP6 inflammasome regulates colonic microbial ecology and risk for colitis. *Cell* 145 (5):745–57. doi: 10.1016/j.cell.2011.04.022; S0092-8674(11)00480-6 [pii].

Fukuda, S., H. Toh, T. D. Taylor, H. Ohno, and M. Hattori. 2012. Acetate-producing bifidobacteria protect the host from enteropathogenic infection via carbohydrate transporters. *Gut Microbes* 3 (5):449–54. doi: 10.4161/gmic.21214.

Gorbach, S. L., J. W. Mayhew, J. G. Bartlett, H. Thadepalli, and A. B. Onderdonk. 1976. Rapid diagnosis of anaerobic infections by direct gas-liquid chromatography of clinical speciments. *Journal of Clinical Investigtion* 57 (2):478–84. doi: 10.1172/JCI108300.

Graham, L. S., L. Krass, M. R. Zariffard, G. T. Spear, and P. Mirmonsef. 2013. Effects of succinic acid and other microbial fermentation products on HIV expression in macrophages. *BioResearch Open Access* 2 (5):385–91. doi: 10.1089/biores.2013.0013.

Hancock, J. F. 2006. Lipid rafts: Contentious only from simplistic standpoints. *Nature Reviews. Molecular Cell Biology* 7 (6):456–62. doi: 10.1038/nrm1925.

Hara, T., D. Kashihara, A. Ichimura, I. Kimura, G. Tsujimoto, and A. Hirasawa. 2014. Role of free fatty acid receptors in the regulation of energy metabolism. *Biochimica et Biophys Acta* 1841 (9):1292–300. doi: 10.1016/j.bbalip.2014.06.002.

Harig, J. M., K. H. Soergel, R. A. Komorowski, and C. M. Wood. 1989. Treatment of diversion colitis with short-chain-fatty acid irrigation. *New England Journal of Medicine* 320 (1):23–8.

Hirota, S. A., J. Ng, A. Lueng, M. Khajah, K. Parhar, Y. Li, V. Lam, M. S. Potentier, K. Ng, M. Bawa, D. M. McCafferty, K. P. Rioux, S. Ghosh, R. J. Xavier, S. P. Colgan, J. Tschopp, D. Muruve, J. A. MacDonald, and P. L. Beck. 2011. NLRP3 inflammasome plays a key role in the regulation of intestinal homeostasis. *Inflammatory Bowel Diseases* 17 (6):1359–72. doi: 10.1002/ibd.21478.

Hung, C. C., C. D. Garner, J. M. Slauch, Z. W. Dwyer, S. D. Lawhon, J. G. Frye, M. McClelland, B. M. Ahmer, and C. Altier. 2013. The intestinal fatty acid propionate inhibits Salmonella invasion through the post-translational control of HilD. *Molecular Microbiology* 87 (5):1045–60. doi: 10.1111/mmi.12149.

Katritch, V., V. Cherezov, and R. C. Stevens. 2013. Structure-function of the G protein-coupled receptor superfamily. *Annual Review of Pharmacology and Toxicology* 53:531–56. doi: 10.1146/annurev-pharmtox-032112-135923.

Kim, M. H., S. G. Kang, J. H. Park, M. Yanagisawa, and C. H. Kim. 2013. Short-chain fatty acids activate GPR41 and GPR43 on intestinal epithelial cells to promote inflammatory responses in mice. *Gastroenterology* 145 (2):396–406 e1–10. doi: 10.1053/j.gastro.2013.04.056.

Le Poul, E., C. Loison, S. Struyf, J. Y. Springael, V. Lannoy, M. E. Decobecq, S. Brezillon, V. Dupriez, G. Vassart, J. Van Damme, M. Parmentier, and M. Detheux. 2003. Functional characterization of human receptors for short chain fatty acids and their role in polymorphonuclear cell activation. *Journal of Biological Chemistry* 278 (28):25481–9. doi: 10.1074/jbc.M301403200.

Liu, L., L. Li, J. Min, J. Wang, H. Wu, Y. Zeng, S. Chen, and Z. Chu. 2012a. Butyrate interferes with the differentiation and function of human monocyte-derived dendritic cells. *Cell Immunology* 277 (1–2):66–73. doi: 10.1016/j.cellimm.2012.05.011.

Liu, Q., T. Shimoyama, K. Suzuki, T. Umeda, S. Nakaji, and K. Sugawara. 2001. Effect of sodium butyrate on reactive oxygen species generation by human neutrophils. *Scandinavian Journal of Gastroenterology* 36 (7):744–50.

Liu, T., J. Li, Y. Liu, N. Xiao, H. Suo, K. Xie, C. Yang, and C. Wu. 2012b. Short-chain fatty acids suppress lipopolysaccharide-induced production of nitric oxide and proinflammatory cytokines through inhibition of NF-kappaB pathway in RAW264.7 cells. *Inflammation* 35 (5):1676–84. doi: 10.1007/s10753-012-9484-z.

Louis, P., G. L. Hold, and H. J. Flint. 2014. The gut microbiota, bacterial metabolites and colorectal cancer. *Nature Reviews. Microbiology* 12 (10):661–72. doi: 10.1038/nrmicro3344.

Lu, R., H. Meng, X. Gao, L. Xu, and X. Feng. 2014. Effect of non-surgical periodontal treatment on short chain fatty acid levels in gingival crevicular fluid of patients with generalized aggressive periodontitis. *Journal of Periodontal Research* 49 (5):574–83.

Macia, L., J. Tan, A. T. Vieira, K. Leach, D. Stanley, S. Luong, M. Maruya, C. Ian McKenzie, A. Hijikata, C. Wong, L. Binge, A. N. Thorburn, N. Chevalier, C. Ang, E. Marino, R. Robert, S. Offermanns, M. M. Teixeira, R. J. Moore, R. A. Flavell, S. Fagarasan, and C. R. Mackay. 2015. Metabolite-sensing receptors GPR43 and GPR109A facilitate dietary fibre-induced gut homeostasis through regulation of the inflammasome. *Nature Communications* 6:6734. doi: 10.1038/ncomms7734.

Mantovani, A., M. A. Cassatella, C. Costantini, and S. Jaillon. 2011. Neutrophils in the activation and regulation of innate and adaptive immunity. *Nature Reviews. Immunology* 11 (8):519–31. doi: 10.1038/nri3024.

Maslowski, K. M., A. T. Vieira, A. Ng, J. Kranich, F. Sierro, D. Yu, H. C. Schilter, M. S. Rolph, F. Mackay, D. Artis, R. J. Xavier, M. M. Teixeira, and C. R. Mackay. 2009. Regulation of inflammatory responses by gut microbiota and chemoattractant receptor GPR43. *Nature* 461 (7268):1282–6.

Millard, A. L., P. M. Mertes, D. Ittelet, F. Villard, P. Jeannesson, and J. Bernard. 2002. Butyrate affects differentiation, maturation and function of human monocyte-derived dendritic cells and macrophages. *Clinical & Experimental Immunology* 130 (2):245–55.

Miller, T. L. and M. J. Wolin. 1996. Pathways of acetate, propionate, and butyrate formation by the human fecal microbial flora. *Applied and Environmental Microbiology* 62 (5):1589–92.

Mills, S. W., S. H. Montgomery, and D. W. Morck. 2006. Evaluation of the effects of short-chain fatty acids and extracellular pH on bovine neutrophil function in vitro. *American Journal of Veterinary Research* 67 (11):1901–7. doi: 10.2460/ajvr.67.11.1901.

Mirmonsef, P., D. Gilbert, M. R. Zariffard, B. R. Hamaker, A. Kaur, A. L. Landay, and G. T. Spear. 2011. The effects of commensal bacteria on innate immune responses in the female genital tract. *American Journal of Reproductive Immunology* 65 (3):190–5. doi: 10.1111/j.1600-0897.2010.00943.x.

Mirmonsef, P., M. R. Zariffard, D. Gilbert, H. Makinde, A. L. Landay, and G. T. Spear. 2012. Short-chain fatty acids induce pro-inflammatory cytokine production alone and in combination with toll-like receptor ligands. *American Journal of Reproductive Immunology* 67 (5):391–400. doi: 10.1111/j.1600-0897.2011.01089.x.

Niederman, R., J. Zhang, and S. Kashket. 1997. Short-chain carboxylic-acid-stimulated, PMN-mediated gingival inflammation. *Critical Reviews in Oral Biology & Medicine* 8 (3):269–90.

Nieman, C. 1954. Influence of trace amounts of fatty acids on the growth of microorganisms. *Bacteriological Reviews* 18 (2):147–63.

Park, J., M. Kim, S. G. Kang, A. H. Jannasch, B. Cooper, J. Patterson, and C. H. Kim. 2015. Short-chain fatty acids induce both effector and regulatory T cells by suppression of histone deacetylases and regulation of the mTOR-S6K pathway. *Mucosal Immunology* 8 (1):80–93. doi: 10.1038/mi.2014.44.

Park, J. S., E. J. Lee, J. C. Lee, W. K. Kim, and H. S. Kim. 2007. Anti-inflammatory effects of short chain fatty acids in IFN-gamma-stimulated RAW 264.7 murine macrophage cells: Involvement of NF-kappaB and ERK signaling pathways. *International Immunopharmacology* 7 (1):70–7.

Perez, D. A., J. P. Vago, R. M. Athayde, A. C. Reis, M. M. Teixeira, L. P. Sousa, and V. Pinho. 2014. Switching off key signaling survival molecules to switch on the resolution of inflammation. *Mediators of Inflammation* 2014:829851. doi: 10.1155/2014/829851.

Pomare, E. W., W. J. Branch, and J. H. Cummings. 1985. Carbohydrate fermentation in the human colon and its relation to acetate concentrations in venous blood. *Journal of Clinical Investigation* 75 (5):1448–54. doi: 10.1172/JCI111847.

Pryde, S. E., S. H. Duncan, G. L. Hold, C. S. Stewart, and H. J. Flint. 2002. The microbiology of butyrate formation in the human colon. *FEMS Microbiology Letters* 217 (2):133–9.

Qiqiang, L., M. Huanxin, and G. Xuejun. 2012. Longitudinal study of volatile fatty acids in the gingival crevicular fluid of patients with periodontitis before and after nonsurgical therapy. *Journal of Periodontal Research* 47 (6):740–9. doi: 10.1111/j.1600-0765.2012.01489.x.

Ramsey, M. M., K. P. Rumbaugh, and M. Whiteley. 2011. Metabolite cross-feeding enhances virulence in a model polymicrobial infection. *PLOS Pathogens* 7 (3):e1002012. doi: 10.1371/journal.ppat.1002012.

Raqib, R., P. Sarker, A. Mily, N. H. Alam, A. S. Arifuzzaman, R. S. Rekha, J. Andersson, G. H. Gudmundsson, A. Cravioto, and B. Agerberth. 2012. Efficacy of sodium butyrate adjunct therapy in shigellosis: A randomized, double-blind, placebo-controlled clinical trial. *BMC Infectious Diseases* 12:111. doi: 10.1186/1471-2334-12-111.

Raqib, R., P. Sarker, P. Bergman, G. Ara, M. Lindh, D. A. Sack, K. M. Nasirul Islam, G. H. Gudmundsson, J. Andersson, and B. Agerberth. 2006. Improved outcome in shigellosis associated with butyrate induction of an endogenous peptide antibiotic. *Proceedings of the National Academy of Sciences of the United States of America* 103 (24):9178–83. doi: 10.1073/pnas.0602888103.

Rodrigues, H. G., F. Takeo Sato, R. Curi, and M. A. Vinolo. 2015. Fatty acids as modulators of neutrophil recruitment, function and survival. *European Journal of Pharmacology* 785:50–8. doi: 10.1016/j.ejphar.2015.03.098.

Roediger, W. E. 1982. Utilization of nutrients by isolated epithelial cells of the rat colon. *Gastroenterology* 83 (2):424–9.

Sandoval, A., F. Trivinos, A. Sanhueza, D. Carretta, M. A. Hidalgo, J. L. Hancke, and R. A. Burgos. 2007. Propionate induces pH(i) changes through calcium flux, ERK1/2, p38, and PKC in bovine neutrophils. *Veterinary Immunology and Immunopathology* 115 (3–4):286–98. doi: 10.1016/j.vetimm.2006.11.003.

Savill, J. and C. Haslett. 1995. Granulocyte clearance by apoptosis in the resolution of inflammation. *Seminars in Cell Biology* 6 (6):385–93.

Schauber, J., C. Svanholm, S. Termen, K. Iffland, T. Menzel, W. Scheppach, R. Melcher, B. Agerberth, H. Luhrs, and G. H. Gudmundsson. 2003. Expression of the cathelicidin LL-37 is modulated by short chain fatty acids in colonocytes: Relevance of signalling pathways. *Gut* 52 (5):735–41.

Serhan, C. N., N. Chiang, and T. E. Van Dyke. 2008. Resolving inflammation: Dual anti-inflammatory and pro-resolution lipid mediators. *Nature Reviews. Immunology* 8 (5):349–61. doi: 10.1038/nri2294.

Serhan, C. N., S. D. Brain, C. D. Buckley, D. W. Gilroy, C. Haslett, L. A. O'Neill, M. Perretti, A. G. Rossi, and J. L. Wallace. 2007. Resolution of inflammation: State of the art, definitions and terms. *FASEB Journal: Official Publication of the Federation of American Societies for Experimental Biology* 21 (2):325–32. doi: 10.1096/fj.06-7227rev.

Sharova, N., C. Swingler, M. Sharkey, and M. Stevenson. 2005. Macrophages archive HIV-1 virions for dissemination in trans. *Embo Journal* 24 (13):2481–9. doi: 10.1038/sj.emboj.7600707.

Shaykhiev, R. and R. Bals. 2007. Interactions between epithelial cells and leukocytes in immunity and tissue homeostasis. *Journal of Leukocyte Biology* 82 (1):1–15. doi: 10.1189/jlb.0207096.

Sina, C., O. Gavrilova, M. Forster, A. Till, S. Derer, F. Hildebrand, B. Raabe, A. Chalaris, J. Scheller, A. Rehmann, A. Franke, S. Ott, R. Hasler, S. Nikolaus, U. R. Folsch, S. Rose-John, H. P. Jiang, J. Li, S. Schreiber, and P. Rosenstiel. 2009. G protein-coupled receptor 43 is essential for neutrophil recruitment during intestinal inflammation. *Journal of Immunology* 183 (11):7514–22. doi: 10.4049/jimmunol.0900063.

Singh, N., A. Gurav, S. Sivaprakasam, E. Brady, R. Padia, H. Shi, M. Thangaraju, P. D. Prasad, S. Manicassamy, D. H. Munn, J. R. Lee, S. Offermanns, and V. Ganapathy. 2014. Activation of Gpr109a, receptor for niacin and the commensal metabolite butyrate, suppresses colonic inflammation and carcinogenesis. *Immunity* 40 (1):128–39. doi: 10.1016/j.immuni.2013.12.007.

Smith, P. M., M. R. Howitt, N. Panikov, M. Michaud, C. A. Gallini, Y. M. Bohlooly, J. N. Glickman, and W. S. Garrett. 2013. The microbial metabolites, short-chain fatty acids, regulate colonic Treg cell homeostasis. *Science* 341 (6145):569–73. doi: 10.1126/science.1241165.

Soga, T., M. Kamohara, J. Takasaki, S. Matsumoto, T. Saito, T. Ohishi, H. Hiyama, A. Matsuo, H. Matsushime, and K. Furuichi. 2003. Molecular identification of nicotinic acid receptor. *Biochemical and Biophysical Research Communications* 303 (1):364–9.

Spiegel, C. A., R. Amsel, and K. K. Holmes. 1983. Diagnosis of bacterial vaginosis by direct gram stain of vaginal fluid. *Journal of Clinical Microbiology* 18 (1):170–7.

Stecher, B. and W. D. Hardt. 2008. The role of microbiota in infectious disease. *Trends in Microbiology* 16 (3):107–14. doi: 10.1016/j.tim.2007.12.008.

Sunkara, L. T., W. Jiang, and G. Zhang. 2012. Modulation of antimicrobial host defense peptide gene expression by free fatty acids. *PLOS ONE* 7 (11):e49558. doi: 10.1371/journal.pone.0049558.

Taggart, A. K., J. Kero, X. Gan, T. Q. Cai, K. Cheng, M. Ippolito, N. Ren, R. Kaplan, K. Wu, T. J. Wu, L. Jin, C. Liaw, R. Chen, J. Richman, D. Connolly, S. Offermanns, S. D. Wright, and M. G. Waters. 2005. (D)-beta-Hydroxybutyrate inhibits adipocyte lipolysis via the nicotinic acid receptor PUMA-G. *Journal of Biological Chemistry* 280 (29):26649–52. doi: 10.1074/jbc.C500213200.

Tan, J., C. McKenzie, M. Potamitis, A. N. Thorburn, C. R. Mackay, and L. Macia. 2014. The role of short-chain fatty acids in health and disease. *Advances in Immunology* 121:91–119. doi: 10.1016/B978-0-12-800100-4.00003-9.

Tecchio, C. and M. A. Cassatella. 2014. Neutrophil-derived cytokines involved in physiological and pathological angiogenesis. *Chemical Immunology and Allergy* 99:123–37. doi: 10.1159/000353358.

Tedelind, S., F. Westberg, M. Kjerrulf, and A. Vidal. 2007. Anti-inflammatory properties of the short-chain fatty acids acetate and propionate: A study with relevance to inflammatory bowel disease. *World Journal of Gastroenterology: WJG* 13 (20):2826–32.

Theriot, C. M., M. J. Koenigsknecht, P. E. Carlson, Jr., G. E. Hatton, A. M. Nelson, B. Li, G. B. Huffnagle, Z. Li J, and V. B. Young. 2014. Antibiotic-induced shifts in the mouse gut microbiome and metabolome increase susceptibility to Clostridium difficile infection. *Nature Communications* 5:3114. doi: 10.1038/ncomms4114.

Trompette, A., E. S. Gollwitzer, K. Yadava, A. K. Sichelstiel, N. Sprenger, C. Ngom-Bru, C. Blanchard, T. Junt, L. P. Nicod, N. L. Harris, and B. J. Marsland. 2014. Gut microbiota metabolism of dietary fiber influences allergic airway disease and hematopoiesis. *Nature Medicine* 20 (2):159–66. doi: 10.1038/nm.3444.

Tunaru, S., J. Kero, A. Schaub, C. Wufka, A. Blaukat, K. Pfeffer, and S. Offermanns. 2003. PUMA-G and HM74 are receptors for nicotinic acid and mediate its anti-lipolytic effect. *Nature Medicine* 9 (3):352–5. doi: 10.1038/nm824.

van Nood, E., A. Vrieze, M. Nieuwdorp, S. Fuentes, E. G. Zoetendal, W. M. de Vos, C. E. Visser, E. J. Kuijper, J. F. Bartelsman, J. G. Tijssen, P. Speelman, M. G. Dijkgraaf, and J. J. Keller. 2013. Duodenal infusion of donor feces for recurrent Clostridium difficile. *New England Journal of Medicine* 368 (5):407–15. doi: 10.1056/NEJMoa1205037.

Vinolo, M. A., E. Hatanaka, R. H. Lambertucci, P. Newsholme, and R. Curi. 2009a. Effects of short chain fatty acids on effector mechanisms of neutrophils. *Cell Biochemistry and Function* 27 (1):48–55.

Vinolo, M. A., G. J. Ferguson, S. Kulkarni, G. Damoulakis, K. Anderson, Y. M. Bohlooly, L. Stephens, P. T. Hawkins, and R. Curi. 2011a. SCFAs induce mouse neutrophil chemotaxis through the GPR43 receptor. *PLOS ONE* 6 (6):e21205. doi: 10.1371/journal.pone.0021205.

Vinolo, M. A., H. G. Rodrigues, E. Hatanaka, C. B. Hebeda, S. H. Farsky, and R. Curi. 2009b. Short-chain fatty acids stimulate the migration of neutrophils to inflammatory sites. *Clinical Science* 117 (9):331–8. doi: 10.1042/CS20080642.

Vinolo, M. A., H. G. Rodrigues, E. Hatanaka, F. T. Sato, S. C. Sampaio, and R. Curi. 2011b. Suppressive effect of short-chain fatty acids on production of proinflammatory mediators by neutrophils. *Journal of Nutritional Biochemistry* 22 (9):849–55. doi: 10.1016/j.jnutbio.2010.07.009.

Vinolo, M. A., H. G. Rodrigues, R. T. Nachbar, and R. Curi. 2011c. Regulation of inflammation by short chain Fatty acids. *Nutrients* 3 (10):858–76. doi: 10.3390/nu3100858.

Vinolo, M. A., S. M. Hirabara, and R. Curi. 2012. G-protein-coupled receptors as fat sensors. *Current Opinion in Clinical Nutrition and Metabolic Care* 15 (2):112–6. doi: 10.1097/MCO.0b013e32834f4598.

Vogt, J. A., P. B. Pencharz, and T. M. Wolever. 2004. L-Rhamnose increases serum propionate in humans. *American Journal of Clinical Nutrition* 80 (1):89–94.

Wolever, T. M., K. B. Schrade, J. A. Vogt, E. B. Tsihlias, and M. I. McBurney. 2002. Do colonic short-chain fatty acids contribute to the long-term adaptation of blood lipids in subjects with type 2 diabetes consuming a high-fiber diet? *American Journal of Clinical Nutrition* 75 (6):1023–30.

Wolever, T. M., R. G. Josse, L. A. Leiter, and J. L. Chiasson. 1997. Time of day and glucose tolerance status affect serum short-chain fatty acid concentrations in humans. *Metabolism: Clinical and Experimental* 46 (7):805–11.

Wong, J. M., R. de Souza, C. W. Kendall, A. Emam, and D. J. Jenkins. 2006. Colonic health: Fermentation and short chain fatty acids. *Journal of Clinical Gastroenterology* 40 (3):235–43.

Yu, X., A. M. Shahir, J. Sha, Z. Feng, B. Eapen, S. Nithianantham, B. Das, J. Karn, A. Weinberg, N. F. Bissada, and F. Ye. 2014. Short-chain fatty acids from periodontal pathogens suppress histone deacetylases, EZH2, and SUV39H1 to promote Kaposi's sarcoma-associated herpesvirus replication. *Journal of Virology* 88 (8):4466–79. doi: 10.1128/JVI.03326-13.

Zaki, M. H., K. L. Boyd, P. Vogel, M. B. Kastan, M. Lamkanfi, and T. D. Kanneganti. 2010a. The NLRP3 inflammasome protects against loss of epithelial integrity and mortality during experimental colitis. *Immunity* 32 (3):379–91. doi: 10.1016/j.immuni.2010.03.003; S1074–7613(10)00086-5 [pii].

Zaki, M. H., P. Vogel, M. Body-Malapel, M. Lamkanfi, and T. D. Kanneganti. 2010b. IL-18 production downstream of the Nlrp3 inflammasome confers protection against colorectal tumor formation. *Journal of Immunology* 185 (8):4912–20. doi: 10.4049/jimmunol.1002046; jimmunol.1002046 [pii].

Zasloff, M. 2002. Antimicrobial peptides of multicellular organisms. *Nature* 415 (6870):389–95. doi: 10.1038/415389a.

Zeng, X., L. T. Sunkara, W. Jiang, M. Bible, S. Carter, X. Ma, S. Qiao, and G. Zhang. 2013. Induction of porcine host defense peptide gene expression by short-chain fatty acids and their analogs. *PLOS ONE* 8 (8):e72922. doi: 10.1371/journal.pone.0072922.

Zimmerman, M. A., N. Singh, P. M. Martin, M. Thangaraju, V. Ganapathy, J. L. Waller, H. Shi, K. D. Robertson, D. H. Munn, and K. Liu. 2012. Butyrate suppresses colonic inflammation through HDAC1-dependent Fas upregulation and Fas-mediated apoptosis of T cells. *American Journal of Physiology. Gastrointestinal and Liver Physiology* 302 (12):G1405–15. doi: 10.1152/ajpgi.00543.2011.

Zumbrun, S. D., A. R. Melton-Celsa, M. A. Smith, J. J. Gilbreath, D. S. Merrell, and A. D. O'Brien. 2013. Dietary choice affects Shiga toxin-producing Escherichia coli (STEC) O157:H7 colonization and disease. *Proceedings of the National Academy of Sciences of theUnited States of America* 110 (23):E2126–33. doi: 10.1073/pnas.1222014110.

17 Omega-3 Fatty Acids and T-Cell Responses

Tim Y. Hou, David N. McMurray, and Robert S. Chapkin

CONTENTS

17.1 Introduction 295
17.2 T-Cell Responses and Inflammation 295
17.3 n-3 Polyunsaturated Fatty Acids 296
17.4 n-3 PUFAs and Phospholipids: Membrane Effects...297
17.5 PUFAs and Eicosanoids 300
17.6 n-3 PUFAs and Pro-Resolving Lipid Mediators 301
17.7 n-3 PUFAs and Nuclear Receptors 302
17.8 n-3 PUFAs and Autoimmune Diseases 302
17.9 n-3 PUFAs and Infection...303
17.10 Concluding Comments...303
Acknowledgments..304
References...304

17.1 INTRODUCTION

T-cell–mediated high-grade and low-grade chronic inflammatory diseases, including obesity and its associated metabolic syndrome, are a global health problem [1–3]. Although pharmaceuticals such as nonsteroidal anti-inflammatory drugs (NSAIDs) and glucocorticoids are available for treatment of high-grade inflammation, they are expensive and often trigger serious side effects [4,5]. Given the high proportion of the population that is afflicted by chronic inflammation, it is important to identify innocuous anti-inflammatory dietary compounds that could ameliorate inflammation and improve overall health in the population. Mounting evidence suggests that n-3 polyunsaturated fatty acids (PUFAs), found in oily fish and fish oil supplements, offer great potential as anti-inflammatory agents or as adjunctive therapies with established drugs [6–18]. The primary bioactive n-3 PUFAs are thought to be eicosapentaenoic acid (EPA, 20:5n-3) and docosahexaenoic acid (DHA, 22:6n-3), which have been shown to attenuate inflammatory responses, biomarkers, and mortality in preclinical models [19–22] and humans [6–17]. From an immunological perspective, the anti-inflammatory properties of EPA and DHA include effects on mediators of both the innate immune response [23–26] and the adaptive immune response. In this chapter, we will review the anti-inflammatory and immunomodulatory mechanisms by which n-3 PUFAs influence T-cell responses.

17.2 T-CELL RESPONSES AND INFLAMMATION

Inflammation is a critical component in the defense of the human host against microbial pathogens and in response to internal danger signals. By creating a microenvironment to eliminate harmful pathogens or damaged cells, the host can then initiate tissue repair and restoration of normal function. Inflammation is characterized by the five classical signs of heat, redness, swelling, pain, and loss of function, and is a complex process involving many cell types and biochemical mediators. Inflammation is an essential feature of both the innate and adaptive immune responses. Although acute inflammation is critical in the host's response against harmful stimuli, unresolved or chronic inflammation can lead to diseases such as rheumatoid arthritis (RA), inflammatory bowel diseases (IBDs), obesity and its related metabolic syndrome, and even cancer. Thus, understanding the contributions of inflammation to the etiology of these diseases, and elucidating the mechanisms by which dietary bioactives can modulate these inflammatory responses are essential prerequisites to the use of diet to treat various chronic inflammatory conditions.

T lymphocytes circulate around the body to survey for foreign antigens and target them for destruction. However, under certain pathophysiological conditions such as autoimmune diseases, the adaptive immune system is unable to differentiate between self and foreign antigens, resulting in aberrant T lymphocyte activation and responses. This could manifest itself in autoimmune diseases such as IBDs (i.e., Crohn's disease, ulcerative colitis [27], and RA). The adaptive immune system is comprised principally of two cell types: (i) B lymphocytes, which are responsible for antibody-mediated (humoral) immunity; and (ii) T lymphocytes, which are responsible for the regulation of humoral and cell-mediated immunity. T lymphocytes can be separated into cytotoxic T lymphocytes (CD8+ or Tc lymphocytes) and helper T lymphocytes (CD4+ or Th lymphocytes). While CD8+ T lymphocytes play an important role in host defense and autoimmune disease, CD4+ T lymphocytes can further differentiate into several unique effector cell types (Th1, Th2, Treg, Th17, etc.), which may have opposing roles in autoimmune and chronic inflammatory diseases [28].

17.3   n-3 POLYUNSATURATED FATTY ACIDS

n-3 PUFAs are characterized by the location of the last double bond in the acyl chain being three carbons from the terminal methyl group. n-3 PUFAs can be synthesized by first converting n-6 PUFA linoleic acid (LA, 18:2n-6) to α-linolenic acid (ALA, 18:3n-3), a step that is catalyzed by the D15-desaturase. ALA is then elongated and desaturated to synthesize EPA and DHA (Figure 17.1

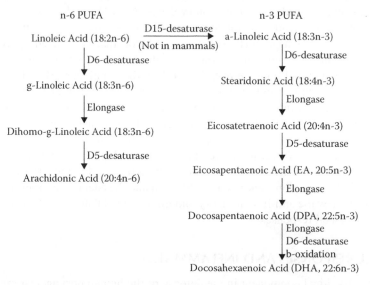

FIGURE 17.1   Biosynthesis of n-6 and n-3 PUFAs. Mammals lack the enzyme required to synthesize α-linoleic acid (ALA, 18:3n-3) from linoleic acid (LA, 18:2n-6). Furthermore, the conversion from ALA into EPA and DHA is not efficient in humans, thus the dietary intake of long-chain n-3 PUFA is required to obtain adequate levels of EPA and DHA.

[29,30]). Even though humans express the desaturases and elongases required for the conversion of ALA into EPA and DHA [31], they lack the D15-desaturase to generate ALA [32–34]. Furthermore, analysis of adult human plasma revealed that only 0.2% of plasma ALA was converted into EPA [31], thus, EPA and DHA are poorly synthesized in humans and must be acquired through diet. Fatty, cold-water fish accumulate EPA and DHA by ingestion of zooplankton and phytoplankton, and they offer one of the main dietary sources of the n-3 PUFAs EPA and DHA.

Human studies have provided a wealth of evidence demonstrating the anti-inflammatory effects of n-3 PUFAs (reviewed in [30,35]). For example, clinical studies have shown n-3 PUFA efficacy in the treatment of patients with ulcerative colitis [36–39] and Crohn's disease [6,40]. n-3 PUFAs have also been shown to reduce disease symptoms and severity in patients with RA [41,42]. Finally, treatment with EPA and DHA reduced adipose tissue and systemic inflammation in severely obese, nondiabetic patients [10]. Although these studies have demonstrated beneficial effects of n-3 PUFA intake, data from the analysis of the U.S. National Health and Nutrition Examination Survey suggested that the U.S. population consumed 0.15 ± 0.03 oz/day of fish high in n-3 PUFAs, with the mean consumption of EPA and DHA at 23 ± 7 mg and 63 mg ± 2 mg/day, respectively [43]. The American Heart Association recommends more than two 3.5 oz servings of (oily) fish per week [44], while the Dietary Guidelines for Americans suggest 8 oz of fish per week, with approximately 250 mg per day of EPA and DHA [45]. Clearly, fish and n-3 PUFA consumption in the U.S. are insufficient, and boosting fish oil intake may be one strategy in the complementary and alternative medicine armamentarium to combat chronic inflammation.

17.4 n-3 PUFAs AND PHOSPHOLIPIDS: MEMBRANE EFFECTS

EPA and DHA are incorporated into the two major classes of phospholipids in the plasma membrane, phosphatidylethanolamine and phosphatidylcholine, mainly at the sn-2 position [46,47]. It has been demonstrated that DHA is highly disordered, adopting various conformations on the subnanosecond time scale [48,49]. By eliminating the double bond of DHA (22:6Δ4,7,10,13,16,19) at the n-3 position to generate n-6 docosapentaenoic acid (DPA, 22:5Δ4,7,10,13,16), the chain dynamics of the fatty acid were reduced [48], demonstrating that the unsaturation at the n-3 position gave unique biophysical properties to EPA and DHA when incorporated into the phospholipids (Figure 17.2).

Studies conducted on human peripheral blood mononuclear cells have suggested that the incorporation of n-3 PUFAs into the plasma membrane alters T-cell activation and IL-2 production [50,51]. More mechanistic studies probing the effects of n-3 PUFAs on CD4+ T-cells have utilized mouse models and immortalized cell lines. When the T-cell receptor on the CD4+ T-cell recognizes a foreign antigen in the major histocompatibility class II on an antigen-presenting cell, major proteomic

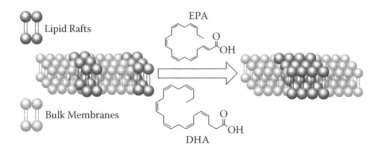

FIGURE 17.2 (See color insert.)   Phospholipid-membrane effects of n-3 PUFA. When highly unsaturated EPA and DHA incorporate into plasma membrane phospholipids, they modify the lateral organization of the lipid bilayer. This results in an alteration in the size/stability of lipid rafts in the plasma membrane, perturbing membrane-regulated signal transduction.

and lipidomic rearrangement occurs at the contact site, creating a supramolecular complex termed the immunological synapse (IS). At the IS, proteins participating in T-cell signaling are enriched to form the central supramolecular activation cluster (cSMAC). Adhesion proteins form the peripheral supramolecular activation cluster (pSMAC) to stabilize the IS formation [52,53]. Additional proteins that can abrogate T-cell activation, such as phosphatases, are excluded from the cSMAC and pSMAC. At the IS, tyrosine kinases Lck and ZAP70 are activated and subsequently phosphorylate the adaptor protein linker for activation of T-cells (LAT), leading to the assembly of the signalsome [54]. The formation and stability of the IS are intimately linked to the actin cytoskeleton [55–57]. T-cell activation can be abolished by disrupting the actin cytoskeleton, highlighting its importance [58–61]. A second important contribution to T-cell activation comes from the lipid-lipid interactions at the plasma membrane. Upon T-cell activation, lipid rafts, nanoscale regions of the plasma membrane enriched with cholesterol, sphingolipids, and saturated fatty acids, accumulate at the IS [47,62–64]. Disruption of lipid rafts with various agents, including methyl-β-cyclodextrin [65], 7-ketocholesterol [66], or n-3 PUFAs such as EPA [discussed below, 62], suppresses T-cell activation.

As described above, the unsaturation at the n-3 position of EPA and DHA gives these long-chain n-3 PUFAs unique biophysical properties when incorporated into the plasma membrane. For example, the highly disordered nature of DHA results in distinct nonraft DHA domains, which could modify the lateral organization of the plasma membrane [67,68]. It is worth noting that the nonraft DHA domain is distinct from lipid rafts due to the highly flexible DHA, which is incompatible with the rigidity of sphingolipids and cholesterol. Experimental evidence from nuclear magnetic resonance (NMR) data supports this model, since EPA and DHA are incorporated into both raft and nonraft domains in a phosphatidylethanolamine/sphingomyelin/cholesterol membrane mixture [69]. Similar results have also been observed *in vivo* by analyzing phospholipids of CD4+ T-cells after isolating the detergent-resistant and soluble membrane fractions [46,47], as well as utilizing lipid-sensitive fluorescent probes [64,70].

Because of the flexibility of n-3 PUFAs, phospholipids containing them are incompatible with the rigid cholesterol. This results in the aggregation of cholesterol in the plasma membrane and the segregation of lipid rafts from the bulk membrane [71]. Thus, one effect of EPA and DHA on lipid rafts is an increase in the size of these nanoscale domains, which have been demonstrated in various cell types such as HEK cells, CD4+ T-cells, and B-cells [64,72,73]. This perturbation in size of lipid rafts leads to alterations in the cellular signaling required for CD4+ T-cell activation and differentiation. Indeed, it has been demonstrated that n-3 PUFAs can alter the size and/or stability of lipid rafts in CD4+ T-cells [46,47,62,64,70], and therefore, downstream T-cell activation. Studies in immortalized Jurkat T-cells demonstrated that n-3 PUFAs changed the localization of signaling proteins necessary for T-cell activation, such as the Src family kinases Lck and Fyn [74], and LAT [75], from detergent-resistant membrane fractions. Using n-3 PUFA-enriched mouse CD4+ T-cells, it was also shown that recruitment and activation of signaling proteins such as PKCγ, LAT, Fas, PLC-γ1, and F-actin were altered [46,64]. Suppression of these early signaling events by n-3 PUFAs results in inhibition of downstream activation signaling in CD4+ T-cells (Figure 17.3a), including mitochondrial translocation [76], IL-2 secretion [46,77–81], and lymphoproliferation [64,78,82].

As mentioned above, IS formation requires tight regulation of the actin cytoskeleton [55–57]. Both lipid-lipid interactions and lipid-protein interactions (i.e., membrane-actin cytoskeleton interactions) contribute to T-cell activation and the formation of the IS. n-3 PUFAs can directly perturb the membrane-actin cytoskeleton (i.e., lipid-protein) interactions by depleting the overall level of PI (4,5)P$_2$ in CD4+ T-cells, resulting in decreased actin cytoskeletal rearrangement upon T-cell activation [83]. The suppressive actin cytoskeletal rearrangement can be rescued by exogenous incubation of n-3 PUFA-enriched CD4+ T-cells with PI (4, 5)P$_2$. It is interesting to note that colonocytes enriched with n-3 PUFAs also exhibited suppressive activation of cytoskeletal remodeling proteins such as PLC-γ1, Rc1, and Cdc42 [84], suggesting that perturbation of membrane-actin cytoskeleton interactions by n-3 PUFAs may occur in other cell types.

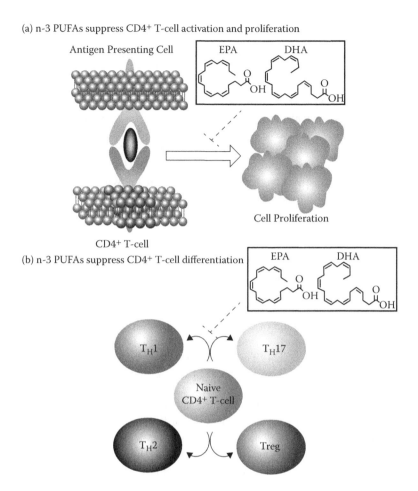

(a) n-3 PUFAs suppress CD4+ T-cell activation and proliferation

Antigen Presenting Cell

EPA DHA

Cell Proliferation

CD4+ T-cell

(b) n-3 PUFAs suppress CD4+ T-cell differentiation

EPA DHA

T_H1

T_H17

Naive
CD4+ T-cell

T_H2

Treg

FIGURE 17.3 n-3 PUFAs attenuate (a) CD4+ T-cell activation and proliferation, and (b) suppress differentiation into proinflammatory T_H1 and T_H17 CD4+ T-cell effector subsets. Note that coreceptors necessary for T-cell activation are not depicted in the diagram for simplicity purposes.

Upon T-cell activation, CD4+ T-cells can differentiate into proinflammatory (Th1 and Th17) and anti-inflammatory (Th2 and Treg) effector subsets in the presence of various cytokines [28]. These effector subsets are typically identified by their master transcriptional regulators and by the cytokines they release into the surrounding microenvironment [28]. In regard to the proinflammatory subsets, numerous reports have demonstrated the suppressive effects of n-3 PUFAs on Th1 [19,21,85–92] and Th17 [19,21,87,93–95] differentiation (Figure 17.3b). The influences of n-3 PUFAs on Th2 [85–88] and Treg differentiation [94,96,97] are not as conclusive. Not surprisingly, CD4+ T-cell differentiation has been linked to plasma membrane properties. Disrupting CD4+ T-cell lipid rafts using methyl-β-cyclodextrin suppressed Ca^{2+} influx upon antigen stimulation in Th1, but not Th2, cells [98]. This may be due, in part, to the different IS architecture between Th1 and Th2 cells. For example, the Th1 IS is characterized by the bull's-eye pattern of the cSMAC surrounded by the pSMAC, while the Th2 IS is multifocal and dependent on the concentration of antigens [99].

Human CD4+ T-cells can also be categorized by their plasma membrane lipid order. Using the probe di-4-ANEPPDHQ, which changes its fluorescence intensities at 570 nm and 620 nm based on the lipid order of its membrane microenvironment, human CD4+ T-cells can be classified as low, intermediate, or high lipid order [100]. Lipid order was associated with a specific effector CD4+ T-cell subset. CD4+ T-cells with intermediate membrane order were associated with IFN-γ production (i.e., Th1 phenotype), while high membrane order was associated with IL-4 production (i.e., Th2 phenotype). Culturing CD4+ T-cells in Th1- or Th2-polarizing conditions can also dictate the membrane order; culturing CD4+ T-cells under Th1 conditions results in intermediate membrane order, while culturing under Th2 conditions results in high membrane order. By reducing the membrane order with 7-ketocholesterol, the number of CD4+ T-cells producing IFN-γ (Th1 cytokine) was increased, indicative of a switch from Th2 (high order) to Th1 (intermediate order) cells. Changes in the membrane phospholipids in CD4+ T-cells can also be observed in clinical pathology. Human patients with systemic lupus erythematosus, Sjorgren's Syndrome, or RA have an increased population of intermediate membrane order CD4+ T-cells, which is associated with the proinflammatory, IFN-γ–producing CD4+ Th1 cells [100,101]. The other proinflammatory CD4+ T effector subset, Th17, is also known to be affected by membrane order. Decreasing glycosphingolipid, a lipid known to be associated with lipid rafts, in CD4+ T-cells resulted in reduced Th17 differentiation [102]. These studies highlight the importance of the plasma membrane in regulating CD4+ T-cell differentiation, and reveal the biochemical mechanism by which phospholipids containing n-3 PUFAs can suppress CD4+ T-cell differentiation.

As one example, the suppression of Th17 CD4+ T-cell differentiation by n-3 PUFAs involves the IL-6-gp130-STAT3 signaling axis. This signaling pathway, consisting of a hexameric signaling complex composed of two IL-6 bound to two membrane-bound IL-6 receptors (mIL-6R) and two glycoprotein 130 (gp130) leads to the phosphorylation of STAT3 and activation of the master regulator of Th17, RORγt. Activation of this pathway regulates the earliest events in Th17 cell differentiation [103–108]. Initial reports demonstrated that n-3 PUFAs suppressed phosphorylation of STAT3 and activation of RORγt CD4+ T-cells [95,109]. This led to the hypothesis that the IL-6-gp130-STAT3 signaling axis was perturbed by n-3 PUFAs, since IL-6R and gp130 were found to associate with lipid rafts. Cholesterol regulated the localization of IL-6R at the plasma membrane [110], while gp130 was localized in lipid rafts of kidney [111] and neuroepithelial [112] cell plasma membranes. n-3 PUFAs decreased surface expression of IL-6R and the association of gp130 with lipid rafts, reducing homodimerization of gp130 and causing decreased downstream STAT3 phosphorylation [93]. This study demonstrated that membrane perturbation induced by n-3 PUFAs suppressed Th17 differentiation by downregulating the IL6-gp130-STAT3 pathway.

17.5 PUFAs AND EICOSANOIDS

Eicosanoids are lipid mediators primarily synthesized from the n-6 PUFA arachidonic acid (AA, 20:4n-6) during an inflammatory response. AA is first released from the membrane phospholipids by phospholipase A_2 and then the free AA becomes the substrate for either cyclooxygenase (COX) to form prostaglandins, lipoxygenase enzymes (LOX) to form 5-, 12-, or 15-hydroxyicosatetraenoic acids and leukotrienes, or cytochrome P450 enzymes to form additional spell out (HETEs). These eicosanoids are synthesized by immune cells such as neutrophils, macrophages, and lymphocytes to act in a paracrine fashion, and are important in the development and resolution of an effective inflammatory response [113–115]. Pharmaceuticals have been developed to block these pathways to combat hyperactive inflammation (e.g. aspirin [116]). Prostaglandin E_2 (PGE$_2$) is thought to suppress CD4+ T-cell activation and proliferation. Additionally, PGE$_2$ has been shown to regulate the Th1/Th2 balance by inhibiting Th1, and promoting Th2 cytokines [117–120]. PGE$_2$ also has been shown to enhance the induction and differentiation of the Treg subset [121], suggesting that PGE$_2$ overall exerts an anti-inflammatory effect on CD4+ T-cells. Recently, however, it has been suggested that the concentration of PGE$_2$ may dictate its pro- and anti-inflammatory effects. Nanomolar concentrations of PGE$_2$ have been shown to promote Th1 and Th17 differentiation [122,123] through the EP2 and EP4 receptors [123]. Blocking the EP4 receptor with an antagonist suppressed Th1 and Th17 differentiation in mouse models of two inflammatory diseases, contact hypersensitivity and experimental autoimmune encephalomyelitis [123]. These observations highlight the complex roles of eicosanoids in regulating CD4+ T-cell activation and differentiation.

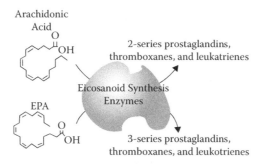

FIGURE 17.4 EPA competes with arachidonic acid for eicosanoid biosynthesis enzymes. This results in a decrease in 2-series prostaglandins, thromboxanes, and leukotrienes, as well as less potent substrates.

EPA and DHA have been demonstrated to suppress the synthesis of AA-derived eicosanoids in animal [124–126] and human studies [50,127–131]. One mechanism by which n-3 PUFAs suppress AA-derived eicosanoids is through direct competition with the enzymes that synthesize AA-derived eicosanoids (Figure 17.4). Since EPA is also a 20-carbon PUFA, it can be a substrate for COX, LOX, and cytochrome P450 enzymes to produce alternative mediators. For example, EPA is converted to PGE_3 by the COX enzyme, resulting in a lipid mediator that is less bioactive compared to PGE_2 [132–134] due to decreased affinity for its receptors [135]. Very little research has been conducted on the effects of these "alternative" eicosanoids on CD4+ T-cell activation and differentiation. Current research supports conflicting views with respect to eicosanoids produced from AA versus EPA. Some have reported that the effects of n-3 PUFAs on CD4+ T-cell proliferation is independent of the shift in eicosanoid species [136–138], while others have shown a more suppressive effect of EPA-derived PGE_3 [139]. One study demonstrated that PGE_3 was equipotent to PGE_2 in suppressing the Th1 cytokines IL-2 and IFN-γ [131], suggesting that the effects of n-3 PUFAs on CD4+ T-cell proliferation and differentiation may not be due to alternative eicosanoids.

17.6   n-3 PUFAs AND PRO-RESOLVING LIPID MEDIATORS

One of the latest discoveries in the field of n-3 PUFAs and immunity is the new class of lipid mediators produced from EPA, the E-series resolvins, and from DHA, the D-series resolvins and protectins (Figure 17.5) [140]. These specialized pro-resolving lipid mediators (SPM) are derived from the COX and LOX pathways, with alternative epimers synthesized in the presence of aspirin [141,142]. These compounds were first described as lipid mediators that participate in the anti-inflammatory and pro-resolving phase of the immune response by suppressing leukocyte activation and reducing leukocyte recruitment and infiltration to the site of inflammation [140].

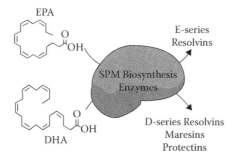

FIGURE 17.5 EPA and DHA are converted into specialized pro-resolving lipid mediators (SPMs) that can exert anti-inflammatory effects on inflammation. These mediators have yet to be examined in the context of CD4+ T-cell biology.

Resolvins and protectins have been shown in mouse models of inflammatory diseases to be protective (reviewed in [140]); however, the direct effect of these SPMs on CD4$^+$ T-cell proliferation and differentiation has not been established. One report demonstrated that human T-cells skewed toward a Th2-, but not Th1-phenotype synthesized protectin D1 (PD1) from DHA using the enzyme 15-lipoxygenase 1 [143]. PD1 was able to suppress the migration of T- and B-cells in a mouse model of peritonitis [143], and to inhibit the secretion of TNF-α and IFN-γ upon stimulation of human peripheral blood mononuclear cells with anti-CD3 and anti-CD28 [143]. On the cellular level, PD1 promoted the aggregation of Fas ligand and lipid rafts in human T-cells, resulting in induction of apoptosis [143]. Collectively, these results demonstrate an additional mechanism by which n-3 PUFAs such as DHA may affect T-cell biology. However, more studies are required to further demonstrate if, and how, these SPMs may affect T-cell activation and differentiation. One study of healthy volunteers fed seven capsules of Lovaza three times a day (17.6 g/day of n-3 PUFAs consisting of 9.7 g/day of EPA and 7.9 g/day of DHA) for approximately 24 days failed to detect these SPMs upon an acute challenge with lipopolysaccharide, suggesting that SPMs do not appear to be modulated by dietary n-3 PUFAs [144].

17.7 n-3 PUFAs AND NUCLEAR RECEPTORS

The best-characterized nuclear receptor that is activated by n-3 PUFAs is peroxisome proliferator-activated receptor-γ (PPARγ). CD4$^+$ T-cells isolated from PPARγ knockout mice exhibited an increase in IFN-γ secretion and lymphoproliferation upon activation [145]. In addition, the differentiation of anti-inflammatory Treg cells was suppressed in PPARγ-null CD4$^+$ T-cells, demonstrating that activation of PPARγ can exert anti-inflammatory effects. X-ray crystallography studies revealed that 4-oxodocosahexaenoic acid was a potent activator of PPARγ [146]. The nonoxidized versions of n-3 PUFAs themselves have been shown to activate PPARγ, but in the micromolar range [147,148]. In a mouse model of mismatched cardiac allograft, where Treg cells are important for the maintenance of transplant tolerance, administration of EPA on the day of the transplantation increased the Treg population in the recipient mouse, resulting in prolonged graft survival [145]. The administration of bisphenol A diglycidyl ether, a PPARγ antagonist, blocked the protective effect of EPA, suggesting a PPARγ-dependent mechanism [149]. In the mouse model of experimental autoimmune encephalomyelitis (EAE), a disease model involving T-cell components [150], EPA ameliorated the severity of EAE and decreased the proinflammatory cytokines IFN-γ and IL-17 produced by CD4$^+$ T-cells isolated from the central nervous system [150]. EPA also induced PPARγ mRNA expression in CNS-infiltrating CD4$^+$ T-cells, suggesting the involvement of PPARγ. Additional nuclear receptors that can be activated or inhibited by n-3 PUFAs to control CD4$^+$ T-cell activation and differentiation have yet to be characterized.

17.8 n-3 PUFAs AND AUTOIMMUNE DISEASES

IBDs are inflammatory conditions affecting the gastrointestinal tract, with Crohn's disease and ulcerative colitis being the major types. While Crohn's disease may manifest in any part of the gastrointestinal tract, ulcerative colitis is restricted to the colon. CD4$^+$ T-cell effector subsets are important in the pathogenesis of these diseases; Th1 and Th17 subsets have been implicated in the development of IBDs [151]. Additionally, proinflammatory eicosanoids have been detected in the intestinal mucosa of human patients with IBD [152,153]. Similarly, RA is an autoimmune disease characterized by recruitment of CD4$^+$ T-cells and increased proinflammatory cytokines [154]. Given that n-3 PUFAs can suppress Th1 and Th17 differentiation, as well as alter the eicosanoid profiles, n-3 PUFAs may be beneficial for the treatment of IBDs and RA.

In animal models of IBDs (mainly colitis models), n-3 PUFAs had beneficial effects on symptoms of colitis. For example, colonic injury and inflammation were reduced by n-3 PUFAs

[19,21,109,155–163]. The beneficial effects of n-3 PUFAs were attributed to suppression of Th1 and Th17 differentiation [19,21,109,157]; decreased secretion of proinflammatory cytokines such as TNF-α, IFN-γ, IL-1β, IL-6, IL-12, and IL-18, and of lipid mediators such as PGE_2 and leukotriene B_4 (LTB_4); and lowered expression of iNOS [155,156,158–163]. In addition, n-3 PUFAs also increased synthesis of anti-inflammatory lipid mediators such as resolvin D1, resolvin D2, and maresin 1 [159–161]. These animal studies highlight the efficacy of n-3 PUFAs in treating IBDs and the pleotropic mechanisms by which n-3 PUFAs suppress gastrointestinal inflammation. Although some clinical studies have demonstrated beneficial effects of n-3 PUFAs on IBDs [15,17,40], meta-analyses have found either no effect [164] or inconclusive results [165]. It is difficult to compare clinical studies due to many variables such as the dose of n-3 PUFAs used, the EPA and DHA content, and the preparation and formulation of n-3 PUFAs.

Similar to animal models of IBDs, rodent studies also demonstrated the beneficial effects of n-3 PUFAs on RA symptoms [166,167]. EPA and DHA reduced symptoms of arthritis induced by collagen, accompanied by the decrease in proinflammatory cytokines IL-1β and IFN-γ and the increase in the Th2 cytokines IL-1α, IL-10, and IL-13, all suggestive of a suppression in the proinflammatory Th1 CD4+ T-cell subsets. Clinical studies in RA patients have documented the ability of n-3 PUFAs to relieve symptoms and reduce the levels of proinflammatory cytokines [168,169]. Although one meta-analysis has concluded that n-3 PUFAs may be effective in alleviating symptoms of RA [170], more carefully designed, larger clinical studies need to be conducted to prove conclusively that n-3 PUFAs are effective in treating autoimmune and inflammatory diseases such as IBD and RA.

17.9 n-3 PUFAs AND INFECTION

In general, n-3 PUFAs exert their anti-inflammatory effects by suppressing CD4+ T-cell activation and differentiation into proinflammatory CD4+ T-cell effector subsets. Thus, it might be expected that n-3 PUFAs would be detrimental to host resistance to infectious diseases, which require pro-inflammatory effector subsets of CD4+ T-cells. In a guinea pig model of infection with virulent *Mycobacterium tuberculosis*, n-3 PUFAs suppressed delayed-type hypersensitivity as measured by the skin test response induced by purified protein derivative of tuberculin (PPD) [171]. Splenocytes isolated from guinea pigs fed n-3 PUFAs for 3 weeks exhibited a reduction in IFN-γ and a concomitant increase in TGF-β mRNA expression levels upon PPD stimulation. Furthermore, guinea pigs fed an n-3 PUFA–enriched diet had significantly higher bacillary loads in the lungs after a low-dose pulmonary challenge with virulent *M. tuberculosis* [171]. The detrimental impact of dietary n-3 PUFAs on resistance to *M. tuberculosis* infection was also recapitulated in a mouse model that can genetically synthesize n-3 PUFAs [172].

Using SMAD3$^{-/-}$ mice exposed to *Helicobacter hepaticus* as a model of colitis, high doses of dietary fish oil (2.25%–6%) exacerbated colonic inflammation and increased postinfection mortality [97]. One study using the dextran sulphate sodium induction of colitis in mice also suggested a detrimental effect of n-3 PUFAs, possibly through modulation of the adiponectin signaling [173]. These studies highlight the immunosuppressive effects of n-3 PUFAs, and the importance of determining the best doses of n-3 PUFAs to impact inflammatory diseases without influencing infection risk.

17.10 CONCLUDING COMMENTS

The n-3 PUFAs EPA and DHA alter differentiation and function of CD4+ T-cells, helping to attenuate inflammation. That n-3 PUFAs are anti-inflammatory is well demonstrated in numerous animal models and in human patients. A number of mechanisms of action by which n-3 PUFAs affect T-cells have been elucidated, many of them involving alterations in membrane composition and in membrane functionality in response to signals. Many questions remain to be answered with regard to how n-3 PUFAs alter CD4+ T-cell biology and the impact that this can have on human inflammatory disease and on susceptibility to infection. Among these questions are:

1. Do EPA and DHA affect CD4+ T-cells to the same degree and by the same molecular mechanisms? Biophysical studies suggest that EPA and DHA differentially perturb the plasma membrane [67,69], and biochemical analyses have shown that EPA and DHA generate distinct metabolites [140]. Thus, the contribution from each individual n-3 PUFA needs to be assessed to understand the relative contributions of EPA and DHA to the treatment of inflammatory diseases.
2. Can n-3 PUFAs be used in combination with other bioactive nutraceuticals to enhance the anti-inflammatory effects? Previous studies have shown that n-3 PUFAs and curcumin, a curcumoid found in the Indian spice turmeric, reduce proliferation of CD4+ T-cells [174] and suppress colonic inflammation by suppressing the proinflammatory transcription regulator NF-κB [175]. This is an example of how nutrients can act in combination in order to modulate T-cell–induced inflammation. Therefore, additional studies should be carried out to elucidate how other anti-inflammatory compounds function in combination to modulate T-cell biology and inflammation.
3. Do n-3 PUFAs suppress the differentiation and activation of other CD4+ T-cell effector subsets, such as Th9 and Th22 cells [176], and modulate their roles in inflammatory diseases?

In summary, although a wealth of studies has demonstrated the usefulness of n-3 PUFAs in targeting CD4+ T-cells to exert anti-inflammatory effects on a series of animal models of inflammatory disorders, clinical studies have yet to yield conclusive results supporting the efficacy of these bioactive molecules. This highlights the need to better understand not only the biochemical and biophysical mechanisms by which n-3 PUFAs affect CD4+ T-cell biology, but also the cellular and physiological mechanisms by which these dietary bioactives work in a pleotropic fashion.

ACKNOWLEDGMENTS

This work was supported in part by the Clinical Science and Translational Research Institute grant program at Texas A&M and NIH grants R35CA197707, CA129444 and P30ES023512.

REFERENCES

1. Loftus, E. V., Jr. (2007) The burden of inflammatory bowel disease in the United States: A moving target? *Clinical Gastroenterology and Hepatology: The Official Clinical Practice Journal of the American Gastroenterological Association.* **5**, 1383–1384.
2. Lumeng, C. N., Maillard, I. and Saltiel, A. R. (2009) T-ing up inflammation in fat. *Nature Medicine.* **15**, 846–847.
3. O'Rourke, R. W. and Lumeng, C. N. (2013) Obesity heats up adipose tissue lymphocytes. *Gastroenterology.* **145**, 282–285.
4. Baigent, C. N. T. C., Bhala, N., Emberson, J., Merhi, A., Abramson, S., Arber, N., Baron, J. A., Bombardier, C., Cannon, C., Farkouh, M. E. et al. (2013) Vascular and upper gastrointestinal effects of non-steroidal anti-inflammatory drugs: Meta-analyses of individual participant data from randomised trials. *Lancet.* **382**, 769–779.
5. van Everdingen, A. A., Jacobs, J. W., Siewertsz Van Reesema, D. R. and Bijlsma, J. W. (2002) Low-dose prednisone therapy for patients with early active rheumatoid arthritis: Clinical efficacy, disease-modifying properties, and side effects: A randomized, double-blind, placebo-controlled clinical trial. *Annals of Internal Medicine.* **136**, 1–12.
6. Belluzzi, A., Boschi, S., Brignola, C., Munarini, A., Cariani, G. and Miglio, F. (2000) Polyunsaturated fatty acids and inflammatory bowel disease. *American Journal of Clinical Nutrition.* **71**, 339S–342S.

7. Bouwens, M., van de Rest, O., Dellschaft, N., Bromhaar, M. G., de Groot, L. C., Geleijnse, J. M., Muller, M. and Afman, L. A. (2009) Fish-oil supplementation induces antiinflammatory gene expression profiles in human blood mononuclear cells. *American Journal of Clinical Nutrition*. **90**, 415–424.

8. Farzaneh-Far, R., Harris, W. S., Garg, S., Na, B. and Whooley, M. A. (2009) Inverse association of erythrocyte n-3 fatty acid levels with inflammatory biomarkers in patients with stable coronary artery disease: The Heart and Soul Study. *Atherosclerosis*. **205**, 538–543.

9. Guebre-Egziabher, F., Debard, C., Drai, J., Denis, L., Pesenti, S., Bienvenu, J., Vidal, H., Laville, M. and Fouque, D. (2013) Differential dose effect of fish oil on inflammation and adipose tissue gene expression in chronic kidney disease patients. *Nutrition*. **29**, 730–736.

10. Itariu, B. K., Zeyda, M., Hochbrugger, E. E., Neuhofer, A., Prager, G., Schindler, K., Bohdjalian, A., Mascher, D., Vangala, S., Schranz, M. et al. (2012) Long-chain n-3 PUFAs reduce adipose tissue and systemic inflammation in severely obese nondiabetic patients: A randomized controlled trial. *American Journal of Clinical Nutrition*. **96**, 1137–1149

11. Mozaffarian, D., Lemaitre, R. N., King, I. B., Song, X., Huang, H., Sacks, F. M., Rimm, E. B., Wang, M. and Siscovick, D. S. (2013) Plasma phospholipid long-chain omega-3 fatty acids and total and cause-specific mortality in older adults: A cohort study. *Annals of Internal Medicine*. **158**, 515–525.

12. Noel, S. E., Newby, P. K., Ordovas, J. M. and Tucker, K. L. (2010) Adherence to an (n-3) fatty acid/fish intake pattern is inversely associated with metabolic syndrome among Puerto Rican adults in the Greater Boston area. *Journal of Nutrition*. **140**, 1846–1854.

13. Snodgrass, R. G., Huang, S., Choi, I. W., Rutledge, J. C. and Hwang, D. H. (2013) Inflammasome-mediated secretion of IL-1beta in human monocytes through TLR2 activation; modulation by dietary fatty acids. *Journal of Immunology*. **191**, 4337–4347.

14. Spencer, M., Finlin, B. S., Unal, R., Zhu, B., Morris, A. J., Shipp, L. R., Lee, J., Walton, R. G., Adu, A., Erfani, R. A. et al. (2013) Omega-3 fatty acids reduce adipose tissue macrophages in human subjects with insulin resistance. *Diabetes*. **62**, 1709–1717.

15. Uchiyama, K., Nakamura, M., Odahara, S., Koido, S., Katahira, K., Shiraishi, H., Ohkusa, T., Fujise, K. and Tajiri, H. (2010) N-3 polyunsaturated fatty acid diet therapy for patients with inflammatory bowel disease. *Inflammatory Bowel Disease*. **16**, 1696–1707.

16. Vedin, I., Cederholm, T., Freund Levi, Y., Basun, H., Garlind, A., Faxen Irving, G., Jonhagen, M. E., Vessby, B., Wahlund, L. O. and Palmblad, J. (2008) Effects of docosahexaenoic acid-rich n-3 fatty acid supplementation on cytokine release from blood mononuclear leukocytes: The OmegAD study. *American Journal of Clinical Nutrition*. **87**, 1616–1622.

17. Weaver, K. L., Ivester, P., Seeds, M., Case, L. D., Arm, J. P. and Chilton, F. H. (2009) Effect of dietary fatty acids on inflammatory gene expression in healthy humans. *Journal of Biological Chemistry*. **284**, 15400–15407.

18. Flock, M. R., Rogers, C. J., Prabhu, K. S. and Kris-Etherton, P. M. (2013) Immunometabolic role of long-chain omega-3 fatty acids in obesity-induced inflammation. *Diabetes/Metabolism Research and Reviews*. **29**, 431–445.

19. Monk, J. M., Jia, Q., Callaway, E., Weeks, B., Alaniz, R. C., McMurray, D. N. and Chapkin, R. S. (2012) Th17 cell accumulation is decreased during chronic experimental colitis by (n-3) PUFA in Fat-1 mice. *Journal of Nutrition*. **142**, 117–124.

20. Monk, J. M., Kim, W., Callaway, E., Turk, H. F., Foreman, J. E., Peters, J. M., He, W., Weeks, B., Alaniz, R. C., McMurray, D. N. et al. (2012) Immunomodulatory action of dietary fish oil and targeted deletion of intestinal epithelial cell PPARdelta in inflammation-induced colon carcinogenesis. *American Journal of Physiology. Gastrointestinal and Liver Physiology*. **302**, G153–G167.

21. Monk, J. M., Turk, H. F., Fan, Y. Y., Callaway, E., Weeks, B., Yang, P., McMurray, D. N. and Chapkin, R. S. (2014) Antagonizing arachidonic acid-derived eicosanoids reduces inflammatory th17 and Th1 cell-mediated inflammation and colitis severity. *Mediators of Inflammation*. **2014**, 917149.

22. Yan, Y., Jiang, W., Spinetti, T., Tardivel, A., Castillo, R., Bourquin, C., Guarda, G., Tian, Z., Tschopp, J. and Zhou, R. (2013) Omega-3 fatty acids prevent inflammation and metabolic disorder through inhibition of NLRP3 inflammasome activation. *Immunity*. **38**, 1154–1163.

23. Marty-Roix, R. and Lien, E. (2013) (De-) oiling inflammasomes. *Immunity*. **38**, 1088–1090.

24. Oh, D. Y., Talukdar, S., Bae, E. J., Imamura, T., Morinaga, H., Fan, W., Li, P., Lu, W. J., Watkins, S. M. and Olefsky, J. M. (2010) GPR120 is an omega-3 fatty acid receptor mediating potent anti-inflammatory and insulin-sensitizing effects. *Cell*. **142**, 687–698.

25. Spite, M., Claria, J. and Serhan, C. N. (2014) Resolvins, specialized proresolving lipid mediators, and their potential roles in metabolic diseases. *Cell Metabolism*. **19**, 21–36.

26. White, P. J. and Marette, A. (2014) Potential role of omega-3-derived resolution mediators in metabolic inflammation. *Immunology and Cell Biology*. **92**, 324–330.

27. Zenewicz, L. A., Antov, A. and Flavell, R. A. (2009) CD4 T-cell differentiation and inflammatory bowel disease. *Trends in Molecular Medicine*. **15**, 199–207.
28. Zhu, J., Yamane, H. and Paul, W. E. (2010) Differentiation of effector CD4 T cell populations (*). *Annual Review of Immunology*. **28**, 445–489.
29. Nakamura, M. T. and Nara, T. Y. (2004) Structure, function, and dietary regulation of delta6, delta5, and delta9 desaturases. *Annual Review of Nutrition*. **24**, 345–376.
30. Calder, P. C. (2015) Marine omega-3 fatty acids and inflammatory processes: Effects, mechanisms and clinical relevance. *Biochimica et Biophysica Acta*. **1851**, 469–484.
31. Pawlosky, R. J., Hibbeln, J. R., Novotny, J. A. and Salem, N., Jr. (2001) Physiological compartmental analysis of alpha-linolenic acid metabolism in adult humans. *Journal of Lipid Research*. **42**, 1257–1265.
32. Watts, J. L. and Browse, J. (2002) Genetic dissection of polyunsaturated fatty acid synthesis in Caenorhabditis elegans. *Proceeding of the National Academy of Sciences of the United States of America*. **99**, 5854–5859.
33. Spychalla, J. P., Kinney, A. J. and Browse, J. (1997) Identification of an animal omega-3 fatty acid desaturase by heterologous expression in Arabidopsis. *Proceeding of the National Academy of Sciences of the United States of America*. **94**, 1142–1147.
34. Meesapyodsuk, D., Reed, D. W., Savile, C. K., Buist, P. H., Ambrose, S. J. and Covello, P. S. (2000) Characterization of the regiochemistry and cryptoregiochemistry of a Caenorhabditis elegans fatty acid desaturase (FAT-1) expressed in Saccharomyces cerevisiae. *Biochemistry*. **39**, 11948–11954.
35. Calder, P. C. (2013) Omega-3 polyunsaturated fatty acids and inflammatory processes: Nutrition or pharmacology? *British Journal of Clinical Pharmacology*. **75**, 645–662.
36. McCall, T. B., O'Leary, D., Bloomfield, J. and O'Morain, C. A. (1989) Therapeutic potential of fish oil in the treatment of ulcerative colitis. *Alimentary Pharmacology and Therapeutics*. **3**, 415–424.
37. Hawthorne, A. B., Daneshmend, T. K., Hawkey, C. J., Belluzzi, A., Everitt, S. J., Holmes, G. K., Malkinson, C., Shaheen, M. Z. and Willars, J. E. (1992) Treatment of ulcerative colitis with fish oil supplementation: A prospective 12 month randomised controlled trial. *Gut*. **33**, 922–928.
38. Stenson, W. F., Cort, D., Rodgers, J., Burakoff, R., DeSchryver-Kecskemeti, K., Gramlich, T. L. and Beeken, W. (1992) Dietary supplementation with fish oil in ulcerative colitis. *Annals of Internal Medicine*. **116**, 609–614.
39. Shimizu, T., Fujii, T., Suzuki, R., Igarashi, J., Ohtsuka, Y., Nagata, S. and Yamashiro, Y. (2003) Effects of highly purified eicosapentaenoic acid on erythrocyte fatty acid composition and leukocyte and colonic mucosa leukotriene B4 production in children with ulcerative colitis. *Journal of Pediatric Gastroenterology and Nutrition*. **37**, 581–585.
40. Belluzzi, A., Brignola, C., Campieri, M., Pera, A., Boschi, S. and Miglioli, M. (1996) Effect of an enteric-coated fish-oil preparation on relapses in Crohn's disease. *New England Journal of Medicine*. **334**, 1557–1560.
41. Miles, E. A. and Calder, P. C. (2012) Influence of marine n-3 polyunsaturated fatty acids on immune function and a systematic review of their effects on clinical outcomes in rheumatoid arthritis. *British Journal of Nutrition*. **107 Suppl 2**, S171–184.
42. Cleland, L. G., Caughey, G. E., James, M. J. and Proudman, S. M. (2006) Reduction of cardiovascular risk factors with longterm fish oil treatment in early rheumatoid arthritis. *Jourmnal of Rheumatology*. **33**, 1973–1979.
43. Papanikolaou, Y., Brooks, J., Reider, C. and Fulgoni, V. L., 3rd. (2014) U.S. adults are not meeting recommended levels for fish and omega-3 fatty acid intake: Results of an analysis using observational data from NHANES 2003–2008. *Nutrition Journal*. **13**, 31.
44. Lloyd-Jones, D. M., Hong, Y., Labarthe, D., Mozaffarian, D., Appel, L. J., Van Horn, L., Greenlund, K., Daniels, S., Nichol, G., Tomaselli, G. F. et al. (2010) Defining and setting national goals for cardiovascular health promotion and disease reduction: The American Heart Association's strategic Impact Goal through 2020 and beyond. *Circulation*. **121**, 586–613.
45. U.S. Department of Agriculture and U.S. Department of Health and Human Services (December 2010) *Dietary Guidelines for Americans*, Washington, DC: U.S. Government Printing Office.
46. Fan, Y. Y., Ly, L. H., Barhoumi, R., McMurray, D. N. and Chapkin, R. S. (2004) Dietary docosahexaenoic acid suppresses T cell protein kinase C theta lipid raft recruitment and IL-2 production. *Journal of Immunology*. **173**, 6151–6160.
47. Fan, Y. Y., McMurray, D. N., Ly, L. H. and Chapkin, R. S. (2003) Dietary (n-3) polyunsaturated fatty acids remodel mouse T-cell lipid rafts. *Journal of Nutrition*. **133**, 1913–1920.
48. Gawrisch, K. and Soubias, O. (2008) Structure and dynamics of polyunsaturated hydrocarbon chains in lipid bilayers-significance for GPCR function. *Chemistry and Physics of Lipids*. **153**, 64–75.

49. Soubias, O. and Gawrisch, K. (2007) Docosahexaenoyl chains isomerize on the sub-nanosecond time scale. *Journal of the American Chemical Society.* **129**, 6678–6679.
50. Meydani, S. N., Endres, S., Woods, M. M., Goldin, B. R., Soo, C., Morrill-Labrode, A., Dinarello, C. A. and Gorbach, S. L. (1991) Oral (n-3) fatty acid supplementation suppresses cytokine production and lymphocyte proliferation: Comparison between young and older women. *Journal of Nutrition.* **121**, 547–555.
51. Thies, F., Nebe-von-Caron, G., Powell, J. R., Yaqoob, P., Newsholme, E. A. and Calder, P. C. (2001) Dietary supplementation with gamma-linolenic acid or fish oil decreases T lymphocyte proliferation in healthy older humans. *Journal of Nutrition.* **131**, 191–1927.
52. Lee, K. H., Dinner, A. R., Tu, C., Campi, G., Raychaudhuri, S., Varma, R., Sims, T. N., Burack, W. R., Wu, H., Wang, J. et al. (2003) The immunological synapse balances T cell receptor signaling and degradation. *Science.* **302**, 1218–1222.
53. Monks, C. R., Freiberg, B. A., Kupfer, H., Sciaky, N. and Kupfer, A. (1998) Three-dimensional segregation of supramolecular activation clusters in T cells. *Nature.* **395**, 82–86.
54. Tybulewicz, V. L. and Henderson, R. B. (2009) Rho family GTPases and their regulators in lymphocytes. *Nature Reviews Immunology.* **9**, 630–644.
55. Gomez, T. S. and Billadeau, D. D. (2008) T cell activation and the cytoskeleton: You can't have one without the other. *Advances in Immunology.* **97**, 1–64.
56. Huang, Y. and Burkhardt, J. K. (2007) T-cell-receptor-dependent actin regulatory mechanisms. *Journal of Cell Science.* **120**, 723–730.
57. Meiri, K. F. (2005) Lipid rafts and regulation of the cytoskeleton during T cell activation. *Philosophical Transactions of the Royal Society of London. Series B Biological Sciences.* **360**, 1663–1672.
58. Campi, G., Varma, R. and Dustin, M. L. (2005) Actin and agonist MHC-peptide complex-dependent T cell receptor microclusters as scaffolds for signaling. *Journal of Experimental Medicine.* **202**, 1031–1036.
59. DeMond, A. L., Mossman, K. D., Starr, T., Dustin, M. L. and Groves, J. T. (2008) T cell receptor microcluster transport through molecular mazes reveals mechanism of translocation. *Biophysical Journal.* **94**, 3286–3292.
60. Yokosuka, T., Sakata-Sogawa, K., Kobayashi, W., Hiroshima, M., Hashimoto-Tane, A., Tokunaga, M., Dustin, M. L. and Saito, T. (2005) Newly generated T cell receptor microclusters initiate and sustain T cell activation by recruitment of Zap70 and SLP-76. *Nature Immunology.* **6**, 1253–1262.
61. Kaizuka, Y., Douglass, A. D., Varma, R., Dustin, M. L. and Vale, R. D. (2007) Mechanisms for segregating T cell receptor and adhesion molecules during immunological synapse formation in Jurkat T cells. *Proceeedings of the National Academy of Sciences of the United States of America.* **104**, 20296–20301.
62. Zech, T., Ejsing, C. S., Gaus, K., de Wet, B., Shevchenko, A., Simons, K. and Harder, T. (2009) Accumulation of raft lipids in T-cell plasma membrane domains engaged in TCR signalling. *EMBO Journal.* **28**, 466–476.
63. Burack, W. R., Lee, K. H., Holdorf, A. D., Dustin, M. L. and Shaw, A. S. (2002) Cutting edge: Quantitative imaging of raft accumulation in the immunological synapse. *Journal of Immunology.* **169**, 2837–2841.
64. Kim, W., Fan, Y. Y., Barhoumi, R., Smith, R., McMurray, D. N. and Chapkin, R. S. (2008) n-3 polyunsaturated fatty acids suppress the localization and activation of signaling proteins at the immunological synapse in murine CD4+ T cells by affecting lipid raft formation. *Journal of Immunology.* **181**, 6236–6243.
65. Xavier, R., Brennan, T., Li, Q., McCormack, C. and Seed, B. (1998) Membrane compartmentation is required for efficient T cell activation. *Immunity.* **8**, 723–732.
66. Rentero, C., Zech, T., Quinn, C. M., Engelhardt, K., Williamson, D., Grewal, T., Jessup, W., Harder, T. and Gaus, K. (2008) Functional implications of plasma membrane condensation for T cell activation. *PLOS ONE.* **3**, e2262.
67. Shaikh, S. R., Kinnun, J. J., Leng, X., Williams, J. A. and Wassall, S. R. (2014) How polyunsaturated fatty acids modify molecular organization in membranes: Insight from NMR studies of model systems. *Biochimica et Biophysica Acta* 1848:211–9.
68. Wassall, S. R. and Stillwell, W. (2008) Docosahexaenoic acid domains: The ultimate non-raft membrane domain. *Chemistry and Physics of Lipids.* **153**, 57–63.
69. Williams, J. A., Batten, S. E., Harris, M., Rockett, B. D., Shaikh, S. R., Stillwell, W. and Wassall, S. R. (2012) Docosahexaenoic and eicosapentaenoic acids segregate differently between raft and nonraft domains. *Biophysical Journal.* **103**, 228–237.
70. Kim, W., Barhoumi, R., McMurray, D. N. and Chapkin, R. S. (2014) Dietary fish oil and DHA downregulate antigen-activated CD4+ T-cells while promoting the formation of liquid-ordered mesodomains. *British Journal of Nutrition.* **111**, 254–260.
71. Wassall, S. R. and Stillwell, W. (2009) Polyunsaturated fatty acid-cholesterol interactions: Domain formation in membranes. *Biochimica et Biophysica Acta.* **1788**, 24–32.

72. Chapkin, R. S., Wang, N., Fan, Y. Y., Lupton, J. R. and Prior, I. A. (2008) Docosahexaenoic acid alters the size and distribution of cell surface microdomains. *Biochimica et Biophysica Acta*. **1778**, 466–471.

73. Rockett, B. D., Teague, H., Harris, M., Melton, M., Williams, J., Wassall, S. R. and Shaikh, S. R. (2012) Fish oil increases raft size and membrane order of B cells accompanied by differential effects on function. *Journal of Lipid Research*. **53**, 674–685.

74. Stulnig, T. M., Berger, M., Sigmund, T., Raederstorff, D., Stockinger, H. and Waldhausl, W. (1998) Polyunsaturated fatty acids inhibit T cell signal transduction by modification of detergent-insoluble membrane domains. *Journal of Cell Biology*. **143**, 637–644.

75. Stulnig, T. M., Huber, J., Leitinger, N., Imre, E. M., Angelisova, P., Nowotny, P. and Waldhausl, W. (2001) Polyunsaturated eicosapentaenoic acid displaces proteins from membrane rafts by altering raft lipid composition. *Journal of Biological Chemistry*. **276**, 37335–37340.

76. Yog, R., Barhoumi, R., McMurray, D. N. and Chapkin, R. S. (2010) n-3 polyunsaturated fatty acids suppress mitochondrial translocation to the immunologic synapse and modulate calcium signaling in T cells. *Journal of Immunology*. **184**, 5865–5873.

77. Jolly, C. A., Jiang, Y. H., Chapkin, R. S. and McMurray, D. N. (1997) Dietary (n-3) polyunsaturated fatty acids suppress murine lymphoproliferation, interleukin-2 secretion, and the formation of diacylglycerol and ceramide. *Journal of Nutrition*. **127**, 37–43.

78. McMurray, D. N., Jolly, C. A. and Chapkin, R. S. (2000) Effects of dietary n-3 fatty acids on T cell activation and T cell receptor-mediated signaling in a murine model. *Journal of Infectious Diseases*. **182 Suppl 1**, S103–S107.

79. Arrington, J. L., McMurray, D. N., Switzer, K. C., Fan, Y. Y. and Chapkin, R. S. (2001) Docosahexaenoic acid suppresses function of the CD28 costimulatory membrane receptor in primary murine and Jurkat T cells. *Journal of Nutrition*. **131**, 1147–1153.

80. Chapkin, R. S., Arrington, J. L., Apanasovich, T. V., Carroll, R. J. and McMurray, D. N. (2002) Dietary n-3 PUFA affect TcR-mediated activation of purified murine T cells and accessory cell function in co-cultures. *Clinical and Experimental Immunology*. **130**, 12–18.

81. Ly, L. H., Smith, R., Switzer, K. C., Chapkin, R. S. and McMurray, D. N. (2006) Dietary eicosapentaenoic acid modulates CTLA-4 expression in murine CD4+ T-cells. *Prostaglandins, Leukotrienes, and Essential Fatty Acids*. **74**, 29–37.

82. Fan, Y. Y., Kim, W., Callaway, E., Smith, R., Jia, Q., Zhou, L., McMurray, D. N. and Chapkin, R. S. (2008) fat-1 transgene expression prevents cell culture-induced loss of membrane n-3 fatty acids in activated CD4+ T-cells. *Prostaglandins, Leukotrienes, and Essential Fatty Acids*. **79**, 209–214.

83. Hou, T. Y., Monk, J. M., Fan, Y. Y., Barhoumi, R., Chen, Y. Q., Rivera, G. M., McMurray, D. N. and Chapkin, R. S. (2012) n-3 polyunsaturated fatty acids suppress phosphatidylinositol 4,5-bisphosphate-dependent actin remodelling during CD4+ T-cell activation. *Biochemical Journal*. **443**, 27–37.

84. Turk, H. F., Monk, J. M., Fan, Y. Y., Callaway, E. S., Weeks, B. and Chapkin, R. S. (2013) Inhibitory effects of omega-3 fatty acids on injury-induced epidermal growth factor receptor transactivation contribute to delayed wound healing. *American Journal of Physiology. Cell Physiology*. **304**, C905–C917.

85. Attakpa, E., Hichami, A., Simonin, A. M., Sanson, E. G., Dramane, K. L. and Khan, N. A. (2009) Docosahexaenoic acid modulates the expression of T-bet and GATA-3 transcription factors, independently of PPARalpha, through suppression of MAP kinase activation. *Biochimie*. **91**, 1359–1365.

86. Johansson, S., Lonnqvist, A., Ostman, S., Sandberg, A. S. and Wold, A. E. (2010) Long-chain polyunsaturated fatty acids are consumed during allergic inflammation and affect T helper type 1 (Th1)- and Th2-mediated hypersensitivity differently. *Clinical and Experimental Immunology*. **160**, 411–419.

87. Kong, W., Yen, J. H. and Ganea, D. (2011) Docosahexaenoic acid prevents dendritic cell maturation, inhibits antigen-specific Th1/Th17 differentiation and suppresses experimental autoimmune encephalomyelitis. *Brain, Behavior, and Immunity*. **25**, 872–882.

88. Sierra, S., Lara-Villoslada, F., Comalada, M., Olivares, M. and Xaus, J. (2006) Dietary fish oil n-3 fatty acids increase regulatory cytokine production and exert anti-inflammatory effects in two murine models of inflammation. *Lipids*. **41**, 1115–1125.

89. Switzer, K. C., Fan, Y. Y., Wang, N., McMurray, D. N. and Chapkin, R. S. (2004) Dietary n-3 polyunsaturated fatty acids promote activation-induced cell death in Th1-polarized murine CD4+ T-cells. *Journal of Lipid Research*. **45**, 1482–1492.

90. Switzer, K. C., McMurray, D. N., Morris, J. S. and Chapkin, R. S. (2003) (n-3) Polyunsaturate fatty acids promote activation-induced cell death in murine T lymphocytes. *Journal of Nutrition*. **133**, 496–503.

91. Zhang, P., Kim, W., Zhou, L., Wang, N., Ly, L. H., McMurray, D. N. and Chapkin, R. S. (2006) Dietary fish oil inhibits antigen-specific murine Th1 cell development by suppression of clonal expansion. *Journal of nutrition*. **136**, 2391–2398.

92. Zhang, P., Smith, R., Chapkin, R. S. and McMurray, D. N. (2005) Dietary (n-3) polyunsaturated fatty acids modulate murine Th1/Th2 balance toward the Th2 pole by suppression of Th1 development. *Journal of Nutrition.* **135**, 1745–1751.
93. Allen, M. J., Fan, Y. Y., Monk, J. M., Hou, T. Y., Barhoumi, R., McMurray, D. N. and Chapkin, R. S. (2014) n-3 PUFAs reduce T-helper 17 cell differentiation by decreasing responsiveness to interleukin-6 in isolated mouse splenic CD4(+) T cells. *Journal of Nutrition.* **144**, 1306–1313.
94. Qin, S., Wen, J., Bai, X. C., Chen, T. Y., Zheng, R. C., Zhou, G. B., Ma, J., Feng, J. Y., Zhong, B. L. and Li, Y. M. (2014) Endogenous n-3 polyunsaturated fatty acids protect against imiquimod-induced psoriasis-like inflammation via the IL-17/IL-23 axis. *Molecular Medicine Reports.* **9**, 2097–2104.
95. Monk, J. M., Hou, T. Y., Turk, H. F., McMurray, D. N. and Chapkin, R. S. (2013) n3 PUFAs reduce mouse CD4+ T-cell ex vivo polarization into Th17 cells. *Journal of Nutrition.* **143**, 1501–1508.
96. Yessoufou, A., Ple, A., Moutairou, K., Hichami, A. and Khan, N. A. (2009) Docosahexaenoic acid reduces suppressive and migratory functions of CD4+CD25+ regulatory T-cells. *Journal of Lipid Research.* **50**, 2377–2388.
97. Woodworth, H. L., McCaskey, S. J., Duriancik, D. M., Clinthorne, J. F., Langohr, I. M., Gardner, E. M. and Fenton, J. I. (2010) Dietary fish oil alters T lymphocyte cell populations and exacerbates disease in a mouse model of inflammatory colitis. *Cancer Research.* **70**, 7960–7969.
98. Balamuth, F., Leitenberg, D., Unternaehrer, J., Mellman, I. and Bottomly, K. (2001) Distinct patterns of membrane microdomain partitioning in Th1 and th2 cells. *Immunity.* **15**, 729–738.
99. Thauland, T. J., Koguchi, Y., Wetzel, S. A., Dustin, M. L. and Parker, D. C. (2008) Th1 and Th2 cells form morphologically distinct immunological synapses. *Journal of Immunology.* **181**, 393–399.
100. Miguel, L., Owen, D. M., Lim, C., Liebig, C., Evans, J., Magee, A. I. and Jury, E. C. (2011) Primary human CD4+ T cells have diverse levels of membrane lipid order that correlate with their function. *Journal of Immunology.* **186**, 3505–3516.
101. McDonald, G., Deepak, S., Miguel, L., Hall, C. J., Isenberg, D. A., Magee, A. I., Butters, T. and Jury, E. C. (2014) Normalizing glycosphingolipids restores function in CD4+ T cells from lupus patients. *Journal of Clinical Investigation.* **124**, 712–724.
102. Zhu, Y., Gumlaw, N., Karman, J., Zhao, H., Zhang, J., Jiang, J. L., Maniatis, P., Edling, A., Chuang, W. L., Siegel, C. et al. (2011) Lowering glycosphingolipid levels in CD4+ T cells attenuates T cell receptor signaling, cytokine production, and differentiation to the Th17 lineage. *Journal of Biological Chemistry.* **286**, 14787–14794.
103. Bettelli, E., Carrier, Y., Gao, W., Korn, T., Strom, T. B., Oukka, M., Weiner, H. L. and Kuchroo, V. K. (2006) Reciprocal developmental pathways for the generation of pathogenic effector TH17 and regulatory T cells. *Nature.* **441**, 235–238.
104. Briso, E. M., Dienz, O. and Rincon, M. (2008) Cutting edge: Soluble IL-6R is produced by IL-6R ectodomain shedding in activated CD4 T cells. *Journal of Immunology.* **180**, 7102–7106.
105. Jones, G. W., Greenhill, C. J., Williams, J. O., Nowell, M. A., Williams, A. S., Jenkins, B. J. and Jones, S. A. (2013) Exacerbated inflammatory arthritis in response to hyperactive gp130 signalling is independent of IL-17A. *Annals of Rheumatic Diseases.* **72**, 1738–1742.
106. Jones, G. W., McLoughlin, R. M., Hammond, V. J., Parker, C. R., Williams, J. D., Malhotra, R., Scheller, J., Williams, A. S., Rose-John, S., Topley, N. et al. (2010) Loss of CD4+ T cell IL-6R expression during inflammation underlines a role for IL-6 trans signaling in the local maintenance of Th17 cells. *Journal of Immunology.* **184**, 2130–2139.
107. Nishihara, M., Ogura, H., Ueda, N., Tsuruoka, M., Kitabayashi, C., Tsuji, F., Aono, H., Ishihara, K., Huseby, E., Betz, U. A. et al. (2007) IL-6-gp130-STAT3 in T cells directs the development of IL-17+ Th with a minimum effect on that of Treg in the steady state. *International Immunology.* **19**, 695–702.
108. Veldhoen, M., Hocking, R. J., Atkins, C. J., Locksley, R. M. and Stockinger, B. (2006) TGFbeta in the context of an inflammatory cytokine milieu supports de novo differentiation of IL-17-producing T cells. *Immunity.* **24**, 179–189.
109. Monk, J. M., Hou, T. Y., Turk, H. F., Weeks, B., Wu, C., McMurray, D. N. and Chapkin, R. S. (2012) Dietary n-3 polyunsaturated fatty acids (PUFA) decrease obesity-associated Th17 cell-mediated inflammation during colitis. *PLOS ONE.* **7**, e49739.
110. Matthews, V., Schuster, B., Schutze, S., Bussmeyer, I., Ludwig, A., Hundhausen, C., Sadowski, T., Saftig, P., Hartmann, D., Kallen, K. J. et al. (2003) Cellular cholesterol depletion triggers shedding of the human interleukin-6 receptor by ADAM10 and ADAM17 (TACE). *Journal of Biological Chemistry.* **278**, 38829–38839.

111. Buk, D. M., Waibel, M., Braig, C., Martens, A. S., Heinrich, P. C. and Graeve, L. (2004) Polarity and lipid raft association of the components of the ciliary neurotrophic factor receptor complex in Madin-Darby canine kidney cells. *Journal of Cell Science*. **117**, 2063–2075.
112. Yanagisawa, M., Nakamura, K. and Taga, T. (2004) Roles of lipid rafts in integrin-dependent adhesion and gp130 signalling pathway in mouse embryonic neural precursor cells. *Genes Cells: Devoted to Molecular & Cellular Mechanisms*. **9**, 801–809.
113. Tilley, S. L., Coffman, T. M. and Koller, B. H. (2001) Mixed messages: Modulation of inflammation and immune responses by prostaglandins and thromboxanes. *Journal of Clinical Investigation*. **108**, 15–23.
114. Mandal, A. K., Zhang, Z., Kim, S. J., Tsai, P. C. and Mukherjee, A. B. (2005) Yin-yang: Balancing act of prostaglandins with opposing functions to regulate inflammation. *Journal of Immunology*. **175**, 6271–6273.
115. Mangino, M. J., Brounts, L., Harms, B. and Heise, C. (2006) Lipoxin biosynthesis in inflammatory bowel disease. *Prostaglandins & Other Lipid Mediators*. **79**, 84–92.
116. Vane, J. R. (1971) Inhibition of prostaglandin synthesis as a mechanism of action for aspirin-like drugs. *Nature: New Biology*. **231**, 232–235.
117. Betz, M. and Fox, B. S. (1991) Prostaglandin E2 inhibits production of Th1 lymphokines but not of Th2 lymphokines. *Journal of Immunology*. **146**, 108–113.
118. Snijdewint, F. G., Kalinski, P., Wierenga, E. A., Bos, J. D. and Kapsenberg, M. L. (1993) Prostaglandin E2 differentially modulates cytokine secretion profiles of human T helper lymphocytes. *Journal of Immunology*. **150**, 5321–5329.
119. Demeure, C. E., Yang, L. P., Desjardins, C., Raynauld, P. and Delespesse, G. (1997) Prostaglandin E2 primes naive T cells for the production of anti-inflammatory cytokines. *European Journal of Immunology*. **27**, 3526–3531.
120. Wu, C. Y., Wang, K., McDyer, J. F. and Seder, R. A. (1998) Prostaglandin E2 and dexamethasone inhibit IL-12 receptor expression and IL-12 responsiveness. *Journal of Immunology*. **161**, 2723–2730.
121. Baratelli, F., Lin, Y., Zhu, L., Yang, S. C., Heuze-Vourc'h, N., Zeng, G., Reckamp, K., Dohadwala, M., Sharma, S. and Dubinett, S. M. (2005) Prostaglandin E2 induces FOXP3 gene expression and T regulatory cell function in human CD4+ T cells. *Journal of Immunology*. **175**, 1483–1490.
122. Boniface, K., Bak-Jensen, K. S., Li, Y., Blumenschein, W. M., McGeachy, M. J., McClanahan, T. K., McKenzie, B. S., Kastelein, R. A., Cua, D. J. and de Waal Malefyt, R. (2009) Prostaglandin E2 regulates Th17 cell differentiation and function through cyclic AMP and EP2/EP4 receptor signaling. *Journal of Experimental Medicine*. **206**, 535–548.
123. Yao, C., Sakata, D., Esaki, Y., Li, Y., Matsuoka, T., Kuroiwa, K., Sugimoto, Y. and Narumiya, S. (2009) Prostaglandin E2-EP4 signaling promotes immune inflammation through Th1 cell differentiation and Th17 cell expansion. *Nature Medicine*. **15**, 633–640.
124. Chapkin, R. S., Akoh, C. C. and Miller, C. C. (1991) Influence of dietary n-3 fatty acids on macrophage glycerophospholipid molecular species and peptidoleukotriene synthesis. *Journal of Lipid Research*. **32**, 1205–1213.
125. Yaqoob, P. and Calder, P. (1995) Effects of dietary lipid manipulation upon inflammatory mediator production by murine macrophages. *Cell Immunology*. **163**, 120–128.
126. Peterson, L. D., Jeffery, N. M., Thies, F., Sanderson, P., Newsholme, E. A. and Calder, P. C. (1998) Eicosapentaenoic and docosahexaenoic acids alter rat spleen leukocyte fatty acid composition and prostaglandin E2 production but have different effects on lymphocyte functions and cell-mediated immunity. *Lipids*. **33**, 171–180.
127. Lee, T. H., Hoover, R. L., Williams, J. D., Sperling, R. I., Ravalese, J., 3rd, Spur, B. W., Robinson, D. R., Corey, E. J., Lewis, R. A. and Austen, K. F. (1985) Effect of dietary enrichment with eicosapentaenoic and docosahexaenoic acids on in vitro neutrophil and monocyte leukotriene generation and neutrophil function. *New England Journal of Medicine*. **312**, 1217–1224.
128. Endres, S., Ghorbani, R., Kelley, V. E., Georgilis, K., Lonnemann, G., van der Meer, J. W., Cannon, J. G., Rogers, T. S., Klempner, M. S., Weber, P. C. et al. (1989) The effect of dietary supplementation with n-3 polyunsaturated fatty acids on the synthesis of interleukin-1 and tumor necrosis factor by mononuclear cells. *New England Journal of Medicine*. **320**, 265–271.
129. Sperling, R. I., Benincaso, A. I., Knoell, C. T., Larkin, J. K., Austen, K. F. and Robinson, D. R. (1993) Dietary omega-3 polyunsaturated fatty acids inhibit phosphoinositide formation and chemotaxis in neutrophils. *Journal of Clinical Investigation*. **91**, 651–660.
130. von Schacky, C., Kiefl, R., Jendraschak, E. and Kaminski, W. E. (1993) n-3 fatty acids and cysteinyl-leukotriene formation in humans in vitro, ex vivo, and in vivo. *Journal of Laboratory and Clinical Medicine*. **121**, 302–309.

131. Trebble, T. M., Wootton, S. A., Miles, E. A., Mullee, M., Arden, N. K., Ballinger, A. B., Stroud, M. A., Burdge, G. C. and Calder, P. C. (2003) Prostaglandin E2 production and T cell function after fish-oil supplementation: Response to antioxidant cosupplementation. *American Journal of Clinical Nutrition.* **78**, 376–382.

132. Goldman, D. W., Pickett, W. C. and Goetzl, E. J. (1983) Human neutrophil chemotactic and degranulating activities of leukotriene B5 (LTB5) derived from eicosapentaenoic acid. *Biochemical and Biophysical Research Communications.* **117**, 282–288.

133. Lee, T. H., Menica-Huerta, J. M., Shih, C., Corey, E. J., Lewis, R. A. and Austen, K. F. (1984) Characterization and biologic properties of 5,12-dihydroxy derivatives of eicosapentaenoic acid, including leukotriene B5 and the double lipoxygenase product. *Journal of Biological Chemistry.* **259**, 2383–2389.

134. Bagga, D., Wang, L., Farias-Eisner, R., Glaspy, J. A. and Reddy, S. T. (2003) Differential effects of prostaglandin derived from omega-6 and omega-3 polyunsaturated fatty acids on COX-2 expression and IL-6 secretion. *Proceedings of the National Academy of Sciences of the United States of America.* **100**, 1751–1756.

135. Wada, M., DeLong, C. J., Hong, Y. H., Rieke, C. J., Song, I., Sidhu, R. S., Yuan, C., Warnock, M., Schmaier, A. H., Yokoyama, C. et al. (2007) Enzymes and receptors of prostaglandin pathways with arachidonic acid-derived versus eicosapentaenoic acid-derived substrates and products. *Journal of Biological Chemistry.* **282**, 22254–22266.

136. Santoli, D., Phillips, P. D., Colt, T. L. and Zurier, R. B. (1990) Suppression of interleukin 2-dependent human T cell growth in vitro by prostaglandin E (PGE) and their precursor fatty acids. Evidence for a PGE-independent mechanism of inhibition by the fatty acids. *Journal of Clinical Investigation.* **85**, 424–432.

137. Calder, P. C., Bevan, S. J. and Newsholme, E. A. (1992) The inhibition of T-lymphocyte proliferation by fatty acids is via an eicosanoid-independent mechanism. *Immunology.* **75**, 108–115.

138. Dooper, M. M., Wassink, L., M'Rabet, L. and Graus, Y. M. (2002) The modulatory effects of prostaglandin-E on cytokine production by human peripheral blood mononuclear cells are independent of the prostaglandin subtype. *Immunology.* **107**, 152–159.

139. Shapiro, A. C., Wu, D. and Meydani, S. N. (1993) Eicosanoids derived from arachidonic and eicosapentaenoic acids inhibit T cell proliferative response. *Prostaglandins.* **45**, 229–240.

140. Serhan, C. N., Chiang, N. and Van Dyke, T. E. (2008) Resolving inflammation: Dual anti-inflammatory and pro-resolution lipid mediators. *Nature Reviews Immunology.* **8**, 349–361.

141. Serhan, C. N., Clish, C. B., Brannon, J., Colgan, S. P., Chiang, N. and Gronert, K. (2000) Novel functional sets of lipid-derived mediators with antiinflammatory actions generated from omega-3 fatty acids via cyclooxygenase 2-nonsteroidal antiinflammatory drugs and transcellular processing. *Journal of Experimantal Medicine.* **192**, 1197–1204.

142. Serhan, C. N., Clish, C. B., Brannon, J., Colgan, S. P., Gronert, K. and Chiang, N. (2000) Antimicroinflammatory lipid signals generated from dietary N-3 fatty acids via cyclooxygenase-2 and transcellular processing: A novel mechanism for NSAID and N-3 PUFA therapeutic actions. *Journal of Physiology and Pharmacology: An Official Journal of the Polish Physiological Society.* **51**, 643–654.

143. Ariel, A., Li, P. L., Wang, W., Tang, W. X., Fredman, G., Hong, S., Gotlinger, K. H. and Serhan, C. N. (2005) The docosatriene protectin D1 is produced by TH2 skewing and promotes human T cell apoptosis via lipid raft clustering. *Journal of Biological Chemistry.* **280**, 43079–43086.

144. Skarke, C., Alamuddin, N., Lawson, J. A., Li, X., Ferguson, J. F., Reilly, M. P. and FitzGerald, G. A. (2015) Bioactive products formed in humans from fish oils. *Journal of Lipid Research.* **56**, 1808–1820.

145. Hontecillas, R. and Bassaganya-Riera, J. (2007) Peroxisome proliferator-activated receptor gamma is required for regulatory CD4+ T cell-mediated protection against colitis. *Journal of Immunology.* **178**, 2940–2949.

146. Amano, Y., Yamaguchi, T., Ohno, K., Niimi, T., Orita, M., Sakashita, H. and Takeuchi, M. (2012) Structural basis for telmisartan-mediated partial activation of PPAR gamma. *Hypertension Research: Official Journal of the Japanese Society of Hypertension.* **35**, 715–719.

147. Kliewer, S. A., Sundseth, S. S., Jones, S. A., Brown, P. J., Wisely, G. B., Koble, C. S., Devchand, P., Wahli, W., Willson, T. M., Lenhard, J. M. et al. (1997) Fatty acids and eicosanoids regulate gene expression through direct interactions with peroxisome proliferator-activated receptors alpha and gamma. *Proceedings of the National Academy of Sciences of the United States of America.* **94**, 4318–4323.

148. Xu, H. E., Lambert, M. H., Montana, V. G., Parks, D. J., Blanchard, S. G., Brown, P. J., Sternbach, D. D., Lehmann, J. M., Wisely, G. B., Willson, T. M. et al. (1999) Molecular recognition of fatty acids by peroxisome proliferator-activated receptors. *Molecular Cell.* **3**, 397–403.

149. Iwami, D., Zhang, Q., Aramaki, O., Nonomura, K., Shirasugi, N. and Niimi, M. (2009) Purified eicos-apentaenoic acid induces prolonged survival of cardiac allografts and generates regulatory T cells. *American Journal of Transplantation: Official Journal of the American Society of Transplantation and the American Society of Transplant Surgeons.* **9**, 1294–1307.

150. Sospedra, M. and Martin, R. (2005) Immunology of multiple sclerosis. *Annual Review of Immunology.* **23**, 683–747.

151. Shale, M., Schiering, C. and Powrie, F. (2013) CD4(+) T-cell subsets in intestinal inflammation. *Immunological Reviews.* **252**, 164–182.

152. Sharon, P. and Stenson, W. F. (1984) Enhanced synthesis of leukotriene B4 by colonic mucosa in inflammatory bowel disease. *Gastroenterology.* **86**, 453–460.

153. Masoodi, M., Pearl, D. S., Eiden, M., Shute, J. K., Brown, J. F., Calder, P. C. and Trebble, T. M. (2013) Altered colonic mucosal Polyunsaturated Fatty Acid (PUFA) derived lipid mediators in ulcerative colitis: New insight into relationship with disease activity and pathophysiology. *PLOS ONE.* **8**, e76532.

154. Gizinski, A. M. and Fox, D. A. (2014) T cell subsets and their role in the pathogenesis of rheumatic disease. *Current Opinion in Rheumatology.* **26**, 204–210.

155. Hudert, C. A., Weylandt, K. H., Lu, Y., Wang, J., Hong, S., Dignass, A., Serhan, C. N. and Kang, J. X. (2006) Transgenic mice rich in endogenous omega-3 fatty acids are protected from colitis. *Proceedings of the National Academy of Sciences of the Unites States of America.* **103**, 11276–11281.

156. Nowak, J., Weylandt, K. H., Habbel, P., Wang, J., Dignass, A., Glickman, J. N. and Kang, J. X. (2007) Colitis-associated colon tumorigenesis is suppressed in transgenic mice rich in endogenous n-3 fatty acids. *Carcinogenesis.* **28**, 1991–1995.

157. Jia, Q., Lupton, J. R., Smith, R., Weeks, B. R., Callaway, E., Davidson, L. A., Kim, W., Fan, Y. Y., Yang, P., Newman, R. A. et al. (2008) Reduced colitis-associated colon cancer in Fat-1 (n-3 fatty acid desaturase) transgenic mice. *Cancer Research.* **68**, 3985–3991.

158. Gravaghi, C., La Perle, K. M., Ogrodwski, P., Kang, J. X., Quimby, F., Lipkin, M. and Lamprecht, S. A. (2011) Cox-2 expression, PGE(2) and cytokines production are inhibited by endogenously synthesized n-3 PUFAs in inflamed colon of fat-1 mice. *Journal of Nutritional Biochemistry.* **22**, 360–365.

159. Marcon, R., Bento, A. F., Dutra, R. C., Bicca, M. A., Leite, D. F. and Calixto, J. B. (2013) Maresin 1, a proresolving lipid mediator derived from omega-3 polyunsaturated fatty acids, exerts protective actions in murine models of colitis. *Journal of Immunology.* **191**, 4288–4298.

160. Bento, A. F., Claudino, R. F., Dutra, R. C., Marcon, R. and Calixto, J. B. (2011) Omega-3 fatty acid-derived mediators 17(R)-hydroxy docosahexaenoic acid, aspirin-triggered resolvin D1 and resolvin D2 prevent experimental colitis in mice. *Journal of Immunology.* **187**, 1957–1969.

161. Ishida, T., Yoshida, M., Arita, M., Nishitani, Y., Nishiumi, S., Masuda, A., Mizuno, S., Takagawa, T., Morita, Y., Kutsumi, H. et al. (2010) Resolvin E1, an endogenous lipid mediator derived from eicosa-pentaenoic acid, prevents dextran sulfate sodium-induced colitis. *Inflammatory Bowel Diseases.* **16**, 87–95.

162. Whiting, C. V., Bland, P. W. and Tarlton, J. F. (2005) Dietary n-3 polyunsaturated fatty acids reduce disease and colonic proinflammatory cytokines in a mouse model of colitis. *Inflammatory Bowel Diseases.* **11**, 340–349.

163. Camuesco, D., Galvez, J., Nieto, A., Comalada, M., Rodriguez-Cabezas, M. E., Concha, A., Xaus, J. and Zarzuelo, A. (2005) Dietary olive oil supplemented with fish oil, rich in EPA and DHA (n-3) polyunsaturated fatty acids, attenuates colonic inflammation in rats with DSS-induced colitis. *Journal of Nutrition.* **135**, 687–694.

164. Lev-Tzion, R., Griffiths, A. M., Leder, O. and Turner, D. (2014) Omega 3 fatty acids (fish oil) for maintenance of remission in Crohn's disease. *Cochrane Database of Systematic Reviews.* **2**, CD006320.

165. De Ley, M., de Vos, R., Hommes, D. W. and Stokkers, P. (2007) Fish oil for induction of remission in ulcerative colitis. *Cochrane Database of Systematic Reviews.* **17**, CD005986.

166. Ierna, M., Kerr, A., Scales, H., Berge, K. and Griinari, M. (2010) Supplementation of diet with krill oil protects against experimental rheumatoid arthritis. *BMC Musculoskeletal Disorders.* **11**, 136.

167. Olson, M. V., Liu, Y. C., Dangi, B., Paul Zimmer, J., Salem, N., Jr. and Nauroth, J. M. (2013) Docosahexaenoic acid reduces inflammation and joint destruction in mice with collagen-induced arthritis. *Inflammation Research: Official Journal of the European Histamine Research Society ... [et al.].* **62**, 1003–1013.

168. Sundrarjun, T., Komindr, S., Archararit, N., Dahlan, W., Puchaiwatananon, O., Angthararak, S., Udomsuppayakul, U. and Chuncharunee, S. (2004) Effects of n-3 fatty acids on serum interleukin-6, tumour necrosis factor-alpha and soluble tumour necrosis factor receptor p55 in active rheumatoid arthritis. *Journal of International Medical Research.* **32**, 443–454.

169. Berbert, A. A., Kondo, C. R., Almendra, C. L., Matsuo, T. and Dichi, I. (2005) Supplementation of fish oil and olive oil in patients with rheumatoid arthritis. *Nutrition.* **21**, 131–136.
170. Goldberg, R. J. and Katz, J. (2007) A meta-analysis of the analgesic effects of omega-3 polyunsaturated fatty acid supplementation for inflammatory joint pain. *Pain.* **129**, 210–223.
171. McFarland, C. T., Fan, Y. Y., Chapkin, R. S., Weeks, B. R. and McMurray, D. N. (2008) Dietary polyunsaturated fatty acids modulate resistance to Mycobacterium tuberculosis in guinea pigs. *Journal of Nutrition.* **138**, 2123–2128.
172. Bonilla, D. L., Fan, Y. Y., Chapkin, R. S. and McMurray, D. N. (2010) Transgenic mice enriched in omega-3 fatty acids are more susceptible to pulmonary tuberculosis: Impaired resistance to tuberculosis in fat-1 mice. *Journal of Infectious Diseases.* **201**, 399–408.
173. Matsunaga, H., Hokari, R., Kurihara, C., Okada, Y., Takebayashi, K., Okudaira, K., Watanabe, C., Komoto, S., Nakamura, M., Tsuzuki, Y. et al. (2008) Omega-3 fatty acids exacerbate DSS-induced colitis through decreased adiponectin in colonic subepithelial myofibroblasts. *Inflammatory Bowel Diseases.* **14**, 1348–1357.
174. Kim, W., Fan, Y. Y., Smith, R., Patil, B., Jayaprakasha, G. K., McMurray, D. N. and Chapkin, R. S. (2009) Dietary curcumin and limonin suppress CD4+ T-cell proliferation and interleukin-2 production in mice. *Journal of Nutrition.* **139**, 1042–1048.
175. Jia, Q., Ivanov, I., Zlatev, Z. Z., Alaniz, R. C., Weeks, B. R., Callaway, E. S., Goldsby, J. S., Davidson, L. A., Fan, Y. Y., Zhou, L. et al. (2011) Dietary fish oil and curcumin combine to modulate colonic cytokinetics and gene expression in dextran sodium sulphate-treated mice. *British Journal of Nutrition.* **106**, 519–529.
176. Raphael, I., Nalawade, S., Eagar, T. N. and Forsthuber, T. G. (2015) T cell subsets and their signature cytokines in autoimmune and inflammatory diseases. *Cytokine.* **74**, 5–17.

18 Novel Immunoregulatory Mediators Produced from Omega-3 Fatty Acids

Patricia R. Souza, Hefin R. Jones, and Lucy V. Norling

Contents

18.1 Host Control of Inflammation 315
18.2 Discovery and Biosynthesis of Novel Omega-3 Derived Lipid Mediators 316
18.3 Microparticles as Novel Sources of Proresolving Lipids 318
18.4 SPMs Signal via G-Protein Coupled Receptors 319
18.5 Active Termination of Inflammation: SPMs and their Actions on Neutrophils 320
    18.5.1 Neutrophil Recruitment 320
    18.5.2 Chemotaxis 321
    18.5.3 Phagocytosis and Microbial Killing 321
    18.5.4 Apoptosis 321
18.6 Molecular and Cellular Effects of Proresolving Lipids on Macrophages 323
18.7 SPMs Help Fight Infection 327
18.8 Conclusion 328
Acknowledgments 328
References 328

18.1 HOST CONTROL OF INFLAMMATION

Inflammation is a protective mechanism initiated following injury or infection that serves to clear invading agents and restore tissue homeostasis. In the initial stages of an inflammatory response, proinflammatory lipid mediators derived from arachidonic acid (AA), including the prostaglandins (PGs) and leukotrienes (LTs), play an essential role to mount the inflammatory response (Palmblad et al. 1988). A controlled inflammatory reaction and its complete termination (termed resolution) are essential for ongoing health. However, excessive inflammation can become deleterious to the host and can progress to chronic inflammation, tissue scarring, and fibrosis. Indeed, uncontrolled inflammation is a hallmark of multiple pathologies, including atherosclerosis and arthritis (Nathan and Ding 2010). This leads to the notion that chronic inflammation could be associated not only with excessive production of proinflammatory mediators but also attributed to a defect in endogenous anti-inflammatory pathways.

Contrary to initial belief, an acute inflammatory response does not simply dissipate due to dilution/degradation of proinflammatory mediators. Extensive work over the last two decades now indicates that the resolving phase of inflammation is not a passive process, but actively "turns-off" via the biosynthesis of endogenous anti-inflammatory and proresolving mediators (Gilroy et al. 2004; Serhan and Savill 2005). By definition, a proresolving mediator is not equivalent to an anti-inflammatory mediator. Anti-inflammatory agents typically block mediators or enzymes involved in the initiation of an inflammatory response whereas proresolving mediators stimulate and activate endogenous pathways that regulate cellular trafficking and enhance tissue restoration to accelerate resolution. Compared to current anti-inflammatories that typically target the initiation phase of the immune response, new therapeutics based on proresolution mediators would accelerate the healing process and the regain of physiological tissue function.

Proresolving mediators are chemically distinct and include proteins (e.g., annexin A1) and peptides (Dalli et al. 2013a), gaseous mediators (e.g., hydrogen sulfide [Caliendo et al. 2010] and carbon monoxide [Dalli et al. 2015; Chiang et al. 2013]), a purine (adenosine [Ehrentraut et al. 2013]), neuromodulator release under the control of the vagus nerve (Mirakaj et al. 2014; Pavlov and Tracey 2012) as well as specialized proresolving lipid mediators (SPMs, i.e., lipoxins, resolvins, protectins, and maresins) (Norling and Serhan 2010). SPMs are the focus of this chapter. Herein, we discuss how SPMs activate innate host defense mechanisms to limit the magnitude of inflammation, contain and efficiently clear microbes, and initiate timely resolution. For comprehensive literature on other important aspects of SPM biology including anti-analgesic actions and wound-repair mechanisms, see recent reviews (Serhan 2014; Serhan, Chiang, and Dalli 2015).

18.2 DISCOVERY AND BIOSYNTHESIS OF NOVEL OMEGA-3 DERIVED LIPID MEDIATORS

Inflammatory exudates were collected from mice during the natural resolution phase of inflammation and profiled for novel lipid mediators using metabololipidomic analyses. A number of autacoids coined specialized proresolving mediators (SPMs) that possess potent anti-inflammatory, proresolving. and protective properties were discovered. These include the omega-3 fatty acid–derived resolvins and protectins as well as the more recently identified maresins. Each of these unique stereospecific mediators is actively generated either within a single cell type (if all the enzymes required for the biosynthesis are expressed) or in some instances via transcellular enzymatic pathways (where one cell makes and releases a component of the biosynthetic cascade that is utilized by a second cell to generate the final product).

The omega-3 fatty acids EPA and DHA are substrates for the biosynthesis of most SPMs.

The generation of resolvins derived DHA, denoted D series resolvins (RvD), involves sequential enzymatic transformations of the substrate. Initially, DHA is converted to 17S-hydroperoxy docosahexaenoic acid (17S-H(p)DHA) by 15-lipoxygenase type I (15-LO) in humans and 12/15-LO in mice. This pivotal biosynthetic intermediate can subsequently be transformed via 5-LO to several chemically distinct bioactive compounds, including RvD1-RvD6 (Figure 18.1). Neutrophils express high levels of 5-LO and are a cellular source of these biosynthetic compounds. Indeed, isolated human neutrophils (with approximately 95% purity, 1% eosinophils, 4% mononuclear cells) can generate RvD2 when incubated with DHA, which was demonstrated using deuterium labeling for tracking the substrate conversion by liquid chromatography tandem mass spectrometry (LC-MS-MS) (Spite et al. 2009). Following 3 weeks of dietary omega-3 fatty acid supplementation, physiologically active levels of the D-series resolvin precursor 17R/S-HDHA together with RvD1 and RvD2 are detected within the plasma of healthy individuals (Mas et al. 2012). Oily fish such as Atlantic salmon are a good source of omega-3 fatty acids and can generate resolvins endogenously, but these are degraded during cooking (Raatz et al. 2011).

Protectin D1 (PD1) was appropriately named from its observed anti-inflammatory and protective actions in neural tissues and systems (Hong et al. 2003). This SPM is distinguished by the presence of a conjugated triene containing structure (Serhan et al. 2006). Somewhat surprisingly, eosinophils, which are traditionally associated with allergic diseases or parasitic infections, have proved to have an important role in the resolution of acute inflammation and to be a source of PD1 biosynthesis from DHA via 12/15-LO (Yamada et al. 2011) (Figure 18.1). Accordingly, when these cells were depleted during acute murine peritonitis the resultant phenotype was a failure to

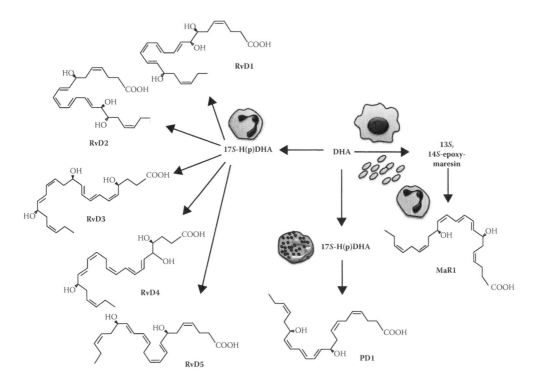

FIGURE 18.1 Biosynthesis of DHA-derived SPMs (D-series resolvins, protectins, and maresins). The generation of SPMs is initiated in resolving inflammatory exudates by neutrophils, eosinophils, platelets, and macrophages. Refer to text for references and further details of biosynthetic pathways.

efficiently resolve the inflammation (Yamada et al. 2011). During the resolution of murine peritonitis, both 17S-HDHA, a known marker of D-series resolvin and protectin biosynthesis, as well as 14S-HDHA accumulated in exudates from endogenous DHA (Serhan et al. 2009). These findings suggested that 14S-HDHA could be an intermediate in a new biosynthetic pathway for SPMs. Resolution-phase macrophages attested to be important in the generation of a novel class of SPMs named maresins (macrophage mediator in resolving inflammation). These include maresin (MaR) 1 (7R, 14S-dihydroxy-docosa-4Z, 8, 10, 12, 16Z, 19Z-hexaenoic acid) (Serhan et al. 2009) and MaR2 (13R, 14S-diHDHA) (Deng et al. 2014). Another biosynthetic route for maresin generation was recently uncovered during human platelet–neutrophil interactions, with platelet 12-LO yielding 13S, 14S-diHDHA that is further transformed by neutrophils to MaR1 (Abdulnour et al. 2014) (Figure 18.1).

Resolvins are also derived from EPA, denoted E-series resolvins (RvE), which involves oxygenation of EPA via cytochrome P450 to produce an intermediate that can be reduced into 18R-hydroxy eicosapentaenoic acid (18R-HEPE). This intermediate can subsequently be transformed by 5-LO rich cells, such as neutrophils to generate RvE1 or RvE2 (Figure 18.2). Importantly, bioactive concentrations of RvE1 are detected in plasma of healthy volunteers 4 hours after fish oil supplementation (1 g EPA and 0.7 g DHA) followed by low dose (160 mg) aspirin (Arita et al. 2005). Even without omega-3 fatty acid supplementation, RvE2 can be detected in plasma of healthy volunteers in the range of 0.53–3.72 ng/mL (Oh et al. 2012). Recent studies indicate that in addition to PD1 biosynthesis, eosinophils produce another mediator of resolution via 12/15-LO, RvE3 (17R/S-di-hydroxy eicosapentaenoic acid) to aid resolution (Isobe et al. 2012) (Figure 18.2). Whether this is a direct effect or involves an intermediate resident cell type such as the macrophage remains to be determined.

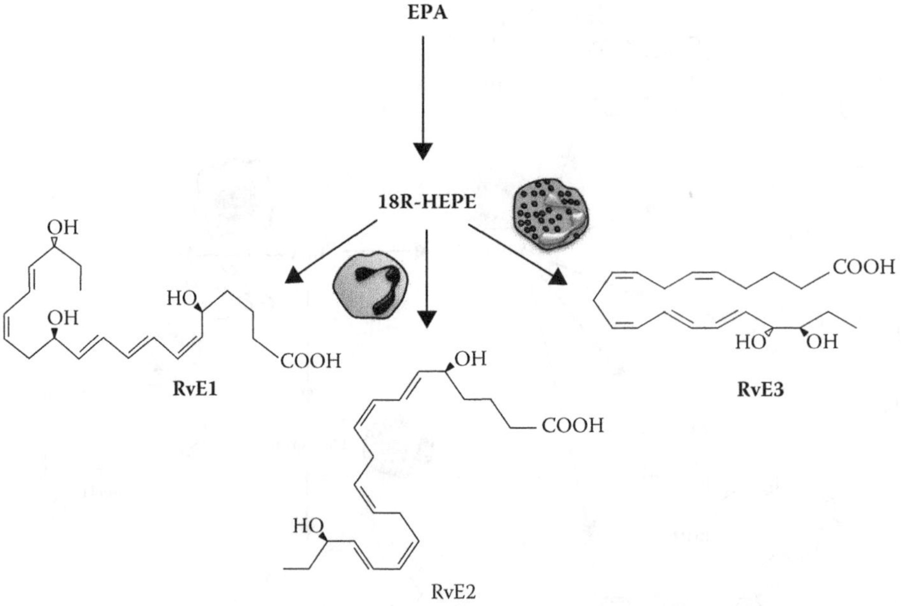

FIGURE 18.2 Biosynthesis of E-series resolvins. EPA provides a substrate for the generation of resolvins during inflammation. Refer to text for references and further details of biosynthetic pathways.

Aspirin, a commonly used anti-inflammatory drug, acetylates COX-2 which blocks prostaglandin biosynthesis yet modifies the catalytic domain of the enzyme in a way that enables it to still function. This unexpected twist in the pharmacology of aspirin yields epimers of the resolvin and protectin intermediates, such as 17*R*-HpDHA, providing substrates for generating so-called aspirin-triggered SPM. In addition to aspirin, statins that are widely used for cholesterol lowering in cardiovascular disease, promote the synthesis of AA-derived aspirin-triggered lipoxins via *S*-nitrosylation of COX-2 (Birnbaum et al. 2006). Therefore, these drugs, which are extensively used to treat a host of ailments, may be efficacious due to their positive impact on the generation of proresolving mediators (and their receptors), initiating the timely resolution of inflammation.

18.3 MICROPARTICLES AS NOVEL SOURCES OF PRORESOLVING LIPIDS

Microparticles (also known as microvesicles and ectosomes) are right-side-out membrane vesicles that bud from the plasma membrane of all eukaryotic cells upon an increase in intracellular calcium (Yanez-Mo et al. 2015). Far from being waste products, these vesicles are a highly evolutionarily conserved mechanism of insoluble, intercellular signaling and participate in a spectrum of physiological and pathophysiological processes. In response to "activating" stimuli or apoptosis, eukaryotic cells rapidly disseminate microparticles that carry membranous and cytosolic proteins (including functional receptors), nucleic acids such as mRNA and miRNA, and bioactive lipids derived from the parent cell. When released, microparticles take both a passive sample of the cell's proteome, transcriptome, and lipidome, and are also actively enriched in certain mediators (Garzetti et al. 2013).

In the context of inflammation, microparticles appear to be two-faced, both exacerbating inflammation and promoting its resolution dependent on their cellular origin and the target cells they interact with. Perhaps paradoxically, the neutrophil microparticle is one of a few populations, which reliably exerts proresolution signals during inflammation (Gasser and Schifferli 2004; Eken et al. 2008; Dalli et al. 2008). While microparticle-exposed phosphatidylserine and the proresolving protein annexin A1 can convey many of these effects, neutrophil microparticles are emerging as sources of proresolving lipid mediators.

Microparticles collected following zymosan-induced peritonitis were found to be vectors of 17- and 14-hydroxy DHA, precursors of D-series resolvins, protectins, and maresins, presenting a role of microparticles in the transcellular biosynthesis of these mediators (Norling et al. 2011). These hydroxy intermediates were found to be esterified within microparticle phospholipids and could be liberated by secreted PLA_2 ($sPLA_2$) for their subsequent conversion. In fact, neutrophil microparticles were shown to increase the production of resolvins D2, D5, E2, MaR1, and PD1, as well as prostaglandins D2 and F2α, in human macrophages during efferocytosis, where the microparticles provided the organic intermediates for their production (Dalli and Serhan 2012).

These structures offer a therapeutic opportunity, as they are inherently anti-inflammatory and proresolving (Dalli et al. 2008; Gasser and Schifferli 2004; Norling et al. 2011), can be readily isolated from peripheral blood human neutrophils, enriched with proresolving lipids and administered to attenuate inflammation. Indeed, AT-RvD1 or lipoxin analog (benzo-LXA_4)–loaded microparticles termed nano-proresolving medicines (NPRMs) enhanced wound closure of dermal keratinocytes and limited PMN infiltration in the temporomandibular joint during ongoing inflammation (Norling et al. 2011). Recent studies have demonstrated tissue regenerative properties of benzo-LXA_4–enriched NPRM, yielding soft tissue and new bone formation in periodontitis (Van Dyke et al. 2015).

18.4 SPMs SIGNAL VIA G-PROTEIN COUPLED RECEPTORS

The anti-inflammatory and proresolving activities of SPMs are mediated via specific G-protein-coupled receptors (GPCRs). Two GPCRs for RvD1 were identified on human leukocytes using a GPCR β-arrestin–coupled system, the LXA_4 and annexin-A1 receptor (ALX/FPR2) and an orphan receptor GPR32 (Krishnamoorthy et al. 2010). In addition to RvD1, AT-RvD1 as well as RvD3 and RvD5 can also signal via GPR32 (Chiang et al. 2012; Dalli et al. 2013b). Nongenomic regulation of FPR2/ALX, but not GPR32, is observed on human neutrophils, with increased expression following activation with proinflammatory stimuli, a process secondary to secretory vesicle mobilization (Norling et al. 2012). On human monocytes, FPR2/ALX and GPR32 are upregulated over a 24–48-hour period following exposure to zymosan particles or GM-CSF (Krishnamoorthy et al. 2010). In the mouse, ALX/FPR2 is encoded by two genes *fpr2/3*, whereas there is no known murine ortholog of GPR32. Transgenic mice overexpressing the ALX receptor display accelerated resolution during peritonitis when the agonists LXA_4 or RvD1 are administered (Krishnamoorthy et al. 2012). Conversely, RvD1 is without effect in mice deficient in *fpr2/3* (Norling et al. 2012; Krishnamoorthy et al. 2012), and these mice exhibit increased disease severity in a model of neutrophil-driven arthritis and experimental sepsis, suggesting this receptor has an endogenous proresolving function (Dufton et al. 2010; Gobbetti et al. 2014). The receptor for RvD2 was newly identified using an unbiased GPCR β-arrestin–based screening strategy, namely GPR18, which is expressed on innate immune cells including PMNs, monocytes, and macrophages (Chiang et al., 2015). Protection from RvD2 in ischemia-reperfusion-initiated acute lung injury was abolished in GPR18 null mice implicating a critical role for this receptor in mediating RvD2's actions (Chiang et al. 2015).

RvE1 acts via two GPCRs, as a full agonist on human chemokine-like receptor 1 (ChemR23) and as a partial agonist on the LTB_4 receptor (BLT1), thus competing with LTB_4 for binding (Arita et al. 2005). Transgenic mice overexpressing ChemR23 reveal an exaggerated response to RvE1, reducing PMN influx, enhancing phagocytosis, and preserving bone during periodontitis (Gao et al. 2013; Herrera et al. 2015). RvE2 blocks LTB_4 signaling to comparable levels as RvE1 yet is less effective at activating ChemR23, suggesting it may not be a full agonist at this receptor (Oh et al. 2012). Other receptors for SPMs are yet to be identified, but are predicted to be high-affinity GPCRs as they exhibit stereoselectivity and are very potent both in *in vitro* assays and experimental models, and, in some instances, bioactions can be blocked with pertussis toxin or cholera toxin.

18.5   ACTIVE TERMINATION OF INFLAMMATION: SPMs AND THEIR ACTIONS ON NEUTROPHILS

Neutrophils are the most abundant cells of the innate immune system and play a vital role in the inflammatory process. Neutrophils and their armamentarium can contribute directly or indirectly to the initiation, development, and resolution of the inflammatory response. Thus, control of when, where, and how neutrophils act is essential for a healthy immune system. Microbial stimuli or damage associated molecular patterns (DAMPs) released from dying cells such as DNA, extracellular ATP or formylated peptides trigger leukocyte recruitment. In response to these stimuli, circulating neutrophils initially tether to endothelial cells, then roll and firmly adhere before transmigrating into the inflamed tissue (Pober and Sessa 2007; Ley et al. 2007). Within the tissue, they become further activated and assist in the elimination of the injurious stimuli (such as bacteria). However, due to the toxic nature of the cell contents, this process may contribute to damage of adjacent tissues and can exacerbate inflammation. So, for an effective host control of inflammation, the recruitment of granulocytes must be limited. Each of the SPMs has a fundamental role in reducing neutrophil influx, which has been demonstrated in murine models of acute and chronic inflammation, as well as using human cells.

18.5.1   Neutrophil Recruitment

RvD1 as well as its aspirin-triggered epimer limit PMN infiltration at nanogram levels in murine peritonitis and block transendothelial migration of human neutrophils in a concentration-dependent manner (Sun et al. 2007). These compounds are potent, with concentrations as low as 10 nM producing an ~50% reduction in PMN transmigration in a static Transwell assay (Serhan et al. 2002; Sun et al. 2007). RvD1 also attenuates PMN-endothelial interactions in settings that mimic the blood flow within the vasculature, namely a "flow chamber assay," where cells are subjected to shear stress. RvD1 significantly blunted initial PMN capture, rolling, and firm adhesion to TNF-α–stimulated endothelium in a concentration-dependent manner (0.1–100 nM) (Norling et al. 2012). Additionally, RvD1 can protect against impairment of endothelial barrier function by attenuating LPS-induced permeability and redistribution of tight junction proteins including ZO-1, occludin, and f-actin (Zhang et al. 2013). RvD2 displays extremely potent bioactivity with doses as low as 10 pg causing approximately 70% reduction in PMN recruitment during acute peritonitis. Mechanistically, RvD2 acts on both the PMN counteracting PAF-mediated L-selectin shedding and CD18 upregulation, and acts on the endothelium, stimulating the vasoactive mediators nitric oxide (NO) and prostacyclin, which are anti-adhesive (Spite et al. 2009).

Functionally, RvE1 (10–100 nM range) induces L-selectin shedding in neutrophils and reduces CD18 expression on both human PMNs and monocytes. At 300 nM, RvE1 reduces expression of P-selectin, a bridging molecule for platelet-leukocyte interactions, by around 35% in human whole blood (Dona et al. 2008). Accordingly, RvE1 reduces leukocyte rolling by approximately 40% in murine venules *in vivo* (Dona et al. 2008). RvE1 also reduces transepithelial migration in a concentration-dependent manner, by inducing the expression of decay-accelerating factor (DAF, also termed CD55), an apically expressed anti-adhesive molecule on the epithelium (Campbell et al. 2007). Similarly. to RvE1, RvE2 also suppresses zymosan-induced PMN infiltration in murine peritonitis (Tjonahen et al. 2006), and can counteract PAF-stimulated surface integrin expression (CD18) in human whole blood PMNs (Oh et al. 2012).

Protectin D1 is also protective by limiting neutrophil recruitment in acute models of inflammation including zymosan-initiated peritonitis (Schwab et al. 2007) and following ischemic kidney injury (Duffield et al. 2006). Doses as low as 1 ng are effective at blocking >90% of further leukocyte infiltration at 4 hours, stopping PMN migration and infiltration into the site *in vivo* (Serhan et al. 2006). Studies were performed to determine whether the actions of PD1 and RvE1 were synergistic or additive by coadministration. Treatment with RvE1 (10 ng) significantly reduced PMN infiltration, although the response was less than that obtained with PD1 (10 ng). In combination, the effect was even greater, implicating an additive effect of PD1 and RvE1 *in vivo* in murine peritonitis. Both MaR1 and MaR2 can potently block the infiltration of neutrophils (Serhan et al. 2012); at 1 ng per mouse these compounds gave a comparable response, reducing neutrophil infiltration in mouse peritonitis by ~40% (Deng et al. 2014).

18.5.2 CHEMOTAXIS

Canonical mediators that promote the directed migration (termed chemotaxis) of neutrophils include LTB_4 and IL-8. This movement is distinct from chemokinesis, where leukocytes locomote yet move in a random direction. For a neutrophil to chemotax, it must first detect a chemical gradient, then become polarized, and then move toward the highest concentration of chemoattractant. Microfluidics chambers were engineered for testing the actions of bioactive lipid mediators on the chemotactic behavior of human neutrophils in real-time. Kasuga and colleagues demonstrated the direct impact of RvD1 on PMNs, which induced a dramatic shape change and ceased directed chemotactic movements towards IL-8 (Kasuga et al. 2008). More recently, a new design in microfluidics chamber was utilized to visualize neutrophil and monocyte intercellular interactions, this novel chamber was coated with elastin to distinguish between phlogistic and nonphlogistic leukocyte behavior (Jones et al. 2012). LXA_4 and RvD1 limited neutrophil and monocyte chemotaxis toward LTB_4 with a reduction in elastase activity following LXA_4 treatment, whereas RvD1 caused a sharp but transient spike in activity (Jones et al. 2012).

Whereas the mechanisms governing neutrophil recruitment and chemotaxis are comprehensively studied, the signals restricting neutrophil migration are less well characterized. To date, the pathways curtailing neutrophil chemotaxis in response to SPMs are yet to be uncovered. Exposure of human PMNs to RvD1 (10 nM) significantly blocked LTB_4-stimulated (10 nM) actin polymerization within 5 minutes (Krishnamoorthy et al. 2010). Yet, PMN treatment with RvD1 is not associated with intracellular calcium mobilization or stimulation of cyclic AMP implying that these canonical second messengers are not downstream of RvD1 receptor activation (Krishnamoorthy et al. 2010). RvE1 abrogates LTB_4-BLT1 signaling via NFκB and thus the production of proinflammatory cytokines and chemokines (Bannenberg et al. 2005; Arita et al. 2007; Haworth et al. 2008).

18.5.3 PHAGOCYTOSIS AND MICROBIAL KILLING

Once neutrophils have migrated to the infected or damaged tissue, their main function is to neutralize and eliminate potentially injurious stimuli, which is one of the more obvious requirements for an inflammatory reaction to resolve. Dispensing with the inciting stimulus will halt further proinflammatory mediator synthesis (e.g., eicosanoids, chemokines, and cytokines) and lead to their catabolism, reducing proinflammatory signaling pathways (Serhan et al. 2007). All members of the SPM family enhance neutrophil phagocytosis. These mediators also stimulate PMN antimicrobial defense mechanisms, increasing microbe ingestion and intracellular reactive oxygen species (ROS) production for killing bacteria/yeast particles. For example, RvE1 can inhibit neutrophil ROS in response to TNF-α and the bacterial peptide, fMLP (Gronert et al. 2004). It should be noted that SPM actions are not by direct antibacterial actions but by enhancing phagocytic activity (Chiang et al. 2012; Serhan et al. 2009; Spite et al. 2009).

18.5.4 APOPTOSIS

Apoptosis is a process of programmed cell death in vertebrates, and a very important step for the resolution of inflammation. Under normal conditions, neutrophils undergo apoptosis once they have phagocytized microbes or cellular debris. Neutrophil apoptosis was first reported in the late 1980s by Savill and colleagues; until that time, it was believed that neutrophils died by the classical mode of cell death (necrosis). Necrotic neutrophils undergo disruption of the plasma membrane and consequently release their cellular contents into the microenvironment in an irreversible manner, causing further tissue damage and inflammatory cell recruitment. In contrast, neutrophils undergoing apoptosis are phenotypically distinct; their cytoplasmic granules are intact, they have a densely condensed nuclei and vacuolated cytoplasm (Savill et al. 1989). Some of the proresolving mediators induce neutrophil apoptosis, including AnxA1 (Perretti and Solito 2004) and LXA_4 (Weinberger et al. 2008). Among the omega-3–derived SPMs, RvE1 induces neutrophil apoptosis either directly or against an antiapoptotic stimulus (El Kebir, Gjorstrup, and Filep 2012 and can upregulate the CC-chemokine receptor 5 (CCR5) on late apoptotic neutrophils, which terminates chemokine signaling (Ariel et al. 2006).

An important consequence of apoptosis is the alteration in expression of surface molecules on the dying cell (e.g., increased expression of phosphatidylserine), known as "find me" and "eat me" signals. Such alterations lead to rapid recognition and phagocytosis of apoptotic cells by macrophages in a process termed efferocytosis (Poon et al. 2014). Over the past few years, it has become clear that the phagocytic clearance of apoptotic cells and bodies (membrane-bound cell fragments that are produced by apoptotic-cell blebbing) can result in powerful anti-inflammatory and immunosuppressive effects. Indeed, the defective clearance of apoptotic cells is closely linked to autoimmunity and persistent inflammatory diseases (Shao and Cohen 2011). The discovery of

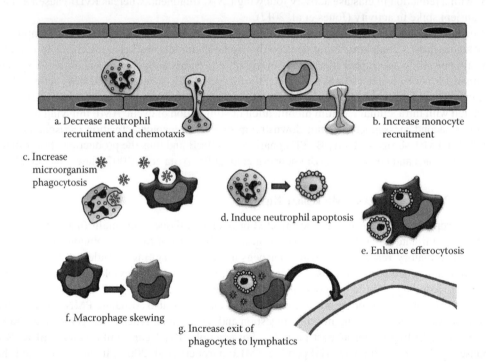

FIGURE 18.3 Key bioactions of SPMs on myeloid cells during inflammatory resolution. During inflammation, a number of endogenous anti-inflammatory and proresolving mediators are generated locally and act via specific GPCRs to initiate resolution. A common feature of SPMs is that they act essentially as brake signals to circumvent neutrophil-mediated tissue injury, by limiting neutrophil adhesion and diapedesis (a). SPMs, including LXA_4, increase monocyte recruitment to aid in microbial/debris clearance (b). These protective mediators also enhance phagocyte function to contain and clear microorganisms (c). Some of the SPMs (e.g., RvE1) can enhance neutrophil apoptosis (d) as well as their subsequent uptake via macrophages (e). Macrophage efferocytosis is known to skew macrophages toward a healing phenotype to assist with the restoration of tissue homeostasis; this process can also be induced by SPMs (f). LXA_4 and RvE1 augment phagocyte egress to the draining lymphatics (g). Refer to main text for references.

SPMs brings new insights that efferocytosis can be induced. Indeed, a common feature of SPMs is that they can enhance macrophage phagocytosis of apoptotic PMNs (Krishnamoorthy et al. 2010; Spite et al. 2009; Sun et al. 2007; Serhan et al. 2009; Abdulnour et al. 2014; Krishnamoorthy et al. 2010). However, as yet, the mechanisms by which SPMs induce efferocytosis are not fully elucidated (see next section). There is also increasing evidence that neutrophils can contribute significantly to the inflammatory process through expression and release of factors that influence the behavior of other cell types, particularly those involved in promoting resolution of inflammation (Fox et al. 2010). For instance, apoptotic neutrophils prompt a switch from a pro- to an anti-inflammatory macrophage phenotype (Fadok et al. 1998; Michlewska et al. 2009), which is a prerequisite for macrophage egress via the lymphatic vessels favoring return to tissue homeostasis (Figure 18.3).

18.6 MOLECULAR AND CELLULAR EFFECTS OF PRORESOLVING LIPIDS ON MACROPHAGES

Macrophages are renowned for exhibiting remarkable plasticity and generate a wide array of responses to a vast spectrum of stimuli. The implication of this is that these cells, which exist in all tissues, can promote both inflammation and its resolution dependent upon timely and appropriate exposure to a variety of mediators. When exposed to lipopolysaccharide, interferon γ or tumor necrosis factor α, macrophages assume a proinflammatory, "classically activated" phenotype, which expresses high levels of IL-12, IL-1, and IL-6; undergoes oxidative burst; and favors micropinocytosis over phagocytosis (Biswas and Mantovani 2010; Bosedasgupta and Pieters 2014). Classical activation of phlogistic monocyte-derived macrophages as well as resident tissue macrophages promotes local tissue damage, recruits additional waves of extravasating neutrophils and monocytes, and pathogen-killing (in the context of nonsterile inflammation).

In addition to promoting inflammation, macrophages are crucial to the resolution process. For appropriate resolution of acute inflammation, macrophage phenotype must undergo a shift toward what Siamon Gordon's group first described as an "alternatively activated" macrophage (Stein et al. 1992). Alternatively activated macrophages are generated *in vitro* in response to IL-4 and IL-13, IL-10, or glucocorticoids, and promote Th2 responses (and are therefore immunoregulatory in the context of a Th1-type inflammatory response). To maintain consistency with the Th1/Th2 nomenclature, classically and alternatively activated macrophages are referred to as M1 and M2 respectively. While in recent years the M1/M2 paradigm was criticized as unrealistically simple, it does however serve as a tool to describe the shift to a proresolution macrophage phenotype. For example, M2 macrophages downregulate the release of proinflammatory cytokines, reactive intermediates, and antigen-presenting apparatus, as well as release the anti-inflammatory cytokines IL-10 and transforming growth factor β (TGF-β) and begin efferocytosing apoptotic neutrophils, a major checkpoint during resolution (Novak and Thorp 2013).

As cytokines have dominated the field of leukocyte signaling during inflammation, the roles of specialized, proresolving lipid mediators in driving resolution have only recently emerged. In the macrophage, lipoxins A_4 and B_4; resolvins E1, E2, D1, D2, and D3; maresins 1 and 2; and protectin D1 have all been shown to promote the efferocytosis and clearance of apoptotic neutrophils (Table 18.1), a function both associated with and stimulatory of an M2 phenotype (Krishnamoorthy et al. 2010; Spite et al. 2009; Sun et al. 2007; Serhan et al. 2009, 2012; Abdulnour et al. 2014; Godson et al. 2000; Oh et al. 2012; McCauley et al. 2014; Deng et al. 2014). RvE1 (via its receptor ChemR23) and the lipoxins (via ALX/FPR2) induce the recruitment of nonphlogistic monocytes into inflamed sites, thereby inflating the pool of macrophages, which can begin clearance of dead neutrophils (Schwab et al. 2007; Herova et al. 2015). LXA$_4$, RvE1, and PD1 promote the efflux of macrophages to draining lymph nodes (restoring the level of macrophages in the tissue to preinflammation levels) and decrease macrophage release of IFN-γ, a cytokine that promotes their M1 polarization (Schwab et al. 2007).

TABLE 18.1
Summary of the Effects of SPMs on Monocyte/Macrophage Phenotype and Function

	LXA$_4$	LXB$_4$	RvE1	RvE2	RvD1	RvD2	RvD3	RvD5	MaR1	MaR2	PD1
↑ Efferocytosis	Godson et al. (2000), Mitchell et al. (2002), Schwab et al. (2007)	Mitchell et al. (2002)	Schwab et al. (2007)	Oh et al. (2012)	McCauley et al. (2014), Lee et al. (2013), Dalli et al. (2013b), Mirakaj et al. (2014)	McCauley et al. (2014), Dalli et al. (2013b), Chiang et al. (2015)	Dalli et al. (2013b)	–	Serhan et al. (2012), Deng et al. (2014), Dalli et al. (2013b)	Deng et al. (2014)	Schwab et al. (2007), Dalli et al. (2013b)
↑ Pathogen phagocytosis	Schwab et al. (2007)	–	Serhan et al. (2009), Schwab et al. (2007), Ohira et al. (2010)	(Oh et al. 2012)	Merched et al. (2008), Krishnamoorthy et al. (2010), Norling et al. (2012), Chiang et al. (2012)	Spite et al. (2009), Chiang et al. (2015)	Dalli et al. (2013b)	Chiang et al. (2012)	Deng et al. (2014)	Deng et al. (2014)	Serhan et al. (2009b), Schwab et al. (2007), Chiang et al. (2012)
↑ Monocyte recruitment	Maddox and Serhan (1996)	Maddox and Serhan (1996)	Schwab et al. (2007)	–	–	–	–	–	–	–	–
↑ Efflux to lymph node	Schwab et al. (2007)	–	Schwab et al. (2007)	–	–	–	–	–	–	–	Schwab et al. (2007)
↓ IFN-γ	Schwab et al. (2007)	–	Schwab et al. (2007)	–	–	–	–	–	–	–	Schwab et al. (2007)

(Continued)

TABLE 18.1 (*Continued*)
Summary of the Effects of SPMs on Monocyte/Macrophage Phenotype and Function

	LXA₄	LXB₄	RvE1	RvE2	RvD1	RvD2	RvD3	RvD5	MaR1	MaR2	PD1
↓ TNF-α	Kure et al. (2010), Ueda et al. (2014)	–	Schif-Zuck et al. (2011)		Titos et al. (2011), Lee et al. (2013), Chiang et al. (2012), Schif-Zuck et al. (2011)	Titos et al. (2011)		Chiang et al. (2012)	Nordgren et al. (2013), Gong et al. (2014)	–	Titos et al. (2011)
↓ IL-6	(Schwab et al. 2007; Ueda et al. 2014)	–	Schwab et al. (2007), Haworth et al. (2008)		Titos et al. (2011), Chiang et al. (2012)	Titos et al. (2011)	Dalli et al. (2013b)	–	Nordgren et al. (2013), Gong et al. (2014)	–	Schwab et al. (2007), Titos et al. (2011)
↓ IL-12	(Kure et al. 2010)	–	–	–	–	–	–	–	–	–	–
↑ IL-10	Schwab et al. (2007)	–	Herova et al. (2015), Schif-Zuck et al. (2011)	(Oh et al. 2012)	Titos et al. (2011), Lee et al. (2013), Schif-Zuck et al. (2011), Chiang et al. (2012)	Titos et al. (2011)	Dalli et al. (2013b)	–		–	Schwab et al. (2007), Titos et al. (2011)
↑ LXA₄	–	–	Haworth et al. (2008)	–	Fredman et al. (2014)	–	–	–		–	–
↑ Arg I	–	–	–	–	Titos et al. (2011)	Titos et al. (2011), Chiang et al. (2015)	–	–		–	Titos et al. (2011)
↑ CD206	–	–	–	–	Titos et al. (2011), Dalli et al. (2013c)	Titos et al. (2011), Chiang et al. (2015)	–	–	Dalli et al. (2013c)	–	Titos et al. (2011)

Although the impact of every proresolving lipid mediator on macrophage function has yet to be fully explored, they seem to generally promote an M2, proresolving and pro-wound healing phenotype (Table 18.1). For example, LXA$_4$ suppresses TNF-α (Kure et al. 2010; Ueda et al. 2014), IL-6 (Schwab et al. 2007; Ueda et al. 2014), and IL-12 release (Kure et al. 2010) while stimulating the release of IL-10 (Schwab et al. 2007). RvE1 is reported to have similar effects on IL-6 and IL-10 (Schwab et al. 2007; Herova et al. 2015; Titos et al. 2011), where the latter is upregulated by RvE2 also (Oh et al. 2012). The DHA derivatives (D-series resolvins and protectins) contribute to inducing this M2 expression fingerprint by downregulating TNF-α and IL-6 and concomitantly upregulating IL-10, arginase I, and CD206 (Schwab et al. 2007; Titos et al. 2011). M1 macrophages treated with either MaR1 (10 nM) or RvD1 (10 nM) showed a significant reduction in CD54 and CD80 expression and a concomitant increase in CD163 and CD206 (Dalli et al. 2013c). Increased CD206 (macrophage mannose receptor) expression may promote the clearance of residual microorganisms and endocytic clearance of noxious glycoproteins released during inflammation, such as myeloperoxidase (Lee et al. 2002; Gazi and Martinez-Pomares 2009). In contrast, elevated arginase activity competes with nitric oxide synthase for arginine, decreasing Th1 cytokine production and increasing matrix deposition and wound healing (Popovic, Zeh, and Ochoa 2007).

Mechanistically, the proresolution effects of SPMs on macrophages are beginning to be uncovered. The proresolving action of LXA$_4$ on macrophages depends on inhibition of NFκB nuclear translocation (Kure et al. 2010). LXA$_4$-mediated phagocytosis signals phosphorylation of key polarity organization molecules: Akt, protein kinase C zeta, and glycogen synthase kinase-3β, which lead to actin cytoskeleton rearrangement and cell polarization (Reville et al. 2006). In terms of lipoxin-stimulated efferocytosis, the signaling molecules PKC and PI3-kinase proved important (Mitchell et al. 2002). Additionally, the $\alpha_v\beta_3$-CD36 complex is required for lipoxin-stimulated efferocytosis, but was deemed independent of the phosphatidylserine receptor (Mitchell et al. 2002). Recently, a proresolving cascade stimulated by RvD1 was deciphered that switches macrophage production from proinflammatory LTB$_4$ to protective LXA$_4$ biosynthesis (Fredman et al. 2014). RvD1 signals via FPR2/ALX, suppresses cytosolic calcium and reduces activation of calcium-sensitive kinase calcium-calmodulin–dependent protein kinase II (CamKII). The inhibition of this kinase reduces activation of signaling molecules p38 and mitogen-activated protein kinase activated protein kinase 2 (MAPKAPK2; MK2), which subsequently reduces ser271 phosphorylation of 5-LO and causes its translocation from the nucleus to the cytosol. This translocation favors LXA$_4$ biosynthesis and limits LTB$_4$ production (Fredman et al. 2014). RvD1 also initiates a selective regulation of transcription factors, microRNAs, and select genes that drive proresolving functions in macrophages (Titos et al. 2011; Recchiuti et al. 2011, 2014). Incubation of resolution-phase macrophages with RvD1 caused a twofold to threefold downregulation in coactivator-associated arginine methyltransferase 1 (CARM1), which plays an important role in macrophage activation as a coactivator of a number of NFκB-dependent genes. Accordingly, RvD1 reduced the expression of downstream genes of CARM1 such as intercellular adhesion molecule 1 (ICAM-1), colony stimulating factor 3 (CSF3), and monocyte inflammatory protein 2 (MIP-2), which are characteristic of a M1 macrophage phenotype (Recchiuti et al. 2014). RvD1 enhances efferocytosis by limiting TNF-α production from macrophages by two distinct NFκB pathways. Firstly, suppressing the nuclear translocation of p65/p50 heterodimer by downregulating IKKβ activity, and secondly promoting the nuclear translocation of p50/p50 homodimer via p105 degradation (Lee et al. 2013). RvD1 also rescues macrophages from oxidative stress-induced apoptosis during efferocytosis via PKA-mediated repression of NOX activation and by upregulating the antiapoptotic proteins Bcl-xL and Bcl-2 (Lee and Surh 2013). Insights into the intracellular signaling downstream of RvE1 were recently determined on macrophages: RvE1 causes phosphoprotein-mediated signaling, involving the PI3-K/Akt pathway leading to downstream enhancement of macrophage phagocytosis (Ohira et al. 2010).

18.7 SPMs HELP FIGHT INFECTION

If infection is not contained and eliminated by phagocytes, it can rapidly progress, leading to sepsis, which is characterized by excessive inflammation, as well as epithelial and endothelial barrier dysfunction, causing immune suppression and multiple-organ failure that can be fatal. Sepsis remains a huge clinical challenge with increasing prevalence and mortality rates. Therefore, new therapeutic strategies that could increase the therapeutic window to afford additional time for further interventions, such as administering antibiotics, are needed. Preclinical animal studies using RvD2 have yielded promising results; administration of RvD2 proved protective in a model of mucosal barrier breakage and leak leading to sepsis, initiated by midgrade cecal ligation and puncture (CLP) (Spite et al. 2009). Following CLP, mice had a severe bacterial burden both locally within the peritoneum and systemically. Treatment with RvD2 immediately postsurgery significantly reduced bacterial levels in both the blood and peritoneal cavity and dramatically limited local PMN influx. Further analysis of septic peritoneal exudates showed a "cytokine storm" of proinflammatory cytokines such as TNF-α, IL-1β, IL-6, and other mediators associated with a detrimental outcome in sepsis, for example IL-10 and IL-17, as well as elevated proinflammatory lipid mediators LTB$_4$ and PGE$_2$. RvD2 significantly blunted overzealous cytokine production and proinflammatory lipid mediators measured 12 hours after CLP. Septic mice exhibited hypothermia 12 hours after CLP and displayed a drastic decrease in activity levels, whereas RvD2-treated mice remained active and their body temperatures were similar to sham-operated control mice. Importantly, the survival rate 7 days post midgrade CLP was doubled with early administration of RvD2. Notably, RvD2 did not display direct bacteriostatic activity but acted on phagocytes to contain and clear bacteria; murine lymph nodes displayed disseminated bacteria in vehicle-treated CLP mice, whereas bacteria-loaded phagocytes could be observed histologically following RvD2 treatment. Corroborative results were obtained with human PMNs *in vitro*, where exposure to RvD2 (1 and 10 nM) increased phagocytosis and killing of *E. coli* (Spite et al. 2009). Endogenous levels of PD1, RvD1, and RvD5 are increased during ongoing infections with *E. coli* (Chiang et al. 2012). Importantly, mice administered with SPMs need much lower doses of antibiotics to fight and clear infection. This offers a possibility to lower antibiotic requirements, which may ultimately help reduce the increased incidence of antibiotic resistance (Chiang et al. 2012). RvE1 also increases survival in a model of pneumonia, by reducing proinflammatory cytokines, decreasing pulmonary PMN numbers, and enhancing clearance of bacteria from mouse lungs (Seki et al. 2010).

SPMs can also enhance clearance of bacteria by stimulating mucosal epithelial cells to produce antimicrobial peptides to minimize the incidence of epithelium-adhering bacteria. Aspirin-triggered lipoxin induces the expression of an antimicrobial peptide, bactericidal permeability increasing protein (BPI), in epithelial cells, which blocks endotoxin-mediated signaling in epithelia (Canny et al. 2002). Also notable was the induction of epithelial alkaline phosphatase (ALPI) expression and enzymatic activity by RvE1. Surface-expressed ALPI was shown to detoxify bacterial LPS and retard growth of *E. coli* (Campbell et al. 2007). Although antimicrobial peptide release is beneficial during bacterial infection, if inappropriately released these cationic peptides can cause host damage. Importantly, RvE1 blocks a positive feed forward loop of LTB$_4$-stimulated release of LL-37 by human PMNs and LXA$_4$ inhibits proinflammatory actions of LL-37, thus limiting unwanted tissue damage (Wan et al. 2011). Thus, contradicting the erroneous belief that resolution may impede host immunity, SPMs enhance innate antimicrobial systems in phagocytes and mucosa to control infection.

Antiviral actions are also reported for SPMs. Infection of the eye with herpes simplex virus (HSV) can lead to visual impairment and even blindness if recurrent infections become chronic and inflammation results in neovascularization of the avascular cornea. Resolvin E1 and PD1 reduced proinflammatory mediators, angiogenic factors, infiltration of PMNs, and pathogenic CD4+ T-cells in the cornea and stimulated IL-10 production following induction of stromal keratitis with HSV, greatly improving the pathology (Rajasagi et al. 2011, 2013). PD1 can also block the replication of the respiratory pathogen H5N1 influenza virus. Mechanistically, PD1 prevents viral RNA export from the nucleus to the cytoplasm by interfering with binding of host nuclear export factors to influenza virus RNAs (Morita et al. 2013). Lipidomic analysis profiling the time course of influenza infection identified 5-LOX metabolites during the pathogenic phase and 12/15-LOX metabolites during the resolution phase (Tam et al. 2013). Interestingly, levels of PD1 were downregulated during severe infection and generation of PD1 inversely correlated with virulence and disease status (Morita et al. 2013). Likewise, dissemination of the H5N1 virus–induced genes associated with lipoxin generation and signaling and sustained inflammation inhibited lipoxin-mediated anti-inflammatory responses allowing the virus to spread to extrapulmonary organs (Cilloniz et al. 2010). Importantly, exogenous administration with PD1 improved survival and pathology of mice with influenza even when current antivirals were ineffective (Morita et al. 2013).

18.8 CONCLUSION

Endogenous SPMs exert multifaceted actions to enhance host defense and activate resolution circuits via specific cell-surface receptors. SPMs limit neutrophil recruitment by counter-regulating their surface adhesion molecules and stimulating the endothelium and epithelium to release anti-adhesive mediators/molecules. SPMs also stimulate phagocyte function to contain and eliminate microbes and viruses to prevent the spread of infection and protect the host from tissue and organ damage. These novel omega-3–derived lipid mediators stimulate endogenous inflammatory control mechanisms to accelerate resolution making them attractive therapeutics for the treatment of inflammatory and infectious diseases.

ACKNOWLEDGMENTS

Our research is funded by the Arthritis Research UK (Career Development Fellowship 19909 to LVN) and studentships from the BBSRC (CASE Studentship BB/K011782/1) to HRJ and the Brazilian Government (238277/2012-7) to PRS.

REFERENCES

Abdulnour, R. E., J. Dalli, J. K. Colby, et al. 2014. Maresin 1 biosynthesis during platelet-neutrophil interactions is organ-protective. *Proc Natl Acad Sci U S A* 111 (46):16526–31. doi: 10.1073/pnas.1407123111.
Ariel, A., G. Fredman, Y. P. Sun, et al. 2006. Apoptotic neutrophils and T cells sequester chemokines during immune response resolution through modulation of CCR5 expression. *Nat Immunol* 7 (11):1209–16.
Arita, M., F. Bianchini, J. Aliberti, et al. 2005. Stereochemical assignment, antiinflammatory properties, and receptor for the omega-3 lipid mediator resolvin E1. *J Exp Med* 201 (5):713–22. doi: 10.1084/jem.20042031.
Arita, M., T. Ohira, Y. P. Sun, et al. 2007. Resolvin E1 selectively interacts with leukotriene B4 receptor BLT1 and ChemR23 to regulate inflammation. *J Immunol* 178 (6):3912–7.
Bannenberg, G. L., N. Chiang, A. Ariel, et al. 2005. Molecular circuits of resolution: Formation and actions of resolvins and protectins. *J Immunol* 174 (7):4345–55.
Birnbaum, Y., Y. Ye, Y. Lin, et al. 2006. Augmentation of myocardial production of 15-epi-lipoxin-a4 by pioglitazone and atorvastatin in the rat. *Circulation* 114 (9):929–35. doi: 10.1161/CIRCULATIONAHA.106.629907.
Biswas, S. K. and A. Mantovani. 2010. Macrophage plasticity and interaction with lymphocyte subsets: Cancer as a paradigm. *Nat Immunol* 11 (10):889–96. doi: 10.1038/ni.1937.
Bosedasgupta, S. and J. Pieters. 2014. Inflammatory stimuli reprogram macrophage phagocytosis to macropinocytosis for the rapid elimination of pathogens. *PLOS Pathog* 10 (1):e1003879. doi: 10.1371/journal.ppat.1003879.
Caliendo, G., G. Cirino, V. Santagada, et al. 2010. Synthesis and biological effects of hydrogen sulfide (H2S): Development of H2S-releasing drugs as pharmaceuticals. *J Med Chem* 53 (17):6275–86. doi: 10.1021/jm901638j.

Campbell, E. L., N. A. Louis, S. E. Tomassetti, et al. 2007. Resolvin E1 promotes mucosal surface clearance of neutrophils: A new paradigm for inflammatory resolution. *FASEB J* 21 (12):3162–70. doi: 10.1096/fj.07-8473com.

Canny, G., O. Levy, G. T. Furuta, et al. 2002. Lipid mediator-induced expression of bactericidal/ permeability-increasing protein (BPI) in human mucosal epithelia. *Proc Natl Acad Sci U S A* 99 (6):3902–7. doi: 10.1073/pnas.052533799.

Chiang, N., G. Fredman, F. Backhed, et al. 2012. Infection regulates pro-resolving mediators that lower antibiotic requirements. *Nature* 484 (7395):524–8. doi: 10.1038/nature11042.

Chiang, N., J. Dalli, R. A. Colas, et al. 2015. Identification of resolvin D2 receptor mediating resolution of infections and organ protection *J Exp Med*. 212(8):1203–17. doi: 10.1084/jem.20150225.

Chiang, N., M. Shinohara, J. Dalli, et al. 2013. Inhaled carbon monoxide accelerates resolution of inflammation via unique proresolving mediator-heme oxygenase-1 circuits. *J Immunol* 190 (12):6378–88. doi: 10.4049/jimmunol.1202969.

Cilloniz, C., M. J. Pantin-Jackwood, C. Ni, et al. 2010. Lethal dissemination of H5N1 influenza virus is associated with dysregulation of inflammation and lipoxin signaling in a mouse model of infection. *J Virol* 84 (15):7613–24. doi: 10.1128/JVI.00553-10.

Dalli, J., A. P. Consalvo, V. Ray, et al. 2013a. Proresolving and tissue-protective actions of annexin A1-based cleavage-resistant peptides are mediated by formyl peptide receptor 2/lipoxin A4 receptor. *J Immunol* 190 (12):6478–87. doi: 10.4049/jimmunol.1203000.

Dalli, J., B. D. Kraft, R. A. Colas, et al. 2015. Proresolving lipid mediator profiles in baboon pneumonia are regulated by inhaled carbon monoxide. *Am J Respir Cell Mol Biol* 53:314–25. doi: 10.1165/rcmb.2014-0299OC.

Dalli, J. and C. N. Serhan. 2012. Specific lipid mediator signatures of human phagocytes: Microparticles stimulate macrophage efferocytosis and pro-resolving mediators. *Blood* 120 (15):e60–72. doi: 10.1182/blood-2012-04-423525.

Dalli, J., J. W. Winkler, R. A. Colas, et al. 2013b. Resolvin D3 and aspirin-triggered resolvin D3 are potent immunoresolvents. *Chem Biol* 20 (2):188–201. doi: 10.1016/j.chembiol.2012.11.010.

Dalli, J., L. V. Norling, D. Renshaw, et al. 2008. Annexin 1 mediates the rapid anti-inflammatory effects of neutrophil-derived microparticles. *Blood* 112 (6):2512–9. doi: 10.1182/blood-2008-02-140533.

Dalli, J., M. Zhu, N. A. Vlasenko, et al. 2013c. The novel 13S,14S-epoxy-maresin is converted by human macrophages to maresin 1 (MaR1), inhibits leukotriene A4 hydrolase (LTA4H), and shifts macrophage phenotype. *FASEB J* 27 (7):2573–83. doi: 10.1096/fj.13-227728.

Deng, B., C. W. Wang, H. H. Arnardottir, et al. 2014. Maresin biosynthesis and identification of maresin 2, a new anti-inflammatory and pro-resolving mediator from human macrophages. *PLOS ONE* 9 (7):e102362. doi: 10.1371/journal.pone.0102362.

Dona, M., G. Fredman, J. M. Schwab, et al. 2008. Resolvin E1, an EPA-derived mediator in whole blood, selectively counterregulates leukocytes and platelets. *Blood* 112 (3):848–55. doi: 10.1182/blood-2007-11-122598.

Duffield, J. S., S. Hong, V. S. Vaidya, et al. 2006. Resolvin D series and protectin D1 mitigate acute kidney injury. *J Immunol* 177 (9):5902–11.

Dufton, N., R. Hannon, V. Brancaleone, et al. 2010. Anti-inflammatory role of the murine formyl-peptide receptor 2: Ligand-specific effects on leukocyte responses and experimental inflammation. *J Immunol* 184 (5):2611–9. doi: 10.4049/jimmunol.0903526.

Ehrentraut, H., E. T. Clambey, E. N. McNamee, et al. 2013. CD73+ regulatory T cells contribute to adenosine-mediated resolution of acute lung injury. *FASEB J* 27(6):2207–19. doi: 10.1096/fj.12-225201.

Eken, C., O. Gasser, G. Zenhaeusern, et al. 2008. Polymorphonuclear neutrophil-derived ectosomes interfere with the maturation of monocyte-derived dendritic cells. *J Immunol* 180 (2):817–24.

El Kebir, D., P. Gjorstrup, and J. G. Filep. 2012. Resolvin E1 promotes phagocytosis-induced neutrophil apoptosis and accelerates resolution of pulmonary inflammation. *Proc Natl Acad Sci U S A* 109 (37):14983–8. doi: 10.1073/pnas.1206641109.

Fadok, V. A., D. L., Bratton, A. Konowal, P. W. Freed, J. Y. Westcott, P. M. Henson. 1998. Macrophages that have ingested apoptotic cells in vitro inhibit proinflammatory cytokine production through autocrine/paracrine mechanisms involving TGF-beta, PGE2, and PAF. *J of Clini Invest* 101(4):890-898.

Fox, S., A. E. Leitch, R. Duffin, C. Haslett, and A. G. Rossi. 2010. Neutrophil apoptosis: Relevance to the innate immune response and inflammatory disease. *J Innate Immun* 2 (3):216–27. doi: 10.1159/000284367.

Fredman, G., L. Ozcan, S. Spolitu, et al. 2014. Resolvin D1 limits 5-lipoxygenase nuclear localization and leukotriene B4 synthesis by inhibiting a calcium-activated kinase pathway. *Proc Natl Acad Sci U S A* 111 (40):14530–5. doi: 10.1073/pnas.1410851111.

Gao, L., D. Faibish, G. Fredman, et al. 2013. Resolvin E1 and chemokine-like receptor 1 mediate bone preservation. *J Immunol* 190 (2):689–94. doi: 10.4049/jimmunol.1103688.

Garzetti, L., R. Menon, A. Finardi, et al. 2013. Activated macrophages release microvesicles containing polarized M1 or M2 mRNAs. *J Leukoc Biol* 95(5):817–825. doi: 10.1189/jlb.0913485.

Gasser, O. and J. A. Schifferli. 2004. Activated polymorphonuclear neutrophils disseminate anti-inflammatory microparticles by ectocytosis. *Blood* 104 (8):2543–8. doi: 10.1182/blood-2004-01-0361.

Gazi, U. and L. Martinez-Pomares. 2009. Influence of the mannose receptor in host immune responses. *Immunobiology* 214 (7):554–61. doi: 10.1016/j.imbio.2008.11.004.

Gilroy, D. W., T. Lawrence, M. Perretti, and A. G. Rossi. 2004. Inflammatory resolution: New opportunities for drug discovery. *Nat Rev Drug Discov* 3 (5):401–16. doi: 10.1038/nrd1383; nrd1383 [pii].

Gobbetti, T., S. M. Coldewey, J. Chen, et al. 2014. Nonredundant protective properties of FPR2/ALX in polymicrobial murine sepsis. *Proc Natl Acad Sci U S A* 111 (52):18685–90. doi: 10.1073/pnas.1410938111.

Godson, C., S. Mitchell, K. Harvey, et al. 2000. Cutting edge: Lipoxins rapidly stimulate nonphlogistic phagocytosis of apoptotic neutrophils by monocyte-derived macrophages. *J Immunol* 164 (4):1663–7.

Gong, J., Z. Y. Wu, H. Qi, et al. 2014. Maresin 1 mitigates LPS-induced acute lung injury in mice. *Br J Pharmacol* 171 (14):3539–50. doi: 10.1111/bph.12714.

Gronert, K., A. Kantarci, B. D. Levy, et al. 2004. A molecular defect in intracellular lipid signaling in human neutrophils in localized aggressive periodontal tissue damage. *J Immunol* 172 (3):1856–61.

Haworth, O., M. Cernadas, R. Yang, et al. 2008. Resolvin E1 regulates interleukin 23, interferon-gamma and lipoxin A4 to promote the resolution of allergic airway inflammation. *Nat Immunol* 9 (8):873–9. doi: 10.1038/ni.1627.

Herova, M., M. Schmid, C. Gemperle, and M. Hersberger. 2015. ChemR23, the receptor for chemerin and resolvin E1, is expressed and functional on M1 but not on M2 macrophages. *J Immunol* 194 (5):2330–7. doi: 10.4049/jimmunol.1402166.

Herrera, B. S., H. Hasturk, A. Kantarci, et al. 2015. Impact of resolvin E1 on murine neutrophil phagocytosis in type 2 diabetes. *Infect Immun* 83 (2):792–801. doi: 10.1128/IAI.02444-14.

Hong, S., K. Gronert, P. Devchand, et al. 2003. Novel docosatrienes and 17S-resolvins generated from docosahexaenoic acid in murine brain, human blood and glial cells: Autacoids in anti-inflammation. *J Biol Chem* 278:14677–87.

Isobe, Y., M. Arita, S. Matsueda, et al. 2012. Identification and structure determination of novel anti-inflammatory mediator resolvin E3, 17,18-dihydroxyeicosapentaenoic acid. *J Biol Chem* 287 (13):10525–34. doi: 10.1074/jbc.M112.340612.

Jones, C. N., J. Dalli, L. Dimisko, et al. 2012. Microfluidic chambers for monitoring leukocyte trafficking and humanized nano-proresolving medicines interactions. *Proc Natl Acad Sci U S A* 109 (50):20560–5. doi: 10.1073/pnas.1210269109.

Kasuga, K., R. Yang, T. F. Porter, et al. 2008. Rapid appearance of resolvin precursors in inflammatory exudates: Novel mechanisms in resolution. *J Immunol* 181 (12):8677–87.

Krishnamoorthy, S., A. Recchiuti, N. Chiang, et al. 2012. Resolvin D1 receptor stereoselectivity and regulation of inflammation and proresolving microRNAs. *Am J Pathol* 180 (5):2018–27. doi: 10.1016/j.ajpath.2012.01.028.

Krishnamoorthy, S., A. Recchiuti, N. Chiang, et al. 2010. Resolvin D1 binds human phagocytes with evidence for proresolving receptors. *Proc Natl Acad Sci U S A* 107 (4):1660–5. doi: 10.1073/pnas.0907342107.

Kure, I., S. Nishiumi, Y. Nishitani, et al. 2010. Lipoxin A(4) reduces lipopolysaccharide-induced inflammation in macrophages and intestinal epithelial cells through inhibition of nuclear factor-kappaB activation. *J Pharmacol Exp Ther* 332 (2):541–8. doi: 10.1124/jpet.109.159046.

Lee, H. N., J. K. Kundu, Y. N. Cha, and Y. J. Surh. 2013. Resolvin D1 stimulates efferocytosis through p50/p50-mediated suppression of tumor necrosis factor-alpha expression. *J Cell Sci* 126 (Pt 17):4037–47. doi: 10.1242/jcs.131003.

Lee, H. N. and Y. J. Surh. 2013. Resolvin D1-mediated NOX2 inactivation rescues macrophages undertaking efferocytosis from oxidative stress-induced apoptosis. *Biochem Pharmacol* 86 (6):759–69. doi: 10.1016/j.bcp.2013.07.002.

Lee, S. J., S. Evers, D. Roeder, et al. 2002. Mannose receptor-mediated regulation of serum glycoprotein homeostasis. *Science* 295 (5561):1898–901. doi: 10.1126/science.1069540.

Ley, K., C. Laudanna, M. I. Cybulsky, et al. 2007. Getting to the site of inflammation: The leukocyte adhesion cascade updated. *Nat Rev Immunol* 7 (9):678–89. doi: 10.1038/nri2156.

Maddox, J. F. and C. N. Serhan. 1996. Lipoxin A4 and B4 are potent stimuli for human monocyte migration and adhesion: Selective inactivation by dehydrogenation and reduction. *J Exp Med* 183 (1):137–46.

Mas, E., K. D. Croft, P. Zahra, et al. 2012. Resolvins D1, D2, and other mediators of self-limited resolution of inflammation in human blood following n-3 fatty acid supplementation. *Clin Chem* 58 (10):1476–84. doi: 10.1373/clinchem.2012.190199.

McCauley, L. K., J. Dalli, A. J. Koh, et al. 2014. Cutting edge: Parathyroid hormone facilitates macrophage efferocytosis in bone marrow via proresolving mediators resolvin D1 and resolvin D2. *J Immunol* 193 (1):26–9. doi: 10.4049/jimmunol.1301945.

Merched, A. J., K. Ko, K. H. Gotlinger, et al. 2008. Atherosclerosis: Evidence for impairment of resolution of vascular inflammation governed by specific lipid mediators. *FASEB J* 22 (10):3595–606. doi: 10.1096/fj.08-112201.

Michlewska, S., I. Dransfield, I. L. Megson, A. G. Rossi. 2009. Macrophage phagocytosis of apoptotic neutrophils is critically regulated by the opposing actions of pro-inflammatory and anti-inflammatory agents: Key role for TNF-alpha. *FASEB J.* 23:844–854.

Mirakaj, V., J. Dalli, T. Granja, et al. 2014. Vagus nerve controls resolution and pro-resolving mediators of inflammation. *J Exp Med* 211 (6):1037–48. doi: 10.1084/jem.20132103.

Mitchell, S., G. Thomas, K. Harvey, et al. 2002. Lipoxins, aspirin-triggered epi-lipoxins, lipoxin stable analogues, and the resolution of inflammation: Stimulation of macrophage phagocytosis of apoptotic neutrophils in vivo. *J Am Soc Nephrol* 13 (10):2497–507.

Morita, M., K. Kuba, A. Ichikawa, et al. 2013. The lipid mediator protectin D1 inhibits influenza virus replication and improves severe influenza. *Cell* 153 (1):112–25. doi: 10.1016/j.cell.2013.02.027.

Nathan, C. and A. Ding. 2010. Nonresolving inflammation. *Cell* 140 (6):871–82. doi: 10.1016/j.cell.2010.02.029; S0092-8674(10)00182-0 [pii].

Nordgren, T. M., A. J. Heires, T. A. Wyatt, et al. 2013. Maresin-1 reduces the pro-inflammatory response of bronchial epithelial cells to organic dust. *Respir Res* 14:51. doi: 10.1186/1465-9921-14-51.

Norling, L. V. and C. N. Serhan. 2010. Profiling in resolving inflammatory exudates identifies novel anti-inflammatory and pro-resolving mediators and signals for termination. *J Intern Med* 268 (1):15–24. doi: 10.1111/j.1365-2796.2010.02235.x.

Norling, L. V., J. Dalli, R. J. Flower, et al. 2012. Resolvin D1 limits polymorphonuclear leukocyte recruitment to inflammatory loci: Receptor-dependent actions. *Arterioscler Thromb Vasc Biol* 32 (8):1970–8. doi: 10.1161/ATVBAHA.112.249508.

Norling, L. V., M. Spite, R. Yang, et al. 2011. Cutting edge: Humanized nano-proresolving medicines mimic inflammation-resolution and enhance wound healing. *J Immunol* 186 (10):5543–7. doi: 10.4049/jimmunol.1003865.

Novak, M. L. and E. B. Thorp. 2013. Shedding light on impaired efferocytosis and nonresolving inflammation. *Circ Res* 113 (1):9–12. doi: 10.1161/CIRCRESAHA.113.301583.

Oh, S. F., M. Dona, G. Fredman, et al. 2012. Resolvin E2 formation and impact in inflammation resolution. *J Immunol* 188 (9):4527–34. doi: 10.4049/jimmunol.1103652.

Ohira, T., M. Arita, K. Omori, et al. 2010. Resolvin E1 receptor activation signals phosphorylation and phagocytosis. *J Biol Chem* 285 (5):3451–61. doi: 10.1074/jbc.M109.044131.

Palmblad, J., R. W. Wannemacher, N. Salem, Jr., et al. 1988. Essential fatty acid deficiency and neutrophil function: Studies of lipid-free total parenteral nutrition in monkeys. *J Lab Clin Med* 111 (6):634–44. 0022-2143(88)90335-6 [pii].

Pavlov, V. A. and K. J. Tracey. 2012. The vagus nerve and the inflammatory reflex–linking immunity and metabolism. *Nat Rev Endocrinol* 8 (12):743–54. doi: 10.1038/nrendo.2012.189.

Perretti, M. and E. Solito. 2004. Annexin 1 and neutrophil apoptosis. *Biochem Soc Trans* 32 (Pt 3):507–10. doi: 10.1042/BST0320507.

Pober, J. S. and W. C. Sessa. 2007. Evolving functions of endothelial cells in inflammation. *Nat Rev Immunol* 7 (10):803–15. doi: 10.1038/nri2171.

Poon, I. K., C. D. Lucas, A. G. Rossi, et al. 2014. Apoptotic cell clearance: Basic biology and therapeutic potential. *Nat Rev Immunol* 14 (3):166–80. doi: 10.1038/nri3607.

Popovic, P. J., H. J. Zeh, 3rd, and J. B. Ochoa. 2007. Arginine and immunity. *J Nutr* 137 (6 Suppl 2):1681S–6.

Raatz, S. K., M. Y. Golovko, S. A. Brose, et al. 2011. Baking reduces prostaglandin, resolvin, and hydroxy-fatty acid content of farm-raised Atlantic salmon (Salmo salar). *J Agric Food Chem* 59 (20):11278–86. doi: 10.1021/jf202576k.

Rajasagi, N. K., P. B. Reddy, A. Suryawanshi, et al. 2011. Controlling herpes simplex virus-induced ocular inflammatory lesions with the lipid-derived mediator resolvin E1. *J Immunol* 186 (3):1735–46. doi: 10.4049/jimmunol.1003456.

Rajasagi, N. K., P. B. Reddy, S. Mulik, et al. 2013. Neuroprotectin D1 reduces the severity of herpes simplex virus-induced corneal immunopathology. *Invest Ophthalmol Vis Sci* 54 (9):6269–79. doi: 10.1167/iovs.13-12152.

Recchiuti, A., M. Codagnone, A. M. Pierdomenico, et al. 2014. Immunoresolving actions of oral resolvin D1 include selective regulation of the transcription machinery in resolution-phase mouse macrophages. *FASEB J* 28 (7):3090–102. doi: 10.1096/fj.13-248393.

Recchiuti, A., S. Krishnamoorthy, G. Fredman, et al. 2011. MicroRNAs in resolution of acute inflammation: Identification of novel resolvin D1-miRNA circuits. *FASEB J* 25 (2):544–60. doi: 10.1096/fj.10-169599.

Reville, K., J. K. Crean, S. Vivers, et al. 2006. Lipoxin A4 redistributes myosin IIA and Cdc42 in macrophages: Implications for phagocytosis of apoptotic leukocytes. *J Immunol* 176 (3):1878–88.

Savill, J. S., A. H. Wyllie, J. E. Henson, et al. 1989. Macrophage phagocytosis of aging neutrophils in inflammation. Programmed cell death in the neutrophil leads to its recognition by macrophages. *J Clin Invest* 83 (3):865–75. doi: 10.1172/JCI113970.

Schif-Zuck, S., N. Gross, S. Assi, et al. 2011. Saturated-efferocytosis generates pro-resolving CD11b low macrophages: Modulation by resolvins and glucocorticoids. *Eur J Immunol* 41 (2):366–79. doi: 10.1002/eji.201040801.

Schwab, J. M., N. Chiang, M. Arita, et al. 2007. Resolvin E1 and protectin D1 activate inflammation-resolution programmes. *Nature* 447 (7146):869–74. doi: 10.1038/nature05877.

Seki, H., K. Fukunaga, M. Arita, et al. 2010. The anti-inflammatory and proresolving mediator resolvin E1 protects mice from bacterial pneumonia and acute lung injury. *J Immunol* 184 (2):836–43. doi: 10.4049/jimmunol.0901809; jimmunol.0901809 [pii].

Serhan, C. N. 2014. Pro-resolving lipid mediators are leads for resolution physiology. *Nature* 510 (7503):92–101. doi: 10.1038/nature13479.

Serhan, C. N. and J. Savill. 2005. Resolution of inflammation: The beginning programs the end. *Nat Immunol* 6:1191–7.

Serhan, C. N., J. Dalli, S. Karamnov, et al. 2012. Macrophage proresolving mediator maresin 1 stimulates tissue regeneration and controls pain. *FASEB J* 26 (4):1755–65. doi: 10.1096/fj.11-201442.

Serhan, C. N., K. Gotlinger, S. Hong, et al. 2006. Anti-inflammatory actions of neuroprotectin D1/protectin D1 and its natural stereoisomers: Assignments of dihydroxy-containing docosatrienes. *J Immunol* 176:1848–59.

Serhan, C. N., N. Chiang, and J. Dalli. 2015. The resolution code of acute inflammation: Novel pro-resolving lipid mediators in resolution. *Semin Immunol* 27(3):200–15. doi: 10.1016/j.smim.2015.03.004.

Serhan, C. N., R. Yang, K. Martinod, et al. 2009. Maresins: Novel macrophage mediators with potent antiinflammatory and proresolving actions. *J Exp Med* 206 (1):15–23. doi: 10.1084/jem.20081880.

Serhan, C. N., S. Hong, K. Gronert, et al. 2002. Resolvins: A family of bioactive products of omega-3 fatty acid transformation circuits initiated by aspirin treatment that counter proinflammation signals. *J Exp Med* 196 (8):1025–37.

Serhan, C. N., S. D. Brain, C. D. Buckley, et al. 2007. Resolution of inflammation: State of the art, definitions and terms. *FASEB J* 21 (2):325–32. doi: 10.1096/fj.06-7227rev.

Shao, W. H. and P. L. Cohen. 2011. Disturbances of apoptotic cell clearance in systemic lupus erythematosus. *Arthritis Res Ther* 13 (1):202. doi: 10.1186/ar3206.

Spite, M., L. V. Norling, L. Summers, et al. 2009. Resolvin D2 is a potent regulator of leukocytes and controls microbial sepsis. *Nature* 461 (7268):1287–91. doi: 10.1038/nature08541.

Stein, M., S. Keshav, N. Harris, et al. 1992. Interleukin 4 potently enhances murine macrophage mannose receptor activity: A marker of alternative immunologic macrophage activation. *J Exp Med* 176 (1):287–92.

Sun, Y. P., S. F. Oh, J. Uddin, et al. 2007. Resolvin D1 and its aspirin-triggered 17R epimer. Stereochemical assignments, anti-inflammatory properties, and enzymatic inactivation. *J Biol Chem* 282 (13):9323–34. doi: 10.1074/jbc.M609212200.

Tam, V. C., O. Quehenberger, C. M. Oshansky, et al. 2013. Lipidomic profiling of influenza infection identifies mediators that induce and resolve inflammation. *Cell* 154 (1):213–27. doi: 10.1016/j.cell.2013.05.052.

Titos, E., B. Rius, A. Gonzalez-Periz, et al. 2011. Resolvin D1 and its precursor docosahexaenoic acid promote resolution of adipose tissue inflammation by eliciting macrophage polarization toward an M2-like phenotype. *J Immunol* 187 (10):5408–18. doi: 10.4049/jimmunol.1100225.

Tjonahen, E., S. F. Oh, J. Siegelman, et al. 2006. Resolvin E2: Identification and anti-inflammatory actions: Pivotal role of human 5-lipoxygenase in resolvin E series biosynthesis. *Chem Biol* 13 (11):1193–202. doi: 10.1016/j.chembiol.2006.09.011.

Ueda, T., K. Fukunaga, H. Seki, et al. 2014. Combination therapy of 15-epi-lipoxin A4 with antibiotics protects mice from Escherichia coli-induced sepsis*. *Crit Care Med* 42 (4):e288–95. doi: 10.1097/CCM.0000000000000162.

Van Dyke, T. E., H. Hasturk, A. Kantarci, et al. 2015. Proresolving nanomedicines activate bone regeneration in periodontitis. *J Dent Res* 94 (1):148–56. doi: 10.1177/0022034514557331.

Wan, M., C. Godson, P. J. Guiry, et al. 2011. Leukotriene B4/antimicrobial peptide LL-37 proinflammatory circuits are mediated by BLT1 and FPR2/ALX and are counterregulated by lipoxin A4 and resolvin E1. *FASEB J* 25 (5):1697–705. doi: 10.1096/fj.10-175687.

Weinberger, B., C. Quizon, A. M. Vetrano, et al. 2008. Mechanisms mediating reduced responsiveness of neonatal neutrophils to lipoxin A4. *Pediatr Res* 64 (4):393–8. doi: 10.1203/PDR.0b013e318180e4af.

Yamada, T., Y. Tani, H. Nakanishi, et al. 2011. Eosinophils promote resolution of acute peritonitis by producing proresolving mediators in mice. *FASEB J* 25 (2):561–8. doi: 10.1096/fj.10-170027.

Yanez-Mo, M., P. R. Siljander, Z. Andreu, et al. 2015. Biological properties of extracellular vesicles and their physiological functions. *J Extracell Vesicles* 4:27066. doi: 10.3402/jev.v4.27066.

Zhang, X., T. Wang, P. Gui, et al. 2013. Resolvin D1 reverts lipopolysaccharide-induced TJ proteins disruption and the increase of cellular permeability by regulating IkappaBalpha signaling in human vascular endothelial cells. *Oxid Med Cell Longev* 2013:185715. doi: 10.1155/2013/185715.

19 Roles of Arginine in Cell-Mediated and Humoral Immunity

Wenkai Ren, Yulong Yin, Beiyan Zhou,
Fuller W. Bazer, and Guoyao Wu

CONTENTS

19.1 Introduction 335
19.2 The Immune Response 336
19.3 Arginine and Cell-Mediated Immunity 338
    19.3.1 Arginine and Th1 Responses 338
    19.3.2 Arginine and Th2 Responses 338
    19.3.3 Arginine and Th9 Responses 339
    19.3.4 Arginine and Th17 Responses 340
    19.3.5 Arginine and Th22 Responses 340
    19.3.6 Arginine and Regulatory T-Cells 340
    19.3.7 Arginine and CD8+ T-Cells 341
    19.3.8 Arginine and $\gamma\delta$ T, NKT, and Tfh Cells 341
19.4 Arginine and Humoral Immunity 342
19.5 Conclusion and Perspectives 342
Acknowledgments 343
References 343

19.1 INTRODUCTION

According to the growth or nitrogen (N) balance of animals, amino acids (AA) have been traditionally classified as nutritionally essential AA (EAA) or nutritionally nonessential AA (NEAA) (see Hou et al. 2015 for review). EAA are those AA that are not synthesized *de novo* or usually are not synthesized in adequate amounts to meet the animal's needs, whereas NEAA are those AA that are synthesized *de novo* in animal cells and thought to be dispensable in diets. Arginine has long been considered an NEAA for adult animals including humans, but has recently been classified as a nutritionally semi-essential AA for young mammals (such as rats, swine, and human infants), as well as males and females of reproductive age (Wu et al. 2014). This is because the rate of arginine utilization is greater than the rate of its synthesis under certain conditions (e.g., early weaning; lactation; pregnancy; spermatogenesis; tissue repair following burns, injury, or infection; heat stress; and cold stress) (Wu et al. 2014; Wu 2009; Ren et al. 2012b). Arginine is a functional AA that can regulate key metabolic pathways to improve the survival, growth, development, lactation, reproduction, and health of animals (Wu et al. 2014; Wu 2010; Ren et al. 2014c).

In mammals, net arginine synthesis occurs through the intestinal-renal axis. Citrulline formed from glutamine and proline via pyrroline-5-carboxylate (P5C) synthase in the mitochondria of enterocytes is utilized for production of arginine primarily in the kidneys via cytosolic argininosuccinate synthase and lyase (Wu and Morris 1998). P5C synthase and N-acetylglutamate (NAG) synthase are the rate-controlling enzymes for the generation of P5C from glutamine, whereas proline oxidase is a major determinant of the intestinal conversion of proline into citrulline (Wu et al. 2004). In humans, pigs, and rats, most dietary arginine is metabolized via the arginase and arginine-glycine amidinotransferase pathways, but the production of nitric oxide (NO) from arginine (accounting for < 1% of dietary arginine used) plays an important role in immune functions (Wu et al. 2009). Three isoforms of nitric oxide synthase (NOS) generate NO from arginine in a cell-specific manner (Wu et al. 2009). The nutritional significance of this metabolic pathway is supported by the observations that dietary supplementation with arginine improves immunity, leading to the killing of pathogens (e.g., bacteria and viruses) (Ren et al. 2012b, 2013f, 2014a,c; Li et al. 2007). At the molecular and cellular levels, arginine activates both cell- and antibody-mediated immune responses in mice (Ren et al. 2013f, 2014a; Shang et al. 2003), humans (Moriguti et al. 2005), chickens (Munir et al. 2009; Perez-Carbajal et al. 2010), pigs (Chen et al. 2012a; Tan et al. 2009), and fish (Pohlenz et al. 2012). This chapter will describe the effects of arginine on immune function and the mechanisms involved.

19.2   THE IMMUNE RESPONSE

The primary role of the immune system is recognition, neutralization, and elimination of bacteria, viruses, and substances that are foreign and harmful for the host (Miles and Calder 2015). Generally, resistance to infectious disease is dependent on two major systems: innate and adaptive immunity. The innate immune system is the first line of host defense in the recognition and elimination of pathogens (Bonaventura et al. 2014; Turvey and Broide 2010). Innate immunity protects the host against all pathogens, and mainly consists of physical barriers (e.g., skin and epithelial cells of the gastrointestinal tract), phagocytes (e.g., monocytes, macrophages, and dendritic cells), polymorphonuclear granulocytes (e.g., neutrophils, eosinophils, and basophils), natural killer cells, platelets, and humoral factors including complement, C-reactive proteins, and lysozyme (Figure 19.1).

The skin contains the epidermis (a thinner outer layer) and the dermis (a thicker layer supporting the epidermis). The mucous membrane, which lines the conjunctivae, as well as the alimentary, respiratory, and urogenital tracts, includes an outer epithelial layer and an underlying layer of connective tissue. The secretions from the mucous membrane have protective roles in immune responses.

The innate immune system provides robust and immediate response to invading pathogens, but is nonspecific and does not confer long-lasting immunity (memory) (Akira et al. 2001; Geremia et al. 2014). When infection cannot be fully cleared by the innate immune system, the adaptive immune system is activated to destroy infectious pathogens (viruses or bacteria). The humoral and cell-mediated immune responses orchestrate adaptive immunity in the host (Ruth and Field 2013). Humoral immunity is the responsibility of B lymphocytes, which produce antibodies targeted to specific antigens, while cell-mediated immunity is associated with T lymphocytes, which activate other immune cells (T helper lymphocytes) and kill infected cells (cytotoxic T lymphocytes) (Siegmund and Zeitz 2011). As opposed to the innate immune response, the adaptive immune system is highly specific and confers long-lasting immunity (Figure 19.2). As antigen-presenting cells, dendritic cells serve as a link between the innate and adaptive immune systems, and are responsible for T-cell activation and induction of the adaptive immune response (Geremia et al. 2014; Bonaventura et al. 2014). There is compelling support for the role of AA in animal health including in immune defense (i.e., dietary arginine, glutamine, and proline are highly beneficial for support of innate immunity and adaptive immunity) (Ren et al. 2013a,b,c,e, 2014b; Li et al. 2007).

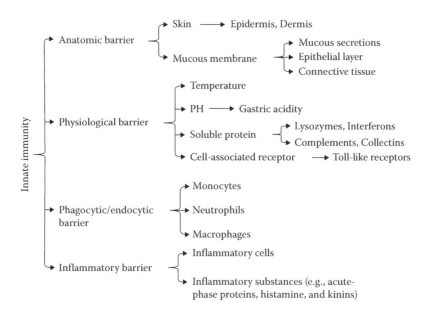

FIGURE 19.1 Innate immunity in humans and animals. Innate immunity includes physical/anatomical, physiological, phagocytic/endocytic, and inflammatory barriers. The skin and the surface of mucous membranes contribute to physical/anatomical barriers. The physiological barriers of innate immunity consists of body temperature, pH (i.e., gastric acidity), and various soluble factors (e.g., lysozymes, interferons, and complements) and cell-associated molecules (e.g., toll-like receptors). Phagocytosis and endocytosis are also components of the innate immune system that includes specialized cells, such as blood monocytes, neutrophils, and tissue macrophages. In response to tissue damage by invading pathogens, a complex set of inflammatory reactions is triggered, including interactions among various inflammatory cells and proinflammatory molecules (i.e., acute-phase proteins and histamine).

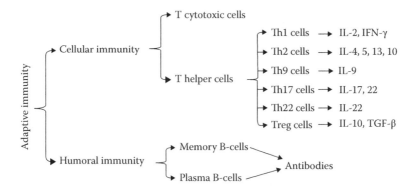

FIGURE 19.2 The adaptive immune system in humans and animals. Two major populations of lymphocytes, B-cells and T-cells, participate in the adaptive immunity. Humoral immunity requires B-cells (plasma or memory B-cells) and specific antibodies, whereas cellular immunity depends on T-cells (T helper (Th) or T cytotoxic cells) and cytokines. T helper cells are further divided into six Th subsets (Th1, Th2, Th9, Th17, Th22, and Treg) based on the cytokines they secrete.

19.3 ARGININE AND CELL-MEDIATED IMMUNITY

19.3.1 ARGININE AND Th1 RESPONSES

Th1 cells are characterized by their production of the signature cytokines interleukin 2 (IL-2) and interferon gamma (IFN-γ). These cells also produce a number of other cytokines including tumor necrosis factor (TNF), lymphotoxin, and granulocyte-macrophage colony-stimulating factor (GM-CSF) (Raphael et al. 2014). The differentiation of Th1 cells requires IL-12, the master transcription factor TBX21 (T-box transcription factor TBX21), and signal transducer and activator of transcription 4 (STAT4) (Chen and Kolls 2013). In addition, IFN-γ/STAT1 signaling, IL-2/STAT5 signaling, and strong T-cell receptor (TCR) signals favor Th1 differentiation (Raphael et al. 2014). Through the production of IFN-γ, Th1 cells are thought to be important for immunity against intracellular pathogens.

An early discovery from *in vitro* studies indicated that Th1 cells can be activated to produce large amounts of NO from arginine because IFN-γ stimulates expression of NOS2 (also known as inducible NOS or iNOS), and the resultant NO inhibits the secretion of IL-2 and IFN-γ by Th1 cells by suppressing IL-12 synthesis (Liew et al. 1991; Cenci et al. 1993; Modolell et al. 1995; Wei et al. 1995; Taylor-Robinson et al. 1994). Furthermore, the induction of NOS2 impairs T-cell proliferation, whereas cytotoxic derivatives of NO (e.g., peroxynitrite) result in apoptosis of T lymphocytes (Bronte et al. 2003). NO does not impair the early events triggered by TCR cross-linking, but acts instead at the level of IL-2 receptor signaling by reducing the phosphorylation and activation of several signaling molecules, including Janus kinases (JAKs) 1 and 3, STAT5, Erk, and Akt (Bronte et al. 2003). Interestingly, in histidine decarboxylase-knockout mice, NO production is essential for regulating IFN-γ production. This notion is supported by the following lines of evidence (Koncz et al. 2007). First, an NO precursor increases concanavalin A (Con A)–induced IFN-γ production by splenocytes. Secondly, the exposure of these cells to N^G-monomethyl-l-arginine and nitronidazole reduces NO production, which inhibits IFN-γ production. Thirdly, pharmacological inhibition of NO production by splenocytes decreases IFN-γ synthesis. Fourthly, arginine enhances the synthesis of Th1 cytokines (IL-2 and IFN-γ) by murine Peyer's patch (PP) Th cells (Kobayashi et al. 1998). Of note, the effects of arginine on Th1 responses depend on the immune status of the host. Generally, arginine inhibits Th1 responses by reducing expression of IL-2, IFN-γ, and TNF-α and, therefore, inflammation in fish (Jiang et al. 2014), pigs (Wu et al. 2013; Chen et al. 2012a), and mice (Quirino et al. 2016; Chatterjee et al. 2006; Yeh et al. 2006) and rats (Chen et al. 2012b; Bonhomme et al. 2013). However, in immunocompromised animals, arginine enhances Th1 responses by increasing the expression of IFN-γ (Shang et al. 2005; Zhu et al. 2012; Emadi et al. 2011; Han et al. 2009). Mice that lack cationic amino acid transporter 2 (CAT2), which is essential for the transport of arginine into immune cells, exhibit a decrease in Th1 responses as indicated by a higher ratio of IL-12 p40:p70 and a lower abundance of the IFN-γ-induced protein 10 (IP-10), in comparison with wild type mice after *Helicobacter pylori* infection (Barry et al. 2011). In vaccine-immunized chickens, arginine does not appear to influence IFN-γ levels in the blood (Szabo et al. 2014). However, in chickens immunized with infectious bursal disease virus vaccine, arginine supplementation increases the concentration of IFN-γ in serum, indicating that arginine promotes a Th1 response (Emadi et al. 2011). Furthermore, Ren et al. (2013d) found that dietary arginine supplementation did not affect concentrations of TNF-α in sera of mice with inactivated *Pasteurella multocida* vaccination, suggesting that arginine does not influence the Th1 response under those experimental conditions (Ren et al. 2013d). In contrast, dietary arginine supplementation promotes the expression of IFN-γ in the jejunum and ileum of normal mice, likely because of its effects on the intestinal microbiota and immune signaling pathways involving activation of NF-κB, MAPK, and PI3K-Akt (Ren et al. 2014a).

19.3.2 ARGININE AND Th2 RESPONSES

Th2 cells are best known for their role in host defense against multicellular parasites and their involvement in allergies because they produce IL-4, IL-5, and IL-13, as well as IL-10 (Vahedi et al.

2013; Raphael et al. 2014). IL-4 can serve as an autocrine factor for Th2 differentiation and can promote the differentiation of B-cells into plasma cells and induce an antibody class switching to IgG1 and IgE, while enhancing the differentiation of dendritic cells (Raphael et al. 2014; Chen and Kolls 2013). IL-5 is critical for eosinophilopoiesis and eosinophil activation, as well as antibody production by activated B-cells (Chen and Kolls 2013). In addition, IL-13 facilitates B-cell activation and maturation, and promotes mucus production (Chen and Kolls 2013; Raphael et al. 2014). As an important immunoregulatory cytokine, IL-10 is best known for its anti-inflammatory role. Available evidence shows that Th2 cell differentiation depends on the cytokine IL-4 and is controlled by the master transcription factors GATA3 and STAT6.

Th2 cytokines (i.e., IL-4 and IL-10) can induce expression of arginase, thereby promoting the hydrolysis of arginine to ornithine and inhibiting the availability of arginine for metabolism by NOS (Liew et al. 1991; Cenci et al. 1993; Modolell et al. 1995). The activation of arginase can also result in a reversible block to T-cell proliferation, and cause activated T lymphocytes to undergo apoptosis (Bronte et al. 2003). The arginase-initiated depletion of arginine in the microenvironment suppresses expression of the CD3 ζ chain, which is the principal signal transduction element of the T-cell receptor (TCR). T lymphocytes with a deficiency of arginine undergo a decrease in proliferation (Bronte et al. 2003), suggesting an important role for arginine in TCR signaling and modulating T-cell function at an early stage of lymphocyte activation. These compelling findings suggest that extracellular arginine is indispensible for Th2 responses in the immune system. In support of this proposition, arginine increases the synthesis of Th2 cytokines (IL-4 and IL-5) by Th cells in murine Peyer's patches (Kobayashi et al. 1998). Additionally, dietary arginine supplementation enhances mRNA levels for Th2 cytokines (IL-4 and IL-10) in the spleen of rats with gut-derived sepsis (Shang et al. 2005). Similar results were observed in severely burned mice (Fan et al. 2010), mice with gut-derived sepsis (Yeh et al. 2006), and rats with subacute peritonitis (Chen et al. 2012b). However, in mice coinfected with malaria and nontyphoidal salmonella serotypes, dietary supplementation with L-arginine or L-citrulline reduced the expression of IL-4 in the ileum (Chau et al. 2013). Likewise, in broiler chickens with lipopolysaccharide-induced inflammation, dietary arginine supplementation reduced the expression of IL-10 in cecal tonsils (Tan et al. 2014b). These inconsistent findings indicate that, like Th1 responses, the roles of arginine in secretion of Th2 cytokines likely depend on the model and the nutritional status of the host.

19.3.3 Arginine and Th9 Responses

The Th9 cell, one of the recently defined subsets of Th cells, preferentially produces its signature cytokine, IL-9 (Zhao et al. 2013b; Schmitt et al. 2014; Pan et al. 2013). There is evidence that the production of IL-9 is promoted by IL-4 and transforming growth factor (TGF-β), and can be further enhanced by IL-1 (Kaplan 2013). In contrast, IFN-γ inhibits IL-9 expression (Zhao et al. 2013b; Schmitt et al. 2014). Th9 cells facilitate immune responses against melanoma and intestinal worms, and are closely associated with the immunopathology of allergies and autoimmune diseases such as systemic lupus erythematosus, experimental autoimmune encephalitis, and systemic sclerosis (Zhao et al. 2013b; Schmitt et al. 2014; Pan et al. 2013).

To our knowledge, there has not been a study to directly explore the effects of arginine on Th9 responses and IL-9 production. However, as stated previously, arginine affects the expression of IL-2, IL-4, and IFN-γ, implicating a possible role for this amino acid in Th9 production and signaling. Dietary arginine supplementation augments the expression of IL-1β in LPS-challenged fish (Jiang et al. 2014) and broiler chickens (Chen et al. 2012a), as well as deoxynivalenol-treated pigs (Wu et al. 2013). Also, arginine administration promotes the expression of TGF-β in rats exposed to exogenous advanced glycosylation end products (Yeh et al. 2012) and in mice with lupus nephritis (Peters et al. 2003a). In contrast, arginine inhibits the expression of TGF-β in rats with glomerulonephritis (Peters et al. 2003b) and patients undergoing stent implantation (Dudek et al. 2002), but has no effects on rats with unilateral urethral obstruction (Ito et al. 2005). These interesting results implicate a role for arginine in influencing Th9 responses, but further evidence from *in vitro* and *in vivo* experiments is needed.

19.3.4 ARGININE AND Th17 RESPONSES

Th17 cells provide protection against viral infection, and are also associated with the development of autoimmune diseases because of the recruitment of cells of the granulocyte lineage, especially neutrophils (Miossec and Kolls 2012). IL-17 is the signature cytokine for Th17 cells, but these cells also secrete IL-17F, IL-21, IL-22, and IL-23. TGF-β, IL-6, IL-1β, and TNF-α promote Th17 differentiation (Wilson et al. 2007). TGF-β promotes Th17 differentiation by suppressing the production of inhibitory cytokines IFN-γ and IL-4, or synergizing with IL-6 to induce expression of the transcription factor retinoic acid receptor–related orphan receptor-γt (RORγt), a key regulator of differentiation of Th17 cells (Ivanov et al. 2007; Shabgah et al. 2014). IL-1β and IL-6, in association with RORγt, IFN-regulatory factor 4 (IRF-4), aryl-hydrocarbon receptor (AHR), and the transcription factor signal transducer and activator of transcription 3 (STAT3), stimulate differentiation of Th17 cells (McGeachy and Cua 2008; Shabgah et al. 2014). Intriguingly, mammalian target of rapamycin (mTOR) signaling, which integrates input from insulin, growth factors, and amino acids, while sensing cellular nutrient and energy levels, also regulates differentiation of Th17 cells and IL-17 gene expression (Nagai et al. 2013; Kim et al. 2013).

Arginine promotes the expression of IL-17A in mononuclear cells in rats exposed to exogenous advanced glycosylation end products (Yeh et al. 2012). However, in the dextran sulfate sodium (DSS)–induced colitis mouse model, reduced availability of arginine was associated with IL-17 production. Further studies have shown that arginine supplementation promotes the colonic expression of IL-17 at 7 days post-DSS treatment, while reducing the expression of IL-17 and TNF-α in the colon at 12 days post-DSS administration in mice (Ren et al. 2014c). These results indicate that the effects of arginine on Th17 responses depend on the model being used. Such actions of arginine may result from Th1 and Th2 responses through mTOR signaling because this amino acid activates mTOR (Yao et al. 2008; Kong et al. 2012).

19.3.5 ARGININE AND Th22 RESPONSES

Traditionally, IL-22 was regarded as the product of Th17 cells; however, recent studies have shown that a distinct subset of CD4+ T-cells in human skin produces IL-22, but not IL-17 or IFN-γ (Trifari et al. 2009). Hence, these cells have been coined "Th22." The development of Th22 cells from naive T-cells requires stimulation by IL-6 and TNF-α or antigens in the context of plasmacytoid dendritic cells, and depends on the aryl hydrocarbon receptor (AHR) (Raphael et al. 2014). To date, there are no available data to indicate the role of arginine in Th22 responses. However, as stated previously, arginine influences the production of IL-6 and TNF-α, which provides a potential mechanism for this amino acid to affect Th22 responses.

19.3.6 ARGININE AND REGULATORY T-CELLS

Regulatory T-cells (Tregs) are important immunoregulators in many inflammatory and autoimmune diseases as they modulate secretion of anti-inflammatory cytokines and the expression of receptors for cytokines (Miyara and Sakaguchi 2007). These cells include thymus-derived or natural Tregs (nTregs) and Treg cells induced via postthymic maturation (iTregs). Tregs express the signature Foxp3 transcription factor, which is critical for their development, lineage commitment, and regulatory functions (Hori et al. 2003; Raphael et al. 2014). The two major cytokines produced by Tregs are IL-10 and TGF-β (Raphael et al. 2014). Different from Th1, Th2, and Th17 cells, which express abundant amounts of glucose transporter 1 (Glut1) on their membranes and are highly glycolytic, Tregs express low levels of Glut1 and have high lipid oxidation rates *in vitro* (Michalek et al. 2011). TGF-β is required for the generation of iTregs because, under the influence of IL-2, TGF-β induces the expression of Foxp3 in a paracrine feedback loop, leading to conversion of naive T-cells (Th0) into iTreg cells (Carrier et al. 2007). This is distinct from Th17 cells for which TGF-β, in the presence of IL-6, activates naive T-cells to express the transcription factors STAT3 and Rorγt and to secrete IL-17.

mTOR signaling is critical for proliferation and differentiation of Treg cells by promoting glycolysis and expression of the transcription factor hypoxia-inducible factor 1α (HIF1α), which binds FoxP3 and targets FoxP3 for proteasomal degradation (Dang et al. 2011; Coe et al. 2014). Tregs increase expression of arginase 1 and NOS2 in actively tolerant skin grafts *in vivo* (Cobbold et al. 2009), providing evidence that Tregs can influence arginine availability and arginine, in turn, may affect responses of Treg cells. In mice infected with *Plasmodium yoelii* 17XL, arginine supplementation does not affect the number of Treg cells (Zhu et al. 2012). In contrast, arginine supplementation lowers the percentage of Foxp3 Treg cells in rats treated with exogenous advanced glycosylation end products (Yeh et al. 2012). A concern with these previous studies is the inconsistent doses of arginine and different composition of other amino acids in the animal diets. In light of the inconsistent evidence from *in vivo* studies, effects of arginine at nutritional and physiological doses on Treg cell responses merit further investigations.

19.3.7   ARGININE AND CD8+ T-CELLS

CD8+ T-cells are cytotoxic T-cells that kill (a) cells infected by pathogens (e.g., viruses), (b) cancer cells, and (c) cells that are damaged by various factors. Unlike CD4+ T-cells, which recognize an MHC class II–presented antigen, CD8+ T-cells are activated by an MHC class I-presented antigen. Upon activation, CD8+ T-cells cause apoptosis in target cells through the release of cytotoxins (perforin, granzymes and granulysin) or via the FasL-Fas pathway. CD8+ T-cells also produce IFN-γ, TNF-α, and IL-2 in response to an immunological challenge (Chen and Kolls 2013).

Results from *in vitro* studies indicate that arginine increases the proliferation of cytotoxic T-cells, the number of CD45RA-negative CD8 positive (memory) T-cells, and the abundance of cell-surface CD8 receptors (CD8R) and CD3 receptors (CD3R) (Ochoa et al. 2001). Dietary arginine supplementation increases the number of CD8+ T-cells at 2 days postinoculation of infectious bursal disease virus (IBDV) in broiler chickens (Tan et al. 2015). Similar results have been reported for weaned pigs after *Escherichia coli* LPS challenge (Zhu et al. 2013). However, for patients with gastric cancer, arginine-enriched nutrition has little effect on CD8+ T-cells, but increases the numbers of CD4+ T-cells and NK cells (Zhao et al. 2013a). Likewise, arginine supplementation does not affect the number of CD8+ cells in whole blood or splenocytes from rats with gut-derived sepsis (Shang et al. 2005). However, interpretation of these results is seriously confounded because the control and experimental diets differed not only in arginine content, but also in other amino acids. Thus, the effects of arginine on CD8+ T-cells require further investigation.

19.3.8   ARGININE AND γδ T, NKT, AND Tfh CELLS

Unlike conventional T-cells (CD4 and CD8), which have a T-cell receptor composed of α and β chains, γδ T-cells are a small subset of T-cells that contain one γ chain and one δ chain. Human γδ T lymphocytes include two subsets: (1) Vδ1T cells, which are located primarily in mucosa-associated lymphoid tissues (e.g., intestine) and play a critical role in the first line of defense against viral, bacterial, and fungal pathogens; and (2) Vδ2T cells, which are present in blood and respond to mycobacteria and solid tumors (Poggi and Zocchi 2014). The γδ T-cells produce IFN-γ, TNF-α, and IL-17 in response to infection (Chen and Kolls 2013). Natural killer (NK) T-cells are a subset of T-cells expressing a TCRαβ and several NK cell markers (e.g., NK1.1). NKT cells recognize antigens presented by the CD1d molecule and produce Th1, Th2, or Th17 cytokines, thereby affecting immune responses against pathogens and the onset of autoimmune diseases (Ghazarian et al. 2014; Chen and Kolls 2013). Follicular helper T-cells (Tfh), which are found in B-cell follicles of secondary lymphoid organs, are antigen-experienced CD4+ T-cells that express B-cell follicle homing receptor CXC chemokine receptor 5. Tfh cells facilitate B-cell activation and antibody production by interacting with ligands on the surface of B-cells (Morita et al. 2011). IL-6 and IL-21 are critical cytokines for the differentiation of Tfh cells, which preferentially produce IL-21 (Nurieva et al. 2008). In turn, IL-21 regulates proliferation, maturation, and class switching of B-cells (Spolski and Leonard 2008).

There is increasing evidence that arginine or the arginine-NO pathway influences the responses of $\gamma\delta$T, NKT, and Tfh cells to immunological challenges. For example, in CAT2$^{-/-}$ mice which cannot transport arginine, DSS treatment increases the number of IL-17-expressing $\gamma\delta$T cells in the colon and mesenteric lymph nodes compared to wild-type mice (Singh et al. 2013). Interestingly, arginine restores NKT cytotoxicity *in vivo* and *in vitro* (Santarelli et al. 2006). Besides NO, polyamines produced from arginine may also modulate proliferation and differentiation of all T lymphocytes (Wu 2013).

19.4 ARGININE AND HUMORAL IMMUNITY

Upon activation, B-cells produce antibodies (e.g., IgA, IgD, IgE, IgG, and IgM), which identify and neutralize foreign pathogens such as bacteria and viruses. Nutrients, including arginine and vitamin A, are critical for B-cell development and proliferation, class switch recombination (a biological mechanism responsible for changes in the production of antibodies by B-cells from one type to another, such as from IgM to IgG), and the generation of antibodies by plasma cells (Ross et al. 2009). Thus, arginine affects humoral immunity in the host and increases IgA secretion by the small intestine of rats with septic peritonitis (Shang et al. 2004). Dietary supplementation of young pigs with arginine enhances concentrations of IgG and IgM in serum compared with unsupplemented controls (Tan et al. 2009). Similar findings have been reported for severely burned mice (Fan et al. 2010). However, when arginine was administrated through parenteral nutrition, no significant changes in intestinal and respiratory tract IgA levels in mice were detected (Fukatsu et al. 2004; Shang et al. 2004). This is likely because there is little uptake of arginine from the vascular system of the gut (Wu 1998).

In vaccine-immunized models, dietary arginine supplementation augments pathogen-specific production of antibodies by B-cells against *Pseudomonas aeruginosa* in mice at 4 and 7 weeks after immunization with detoxified *Pseudomonas* exotoxin A linked with the outer membrane proteins I and F (Shang et al. 2003). Likewise, dietary arginine supplementation increases serum IgG antibodies against pneumococcal polysaccharide serotypes 5 in older people after vaccination against *Streptococcus pneumonia* (Moriguti et al. 2005). Also, in mice immunized with an inactivated *Pasteurella multocida* vaccine, the antibody titers against *Pasteurella multocida* after arginine supplementation are much higher than those in the vaccine-oil adjuvant mice, and even at 36 hours postinfection with *P. multocida* serotype A (Ren et al. 2013d). However, effects of arginine on antibody production vary among animal models challenged with pathogen-induced infections. For example, in mice challenged with influenza virus A/Port Chalmers/1/73 (H3N2), dietary arginine supplementation has little effect on antibody titers to influenza in serum at day 31 postchallenge (Suarez Butler et al. 2005). In contrast, dietary arginine supplementation decreases mucosal secretory IgG concentrations in broiler chickens subjected to a coccidial challenge (Tan et al. 2014a). However, dietary arginine supplementation increases antibody titers in serum against infectious bursal disease virus in broiler chickens infected with bursal disease virus (Tan et al. 2015). Further research is required to understand the complex roles of arginine in modulating humoral immunity in animals with various pathogen-induced diseases.

19.5 CONCLUSION AND PERSPECTIVES

A deficiency of arginine in the diet severely impairs immunity in mammals, birds, and fish (Li et al. 2007). Over the past decade, there has been rapid progress toward increasing understanding of the roles of arginine in regulating the production of cytokines by T-cells and antibodies by B-cells to modulate both innate and adaptive immunities (Figure 19.3). In innate immunity, arginine influences the expression of toll-like receptors and antimicrobials (Ren et al. 2014a), the phagocytic activity of immunologically activated macrophages (Rutherfurd-Markwick et al. 2013), antioxidatant enzymes (e.g., superoxide dismutase and glutathione peroxidase) (Jobgen et al. 2009a,b),

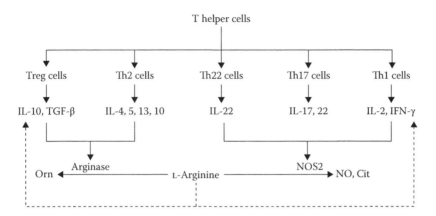

FIGURE 19.3 The interaction between Th cells and arginine metabolism in humans and animals. Arginine is metabolized by inducible nitric oxide synthase (NOS2) to generate NO and citrulline (Cit), or by arginase to form ornithine (Orn) and polyamines. Proinflammatory cytokines released by Th1, Th17, and Th22 cells promote the activity of NOS2, while anti-inflammatory cytokines from Th2 and Treg cells activate arginase for conversion of arginine to ornithine and polyamines. Arginine also affects the production of cytokines from all Th subsets, depending on the animal model (shown by the dotted line).

low-molecular-weight antioxidants (e.g., glutathione) (Ren et al. 2012a), tight junction proteins (Ren et al. 2014c), and other mediators (e.g., NO, creatine, and polyamines) (Wu 2009, 2010; Li et al. 2007). In adaptive immunity, arginine affects the responses of Th cells to antigens, the activity of cytotoxic T cells, and the production of antibodies against specific pathogens. There is considerable evidence that the effects of arginine on innate and adaptive immunities depend on a variety of physiological and pathological factors, including dietary provision of protein, amino acids, fatty acids, carbohydrates, vitamins, and minerals. In this context, balanced nutrition is a foundation for arginine to exert its beneficial actions on the immune system to protect the host from invading pathogens. Thus, arginine is truly a functional amino acid (Wu 2010) and must be provided in diets to improve health and well-being in humans and animals (Hou et al. 2015). The concept of dietary essentiality of arginine in both young and adult animals and humans represents a new paradigm shift in nutritional immunology.

ACKNOWLEDGMENTS

This study was jointly supported by the Chinese Academy of Science STS Project (KFJ-EW-STS-063 to YL Yin), Key Projects in the National Science & Technology Pillar Program (2013BAD21B04 to YL Yin), Agriculture and Food Research Initiative Competitive Grants (2014-67015-21770 and 2015-67015-23276 to G. Wu and F.W. Bazer) from the USDA National Institute of Food and Agriculture, a Hatch project from Texas A&M AgriLife Research (H-8200 to G. Wu), the American Diabetes Association (1-13-JF-59 to B. Zhou), and the National Institute of Health/National Institute of Diabetes and Digestive and Kidney Diseases (NIH/NIDDK 1R01DK098662 to B. Zhou). The corresponding author of this chapter is Guoyao Wu (g-wu@tamu.edu).

REFERENCES

Akira S, Takeda K, Kaisho T (2001) Toll-like receptors: Critical proteins linking innate and acquired immunity. *Nat Immunol* 2 (8):675–680. doi:10.1038/90609.
Barry DP, Asim M, Scull BP, Piazuelo MB, de Sablet T, Lewis ND, Coburn LA, Singh K, Ellies LG, Gobert AP, Chaturvedi R, Wilson KT (2011) Cationic amino acid transporter 2 enhances innate immunity during Helicobacter pylori infection. *PLOS ONE* 6 (12):e29046. doi:10.1371/journal.pone.0029046.
Bonaventura P, Benedetti G, Albarede F, Miossec P (2014) Zinc and its role in immunity and inflammation. *Autoimmun Rev* 14 (4):277–285. doi:10.1016/j.autrev.2014.11.008.

Bonhomme S, Belabed L, Blanc MC, Neveux N, Cynober L, Darquy S (2013) Arginine-supplemented enteral nutrition in critically ill diabetic and obese rats: A dose-ranging study evaluating nutritional status and macrophage function. *Nutrition* 29 (1):305–312. doi:10.1016/j.nut.2012.07.005.

Bronte V, Serafini P, Mazzoni A, Segal DM, Zanovello P (2003) L-arginine metabolism in myeloid cells controls T-lymphocyte functions. *Trends Immunol* 24 (6):302–306.

Carrier Y, Yuan J, Kuchroo VK, Weiner HL (2007) Th3 cells in peripheral tolerance. I. Induction of Foxp3-positive regulatory T cells by Th3 cells derived from TGF-beta T cell-transgenic mice. *J Immunol* 178 (1):179–185.

Cenci E, Romani L, Mencacci A, Spaccapelo R, Schiaffella E, Puccetti P, Bistoni F (1993) Interleukin-4 and interleukin-10 inhibit nitric oxide-dependent macrophage killing of Candida albicans. *Eur J Immunol* 23 (5):1034–1038. doi:10.1002/eji.1830230508.

Chatterjee S, Premachandran S, Bagewadikar RS, Bhattacharya S, Chattopadhyay S, Poduval TB (2006) Arginine metabolic pathways determine its therapeutic benefit in experimental heatstroke: Role of Th1/Th2 cytokine balance. *Nitric Oxide* 15 (4):408–416. doi:10.1016/j.niox.2006.04.003.

Chau JY, Tiffany CM, Nimishakavi S, Lawrence JA, Pakpour N, Mooney JP, Lokken KL, Caughey GH, Tsolis RM, Luckhart S (2013) Malaria-associated L-arginine deficiency induces mast cell-associated disruption to intestinal barrier defenses against nontyphoidal Salmonella bacteremia. *Infect Immun* 81 (10):3515–3526. doi:10.1128/IAI.00380-13.

Chen K, Kolls JK (2013) T cell-mediated host immune defenses in the lung. *Annu Rev Immunol* 31:605–633. doi:10.1146/annurev-immunol-032712-100019.

Chen Y, Chen D, Tian G, He J, Mao X, Mao Q, Yu B (2012a) Dietary arginine supplementation alleviates immune challenge induced by Salmonella enterica serovar Choleraesuis bacterin potentially through the Toll-like receptor 4-myeloid differentiation factor 88 signalling pathway in weaned piglets. *Br J Nutr* 108 (6):1069–1076. doi:10.1017/S0007114511006350.

Chen YH, Lee CH, Hsu LS, Hsiao CC, Lo HC (2012b) Appropriate dose of parenteral arginine enhances immunity of peripheral blood cells and splenocytes in rats with subacute peritonitis. *JPEN J Parenter Enteral Nutr* 36 (6):741–749. doi:10.1177/0148607111429793.

Cobbold SP, Adams E, Farquhar CA, Nolan KF, Howie D, Lui KO, Fairchild PJ, Mellor AL, Ron D, Waldmann H (2009) Infectious tolerance via the consumption of essential amino acids and mTOR signaling. *Proc Natl Acad Sci U S A* 106 (29):12055–12060. doi:10.1073/pnas.0903919106.

Coe DJ, Kishore M, Marelli-Berg F (2014) Metabolic regulation of regulatory T cell development and function. *Front Immunol* 5:590. doi:10.3389/fimmu.2014.00590.

Dang EV, Barbi J, Yang HY, Jinasena D, Yu H, Zheng Y, Bordman Z, Fu J, Kim Y, Yen HR, Luo W, Zeller K, Shimoda L, Topalian SL, Semenza GL, Dang CV, Pardoll DM, Pan F. (2011) Control of T(H)17/T(reg) balance by hypoxia-inducible factor 1. *Cell* 146 (5):772–784. doi:10.1016/j.cell.2011.07.033.

Dudek D, Heba G, Bartus S, Partyka L, Dembinska-Kiec A, Huk J, Legutko J, Dubiel JS (2002) Effects of L-arginine supplementation on endothelial function after stent implantation. *Kardiol Pol* 57 (11):389–397; discussion 398.

Emadi M, Jahanshiri F, Kaveh K, Hair-Bejo M, Ideris A, Alimon AR (2011) Nutrition and immunity: The effects of the combination of arginine and tryptophan on growth performance, serum parameters and immune response in broiler chickens challenged with infectious bursal disease vaccine. *Avian Pathol* 40 (1):63–72. doi:10.1080/03079457.2010.539590.

Fan J, Meng Q, Guo G, Xie Y, Li X, Xiu Y, Li T, Ma L (2010) Effects of early enteral nutrition supplemented with arginine on intestinal mucosal immunity in severely burned mice. *Clin Nutr* 29 (1):124–130. doi:10.1016/j.clnu.2009.07.005.

Fukatsu K, Ueno C, Maeshima Y, Hara E, Nagayoshi H, Omata J, Mochizuki H, Hiraide H (2004) L-arginine-enriched parenteral nutrition affects lymphocyte phenotypes of gut-associated lymphoid tissue. *JPEN J Parenter Enteral Nutr* 28 (4):246–250.

Geremia A, Biancheri P, Allan P, Corazza GR, Di Sabatino A (2014) Innate and adaptive immunity in inflammatory bowel disease. *Autoimmun Rev* 13 (1):3–10. doi:10.1016/j.autrev.2013.06.004.

Ghazarian L, Simoni Y, Magalhaes I, Lehuen A (2014) Invariant NKT cell development: Focus on NOD mice. *Curr Opin Immunol* 27:83–88. doi:10.1016/j.coi.2014.02.004.

Han J, Liu YL, Fan W, Chao J, Hou YQ, Yin YL, Zhu HL, Meng GQ, Che ZQ (2009) Dietary L-arginine supplementation alleviates immunosuppression induced by cyclophosphamide in weaned pigs. *Amino Acids* 37 (4):643–651. doi:10.1007/s00726-008-0184-9.

Hori S, Nomura T, Sakaguchi S (2003) Control of regulatory T cell development by the transcription factor Foxp3. *Science* 299 (5609):1057–1061. doi:10.1126/science.1079490.

Hou YQ, Yin YL, Wu G (2015) Dietary essentiality of "nutritionally nonessential amino acids" for animals and humans. *Exp Biol Med* 240:997–1007.

Ito K, Chen J, Seshan SV, Khodadadian JJ, Gallagher R, El Chaar M, Vaughan ED, Jr., Poppas DP, Felsen D (2005) Dietary arginine supplementation attenuates renal damage after relief of unilateral ureteral obstruction in rats. *Kidney Int* 68 (2):515–528. doi:10.1111/j.1523-1755.2005.00429.x.

Ivanov, II, Zhou L, Littman DR (2007) Transcriptional regulation of Th17 cell differentiation. *Semin Immunol* 19 (6):409–417. doi:10.1016/j.smim.2007.10.011.

Jiang J, Shi D, Zhou XQ, Hu Y, Feng L, Liu Y, Jiang WD, Zhao Y (2014) In vitro and in vivo protective effect of arginine against lipopolysaccharide induced inflammatory response in the intestine of juvenile Jian carp (Cyprinus carpio var. Jian). *Fish Shellfish Immunol* 42 (2):457–464. doi:10.1016/j.fsi.2014.11.030.

Jobgen W, Fu WJ, Gao H, Li P, Meininger CJ, Smith SB, Spencer TE, Wu G (2009a) High fat feeding and dietary L-arginine supplementation differentially regulate gene expression in rat white adipose tissue. *Amino Acids* 37:187–198.

Jobgen WJ, Meininger CJ, Jobgen SC, Li P, Lee MJ, Smith SB, Spencer TE, Fried SK, Wu G (2009b) Dietary L-arginine supplementation reduces white-fat gain and enhances skeletal muscle and brown fat masses in diet-induced obese rats. *J Nutr* 139:230–237.

Kaplan MH (2013) Th9 cells: Differentiation and disease. *Immunol Rev* 252 (1):104–115. doi:10.1111/imr.12028.

Kim JS, Sklarz T, Banks LB, Gohil M, Waickman AT, Skuli N, Krock BL, Luo CT, Hu W, Pollizzi KN, Li MO, Rathmell JC, Birnbaum MJ, Powell JD, Jordan MS, Koretzky GA (2013) Natural and inducible TH17 cells are regulated differently by Akt and mTOR pathways. *Nat Immunol* 14 (6):611–618. doi:10.1038/ni.2607.

Kobayashi T, Yamamoto M, Hiroi T, McGhee J, Takeshita Y, Kiyono H (1998) Arginine enhances induction of T helper 1 and T helper 2 cytokine synthesis by Peyer's patch alpha beta T cells and antigen-specific mucosal immune response. *Biosci Biotechnol Biochem* 62 (12):2334–2340. doi:10.1271/bbb.62.2334.

Koncz A, Pasztoi M, Mazan M, Fazakas F, Buzas E, Falus A, Nagy G (2007) Nitric oxide mediates T cell cytokine production and signal transduction in histidine decarboxylase knockout mice. *J Immunol* 179 (10):6613–6619.

Kong X, Tan B, Yin Y, Gao H, Li X, Jaeger LA, Bazer FW, Wu G (2012) L-Arginine stimulates the mTOR signaling pathway and protein synthesis in porcine trophectoderm cells. *J Nutr Biochem* 23 (9):1178–1183. doi:10.1016/j.jnutbio.2011.06.012.

Li P, Yin YL, Li D, Kim SW, Wu G (2007) Amino acids and immune function. *Br J Nutr* 98 (2):237–252. doi:10.1017/S000711450769936X.

Liew FY, Li Y, Severn A, Millott S, Schmidt J, Salter M, Moncada S (1991) A possible novel pathway of regulation by murine T helper type-2 (Th2) cells of a Th1 cell activity via the modulation of the induction of nitric oxide synthase on macrophages. *Eur J Immunol* 21 (10):2489–2494. doi:10.1002/eji.1830211027.

McGeachy MJ, Cua DJ (2008) Th17 cell differentiation: The long and winding road. *Immunity* 28 (4):445–453. doi:10.1016/j.immuni.2008.03.001.

Michalek RD, Gerriets VA, Jacobs SR, Macintyre AN, MacIver NJ, Mason EF, Sullivan SA, Nichols AG, Rathmell JC (2011) Cutting edge: Distinct glycolytic and lipid oxidative metabolic programs are essential for effector and regulatory CD4+ T cell subsets. *J Immunol* 186 (6):3299–3303. doi:10.4049/jimmunol.1003613.

Miles EA, Calder PC (2015) Fatty acids, lipid emulsions and the immune and inflammatory systems. *World Rev Nutr Diet* 112:17–30. doi: 10.1159/000365426.

Miossec P, Kolls JK (2012) Targeting IL-17 and TH17 cells in chronic inflammation. *Nat Rev Drug Discov* 11 (10):763–776. doi: 10.1038/nrd3794.

Miyara M, Sakaguchi S (2007) Natural regulatory T cells: Mechanisms of suppression. *Trends Mol Med* 13 (3):108–116. doi: 10.1016/j.molmed.2007.01.003.

Modolell M, Corraliza IM, Link F, Soler G, Eichmann K (1995) Reciprocal regulation of the nitric oxide synthase/arginase balance in mouse bone marrow-derived macrophages by TH1 and TH2 cytokines. *Eur J Immunol* 25 (4):1101–1104. doi: 10.1002/eji.1830250436.

Moriguti JC, Ferriolli E, Donadi EA, Marchini JS (2005) Effects of arginine supplementation on the humoral and innate immune response of older people. *Eur J Clin Nutr* 59 (12):1362–1366. doi: 10.1038/sj.ejcn.1602247.

Morita R, Schmitt N, Bentebibel SE, Ranganathan R, Bourdery L, Zurawski G, Foucat E, Dullaers M, Oh S, Sabzghabaei N, Lavecchio EM, Punaro M, Pascual V, Banchereau J, Ueno H (2011) Human blood CXCR5(+)CD4(+) T cells are counterparts of T follicular cells and contain specific subsets that differentially support antibody secretion. *Immunity* 34 (1):108–121. doi: 10.1016/j.immuni.2010.12.012.

Munir K, Muneer MA, Masaoud E, Tiwari A, Mahmud A, Chaudhry RM, Rashid A (2009) Dietary arginine stimulates humoral and cell-mediated immunity in chickens vaccinated and challenged against hydropericardium syndrome virus. *Poult Sci* 88 (8):1629–1638. doi: 10.3382/ps.2009-00152.

Nagai S, Kurebayashi Y, Koyasu S (2013) Role of PI3K/Akt and mTOR complexes in Th17 cell differentiation. *Ann N Y Acad Sci* 1280:30–34. doi: 10.1111/nyas.12059.

Nurieva RI, Chung Y, Hwang D, Yang XO, Kang HS, Ma L, Wang YH, Watowich SS, Jetten AM, Tian Q, Dong C (2008) Generation of T follicular helper cells is mediated by interleukin-21 but independent of T helper 1, 2, or 17 cell lineages. *Immunity* 29 (1):138–149. doi: 10.1016/j.immuni.2008.05.009.

Ochoa JB, Strange J, Kearney P, Gellin G, Endean E, Fitzpatrick E (2001) Effects of L-arginine on the proliferation of T lymphocyte subpopulations. *JPEN J Parenter Enteral Nutr* 25 (1):23–29.

Pan HF, Leng RX, Li XP, Zheng SG, Ye DQ (2013) Targeting T-helper 9 cells and interleukin-9 in autoimmune diseases. *Cytokine Growth Factor Rev* 24 (6):515–522.

Perez-Carbajal C, Caldwell D, Farnell M, Stringfellow K, Pohl S, Casco G, Pro-Martinez A, Ruiz-Feria CA (2010) Immune response of broiler chickens fed different levels of arginine and vitamin E to a coccidiosis vaccine and Eimeria challenge. *Poult Sci* 89 (9):1870–1877. doi: 10.3382/ps.2010-00753.

Peters H, Border WA, Ruckert M, Kramer S, Neumayer HH, Noble NA (2003a) L-arginine supplementation accelerates renal fibrosis and shortens life span in experimental lupus nephritis. *Kidney Int* 63 (4):1382–1392. doi: 10.1046/j.1523-1755.2003.00881.x.

Peters H, Daig U, Martini S, Ruckert M, Schaper F, Liefeldt L, Kramer S, Neumayer HH (2003b) NO mediates antifibrotic actions of L-arginine supplementation following induction of anti-thy1 glomerulonephritis. *Kidney Int* 64 (2):509–518. doi: 10.1046/j.1523-1755.2003.00112.x.

Poggi A, Zocchi MR (2014) Gammadelta T lymphocytes as a first line of immune defense: Old and new ways of antigen recognition and implications for cancer immunotherapy. *Front Immunol* 5:575. doi: 10.3389/fimmu.2014.00575.

Pohlenz C, Buentello A, Criscitiello MF, Mwangi W, Smith R, Gatlin DM, 3rd (2012) Synergies between vaccination and dietary arginine and glutamine supplementation improve the immune response of channel catfish against Edwardsiella ictaluri. *Fish Shellfish Immunol* 33 (3):543–551. doi: 10.1016/j.fsi.2012.06.005.

Quirino IE, Carneiro MB, Cardoso VN, das Gracas Carvalho Dos Santos R, Vieira LQ, Fiuza JA, Alvarez-Leite JI, de Vasconcelos Generoso S, Correia MI (2016) Arginine supplementation induces arginase activity and inhibits TNF-alpha synthesis in mice spleen macrophages after intestinal obstruction. *JPEN J Parenter Enteral Nutr* 40 (3):417–422. doi: 10.1177/0148607114546374.

Raphael I, Nalawade S, Eagar TN, Forsthuber TG (2014) T cell subsets and their signature cytokines in autoimmune and inflammatory diseases. *Cytokine* 74 (1):5–17. doi: 10.1016/j.cyto.2014.09.011.

Ren W, Chen S, Yin J, Duan J, Li T, Liu G, Feng Z, Tan B, Yin Y, Wu G (2014a) Dietary arginine supplementation of mice alters the microbial population and activates intestinal innate immunity. *J Nutr* 144 (6):988–995. doi: 10.3945/jn.114.192120.

Ren W, Duan J, Yin J, Liu G, Cao Z, Xiong X, Chen S, Li T, Yin Y, Hou Y, Wu G (2014b) Dietary L-glutamine supplementation modulates microbial community and activates innate immunity in the mouse intestine. *Amino Acids* 46 (10):2403–2413. doi: 10.1007/s00726-014-1793-0.

Ren W, Li Y, Yu X, Luo W, Liu G, Shao H, Yin Y (2013a) Glutamine modifies immune responses of mice infected with porcine circovirus type 2. *Br J Nutr* 110 (6):1053–1060. doi: 10.1017/S0007114512006101.

Ren W, Liu S, Chen S, Zhang F, Li N, Yin J, Peng Y, Wu L, Liu G, Yin Y, Wu G (2013b) Dietary L-glutamine supplementation increases Pasteurella multocida burden and the expression of its major virulence factors in mice. *Amino Acids* 45 (4):947–955. doi: 10.1007/s00726-013-1551-8.

Ren W, Wu M, Luo W, Huang R, Yin Y, Li Y, Li T, Yu X (2013c) Dietary supplementation with proline confers a positive effect in both porcine circovirus-infected pregnant and non-pregnant mice. *Br J Nutr* 110 (8):1492–1499. doi: 10.1017/S0007114513000652.

Ren W, Yin J, Wu M, Liu G, Yang G, Xion Y, Su D, Wu L, Li T, Chen S, Duan J, Yin Y, Wu G (2014c) Serum amino acids profile and the beneficial effects of L-arginine or L-glutamine supplementation in dextran sulfate sodium colitis. *PLOS ONE* 9 (2):e88335. doi: 10.1371/journal.pone.0088335.

Ren W, Yin Y, Liu G, Yu X, Li Y, Yang G, Li T, Wu G (2012a) Effect of dietary arginine supplementation on reproductive performance of mice with porcine circovirus type 2 infection. *Amino Acids* 42 (6):2089–2094. doi: 10.1007/s00726-011-0942-y.

Ren W, Zou L, Li N, Wang Y, Liu G, Peng Y, Ding J, Cai L, Yin Y, Wu G (2013d) Dietary arginine supplementation enhances immune responses to inactivated pasteurella multocida vaccination in mice. *Br J Nutr* 109 (5):867–872. doi: 10.1017/S0007114512002681.

Ren WK, Yin J, Zhu XP, Liu G, Li NZ, Peng YY, Yin YL (2013e) Glutamine on intestinal inflammation: A mechanistic perspective. *Eur J Inflamm* 11 (2):315–326.

Ren WK, Yin YL, Liu G, Yu XL, Li YH, Yang G, Li TJ, Wu GY (2012b) Effect of dietary arginine supplementation on reproductive performance of mice with porcine circovirus type 2 infection. *Amino Acids* 42 (6):2089–2094. doi: Doi 10.1007/S00726-011-0942-Y.

Ren WK, Zou LX, Li NZ, Wang Y, Liu G, Peng YY, Ding JN, Cai LC, Yin YL, Wu GY (2013f) Dietary arginine supplementation enhances immune responses to inactivated Pasteurella multocida vaccination in mice. *B J Nutr* 109 (5):867–872. doi: Doi 10.1017/S0007114512002681.

Ross AC, Chen Q, Ma Y (2009) Augmentation of antibody responses by retinoic acid and costimulatory molecules. *Semin Immunol* 21 (1):42–50. doi: 10.1016/j.smim.2008.08.004.

Ruth MR, Field CJ (2013) The immune modifying effects of amino acids on gut-associated lymphoid tissue. *J Anim Sci Biotechnol* 4(1):27. doi: 10.1186/2049-1891-4-27.

Rutherfurd-Markwick KJ, Hendriks WH, Morel PC, Thomas DG (2013) The potential for enhancement of immunity in cats by dietary supplementation. *Vet Immunol Immunopathol* 152 (3–4):333–340. doi: 10.1016/j.vetimm.2013.01.007.

Santarelli L, Bracci M, Mocchegiani E (2006) In vitro and in vivo effects of mercuric chloride on thymic endocrine activity, NK and NKT cell cytotoxicity, cytokine profiles (IL-2, IFN-gamma, IL-6): Role of the nitric oxide-L-arginine pathway. *Int Immunopharmacol* 6 (3):376–389. doi: 10.1016/j.intimp.2005.08.028.

Schmitt E, Klein M, Bopp T (2014) Th9 cells, new players in adaptive immunity. *Trends Immunol* 35 (2):61–68. doi: 10.1016/j.it.2013.10.004.

Shabgah AG, Fattahi E, Shahneh FZ (2014) Interleukin-17 in human inflammatory diseases. *Postepy Dermatol Alergol* 31 (4):256–261. doi: 10.5114/pdia.2014.40954.

Shang HF, Hsu CS, Yeh CL, Pai MH, Yeh SL (2005) Effects of arginine supplementation on splenocyte cytokine mRNA expression in rats with gut-derived sepsis. *World J Gastroenterol* 11 (45):7091–7096.

Shang HF, Tsai HJ, Chiu WC, Yeh SL (2003) Effects of dietary arginine supplementation on antibody production and antioxidant enzyme activity in burned mice. *Burns* 29 (1):43–48.

Shang HF, Wang YY, Lai YN, Chiu WC, Yeh SL (2004) Effects of arginine supplementation on mucosal immunity in rats with septic peritonitis. *Clin Nutr* 23 (4):561–569. doi: 10.1016/j.clnu.2003.10.005.

Siegmund B, Zeitz M (2011) Innate and adaptive immunity in inflammatory bowel disease. *World J Gastroenterol* 17 (27):3178–3183. doi: 10.3748/wjg.v17.i27.3178.

Singh K, Coburn LA, Barry DP, Asim M, Scull BP, Allaman MM, Lewis ND, Washington MK, Rosen MJ, Williams CS, Chaturvedi R, Wilson KT (2013) Deletion of cationic amino acid transporter 2 exacerbates dextran sulfate sodium colitis and leads to an IL-17-predominant T cell response. *Am J Physiol Gastrointest Liver Physiol* 305 (3):G225–240. doi: 10.1152/ajpgi.00091.2013.

Spolski R, Leonard WJ (2008) Interleukin-21: Basic biology and implications for cancer and autoimmunity. *Annu Rev Immunol* 26:57–79. doi: 10.1146/annurev.immunol.26.021607.090316.

Suarez Butler MF, Langkamp-Henken B, Herrlinger-Garcia KA, Klash AE, Szczepanik ME, Nieves C, Jr., Cottey RJ, Bender BS (2005) Arginine supplementation enhances mitogen-induced splenocyte proliferation but does not affect in vivo indicators of antigen-specific immunity in mice. *J Nutr* 135 (5):1146–1150.

Szabo J, Andrasofszky E, Tuboly T, Bersenyi A, Weisz A, Hetenyi N, Hullar I (2014) Effect of arginine or glutamine supplementation on production, organ weights, interferon gamma, interleukin 6 and antibody titre of broilers. *Acta Vet Hung* 62 (3):348–361. doi: 10.1556/AVet.2014.017.

Tan B, Li XG, Kong X, Huang R, Ruan Z, Yao K, Deng Z, Xie M, Shinzato I, Yin Y, Wu G (2009) Dietary L-arginine supplementation enhances the immune status in early-weaned piglets. *Amino Acids* 37 (2):323–331. doi: 10.1007/s00726-008-0155-1.

Tan J, Applegate TJ, Liu S, Guo Y, Eicher SD (2014a) Supplemental dietary L-arginine attenuates intestinal mucosal disruption during a coccidial vaccine challenge in broiler chickens. *Br J Nutr* 112 (7):1098–1109. doi: 10.1017/S0007114514001846.

Tan J, Liu S, Guo Y, Applegate TJ, Eicher SD (2014b) Dietary L-arginine supplementation attenuates lipopolysaccharide-induced inflammatory response in broiler chickens. *Br J Nutr* 111 (8):1394–1404. doi: 10.1017/S0007114513003863.

Tan JZ, Guo YM, Applegate TJ, Du EC, Zhao X (2015) Dietary L-arginine modulates immunosuppression in broilers inoculated with an intermediate strain of infectious bursa disease virus. *J Sci Food Agric* 95 (1):126–135. doi: 10.1002/jsfa.6692.

Taylor-Robinson AW, Liew FY, Severn A, Xu D, McSorley SJ, Garside P, Padron J, Phillips RS (1994) Regulation of the immune response by nitric oxide differentially produced by T helper type 1 and T helper type 2 cells. *Eur J Immunol* 24 (4):980–984. doi: 10.1002/eji.1830240430.

Trifari S, Kaplan CD, Tran EH, Crellin NK, Spits H (2009) Identification of a human helper T cell population that has abundant production of interleukin 22 and is distinct from T(H)-17, T(H)1 and T(H)2 cells. *Nat Immunol* 10 (8):864–871. doi: 10.1038/ni.1770.

Turvey SE, Broide DH (2010) Innate immunity. *J Allergy Clin Immunol* 125 (2 Suppl 2):S24–32. doi: 10.1016/j. jaci.2009.07.016.

Vahedi G, A CP, Hand TW, Laurence A, Kanno Y, O'Shea JJ, Hirahara K (2013) Helper T-cell identity and evolution of differential transcriptomes and epigenomes. *Immunol Rev* 252 (1):24–40. doi: 10.1111/ imr.12037.

Wei XQ, Charles IG, Smith A, Ure J, Feng GJ, Huang FP, Xu D, Muller W, Moncada S, Liew FY (1995) Altered immune responses in mice lacking inducible nitric oxide synthase. *Nature* 375 (6530):408–411. doi: 10.1038/375408a0.

Wilson NJ, Boniface K, Chan JR, McKenzie BS, Blumenschein WM, Mattson JD, Basham B, Smith K, Chen T, Morel F, Lecron JC, Kastelein RA, Cua DJ, McClanahan TK, Bowman EP, de Waal Malefyt R (2007) Development, cytokine profile and function of human interleukin 17-producing helper T cells. *Nat Immunol* 8 (9):950–957. doi: 10.1038/ni1497.

Wu G (1998) Intestinal mucosal amino acid catabolism. *J Nutr* 128:1249–1252.

Wu G (2009) Amino acids: Metabolism, functions, and nutrition. *Amino Acids* 37 (1):1–17. doi: 10.1007/ s00726-009-0269-0.

Wu G (2010) Functional amino acids in growth, reproduction, and health. *Adv Nutr* 1 (1):31–37. doi: 10.3945/ an.110.1008.

Wu G (2013) Arginine and immune function. In: *Diet, Immunity, and Inflammation*, edited by P.C. Calder and P. Yaqoob, Cambridge: Woodhead Publishing. pp. 523–543.

Wu G, Bazer FW, Dai Z, Li D, Wang J, Wu Z (2014) Amino Acid nutrition in animals: Protein synthesis and beyond. *Annu Rev Anim Biosci* 2:387–417. doi: 10.1146/annurev-animal-022513-114113.

Wu G, Bazer FW, Davis TA, Kim SW, Li P, Rhoads JM, Carey Satterfield M, Smith SB, Spencer TE, Yin Y (2009) Arginine metabolism and nutrition in growth, health and disease. *Amino Acids* 37 (1):153–168. doi: 10.1007/s00726-008-0210-y.

Wu G, Knabe DA, Kim SW (2004) Arginine nutrition in neonatal pigs. *J Nutr* 134 (10 Suppl):2783S–2790S; discussion 2796S-2797S.

Wu G, Morris SM Jr (1998) Arginine metabolism: Nitric oxide and beyond. *Biochem J* 336:1–17.

Wu L, Wang W, Yao K, Zhou T, Yin J, Li T, Yang L, He L, Yang X, Zhang H, Wang Q, Huang R, Yin Y (2013) Effects of dietary arginine and glutamine on alleviating the impairment induced by deoxynivalenol stress and immune relevant cytokines in growing pigs. *PLOS ONE* 8 (7):e69502. doi: 10.1371/journal. pone.0069502.

Yao K, Yin YL, Chu W, Liu Z, Deng D, Li T, Huang R, Zhang J, Tan B, Wang W, Wu G (2008) Dietary arginine supplementation increases mTOR signaling activity in skeletal muscle of neonatal pigs. *J Nutr* 138 (5):867–872.

Yeh CL, Hsu CS, Chiu WC, Hou YC, Yeh SL (2006) Dietary arginine enhances adhesion molecule and T helper 2 cytokine expression in mice with gut-derived sepsis. *Shock* 25 (2):155–160. doi: 10.1097/01. shk.0000189842.01601.f2.

Yeh CL, Hu YM, Liu JJ, Chen WJ, Yeh SL (2012) Effects of supplemental dietary arginine on the exogenous advanced glycosylation end product-induced interleukin-23/interleukin-17 immune response in rats. *Nutrition* 28 (10):1063–1067. doi: 10.1016/j.nut.2012.01.014.

Zhao H, Zhao H, Wang Y, Jing H, Ding Q, Xue J (2013a) Randomized clinical trial of arginine-supplemented enteral nutrition versus standard enteral nutrition in patients undergoing gastric cancer surgery. *J Cancer Res Clin Oncol* 139 (9):1465–1470. doi: 10.1007/s00432-013-1466-5.

Zhao P, Xiao X, Ghobrial RM, Li XC (2013b) IL-9 and Th9 cells: Progress and challenges. *Int Immunol* 25 (10):547–551. doi: 10.1093/intimm/dxt039.

Zhu HL, Liu YL, Xie XL, Huang JJ, Hou YQ (2013) Effect of L-arginine on intestinal mucosal immune barrier function in weaned pigs after Escherichia coli LPS challenge. *Innate Immun* 19 (3):242–252. doi: 10.1177/1753425912456223.

Zhu X, Pan Y, Li Y, Cui L, Cao Y (2012) Supplement of L-Arg improves protective immunity during early-stage Plasmodium yoelii 17XL infection. *Parasite Immunol* 34 (8–9):412–420. doi: 10.1111/j.1365-3024.2012.01374.x.

20 Nitric Oxide and the Immune System

Fernanda Salomao Costa, Anil Kulkarni, Alamelu Sundaresan, Davide Cattano, and Marie-Francoise Doursout

CONTENTS

20.1 Introduction: NO and NOS 349
20.2 Nitric Oxide and the Immune System..350
20.3 Role of Nitric Oxide in Autoimmune Diseases..352
20.4 Nitric Oxide and Vascular Diseases 352
    20.4.1   NO and Endothelial Dysfunction..352
    20.4.2   NO and Inflammation 353
20.5 Diet and Nitric Oxide...353
20.6 Nitric Oxide and Pharmaceuticals 354
References...354

20.1 INTRODUCTION: NO AND NOS

Although the importance of nitric oxide (NO) on the immune system is well known (Bogdan 2001, 2015), its mechanisms remain poorly described due to the involvement of different proteins and pathways and many interactions among these. NO is a free radical produced by the enzyme nitric oxide synthase (NOS) from the amino acid L-arginine. NO regulates some of the most important functions in the body, including blood pressure, neurotransmission, platelet aggregation, and the immune response (Murad et al. 2011). NO is a gas, is often short lived, and acts locally to its site of production. However, the vast range of functions of NO can be explained partly by its ability to form complexes by associating with thiol groups on peptides and proteins, for example glutathione and hemoglobin, and then disassociating from these complexes, allowing it to act at sites distal from its formation.

There are three ubiquitous NOS isoforms that have been characterized in mammalian tissues, encoded by different genes: neuronal NOS (nNOS), endothelial NOS (eNOS), and inducible NOS (iNOS), each one with different targets (Nathan 1992) (Figure 20.1). NOS proteins are heme proteins, and all three isoforms need calmodulin to be activated; NO formation is a Ca^{2+}-dependent reaction. NOS enzymes carry out the oxidation of the semi-essential amino acid L-arginine, catalyzing a 5-electron oxidation of the guanidine nitrogen of L-arginine to produce NO and citrulline (Figure 20.1). The NO metabolites nitrate and nitrite are stable and long lived, and may be NO storage pools. Nitrite and nitrate can be easily determined using the Griess reaction that measures the combined concentrations of both anions (termed NOx).

Neuronal NOS (nNOS) was the first NOS isoform to be described. It is expressed in central and peripheral neurons and also in some other cell types, such as in skeletal muscle cells. Its functions include synaptic plasticity in the central nervous system (CNS), central regulation of blood pressure, smooth muscle relaxation, and vasodilatation via peripheral nitrergic nerves (Förstermann et al. 2012). It has been shown that nNOS also plays an important role in glomerular (Blantz et al. 2002) and gastric function (Takahashi 2003).

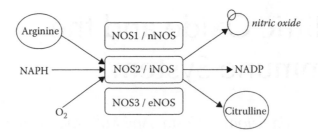

FIGURE 20.1 The nitric oxide synthase (NOS) enzymes.

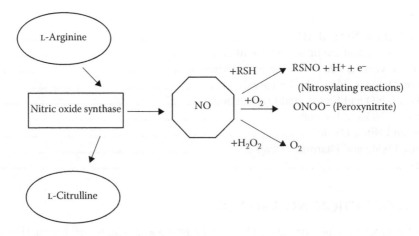

FIGURE 20.2 Scheme of peroxynitrite production from NO during inflammation.

Inducible NOS (iNOS) is induced in response to inflammatory cytokines and bacterial lipopoly-saccharide (LPS) in macrophages, neutrophils, hepatocytes, and other cells (MacMicking et al. 1997). Macrophages stimulated with LPS produce NO and CO by concomitant transcriptional activation of iNOS and heme oxygenase-1 (HO-1), and inhibition of iNOS activity by N-monomethyl-L-arginine significantly suppressed LPS induction of HO-1 without affecting the iNOS protein level. Large amounts of NO produced through iNOS play a significant role in killing invading microbes. NO can activate the apoptotic signal cascade in some situations, whereas it protects cells against spontaneous and induced apoptosis. Overproduction of NO is involved in pathogenesis of various inflammatory diseases (Nathan 1992). There is evidence of an association between increases in iNOS activity and peroxynitrite levels (Figure 20.2), the latter being considered as a biomarker of inflammatory disease (Ascenzi et al. 2010).

Endothelial NOS (eNOS) is responsible for the production of most of systemic NO (Knowles and Moncada 1994). In disease states such as atherosclerosis, hypoxic conditions combined with an oxidative environment can limit eNOS-derived NO production (Knowles and Moncada 1994; Stuehr 1999). Overall, altered NO production is an early event in the progression to poor vascular health outcomes, as in the cardiovascular system; thus its detection and measurement remains a valid indicator to preview patient health.

20.2 NITRIC OXIDE AND THE IMMUNE SYSTEM

The innate immune system is an ancient first line of defense against foreign organisms (Hoffmann et al. 1999). In contrast to the genetic rearrangements and clonal selection processes that underlie adaptive immunity, innate immunity relies on the functions of germ-line encoded gene products.

TABLE 20.1

Sources of NO and Related Effector Functions

Cellular Source of NO	Category of Response	Effector Function
Macrophages, microglia, neutrophils, eosinophils, fibroblasts, endothelial cells, epithelial cells	Antimicrobial activity	Killing or reduced replication of infectious agents (viruses, bacteria, protozoa, fungi, and helminths)
Macrophages, eosinophils	Antitumor activity	Killing or growth inhibition of tumor cells
Macrophages, microglia,astroglia, keratinocytes, mesangial cells	Tissue damage (immunopathology)	Necrosis or fibrosis of the parenchyma
Macrophages ("suppressor phenotype")	Anti-inflammatory— immunosuppressive effect	Immunoregulatory functions: inhibition of T- and B-cell profileration, leukocyte recruitment (adhesion, extravasation, chemotaxis), antibody production by CD5$^+$ B-cells, autoreactive T- and B-cell diversification
Macrophages,T-cells,endothelial cells, fibroblasts	Modulation of the immune response	Up- and downregulation (e.g., of: IL-1, IL-6, IL-8, IL-10, IL-12, IL-18, IFN-γ, TNF, TGF-β, G-CSF, VEG, MIP-1α, MIP-2, MCP-1)
Macrophages	Modulation of the immune response	Induction and differentiation of Th1 cells; supresion of Th1 (and Th2) cell responses; supresion of tolerogenic T-cell responses

NO is a highly reactive molecule with innate immune functions, as well as roles in responses to hypoxia and CNS development (Dawson et al. 1991; Bredt and Snyder 1994; Gibbs and Truman 1998; Bogdan 2001, 2015). NO plays an important role in different immune cells, including T lymphocytes, dendritic cells, natural killer cells, and mast cells, cell types belonging to both innate and adaptive immunity (Table 20.1). iNOS activity is responsible for most NO-mediated immune effects, which apart from releasing NO, provokes the depletion of local arginine (together with arginase) in macrophages or other host cells promoting growth inhibition and death of the parasites. Because NO can diffuse across cell membranes, it has an antimicrobial activity and can act in cells that do not express iNOS. For example, there is evidence that the diffusion of NO from phagocytes at the site of infection promotes equally effective parasite killing in both NO-producing cells and bystander cells.

Macrophages are divided into two major phenotypic categories (M1 and M2) depending on their activation status and inflammatory tone. Once differentiated, M1 macrophages trigger a Th1-mediated immune response; M1 macrophages secrete large amounts of NO to kill intracellular pathogens and to exert cytotoxicity toward tumor cells, killing tumor clones. Later in the response, tumor-reprogrammed macrophages produce low levels of NO/reactive nitrogen species (RNS), which permits cancer growth and spreading (Srisook et al. 2005). M2 macrophages express high levels of arginase-I, which competes with iNOS for their common substrate L-arginine, thus preventing NO generation. In cancer, it is known that high concentrations of NO impair T-cell functions by blocking the signaling cascade downstream of IL-2 binding (Predonzani et al. 2015). In contrast, lower concentrations of NO have been shown to promote Th1 differentiation by selectively upregulating IL-12 receptor beta 2. Dendritic cells (DCs) act as sources of NO during a variety of infections. Natural killer (NK) cells are important cells of the innate immune system, contributing to host defense towards bacteria, viruses, and parasites. Moreover, NKs actively participate in tumor surveillance and rejection of transplanted organs. However, the role of NO in NK cell activation and action is not completely understood. It was proposed that endogenous NO generation by eNOS prevents NK cells from activation-induced apoptosis, providing self-protection (Cifone et al. 2001). Mast cells are highly specialized secretory cells distributed widely throughout the tissues, particularly in proximity to blood vessels, nerves, and epithelial surfaces (Metcalfe et al. 1997; Williams and Galli 2000). The action of NO on mast cells is time-dependent, requiring several hours, and is non-cGMP mediated, most probably involving chemical modification of proteins. A combination of *in vitro* and *in vivo* studies reveal inhibitory actions of NO on mast cell degranulation and mediator release, and mast cell–dependent inflammatory events including vasodilatation, and leukocyte-endothelial cell adhesion. In inflammatory diseases, such as asthma, human and animal studies reveal possible proinflammatory and protective roles for NO, but overall the weight of evidence indicates a beneficial immunologic role for NO (Table 20.1). Future research directions in inflammation and asthma are likely to cover the regulatory and signaling effects of NO on mast cells, T-cells and other key cells, and the effects of NO donors and NOS inhibitors on disease severity and progression.

20.3   ROLE OF NITRIC OXIDE IN AUTOIMMUNE DISEASES

An autoimmune disease is characterized by a chronic inflammatory state and a dysregulation of immune tolerance, a complex process involving both genetic and environmental factors. In an effort to promote an effective immune response in the control of infectious diseases, NO (mainly iNOS mediated) may be involved in the breakdown of immunity, triggering chronic inflammatory disorders or contributing to autoimmune diseases (Singh et al. 2000). NO has recently been shown to act as a potent cytotoxic effector molecule as well as to play an important role in the pathogenesis of organ-specific autoimmunity. NO may also modulate autoimmunity by altering the Th1/Th2 balance (Hooper et al. 1995).

20.4   NITRIC OXIDE AND VASCULAR DISEASES

20.4.1   NO AND ENDOTHELIAL DYSFUNCTION

The endothelial cells of the vascular system are responsible for many biological activities that maintain vascular homeostasis. Responding to a variety of chemical and physical stimuli, the endothelium elaborates a host of vasoactive agents. One of these agents, originally termed endothelium-derived relaxing factor, is now accepted to be NO, and it influences both cellular constituents of the blood and vascular smooth muscle (Furchgott et al. 1999; Ignarro et al. 2002). A principal intracellular target for NO is guanylate cyclase, which, when activated, increases the intracellular concentration of cyclic guanosine monophosphate (cGMP), which in turn activates protein kinase G. Acting by this pathway, NO induces relaxation of vascular smooth muscle and inhibits platelet activation and aggregation. Derangements in endothelial production of NO are implicated as both a cause and a consequence of vascular diseases, including hypertension, atherosclerosis, and coronary artery disease (Moncada and Higgs 2006). According to the World Health Organization (WHO), cardiovascular disease is the number one killer of both men and women in the U.S., representing a staggering 40% of all deaths. One million people die each year and more than 6 million are hospitalized in the U.S. as a result of cardiovascular disease. Ischemic heart diseases alone cause nearly 20% of all deaths. Development of heart disease involves a dysfunctional endothelium; this occurs early and is easily found in patients with diabetes, hypertension, and obesity, and in smokers (Lundberg et al. 2009). An enhanced inactivation and/or reduced synthesis of NO is seen, in conjunction with risk factors for cardiovascular disease. This condition (i.e., endothelial dysfunction) can promote vasospasm, thrombosis, vascular inflammation, and proliferation of vascular smooth muscle cells. Vascular oxidative stress with an increased production of reactive oxygen species (ROS) contributes to mechanisms of vascular dysfunction. Oxidative stress is mainly caused by an imbalance between the activity of endogenous pro-oxidative enzymes (such as NADPH oxidase, xanthine oxidase, and the mitochondrial respiratory chain) and anti-oxidative enzymes (such as superoxide dismutase, glutathione peroxidase, heme oxygenase, thioredoxin peroxidase/peroxiredoxin, catalase, and paraoxonase) in favor of the former. Also, small molecular weight antioxidants may play a role in the defense against oxidative stress. Increased ROS concentrations reduce the amount of bioactive NO by chemical inactivation to form toxic peroxynitrite (Förstermann 2010) (Figure 20.2). Peroxynitrite, in turn, can "uncouple" eNOS to become a dysfunctional superoxide-generating enzyme that contributes to vascular oxidative stress. Oxidative stress and endothelial dysfunction can promote atherogenesis. Drugs in clinical use such as ACE inhibitors, AT(1) receptor blockers, and statins have pleiotropic actions that can improve endothelial function. Also, there may be a role for dietary polyphenolic antioxidants, which can reduce oxidative stress, and for the antioxidant vitamins C and E, although clinical trials have failed to show an improved cardiovascular outcome with the latter.

20.4.2 NO and Inflammation

NO is produced as part of the inflammatory response, and so elevated NO metabolites are seen in inflammatory conditions such as in the inflammatory bowel diseases (IBDs) in which iNOS activity is related to disease activity. In tissues suffering chronic inflammation, such as inflamed bowel tissue in patients with ulcerative colitis, iNOS can generate high concentrations of NO that promote carcinogenesis by inhibiting apoptosis, enhancing prostaglandin formation, and promoting angiogenesis (Saijo et al. 2009). As NO can act distal from the site where it is produced, it is also possible to see the consequences of inflammation in extra-bowel tissues, because of IBD. These effects may involve NO or its metabolic peroxynitrite. For example, studies showed increases in platelet aggregation and tromboembolic events, as a consequence of IBD. Thus, it is not clear if NO is protective or harmful, since it has different actions depending upon its cellular origin, site of production, concentration, and target.

20.5 DIET AND NITRIC OXIDE

Because NO is synthesized from the amino acid L-arginine, dietary recommendations for boosting NO might include protein-rich meat and poultry. However, much dietary arginine is metabolized in the enterocytes limiting its availability as a NOS. Also dietary arginine would need to be targeted to sites where specific NOS isoforms activities were desired. Another dietary source of NO could be nitrites and nitrates (Bryan and Ivy 2015; Milkowski et al. 2010). Many plant foods, particularly beets and leafy greens like kale, Swiss chard, arugula, and spinach, are rich in nitrates and nitrites. Coupled with its abundance of protective potassium, it is not surprising that a plant-based diet is associated with lower blood pressure and reduced risk of stroke, heart attack, diabetes, and a variety of other health concerns (Zand et al. 2009). Plant rich diets like the Mediterranean diet and the Japanese diet contain significant amounts of nitrate.

The amount of nitrate in plants is a consequence of multiple factors, such as genotype, soil conditions, growth conditions, and storage and transport conditions. Nitrate is converted in nitrite by the action of nitrate reductase enzymes in anaerobic bacteria in the oral microbiota. In the absence of oxygen these bacteria use nitrate as an alternative electron acceptor to gain adenosine triphosphate. The nitrite produced is concentrated in the salivary gland, making saliva 1,000 times richer in nitrite than blood. In the stomach, nitrite-rich saliva meets the acidic gastric juice, nitrite is protonated to form nitrous acid (HNO_2), which then decomposes to NO and other nitrogen metabolites that are absorbed and transported throughout the body. Because of the benefits of NO in many physiologic functions, it has been discussed how to increase NO bioavailability through supplementation with NO-rich or NO-active food (Hord et al. 2009). It is known that the oral administration of nitrate and nitrite is efficient at promoting NO production (Lundberg et al. 2009). Some dietary supplements have been formulated based on these ideas.

Long-term consumption of diets containing high levels of nitrate and nitrite may have important implications for providing health benefits by ensuring high concentrations of nitrogen oxides as a "reserve" for tissue defense and homeostasis in stress and disease. Another important and very old application of nitrate in diet is as a preservative. Nitrite is able to inhibit outgrowth of *Clostridium botulinum* spores in nonrefrigerated meat products. Also, nitrate has the capacity to inhibit growth of *Listeria monocytogenes*, *E. coli*, *Staphylococcus aureus*, and *Bacillus cereus* in processed meats. Nitrate can protect the body from foodborne pathogens such as *Escherichia coli* 0157:H7 and salmonella by enhancing gastric fluid, when nitrate is converted to nitrous acid and other nitrogen oxides. The WHO acceptable daily intake for nitrate (0–3.7 mg/kg body weight) translates into an equivalent of 222 mg nitrate for a 60 kg adult. The conclusions of the European Food Safety Authority is that the benefits of vegetable and fruit consumption outweigh any perceived risk of developing cancer from the consumption of nitrate and nitrite in these foods.

NO has become of interest in sports nutrition and is being used in sport supplements and drinks. This is because NO seems to enhance performance by improving muscular efficiency at various levels. This is a natural response to exercise in the body, that is lost when endothelial cells lose the ability to produce NO, leading to endothelial dysfunction. On the other hand, physical activities are good in preventing age-related NO decrease, proved by studying old athletes.

20.6 NITRIC OXIDE AND PHARMACEUTICALS

There are three classes of pharmaceutical agents related to NO. Organic nitrates such as nitroglycerin are used for the treatment of acute angina, while inhaled NO therapy is used in neonates for treatment of pulmonary hypertension because of underdeveloped lungs. Finally phosphodiesterase inhibitors such as sildenafil are used to treat erectile dysfunctional. Some of these increase NO while some act on downstream second messengers of NO. There is currently much research in how to apply NO in other disease situations like pulmonary hypertension and ventilator-induced lung injury (Lundberg et al. 2009). Very low doses of dietary nitrite attenuated proteinuria, preventing renal histological damage induced by chronic administration of a NOS inhibitor (Kanematsu et al. 2008). There is research on NO in organ transplantation and ischemia. Future discoveries in NO biology and therapeutics will bring new treatments and an important reduction in healthcare costs.

REFERENCES

Ascenzi P, di Masi A, Sciorati C, Clementi E. 2010. Peroxynitrite: An ugly biofactor? *Biofactors* 36:264–73.
Blantz RC, Deng A, Lortie M, Munger K, Vallon V, Gabbai FB, Thomson SC. 2002. The complex role of nitric oxide in the regulation of glomerular utrafiltration. *Kidney Int.* 61:782–5.
Bogdan C. 2001. Nitric oxide and the immune response. *Nat. Immunol.* 2:907–16.
Bogdan C. 2015. Nitric oxide synthase in innate and adaptive immunity: An update. *Trends Immunol.* 36:161–78.
Bredt DS, Snyder SH. 1994. Nitric oxide: A physiologic messenger molecule. *Annu. Rev. Biochem.* 63:175–95.
Bryan NS, Ivy JL. 2015. Inorganic nitrite and nitrate: Evidence to support consideration as dietary nutrients. *Nutr. Res.* 35:643–54.
Chung H, Choi B, Kwon Y, Kim Y. 2008. Interactive Relations between Nitric Oxide (NO) and Carbon Monoxide (CO): Heme Oxygenase-1/CO Pathway Is a Key Modulator in NO-Mediated Antiapoptosis and Anti-inflammation. *Meth. Enzymol.* 441:329–38.
Cifone MG1, Ulisse S, Santoni A. 2001. Natural killer cells and nitric oxide. *Int. Immunopharmacol.* 1:1513–24.
Dawson TM, Bredt DS, Fotuhi M, Hwang PM, Snyder SH. 1991. Nitric oxide synthase and neuronal NADPH diaphorase are identical in brain and peripheral tissues. *Proc. Natl. Acad. Sci. USA* 88:7797–801.
Förstermann U. 2010. Nitric oxide and oxidative stress in vascular disease. *Pflugers Arch.* 459:923–39.
Förstermann U, Sessa WC. 2012. Nitric oxide synthases: Regulation and function. *Eur. Heart J.* 33:829–37.

Furchgott RF. 1999. Endothelium-derived relaxing factor: Discovery, early studies, and identification as nitric oxide. *Biosci. Rep.* 19:235–51.

Gibbs SM, Truman JW. 1998. Nitric oxide and cyclic GMP regulate retinal patterning in the optic lobe of Drosophila. *Neuron* 20:83–93.

Hoffmann JA, Kafatos FC, Janeway CA, Ezekowitz RA. 1999. Phylogenetic perspectives in innate immunity. *Science* 284:1313–8.

Hooper DC, Ohnishi ST, Kean R, Numagami Y, Dietzschold B, Koprowski H. 1995. Local nitric oxide production in viral and autoimmune diseases of the central nervous system. *Proc. Natl. Acad. Sci. USA* 92:5312–6.

Hord GN, Tang Y, Bryan NS. 2009. Food sources of nitrates and nitrites: The physiologic context for potential health benefits. *Am. J. Clin. Nutr.* 90:1–10

Ignarro LJ. 2002. Nitric oxide as a unique signaling molecule in the vascular system: A historical overview. *J. Physiol. Pharmacol.* 53:503–14

Kanematsu Y, Yamaguchi K, Ohnishi H, Motobayashi Y, Ishizawa K, Izawa Y, Kawazoe K, Kondo S, Kagami S, Tomita S, Tsuchiya K, Tamaki T. 2008. Dietary doses of nitrite restore circulating nitric oxide level and improve renal injury in L-NAME-induced hypertensive rats. *Am. J. Physiol. Renal. Physiol.* 295:F1457–62.

Knowles RG, Moncada S. 1994. Nitric oxide synthases in mammals. *Biochem. J.* 298: 249–58.

Lundberg JO, Gladwin MT, Ahluwalia A, Benjamin N, Bryan NS, Butler A, Cabrales P, Fago A, Feelisch M, Ford PC, Freeman BA, Frenneau M, Friedman J, Kelm M, Kevil CG, Kim-Shapiro DB, Kozlov AV, Lancaster Jr JR, Lefer DJ, McColl K, McCurry K, Patel R, Petersson J, Rassaf T, Reutov VP, Richter-Addo GB, Schechter A, Shiva S, Tsuchiya K, van Faassen EE, Webb AJ, Zuckerbraun BS, Zweier JL, Weitzberg E. 2009. Nitrate and nitrite in biology, nutrition and therapeutics. *Nat. Chem. Biol.* 5: 865–9.

MacMicking J, Xie QW, Nathan C. 1997. Nitric oxide and macrophage function. *Annu. Rev. Immunol.* 15:323–50.

Metcalfe DD, Baram D, Mekori YA. 1997. Mast cells. *Physiol. Rev.* 77:1033–79.

Milkowski A, Garg HK, Coughlin JR, Bryan NS. 2010. Nutritional epidemiology in the context of nitric oxide biology: A risk–benefit evaluation for dietary nitrite and nitrate. *Nitric Oxide* 22:110–9.

Moncada S, Higgs EA. 2006. The discovery of nitric oxide and its role in vascular biology. *Brit. J. Pharmacol.* 147 (Suppl 1):S193–201.

Murad F. 2011. Nitric oxide: The coming of the second messenger. *Rambam Maimonides Med. J.* 2:e0038.

Nathan C. 1992. Nitric oxide as a secretory product of mammalian cells. *FASEB J.* 6: 3051–64.

Predonzani A, Calì B, Agnellini AHR, Molon B. 2015. Spotlights on immunological effects of reactive nitrogen species: When inflammation says nitric oxide. *World J. Exp. Med.* 5:64–76.

Saijo F, Milsom AB, Bryan SN, Bauer SM, Vowinkel T, Ivanovic M, Andry C, Granger DN, Rodriguez J, Feelisch M. 2009. On the dynamics of nitrite, nitrate and other biomarkers of nitric oxide production in inflammatory bowel disease. *Nitric Oxide* 22:155–67.

Singh VK, Mehrotra S, Narayan P, Pandey CM, Agarwal SS. 2000. Modulation of autoimmune diseases by nitric oxide. *Immunol. Res.* 22:1–19.

Srisook K, Kim C, Cha YN. 2005. Cytotoxic and cytoprotective actions of O_2-and NO (ONOO-) are determined both by cellular GSH level and HO activity in macrophages. *Methods Enzymol.* 396:414–24.

Stuehr DJ. 1999. Mammalian nitric oxide synthases. *Biochim. Biophys. Acta* 1411: 217–30.

Takahashi T. 2003. Pathophysiological significance of neuronal nitric oxide synthase in the gastrointestinal tract. *J. Gastroenterol.* 38:421–30.

Williams CM, Galli SJ. 2000. The diverse potential effector and immunoregulatory roles of mast cells in allergic disease. *J. Allergy Clin. Immunol.* 105:847–59.

Zand J, Lanza F, Garg HK, Bryan NS. 2009. All-natural nitrite and nitrate containing dietary supplement promotes nitric oxide production and reduces triglycerides in humans. *Nutr. Res.* 31:262–2.

21 Glutamine and the Immune System

Vinicius Fernandes Cruzat and Philip Newsholme

CONTENTS

21.1 Introduction...357
21.2 Glutamine Metabolism Is Important for Cell Function 358
21.3 Metabolic Fates of Glutamine in Immune Cells..360
    21.3.1 Glutamine and Neutrophil Metabolic Requirements...360
    21.3.2 Glutamine and Macrophage Metabolic Requirements 361
    21.3.3 Glutamine and Lymphocyte Metabolic Requirements 362
21.4 Glutamine in the Context of Exercise 363
21.5 Provision of Glutamine for Recovery: From the Bench to Bedside 366
    21.5.1 The Parenteral Supply of Glutamine 366
    21.5.2 New Perspectives in Enteral Glutamine..368
21.6 Conclusion 369
References..369

21.1 INTRODUCTION

Glutamine is recognized as a crucial and versatile amino acid for cell survival and growth, playing an important role in metabolism. Moreover, compared to all other amino acids in the body, glutamine is present at the highest extracellular concentration, and is considered the most abundant free amino acid. In fact, in addition to glucose, glutamine represents a primary nutrient for maintenance of the body's homeostasis (Newsholme et al. 2003a).

Because it can be synthesized and released from many tissues, glutamine is classified as nutritionally nonessential. However, in some catabolic conditions such as sepsis, recovery from burns or surgery, as well as in high-intensity exercise, glutamine availability can be compromised due to the increased requirements, especially from the rapidly dividing cells of the immune system and other leukocytes (Newsholme 2001; Cruzat et al. 2014c). For this reason, glutamine is considered as a "fuel for the immune system," and a low concentration may impact on defense mechanisms, resulting in poor clinical outcomes and increased risk of mortality (Rodas et al. 2012). Thus, glutamine supplementation has been widely studied in order to gain insight into optimal routes for glutamine provision, amounts, and metabolism.

Eric Newsholme's laboratory at the University of Oxford was the first to demonstrate glutamine utilization by lymphocytes and macrophages; this work was published in a series of papers in the 1980s (Ardawi and Newsholme 1982, 1983; Newsholme et al. 1986; Newsholme, Gordon, and Newsholme 1987). The mechanisms underlying the diverse actions of glutamine are only now becoming clear and are discussed in the present chapter.

21.2   GLUTAMINE METABOLISM IS IMPORTANT FOR CELL FUNCTION

Glutamine ($C_5H_{10}N_2O_3$) is present at ten- to hundredfold in excess of any other free amino acid in the blood. *In vitro* studies demonstrated that glutamine could not be replaced by glutamic acid or glucose or other amino acids, when cell function and viability were tested. Glutamine can be utilized for a wide variety of functions via many metabolic pathways. Glutamine oxidation can lead to the production of ATP, nicotinamide adenine dinucleotide phosphate (NADPH), and CO_2, while the amide nitrogen atom can be utilized for biosynthetic purposes, including synthesis of purines, pyrimidines, and amino sugars (Newsholme et al. 2003b). Moreover, glutamine plays crucial roles in cellular defense mediated by glutathione (GSH), heat shock proteins (HSPs), and the hexosamine biosynthetic pathway (HBP), required for maintaining cellular integrity and function.

At physiological pH, the carboxyl group of glutamine carries a negative charge, whereas the amino group is protonated, resulting in a molecule with a net charge of 0, thus classifying glutamine as a neutral amino acid. The side-chain amide group is easily removed by various enzymatic reactions and even by spontaneous hydrolysis at room temperature. These particular biochemical characteristics confer to L-glutamine the ability to be highly hydrophilic and a preferred substrate for cells requiring a source of L-glutamate and/or ammonium ion (NH_4^+) for physiologic purposes (Young and Ajami 2001).

Hlaziwetz and Habermann in 1873 first described glutamine as a molecule with important biological properties and a structural component of proteins. Subsequently, it was shown that free glutamine is abundant in certain plants, but relatively little was known about the metabolism of glutamine until the 1930s. The number of studies reporting the importance of glutamine metabolism increased significantly following the early work of Sir Hans Adolf Krebs (1900–1981) (Krebs 1935), who was responsible for many important discoveries in metabolic biochemistry and physiology in the twentieth century (he jointly received the Nobel Prize in Physiology or Medicine in 1953) (Meister 1956).

In culture, cells utilize glutamine in a greater amount than any other amino acid (Eagle et al. 1956; Curi et al. 2005a). Eagle and colleagues observed structural degeneration followed by cell death in isolated mouse fibroblasts cultivated in the absence of glutamine (Eagle 1959). Further work at that stage was hampered partly because glutamine was classified as a nonessential amino acid, but also because it was difficult to measure the levels in plasma and tissues.

Throughout the 1960s, 1970s, and 1980s, the University of Oxford was the location for several of the key researchers that have shaped our current understanding of the regulation of energy, glucose, fatty acid, ketone body, and amino acid metabolism in health and disease (such as diabetes, inflammatory diseases, and cancer). Hans Krebs, Philip Randle, Derek Williamson, and Eric Newsholme all worked on metabolic regulation utilizing different research models, from isolated cells *in vitro*, to human and *in vivo* experiments. Studies with various cell types, such as HeLa cells (Eagle 1959), lymphocytes (Ardawi and Newsholme 1982), macrophages (Newsholme et al. 1986), and enterocytes (Yamauchi et al. 2002) demonstrated the importance of glutamine for cell division, function, and maintenance of intermediary metabolism. These studies raised the profile for glutamine in publications, which averaged two or three per year in the late 1960s and early 1970s but reached well in excess of 1,000 publications in 2014.

There are many enzymes that are involved in glutamine metabolism. Glutamine is synthesized in specialized tissues and organs including skeletal muscle and brain, from glutamate, depending on ATP availability. Glutamine synthetase (GS) promotes glutamine synthesis from glutamate. Glutamate in turn is synthesized from 2-oxoglutarate and NH_4^+. Hence, the synthesis of glutamine provides an efficient mechanism for nitrogen export and transport, as well as ammonia (NH_3) removal. Glutamine hydrolysis occurs through the action of the glutaminase (GLS) enzyme, releasing NH_4^+ and glutamate (Newsholme et al. 2003a) (Figure 21.1).

Glutamine and the related amino acid glutamate are 5-carbon amino acids (Figure 21.1). Glutamate is a molecule with two carboxyl groups, conferring a net negative charge. This

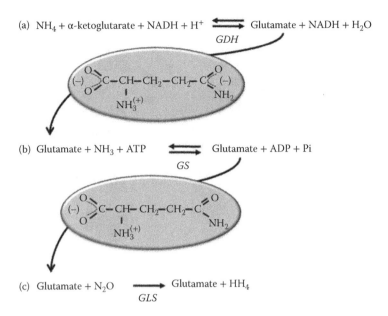

(a) $NH_4 + \alpha\text{-ketoglutarate} + NADH + H^+ \rightleftharpoons$ Glutamate $+ NADH + H_2O$

GDH

(b) Glutamate $+ NH_3 + ATP \rightleftharpoons$ Glutamate $+ ADP + Pi$

GS

(c) Glutamate $+ N_2O \longrightarrow$ Glutamate $+ HH_4$

GLS

FIGURE 21.1 Biochemistry of glutamine and glutamate. (a) Chemical structure of glutamate and its synthesis through glutamate dehydrogenase (GDH); (b) chemical structure of glutamine and its synthesis through glutamine synthetase (GS); (c) degradation of glutamine through glutaminase (GLS).

biochemical difference between glutamate and glutamine partially accounts for the transport of these two amino compounds across the cell membranes through different transport systems, at substantially different rates (glutamine at a much higher rate) altering cell function in markedly different ways (Newsholme et al. 2003b). The intracellular glutamate supply (very important for cellular metabolism, as described below) will occur through glutamine availability.

Cells of the immune system, the kidney, and the intestine are considered predominantly glutamine-consuming (van de Poll et al. 2004) (Figure 21.2). In response to starvation or a high protein diet or even high catabolic situations or diseases, such as sepsis and uncontrolled diabetes, glutaminase activity increases, since under these situations there is a heightened catabolism of amino acids, whether derived from muscle stores or from dietary sources (Cruzat et al. 2014c, Labow, Souba, and Abcouwer 2001).

Increased glutaminase activity and increased glutamine catabolism are partly to support increased gluconeogenesis in the kidney and liver, which depends on precursors derived from the carbon skeleton of glutamine, delivering additional nitrogen to the urea cycle for disposal. On the other hand, the skeletal muscles, the lungs, the liver, and the brain exhibit a higher capacity for glutamine synthesis by means of glutamine synthetase, and therefore may be considered predominantly glutamine-synthesizing tissues (Antonio and Street 1999; Frayn et al. 1991) (Figure 21.2). All tissues are important for glutamine metabolism and homeostasis; however, the liver and skeletal muscle play key roles in the maintenance of glutamine availability (Figure 21.2).

Glutamine concentration in the blood can be altered in catabolic situations, such as sepsis (Newsholme 2001; Cruzat et al. 2014c), infections (Rogero et al. 2008a), surgery (Rodas et al. 2012), trauma (Flaring et al. 2003), and intense and prolonged physical exercise (Cruzat and Tirapegui 2009; Newsholme et al. 2011). This effect may compromise cell function, especially within the immune system. Importantly in some catabolic situations, which includes diabetes (Menge et al. 2010; Tsai et al. 2012), metabolic syndrome, and especially exhaustive physical exercise (Petry et al. 2014), plasma glutamine may be reduced from around 500–700 to 300–400 µM with possible impact in immune cells (Hiscock and Pedersen 2002). Immune cells generally perform well over these ranges of plasma glutamine in terms of proliferation and function (Cruzat, Krause, and

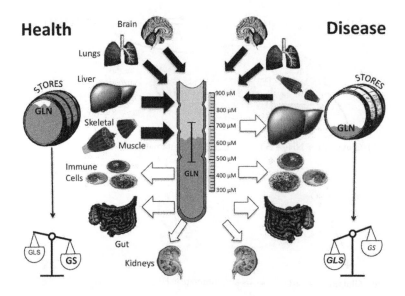

FIGURE 21.2 Glutamine metabolism in health and disease. Tissues such as brain, lungs, liver, skeletal muscle, and the gut exhibit enzymes that control both glutamine synthesis and degradation, named glutamine synthetase (GS) and glutaminase (GLS), respectively. Cells of the immune system and kidneys do not exhibit GS, only GLS. In a healthy or fed state, glutamine stores are in equilibrium in plasma and tissues, maintained constantly mainly by the liver and skeletal muscles, two major stores of glutamine in the body. Under disease states or catabolic situations, glutaminemia is affected. However, even in catabolic situations, plasma glutamine can be maintained by glutamine stores, which fall since the liver consumes the amino acid to generate glucose among other functions, and immune cells, kidney, and the gut increase their consumption. Moreover, due to the catabolic process, muscle cells reduce their capacity to release glutamine.

Newsholme 2014). However, glutamine stores, especially in the liver and skeletal muscle, may fall in catabolic situations, altering immune competence (Cruzat et al. 2014c, Newsholme et al. 2011; Rogero et al. 2008a, Cruzat, Rogero, and Tirapegui 2010). This may have an impact in clinical outcome, recovery, and, in critically ill patients, increase the risk of mortality (Rodas et al. 2012).

21.3 METABOLIC FATES OF GLUTAMINE IN IMMUNE CELLS

Lymphocytes, macrophages, and neutrophils play crucial roles in the immune and inflammatory responses (see also Chapter 1). This system is of fundamental importance not only in preventing or limiting infection (immune activation), but also in the overall process of repair and recovery from injury (wound healing and resolution of inflammation). Although glucose is a vital metabolite, and a main fuel for a large number of cells in the body, in the early/mid 1980s it was established that immune cells such as lymphocytes and macrophages could utilize glutamine at high rates similar to or greater than glucose (Curi, Newsholme, and Newsholme 1986; Newsholme, Newsholme, and Curi 1987). Currently, it is clear that immune cells have a high dependence on glutamine availability.

21.3.1 GLUTAMINE AND NEUTROPHIL METABOLIC REQUIREMENTS

Acting as antibacterial effector cells, neutrophils are part of the first line of defense cells. When encountering pathogens, neutrophils engage in phagocytosis of bacteria either directly or in cooperation with antigen-specific defenses. Neutrophils are critical for defense against several different pathogens, from viruses to multicellular parasites that cause potentially lethal infections. The capacity to recognize and kill invaders largely depends on protein factors derived from activation of

inflammation and degranulation of specialized cells. However, neutrophils are additionally associated with extracellular structures, composed of decondensed chromatin and antimicrobial factors,
also called neutrophil extracellular traps (NETs). The action of NETs requires the synthesis of
reactive oxygen species (ROS), the enzyme myeloperoxidase (MPO), and neutrophil elastase (NE),
found in azurophil granules (Branzk et al. 2014). Once activated, NE is released into the cytosol
and translocates to the nucleus, where it cleaves histones so releasing chromatin from its condensed
form. Although these steps may occur independent of enzymatic activity, their combination is essential to constitute an important trigger for timely cell rupture and NET release (Papayannopoulos
et al. 2010). The process of ROS production and release is dependent on activation of the NADPH
oxidase 2 enzyme (NOX2), increasing the synthesis of superoxide (O_2^-) from molecular oxygen
(Rodrigues-Krause et al. 2013). NADPH oxidase generated O_2^- is rapidly removed by superoxide
dismutase (SOD) activity resulting in the synthesis of hydrogen peroxide (H_2O_2). ROS are also
produced by the release of MPO to generate hypochlorous acid (HOCl) in the presence of chloride.
HOCl acts as a potent oxidant and sterilizing factor (Tidball 2005). However, secondary damage to
cells may occur as described for exercise and loading/unloading muscle tissues (Dong et al. 2011).

The primary metabolic substrates for neutrophil survival and activation are glucose and glutamine. However, when compared to other cell types, such as macrophages and lymphocytes, neutrophils consume glutamine at the highest rates (Pithon-Curi, De Melo, and Curi 2004; Pithon-Curi,
Trezena et al. 2002). Much of the glutamine is converted to glutamate, aspartate (via Krebs cycle
activity), and lactate, and under appropriate conditions, CO_2. Glutamine and glutamate are critical
for generation of essential compounds in leukocytes, including glutathione. However, via malate
generation and action of malic enzymes neutrophils may generate substantial quantities of NADPH
required for superoxide production, increasing antimicrobial activity. Indeed, 2 mmol/L extracellular glutamine (two- to threefold physiological levels) was able to attenuate the adrenaline-induced
inhibition of superoxide production (Garcia et al. 1999). On the other hand, the hormonal responses
mediated by adrenaline in "stressed" postoperative patients (whose glutamine concentration may be
reduced) are associated with inhibitory effects on neutrophil O_2^- generating capacity, lowering the
oxidative burst against pathogens. However, once incubated in 2 mmol/L extracellular glutamine
in vitro, the O_2^- generating capacity of the neutrophils was restored. Glutamine can additionally
regulate components of the NADPH-oxidase complex increasing the expression of gp91[phox], p22[phox],
and p47[phox] in neutrophils (Pithon-Curi, Levada et al. 2002) and other cell types (Newsholme et al.
2012).

21.3.2 GLUTAMINE AND MACROPHAGE METABOLIC REQUIREMENTS

The macrophage is one of the principal cells of the mononuclear phagocyte system and is found in
lymphoid tissue, peritoneal, pleural, and pericardial cavities, and within tissues. In addition to their
phagocytic activity, macrophages are capable of secreting a large number of compounds including
nitric oxide (NO), H_2O_2, and proinflammatory cytokines (for a review see Tidball [2005] and Wink
et al. [2011]).

Nitric oxide is a known secretory effector of macrophage antibacterial and antitumor activity (see also Chapter 20). Recent evidence has also implicated NO in the pathogenesis of many
immune-mediated diseases including glomerulonephritis, arthritis, and many allergic skin and lung
reactions. Nitric oxide production occurs via a 5-electron oxidation of L-arginine producing NO and
citrulline. The synthesis of NO has been reported in many cell types including macrophages, neutrophils, endothelial cells, and hepatocytes. A number of nitric oxide synthase (NOS) isoforms are
known to exist in various cells: endothelial constitutive (135 kDa), neuronal constitutive (150–160
kDa), and inducible (130 kDa).

Macrophage NO synthesis occurs via the NADPH-dependent inducible NOS (iNOS) enzyme
located in the cell cytosol. iNOS is expressed in a number of cell types including macrophages,
neutrophils, lung fibroblasts, and epithelial cells. It is widely accepted that iNOS activity depends

upon the presence of L-arginine and the source of this L-arginine is primarily exogenous. However, the importance of extracellular L-arginine *in vivo* is more difficult to quantify. The concentration of L-arginine in blood is approximately 0.08–0.10 mM (compared with 0.4 mM in most types of tissue culture media). Activated macrophages can secrete arginase, thus depleting local exogenous L-arginine concentration *in vivo* and *in vitro*. Alternative sources of L-arginine could be intracellular protein degradation or endogenous synthesis. The major sites of L-arginine synthesis in terrestrial vertebrates are liver (as part of the urea cycle) and kidney where arginine is synthesized from citrulline and released into the circulation. The synthesis of L-arginine from citrulline has been demonstrated for macrophages. The synthesis of citrulline from glutamine in turn has been demonstrated in enterocytes and liver, and more recently in macrophages (Murphy and Newsholme 1998). Thus, glutamine can generate arginine when required in macrophages. Macrophages also can metabolize arginine via arginase to generate urea and ornithine. Indeed, the macrophage phenotypes M1 and M2, where M1 is proinflammatory and M2 much less inflammatory, are associated with high levels of NO synthesis (M1) or much lower levels of NO generation (M2). Glutamine can also be used for macrophage glutathione synthesis and for NADPH production, as described for the neutrophil.

With respect to cytokine production, Yassad et al. (1997) and Murphy and Newsholme (1999) demonstrated that enhancement of interleukin (IL)-6 and tumor necrosis factor-alpha (TNF-α) secretion, respectively, by LPS stimulated macrophages, was dependent on extracellular glutamine availability. TNF-α, IL-1β, and IL-6 are quantitatively the most important cytokines produced by LPS-stimulated macrophages (Cruzat et al. 2014b). Murphy and Newsholme (1999) also demonstrated that in addition to murine macrophage TNF-α production, the production of the quantitatively important human monocyte-derived cytokine, IL-8, was also dependent upon the availability of extracellular glutamine.

21.3.3 GLUTAMINE AND LYMPHOCYTE METABOLIC REQUIREMENTS

Lymphocytes can recognize antigenic structures via their cell-surface receptors (antibody-based B-cell receptors and T-cell receptors), undergoing clonal amplification and cellular differentiation, and production of antibodies as appropriate (Cooper and Alder 2006). T lymphocytes mature in the thymus. On the other hand, B lymphocytes mature in the bone marrow and are able to produce antibodies. However, functions of both types of lymphocytes require energy and place a considerable metabolic burden on the organism, especially in conditions of infection, inflammation, and stress (Newsholme 2001). This results in increased utilization of glutamine, glucose, and some fatty acids.

Up until the early 1980s, it was believed that lymphocytes obtained most of their energy by metabolism and oxidation of glucose (Newsholme et al. 1999). Under stress and inflammation situations, activated lymphocytes (T and B) switch their metabolic requirements to enhance their function. Thus, large amounts of the glucose consumed are converted to lactate via lactate dehydrogenase (LDH), regenerating NAD+, important for the glycolytic enzyme glyceraldehdye-3-phosphate dehydrogenase (GAPDH) (Newsholme et al. 2003a). Lactate production through LDH activity generates 2 ATP per mol of glucose consumed; therefore, activated cells increase their demand for the substrate. The metabolic switch is associated with the fact that mitochondrial respiration supplies the substrates for the biosynthesis of nucleotides, amino acids, proteins, and lipids, but the main source of ATP for the cell is through the glycolytic pathway under these conditions (Newsholme et al. 1986). In fact, T-cells enhance their rate of glycolysis under stress situations and increase demand for glutamine (Ardawi and Newsholme 1983).

Importantly, the high flux rate through glycolysis and the pathway of glutamine utilization allows the cells to make rapid changes to intracellular pathways, as well as enzyme activity and regulation, crucial for lymphocyte proliferation. In this context, glutamine is required for energy generation and may promote synthesis of lipids, polyamines, and amino acids. The rate of glutamine utilization by these cells is either similar to or greater than that of glucose (Newsholme, Gordon,

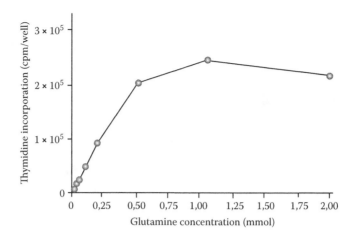

FIGURE 21.3 Lymphocyte proliferation is dependent on extracellular glutamine concentration. Lymphocytes obtained from rat spleens were incubated *in vitro* in RPMI medium–containing antibiotics. They were exposed to the T-cell mitogen concanavalin A at the start of the incubation in a medium containing various extracellular glutamine concentrations. Proliferation is expressed as an increase in radioactively labelled thymidine incorporation into DNA during the last 18 hours of a 66-hour incubation (From Yaqoob, P, and P. C. Calder, *Nutrition,* 13 (7–8), 1997.)

and Newsholme 1987; Pithon-Curi, De Melo, and Curi 2004). Changes in metabolism occur after ligation of the T-cell receptor and the costimulatory molecule CD28; these changes are regulated by phosphoinositide 3-kinase (PI3K) and Akt, which result in the activation of the mammalian target of rapamycin (mTOR), critical for energy utilization and stimulation of biosynthetic pathways (Lochner, Berod, and Sparwasser 2015).

Understanding the regulation of the bioenergetics of leukocytes, especially lymphocytes, by nutrients such as glutamine may lead to novel strategies to modulate immune cell function and cytokine production, both *in vitro* and *in vivo* (Keane et al. 2015). Glutamine may impact expression of key lymphocyte cell surface markers, such as CD25, CD45RO, CD71, and the production of cytokines, such as interferon-gamma (IFN-γ), TNF-α, and IL-6 (Roth et al. 2002; Curi et al. 2005a, Curi et al. 2005b, Hiscock et al. 2003).

Extracellular glutamine concentration also regulates T lymphocyte proliferation (Figure 21.3), which is particularly important in host defense. In general, leukocytes are highly dependent on liver and skeletal muscle generation of glutamine, because they can release the amino acid into the bloodstream to satisfy immune metabolic requirements. For example, glutamine replacement induced an increase in lymphocyte proliferation (T and B) (Cruzat et al. 2014a). Furthermore, glutamine has been reported to support the potential of lymphokine activated killer (LAK) cells, affecting tumors arising from solid organs (Juretic et al. 1994), and the ability of cells to produce cytokines. Differentiated B lymphocytes are also dependent on glutamine availability, maintaining antibody production and secretion (Newsholme 2001). Undoubtedly, glutamine is crucial for lymphocytes, and cannot be replaced by other amino acids.

21.4 GLUTAMINE IN THE CONTEXT OF EXERCISE

Although regular moderate-intensity exercise is essential for the general population to maintain health and reduce the risk of chronic diseases, athletes engaged in intense, prolonged, or exhaustive physical exercise are more susceptible to the adverse effects of high-intensity exercise. Such effects include high rates of protein catabolism, a proinflammatory profile, accompanied by muscle damage, soreness, chronic oxidative stress (Finaud, Lac, and Filaire 2006), and immune suppression (Gleeson 2007; Tanskanen, Atalay, and Uusitalo 2010) (Figure 21.4).

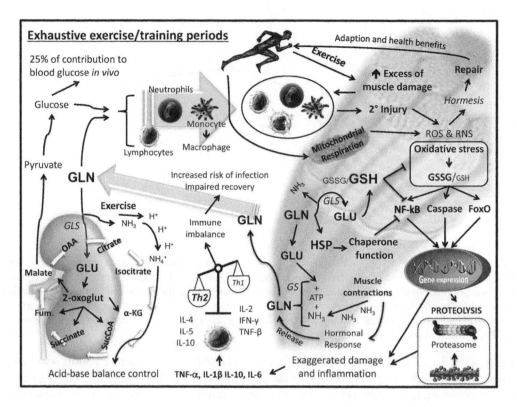

FIGURE 21.4 Glutamine metabolism in the context of exercise immunology. Exhaustive exercise training induces excessive muscle damage promoting immune cell infiltration and inflammation, which chronically promotes oxidative stress leading to proteolysis. Moreover, disturbances in the immunologic system
can create the open window effect for microorganisms via a shift from Th1 to Th2 phenotype during the
differentiation of naive T helper cells. Hence, a decrease in immune capacity and an increase in infection
rate postexercise are mainly related to the suppression of Th1 responses and are less influenced by changes in
humoral immunity. In this scenario, the kidneys increase the glutamine (GLN) uptake to maintain the acid-
base balance and importantly contribute to the homeostatic control of glucose. Both glucose and glutamine are
required for immune cell function. Abbreviations: glutathione (GSH), heat shock proteins (HSP), glutamate
(GLU), glutaminase (GLS), ammonia (NH_3), ammonium ion (NH_4), hydrogen ions (H^+), nuclear factor-kappa
B pathway (NF-κB), Forkhead box O (FoxO), reactive oxygen species (ROS), reactive nitrogen species (RNS),
interleukin (IL), tumor necrosis factor alpha and beta (TNF-α and TNF-β, respectively), interferon-gamma
(IFN-γ), oxaloacetate (OAA), alpha-ketoglutarate (α-KG), succinyl CoA (SucCoA), fumarate (Fum).

Studies have reported the harmful side effects of so-called overtraining syndrome and increased
upper respiratory tract infection (URTI) promoted by exhaustive physical exercise (Gleeson 2007;
Gleeson, Nieman, and Pedersen 2004; Kreher and Schwartz 2012), but the exact prevalence and
incidence in the elite sports field is unknown. Many elite athletes, including adolescents, show
immune suppression, which can be related to the development of overtraining syndrome (Kreher
and Schwartz 2012; Matos, Winsley, and Williams 2011; Meeusen et al. 2013). These disturbances
in the immune system leave an open window for pathogens, and the most reported issue is URTI.
Humoral or cell-mediated immunity responses depend on the type of cytokines that are released by
activated T helper cells. The T lymphocyte response can be classed as type 1 (Th1) or type 2 (Th2),
depending on which cytokines they predominantly synthesize.

The Th1 response typically produces cytokines such as IFN-γ and TNF, which activate macrophages, natural killer cells (NK), and T cytotoxic cells, providing protection against intracellular
pathogens such as viruses. On the other hand, the Th2 response mainly produces interleukins, such
as IL-4, IL-5, IL-10, which are necessary for humoral immunity activity and other functions related

to eosinophils and IgE-mediated allergic reactions (Walsh et al. 2011). Studies have shown that overtraining syndrome enhances Th2 cell responses and induces a shift from Th1 to Th2 during the differentiation of naive T helper cells (Pillon et al. 2013; Dong et al. 2011). Hence, a decrease in immune capacity and an increase in infection rate postexercise are mainly related to the suppression of Th1 responses and are less influenced by changes in humoral immunity (Figure 21.4).

Given the importance of glutamine to the body's defenses, especially to cells of the immune system, in the last 20 to 30 years, many studies have associated a decrease in plasma and tissue concentrations of glutamine with impaired immune function induced by exhaustive physical exercise. At the beginning of an exercise session, the active skeletal muscles promote an accelerated glutamine and alanine release, which increases the plasma concentration of amino acids. This transient increase is driven by the high synthesis of NH_3, promoted by the increased energy demand for ATP during muscle contraction. During the exercise session, mainly when it's performed for more than 1 or 2 hours, a subsequent decrease in plasma glutamine can be observed (Parry-Billings et al. 1992). These levels may remain lower for approximately 2 to 4 hours after the end of exercise (Gleeson 2008; Parry-Billings et al. 1991).

As a catabolic stimulus, high-output exercise (i.e., high-intensity or long-term strenuous exercises) may decrease the body glutamine pool (Santos, Caperuto, and Costa Rosa 2007; Cruzat and Tirapegui 2009). Glutamine availability is largely dependent on exercise duration and intensity. Plasma catabolic hormones, such as adrenocorticotropic hormone (ACTH) and cortisol, stimulate protein breakdown. This promotes the release of glutamine from stores, especially from the liver and skeletal muscles (Cruzat and Tirapegui 2009), and also increased gluconeogenesis and renal uptake (Gleeson 2008). Increased kidney glutamine uptake is required to counteract acidosis induced by exercise; NH_3 is cleaved from glutamine by the action of phosphate-dependent glutaminase, and the NH_3 is exported to the lumen of the collecting tubule where it combines with exported H^+ to form NH_4^+, which is excreted to the urine (Figure 21.4) (Gstraunthaler et al. 2000).

On the other hand, glutamate is converted via formation of intermediary substrates of the Krebs cycle (e.g., 2-oxoglutarate, succinate, fumarate, malate and oxaloacetate to phosphoenolpyruvate, or even malate to pyruvate directly), and then contributes to gluconeogenesis. Importantly, glucose produced by this pathway provides up to 25% of circulating plasma glucose *in vivo*, essential to the capacity to support long periods of exercise stress (Newsholme et al. 2003a). Despite the crucial role of glutamine in kidney metabolism, there was no effect of the exogenous supply of glutamine on blood acid-base balance or time to fatigue in cycling at 100% VO_2max (Haub et al. 1998; Gleeson 2008). When healthy, recreationally active subjects performed a high-intensity incremental cycle ergometer test following 7 days of high protein diet (1.8 to 2.2 g/kg/day, mainly consisting of grain products, chicken, red meat, and eggs); capillary and urine pH were less alkaline than the normal protein diet group (1.0 g/kg/day) (Hietavala et al. 2014).

Immune cells consume high amounts of glutamine, especially under exercise situations, since these cells do not possess GS, the key enzyme for glutamine synthesis. Exercise stimulates glutamine release from tissues into the bloodstream to satisfy immune metabolic requirements, but lower concentration of ATP/ADP and glutamate can inhibit the action of GS. Indeed, this process eventually reduces NH_3 removal in the form of glutamine, leading to hyperammonemia and fatigue (Newsholme 2001; Bassini-Cameron et al. 2008; Cruzat and Tirapegui 2009). Usually, this effect can be observed in exercise situations accompanied by the release into the bloodstream of substances arising from muscle damage and inflammation (Sluka and Rasmussen 2010; Cruzat, Rogero, and Tirapegui 2010). This suggests an important link between glutamine availability, muscle damage, and the immune-inflammatory response.

Lower glutamine availability associated with a high inflammatory response induced by exhaustive exercise may reduce cell antioxidant concentrations, such as GSH (Newsholme et al. 2011; Cruzat and Tirapegui 2009). This effect ultimately favors chronic oxidative stress. As a cause or consequence, oxidative stress can promote DNA damage and trigger the redox pathways for transcriptional activation. Several proteins, such as the classical nuclear factor-kappa B pathway (NFκB), and the proteolytic mechanism mediated by Forkhead box O (FoxO), among others (e.g., caspase cascade), are extremely sensitive to the redox status of the cells (Figure 21.4) (Tisdale 2009; Radak et al. 2013). For instance, athletes diagnosed with overtraining syndrome and involved in exhaustive exercise show high oxidative stress parameters in plasma (Tanskanen, Atalay, and Uusitalo 2010) and in immune cells, such as lymphocytes (Turner et al. 2011). Despite the fact that exhaustive periods of training dramatically increase kidney and immune cell uptake of glutamine, plasma concentration is tightly and constantly regulated between tissues through the solute carrier (SLC) family of amino acid transporters (Pochini et al. 2014).

Glutaminase activity increases in chronic diseases, such as diabetes, or even during acute stresses like starvation or high protein diets, whereas decreased activity of the enzyme occurs with the feeding of low protein diets, both without major changes in plasma glutamine concentration (Labow, Souba, and Abcouwer 2001; Watford 2000). In intensive care unit (ICU) patients, for example, glutamine supplementation (20–25 g/day) improved survival and shortened ICU stay, and plasma glutamine was an independent predictor of mortality (Wernerman 2008; Novak et al. 2002). In nonsurviving septic patients, glutamine in tissues was reduced by 90%, serving as a reliable prognostic marker, and yet no significant changes in glutamine were observed in plasma (Roth et al. 1982).

21.5 PROVISION OF GLUTAMINE FOR RECOVERY: FROM THE BENCH TO BEDSIDE

L-glutamine is composed of 41% carbon, 33% oxygen, 19% nitrogen, and 7% hydrogen by mass. Glutamine is one of the twenty proteinogenic amino acids, and accounts for 5%–6% of bound amino acids in proteins (Roth 2008). Although glutamine can be directly obtained from the diet, its endogenous synthesis may occur from other amino acids, such as the branched-chain amino acids (Newsholme et al. 2014). Thus, in a health context, glutamine is considered a nonessential amino acid commonly supplied to the blood by synthesis from precursors in tissues, especially the skeletal muscle. In healthy humans of approximately 70 kg body weight, 70 to 80 g of glutamine can be found distributed in a number of body tissues, and the endogenous production of glutamine, as estimated by isotopic techniques, is 40–80 g/24 h (Wernerman 2008). In human blood plasma or serum, the normal glutamine concentration is between 500 and 700 µmol/L, and in the intracellular environment can be from 2 to 20 mM (D'Souza and Powell-Tuck 2004; Newsholme et al. 2011). On the other hand, the rationale for the treatment with glutamine supplementation in disease or catabolic conditions is based on compromised blood concentration and lower glutamine synthesis and release rates, especially from skeletal muscle.

21.5.1 THE PARENTERAL SUPPLY OF GLUTAMINE

Different preparations of L-glutamine supplementation can be used for nutritional supplementation, and the application partially depends on the patient catabolic situation. Given parenterally, by itself or as part of a total parenteral nutrition (TPN) formulation, L-glutamine supplementation results in normalization of plasma glutamine concentrations (Flaring et al. 2003; Mondello et al. 2010; Furst, Alteheld, and Stehle 2004). The results of studies of clearance and distribution kinetics may vary according to renal flux and other tissue uptake (Berg et al. 2007); therefore, the dosage of glutamine may be guided by regular measurement of its plasma concentration. Most studies with postoperative patients show that a daily i.v. L-glutamine dosage of 20–30 g or 0.3–0.5 g/kg body weight can reduce the decrease in blood glutamine and also glutamine in tissues such as liver and skeletal muscle (Roth 2008; Weitzel and Wischmeyer 2010).

Free L-glutamine has limited solubility in water and is an unstable amino acid in aqueous solution (hydrolysis will degrade glutamine by approximately 5% per day at 37°C). Moreover, the amino acid cannot be heat sterilized, since it will be degraded. To reduce precipitation, glutamine concentrations in soluble solutions should not exceed 1%–2%, creating a problem for offering adequate amounts of the amino acid to critically ill patients. For these reasons, L-glutamine in its free form was not included in the crystalline amino acid solutions for parenteral use until the dipeptide forms (glycyl-glutamine; alanyl-glutamine) were introduced in the 1990s (Wernerman 2008; Furst, Alteheld, and Stehle 2004). The L-glutamine dipeptides are stable during heat steril-ization and highly soluble, and are therefore suitable constituents of liquid nutrition preparations. Current industrial production levels of L-glutamine dipeptides have allowed for their routine use in clinical nutrition.

Because several different types of peptides containing L-glutamine can be synthesized with a high range of solubility, two types received more attention, L-glycyl-L-glutamine (with solubil-ity of 154 g/L H_2O at 20°C) and L-alanyl-L-glutamine (with solubility of 568 g/L H_2O at 20°C). Several clinical and experimental studies have shown that glutamine-containing dipeptides added to parenteral formulas improve the clinical conditions of individuals with transplanted bone mar-row (Ziegler et al. 1992), attenuating reduction in GSH (Flaring et al. 2003), diminishing muscular atrophy during metabolic stress following surgery (Estivariz et al. 2008), reducing the rate of hospi-tal infection (Grau et al. 2011), promoting immune function (Exner et al. 2003), and improving the nitrogen balance (Mondello et al. 2010), thereby lowering overall hospital costs (Dechelotte et al. 2006), length of stay, and mortality (Weitzel and Wischmeyer 2010; Klassen et al. 2000; Rodas et al. 2012).

In a healthy state, the elimination half-life for L-alanyl-L-glutamine is about 2.4 min, while for L-glycyl-L-glutamine, it is nearly 8.6 min. Both dipeptides are readily hydrolyzed after their bolus injection, resulting in their amino acids being released in the free form to tissues and organs (Figure 21.5) (Albers et al. 1988; Matthews, Battezzati, and Furst 1993; Furst, Alteheld, and Stehle 2004). Despite some differences in the immunological results between the administration of

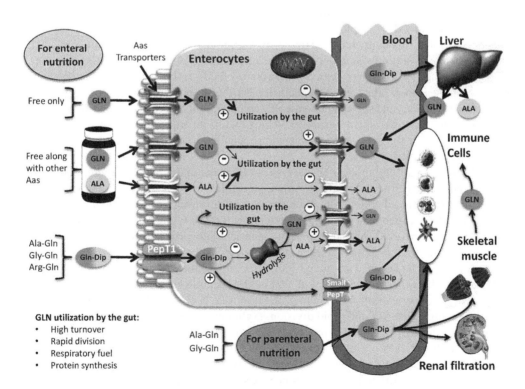

FIGURE 21.5 Handling of different formulations of glutamine provided enterally or parenterally.

L-alanyl-L-glutamine and L-glycyl-L-glutamine, the former is more often used and is available as an integral part of routine clinical practice (Spittler et al. 2001; Exner et al. 2003). This is possibly due to the fact that, although both solutions are well tolerated and effectively reduce the length of hospital stay (Roth 2008), alanyl-glutamine is more closely associated with lower infectious complication rate (Wang et al. 2010; Bollhalder et al. 2013). Nevertheless, further studies are needed to better determine the different physiological effects of glutamine dipeptides administered intravenously and the impact on clinical outcomes.

In general, glutamine dipeptide supply is an important therapeutic strategy in a number of clinical situations, and should be provided immediately after the catabolic insult to initially reverse and stabilize the dramatic fall glutamine in the blood and tissues and its consequences for the whole body. However, as previously mentioned, plasma-free glutamine concentration may not always reflect body glutamine status. Even with normal plasma glutamine levels, severe intracellular glutamine depletion may occur (Wernerman 2008; Novak et al. 2002; Roth et al. 1982). Importantly, the infusion of these dipeptides is mostly well tolerated and reports of complaints or side effects are low (Wang et al. 2010; Roth 2008; Bollhalder et al. 2013).

21.5.2 NEW PERSPECTIVES IN ENTERAL GLUTAMINE

Enteral L-glutamine routes are more physiologically relevant and may stimulate metabolic generation of other amino acid derivatives, such as citrulline (Cynober 2013) and arginine (Krause and de Bittencourt 2008). Both these have important immunological roles but both may be compromised in catabolic situations. In this regard, the L-arginyl-L-glutamine (Arg-Gln) dipeptide has been tested in enteral nutrition. In a mouse hyperoxia model, Arg-Gln attenuated lung injury and inflammatory parameters, including effects on MPO, LDH, and inflammatory cytokines such as IL-6 and C-X-C motif ligand 1/keratinocyte-derived chemokine (Ma et al. 2012). Some of these effects were also observed in intestinal cells using the same animal model of hyperoxia-induced inflammation and neutrophil activation (Li et al. 2012); these effects were associated with restoration of NF-κB. Despite this, the daily dose employed in those studies was higher (5 g/kg/day), levels difficult for humans. Thus, more studies are required to confirm the promising results using more relevant doses.

The efficiency of oral provision of glutamine dipeptides could be the result of its transport into enterocytes through the glycopeptide transport protein-1 (PepT-1) (Figure 21.5). Although transporters of free amino acids exhibit substrate specificity, PepT-1 can potentially transport up to 400 common di- and tripeptides, and some peptidomimetic compounds (Gilbert, Wong, and Webb 2008). An interesting characteristic of this transport protein is that di- or tripeptides can be transported into the cell by PepT-1 for the same energy expenditure required to transport a single free amino acid (Gilbert, Wong, and Webb 2008).

Initial studies in animal models have shown an increase in the plasma glutamine concentration between 30 to 120 minutes after oral supplementation with free and dipeptide forms of L-glutamine (Rogero et al. 2004). However, the concentration and the area under the curve of the dipeptide tend to be higher when compared to the free form of L-glutamine due to the PepT-1 and other mechanisms involved in the transport of dipeptides (Rogero et al. 2006; Gilbert, Wong, and Webb 2008). The result is an increased systemic release of L-glutamine and L-alanine deriving from acute supplementation with alanyl-glutamine, consequently promoting a higher release into tissues, such as the liver (Petry et al. 2015), the immune system (Cruzat et al. 2014a), the kidneys (Alba-Loureiro et al. 2010), and skeletal muscle (Petry et al. 2014). Since enterocytes are cells with high turnover and rapid division, L-glutamine hydrolysis and utilization provides a preferred respiratory fuel and a precursor for protein synthesis (Figure 21.5) (Ueno et al. 2011). In fact, the efficacy of oral interventions with free L-glutamine are frequently questioned due to the high consumption by the small intestine. However, studies in animal models exposed to different catabolic situations and infection have shown that oral supplementation with alanyl-glutamine or free L-glutamine along with free L-alanine may reestablish total glutamine levels, and antioxidant and HSP responses (Cruzat et al. 2014c, Cruzat, Petry, and Tirapegui 2009). Although the precise mechanisms are still unknown, it is clear that L-glutamine and L-alanine work in parallel. L-alanine is rapidly metabolized via alanine aminotransferase to pyruvate, with concomitant production of glutamate from 2-oxoglutarate, which contributes to antioxidant defense, such as GSH production. Thus, the presence of L-alanine in the dipeptide or in its free form can spare glutamine metabolism in order for the latter to be used by high-demand tissues under immune insults (Cruzat et al. 2014c, Cruzat and Tirapegui 2009). Other different combinations of free amino acids need to be tested; however, based on currently available studies, alanyl-glutamine and L-glutamine in its free form, in conjunction with other amino acids, or even proteins with a high glutamine content such as wheat protein, can enhance whole body glutamine status (Harris et al. 2012; Rogero et al. 2008b).

21.6 CONCLUSION

Crucial experiments performed approximately 30 years ago at the University of Oxford demonstrated the unique roles and properties of glutamine with respect to immune cell metabolism and function. Subsequent studies revealed that glutamine deficiency increased the mortality of animals subjected to bacterial stress. In critically ill patients, parenteral glutamine reduced both nitrogen loss and mortality. Glutamine administration in animal studies was able to act on the intestinal mucosa, decreasing intestinal permeability and preventing the translocation of bacteria. Glutamine is clearly an important metabolic substrate of rapidly proliferating cells and has multiple effects on the immune system, on intestinal function, and on protein metabolism. Mechanisms of action potentially include improvement in the cellular redox state through the GSH antioxidant system, heat shock protein expression and concentration, and gene expression related to cell survival. Strategies to correct glutamine deficiency, particularly in nonacute situations such as chronic disease and stress, are under investigation, perhaps revealing metabolic targets for future therapeutic interventions.

REFERENCES

Alba-Loureiro, T. C., R. F. Ribeiro, T. M. Zorn, and C. J. Lagranha. 2010. Effects of glutamine supplementation on kidney of diabetic rat. *Amino Acids* 38 (4):1021–1030.
Albers, S., J. Wernerman, P. Stehle, E. Vinnars, and P. Furst. 1988. Availability of amino acids supplied intravenously in healthy man as synthetic dipeptides: Kinetic evaluation of L-alanyl-L-glutamine and glycyl-L-tyrosine. *Clin Sci (Lond)* 75 (5):463–468.
Antonio, J., and C. Street. 1999. Glutamine: A potentially useful supplement for athletes. *Can J Appl Physiol* 24 (1):1–14.
Ardawi, M. S., and E. A. Newsholme. 1982. Maximum activities of some enzymes of glycolysis, the tricarboxylic acid cycle and ketone-body and glutamine utilization pathways in lymphocytes of the rat. *Biochem J* 208 (3):743–748.
Ardawi, M. S., and E. A. Newsholme. 1983. Glutamine metabolism in lymphocytes of the rat. *Biochem J* 212 (3):835–842.
Bassini-Cameron, A., A. Monteiro, A. Gomes, J. P. Werneck-de-Castro, and L. Cameron. 2008. Glutamine protects against increases in blood ammonia in football players in an exercise intensity-dependent way. *Br J Sports Med* 42 (4):260–266.
Berg, A., A. Norberg, C. R. Martling, L. Gamrin, O. Rooyackers, and J. Wernerman. 2007. Glutamine kinetics during intravenous glutamine supplementation in ICU patients on continuous renal replacement therapy. *Intensive Care Med* 33 (4):660–666.
Bollhalder, Lea, Alena M. Pfeil, Yuki Tomonaga, and Matthias Schwenkglenks. 2013. A systematic literature review and meta-analysis of randomized clinical trials of parenteral glutamine supplementation. *Clin Nutr* 32 (2):213–223.
Branzk, N., A. Lubojemska, S. E. Hardison, Q. Wang, M. G. Gutierrez, G. D. Brown, and V. Papayannopoulos. 2014. Neutrophils sense microbe size and selectively release neutrophil extracellular traps in response to large pathogens. *Nat Immunol* 15 (11):1017–1025.

Cooper, M. D., and M. N. Alder. 2006. The evolution of adaptive immune systems. *Cell* 124 (4):815–822.

Cruzat, V. F., A. Bittencourt, S. P. Scomazzon, J. S. Leite, P. I. de Bittencourt, Jr., and J. Tirapegui. 2014a. Oral free and dipeptide forms of glutamine supplementation attenuate oxidative stress and inflammation induced by endotoxemia. *Nutrition* 30 (5):602–611.

Cruzat, V. F., K. N. Keane, A. L. Scheinpflug, R. Cordeiro, M. J. Soares, and P. Newsholme. 2014b. Alanyl-glutamine improves pancreatic beta-cell function following ex vivo inflammatory challenge. *J Endocrinol* 224 (3):261–271.

Cruzat, V. F., M. Krause, and P. Newsholme. 2014. Amino acid supplementation and impact on immune function in the context of exercise. *J Int Soc Sports Nutr* 11 (1):61.

Cruzat, V. F., L. C. Pantaleao, J. Donato, Jr., P. I. de Bittencourt, Jr., and J. Tirapegui. 2014c. Oral supplementations with free and dipeptide forms of L-glutamine in endotoxemic mice: Effects on muscle glutamine-glutathione axis and heat shock proteins. *J Nutrl Biochem* 25 (3):345–352.

Cruzat, V. F., E. R. Petry, and J. Tirapegui. 2009. Glutamine: Biochemical, metabolic, molecular aspects and supplementation. *Revista Brasileira de Medicina do Esporte* 15 (5):392–397.

Cruzat, V. F., M. M. Rogero, and J. Tirapegui. 2010. Effects of supplementation with free glutamine and the dipeptide alanyl-glutamine on parameters of muscle damage and inflammation in rats submitted to prolonged exercise. *Cell Biochem Funct* 28 (1):24–30.

Cruzat, V. F., and J. Tirapegui. 2009. Effects of oral supplementation with glutamine and alanyl-glutamine on glutamine, glutamate, and glutathione status in trained rats and subjected to long-duration exercise. *Nutrition* 25 (4):428–435.

Curi, R., C. J. Lagranha, S. Q. Doi, D. F. Sellitti, J. Procopio, and T. C. Pithon-Curi. 2005a. Glutamine-dependent changes in gene expression and protein activity. *Cell Biochem Funct* 23 (2):77–84.

Curi, R., C. J. Lagranha, S. Q. Doi, D. F. Sellitti, J. Procopio, T. C. Pithon-Curi, M. Corless, and P. Newsholme. 2005b. Molecular mechanisms of glutamine action. *J Cell Physiol* 204 (2):392–401.

Curi, R., P. Newsholme, and E. A. Newsholme. 1986. Intracellular distribution of some enzymes of the glutamine utilization pathway in rat lymphocytes. *Biochem Biophys Res Commun* 138 (1):318–322.

Cynober, L. 2013. Citrulline: Just a biomarker or a conditionally essential amino acid and a pharmaconutrient in critically ill patients? *Crit Care* 17 (2):122.

D'Souza, R., and J. Powell-Tuck. 2004. Glutamine supplements in the critically ill. *J R Soc Med* 97 (9): 425–427.

Dechelotte, P., M. Hasselmann, L. Cynober, B. Allaouchiche, M. Coeffier, B. Hecketsweiler, V. Merle, M. Mazerolles, D. Samba, Y. M. Guillou, J. Petit, O. Mansoor, G. Colas, R. Cohendy, D. Barnoud, P. Czernichow, and G. Bleichner. 2006. L-alanyl-L-glutamine dipeptide-supplemented total parenteral nutrition reduces infectious complications and glucose intolerance in critically ill patients: The French controlled, randomized, double-blind, multicenter study. *Crit Care Med* 34 (3):598–604.

Dong, J., P. Chen, R. Wang, D. Yu, Y. Zhang, and W. Xiao. 2011. NADPH oxidase: A target for the modulation of the excessive oxidase damage induced by overtraining in rat neutrophils. *Intl J Biol Sci* 7 (6):881–891.

Eagle, H. 1959. Amino acid metabolism in mammalian cell cultures. *Science* 130 (3373):432–437.

Eagle, H., V. I. Oyama, M. Levy, C. L. Horton, and R. Fleischman. 1956. Growth response of mammalian cells in tissue culture to L-glutamine and L-glutamic acid. *J Biol Chem* 218 (2):607–616.

Estivariz, C. F., D. P. Griffith, M. Luo, E. E. Szeszycki, N. Bazargan, N. Dave, N. M. Daignault, G. F. Bergman, T. McNally, C. H. Battey, C. E. Furr, L. Hao, J. G. Ramsay, C. R. Accardi, G. A. Cotsonis, D. P. Jones, J. R. Galloway, and T. R. Ziegler. 2008. Efficacy of parenteral nutrition supplemented with glutamine dipeptide to decrease hospital infections in critically ill surgical patients. *JPEN J Parenter Enteral Nutr* 32 (4):389–402.

Exner, R., D. Tamandl, P. Goetzinger, M. Mittlboeck, R. Fuegger, T. Sautner, A. Spittler, and E. Roth. 2003. Perioperative GLY-GLN infusion diminishes the surgery-induced period of immunosuppression: Accelerated restoration of the lipopolysaccharide-stimulated tumor necrosis factor-alpha response. *Ann Surg* 237 (1):110–115.

Finaud, J., G. Lac, and E. Filaire. 2006. Oxidative stress: Relationship with exercise and training. *Sports Med* 36 (4):327–358.

Flaring, U. B., O. E. Rooyackers, J. Wernerman, and F. Hammarqvist. 2003. Glutamine attenuates post-traumatic glutathione depletion in human muscle. *Clin Sci (Lond)* 104 (3):275–282.

Frayn, K. N., K. Khan, S. W. Coppack, and M. Elia. 1991. Amino acid metabolism in human subcutaneous adipose tissue in vivo. *Clin Sci (Lond)* 80 (5):471–474.

Furst, P., B. Alteheld, and P. Stehle. 2004. Why should a single nutrient—glutamine—improve outcome? The remarkable story of glutamine dipeptides. *Clinical Nutrition*:3–15.

Garcia, C., T. C. Pithon-Curi, M. de Lourdes Firmano, M. Pires de Melo, P. Newsholme, and R. Curi. 1999. Effects of adrenaline on glucose and glutamine metabolism and superoxide production by rat neutrophils. *Clin Sci (Lond)* 96 (6):549–555.

Gilbert, E. R., E. A. Wong, and K. E. Webb, Jr. 2008. Board-invited review: Peptide absorption and utilization: Implications for animal nutrition and health. *J Anim Sci* 86 (9):2135–2155.

Gleeson, M. 2007. Immune function in sport and exercise. *J Appld Physiol* 103 (2):693–699.

Gleeson, M., D. C. Nieman, and B. K. Pedersen. 2004. Exercise, nutrition and immune function. *J Sports Sci* 22 (1):115–125.

Gleeson, M. 2008. Dosing and efficacy of glutamine supplementation in human exercise and sport training. *J Nutr* 138 (10):2045S–2049S.

Grau, T., A. Bonet, E. Minambres, L. Pineiro, J. A. Irles, A. Robles, J. Acosta, I. Herrero, V. Palacios, J. Lopez, A. Blesa, P. Martinez, and Nutrition Working Group Semicyuc Spain Metabolism. 2011. The effect of L-alanyl-L-glutamine dipeptide supplemented total parenteral nutrition on infectious morbidity and insulin sensitivity in critically ill patients. *Crit Care Med* 39 (6):1263–1268.

Gstraunthaler, G., T. Holcomb, E. Feifel, W. Liu, N. Spitaler, and N. P. Curthoys. 2000. Differential expression and acid-base regulation of glutaminase mRNAs in gluconeogenic LLC-PK(1)-FBPase(+) cells. *Am J Physiol Renal Physiol* 278 (2):F227–F237.

Harris, R. C., J. R. Hoffman, A. Allsopp, and N. B. Routledge. 2012. L-glutamine absorption is enhanced after ingestion of L-alanylglutamine compared with the free amino acid or wheat protein. *Nutr Res* 32 (4):272–277.

Haub, M. D., J. A. Potteiger, K. L. Nau, M. J. Webster, and C. J. Zebas. 1998. Acute L-glutamine ingestion does not improve maximal effort exercise. *J Sports Med Phys Fitness* 38 (3):240–244.

Hietavala, E. M., J. R. Stout, J. J. Hulmi, H. Suominen, H. Pitkanen, R. Puurtinen, H. Selanne, H. Kainulainen, and A. A. Mero. 2014. Effect of diet composition on acid-base balance in adolescents, young adults and elderly at rest and during exercise. *Eur J Clin Nutr.* 69 (3):399–404.

Hiscock, N., E. W. Petersen, K. Krzywkowski, J. Boza, J. Halkjaer-Kristensen, and B. K. Pedersen. 2003. Glutamine supplementation further enhances exercise-induced plasma IL-6. *J Appl Physiol* 95 (1):145–148.

Hiscock, N., and B. K. Pedersen. 2002. Exercise-induced immunodepression– plasma glutamine is not the link. *J Appl Physiol* 93 (3):813–822.

Juretic, A., G. C. Spagnoli, H. Horig, R. Babst, K. von Bremen, F. Harder, and M. Heberer. 1994. Glutamine requirements in the generation of lymphokine-activated killer cells. *Clin Nutr* 13 (1):42–49.

Keane, K. N., E. K. Calton, V. F. Cruzat, M. J. Soares, and P. Newsholme. 2015. The impact of cryopreservation on human peripheral blood leukocyte bioenergetics. *Clin Sci (Lond).* 128 (10):723–733.

Klassen, P., M. Mazariegos, N. W. Solomons, and P. Furst. 2000. The pharmacokinetic responses of humans to 20 g of alanyl-glutamine dipeptide differ with the dosing protocol but not with gastric acidity or in patients with acute Dengue fever. *J Nutr* 130 (2):177–182.

Krause, M.S., and P.I.H. Jr. de Bittencourt. 2008. Type 1 diabetes: Can exercise impair the autoimmune event? The L-arginine/glutamine coupling hypothesis. *Cell Biochem Funct* 26 (4):406–433.

Krebs, H. A. 1935. Metabolism of amino-acids: The synthesis of glutamine from glutamic acid and ammonia, and the enzymic hydrolysis of glutamine in animal tissues. *Biochem J* 29 (8):1951–1969.

Kreher, J. B., and Schwartz J. B. 2012. Overtraining syndrome: A practical guide. *Sports Health* 4 (2):128–138.

Labow, B. I., W. W. Souba, and S. F. Abcouwer. 2001. Mechanisms governing the expression of the enzymes of glutamine metabolism—Glutaminase and glutamine synthetase. *J Nutr* 131 (9 Suppl):2467S–2474S; discussion 2486S–2487S.

Li, N., L. Ma, X. Liu, L. Shaw, S. Li Calzi, M. B. Grant, and J. Neu. 2012. Arginyl-glutamine dipeptide or docosahexaenoic acid attenuates hyperoxia-induced small intestinal injury in neonatal mice. *J Pediatr Gastroenterol Nutr* 54 (4):499–504.

Lochner, M., L. Berod, and T. Sparwasser. 2015. Fatty acid metabolism in the regulation of T cell function. *Trends Immunol.* 36 (2):81–91.

Ma, L., N. Li, X. Liu, L. Shaw, S. Li Calzi, M. B. Grant, and J. Neu. 2012. Arginyl-glutamine dipeptide or docosahexaenoic acid attenuate hyperoxia-induced lung injury in neonatal mice. *Nutrition* 28 (11–12):1186–1191.

Matos, N. F., R. J. Winsley, and C. A. Williams. 2011. Prevalence of nonfunctional overreaching/overtraining in young English athletes. *Med Sci Sports Exerc* 43 (7):1287–1294.

Matthews, D. E., A. Battezzati, and P. Furst. 1993. Alanylglutamine kinetics in humans. *Clin Nutr* 12 (1): 57–58.

Meeusen, R., M. Duclos, C. Foster, A. Fry, M. Gleeson, D. Nieman, J. Raglin, G. Rietjens, J. Steinacker, and A. Urhausen. 2013. Prevention, diagnosis, and treatment of the overtraining syndrome: Joint consensus statement of the European College of Sport Science and the American College of Sports Medicine. *Med Sci Sports Exerc* 45 (1):186–205.

Meister, A. 1956. Metabolism of glutamine. *Physiol Rev* 36 (1):103–127.

Menge, B. A., H. Schrader, P. R. Ritter, M. Ellrichmann, W. Uhl, W. E. Schmidt, and J. J. Meier. 2010. Selective amino acid deficiency in patients with impaired glucose tolerance and type 2 diabetes. *Regul Pept* 160 (1–3):75–80.

Mondello, S., D. Italiano, M. S. Giacobbe, P. Mondello, G. Trimarchi, C. Aloisi, P. Bramanti, and E. Spina. 2010. Glutamine-supplemented total parenteral nutrition improves immunological status in anorectic patients. *Nutrition* 26 (6):677–681.

Murphy, C., and P. Newsholme. 1998. Importance of glutamine metabolism in murine macrophages and human monocytes to L-arginine biosynthesis and rates of nitrite or urea production. *Clin Sci (Lond)* 95 (4):397–407.

Murphy, C., and P. Newsholme. 1999. Macrophage-mediated lysis of a beta-cell line, tumour necrosis factor-alpha release from bacillus Calmette-Guerin (BCG)-activated murine macrophages and interleukin-8 release from human monocytes are dependent on extracellular glutamine concentration and glutamine metabolism. *Clin Sci (Lond)* 96 (1):89–97.

Newsholme, E. A., P. Newsholme, and R. Curi. 1987. The role of the citric acid cycle in cells of the immune system and its importance in sepsis, trauma and burns. *Biochem Soc Symp* 54:145–162.

Newsholme, P. 2001. Why is L-glutamine metabolism important to cells of the immune system in health, postinjury, surgery or infection? *J Nutr* 131 (9 Suppl):2515S–22S; discussion 2523S–2524S.

Newsholme, P., V. Cruzat, F. Arfuso, and K. Keane. 2014. Nutrient regulation of insulin secretion and action. *J Endocrinol* 221 (3):R105–R120.

Newsholme, P., R. Curi, S. Gordon, and E. A. Newsholme. 1986. Metabolism of glucose, glutamine, long-chain fatty-acids and ketone-bodies by murine macrophages. *Biochem J* 239 (1):121–125.

Newsholme, P., R. Curi, T. C. Pithon Curi, C. J. Murphy, C. Garcia, and M. Pires de Melo. 1999. Glutamine metabolism by lymphocytes, macrophages, and neutrophils: Its importance in health and disease. *J Nutr Biochem* 10 (6):316–324.

Newsholme, P., S. Gordon, and E. A. Newsholme. 1987. Rates of utilization and fates of glucose, glutamine, pyruvate, fatty acids and ketone bodies by mouse macrophages. *Biochem J* 242 (3):631–636.

Newsholme, P., M. Krause, E. A. Newsholme, S. J. Stear, L. M. Burke, and L. M. Castell. 2011. BJSM reviews: A to Z of nutritional supplements: Dietary supplements, sports nutrition foods and ergogenic aids for health and performance—Part 18. *Br J Sports Med* 45 (3):230–232.

Newsholme, P., M. M. Lima, J. Procopio, T. C. Pithon-Curi, S. Q. Doi, R. B. Bazotte, and R. Curi. 2003a. Glutamine and glutamate as vital metabolites. *Braz J Med Biol Res* 36 (2):153–163.

Newsholme, P., J. Procopio, M. M. Lima, T. C. Pithon-Curi, and R. Curi. 2003b. Glutamine and glutamate—Their central role in cell metabolism and function. *Cell Biochem Funct* 21 (1):1–9.

Newsholme, P., E. Rebelato, F. Abdulkader, M. Krause, A. Carpinelli, and R. Curi. 2012. Reactive oxygen and nitrogen species generation, antioxidant defenses, and beta-cell function: A critical role for amino acids. *J Endocrinol* 214 (1):11–20.

Novak, F., D. K. Heyland, A. Avenell, J. W. Drover, and X. Su. 2002. Glutamine supplementation in serious illness: A systematic review of the evidence. *Crit Care Med* 30 (9):2022–2029.

Papayannopoulos, V., K. D. Metzler, A. Hakkim, and A. Zychlinsky. 2010. Neutrophil elastase and myeloperoxidase regulate the formation of neutrophil extracellular traps. *J Cell Biol* 191 (3):677–691.

Parry-Billings, M., R. Budgett, Y. Koutedakis, E. Blomstrand, S. Brooks, C. Williams, P. C. Calder, S. Pilling, R. Baigrie, and E. A. Newsholme. 1992. Plasma amino acid concentrations in the overtraining syndrome: Possible effects on the immune system. *Med Sci Sports Exerc* 24 (12):1353–1358.

Parry-Billings, M., B. Leighton, G. D. Dimitriadis, J. Bond, and E. A. Newsholme. 1991. The effect of catecholamines on the metabolism of glutamine by skeletal muscle of the rat. *Biochem Soc Trans* 19 (2):130S.

Petry, E. R., V. F. Cruzat, T. G. Heck, J. S. Leite, P. I. Homem de Bittencourt, Jr., and J. Tirapegui. 2014. Alanyl-glutamine and glutamine plus alanine supplements improve skeletal redox status in trained rats: Involvement of heat shock protein pathways. *Life Sci* 94 (2):130–136.

Petry, E. R., V. F. Cruzat, T. G. Heck, P. I. Homem de Bittencourt, Jr., and J. Tirapegui. 2015. L-glutamine supplementations enhance liver glutamine-glutathione axis and heat shock factor-1 expression in endurance-exercise trained rats. *Int J Sport Nutr Exerc Metab.* 25 (2):188–197.

Pillon, N. J., P. J. Bilan, L. N. Fink, and A. Klip. 2013. Cross-talk between skeletal muscle and immune cells: Muscle-derived mediators and metabolic implications. *Am J Physiol Endocrinol Metab* 304 (5):E453–E465.

Pithon-Curi, T. C., M. P. De Melo, and R. Curi. 2004. Glucose and glutamine utilization by rat lymphocytes, monocytes and neutrophils in culture: A comparative study. *Cell Biochem Funct* 22 (5):321–326.

Pithon-Curi, T. C., A. C. Levada, L. R. Lopes, S. Q. Doi, and R. Curi. 2002. Glutamine plays a role in super-oxide production and the expression of p47(phox), p22(phox) and gp91(phox) in rat neutrophils. *Clin Sci(Lond)* 103 (4):403–408.

Pithon-Curi, T. C., A. G. Trezena, W. Tavares-Lima, and R. Curi. 2002. Evidence that glutamine is involved in neutrophil function. *Cell Biochem Funct* 20 (2):81–86.

Pochini, L., M. Scalise, M. Galluccio, and C. Indiveri. 2014. Membrane transporters for the special amino acid glutamine: Structure/function relationships and relevance to human health. *Front Chem* 2:61.

Radak, Z., Z. Zhao, E. Koltai, H. Ohno, and M. Atalay. 2013. Oxygen consumption and usage during physical exercise: The balance between oxidative stress and ROS-dependent adaptive signaling. *Antioxid Redox Signal* 18 (10):1208–1246.

Rodas, P. C., O. Rooyackers, C. Hebert, A. Norberg, and J. Wernerman. 2012. Glutamine and glutathione at ICU admission in relation to outcome. *Clin Sci (Lond)* 122 (12):591–597.

Rodrigues-Krause, J., M. Krause, G. D. Cunha, D. Perin, J. B. Martins, C. L. Alberton, M. I. Schaun, P. I. De Bittencourt, Jr., and A. Reischak-Oliveira. 2014. Ballet dancers cardiorespiratory, oxidative and muscle damage responses to classes and rehearsals. *Eur J Sport Sci* 14 (3):199–208.

Rogero, M. M., P. Borelli, M. A. Vinolo, R. A. Fock, I. S. D. Pires, and J. Tirapegui. 2008a. Dietary gluta-mine supplementation affects macrophage function, hematopoiesis and nutritional status in early weaned mice. *Clin Nutr* 27 (3):386–397.

Rogero, M. M., J. Tirapegui, R. G. Pedrosa, I. A. de Castro, and I. S. D. Pires. 2006. Effect of alanyl-glutamine supplementation on plasma and tissue glutamine concentrations in rats submitted to exhaustive exercise. *Nutrition* 22 (5):564–71.

Rogero, M. M., J. Tirapegui, R. G. Pedrosa, I. S. D. Pires, and I. A. de Castro. 2004. Plasma and tissue gluta-mine response to acute and chronic supplementation with L-glutamine and L-alanyl-L-glutamine in rats. *Nutr Res* 24 (4):261–270.

Rogero, M. M., J. Tirapegui, M. A. Vinolo, M. C. Borges, I. A. de Castro, I. S. Pires, and P. Borelli. 2008b. Dietary glutamine supplementation increases the activity of peritoneal macrophages and hemopoiesis in early-weaned mice inoculated with Mycobacterium bovis bacillus Calmette-Guerin. *J Nutr* 138 (7):1343–1348.

Roth, E. 2008. Nonnutritive effects of glutamine. *J Nutr* 138 (10):2025S–2031S.

Roth, E., J. Funovics, F. Muhlbacher, M. Schemper, W. Mauritz, P. Sporn, and A. Fritsch. 1982. Metabolic disorders in severe abdominal sepsis: Glutamine deficiency in skeletal muscle. *Clin Nutr* 1 (1):25–41.

Roth, E., R. Oehler, N. Manhart, R. Exner, B. Wessner, E. Strasser, and A. Spittler. 2002. Regulative potential of glutamine—Relation to glutathione metabolism. *Nutrition* 18 (3):217–221.

Santos, R. V., E. C. Caperuto, and L. F. Costa Rosa. 2007. Effects of acute exhaustive physical exercise upon glutamine metabolism of lymphocytes from trained rats. *Life Sci* 80 (6):573–578.

Sluka, K. A., and L. A. Rasmussen. 2010. Fatiguing exercise enhances hyperalgesia to muscle inflammation. *Pain* 148 (2):188–197.

Spittler, A., T. Sautner, A. Gornikiewicz, N. Manhart, R. Oehler, M. Bergmann, R. Fugger, and E. Roth. 2001. Postoperative glycyl-glutamine infusion reduces immunosuppression: Partial prevention of the surgery induced decrease in HLA-DR expression on monocytes. *Clin Nutr* 20 (1):37–42.

Tanskanen, M., M. Atalay, and A. Uusitalo. 2010. Altered oxidative stress in overtrained athletes. *J Sports Sci* 28 (3):309–317.

Tidball, J. G. 2005. Inflammatory processes in muscle injury and repair. *Am J Physiol Regul Integr Comp Physiol* 288 (2):R345–353.

Tisdale, M. J. 2009. Mechanisms of cancer cachexia. *Physiol Rev* 89 (2):381–410.

Tsai, P. H., C. L. Yeh, J. J. Liu, W. C. Chiu, and S. L. Yeh. 2012. Effects of dietary glutamine on inflammatory mediator gene expressions in rats with streptozotocin-induced diabetes. *Nutrition* 28 (3):288–293.

Turner, J. E., J. A. Bosch, M. T. Drayson, and S. Aldred. 2011. Assessment of oxidative stress in lymphocytes with exercise. *J Appl Physiol (1985)* 111 (1):206–211.

Ueno, P. M., R. B. Oria, E. A. Maier, M. Guedes, O. G. de Azevedo, D. Wu, T. Willson, S. P. Hogan, A. A. Lima, R. L. Guerrant, D. B. Polk, L. A. Denson, and S. R. Moore. 2011. Alanyl-glutamine promotes intestinal epithelial cell homeostasis in vitro and in a murine model of weanling undernutrition. *Am J Physiol Gastrointest Liver Physiol* 301 (4):G612–622.

van de Poll, M. C. G., P. B. Soeters, N. E. P. Deutz, K. C. H. Fearon, and C. H. C. Dejong. 2004. Renal metabolism of amino acids: Its role in interorgan amino acid exchange. *Am J Clin Nutr* 79 (2):185–197.

Walsh, N. P., M. Gleeson, D. B. Pyne, D. C. Nieman, F. S. Dhabhar, R. J. Shephard, S. J. Oliver, S. Bermon, and A. Kajeniene. 2011. Position statement. Part two: Maintaining immune health. *Exerc Immunol Rev* 17:64–103.

Wang, Y., Z. M. Jiang, M. T. Nolan, H. Jiang, H. R. Han, K. Yu, H. L. Li, B. Jie, and X. K. Liang. 2010. The impact of glutamine dipeptide-supplemented parenteral nutrition on outcomes of surgical patients: A meta-analysis of randomized clinical trials. *JPEN J Parenter Enteral Nutr* 34 (5):521–529.

Watford, M. 2000. Glutamine and glutamate metabolism across the liver sinusoid. *J Nutr* 130 (4S Suppl): 983S–987S.

Weitzel, L. R., and P. E. Wischmeyer. 2010. Glutamine in critical illness: The time has come, the time is now. *Crit Care Clin* 26 (3):515–25, ix–x.

Wernerman, J. 2008. Clinical use of glutamine supplementation. *J Nutr* 138 (10):2040S–2044S.

Wink, D. A., H. B. Hines, R. Y. Cheng, C. H. Switzer, W. Flores-Santana, M. P. Vitek, L. A. Ridnour, and C. A. Colton. 2011. Nitric oxide and redox mechanisms in the immune response. *J Leukoc Biol* 89 (6):873–891.

Yamauchi, K., T. Komatsu, A. D. Kulkarni, Y. Ohmori, H. Minami, Y. Ushiyama, M. Nakayama, and S. Yamamoto. 2002. Glutamine and arginine affect Caco-2 cell proliferation by promotion of nucleotide synthesis. *Nutrition* 18 (4):329–333.

Yaqoob, P., and P. C. Calder. 1997. Glutamine requirement of proliferating T lymphocytes. *Nutrition* 13 (7–8):646–651.

Yassad, A., A. Lavoinne, A. Bion, M. Daveau, and A. Husson. 1997. Glutamine accelerates interleukin-6 production by rat peritoneal macrophages in culture. *FEBS Lett* 413 (1):81–84.

Young, V. R., and A. M. Ajami. 2001. Glutamine: The emperor or his clothes? *J Nutr* 131 (9 Suppl): 2449S–2459S; discussion 2486S–2487S.

Ziegler, T. R., L. S. Young, K. Benfell, M. Scheltinga, K. Hortos, R. Bye, F. D. Morrow, D. O. Jacobs, R. J. Smith, J. H. Antin et al. 1992. Clinical and metabolic efficacy of glutamine-supplemented parenteral nutrition after bone marrow transplantation. A randomized, double-blind, controlled study. *Ann Intern Med* 116 (10):821–828.

22 Glutathione, Immunity, and Infection

Enrique Vera Tudela, Manpreet Singh,
and Vishwanath Venketaraman

CONTENTS

22.1 Introduction 375
22.2 Functions and Synthesis of GSH 376
    22.2.1 Overview of the Functions of GSH 376
    22.2.2 GSH Synthesis 376
22.3 The Immune System: An Overview 377
22.4 GSH and the Innate Immune System 378
    22.4.1 Macrophages and NO 378
    22.4.2 GSNO: More Potent Than NO Alone 378
    22.4.3 GSH and Dendritic Cells 379
    22.4.4 GSH and Natural Killer (NK) Cells 380
22.5 GSH and the Adaptive Immune System 381
    22.5.1 GSH and T Helper Cells 381
    22.5.2 GSH in HIV Infection 381
    22.5.3 GSH and Tregs 382
    22.5.4 GSH in Tuberculosis 382
    22.5.5 GSH in Type II Diabetes Mellitus 383
22.6 GSH and Other Bacteria 383
22.7 Summary 383
References 384

22.1 INTRODUCTION

To eliminate an infection, the immune system must be exquisitely efficient (see Chapters 1 and 2). The number of pathogens to which the human body is subjected is vast. At any given moment, there are countless organisms living, multiplying, and evolving alongside us. Most of these microbes do not cause disease to a healthy individual. However, some microbes are very pathogenic and can potentially cause disease. Fortunately, the immune system is highly evolved to deal with the vast majority of both pathogenic and nonpathogenic microbes. The immune system is elaborately composed of highly specialized cells whose sole function is trapping and containing virulent organisms. Because pathogenic microorganisms evolve at a much faster rate than humans, they are well adapted to avoiding the power of the host immune system. In this chapter, we present the role of reduced glutathione (GSH) in the immune system and infection. A tripeptide antioxidant with a best-recognized role in redox homeostasis, GSH has a wide-ranging role in immunity. Its varied functions affect essentially every cell of the immune system. Understanding the complexities by which GSH directly and indirectly influences immunity is an important area of study. To a large extent, it appears that decreasing the levels of GSH in immune cells is a powerful mechanism by which bacteria and viruses have evolved to avoid the effector mechanisms of the immune system (Herzenberg et al. 1997). Some pathogens, such as mycobacteria and the human immunodeficiency virus (HIV), survive predominantly inside immune cells. As discussed later, compromised levels of GSH aid these microbes in surviving intracellularly through a multitude of mechanisms. The chapter starts by describing the function of GSH in physiological processes. We then introduce several key ways by which GSH allows for increased control of intracellular infections through its influence on cells of the innate immune system, followed by a discussion of the immune-stimulating effects of GSH supplementation in T-cells, leading to improved control of *M. tuberculosis* infection inside monocytes and macrophages. Finally, we consider GSH in the context of Gram-negative and Gram-positive bacteria.

22.2 FUNCTIONS AND SYNTHESIS OF GSH

Human cells carry out a vast number of chemical reactions during their lifetime. Intracellular chemical reactions constantly leave produce reactive molecules that, left unchecked, would damage and even destroy the cellular environment. These reactive intermediates are neutralized through naturally occurring antioxidant molecules. GSH is an intracellular hydrosoluble antioxidant, composed of three amino acids: glycine, cysteine, and glutamate. It is ubiquitous in eukaryotes. Two forms of GSH exist in the cell cytoplasm: a reduced form, sometimes also called free form (rGSH), and an oxidized form called glutathione disulfide (GSSG). The reduced form of the amino acid cysteine contains a thiol group that bestows it with antioxidant activity only displayed by rGSH. During times of increased oxidative stress, rGSH works to neutralize reactive oxygen species (ROS) by means of its reactive sulfhydryl group. Once oxidized, thiol groups from two GSH molecules combine to form GSSG, which does not in itself hold any reducing power. There are enzymes, which will be discussed later, that reduce GSSG back to its antioxidant form, and the cycle starts anew. In this way, reactive byproducts of biochemical reactions are prevented from obliterating the cell's internal environment.

22.2.1 OVERVIEW OF THE FUNCTIONS OF GSH

As an agent against oxidative stress, GSH is indispensable if the cell is to maintain stability. Besides this key role in maintaining redox homeostasis, GSH is important for sustaining the normal function of the immune system. Decreased levels of GSH have been implicated in increased pathogenesis in many disease states and in infections (Morris et al. 2013c). Several studies have documented that different pathways imperative in protecting the host from various pathogens are disrupted when levels of GSH decrease. How GSH works to enhance the immune system can be quite complex, much like the immune system itself. It plays a key role as a major regulator of cytokine levels, which in turn regulates the host's response to trauma and infection (Morris et al. 2013c). As we will see, a decrease in GSH levels correlates with the demise of CD4+ T-cells in HIV infection, disrupting the cytokine equilibrium and promoting HIV progression (Herzenberg et al. 1997). Decreased levels of GSH are also correlated with activation of NF-κB (Lou and Kaplowitz 2007). This is fundamental in activating transcription of an HIV provirus (Hiscott, Kwon, and Génin 2001). GSH serves as a first line of defense against oxidative stress and is indispensable in its ability to restore redox balance and maintain stable immune cell functions.

22.2.2 GSH SYNTHESIS

GSH is a tripeptide. It can be synthesized de novo. Two steps are required for this process, and both are adenosine triphosphate (ATP) dependent (Alberts 2015). The first step is catalyzed by glutamate cysteine ligase (GCL). GCL covalently couples glutamate and cysteine to form γ-glutamylcysteine. The second step is catalyzed by the enzyme GSH synthetase (GSS). GSS links glycine to the γ-glutamylcysteine dipeptide formed by GCL. This leads to the formation of the functional GSH tripeptide. GSH levels are regulated by γ-glutamyltranspeptidase 1 (GGT) via a negative feedback mechanism.

GGT is a membrane-bound enzyme that enhances the disintegration of rGSH into cysteinyl-glycine and glutamate, making them available as raw materials that can be reused for synthesis of new GSH molecules (Dayaram et al. 2006).

During the process of detoxifying ROS, two molecules of GSH get converted to GSSG. This must then be reduced so GSH can be regenerated in the cell. This process involves three enzymes, one of which is GSH reductase (GSR). GSR reduces GSSG to rGSH using NADPH as a cofactor. During this process, NADPH gets oxidized to $NADP^+$.

22.3 THE IMMUNE SYSTEM: AN OVERVIEW

The innate immune system is the first line of defense against infections. It is preformed, nonspecific, and has a rapid onset with no memory generation. Components of innate immunity include the skin, antimicrobial peptides, natural killer (NK) cells, and phagocytic cells such as neutrophils and macrophages. The most abundant cells are the phagocytes, which internalize pathogens for intracellular killing (Owen et al. 2013). The destruction of the internalized pathogens is facilitated by ROS and reactive nitrogen intermediates (RNI). ROS include superoxide, hydroxyl radicals, singlet oxygen, and hydrogen peroxide, all oxygen derivatives. RNIs are metabolites of nitric oxide (NO), a potent reactive species with highly destructive potential (see Chapters 19 and 20). Although innate immunity is effective, it is not always sufficient to control microbial infections. For instance, certain organisms such as *M. tuberculosis*(*M. tb*) possess catalase, an enzyme that degrades hydrogen peroxide to render it ineffective (Owen et al. 2013). In such cases, the adaptive immune system must be recruited.

Beyond the cells and processes of the innate immune system, cells of adaptive immunity are highly specialized to counter the sophisticated mechanisms utilized by many pathogens. The adaptive immune system consists of T-cells and B-cells. Unlike the innate immune cells, these are not preformed and develop only after encountering a pathogen. They are very specific in their interactions with such pathogens, and they exhibit a characteristic memory, ascribing to them the ability to quickly increase in numbers upon future encounters, halting any significant pathogenic activity (Kindt et al. 2007).

The T-cells are associated with one of two markers: CD4 or CD8. Early in the development of T-cells, progenitor T-cells in the bone marrow migrate to the thymus to mature. The earliest T-cells express CD3, and after undergoing various steps of selection they become $CD4^+$ or $CD8^+$ T-cells (Owen et al. 2013). $CD4^+$ T-cells can be further divided into helper T-cells (Th) subsets, named Th1 or Th2, which develop depending on the signals they receive via polarizing cytokines. The Th1 subset produces cytokines that can significantly elevate inflammation, such as interleukin 2 (IL-2) and interferon gamma (IFN-γ). In contrast, the Th2 subset produces interleukin 4 (IL-4), interleukin 5 (IL-5), interleukin 6 (IL-6), and interleukin 10 (IL-10) (Kindt et al. 2007). T helper cells also secrete cytokines important for the stimulation of a B-cell response. It was once thought that Th2 subset of T-cells were the only major player in B-cell activation since most of the cytokines they secrete are involved in various stages of B-cell proliferation. We now know, however, that the influence of Th1 T-cells is just as much a part of this process. B-cells, while they share their importance with T-cells, are in some respect simpler cells. The primary function of the B-cell is to secrete antibodies. Antibodies are highly sensitive proteins that bind to surface molecules of pathogenic species, allowing the immune system to recognize their presence. T-cells and B-cells depend on each other to reach their full immunological potential. Cytokines secreted by T-cells help activate B-cells, and vice versa. The astounding power of the memory response is, in fact, only possible with appropriate interactions between these two cell types (Romagnani 2000).

22.4   GSH AND THE INNATE IMMUNE SYSTEM

22.4.1   MACROPHAGES AND NO

Macrophages are prominent phagocytic cells. They exhibit an inherent flexibility that allows them to alter their mechanisms of action according to the demands of the immune system. Macrophages are activated in response to infection, often by signals from antigen-specific immune cells. Direct contact with lipopolysaccharides (LPS) from Gram-negative bacteria will often be enough for activation, as will cytokines, such as interferon gamma (IFN-γ), released from distant cells (Trinchieri 1997). Once activated, macrophages can induce overpowering cellular damage. One mechanism commonly employed to exert such cytotoxic effects on the target pathogen is through the release of NO, which is so damaging to cell components that it leads to growth arrest, energy depletion, and death of the target cell (Fang and Vazquez-Torres 2002). GSH, hydrogen peroxide, and superoxide radicals enhance the cytotoxic and antimicrobial effects of NO (Morris et al. 2013b). A reactive gaseous metabolite that can readily cross cell membranes, NO has a short half-life that allows for a primarily local effect by which it is able to serve many roles in human physiology, including that of neurotransmitter, vasodilator, and many others (Owen et al. 2013). Given its properties, perhaps it is not surprising that NO is an effector molecule of the immune system. Numerous cells and tissues produce NO by an enzyme called NO synthase (NOS), which catalyzes a deamination reaction of the amino acid arginine (Alberts 2015). The importance of NO to macrophage activity is evidenced by the fact that levels of NOS in macrophages are not constant. Individuals with chronic disease or infection, such as tuberculosis (TB) and AIDS, show a higher expression of NOS when compared to healthy individuals. Studies comparing the levels among different populations indicate that an abundance of NOS in human macrophages varies among geographic regions as well. Healthy individuals in regions of Tanzania where malaria is endemic show a higher level of NOS when compared with healthy individuals in the United States (Butler and Nicholson 2003). The immunological benefit of NO can become a liability. An overproduction of NO is undoubtedly toxic. Past a safe threshold, NO leads to damage to the endothelial tissue of the vascular system (Palmer et al. 1992). NO has been shown to play a role in vascular collapse and is a potent factor in the mortality associated with septic shock (Kuhl and Rosen 1998). How is it that the human body can cope with daily high levels of NO in response to pathogens and injuries? Interestingly, intracellular NO levels are downregulated through a negative feedback loop by the same chemical species that enhances its effect: GSH (Jung et al. 2013).

22.4.2   GSNO: MORE POTENT THAN NO ALONE

While an unquestionably powerful antimicrobial agent, the limitations of NO are clear. A short half-life limits its effects while protecting host cells from widespread, uncontrolled destruction. As it turns out, host cells have evolved a particularly useful method of keeping NO in reserve for immediate, long-lasting effects, slow-release effects. In a process known as S-nitrosylation, GSH reacts with NO to form S-nitrosoglutathione (GSNO) (Venketaraman et al. 2005). GSNO acts as an NO donor, releasing it as needed by the cell. By virtue of GSNO, NO can be better spread throughout the body (Venketaraman et al. 2005). This innovative use of GSH proves particularly powerful during an infection, where macrophage activation utilizes massive quantities of NO (Fang and Vazquez-Torres 2002). The superior functions of GSNO are well evidenced, with studies indicating it has a cidal effect on *M. tuberculosis* (Dayaram et al. 2006). GSNO has also been found to protect against oxidative stress caused by peroxynitrite in the brain, as well as apoptosis induced by oxidative stress through induction of cyclic GMP-mediated synthesis of thioredoxin (Chiueh 2002). Both the destructive and protective functions of GSNO represent a more potent and stable mechanism through which the cell can utilize the powerful effects of NO in the immune system.

22.4.3 GSH and Dendritic Cells

Like macrophages, dendritic cells (DCs) are one of the most immediate effectors of innate immunity. Among the antigen presenting cells (APCs), they have the best intrinsic ability to trigger the host adaptive system. As phagocytic cells, they act through a myriad of signals to activate both the innate and adaptive immune systems (Kindt et al. 2007). The role of GSH in DCs is also important. Treating DCs infected with *M. tuberculosis* with GSH, for instance, seems to improve the control of intracellular growth of *M. tuberculosis* (Morris et al. 2013a). There are numerous ways by which this process occurs.

When *M. tuberculosis* infects the DC, the cell increases its production of IL-10 by threefold, having several downstream effects (Morris et al. 2013a). To begin with, IL-10 inhibits migration of APCs to the lymph nodes, where they can encounter antigens and employ their best antimicrobial strategies. IL-10 also induces the differentiation of T helper cells into the Th2 subset, with increased survival of the mycobacteria within the DC. The Th2 subset of Th cells increases production of IL-4 and IL-5, and the subsequent activation of B-cells amplifies the response, further allowing the bacteria to survive within the DC (Morris et al. 2013a).

Studies interested in the link between *M. tuberculosis*–infected DCs and GSH depletion found a reversal of this process with GSH supplementation, with an induction in the production of IL-12, a key cytokine triggering the differentiation of T helper cells to the Th1 subset, which is closely related to inhibition of *M. tuberculosis* (Morris et al. 2013a). Furthermore, GSH appears to increase expression of costimulatory molecules in DCs. Following infection, host DCs will reduce their expression of CD80 and CD86, in essence preventing T-cell stimulation and activation (Morris et al. 2013a). Binding of CD28 molecules on the cell surface of T-cells with their corresponding ligands CD80 and CD86 on the DC surface is critical for inducing T-cell stimulation and activation (Shi et al. 2008). Without these signals, the infection remains undetected. Importantly, GSH supplementation induces a 2.5-fold increase in the expressions of costimulatory molecules on the cell surface of DCs (Figure 22.1) (Morris et al. 2013a). Finally, GSH enhances the ability of DCs to induce proliferation of T-cells. In particular, DC cells treated with N-acetyl-cysteine (NAC), a reservoir for sulfhydryl groups used to study the effects of GSH, appear to induce increased proliferation of T-cells (Morris et al. 2013a). Moreover, NAC treatment can directly enhance the proliferative capacity of T-cells. The effects of GSH on DCs therefore result in increased expressions of costimulatory molecules and IL-12, as well as downregulation in the synthesis of IL-1 and IL-10 (Figure 22.1) (Morris et al. 2013a). From these studies, it is clear that GSH treatment provides DCs with an advantage in the defense against *M. tuberculosis*.

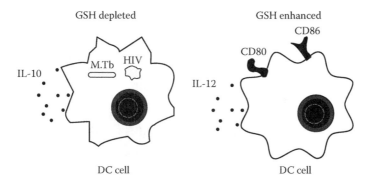

FIGURE 22.1 The effects of GSH treatment on DCs infected with *M. tuberculosis*. Costimulatory molecules CD80/CD86 are increased on the surface of DCs upon GSH treatment, enhancing cell stimulation and activation while inducing a switch in cytokine production from IL-10 to IL-12, thus stimulating a stronger Th1 cell response.

22.4.4 GSH AND NATURAL KILLER (NK) CELLS

During infection, NK cells act as inflammatory cytokine-producing cytotoxic lymphocytes (Freeman et al. 2015). They are especially equipped for protection against tumor formation and intracellular infection, as evident from literature on coculture studies conducted with *M. tuberculosis*–infected monocytes and NK cells (Guerra et al. 2012). As *M. tuberculosis* growth is overwhelmed by the infiltration of macrophages to the site of infection, a stasis effect occurs wherein the bacteria remain in a dormant state, but are not killed. It appears GSH has an important role in this process. The stasis effect on the growth of *M. tuberculosis* largely diminishes when NK cells are treated with agents that lower the levels of GSH, such as buthionine sulfoximine (BSO). As much as a fivefold increase in the intracellular growth of *M. tuberculosis* can be accounted for by GSH depletion in NK cells (Guerra et al. 2012).

The effect of GSH on NK cells is clearly quite significant, and is mediated through different pathways. NK cells, like many cells, express inhibitory receptors on their surface. These receptors act as signals that the system is not on alarm. The killer-cell immunoglobulin-like receptors (KIR), so called because of their evolutionary relationship to the immunoglobulin superfamily, can be exploited by virally infected and tumor cells, compromising their function by keeping the NK cell unaware of the ongoing threat in the external environment. NK cells also express killer activated receptors (KARs) that mediate the recognition and destruction of aberrant cells, making the process especially sensitive to detecting alarm signals initiated by other immune cells. Herein exists one of the beneficial effects of GSH. With costimulation by IL-2 and IL-12, GSH can successfully overcome the exploitation of KIRs by infected cells (Guerra et al. 2012). Increasing GSH levels in NK cells from healthy subjects upregulates the expression of KARs, thereby allowing the NK cell to recognize the infection and act accordingly (Figure 22.2) (Guerra et al. 2012).

The second mechanism by which GSH enhances NK cells is also noteworthy. In addition to KIRs and KARs, NK cells express a number of other molecules on their surface that enhance their antimicrobial abilities. One of these is FasL, which is largely characteristic of CTLs but also expressed on NK cells (Owen et al. 2013). FasL binds to Fas on compromised cells and induces apoptosis in aberrant cells such as those infected with *M. tuberculosis* or compromised by cancer. Another receptor called CD40L is also present on NK cells and activates APCs to carry out very important steps in the thwarting of infections, such as cytokine release and B-cell activation. While a causative mechanism has yet to be elucidated, treating NK cells with GSH is highly correlated with increased expression of FasL and CD40L and inhibition of *M. tuberculosis* growth (Figure 22.2) (Guerra et al 2012).

As a side note, KIRs are also expressed by T lymphocytes, where they can facilitate the development of autoimmune responses (Björkström et al. 2012). The redundancy can be exploited by mechanisms that enhance the production of GSH, preventing a harmful attack on the body against itself.

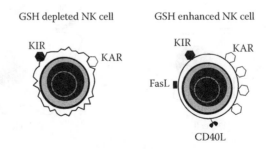

FIGURE 22.2 GSH and NK cells. Treatment of NK cells with GSH upregulates the expression of KARs, overpowering compromised functions of KIRs on the NK cell surface. Increased surface expression of FasL and CD40L with GSH treatment further enhances the effector activities of the NK cells.

22.5   GSH AND THE ADAPTIVE IMMUNE SYSTEM

22.5.1   GSH AND T HELPER CELLS

T helper cells are regulators of the type of adaptive response the immune system will develop. Cytokines produced by DCs, macrophages, and NK cells work in concert to direct a T-cell response during infection. In *M. tuberculosis*, and HIV and other viral infections, a Th1 response should predominate with an increase in proinflammatory cytokines (Romagnani 2000). GSH deficiency or depletion appears to decrease production of proinflammatory cytokines while redirecting the immune system to a Th2-mediated response, one poorly suited for dealing with intracellular invasion (Vera Tudela and Singh 2014) (Figure 22.3). However, GSH treatment has the opposite effect, leading to increased production of proinflammatory cytokines like IL-12, IL-2, and IFN-γ (Figure 22.4) (Herzenberg et al. 1997). Meanwhile, IL-10, IL-4, and IL-6 would likely be decreased. The mechanisms by which GSH induces such effects are largely unknown.

22.5.2   GSH IN HIV INFECTION

The recognition of GSH as a powerful activator of adaptive immunity can be seen best in the context of the challenge facing an estimated 35 million people worldwide: HIV (Fettig et al. 2014). Aptly named due to its potent effect on reducing the power of the immune system, HIV can lead to an abrupt collapse of the defenses of the host. The success of antiretroviral treatments has reduced the deaths from HIV since its discovery in 1985, and the role of GSH supplementation in HIV infection has promising implications. While many oxidative pathways, including those associated with other pathogens, deplete the levels of GSH, there are compensatory mechanisms that replenish it, returning the state to its homeostatic levels (Lushchak 2012). Usually, these are enough. However, the levels of immunosuppression resulting from HIV infection are drastic and the built-in mechanisms for repleting GSH are largely insufficient. HIV infection, whether directly or indirectly, diminishes the ability of GSH to restore homeostasis. HIV infection leads to massive free radical production in the body, depleting the levels of GSH and maintaining a state of oxidative stress (Morris et al. 2012). HIV also depletes GCL, the rate-limiting step in *de novo* synthesis of intracellular GSH (Morris et al. 2012). Chronic infection with HIV appears to lead to a chronic state of inflammation and elevated free radical formation, which may also promote elevated expression of GSR (Morris et al. 2012). Evidence suggests the depletion of GCL may be attributed to HIV-induced overexpression of TGF-β (Lotz and Seth 1993). Furthermore, TGF-β can also enhance the degradation of GCL (Morris et al. 2012). Thus, through misdirecting cytokine production and GSH depletion, it appears

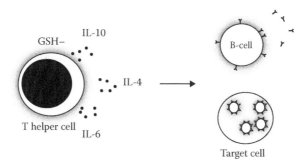

FIGURE 22.3   GSH depletion and adaptive immunity in HIV infection. HIV redirects T helper cells to produce cytokines that augment a B-cell response inappropriate for HIV destruction. With depletion of GSH and increased production of IL-10, IL-4, and IL-6, the immune response is poorly equipped to destroy intracellular virus particles.

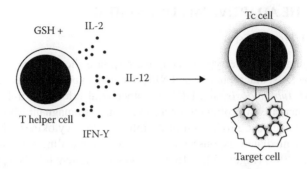

FIGURE 22.4 GSH supplementation and adaptive immunity ion HIV infection. GSH supplementation reverses the effects induced by HIV, allowing the immune system to mount a more robust Th1 response that can appropriately destroy infected cells, giving the host cells an advantage over the virus.

HIV induces a continuous cycle of oxidative stress that further compromises the immune system of the host.

Supplementation with liposome-formulated GSH may reverse these outcomes. The effects of GSH on NK cells, DCs, and T-cells, described in the previous sections, all appear to aid the immune system in HIV infection much as they do in *M. tuberculosis* infection. Because GSH can downregulate production of TGF-β3, it can restore the *de novo* synthesis of GCL, also effective in thwarting tuberculosis infection (Morris et al. 2012). Inhibiting TGF-β3 expression in general has an immune-stimulating effect: enhancing the production of proinflammatory cytokines, particularly through the action of IL-12, is a powerful mechanism to improve control of intracellular infections (Venketaraman 2011).

22.5.3 GSH and Tregs

While T helper cells are the best known (and best understood) T-cells, GSH enhancement in other T-cell subsets has led to promising discoveries. Regulatory T-cells (Tregs) have important functions in immunity. They produce cytokines that increase the differentiation of T helper cells to Th2, increasing production of IL-10 and TGF-β (Garba et al. 2002). Indeed, levels of these cytokines produced from monocytes derived from infection with *M. tuberculosis* are highly correlated to a higher mycobacterial growth rate (Trinchieri 1997). Just as GSH decreases the production of IL-10 in DCs, it appears to have a similar affect in Tregs (Morris et al. 2013). NAC-supplemented Treg cultures show a downregulation in the levels of IL-10 and TGF-β (Morriset al. 2013).

22.5.4 GSH in Tuberculosis

After alveolar macrophages internalize mycobacterium bacilli following droplet inhalation, *M. tuberculosis* infection escapes the normal bactericidal mechanisms employed by the macrophage, enhancing its survival. The control of TB has been complicated by evolution of multidrug-resistant strains and an increase in coinfection with HIV. To successfully control *M. tuberculosis* innate and adaptive immune responses are both important. Decreased GSH levels may help the mycobacteria survive. During active TB infection, blood samples show a significant decrease in GSH levels in blood components including peripheral blood mononuclear cells (PBMCs), red blood cells (RBCs) and plasma, especially with concurrent HIV infection (Venketaraman et al. 2006). Like in HIV, a decrease in proinflammatory cytokines and GSH synthesis allows *M. tuberculosis* to survive intracellularly.

As mentioned earlier, GSNO can act as a reserve of potent bactericidal NO. GSH has a role in enhancing Th1 CD4+ T lymphocyte activation of macrophages via IFN-γ, and through receptor mediated cell death using FASL/CD40L by NK cells. Additionally, GSH may have other functions. In mycobacteria infection, GSH can itself be an innate effector of the immune system (Connell and Venketaraman 2009). How can GSH, a molecule with potent antioxidant roles in cellular physiology, act as a bacteriostatic agent directly? Interestingly, the GSH molecule is structurally not much different from prototypical chemotherapeutics on the market today (Connell and Venketaraman 2009). Structural similarities exist between GSH and antibiotic precursors of penicillin produced in fungi; a beta lactam form of GSH, named glutacilin, is a conceivable conversion product (Connell and Venketaraman 2009). Another possibility is an imbalance in levels of GSH and bacterial alternative thiol containing antioxidants, such as mycothiol. Unlike GSNO, GSH can inhibit bacterial infection without killing the bacteria (Connell and Venketaraman 2009).

22.5.5 GSH in Type II Diabetes Mellitus

Retrospective studies show that individuals with type II diabetes mellitus (T2DM) appear two to three times more susceptible to *M. tuberculosis* infection than those without this condition (Lagman et al. 2015). Experiments have documented increased free radical production in red blood cells from patients with T2DM, which may be due to a substantial decrease in the level of the enzymes of GSH biosynthesis in T2DM (Lagman et al. 2015). The mechanism thought to be responsible appears at least in part relate to the actions of TGF-β, which is also found in increased levels in individuals with T2DM (Herder et al. 2009). A concurrent decrease in GSH-synthetic enzymes is quite suggestive of a causative link, albeit not yet well established. As mentioned previously, GGT is a membrane-bound enzyme that acts in a recycling pathway for GSH. Further observations suggest decreased levels of GGT in red blood cells from T2DM individuals, further indicating the significance of GSH depletion in the connection between T2DM and *M. tuberculosis* infection (Lagman et al. 2015).

22.6 GSH AND OTHER BACTERIA

Unlike in eukaryotes, GSH is not ubiquitous in prokaryotes (Masip, Veeravalli, and Georgiou 2006). With the exception of cyanobacteria and proteobacteria, most bacterial species utilize alternative thiols in the place of GSH (Masip, Veeravalli, and Georgiou 2006). The mechanism by which some bacterial species synthesize GSH varies. In *E. coli*, the inducing factor for GSH synthesis is oxidative stress (Carmel-Harel and Storz 2000). Importantly, other bacteria use GSH to aid infection and virulence. *Francisella tularensis*, for instance, obtains GSH from the cytosol of macrophages, allowing it to acquire cysteine for intracellular growth and survival (Alkhuder et al. 2009). *Treponema denticola* utilizes GSH to synthesize hydrogen sulfide, which is deleterious to the surrounding tissues such as gums (Chu et al. 2002). *Streptococcus pyogenes* may require GSH to combat oxidative stress, increasing its virulence (Brenot et al. 2004).

22.7 SUMMARY

Mammalian cells rely on the antioxidant properties of GSH to carry out a number of redox reactions without irreversibly disrupting the equilibrium. The immune system relies on cells and cytokines to function properly, and aptly adapts itself to the demands of the host to abolish threats to itself, be it in the form of injury, infection, or cancer. Throughout this chapter, the role of GSH was discussed with emphasis on its significance and functions in infection and immunity. A variety of evidence indicates that decreased GSH levels are significantly correlated with decreased immunity in a variety of infections, *M. tuberculosis* and HIV prime among them. In T2DM, depleted GSH levels may increase the susceptibility to *M. tuberculosis* infection, where decreases in the important GSH-synthetic enzymes GCL, GSS, and GGT are likely responsible. GSH supplementation can be a powerful instrument in strengthening the immune system against infection. Macrophages rely on production of NO to combat phagocytosed entities, but a short half-life limits its potential antimicrobial defense. GSNO, a complex formed from GSH and NO, can act for longer and may be better than NO alone. GSH is directly toxic to mycobacteria and can serve as an effector mechanism by which macrophages and DCs can better control *M. tuberculosis* infection. GSH also has immune-enhancing effects on NK and T-cells, with concurrently improved control of *M. tuberculosis* infection inside phagocytic cells. In NK cells, GSH upregulates the expression of KARs, overcoming compromised KIR receptors that would keep the pathogen from being recognized. In T-cells, GSH regulates cytokine levels produced by the T helper cell lineage to support a strong Th1 response necessary for dealing with intracellular pathogens like HIV and *M. tuberculosis*. In T2DM, GSH restores the innate immune response to *M. tuberculosis*, conceivably through restoration of appropriate enzyme levels important for GSH synthesis. It is evident that GSH plays a part in numerous immunological pathways and processes. Further understanding of the molecular mechanisms by which GSH enhances the immune system will have powerful applications in the future of healthcare and medicine.

REFERENCES

Alberts, B. (2015). *Molecular Biology of the Cell* (6th ed.). New York, NY: Garland Science, Taylor & Francis.

Alkhuder, K., K. L. Meibom, I. Dubail, M. Dupuis, and A. Charbit (2009). Glutathione provides a source of cysteine essential for intracellular multiplication of Francisella tularensis. *PLoS Pathog* 5, e1000284.

Björkström, N. K., V. Béziat, F. Cichocki, L. L. Liu, J. Levine, S. Larsson, R. A. Koup, S. K. Anderson, H.-G. Ljunggren, and K.-J. Malmberg (2012). CD8 T cells express randomly selected KIRs with distinct specificities compared with NK cells. *Blood* 120, 3455–3465.

Brenot, A., K. Y. King, B. Janowiak, O. Griffith, and M. G. Caparon (2004). Contribution of glutathione peroxidase to the virulence of Streptococcus pyogenes. *Infect Immun* 72, 408–413.

Butler, A. and R. Nicholson (2003). *Life, Death, and Nitric Oxide*. Cambridge: RSC.

Carmel-Harel, O. and G. Storz (2000). Roles of the glutathione- and thioredoxin-dependent reduction systems in the Escherichia coli and Saccharomyces cerevisiae responses to oxidative stress. *Annu Rev Microbiol* 54, 439–461.

Chiueh, C. C. (2002). S-nitrosoglutathione (GSNO) mediates brain response to hypoxia. *Pediatr Res* 51, 414.

Chu, L., Z. Dong, X. Xu, D. L. Cochran, and J. L. Ebersole (2002). Role of glutathione metabolism of Treponema denticola in bacterial growth and virulence expression. *Infect Immun* 70, 1113–1120.

Connell, N. D. and V. Venketaraman (2009). Control of mycobacterium tuberculosis infection by glutathione. *Recent Pat Antiinfect Drug Discov* 4, 214–226.

Dayaram, Y. K., M. T. Talaue, N. D. Connell, and V. Venketaraman (2006). Characterization of a glutathione metabolic mutant of Mycobacterium tuberculosis and its resistance to glutathione and nitrosoglutathione. *J Bacteriol* 188, 1364–1372.

Fang, F. C. and A. Vazquez-Torres (2002). Nitric oxide production by human macrophages: There's no doubt about it. *Am J Physiol Lung Cell Mol Physiol* 282, L941–L943.

Fettig, J., M. Swaminathan, C. S. Murrill, and J. E. Kaplan (2014). Global epidemiology of HIV. *Infect Dis Clin North Am* 28, 323–337.

Freeman, B. E., H. P. Raué, A. B. Hill, and M. K. Slifka (2015). Cytokine-mediated activation of NK cells during viral infection. *J Virol* 89, 7922–7931.

Garba, M. L., C. D. Pilcher, A. L. Bingham, J. Eron, and J. A. Frelinger (2002). HIV antigens can induce TGF-beta(1)-producing immunoregulatory CD8(+) T cells. *J Immunol* 168(5), 2247–2254.

Guerra, C., K. Johal, D. Morris, S. Moreno, O. Alvarado, D. Gray, M. Tanzil, D. Pearce, and V. Venketaraman (2012). Control of Mycobacterium tuberculosis growth by activated natural killer cells. *Clin Exp Immunol* 168, 142–152.

Herder, C., A. Zierer, W. Koenig, M. Roden, C. Meisinger, and B. Thorand (2009). Transforming growth factor-beta1 and incident type 2 diabetes: Results from the MONICA/KORA case-cohort study, 1984–2002. *Diabetes Care* 32, 1921–1923.

Herzenberg, L. A., S. C. DeRosa, J. G. Dubs, M. Roederer, M. T. Anderson, S. W. Ela, S. C. Deresinski, and L. A. Herzenberg (1997). Glutathione deficiency is associated with impaired survival in HIV disease. *Proc Natl Acad Sci U S A* 94, 1967–1972.

Hiscott, J., H. Kwon, and P. Génin (2001). Hostile takeovers: Viral appropriation of the NF-kappaB pathway. *J Clin Invest* 107, 143–151.

Jung, J.-Y., R. Madan-Lala, M. Georgieva, J. Rengarajan, C. D. Sohaskey, F.-C. Bange, and C. M. Robinson (2013). The intracellular environment of human macrophages that produce nitric oxide promotes growth of mycobacteria. *Infect Immun* 81, 3198–3209.

Kindt, T. J., R. A. Goldsby, B. A. Osborne, and J. Kuby (2007). *Kuby Immunology* (6th ed.). New York, NY: W.H. Freeman.

Kuhl, S. J. and H. Rosen (1998). Nitric oxide and septic shock. From bench to bedside. *West J Med* 168, 176–181.

Lagman, M., J. Ly, T. Saing, M. Kaur Singh, E. Vera Tudela, D. Morris, P. T. Chi, C. Ochoa, A. Sathananthan, and V. Venketaraman (2015). Investigating the causes for decreased levels of glutathione in individuals with type II diabetes. *PLOS ONE* 10, e0118436.

Lotz, M. and P. Seth (1993). TGF beta and HIV infection. *Ann N Y Acad Sci* 685, 501–511.

Lou, H. and N. Kaplowitz (2007). Glutathione depletion down-regulates tumor necrosis factor alpha-induced nf-kappab activity via ikappab kinase-dependent and -independent mechanisms. *J Biol Chem* 282, 29470–29481.

Lushchak, V. I. (2012). Glutathione homeostasis and functions: Potential targets for medical interventions. *J Amino Acids* 2012, 736837

Masip, L., K. Veeravalli, and G. Georgiou (2006). The many faces of glutathione in bacteria. *Antioxid Redox Signal* 8, 753–762.

Morris, D., B. Gonzalez, M. Khurasany, C. Kassissa, J. Luong, S. Kasko, S. Pandya, M. Chu, P.-T. Chi, S. Bui, C. Guerra, J. Chan, and V. Venketaraman (2013a). Characterization of dendritic cell and regulatory T cell functions against mycobacterium tuberculosis infection. *Biomed Res Int* 2013, 402827.

Morris, D., C. Guerra, C. Donohue, H. Oh, M. Khurasany, and V. Venketaraman (2012). Unveiling the mechanisms for decreased glutathione in individuals with HIV infection. *Clin Dev Immunol* 2012, 734125.

Morris, D., C. Guerra, M. Khurasany, F. Guilford, B. Saviola, Y. Huang, and V. Venketaraman (2013b). Glutathione supplementation improves macrophage functions in HIV. *J Interferon Cytokine Res* 33, 270–279.

Morris, D., T. Nguyen, J. Kim, C. Kassissa, M. Khurasany, J. Luong, S. Kasko, S. Pandya, M. Chu, P. T. Chi, J. Ly, M. Lagman, and V. Venketaraman (2013c). An elucidation of neutrophil functions against mycobacterium tuberculosis infection. *Clin Dev Immunol* 2013, 959650.

Owen, J. A., J. Punt, S. A. Stranford, P. P. Jones, and J. Kuby (2013). *Kuby immunology* (7th ed.). New York, NY: W.H. Freeman.

Palmer, R. M., L. Bridge, N. A. Foxwell, and S. Moncada (1992). The role of nitric oxide in endothelial cell damage and its inhibition by glucocorticoids. *Br J Pharmacol* 105, 11–12.

Romagnani, S. (2000). T-cell subsets (Th1 versus Th2). *Ann Allergy Asthma Immunol* 85, 9–18.

Shi, Z., M. Rifa'i, Y. H. Lee, H. Shiku, K. I. Isobe, and H. Suzuki (2008). Importance of CD80/CD86-CD28 interactions in the recognition of target cells by CD8+CD122+ regulatory T cells. *Immunology* 124, 121–128.

Trinchieri, G. (1997). Cytokines acting on or secreted by macrophages during intracellular infection (IL-10, IL-12, IFN-gamma). *Curr Opin Immunol* 9, 17–23.

Venketaraman, V. (2011). Role of cytokines and chemokines in *HIV infection. In HIV and AIDS—Updates on Biology, Immunology, Epidemiology and Treatment Strategies,* Dumais, N. (Ed.).

Venketaraman, V., Y. K. Dayaram, M. T. Talaue, and N. D. Connell (2005). Glutathione and nitrosoglutathione in macrophage defense against mycobacterium tuberculosis. *Infect Immun* 73, 1886–1889.

Venketaraman, V., T. Rodgers, R. Linares, N. Reilly, S. Swaminathan, D. Hom, A. C. Millman, R. Wallis, and N. D. Connell (2006). Glutathione and growth inhibition of mycobacterium tuberculosis in healthy and HIV infected subjects. *AIDS Res Ther* 3, 5.

Vera Tudela, E. and M. Singh (2014). Cytokine levels in plasma samples of individuals with HIV infection. *Austin J Clin Immunol* 1, 5.

23 Dietary Nucleotides and Immunity

Luis Fontana, Olga Martínez-Augustin, and Ángel Gil

CONTENTS

23.1 Introduction 387
23.2 Sources of Dietary Nucleotides 388
23.3 Digestion, Absorption, and Metabolic Fate of Dietary Nucleotides 388
    23.3.1 Absorption of Dietary Nucleotides 388
    23.3.2 Nucleotide Degradation 389
        23.3.2.1 Purine Nucleotide Catabolism 389
        23.3.2.2 Pyrimidine Nucleotide Catabolism 389
        23.3.2.3 Undegraded Bases 390
23.4 Role of Dietary Nucleotides in Immunity 391
    23.4.1 Nucleotide Effects on Lymphocyte Maturation, Activation, and Proliferation 392
    23.4.2 Dietary Nucleotides and Lymphocyte Subpopulations 394
    23.4.3 Modulation of the Macrophage Phagocytic Activity by Dietary Nucleotides 394
    23.4.4 Nucleotide Modulation of the Delayed Hypersensitivity and Allograft and
        Tumor Responses 395
    23.4.5 Modulation of Immunoglobulin Production by Nucleotides 395
    23.4.6 Dietary Nucleotides and Defense against Infection 398
23.5 Nucleotides and Intestinal Inflammation 398
23.6 Potential Mechanism of Action of Dietary Nucleotides 399
References 401

23.1 INTRODUCTION

Nucleotides are ubiquitous, low molecular weight intracellular compounds with considerable structural diversity. They comprise three joined structures: a nitrogenous base, a pentose sugar, and at least one phosphate group. The most common nucleotides can be divided into two groups, purines and pyrimidines, based on the structure of the nitrogenous base. The pentose sugar that binds the base and phosphate within the compound is either ribose or deoxyribose. Ribonucleotides signify those purine or pyrimidine nucleotides linked by ribose, where the purine bases are adenine (A), guanine (G), or inosine (I), while the pyrimidine bases are cytosine (C), uracil (U), or thymine (T). Nucleotides, primarily as components of nucleoproteins, but also as free nucleotides and nucleic acids, are naturally present in all foods of animal and vegetable origin, although their concentration varies greatly between foods (Gil 2002). The nutritional requirement for nucleotides in humans has long been recognized, but nucleotides have not generally been regarded as essential given that *de novo* synthesis and salvage pathways exist in animals, including humans (Traut 2014). Accordingly, the requirement in humans is categorized as "conditionally essential" (van Buren and Rudolph 1997; Carver 1999). The essentiality of ribonucleotides is apparent during the following conditions: rapid growth, malnutrition, infection, or injury (Rudolph et al. 1990; Uauy et al. 1996; Carver 1999). This chapter reviews what is known about nucleotides, immunity, and infection, and draws from studies in both experimental animal models and in human infants.

23.2 SOURCES OF DIETARY NUCLEOTIDES

Exogenous nucleotides are widely distributed in foods, especially those containing cellular elements and nucleoproteins (proteins conjugated with nucleic acids). Such foods include organ meats and seafood (Kojima 1974; Clifford and Story 1976; Barness 1994). Muscle protein is thought to be a relatively poor source of nucleotides as it is comprised mainly of actin-myosin protein (Devresse 2000). Human breast milk has been shown to contain significant concentrations of nucleotides, with profiles and concentrations substantially different from bovine milk (Gil and Sanchez-Medina 1982; Oddy 2002). Numerous studies on preterm and full-term neonates reliant on infant formulas containing supplemental nucleotides as the only alimentary source have demonstrated clear benefits in relation to improved immunity (see meta-analysis by Gutiérrez-Castrellón et al. 2007). Given that single-cell proteins (SCPs) have nucleic acid levels that are around seven times higher than meats (Ingledew 1999), yeasts provide a good source of nucleotides (Tibetts 1999; Li et al. 2007). Thus, industrially produced baker's yeast or brewer's yeast (*Saccharomyces cerevisiae*) has been shown to provide a particularly good source for commercial production of supplemental nucleotides. Commercially available 5'-nucleotides for supplemental use, or addition to infant formulae, include, in particular, AMP (adenosine 5'-monophosphate), GMP (guanine 5'-monophosphate), IMP (inosine 5'-monophosphate), UMP (uracil 5'-monophosphate), and CMP (cytosine 5'-monophosphate).

23.3 DIGESTION, ABSORPTION, AND METABOLIC FATE OF DIETARY NUCLEOTIDES

The absorption and degradation of nucleotides as well as their dephosphorylated forms, nucleosides, have been well established in a diverse range of species, including humans. Uric acid, obtained by oxidation of xanthine, is the final product of purine metabolism in humans, primates, birds, some reptiles, and the majority of insects—such species are referred to as *uricotelics*, since they all excrete uric acid into the urine. In other mammals, given the name *allantoinotelics*, uric acid is degraded by the enzyme uricase (urate oxygen oxidoreductase) to allantoin and carbon dioxide. Moreover, a number of teleostean fish excrete allantoic acid, as allantoin is hydrolyzed by allantoin amidohydrolase. Selacean fish, dipneusta, as well as some teleosteans and batracians, can degrade allantoic acid by allantoate ureohydrolase rendering two molecules of urea and one molecule of glyoxilic acid; (Gil 1984). As a uricotelic species, the products of pyrimidine nucleotide catabolism are harmless (e.g., beta-aminoisobutyrate) or indeed beneficial (e.g., carnosine, anserine, and beta-alanine). While urate (uric acid) is always produced in the body and excreted via the urine, very high intakes of purine nucleotides and purine-rich foods contribute to high serum levels, which can in turn lead to hyperuricemia (excess uric acid in the blood). This condition may cause the precipitation of urate crystals in the blood, tissue, and joints (gout). These mechanisms are described below.

23.3.1 ABSORPTION OF DIETARY NUCLEOTIDES

The three principal features of nucleotide metabolism in humans are (a) *de novo* synthesis from metabolites such as glutamine, aspartate, and glycine, particularly in the liver; (b) salvage from RNA and DNA degradation; and (c) exogenous intake from dietary sources (Grimble and Westwood 2001). There are many factors that control the relative importance of each of these processes in maintaining the body's pool of nucleotides and nucleosides, and the relative contribution of *de novo* and salvage pathways appears to vary both in different tissues and at different phases of the cell cycle (Fairbanks et al. 1999; Grimble et al. 2000; Grimble and Westwood 2001). The exogenous supply of nucleotides is thought to be particularly important in the case of high turnover tissues and cells, such as those growing rapidly or those associated with immunity.

Enterocytes, the terminally differentiated cells of the intestinal epithelium, may be particularly dependent on an exogenous supply of nucleotides in the diet, although hepatic *de novo* synthesis may provide some additional support (Grimble 1996).

Dietary nucleotides have a limited capacity for absorption in the intestinal tract (Sanderson and He 1994), possibly as a result of the lack of a nucleotide transport system and the presence of negatively charged phosphate groups, which hinder absorption (Mateo 2005). However, following dephosphorylation and conversion to nucleosides, they are well absorbed and metabolized. As a result, nucleosides are the major bioavailable form of purines and pyrimidines absorbed into gut epithelial cells. Both purine and pyrimidine nucleosides are actively absorbed through four concentrative gut Na^+-dependent transporters, and they are also absorbed passively through two equilibrative transporters, which exhibit different specificities for purine and pyrimidine derivatives (Ngo et al. 2001; Scharrer et al. 2002). Based on studies on rats, uptake appears to be dependent on diffusion and specific sodium ion–dependent, carrier-mediated mechanisms (Bronk and Hastewell 1987) and more than 90% of dietary and endogenous nucleosides and bases are taken up in the enterocyte (Salati et al. 1984; Uauy 1989). Metabolites are then available to the various salvage pathways that result in the resynthesis of nucleotides for the body's specific required pool (Rolfes 2006).

23.3.2 Nucleotide Degradation

The following subsection is based on material from Swanson et al. (2006) and Angstadt (1997).

23.3.2.1 Purine Nucleotide Catabolism

In the degradation of purine nucleotides, phosphate and ribose are removed first, then the nitrogenous bases are oxidized. The end product of purine catabolism in humans is uric acid, which is excreted in urine via the kidneys. Owing to the presence of the enzyme urate oxidase in most other mammals, the more soluble allantoin is the end product.

Guanine nucleotides are hydrolyzed to the nucleoside guanosine, which undergoes phosphorolysis to guanine and ribose 1-P. However, since intracellular nucleotidases are not very active against AMP in humans, AMP is deaminated by the enzyme adenylate (AMP) deaminase to IMP. In the catabolism of purine nucleotides, IMP is further degraded by hydrolysis with nucleotidase to inosine and then phosphorolysis to hypoxanthine.

Both adenine and guanine nucleotides converge at the common intermediate xanthine. Hypoxanthine, representing the original adenine, is oxidized to xanthine by the enzyme xanthine oxidase. Guanine is deaminated, with the amino group released as ammonia, to xanthine. If this process is occurring in tissues other than liver, most of the ammonia will be transported to the liver as glutamine for ultimate excretion as urea.

Xanthine, like hypoxanthine, is oxidized by oxygen and xanthine oxidase with the production of hydrogen peroxide. In humans, the urate is excreted and the hydrogen peroxide is degraded by catalase. Xanthine oxidase is present in significant concentration only in the liver and intestine. The pathway to the nucleosides, possibly to the free bases, is present in many tissues.

These catabolic pathways for purine nucleotides are shown in Figure 23.1.

23.3.2.2 Pyrimidine Nucleotide Catabolism

Pyrimidines, in contrast to purines, undergo ring cleavage and the usual end products of catabolism are beta-amino acids, ammonia, and carbon dioxide. Pyrimidines sourced either from nucleic acids or the body's energy pool are catabolized by nucleotidases and pyrimidine nucleoside phosphorylase

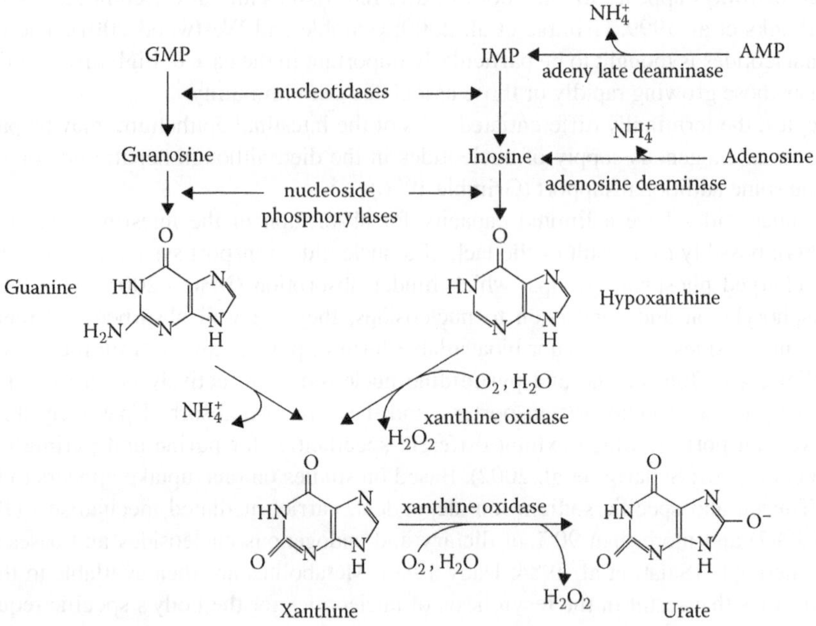

FIGURE 23.1 Typical catabolic pathways of purine nucleotides in humans.

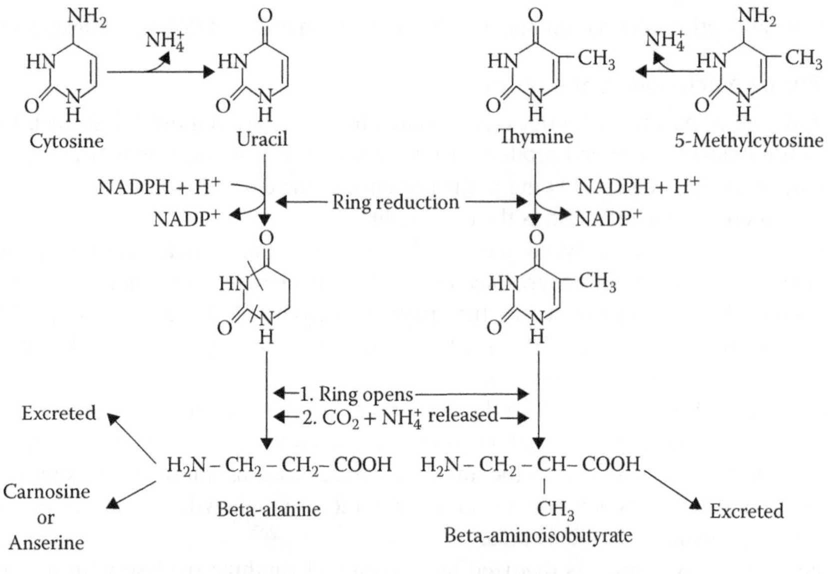

FIGURE 23.2 Typical catabolic pathways of pyrimidine nucleotides in humans.

to yield the free bases. The 4-amino group of both cytosine and 5-methyl cytosine is released as ammonia. These pathways of pyrimidine nucleotide catabolism are shown in Figure 23.2.

23.3.2.3 Undegraded Bases

Purine and pyrimidine bases that are not degraded are recycled through a range of salvage pathways and are so resynthesized as nucleotides (Rolfes 2006). This recycling, however, is not sufficient to meet total body requirements under all conditions and, accordingly, some *de novo* synthesis is essential. *De novo* synthesis of both purine and pyrimidine nucleotides occurs from readily available components (Traut 2014).

23.4 ROLE OF DIETARY NUCLEOTIDES IN IMMUNITY

Although nucleotide deficiency has not been related to any particular disease, dietary nucleotides have been reported to be beneficial for infants, since they positively influence lipid metabolism and immunity, as well as tissue growth, development, and repair (Carver and Walker 1995; Sanchez-Pozo et al. 1999; Gil 2001). Taken together, the existing evidence indicates that dietary nucleotides may enhance the maturation of the immune and gastrointestinal tracts in infants (Carver and Stromquist 2006).

Rapidly proliferating tissues, such as the immune system or the intestine, are not able to fulfill the needs of cell nucleotides exclusively by *de novo* synthesis and they preferentially utilize the salvage pathway, recovering nucleosides and nucleobases from blood and diet. In accordance to this, the intestine is able to hydrolyze RNA and free nucleotides to nucleosides, which are efficiently absorbed by the enterocytes, with the exception of cytidine (Figures 23.3 and 23.4) (Gil et al. 2007). An exogenous supplement of these compounds through the diet may be essential to sustain intestinal growth and to maintain the cellular function in these tissues (Carver and Walker 1995; Uauy et al. 1996).

Nowadays it is well known that the gastrointestinal tract has not only the role of absorbing nutrients but also of protecting the body from potentially pathologic organisms while, at the same time, ensuring tolerance to commensal bacteria, food antigens, and self-antigens (Mason et al. 2008). The protective defenses of the gastrointestinal tract include physical barriers (glycocalyx and intestinal epithelium), antimicrobial compounds, and specialized immune responses (Mason et al. 2008). A significant proportion of the gastrointestinal tract comprises immune cells (mainly T and B lymphocytes, macrophages, and dendritic cells) (see Chapter 2), and even intestinal epithelial cells produce immunomodulatory molecules such as cytokines to regulate the immune function (Walker 1996).

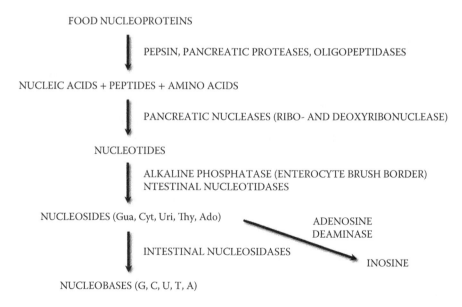

FIGURE 23.3 Digestion of dietary nucleotides. A, adenine; Ado, adenosine; C, cytidine; Cyt, cytosine; DNA, deoxyribonucleic acid; G, guanine; Gua, guanosine; RNA, ribonucleic acid; T, thymine; Thy, thymidine; U, uracil; Uri, uridine.

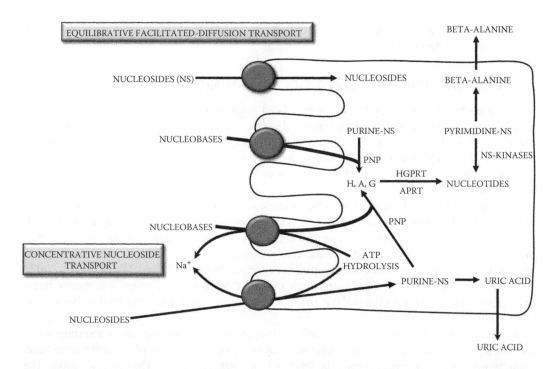

FIGURE 23.4 Absorption of dietary nucleotides. Equilibrative and concentrative nucleoside transporters are responsible for the absorption of nucleosides and, to a lesser extent, nucleobases. Inside the enterocyte, pyrimidine nucleotides are directly synthesized after phosphorylation of pyrimidine nucleosides, namely uridine. This reaction is catalyzed by nucleoside-kinases. In turn, purine nucleosides are first degraded to free bases by the purine phoshorylase (PNP), and then they enter the salvage pathway in which the hypoxanthine-guanine phosphoribosyltransferase (HGPRT) catalyzes the synthesis of nucleotides. Purine nucleosides can also be degraded to uric acid in the enterocyte. A, adenine; ATP, adenosinetriphosphate; G, guanine; H, hipoxantine; NS, nucleosides.

The newborn immune system is relatively immature at least during the first year of life when the levels of IgA and IgG to viral or bacterial pathogens are reduced (Schaller et al. 2007). The delay in innate; acquired immune function in newborns is, however, compensated by in utero transfer of specific IgG and with specific factors present in human milk among which lipids, mucin, oligosaccharides, pathogen-specific antibodies, or nucleotides are included (Schaller et al. 2007). These nutrients influence the maturation of immune cells especially at weanling.

The development and maintenance of the immune tolerance starts very early in life, even prenatally. Tolerance is characterized by the polarization of T helper (Th) cells towards Th2 and T regulatory (Treg) phenotypes, together with a suppression of the Th1 response (Mason et al. 2008; Calder et al. 2006). Oral tolerance is characterized by the production of TGF-β and IL-10 by Treg cells, and IL-3, IL-4, IL-5, and IL-13 by Th2 lymphocytes. The production of TGF-β, IL-4, and IL-5 increases the production of secretory IgA (sIgA).

23.4.1 NUCLEOTIDE EFFECTS ON LYMPHOCYTE MATURATION, ACTIVATION, AND PROLIFERATION

The terminal deoxynucleotidyl transferase (TdT) enzyme has been referred as an index of lymphocyte immaturity (Drexler et al. 1993). Mice fed a nucleotide-free diet have shown a higher percentage of TdT-positive cells proceeding from the thymus and the spleen than those fed a diet supplemented with RNA, adenine, or uracil, suggesting that dietary nucleotides could stimulate the maturation of lymphoid cells (Kulkarni et al.1989). The suggested mechanism proposes that dietary nucleotides exert a predominant effect upon the initial phase of antigen processing and lymphocyte proliferation suppressing the uncommitted T lymphocytes responses, as demonstrated by higher levels of TdT for undifferentiated lymphocytes in primary lymphoid organs in mice fed a nucleotide-free diet (Kulkarni et al. 1989). On the other hand, a regulatory role of dietary nucleotides in immunohematopoiesis has also been proposed (Jyonouchi et al. 1994).

There is considerable evidence demonstrating that exogenous nucleotides increase the proliferative response to T-cell dependent mitogens (PHA, ConA, and PWM), whereas no effects are seen when B-cell–dependent mitogens are used; this has been reviewed extensively in previous works (Carver et al. 1995; Gil 2001; Kulkarni et al. 1989; Jyonouchi et al. 1994; Gil et al. 1997; Rueda and Gil 2000).

In animal models stimulated with allogenic spleen cells, dietary nucleotides enhance the lymphoproliferative response, particularly during the recovery of protein-energy malnutrition, and it has also been reported that in nucleotide-starved rats the parenteral administration of a mixture of nucleotides and nucleosides (OG-VI) resulted in an increase in the proliferative response of spleen cells to the mitogen ConA. It has also been demonstrated that Balb/c and DBA/2 mice present an increase in the popliteal lymph node blastogenic response to antigens, allogens, and mitogens when they are fed with a diet supplemented with a mixture of nucleosides and nucleotides (Gil 2001; Kulkarni et al. 1989; Gil et al. 1997; Rueda and Gil 2000).

Holen et al. (2006) stimulated peripheral blood mononuclear cells (PBMCs) from healthy individuals with influenza virus antigen in the presence of DNA, RNA, dAMP, dCMP, dGMP, dUMP, or TMP. Specific nucleotide derivatives alone did not affect the growth of PBMCs. However, the nucleotide derivatives influenced immune cell growth and cytokine secretion when cocultured with specific antigen. DNA, RNA, dAMP, dCMP, and dUMP increased influenza virus antigen-induced immune cell proliferation. In contrast, dGMP and TMP inhibited the antigen-induced growth response (Holen et al. 2006). RNA and dAMP cocultured with virus antigen significantly increased PBMC secretion of IFN-γ, IL-10, and TNF-α. DNA increased virus antigen-induced immune cell secretion of IFN-γ only, whereas dUMP increased secretion of IL-10 only. Finally, dGMP completely inhibited virus-triggered IFN-γ secretion (Holen et al. 2006).

The effects of dietary nucleotides have been studied by Kulkarni et al. (2002) *in in vivo* and *in vitro* models of microgravity, which have adverse effects on the immune system. Popliteal lymph node response was significantly suppressed in mice subjected to experimental microgravity, and was restored by diets supplemented with either RNA or uracil. Splenocytes isolated from these mice had decreased PHA-stimulated proliferation and IL-2 and IFN-γ levels, and these effects were restored by RNA and uracil diets. Also, splenocytes cultured in microgravity conditions showed an inhibited PHA response, and uridine as well as a mixture of nucleosides and nucleotides restored the proliferative responses. Nucleotide supplementation, especially uridine, was also able to influence cell surface markers, indicating that the lymphocytes had acquired an activated phenotype (Kulkarni et al. 2002).

The effects of dietary nucleotides in newborn term infants was investigated in a double-blind study carried out by Buck et al. (2004), in which 477 subjects were enrolled. The children were divided into three different groups depending on the diet: infant formula with or without nucleotides, or human milk. In contrast with the studies mentioned above, these authors found that during the first year of age there were no changes in the total number of T-cells, B-cells, or NK cells in the bloodstream. Nevertheless T-cell subsets were affected (see below) (Buck et al. 2004). On the other hand, high levels of Tc1 and total IFN-γ-producing cells were found in nucleotide-fed infants. The effect of these cells could be beneficial, as increases in IFN-γ correlate with proliferative responses (Buck et al. 2004). These data suggest that nucleotides, as semiessential nutrients, could have a role in lymphocyte proliferation in several conditions like inflammation or immunosuppression but not in normal conditions.

23.4.2 Dietary Nucleotides and Lymphocyte Subpopulations

Differences in T and B lymphocyte subpopulations between mice fed diets containing nucleotides or not have been described (Buck et al. 2004; Manzano et al. 2003). Manzano et al. have reported that dietary nucleotides affect maturation and differentiation of intestinal lymphocytes that usually takes place at weanling (Manzano et al. 2003). These authors found that nucleotides exert selective effects on the different lymphocyte subsets (Peyer's patches, intraepithelial, and lamina propria). In general, nucleotides promote the development of T helper lymphocytes, and consequently the maturation and differentiation of B-cells. These effects would in part explain the positive modulation that nucleotides exert on immunoglobin production (see the "Modulation of Immunoglobin Production by Nucleotides" section below).

Jyonouchi et al. have described that dietary nucleotides modulate antigen-specific type 1 and type 2 T-cell responses in both C57BL/6 and BALB/cJ mice (Jyonouchi et al. 2000, 2001). The same authors challenged BALB/cJ mice with ovalbumin (OVA) plus incomplete Freund's adjuvant, a combination that predominantly induces Th2 response in these mice. Dietary ribonucleotides increased the OVA-specific Th1 cells after the primary antigen challenge and decreased OVA-specific Th2 cells after the secondary challenge. Costimulatory molecule (CD86 and CD154) expression and the activation state of total Th and cytotoxic cells were not affected in the regional draining lymph node. These results suggest that dietary ribonucleotides may modulate OVA-specific Th1/Th2 responses without nonspecific activation of T-cells (Jyonouchi et al. 2003).

The effects of dietary nucleotides on lymphocyte subset populations in preterm and full-term infants have been reported: there was a higher percentage of blood CD4+ cells in preterm children fed a nucleotide-supplemented formula compared with those fed the standard formula at 10 days of life (Navarro et al. 1999). As mentioned above, Buck et al. investigated the effects of dietary ribonucleotides on the immune cell phenotype and function of infants in their first year of life (Buck et al. 2004). These authors found increases in the percentage of memory/effector T-cell populations and changes in NK cell subtypes in infants fed a nucleotide-supplemented formula compared with infants fed the same formula without nucleotides. The observed increase in memory T-cells correlated with higher vaccine antibody titers and improved cell-mediated immune responses. Furthermore, in this study, the increase in memory/effector T-cell populations was associated with an increase in Tc and Th2 cells, and with a decrease in the population of naive lymphocytes. The increase in the proportion of Th2 cells in the nucleotide-fed group could enhance the systemic and immune mucosal response. Decreases in naive T-cell populations and increases in memory T-cells characterize normal immune maturation/development and normal responses to vaccinations and infections. It is interesting to mention that the observed changes made the immune system of the nucleotide-fed children more similar to that of the breastfed children. Therefore, these results provide evidence that formula supplemented with levels of nucleotides similar to those found in human milk (72 mg/L) may facilitate maturation and immunoregulatory shifts in some lymphocyte populations. These shifts might support increased antibody responses and immune cell protection. The changes in NK cell subsets may also enhance innate immune responses against tumors and/or intracellular pathogens.

23.4.3 Modulation of the Macrophage Phagocytic Activity by Dietary Nucleotides

A number of reports have related dietary nucleotides and macrophage activity. In mice inoculated with *Staphylococcus aureus*, the phagocytosis of microorganisms was lower in those who were fed on a nucleotide-free diet than in those fed on a diet supplemented with RNA or adenine. Dietary nucleotides enhanced the interaction of macrophages and T-cells, explaining the higher susceptibility of mice fed a nucleotide-free diet to *Candida* infection (Kulkarni et al. 1989).

23.4.4 NUCLEOTIDE MODULATION OF THE DELAYED HYPERSENSITIVITY AND ALLOGRAFT AND TUMOR RESPONSES

Early studies showed that mice fed a nucleotide-free diet and previously challenged with an intravenous stimulus of sheep red blood cells (SRBCs) exhibited a delayed cutaneous response when these cells were injected in the mice legs. An increase in the delayed hypersensitivity response to SRBCs and to DNFB in BALB/c and DBA/2 mice fed a diet supplemented with a mixture of nucleotides and nucleosides has been reported (Carver and Walker 1995; Kulkarni et al. 1989; Rueda and Gil 2000). One of the most studied models to ascertain the influence of dietary nucleotides on immunity is the evaluation of the response of the host against allografts. The duration of heart allografts implanted on the ear of mice was shown to increase when the diet was devoid of nucleotides, suggesting an impaired immune response; the addition of yeast RNA to the diet resulted in a reduced period of allograft survival. Likewise, the use of cyclosporine as an immunosuppressive agent in mice had a synergic effect when combined with a nucleotide-free diet leading to a higher period of allograft survival (Kulkarni et al. 1989). Also, administration of a nucleoside/nucleotide-free diet to rats subjected to transplantation of fetal small intestine without vascular anastomosis resulted in less graft rejection and lower plasma IL-2 levels (Ogita et al. 2004b). However, no differences were seen when mice were inoculated with a fibrosarcoma or the LSTRA syngeneic lymphoma, which is highly aggressive (Navarro et al. 1996).

Natural killer (NK) cells are one of the main populations involved in the immune response against transformed cells. The activity of NK cells is increased in mice fed a diet supplemented with nucleotides in respect to those fed a diet without nucleotides. Likewise, Carver has shown in human newborns that NK cell activity at the second month of life is increased in infants fed formula supplemented with nucleotides (Carver and Walker 1995).

23.4.5 MODULATION OF IMMUNOGLOBULIN PRODUCTION BY NUCLEOTIDES

Experiments carried out in mice fed a nucleotide-free diet for 3 weeks have shown a profound decrease of specific antibody response to T-cell–dependent antigens and a retained response to T-cell–independent antigens and lipopolysaccharides (Jyonouchi et al. 1994). Likewise, a mono-nucleotide-nucleoside mixture used in experimental total parenteral nutrition restored the humoral immune responses to T-cell dependent antigens in mice fed a nucleotide-free diet. However, this solution did not show any effect on the *in vitro* specific antibody production in response to T-cell–dependent antigens. Our group reported in BALB/c mice that the addition of nucleotide mixtures to a nucleotide-free diet resulted in an increase in the response of hemolytic IgG-forming cells induced by previous immunization with sheep erythrocytes; when the diet was supplemented with single nucleotides, AMP, GMP, or UMP increased the IgG response whereas CMP and IMP had no effect. GMP was the only nucleotide that increased the hemolytic IgM-forming cell response. A study using ovalbumin-specific T-cell receptor transgenic mice indicated that dietary nucleotides increase mucosal IgA response against specific antigens by increasing the production of transforming growth factor beta by intestinal epithelial cells and the proportion of TCRγδ IELs (Nagafuchi et al. 2002). Although previous studies have demonstrated the effect of dietary nucleotides on the differentiation of enterocytes, this study provides further evidence for the involvement of the enterocyte-mediated immune response in the effect of these compounds (Nagafuchi et al. 2002). In agreement with this, a study carried out in Caco-2 cells showed that exogenous nucleotides modify the expression and activity of transcription factors involved in immune response and inflammation (Ortega et al. 2011).

Our group has done a series of studies to determine the influence of dietary nucleotide supplementation to infant formulas on the levels of circulating antibodies in preterm infants. Total serum IgM and IgA levels increased significantly for the first 3 months of life, whereas no differences were detected for serum IgG; levels of IgE were undetectable (Gil et al. 1997; Navarro et al. 1996)

(Figure 23.5). The aforementioned increase in serum IgA has also been reported by Yau et al. in healthy full-term infants fed a nucleotide-supplemented formula (Yau et al. 2003).

The effect of dietary nucleotides on the antibody response to specific food antigens has been also studied in children. A study with preterm infants showed higher concentration of specific IgG against α-casein and β-lactoglobulin for the first month of life in newborns fed a low-birth-weight-infant nucleotide-supplemented formula (Martinez-Augustin et al. 1997). Nevertheless, no differences were observed in the serum levels of these specific immunoglobulins, nor in those of total immunoglobulins when malnourished children were fed with formulas supplemented with nucleotides (Martinez-Augustin et al. 1997).

Finally, several studies have demonstrated that dietary nucleotides enhance infants' responses to bacterial antigens and to vaccination (see Table 23.1). Thus, Pickering et al. (1998) showed that dietary nucleotides may modulate the immune response in normal infants, enhancing the production of specific IgG against low response antigens, namely *H. influenzae* type b, a bacterium responsible for meningitis episodes in early infancy (Pickering et al. 1998). On the other

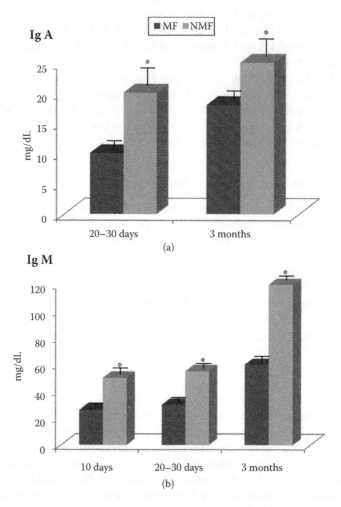

FIGURE 23.5 Nucleotides and humoral responses in preterm infants. Nucleotides increase the serum levels of IgA (a) and IgM (b) in preterm infants fed a nucleotide-supplemented milk formula (NMF) compared to those fed a control milk formula (MF). *$P < 0.05$ MF vs. NMF. (From *Neonatal Hematology and Immunology III*, Gil, A. et al., Role of dietary nucleotides in the modulation of the immune response, 139–144, 1997, with permission from Elsevier, and Navarro, J. et al., *Immunol Lett* 53, 141–145, 1996.)

TABLE 23.1

Effects of Dietary Nucleotides on Infant Immunity

Observed Effects of Nucleotides	Reference
In vitro analysis of specific blood cell populations for functional capacity:	
Increase in the number of T memory/effector cells in the first year of life	Buck et al. (2004)
Lower levels of cytokine-producing T-cells (Tc1 and Th2 cells and total IFN-γ production) in the first year of life	Buck et al. (2004)
Decrease in naive T-cells in children in the first year of life	Buck et al. (2004)
Increased IL-2 production	Carver et al. (1991)
Increased NK cell activity	Carver et al. (1991)
Analysis of *in vivo* responses to antigenic challenge, measuring changes in serum or mucosal antibody concentrations:	
Antibody concentration or production	
Higher IgA and IgM production at 3 months of age	Navarro et al. (1999)
	Maldonado et al. (2001)
Higher serum IgA	Yau et al. (2003)
Higher antibodies against β-lactoglobulin at 1month of life	Martinez-Augustin et al. (1997)
Serum vaccine-specific antibodies	
Higher Hib antibodies at 7 and 12 months	Pickering et al. (1998)
	Ostrom et al. (2002)
Higher diphtheria antibodies at 7 months	Pickering et al. (1998)
	Hawkes et al. (2006)
Higher oral polio virusVN1 antibodies at 7 and 12 months	Schaller et al. (2007)
	Ostrom et al. (2002)
Higher tetanus antibodies at 7 months	Hawkes et al. (2006)
Analysis of the incidence or severity of infection following challenge with live or attenuated pathogens further supported by assessments *in vitro* or *in vivo*:	
Decreased diarrhea incidence	Yau et al. (2003)
	Pickering et al. (1998)
	Brunser et al. (1994)
	Merolla and Gruppo Pediatri Sperimentatori (2000)
	Lama More et al. (1998)
Fewer symptoms of upper respiratory disease after 3 and 7 months	Navarro et al. (1996)
	Hawkes et al. (2006)

Hib, Haemophilus influenzae; IFN, interferon; IL, interleukin; NK, natural killer.

hand, Schaller et al. (2004) explored the effects of ribonucleotide supplementation on antibody responses in children subjected to routine infant immunizations (Schaller et al. 2004). Infants fed a nucleotide-supplemented formula had significantly higher poliovirus type 1 neutralizing antibody responses than did infants fed a nucleotide-free formula (Schaller et al. 2004). Another study demonstrated higher responses to tetanus toxoid (Hawkes et al. 2006), and a thorough study by Buck et al. (2004) showed that ribonucleotide feeding increases antibodies responses to Hib and to poliovirus, making them more similar to those of breast-fed children (Buck et al. 2004).

More recently, the above-mentioned studies and others were systematically reviewed by Gutiérrez-Castrellón et al. (2007), concluding that there is sufficient evidence to support the addition of nucleotides to infant formulas, the two main benefits being the improved maturation of the immune system and the decrease in the incidence of diarrhea (Gutiérrez-Castrellón et al. 2007).

23.4.6 Dietary Nucleotides and Defense against Infection

Animals injected intravenously with *Candida albicans* or *Staphylococcus aureus* and fed a nucleotide-free diet had a significantly lower survival rate than mice fed RNA, adenine, or uracil-supplemented diets. On the other hand, intraperitoneal administration of a nucleoside-nucleotide mixture for 14 days to mice was associated with reduced translocation of Gram-negative enterics to the mesenteric lymph nodes and spleen in comparison to control animals. The extent of the damaged mucosa was greater in controls, and these animals were more susceptible to the lethal effects of the lipopolysaccharide from *E. coli*, which suggests that dietary nucleotides may block bacterial translocation by preventing endotoxin-induced mucosal damage (Carver and Walker 1995; Gil 2001; Kulkarni et al. 1989).

One of the potential mechanisms by which nucleotides reduce the incidence of infection is the modulation of the intestinal microbiota. Our group reported for the first time that nucleotide supplementation to an infant formula reduced the counts of enterobacteria and increased the counts of bifidobacteria in the fecal microbiota (Gil and Uauy 1995; Uauy et al. 1996). These results suggested that nucleotides could act as prebiotics favoring the proliferation of the beneficial flora and inhibiting that of potential pathogens. A more recent study corroborates this, indicating that nucleotide supplementation of infant formulas decrease the ratio of *Bacteroides-Porphyromonas-Prevotella* group to *Bifidobacterium* species (Shingal et al. 2008). These results support clinical findings showing a low incidence of acute diarrhea in infants fed nucleotide-supplemented formula in developing (Brunser et al. 1994) and developed countries (Pickering et al. 1998).

Yau et al. (2003) investigated the effects of an infant formula fortified with nucleotides on the incidence of diarrhea, respiratory tract infections, and immune responses in healthy term infants (Yau et al. 2003). Compared with infants that received a nucleotide-free diet, those fed the supplemented formula had a significantly lower risk (25%) of diarrhea between 8 and 28 weeks. In contrast, the group of infants fed the nucleotide formula showed an increased risk of upper respiratory tract infections.

23.5 NUCLEOTIDES AND INTESTINAL INFLAMMATION

Intestinal inflammation is the hallmark of a range of diseases including inflammatory bowel disease. Because of the effect of nucleotides on immunity, intestinal healing, and proliferation, several studies have assessed their effect on intestinal inflammation in animal models. The first studies, in which nucleotide mixtures were administered to rats with DSS-induced colitis (Sukumar et al. 1998, 1999), described an exacerbation of the inflammatory reaction. In accordance with this, the administration of nucleoside-nucleotide-free diets was described to suppress cytokine production and to protect colonic mucosa in TNBS-induced colitis in rats (Adjei et al. 1996, 1997). These results are in agreement with the fact that the administration of nucleoside-nucleotide–free diets to Lewis rats reduced acute rejection of allogenic transplants. These rats received a 2-cm jejunum transplant from a donor Fischer rat into their abdominal wall (Ogita et al. 2004a,b). As a consequence, a proinflammatory effect of nucleotide mixtures is deduced, while nucleoside-nucleotide–free diets are considered to have immunosuppressive effects.

There is not a clear explanation for the proinflammatory role of dietary nucleotides, and specific studies are lacking, but nucleotides have been shown to be mediators of the purinergic system that plays an important role in maintaining gut homeostasis by regulating a variety of functions including secretion/absorption, immune/inflammatory, and nervous functions (Kolachala et al. 2008; Antonioli et al. 2013). In this sense, extracellular nucleotides liberated from different cell types in stress conditions have been shown to alert the immune system to tissue injury or inflammation. In fact, released nucleotides and their derivatives, such as ATP, ADP, UTP, UDP-glucose, and adenosine, would act as ligands of purinergic receptors (P1 and P2). In general, these receptors work in an autocrine mode. Under normal conditions, low concentrations of nucleotides are present in body fluids and tissues, but during inflammation, large amounts of extracellular nucleotides are rapidly released into the extracellular environment at the site of inflammation, increasing nucleotide concentrations rapidly. For example, released ATP can stimulate P2 (for nucleoside tri-/diphosphate) receptors and is rapidly metabolized by ectonucleotidase into adenosine, that in turn acts on P1 (for adenosine and AMP) receptors and/or is recaptured by nucleoside transporters. Thus, the occurrence of purinergic signals depends on the integrated activity of enzymes and transporters deputed to finely modulate the magnitude and duration of purinergic responses, driving the shift from ATPergic (mainly proinflammatory) to adenosinergic responses, which predominantly ameliorate inflammation (Antonioli et al. 2013). The importance of the purinergic receptor system in the intestinal inflammatory response is illustrated by the fact that some of these receptors like PA(2A), P2X7, P2Y(2), and P2Y(6) are overexpressed in IBD patients or colitic animals and, for example, P2X7-deficient mice do not develop experimental colitis (Neves et al. 2011; Ochoa-Cortes et al. 2014). Furthermore, the release of ATP by damaged intestinal epithelial cells, commensal bacteria, macrophages, platelets, or neutrophils induces the generation of proinflammatory Th17 cells and the activation of mast cells, which in turn produce proinflammatory cytokines, chemokines, and other inflammatory mediators like leukotrienes and histamine (Kurashima et al. 2015). The consequence of the increased extracellular ATP levels is therefore a proinflammatory signal, but also a protective one, since it can help prevent infections by stimulating the immune system. In fact, ATP release has been shown to result from TLR stimulation by intestinal bacteria, and a protective role has been attributed to this phenomenon (Kurashima et al. 2015). After exonucleotidase metabolism ATP is degraded to AMP and adenosine, which interact with P1 receptors such as PA(2A) and PA(3), and which are involved in both the promotion and the resolution of inflammatory responses (Colgan and Eltzschig 2012; Ye and Rajendran 2009). The fact that PA(2A) knockout mice show an exacerbated colonic inflammatory response to infection, while PA(2A) and PA(3) selective agonists ameliorate intestinal inflammation, together with the need for PA(A2) and PA(3) receptor expression on T-cells and myeloid cells for the inhibition of intestinal inflammation (Ye and Rajendran 2009), indicates the importance of these receptors in the development and resolution of intestinal inflammation.

Dietary nucleotides are in direct contact with the intestinal epithelium and the lamina propria, where cells express purinergic receptors; therefore, although not directly demonstrated to our knowledge, it would be reasonable to think that the proinflammatory effects of nucleotide mixtures and the anti-inflammatory effects of nucleoside-nucleotide–free diets could be directly related to the stimulation of the purinergic receptor system.

It is interesting to point out that in models of ileitis induced by indomethacin, the intraperitoneal administration of nucleotides exerts anti-inflammatory effects (Veerabagu et al. 1996). Furthermore, the intraperitoneal administration of inosine (monophosphate disodium salt) has also been shown to attenuate TNBS-induced colitis in rats (Rahimian et al. 2010), an effect that is mediated by PA(2A) receptors. Therefore, it would be possible that the precise effect of nucleotides would depend on the luminal/apical or intraperitoneal/basolateral administration.

23.6 POTENTIAL MECHANISM OF ACTION OF DIETARY NUCLEOTIDES

It has been proposed that dietary nucleotides exert effects upon cellular immune function by acting on the T helper/inducer population with the predominant effect on the initial phase of antigen processing and lymphocyte proliferation. The suggested mechanism would be the suppression of uncommitted T lymphocyte responses as demonstrated by higher activities of deoxynucleotidyl transferase, a marker of undifferentiated lymphocytes, in primary lymphoid organs of mice fed a nucleotide-free diet (Kulkarni et al. 1989).

Another hypothesis is that exogenous nucleotides may modulate T helper (Th) cell-mediated antibody production (Jyonouchi et al. 1994), favoring the balance of T-cell differentiation to Th-2 cells, which are mainly involved in the B-cell response and in the suppression of proinflammatory reactions induced by Th-1 cells.

The molecular mechanisms by which dietary nucleotides modulate the immune system are practically unknown. It has been suggested that the small intestine should play a key role in the regulatory effects of nucleotides upon the immune response. The gut-associated lymphoid tissue can initiate and regulate T-cell development and may act as a thymus analog (Walker 1996). Dietary nucleotides have been shown to enhance the production and the genetic expression of IL-6 and IL-8 by fetal small intestinal explants when challenged with IL-1β, the response being nucleotide concentration dependent. Furthermore, the addition of AMP to the culture medium resulted in the suppression of crypt cell proliferation followed by the restoration of differentiation and the induction of apoptosis across the human small intestinal epithelium (Sanchez-Pozo et al. 1999). Dietary nucleotides may influence the protein biosynthesis by regulating the intracellular nucleotide pool. In addition, signal transduction mediated by the interaction of exogenous nucleosides and their receptors may also contribute to modulate the expression of a number of genes, some of which can directly affect the levels of intestinal cytokines (Figure 23.6).

Nucleotides have been reported to modulate the gene expression of enzymes involved in their own metabolism, such as the purine salvage enzymes hypoxanthine-guanine phosphoribosyl transferase and adenine phosphoribosyl transferase in the small intestine and proximal colon (Leleiko et al. 1987; Leleiko and Walsh 1995). Recently, exogenous nucleosides have been shown to affect the expression and activity of several transcription factors involved in cell growth, differentiation, apoptosis, and in immune response and inflammation in Caco-2 cells. In fact, the addition of nucleosides to the medium increased the expression and activity of the general transcription factor CCAAT displacement protein (CUX1), and decreased the expression and activity of the general upstream stimulatory factor 1 (USF1), glucocorticoid receptor (NR3C1), and nuclear factor kappa B (NF-κB) (Ortega et al. 2011).

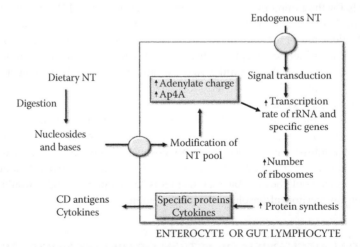

FIGURE 23.6 Potential mechanisms of action of dietary nucleotides. Dietary nucleotides, mainly absorbed as nucleosides in the gut, may influence enterocyte and lymphocyte protein biosynthesis by regulating the intracellular nucleotide pool. In addition, signal membrane transduction mediated by the interaction of exogenous nucleosides and their receptors may also contribute to modulate the expression of a number of genes, some of which can directly affect the levels of intestinal cytokines. NT, = nucleotides; rRNA, = ribosomal ribonucleic acid.

REFERENCES

Adjei, A. A., Ameho, C. K., Harrison, E. K. et al. 1997. Nucleoside-nucleotide-free diet suppresses cytokine production and contact sensitivity responses in rats with trinitrobenzene sulphonic acid-induced colitis. *Am J Med Sci* 314:89–96.

Adjei, A. A., Morioka, T., Ameho, C. K. et al. 1996. Nucleoside-nucleotide free diet protects rat colonic mucosa from damage induced by trinitrobenzene sulphonic acid. *Gut* 39:428–433.

Angstadt, C. N. 1997. Purine and pyrimidine metabolism. NetBiochem website: http://library.med.utah.edu/ NetBiochem/pupyr/pp.htm#Pu%20Catab (Last modified 12 April 1997).

Antonioli, L., Colucci, R., Pellegrini, C. et al. 2013. The role of purinergic pathways in the pathophysiology of gut diseases: pharmacological modulation and potential therapeutic applications. *Pharmacol Therapeut* 139:157–188.

Barness, L. 1994. Dietary source of nucleotides-from breast milk to weaning. *J Nutr* 124:128–130.

Bronk, J. R., and Hastewell, J.G. 1987. The transport of pyrimidines into tissue rings cut from rat small intestine. *J Physiol* 382:475–488.

Brunser, O., Espinoza, J., Araya, M. et al. 1994. Effect of dietary nucleotide supplementation on diarrhoeal disease in infant. *Acta Paediatr* 83:188–191.

Buck, R. H., Thomas, D. L., Winship, T. R. et al. 2004. Effect of dietary ribonucleotides on infant immune status. Part 2: Immune cell development. *Pediatr Res* 56:891–900.

Calder, P. C., Krauss-Etschmann, S., de Jong, E. C. et al. 2006. Early nutrition and immunity—Progress and perspectives. *Br J Nutr* 96:774–790.

Carver, J. D. 1999. Dietary nucleotides: Effects on the immune and gastrointestinal systems. *Acta Paediatr Suppl* 88:83–88.

Carver, J. D., and Stromquist, C. I. 2006. Dietary nucleotides and preterm infant nutrition. *J Perinatol* 26:443–444.

Carver, J. D., and Walker, W. A. 1995. The role of nucleotides in human nutrition. *J Nutr Biochem* 6:58–72.

Carver, J. D., Pimentel, B., Cox, W. I., and Barness, L. A. 1991. Dietary nucleotide effects upon immune function in infants. *Pediatrics* 883:359–363.

Clifford, A. J., and Story, D. L. 1976. Levels of purines in foods and their metabolic effect in rats. *J Nutr* 106:435–442.

Colgan, S. P., and Eltzschig, H. K. 2012. Adenosine and hypoxia-inducible factor signaling in intestinal injury and recovery. *Annu Rev Physiol* 74:153–175.

Devresse, B. 2000. A forgotten but key nutrient for the immune system: Nucleotides. A review and current advances. Paper presented at the V Congreso Ecuatoriano de Acuicultura, enfocando los retos del 2000. 28–30 October 1999, Guayaquil, Ecuador.

Drexler, H. G., Sperling, C., and Ludwig, W. D. 1993. Terminal deoxynucleotidyl transferase (TdT) expression in acute myeloid leukemia. *Leukemia* 7:1142–1150.

Fairbanks, L. D., Rückemann, K., Qiu, Y. et al. 1999. Methotrexate inhibits the first committed step of purine biosynthesis in mitogen-stimulated human T-lymphocytes: A metabolic basis for efficacy in rheumatoid arthritis? *Biochem J* 342(Pt 1):143–152.

Gil, A. 1984. *Nucléotidos en la leche humana. Fundamento para su empleo en leches infantiles* [Human milk nucleotides. Basis for their use in infant formulae]. Granada, Spain.

Gil, A. 2001. New additions to infant formulas. In *Pediatric Gastroenterology and Nutrition in Clinical Practice*, ed. C. Liftschitz, 113–135. New York, NY: Marcel Dekker.

Gil, A. 2002. Modulation of the immune response mediated by dietary nucleotides. *Eur J Clin Nutr* 56 (Suppl 3):S1–S4.

Gil, A. and F. Sanchez-Medina. 1982. Acid-soluble nucleotides of human milk at different stages of lactation. *J Dairy Res* 49:301–307.

Gil, A. and R. Uauy. 1995. Nucleotides and related compounds in human and bovine milks. In *Handbook of Milk Composition*, ed. R. G. Jensen, 436–437. San Diego, CA: Academic Press.

Gil, A., Gómez-León, C., and Rueda, R. 2007. Exogenous nucleic acids and nucleotides are efficiently hydro-lysed and taken up as nucleosides by intestinal explants from suckling piglet. *Br J Nutr* 98:285–291.

Gil, A., Martínez-Augustín, O., and Navarro, J. 1997. Role of dietary nucleotides in the modulation of the immune response. In *Neonatal Hematology and Immunology III*, eds. J. A. Bellanti, R. Bracci, G. Prindull, and M. Xanthou, 139–144. Amsterdam: Elsevier Science.

Grimble, G. K. 1996. Why are dietary nucleotides essential nutrients? *Br J Nutr* 76:475–478.

Grimble, G. K., and Westwood, O. M. 2001. Nucleotides as immunomodulators in clinical nutrition. *Curr Opin Clin Nutr Metab Care* 4:57–64.

Grimble, G. K., Malik, S. B., and Boza, J. J. 2000. Methods for measuring tissue RNA turnover. *Curr Opin Clin Nutr Metab Care* 3:399–408.

Gutiérrez-Castrellón, P., Mora-Magaña, I., Díaz-García, L. et al. 2007. Immune response to nucleotide-supplemented infant formulae: Systematic review and meta-analysis. *Br J Nutr* 98(Suppl 1):S64–S67.

Hawkes, J. S., Gibson, R. A., Roberton, D., and Makrides, M. 2006. Effect of dietary nucleotide supplementation on growth and immune function in term infants: A randomized controlled trial. *Eur J Clin Nutr* 60:254–264.

Holen, E., Bjørge, O. A., and Jonsson, R. 2006. Dietary nucleotides and human immune cells. II. Modulation of PBMC growth and cytokine secretion. *Nutrition* 22:90–96.

Ingledew, W. M. 1999. Yeast-could you base a business on this bug? In: Lyons TP, Jacques KA (Eds). *Biotechnology in the Feed Industry*. Proc. of Alltech' s 15th Annual Symposium, pp. 27-47. Nottingham University Press, Nottingham, UK.

Jyonouchi, H., Sun, S., Winship, T., and Kuchan, M. J. 2000. Dietary nucleotides modulate antigen-specific type 1 and type 2 cell responses in young C57BL/6 mice. *Nutrition* 16:442–446.

Jyonouchi, H., Sun, S., Winship, T., and Kuchan, M. J. 2001. Dietary nucleotides modulate type 1 and type 2 T-helper cell responses against ovalbumin in young BALB/cJ mice. *J Nutr* 131:1165–1170.

Jyonouchi, H., Sun, S., Winship, T., and Kuchan, M. J. 2003. Dietary ribonucleotides increase antigen-specific type 1 T-helper cells in the regional draining lymph nodes in young BALB/cJ mice. *Nutrition* 19:41–46.

Jyonouchi, H., Zhang-Shanbhag, L., Tomita, Y., and Yokoyama, H. 1994. Nucleotide-free diet impairs T-helper cell functions in antibody production in response to T-dependent antigens in normal C57BL/6 mice. *J Nutr* 124:475–484.

Kojima, K. 1974. Safety evaluation of disodium 5'-inosinate, disodium 5'-guanylate and disodium 5'-ribonucleate. *Toxicology* 2:185–206.

Kolachala, V. L., Bajaj, R., Chalasani, M., and Sitaraman, S. V. 2008. Purinergic receptors in gastrointestinal inflammation. *Am J Physiol-Gastr L* 294:G401–G410.

Kulkarni, A. D., Yamauchi, K., Hales, N. W. et al. 2002. Nutrition beyond nutrition: Plausibility of immunotrophic nutrition for space travel. *Clin Nutr* 21:231–238.

Kulkarni, A., Fanslow, W., Higley, H., Pizzini, R., Rudolph, F., and Van Buren, C. 1989. Expression of immune cell surface markers in vivo and immune competence in mice by dietary nucleotides. *Transplant Proc* 21:121–124.

Kurashima, Y., Kiyono, H., and Kunisawa, J. 2015. Pathophysiological role of extracellular purinergic mediators in the control of intestinal inflammation. *Mediators Inflamm* 2015:427125. doi:10.1155/2015/427125.

Lama More, R. A., and Gil-Alberdi González, B. 1998. Effect of nucleotides as dietary supplement on diarrhea in healthy infants. *An Esp Pediatr* 48:371–375.

Leleiko, N. S., and Walsh, M. J. 1995. Dietary purine nucleotides and the gastrointestinal tract. *Nutrition* 11:725–730.

Leleiko, N. S., Martin, B. A., Walsh, M. J. et al. 1987. Tissue-specific gene expression results from a purine- and pyrimidine-free diet and 6-mercaptopurine in the rat small intestine and colon. *Gastroenterology* 93:1014–1020.

Li, P., Lawrence, A. L., Castille, F. L., and Gatlin, D. M. 2007. Preliminary evaluation of a purified nucleotide mixture as a dietary supplement for Pacific white shrimp Litopenaeus vannamei (Boone). *Aquaculture Research* 38:887–890.

Maldonado, J., Navarro, J., Narbona, E., and Gil, A. 2001. The influence of dietary nucleotides on humoral and cell immunity in the neonate and lactating infant. *Early Hum Dev* 65(Suppl):S69–S74.

Manzano, M., Abadía-Molina, A. C., García-Olivares, E. et al. 2003. Dietary nucleotides accelerate changes in intestinal lymphocyte maturation in weanling mice. *J Pediatr Gastroenterol Nutr* 37: 453–461.

Martínez-Augustin, O., Boza, J. J., Del Pino, J. I. et al. 1997. Dietary nucleotides might influence the humoral immune response against cow's milk proteins in preterm neonates. *Biol Neonate* 71:215–223.

Martínez-Augustin, O., Boza, J. J., Navarro, J., Martínez-Valverde, A., Araya, M., and Gil, A. 1997. Dietary nucleotides may influence the humoral immunity in immunocompromised children. *Nutrition* 13:465–9.

Mason, K. L., Huffnagle, G. B., Noverr, M. C., and Kao, J. Y. 2008. Overview of gut immunology. *Adv Exp Med Biol* 635:1–14.

Mateo, C. D. 2005. Aspects of nucleotide nutrition in pigs. PhD diss. South Dakota State University, USA.

Merolla, R., and Gruppo Pediatri Sperimentatori. 2000. Evaluation of the effects of a nucleotide-enriched formula on the incidence of diarrhea. Italian multicenter national study. *Minerva Pediatr.* 52:699–711.

Nagafuchi, S., Totsuka, M., Hachimura, S. et al. 2002. Dietary nucleotides increase the mucosal IgA response and the secretion of transforming growth factor beta from intestinal epithelial cells in mice. *Cytotechnology* 40:49–58.

Navarro, J., Maldonado, J., Narbona, E. et al. 1999. Influence of dietary nucleotides on plasma immunoglobulin levels and lymphocyte subsets of preterm infants. *Biofactors* 10:67–76

Navarro, J., Ruiz-Bravo, A., Jiménez-Valera, M., and Gil, A. 1996. Modulation of antibody-forming cell and mitogen-driven lymphoproliferative responses by dietary nucleotides in mice. *Immunol Lett* 53:141–145.

Neves, A. R., Yoshimoto, A. N., Bernardazzi, C. et al. 2011. Overexpression of ATP-activated P2X7 receptors on immune and non-immune cells of the intestinal mucosa is implicated in the pathogenesis of crohn's disease. *Gastroenterology* 140:S475–S475.

Ngo, L. Y., Patil, S. D., and Unadkat, J. D. 2001. Ontogenic and longitudinal activity of Na+-nucleoside transporters in the human intestine. *Am J Physiol Gastrointest Liver Physiol* 280:G475–G481.

Ochoa-Cortes, F., Linan-Rico, A., Jacobson, K. A., and Christofi, F. L. 2014. Potential for developing purinergic drugs for gastrointestinal diseases. *Inflamm Bowel Dis* 20:1259–1287.

Oddy, W. H. 2002. The impact of breastmilk on infant and child health. *Breastfeed Rev* 10:5–18.

Ogita, K., Suita, S., Taguchi, T., and Uesugi, T. 2004a. Immunosuppressive effect of nucleoside-nucleotide-free diet in rat allogeneic small intestinal transplantation. *Transplant Proc* 36:329–330.

Ogita, K., Suita, S., Taguchi, T., Nakamura, M., and Uesugi, T. 2004b. Effect of a nucleoside/nucleotide-free diet in rat allogenic small intestinal transplantation. *Pediatr Surg Int* 20:5–8.

Ortega, A., Gil, A., and Sánchez-Pozo, A. 2011. Exogenous nucleosides modulate expression and activity of transcription factors in Caco-2 cells. *J Nutr Biochem* 22:595–604.

Ostrom, K. M., Cordle, C. T., Schaller, J. P. et al. 2002. Immune status of infants fed soy-based formulas with or without added nucleotides for 1 year. Part 1: Vaccine responses, and morbidity. *J Pediatr Gastroenterol Nutr* 34:137–44.

Pickering, L. K., Granoff, D. M, Erickson, J. R. et al. 1998. Modulation of the immune system by human milk and infant formula containing nucleotides. *Pediatrics* 101:242–249.

Rahimian, R., Fakhfouri, G., Daneshmand, A. et al. 2010. Adenosine A2A receptors and uric acid mediate protective effects of inosine against TNBS-induced colitis in rats. *Eur J Pharmacol* 649:376–381.

Rolfes, R. J. 2006. Regulation of purine nucleotide biosynthesis: In yeast and beyond. *Biochem Soc Trans* 34(Pt 5):786–790.

Rudolph, F. B., Kulkarni, A. D., Fanslow, W. C., Pizzini, R. P., Kumar, S. and Van Buren, C. T. 1990. Role of RNA as a dietary source of pyrimidines and purines in immune function. *Nutrition* 6:45–52.

Rueda, R., and Gil, A. 2000. Influence of dietary compounds on intestinal immunity. *Microb Ecol Health Dis* 12(Suppl 2):146–156.

Salati, L. M, Gross, C. J, Henderson, L. M., and Savaiano, D. A. 1984. Absorption and metabolism of adenine, adenosine-5'-monophosphate, adenosine and hypoxanthine by the isolated vascularly perfused rat small intestine. *J Nutr* 114:753–760.

Sánchez-Pozo, A., Rueda, R., Fontana L., and Gil, A. 1999. Dietary nucleotides and cell growth. In *Trends in Comparative Biochemistry and Physiology*, ed. S. G. Pandalai, 99–111. Trivandrum: Transworld Research Network.

Sanderson, I. R., and He, Y. 1994. Nucleotide uptake and metabolism by intestinal epithelial cells. *J Nutr* 124(Suppl 1):131S–137S.

Schaller, J. P., Buck, R. H., and Rueda, R. 2007. Ribonucleotides: Conditionally essential nutrients shown to enhance immune function and reduce diarrheal disease in infants. *Semin Fetal Neonatal Med* 12:35–44.

Schaller, J. P., Kuchan, M. J., Thomas, D. L. et al. 2004. Effect of dietary ribonucleotides on infant immune status. Part 1: Humoral responses. *Pediatr Res* 56:883–890.

Scharrer, E., Rech, K. S., and Grenacher, B. 2002. Characteristics of Na+-dependent intestinal nucleoside transport in the pig. *J Comp Physiol B* 172:309–314

Shingal, A., Macfarlane, G., Macfarlane, S. et al. 2008. Dietary nucleotides and fecal microbiota in formula-fed infants: A randomized controlled trial. *Am J Clin Nutr* 87:1785–1792.

Sukumar, P., Loo, A., Adolphe, R., Nandi, J., Oler, A., and Levine, R. A. 1999. Dietary nucleotides augment dextran sulfate sodium-induced distal colitis in rats. *J Nutr* 129:1377–1381.

Sukumar, P., Loo, A., Adolphe, R., Nandi, J., Oler, A., and Levine, R. A. 1998. Dietary nucleotides augment rat colonic myeloperoxidase and interleukin-1 beta in rectal dialysate in dextran sulfate-induced colitis. *Gastroenterology* 114:A1094–A1094.

Swanson, T. A., Kim, S. I., Glucksman, M. J., and Marks, D. B. 2007. Nucleotide and porphyrin metabolism. In *Biochemistry and Molecular Biology (Fourth Edition)*. Chapter 18, 281–282. Philadelphia, PA: Wolters Kluwer Health/Lippincott Williams & Wilkins.

Tibbets, G. W. 1999. Nucleotides from yeast extract: Potential to replace animal protein sources in food animal diets. In *Biotechnology in the Feed Industry. Proceedings of Alltech's 15th Annual Symposium*, eds. T. P. Lyons, and K. A. Jacques KA, 435–443. Nottingham: Nottingham University Press.

Traut, T. 2014. *Nucleotide Synthesis de Novo*. Hoboken, NJ: John Wiley & Sons.

Uauy, R. 1989. Dietary nucleotides and requirements in early life. In *Textbook of Gastroenterology and Nutrition in Infancy*, ed. E. Lebenthal, Vol. 2, 265–280. New York, NY: Raven Press.

Uauy, R., Quan, R., and Gil, A. 1996. Nucleotides in infant nutrition. In *Nutritional and Biological Significance of Dietary Nucleotides and Nucleic Acids,* eds. A. Gil, and R. Uauy, 169–180. Barcelona: Doyma.

Van Buren, C. T., and Rudolph, F. 1997. Dietary nucleotides: A conditional requirement. *Nutrition* 13:470–472.

Veerabagu, M. P., Meguid, M. M., Oler, A., and Levine, R. A. 1996. Intravenous nucleosides and a nucleotide promote healing of small bowel ulcers in experimental enterocolitis. *Digest Dis Sci* 41:1452–1457.

Walker, W. A. 1996. Exogenous nucleotides and gastrointestinal immunity. *Transplant Proc* 28:2438–2441.

Yau, K. I. T, Huang, C. B, Chen, W. et al. 2003. Effect of nucleotides on diarrhea and immune responses in healthy term infants in Taiwan. *J Pediatr Gastroenterol Nutr* 36:37–43.

Ye, J. H. Q., and Rajendran, V. M. 2009. Adenosine: An immune modulator of inflammatory bowel diseases. *World J Gastroenterol* 15:4491–4498.

24 Gangliosides and Immune Regulation

Ricardo Rueda, Esther Castanys-Muñoz,
and Enrique Vázquez

CONTENTS

24.1 Introduction...405
24.2 Definition and Description of Gangliosides...406
24.3 Sources and Quantification of Gangliosides..406
24.4 Overview of the Functions of Gangliosides...409
    24.4.1 Gangliosides as Lipid Raft Constituents..409
    24.4.2 Gangliosides and Cancer 410
    24.4.3 Gangliosides and Neural Development and Function 411
    24.4.4 Gangliosides and Neurodegenerative Disorders...412
    24.4.5 Gangliosides and Inflammation 413
    24.4.6 Gangliosides and Metabolic Syndrome 413
    24.4.7 Gangliosides and Autophagy 414
    24.4.8 Gangliosides and Immunity...414
24.5 Ganglioside Effects on Immune Function 414
24.6 Bifidogenic Effect of Gangliosides 417
24.7 Summary and Future Trends..418
References...419

24.1 INTRODUCTION

This chapter focuses on describing the role of dietary gangliosides in modulation of the immune response, prevention of infection, and regulation of inflammation. It will begin with an overview of the structures and most commonly used nomenclature for gangliosides, followed by a brief description of the quantification methods used. Next, dietary sources of gangliosides will be described, with special focus on milk. Differences in the concentration and distribution of gangliosides between human and bovine milk will be described, as well as information on ganglioside composition in infant formulas. Then, an overview on the wide range of biological functions performed by gangliosides will be presented, including both physiological and pathological settings. Their role as receptors in cell-cell recognition and in lipid raft formation and maintenance will be mentioned. Then, their implication in tumor progression and metastasis will be presented. Their importance in neural development and function, as well as their role in central nervous system pathologies will also be reviewed. The implication of gangliosides in obesity and diabetes will be explained, followed by their anti-inflammatory role. Their recent role as autophagy mediators will be briefly considered. We will then extend on the importance of gangliosides in immunity, both in preventing infections and in modulating the immune system. Their direct effects on the intestinal immune system and consequences on the systemic immune system are considered. We will also evaluate their role as prebiotics, modulating gut microbiota. Finally, current literature regarding the use of dietary gangliosides in clinical situations will be reviewed.

24.2   DEFINITION AND DESCRIPTION OF GANGLIOSIDES

Gangliosides are negatively charged glycosphingolipids, built on the hydrophobic core of ceramide, which is decorated with a hydrophilic oligosaccharide chain, bearing one or more sialic acid residues plus a number of sugars including glucose, galactose, N-acetylglucosamine, and N-acetylgalactosamine (Wiegandt 1982). Ceramide consists of a sphingosine base linked to a fatty acid via an amide bond. The fatty acid is usually saturated, with a chain length of more than 14 carbons.

Different nomenclature systems are currently in use for gangliosides. Svennerholm developed a shorthand nomenclature, which is most frequently used (Svennerholm 1963). His system is based on two letters and one subscript number. The first letter indicates the series, depending on the carbohydrate core and metabolic pathway (G = ganglio series). The second letter refers to the number of sialic acid residues (M, D, T, Q, P, H, S for one, two, three, four, five, or, exceptionally, six or seven residues). The subscript corresponds to five minus the number of neutral monosaccharide residues present in the molecule. Attempts to develop more systematic and comprehensive approaches, such as the IUPAC system, are less frequently applied because of their complexity (Chester 1998).

Gangliosides are constituents of vertebrate plasma membranes, associated with the lipid leaflet through the ceramide, with the glycan moiety exposed to the external milieu. The carbohydrate portion normally functions as a receptor, antigen, and/or ligand in biological functions (Schnaar et al. 2014). Gangliosides are ubiquitously distributed in most vertebrate tissues and body fluids, even when they are more abundantly expressed in the brain. In general, they are isolated from these sources by chloroform-methanol extraction and solvent partition. Quantitative estimation of gangliosides is usually based on the sialic acid moiety, using the lipid-bound sialic acid (LBSA) colorimetric determination. Quantification can be achieved by high-performance liquid chromatography or mass spectrometry, providing suitable standards are available (Huang et al. 2014).

24.3   SOURCES AND QUANTIFICATION OF GANGLIOSIDES

The average ganglioside content in any human diet remains difficult to assess, except for milk, although there are data available for the sphingolipid content in foods. The total amount of sphingolipids in food varies considerably, from micromoles/kg in fruits, to several millimoles/kg in rich sources such as dairy products, eggs, and soybeans (Vesper et al. 1999). Daily intake of sphingolipids was estimated to be 0.3–0.4 g (Vesper et al. 1999). Gangliosides make up a small percentage of sphingolipid intake, and it is difficult to assess and calculate the actual ganglioside content of a diet (McJarrow et al. 2009). They are found in animal sources (i.e., egg yolk, meat, and milk). Currently, there is no literature to support optimal intake levels for either healthy individuals or individuals with various diseases. One study evaluated the ganglioside intake in a healthy population, consuming a well-balanced diet consisting of meat, fish, and dairy products. According to their results, individuals consumed less than 200 mg/d (Pham et al. 2011).

Ganglioside composition has been studied mainly in milk and dairy products. In milk, gangliosides are almost exclusively associated with the milk-fat globule membrane (MFGM), which is derived from the apical plasma membrane of the apocrine secretory cells in the lactating mammary gland (Keenan 1974). Initially, gangliosides were studied in bovine milk, with GD3 and GM3 as the major species (Bushway and Keenan 1978). Results from studies evaluating bovine milk, as well as milk from goats and ewes, have described differences in ganglioside concentrations between species and stages of lactation, as well as seasonal variations (Puente et al. 1992; Puente et al. 1994; Puente et al. 1995; Puente et al. 1996). The predominant ganglioside in bovine milk is GD3, constituting up to 60%–70%, with GM3 and GT3 comprising the majority of the remainder (Laegreid et al. 1986; Lee et al. 2013; Puente et al. 1992).

Human milk contains a higher concentration of gangliosides than bovine milk, the total amount being higher in colostrum compared to mature milk (Martin-Sosa et al. 2004; Pan and Izumi 1999). Individual ganglioside concentrations also vary according to stage of lactation. In fact, the relative concentrations of GM3 and GD3 change between colostrum (days 1–5) and mature milk. GD3 was the most abundant ganglioside in human milk at the beginning of lactation, while GM3 was more predominant toward later stages (Giuffrida et al. 2014; Martin-Sosa et al. 2004; Rueda 2007). The relatively high concentration of gangliosides, together with the changes along lactation may reflect their importance for neonatal development (Rueda 2013). Besides GM3 and GD3, four other gangliosides, possibly from the c-series, were detected in human milk (Pan and Izumi 1999). Highly polar gangliosides, probably polysialogangliosides or complex gangliosides with branched oligosaccharide chains, have also been described (Rueda et al. 1995).

Milk from mothers delivering preterm was reported to differ in the relative concentration of individual gangliosides compared to those delivering full-term (Rueda et al. 1996). In addition, changes in fatty acid composition in human milk gangliosides through lactation have been described (Martin-Sosa et al. 2004), as well as differences in fatty acid composition between bovine and human milk gangliosides (Bode et al. 2004). These studies are of interest, considering that fatty acid composition of gangliosides is usually neglected in structural characterization studies. Nevertheless, their fatty acids determine, together with the oligosaccharide portion, the diverse physiological effects exerted by gangliosides (Bode et al. 2004).

Studies evaluating the concentration of gangliosides in human milk have estimated the mean intake of total ganglioside in infants. This would range from 5.5 mg/day to 8.6 mg/day within the 30 to 120 days postpartum period in infants fed human milk exclusively (Giuffrida et al. 2014). So far, there is little evidence to suggest that maternal diet influences the amount and profile of gangliosides in milk (McJarrow et al. 2009). The importance of nutrition during pregnancy for optimal growth and development of the fetus is nevertheless well known. Considering that dietary or exogenous gangliosides are able to cross the placenta and be assimilated in fetal brain tissues, the idea of supplementing maternal diet with gangliosides to promote an optimum supply during gestation has been suggested (Palmano et al. 2015).

Quantitative data of ganglioside concentrations in complex mixtures is still scarce, given that their chemical nature renders them difficult to analyze (Lacomba et al. 2009). In biological samples, gangliosides are usually quantified as lipid-bound to sialic acid (LBSA) as a surrogate parameter (Rueda 2007). Table 24.1 shows the reported average amount of total gangliosides and of GD3 plus GM3, expressed as LBSA and actual concentration, for different periods of human lactation. The average value of GD3 plus GM3 in human milk, weighted according to the number of samples, was of 13.2 mg/L considering colostrum, transitional, and mature human milk, or 11.1 mg/L when only mature human milk is considered (Rueda 2007).

Recently, quantitative mass spectrometry techniques have been developed. One in particular has been validated to quantify gangliosides in human milk using liquid chromatography coupled with electrospray ionization high-resolution mass spectrometry (LC/ESI-HR-MS). The method was applied to a large human milk sample set to determine the content of gangliosides up to 120 days postpartum. According to the observations, total ganglioside content in human milk ranged from 8.1 to 10.7 µg/mL (Table 24.1) (Giuffrida et al. 2014). Other investigations of gangliosides in bovine milk used ultra-high-performance liquid chromatography tandem MS, and focused on quantifying the specific amounts of gangliosides in bovine milk over lactation. This work showed considerable amounts of gangliosides at day two (GM3, 0.98 mg/L; GD3, 15.2 mg/L), which decreased rapidly by two weeks (GM3, 0.15 mg/L; GD3, 3.3 mg/L) and farther at three months (GM3, 0.15 mg/L; GD3, 3.3 mg/L). Moreover, the authors suggested that gangliosides were preferentially concentrated in side streams such as buttermilk as a result of the dairy processing procedure (Lee et al. 2013).

Considering the potential importance of gangliosides for wide range of functions, the composition of gangliosides and other sialoglycoconjugates in infant formulas has been studied and compared to that of human milk (Pan and Izumi 2000; Sanchez-Diaz et al. 1997). Since bovine milk is the base to manufacture infant formula, the ganglioside distribution is similar in both. However, both the pattern and content of gangliosides in human milk and infant formula differed considerably. In infant formulas, GD3 is the main species detected, and total ganglioside

TABLE 24.1

Ganglioside Concentrations (Total, GM3, and GD3) at Different Stages of Human Lactation

Author	Method	Period of Lactation	n	Total Gangliosides (mg LBSA/L)	GM3 (%)	GD3 (%)	GM3 (mg LBSA/L)	GD3 (mg LBSA/L)	GM3 (mg/L)	GD3 (mg/L)	GM3 + GD3 (mg/L)
Takamizawa et al. (1986)	LBSA	Colostrum	6	5.77	9.05	70.52	0.51	4.07	1.98	10.39	12.37
		Transitional milk	5	4.50	18.02	62.02	0.73	2.85	2.85	7.26	10.11
		Mature milk	6	4.04	60.82	20.30	2.38	0.88	9.24	2.23	11.47
Rueda et al. (1995)	LBSA	Colostrum	4	2.59	6.38	46.20	0.17	1.13	0.65	2.89	3.54
		Transitional milk	7	5.03	13.04	36.81	0.76	2.02	2.97	5.16	8.13
		Mature milk	7	1.79	44.23	15.30	0.62	0.38	2.42	0.96	3.38
Pan and Izumi (1999)	LBSA	Colostrum	16	9.82	3.13	48.19	0.31	4.73	1.19	12.07	13.25
		Transitional milk	35	9.08	26.73	33.97	2.45	3.08	9.53	7.84	17.37
		Mature milk	10	8.02	35.76	24.71	2.88	1.08	11.18	5.05	16.23

Author	Method	Period of Lactation	n	Total Gangliosides (µg/mL)	GM3 (µg/mL)	GD3 (µg/mL)	GM3/GD3
Giuffrida et al. (2014)	LC ESI-HR-MS	0–11 days	450	8.1	4.3 ± 0.9	3.8 ± 0.4	1.1
		30 days	450	9.1	7.4 ± 0.2	1.7 ± 0.2	4.3
		60 days	450	10.0	9.1 ± 0.3	0.9 ± 0.1	10.1
		120 days	450	10.7	9.8 ± 0.3	0.9 ± 0.1	10.9

Source: Adapted from Giuffrida, F. et al., *Lipids* 49 (10):997–1004, 2014; Rueda, R.. In P. C. Calder and P. Yaqoob (ed.), *Diet, Immunity and Inflammation*, Cambridge, Woodhead Publishing Limited, 2013.

Molecular weights: Sialic acid=309; milk GM3=1198.5; milk GD3=1577. Colostrum: 1–5 days; transitional milk: 6–17 days; mature milk: more than 18 days. Results for LBSA (lipid-bound sialic acid) quantification are presented, expressed as mg LBSA/L and as mg/L. Data from quantitative mass spectrometry techniques are expressed as µg/mL.

content is remarkably lower than that of human milk. Our group described the content of total sialic acids (SAs) and gangliosides, measured as LBSA, in a series of starter infant formulas from different brands and countries, comparing it to the human milk content reported in the literature (Martin et al. 2008). SA content in the different formulas, measured as Neu5Ac, varied from 11 to 35 mg/100 mL (mean 19.4 ± 0.6 mg/100 mL). Those formulas claiming exogenous addition of SA had higher concentrations than the rest. Even in fortified formulas, the content of SA remained below that of human milk, which varies from 120–150 mg/100 mL in colostrum to 30–45 mg/100 mL in mature milk (Martin et al. 2007). Formulas were indeed reported to contain less than 25% the content of mature milk SA, with most of it (around 70%) bound to glycoproteins (Wang et al. 2001). LBSA content of the analyzed commercial formulas was on average 0.24 ± 0.10 mg/100 mL, ranging from 0.09–0.53/100 mL (Martin et al. 2007). According to these data, total SA and LBSA contents in commercial formulas remain far below those in human milk. Considering the crucial role that both molecules may play in the development of the newborn, the supplementation of infant formula may be important for the developmental needs of the neonate.

24.4 OVERVIEW OF THE FUNCTIONS OF GANGLIOSIDES

Gangliosides are important components of membranes, involved in the regulation of their organization and function (Sonnino and Prinetti 2010). Due to their localization in the plasma membrane, gangliosides act as receptors in cell-cell recognition systems, interacting through the carbohydrate moiety with glycan-binding proteins on opposing cells. They act thus as regulators of a wide range of normal physiological functions in the immune system, nervous system, and metabolism, but also in pathological events like cancer progression and metastasis (Lopez and Schnaar 2009) (Figure 24.1).

24.4.1 GANGLIOSIDES AS LIPID RAFT CONSTITUENTS

Gangliosides have a key role in the formation and stabilization of membrane raft domains, which serve as platforms for cellular signaling, cell-cell communication, and viral entry. Their enrichment in lipid rafts provides indications of how they may affect cell function. Gangliosides can modulate lipid rafts, thus influencing biological processes, such as immune function, neuronal signaling, cancer cell growth, entry of pathogens through the gut barrier, and insulin resistance in metabolic disorders (Yaqoob and Shaikh 2010). Their presence in raft domains in tissues such as the brain, small intestine, and adipose tissue may be critical for normal development and function, although they also appear to be involved in pathological processes (Yaqoob and Shaikh 2010). Normal composition of gangliosides is essential for the maintenance of lipid rafts, and gangliosides are involved in the maintenance and repair of nervous tissues (Furukawa et al. 2011; Ohmi et al. 2011). Raft architecture is affected by ganglioside deficiency, which in turn is linked to inflammation and the pathogenesis of neural diseases (Ohmi et al. 2012; Schengrund 2015).

Gangliosides act as receptors in cell-cell recognition, interacting with glycan binding proteins (lectins). Sialic-acid-binding immunoglobulin-like lectins (Siglecs) are a family of animal lectins that recognize sialic acids bound to glycans. Through interaction with Siglec-7, gangliosides regulate natural killer (NK) cell cytotoxicity. They also act as receptors for Siglec-4 (myelin-associated glycoprotein), thus modulating myelin-axon interactions and axonal regeneration after injury. They regulate inflammation through interactions with E-selectin (Lopez and Schnaar 2009). In addition, they interact laterally with other membrane lipids and proteins, regulating cell signaling through interaction with insulin, epidermal growth factor (EGF), and vascular endothelial growth factor receptors (VEGF) (Prinetti et al. 2009).

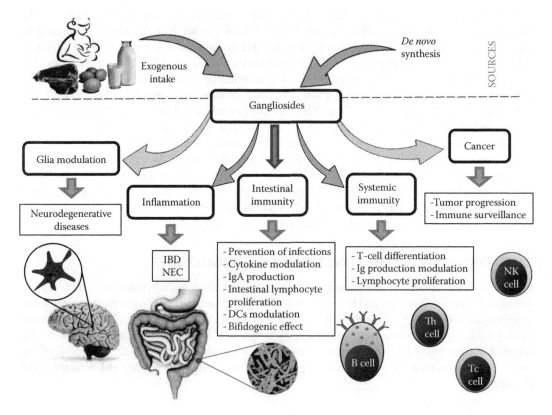

FIGURE 24.1 (See color insert.) Summary of the roles of gangliosides related to immune function and inflammation. Gangliosides can derive from *de novo* synthesis or exogenous intake from the diet. Gangliosides are important components of lipid rafts, which account for a wide range of biological functions; they are involved in: glia modulation, inflammation, intestinal immunity, microbiota regulation, systemic immunity, and cancer.

24.4.2 Gangliosides and Cancer

In addition to their important functions in normal physiological processes, gangliosides also play a role in pathological processes like tumor malignancy and metastasis. Among the multiple factors affecting tumor formation, gangliosides may act as both inhibitory and stimulating molecules. The regulation of growth factors by gangliosides has important consequences for cancer progression and metastasis (Lopez and Schnaar 2009). A number of cancers are characterized by activated EGF, and a crucial factor for tumor progression is the growth of new blood vessels. Tumor cells release VEGF, which stimulates VEGF receptors, resulting in proliferation and migration of vascular endothelial cells (Krengel and Bousquet 2014). Gangliosides can affect signaling by the EGF and VEGF (i.e., GM3 ganglioside has an inhibitory effect on cancer development and progression by inhibiting the activation of EGF receptors) (Hakomori and Handa 2015). In fact, the expression of monosialyl gangliosides such as GM2 and GM1 tended to suppress tumor growth and metastatic potential (Dong et al. 2010). The expression of disialyl gangliosides, on the other hand, has been generally reported to enhance tumor progression and invasion. GD3 and GD2 are highly expressed in melanomas and cell lung cells, as well as in osteosarcomas, where they increase cell growth and invasion (Furukawa et al. 2012). GD3 has been identified as a melanoma-specific antigen, and it has been suggested to be involved in the transformation of melanocytes into melanomas, and the promotion of metastasis (Krengel and Bousquet 2014).

In addition, tumor-associated gangliosides may act as suppressors of the antitumor immune response, downregulating the activity of T- and B-cells, NK cytotoxicity, and dendritic cells, among others. For instance, T-cell dysfunction is promoted by GM2 (Krengel and Bousquet 2014). Gangliosides synthesized by cancer cells may modify the immunological environment, promoting an alteration of T-cell responses toward Th-2, thus contributing to immunosuppression (Crespo et al. 2006). Besides, shedding of gangliosides constitutes an important factor to evade tumor destruction by local immune cells (McKallip et al. 1999). Gangliosides are shed from tumors in great quantities, and could interact with proteins or be incorporated into the membrane of other cells, altering signaling events or cell-cell interactions with healthy cells. They have been shown to inhibit the *in vitro* generation and differentiation of dendritic cells from progenitors (Peguet-Navarro et al. 2003; Shurin et al. 2001). Tumor-associated gangliosides could hence contribute to cancer progression through multiple mechanisms (Krengel and Bousquet 2014).

Many gangliosides associated with tumors are found in normal healthy tissues, but overexpressed in tumors, whereas others are only present in cancer cells. Such is the case of sialic-acid NeuGc, which is found in melanoma and breast cancer (Amon et al. 2014). Gangliosides are considered potential molecules for anticancer therapy, and a promising approach is the treatment with monoclonal antibodies recognizing tumor-associated markers (Couzin-Frankel 2013).

24.4.3 Gangliosides and Neural Development and Function

Gangliosides are essential for normal neural development and function. They play a remarkable role in neuronal growth, migration, and maturation; neuritogenesis; synaptogenesis; and myelination. In addition, they are involved in synaptic transmission (McJarrow et al. 2009). Animal studies exploring the effects of feeding gangliosides or cholesterol (or sialic acid, which is a key component of gangliosides) during early development suggested that they could influence brain development (Carlson 2009). Park et al. demonstrated that gangliosides and phospholipids added to the diet increased the ganglioside content in several tissues throughout the body, including the brain (Park et al. 2005b). Recently, early supplementation with phospholipids and gangliosides in pigs has shown beneficial effects, both in terms of brain and cognitive development (Liu et al. 2014). A pilot study in humans reported beneficial effects on the cognitive development of healthy infants (0–6 months) by supplementing infant formula with complex milk lipids, and the benefits appear to be related to increased ganglioside levels in serum (Gurnida et al. 2012). Other studies evaluated the potential for bovine milk–derived glycomacropeptide as an exogenous source of sialic acid to increase sialylation in brain glycoproteins and positively influence cognitive outcomes in animal models (Wang et al. 2007).

A role for gangliosides in regulating microglia morphology has been proposed. Microglia are vital for CNS homeostasis due to their plasticity and ability to respond to a wide range of challenges. In addition, they perform a structural role, and are involved in synaptic plasticity (Nayak et al. 2014). As immunological competent cells, they are considered key players in brain inflammation. Park et al. described that mixtures of brain gangliosides, and GM1, induced typical ramification in cultured rat microglia, whereas GD1a and GT1b did not (Park et al. 2008). Gangliosides were described to regulate the expression and release of B-cell activating factor (BAFF) expressed in microglia. BAFF is a member of the tumor necrosis factor (TNF) superfamily, with a crucial role in B-cell differentiation, survival, and regulation of immunoglobulin (Ig) production (Kim et al. 2009).

Gangliosides can activate immune cells in the brain, regulating the production of inflammatory mediators. They enhance cell surface expression of TLR2 in microglia, while reducing TLR4. The authors suggest that both TLR2 and TLR4 are involved in gangliosides-stimulated inflammatory responses in the brain (Figure 24.1) (Yoon et al. 2008).

Supplementation with gangliosides was shown to be important for retinal development, as inferred from animal studies. Supplementation with gangliosides and PUFAs induced changes in the phospholipid composition of rat retina. Such changes may affect light adaptation and signaling, and could thus lead to enhanced development of retinal function in neonates. Behavior, memory, and learning were not investigated (Park et al. 2005a).

In addition, deficiency of b-series gangliosides has been linked to neurogenesis deficits and behavioral changes, which indicates that b-series gangliosides are required for the maintenance of the neural stem cell pool (Wang et al. 2014).

24.4.4 GANGLIOSIDES AND NEURODEGENERATIVE DISORDERS

Ganglioside content undergoes drastic changes with age (Yu et al. 2009), which led to investigations of their influence on brain function during aging. In fact, modifications in ganglioside expression in lipid rafts with age has been suggested as a contributor to neurodegeneration leading to certain types of dementia or Alzheimer's disease (AD) (Schengrund 2015; Yaqoob and Shaikh 2010). Alterations in membrane ganglioside composition affect secretase activities, thus modulating the processing of amyloid precursor protein (APP) and generation of amyloid β peptide (Aβ). Alternatively, membrane gangliosides can directly interact with Aβ and modulate its aggregation (Walter and van Echten-Deckert 2013). In fact, GM1 in lipid rafts has been suggested as the possible origin for Aβ accumulation. GM1 promotes conformational changes in Aβ, and the unique GM1-bound form of Aβ would favor Aβ polymerization (Ledeen and Wu 2015; van Echten-Deckert and Walter 2012). It has been suggested that a depletion in ganglioside levels may result in neurodegeneration (Furukawa et al. 2015). Thus, factors altering GM1 expression may affect the onset of neuronal problems. Aging and insulin resistance induce brain insulin resistance, which was accompanied by increased assembly of Aβ fibrils on the surface of neurons, due to a rise in GM1 clustering in the membrane lipid rafts (Yamamoto et al. 2012). Leptin also inhibited GM1 expression in lipid rafts, and Aβ assembly in neurons (Yamamoto et al. 2014).

Ganglioside administration has shown therapeutic benefits for neurologic diseases (Ryan et al. 2013). The fact that GM1 could form complexes with Aβ, hence preventing its deposition and oligomerization, would account for the beneficial effects observed in the treatment of neurologic diseases with exogenous gangliosides (Aureli et al. 2015).

Parkinson's disease (PD) is characterized by a progressive loss of dopaminergic neurons in the substantia nigra region of the midbrain. About one third of the individuals affected will eventually develop dementia in the final stages. Several studies have implicated gangliosides in PD (Schengrund 2015). GM1 was shown to bind to α-synuclein, inducing a conformational change that inhibited its ability to aggregate and form insoluble fibers, thereby altering normal neuronal function (Martinez et al. 2007). Alterations in intracellular GM1 may thus be a contributing factor for PD (Ariga 2014). Studies reported positive effects of GM1 in treating symptoms of PD. GM1 protects against nigrostriatal toxicity and associated motor symptoms in monkeys, restoring cognitive and motor function, and preventing decline in function (Pope-Coleman and Schneider 1998; Pope-Coleman et al. 2000). Parkinson's patients showed a significant improvement following GM1 treatment (Schneider et al. 2013).

Huntington's disease (HD) is a genetic disorder caused by the expansion of a polyglutamine repeat tract, in the protein huntingtin (htt). Patients with HD exhibit progressive motor, cognitive, and psychiatric dysfunction. Several studies have reported decreased concentration of brain gangliosides in patients with HD and in animal models of HD (Ariga 2014). The expression of genes encoding glycosyltransferases, as well as ganglioside metabolic pathways, were shown to be affected in patients with HD (Desplats et al. 2007). Reduced synthesis of GM1 was found to occur in several models of HD (Maglione et al. 2010). In addition, high levels of GD3 were found in human HD, which may be indicative of apoptotic neurodegeneration. Alterations in the metabolism of gangliosides such as GM1 and GD3 may play a role in mediating the pathogenesis of HD (Ariga 2014). The administration of GM1 restores ganglioside levels in HD cells and promotes activation of protein kinase B (AKT), leading to decreased mutant htt toxicity and increased survival of HD cells (Maglione et al. 2010).

These results provide the rationale for considering dietary ganglioside supplementation in patients with neurodegenerative disorders. Ganglioside supplementation may bear special importance during the onset and early stages of the diseases, when nutritional interventions are more likely to show positive effects.

24.4.5 GANGLIOSIDES AND INFLAMMATION

Inflammation has emerged as a leading cause for several brain diseases. Brain-derived gangliosides can induce the production of inflammatory mediators in brain microglia and astrocytes. While some reports have suggested that they may promote inflammation in the brain through modulation of TLR expression (Yoon et al. 2008), other studies propose ganglioside deficiency as the trigger for inflammatory reactions and neurodegeneration through complement activation (Ohmi et al. 2009). Recent reports further support that depletion of gangliosides results in inflammation of CNS and neurodegeneration (Furukawa et al. 2015).

An anti-inflammatory role for gangliosides in the intestines has also been proposed. Gangliosides were suggested to modulate vasoactive mediators and to suppress proinflammatory signals. Indeed, levels of GM3 and GD3 are decreased in inflammation, while low levels of GM3 are associated with higher production of proinflammatory signals (Miklavcic et al. 2012). This protective effect of gangliosides may be particularly relevant for the prevention of necrotizing enterocolitis (NEC), a gastrointestinal disorder primarily affecting preterm infants (Schnabl et al. 2009b). In fact, ganglioside GD3 has been suggested to play an important immunodulatory role in reducing the incidence and severity of NEC in an *in vivo* animal model, by reducing proinflammatory cytokines and increasing anti-inflammatory mediators (Xu et al. 2013). This anti-inflammatory role of gangliosides could be attributed to the ability of dietary gangliosides to modify the composition of the brush border membrane in the intestinal mucosa (Park et al. 2005b; Schnabl et al. 2009a). Dietary gangliosides (GM3 and GD3) were found to protect rat intestinal epithelium from lipolysaccharide (LPS)-induced inflammation via sustained stability of gut-occluding tight junction protein, enhanced intestinal IL-10 production, and reduced generation of inflammatory intermediates (eicosanoids and cytokines) (Park et al. 2007; Park et al. 2010). GM3 has been suggested to exert its anti-inflammatory role by suppressing the expression of inflammatory molecules such as ICAM-1 and VCAM-1 in endothelial cells, thus reducing monocyte adhesion to endothelial cells stimulated by VEGF (Kim et al. 2014). A recent report suggests a protective role for GM1 and GD1a gangliosides in LPS-triggered inflammation in epithelial cells, by preventing TLR4 translocation into lipid rafts (Nikolaeva et al. 2015).

24.4.6 GANGLIOSIDES AND METABOLIC SYNDROME

A link between gangliosides and the pathophysiology of obesity-related diseases has been established. Studies by Tanabe et al. described an increase of a-series gangliosides downstream of GM3 (GM2, GM1, and GD1a) in the adipose tissue of obese mice (Tanabe et al. 2009). Recently, it was suggested that b-series gangliosides in lipid rafts would regulate leptin secretion from adipose tissues (Ji et al. 2015). Moreover, gangliosides are implicated in insulin resistance. Insulin resistance involves changes in the dynamics and organization of lipid raft domains, with GM3 suggested as a key ganglioside involved in altered insulin signaling (Inokuchi 2014; Langeveld and Aerts 2009). The link between chronic low-grade inflammation in obesity and metabolic syndrome might directly involve gangliosides in a membrane microdomain-related mechanism (Yaqoob and Shaikh 2010). In fact, metabolic disorders have been proposed to be membrane microdomain disorders, caused by altered expression of gangliosides (Inokuchi 2014).

24.4.7 GANGLIOSIDES AND AUTOPHAGY

Gangliosides have been increasingly recognized as mediators in processes important for cell survival, such as autophagy. Autophagy is a catabolic pathway, involved in the lysosomal degradation and recycling of proteins and organelles, of remarkable importance for maintaining homeostasis. It has been suggested that gangliosides could participate in the early phases of autophagy due to their molecular interaction with key molecules involved in autophagosome biogenesis and maturation (Tommasino et al. 2015). Actually, GD3 was reported to have a role in the initial phases of autophagy; it is recruited into the autophagosome via molecular interaction with autophagy-associated molecules. It would participate in the maturation of the autophagosome into autolysosome, contributing to the remodeling of the membrane curvature and fluidity (Matarrese et al. 2014).

24.4.8 GANGLIOSIDES AND IMMUNITY

The importance of gangliosides in immunity will be further extended in Section 24.5. Briefly, they can modulate the development or behavior of cells of the immune system (Ebel et al. 1992; Yuasa et al. 1990). Dietary gangliosides perform a remarkable role in promoting the development of intestinal immunity and oral tolerance in the neonate, thus contributing to prevent infections in early infancy (Rueda 2007).

Gangliosides can act as "unintended" target receptors for the adhesion of bacterial toxins, bacteria, or viruses. Enterotoxins from *Escherichia coli* and *Vibrio cholera* interact with GM1 gangliosides, which possess the ability to inactivate them (Laegreid and Otnaess 1987; Otnaess et al. 1983). *Helicobacter pylori* vacuolating cytotoxin could also be neutralized by GM1, by binding directly and preventing the cytotoxin internalization (Wada et al. 2010). Several studies reported the role of cell surface gangliosides as receptors for bacterial adhesion in specific tissues (Hata et al. 2004; Idota and Kawakami 1995). More recently, *in vitro* experiments suggested that gangliosides GM3, GD3, and GM1, at the concentrations found in human milk or infant formula, were able to interfere with the adhesion of several pathogenic bacteria involved in severe neonatal diarrhea episodes (Salcedo et al. 2013). The infection with certain human rotaviruses, the leading cause of severe gastroenteritis in infants, takes place through binding to cell surface GM1 glycan (Fleming et al. 2014; Martinez et al. 2013). Other studies described the implication of gangliosides in the interaction between host and pathogens such as *Campylobacter jejuni* and HIV (Day et al. 2012; Izquierdo-Useros et al. 2014; Puryear et al. 2012). A role for gangliosides in the prevention of parasitic infections was also suggested. In particular, it was reported that gangliosides supplemented into the diet had a protective effect against *Giardia muris* infection *in vitro* and decreased the survival of *G. lamblia* trophozoites *in vitro* (Suh et al. 2004). Dietary gangliosides act as putative decoys, interfering with pathogen binding.

In addition, evidence has accumulated suggesting that MFGM compounds, rich in gangliosides, may be involved in defense against pathogens. In particular, MFGM compounds were reported to adhere to enterotoxigenic *E. coli* strains (Sanchez-Juanes et al. 2009), and to inhibit the infectivity of rotavirus *in vitro* (Fuller et al. 2013). Recently, a clinical trial has shown that formula supplemented with MFGMs decreases the incidence of acute otitis media infections, to a level similar to breastfed infants (Timby et al. 2015). This evidence suggests that gangliosides could reduce the infection capacity of pathogens in the neonate.

24.5 GANGLIOSIDE EFFECTS ON IMMUNE FUNCTION

One of the most established functions of gangliosides is their role as immunomodulating agents. Figure 24.1 illustrates a summary of these roles. GD1α and GD1 were characteristically detected in Th2 and Th1 lymphocyte subpopulations, acting as differentiation markers (Ebel et al. 1992). Several studies suggested that gangliosides could be involved in the activation of T-cells (Yuasa et al. 1990) and in the differentiation of different lymphocyte subpopulations (Ebel et al. 1992; Nakamura et al. 1995; Nashar et al. 1996; Taga et al. 1995). In fact, anti-GD3 antibodies deliver a potent costimulatory signal for antigen-induced proliferation of CD4$^+$ T lymphocytes (Schlaak et al. 1995). T-cell activation via GD3 results in phospholipase C-γ phosphorylation and initiation of Ca^{2+} flux (Ortaldo et al. 1996). These data suggest another mechanism of T-cell activation via a single, nonprotein surface moiety. Given that GD3 is one of the most important gangliosides in human milk and has been involved in the mechanism of T-lymphocyte activation, the supplementation of milk formulas with this ganglioside may contribute to the proliferation, activation, and differentiation of immune cells, especially those from the intestine in the neonate (Rueda 2013).

To understand the role of gangliosides in differentiation, maturation, and activation of T-cells, it is necessary to evaluate ganglioside composition in lipid rafts. Indeed, gangliosides GM1 and GM3 define different type of rafts, segregating differently in the polarized human T-cells (Inokuchi et al. 2013). The activation of individual T-cell subsets requires different types of gangliosides (Nagafuku et al. 2012). In particular, CD4$^+$ T-cells preferentially express a-series gangliosides (the simplest being GM3), whereas CD8$^+$ T-cells express very high levels of o-series gangliosides. These results suggest that CD4$^+$ and CD8$^+$ T-cell subsets require a-series and o-series ganglioside expression, respectively, to undergo activation upon TCR (T-cell antigen receptor) ligation. This different ganglioside pattern may define the immune function of each T-cell subset (Inokuchi et al. 2015). The authors suggest their findings may constitute a new strategy to treat allergic inflammation, targeting helper T-cells to control ganglioside expression in lipid rafts.

In addition to the regulatory role of gangliosides in T-cell differentiation, they exhibit a direct role in effector functions, such as modulation of Ig production. Indeed, gangliosides have been reported to either enhance or inhibit Ig production in different types of cells. GM1 increased Ig production in human plasma cells lines (Kimata 1994). In human B-cell lines, GM2 inhibited Ig production, by reducing the production of IL-10 and TNF-α (Kimata and Yoshida 1996). Other studies reported that ganglioside GQ1b enhanced Ig production of B-cells, by promoting IL-6 and IL-10 production of T-cells (Kanda and Tamaki 1998). In contrast, GD1b had an inhibitory effect, by reducing IL-6 and IL-10 production in CD4$^+$ T-cells (Kanda and Tamaki 1999). Ganglioside GD1a enhanced IgG, IgM, and IgA production by human peripheral mononuclear cells (PBMCs). It enhanced IL-6 and IL-10 production of monocytes, hence indirectly increasing B-cell Ig production (Kanda and Watanabe 2000). Thus, the role of gangliosides in modulating Ig production is complex, acting as either immunosuppressant or enhancer, depending on specific gangliosides species.

Similarly, gangliosides modulate the proliferation of several classes of immune cells *in vitro*, either acting as enhancers or inhibitors. They were shown to enhance the proliferation in human plasma cell lines and B-cells (Kimata 1994; Kimata and Yoshida 1994). In contrast, they were reported to inhibit the proliferation of T and B lymphocytes, T helper cells, and natural killer cells. The mechanisms are not fully understood, although it was described that brain-derived gangliosides bound to IL-2, thus preventing the cytokine binding to its receptor and blocking T-cell division (Irani et al. 1996). The interaction of tumor-derived gangliosides with both IL-2 and IL-4 was reported, thus inhibiting T-cell and T helper proliferation respectively (Chu and Sharom 1995; Lu and Sharom 1995).

Besides their systemic effects, gangliosides exert a direct influence on the immune system through the interaction with the gut associated lymphoid gut tissue (GALT). GALT is the largest immune organ in the body, comprising Peyer's patches, isolated lymphoid follicles, and nonaggregated cells in the lamina propria and intraepithelial lymphocytes (see Chapter 2). It is an essential component of immune defense, protecting the body from foreign antigens and pathogens, while allowing tolerance to commensal bacteria and dietary antigens (Wershil and Furuta 2008). The development of the local immune system in the gastrointestinal tract is relatively independent of systemic immunity. The interaction of different factors, such as intestinal microbiota and nutrients at the local level, may influence the inner regulatory mechanisms of the intestinal immune function, especially during the first year of life. Given that gangliosides in human milk are able to modulate some immunological parameters at the intestine, they would contribute to the proliferation, activation, and differentiation of intestinal cells, which would be particularly important in the neonate.

Unlike primary immune organs such as the spleen or thymus, an important part of GALT is a diffuse system with high numbers of immune cells integrated in the intestinal mucosa, even representing about 25% of the total mucosa mass. Consequently, factors affecting GALT development could therefore modify intestinal development.

The changes in the ganglioside content of mammalian milk during lactation may suggest their role in physiological processes that take place during early phases of infant development (Rueda and Gil 1998; Rueda et al. 1998a). Given that a high concentration of GD3 has been detected in developing tissues (Ando 1983), as well as in human colostrum, it could reflect a biological role in the development of organs (i.e., the neonatal intestine) (Rueda 2013). As mentioned above, human milk contains a significant amount of highly polar gangliosides (Rueda et al. 1995). This type of ganglioside has been detected in developing tissues (i.e., the embryonic chicken brain, syncytiotrophoblast, amnion, and placenta) (Rueda and Gil 1998). Since they are present in amniotic fluid (Rueda et al. 1993), which is in contact with developing tissues, they may thus originate by shedding from these tissues (Ladisch et al. 1983; Li and Ladisch 1991). The role of these highly complex gangliosides in developing tissues remains unknown, although it has been suggested that they act as mediators of certain types of cell-cell interactions during the early stages of mammalian development (Friedman et al. 1983). The complex gangliosides in human milk could thus be shed by the lactating mammary gland, playing an important role in this organ or in developing infant tissues, the small intestine in particular, during early life. Characteristic expression of complex gangliosides (i.e. GD1α) during lactation in the murine mammary gland and in the milk-fat globule has been described (Momoeda et al. 1995).

Dietary gangliosides play an important role in the regulation of intestinal immunity (Figure 24.1). In fact, in a model of weaning mice, gangliosides positively modulated the percentages of Th1 and Th2 lymphocyte subsets in the small intestine (Vazquez et al. 2001). Animals fed gangliosides showed an earlier development in cytokine-secreting cells. In addition, they showed a higher number of Th1 and Th2 cytokine secreting lymphocytes in lamina propia and Peyer's patches after four weeks of feeding (Vazquez et al. 2001). Dietary gangliosides also increased the numbers of intestinal IgA secreting cells (Vazquez et al. 1999) and the luminal content of secretory IgA in weaning mice (Vazquez et al. 2000), which represents the main mechanism of defense against microorganisms entering the gastrointestinal tract. These results are in accordance with previous publications showing that different gangliosides modulate the production of immunoglobulins in a positive way (Kanda 1999; Kanda and Tamaki 1998). The influence of gangliosides in intestinal lymphocyte proliferation *in vitro* has also been reported (Vazquez et al. 2002). Gangliosides induce different effects on intestinal lymphocyte proliferation depending on the presence and concentration of specific structures, suggesting that dietary gangliosides may influence the development of intestinal immunity by either stimulating or inhibiting proliferative or inhibitory responses in intestinal lymphocytes during early infancy.

Gangliosides also exert modulating effects on dendritic cells, key cells with a pivotal role in orchestrating appropriate tolerogenic or immunogenic responses. GD3 and GM3 were described to inhibit dendritic cell maturation and effector functionalities, albeit to different extents. The combined action of both GD3 and GM3 may prevent excessive immune responses against the large amounts of antigen the newborn encounters during the first weeks of life. They would hence promote adequate tolerance against harmless antigens. Given that GD3 has a greater inhibitory potential and is present at higher levels during early stages of lactation, it could be inferred that the immune-regulating effect of the ganglioside milk fraction would be more notable at the beginning of lactation (Brønnum et al. 2005).

Ganglioside treatment was reported to induce a state of tolerance to TLR signaling, leading to blunted activation of innate immune responses (Shen et al. 2008). Ganglioside-exposed dendritic cells promote regulatory T-cell activity that may have long-lasting effects on the development of tumor-specific immune responses (Jales et al. 2011). Even though these results were reported in the context of tumor studies, they may also suggest a role for dietary gangliosides promoting regulatory responses when contacting dendritic cells at the intestinal level.

Considering the important role of gangliosides in the differentiation and modulation of the intestinal immune system, their addition to infant formulas may present several advantages for formula-fed infants (Rueda 2013). Our group also studied tolerance-related parameters (incidence and duration of diarrhea, fecal color and consistency) in piglets fed a control or prototype formulas containing fructooligosaccharides and a higher content of sialic acid, gangliosides, and phospholipids (Ramirez et al. 2008). The incidence of diarrhea was not significantly different among the different study groups, but its duration was shorter in piglets fed the prototype formulas than in those fed control formulas. These results support a role for gangliosides on promoting development of intestinal immunity and oral tolerance in the neonate, and, as a consequence, on preventing infection.

24.6 BIFIDOGENIC EFFECT OF GANGLIOSIDES

The interaction between glycolipids and infant intestinal microbiota has been shown in several publications. First, the excretion of glycolipids in the feces of breastfed newborns and children was reported (Larson et al. 1987). Authors then demonstrated that several bacteria possessed extracellular glycosidases to degrade intestinal glycolipids (Falk et al. 1990; Larson et al. 1988). Later, our clinical study showed that the addition of gangliosides to infant formula, in concentrations similar to those in human milk, modified the intestinal microflora of preterm newborns, increasing *Bifidobacteria* counts while reducing those of *E. coli*. Feces from infants fed the ganglioside supplemented formula contained lower counts of *E. coli* than those from infants fed control formula, with significant differences at 7 days postpartum. After thirty days postpartum, the counts of fecal bifidobacteria were higher in infants fed the ganglioside-supplemented formula (Rueda et al. 1998b). These data suggest that supplementation of infant formula with gangliosides produces a growth-promoting effect of bifidobacteria and pointed to a prebiotic role of gangliosides. However, the ability of bifidobacteria to catabolize gangliosides from milk has not been explored, and the fate of digested milk gangliosides remains difficult to interpret. A more recent study has evaluated the capacity of bifidobacteria to consume milk gangliosides *in vitro*, and the results obtained further support a prebiotic effect for milk gangliosides on bifidobacteria in humans, especially in breastfed infants (Lee et al. 2014). The authors hypothesized that gut bacteria may contribute to the chemical modulation of ingested gangliosides. According to their results, *B. infantis*, *B. bifidum,* and *B. breve* can consume bovine milk ganglioside as the sole carbon source *in vitro*. Analysis of the milk gangliosides remaining after incubation with *Bifidobacterium* species by nano-HPLC Chip QTOF showed that *B. infantis* and *B. bifidum* can catabolize significant amounts of GM3 and GD3; *B. infantis* consumed 63% of GD3 and *B. bifidum* consumed 100%. In contrast, *B. longum, B. adolescentis*, and *B. lactis* degraded ganglioside to a lower extent (30%, 28%, and 48%, respectively) (Lee et al. 2014). It is probable that species of bifidobacteria utilize milk gangliosides as carbon sources by cleaving the glycan parts of the molecule with glycosylhydrolases. The release of free sialic acid in the intestinal tract may change the glycolipid profile in the gut's intestinal epithelial cells and feces. Gangliosides would thus exert a selective prebiotic activity on specific bifidobacteria in infants (Lee et al. 2014). They can therefore influence the immune system not only directly, but also indirectly, by acting as prebiotics favoring the growth of beneficial bacteria.

Besides their role as prebiotics, an additional action could be speculated. Gangliosides modulate dendritic cells, which are implicated in the maintenance of tolerance toward commensal microbiota. Gangliosides could thus be further involved in favoring beneficial bacteria through their interaction with dendritic cells (Rescigno 2011).

24.7   SUMMARY AND FUTURE TRENDS

The role of dietary gangliosides was tested in preterm infants by supplementing infant formula with gangliosides, at concentrations similar to those in human milk. The ganglioside-supplemented formula modified the intestinal microflora of preterm newborns, increasing *Bifidobacteria* counts while reducing *E. coli*. These results suggest that gangliosides at the concentrations found in human milk may significantly modulate the intestinal microbiota of the newborn. However, the mechanisms involved and the relevance of such findings remain to be further elucidated (Rueda 2007, 2013; Rueda et al. 1998b). Gangliosides are able to modulate gut microbiota, toward a more beneficial profile enriched in *Bifidobacterium* (Rueda et al. 1998b). Resident bifidobacteria can metabolize them, which further supports their role as prebiotics (Lee et al. 2014). They may thus act as a contributing factor for the establishment of a protective and balanced microbiota from early infancy. In recent years, accumulating evidence demonstrates the microbiota as a key factor influencing host health. Gut microbiota provides the host with nutrients, but also with a whole range of metabolic activities that would not be accessible otherwise. It exerts a direct action on gut mucosa and enteric nervous system, but the effects go beyond the GI tract, as it influences the function of distal organs and systems (Clarke et al. 2014). The influence of microbiota on health is continuous throughout life. Variations and changes in gut microbiota influence physiology and can contribute to diseases ranging from inflammation to obesity. Microbiota can also communicate with the CNS, hence influencing brain function and behavior (Cryan and Dinan 2012). It is noteworthy that alterations in microbiota during early life have been associated with increased risk of health disorders during childhood and later in life (Arrieta et al. 2014). Given the bifidogenic effect of gangliosides, they may constitute an interesting ingredient to modulate the microbiota toward a beneficial one, especially during early life stages. Besides, milk gangliosides showed beneficial effects in modulating the immune functionality of GALT. Their interaction with dendritic cells may promote suitable tolerance against harmless antigens, which would be crucial for the neonate (Brønnum et al. 2005).

The role of gangliosides in preventing inflammation at the intestinal level suggests that dietary gangliosides may be beneficial in clinical situations involving inflammation (Miklavcic et al. 2012). This may be particularly relevant for the treatment and prevention of inflammatory bowel diseases (IBDs) and NEC, the leading cause (25%) for preterm mortality. Considering that NEC has a lower incidence in breastfed infants than formula-fed ones, it may seem feasible to attribute to gangliosides some of the beneficial effects of breast milk in NEC. However, better effects of bovine colostrum compared to ganglioside-enriched formulas were reported, regarding the stimulation of intestinal function and induction of NEC resistance in a piglet model of preterm infants. These observations would suggest a synergistic effect of several bioactives in milk (Moller et al. 2010). Gangliosides nevertheless could be, either alone or in combination with other bioactives, considered an interesting ingredient in formulas for newborns in the neonatal intensive care unit.

The potential role of gangliosides in neurodevelopment has been explored in depth during the past decades. Many reports support that dietary gangliosides, together with other complex lipids, may be important for brain development early in life. Recently, Liu et al. reported that dietary gangliosides improved spatial learning and affected brain growth and composition in neonatal piglets (Liu et al. 2014). Long-term oral administration of complex milk lipids enriched in gangliosides have been described to improve cognitive function in rats (Guan et al. 2015; Guillermo et al. 2015; Vickers et al. 2009). Only one human study has been conducted to assess the influence of a ganglioside-supplemented infant formula on cognitive functions of normal healthy infants. This pilot study showed that ganglioside supplementation had beneficial effects on cognitive development in healthy infants aged 0–6 months (Gurnida et al. 2012).

MFGM has gained interest as a biologically active fraction with potential beneficial health effects. Several components of MFGM have been reported to be essential for brain development, gangliosides among them (McJarrow et al. 2009). In fact, clinical trials have shown that formula supplemented with MFGM reduced differences in cognitive development between formula-fed and breastfed infants (Timby et al. 2014), and decreased the risk of infection (Timby et al. 2015). Some authors suggest that maternal dietary ganglioside supplementation during pregnancy may promote long-term effects on fetal brain development and improve cognitive function from early neural development (Ryan et al. 2013). The available results, although not conclusive, suggest that the intake of gangliosides during pregnancy may provide a mechanism to enhance brain development during the critical early stages (Ryan et al. 2013).

Gangliosides, as major components of raft domains, perform important functions regulating signaling pathways in lipid rafts, and this accounts for the wide range of biological functions they perform (Figure 24.1). As a consequence, disruption in ganglioside composition affects the maintenance of lipid rafts, which may be the trigger of severe neurodegenerative diseases (Ariga 2014; Schengrund 2015). Understanding the mechanism of action of gangliosides and their role in lipid raft maintenance may lead to new therapies and disease prevention in neurodegenerative diseases such as AD (Ariga 2014). This would decrease the burden caused by these diseases and enhance the quality of life for the aging population (Schengrund 2010). In addition, gangliosides can modulate microglia and regulate the production of proinflammatory mediators in the brain. They could hence be considered for the prevention and treatment of neurodegenerative disorders with a proinflammatory origin.

Finally, gangliosides play an important role preventing the infection by several pathogens, acting as unintended target receptors (Rueda 2007). However, their role in immunity extends beyond a merely protective role, as they influence both systemic and intestinal immunity. At the systemic level, they contribute to the proliferation, activation, and differentiation of immune cells. In the intestine, they regulate the production of cytokines and IgA. In addition, by modulating dendritic cells, they contribute to immune tolerance. Their impact on the immune system could be further extended, if we consider their role as substrates for the microbiota (Rueda 2013).

Despite the numerous publications in the scientific literature regarding the biological effects of gangliosides and their mechanism of action, human studies to demonstrate their clinical relevance when incorporated with the diet are still largely missing. In particular, well-designed clinical trials are needed to provide further understanding of their immune outcomes, in order to support their use in clinical practice in the future.

REFERENCES

Amon, R., E. M. Reuven, S. Leviatan Ben-Arye, and V. Padler-Karavani. 2014. Glycans in immune recognition and response. *Carbohydr Res* 389:115–22.

Ando, S. 1983. Gangliosides in the nervous system. *Neurochem Int* 5 (5):507–37.

Ariga, T. 2014. Pathogenic role of ganglioside metabolism in neurodegenerative diseases. *J Neurosci Res* 92 (10):1227–42.

Arrieta, M. C., L. T. Stiemsma, N. Amenyogbe, E. M. Brown, and B. Finlay. 2014. The intestinal microbiome in early life: Health and disease. *Front Immunol* 5:427.

Aureli, M., L. Mauri, M. G. Ciampa, et al. 2016. GM1 Ganglioside: Past studies and future potential. *Mol Neurobiol* 53 (3):1824–42.

Bode, L., C. Beermann, M. Mank, G. Kohn, and G. Boehm. 2004. Human and bovine milk gangliosides differ in their fatty acid composition. *J Nutr* 134 (11):3016–20.

Brønnum, H., T. Seested, L. I. Hellgren, S. Brix, and H. Frøkiær. 2005. Milk-derived GM3 and GD3 differentially inhibit dendritic cell maturation and effector functionalities. *Scand J Immunol* 61 (6):551–7.

Bushway, A. A., and T. W. Keenan. 1978. Composition and synthesis of three higher ganglioside homologs in bovine mammary tissue. *Lipids* 13 (1):59–65.

Carlson, S. E. 2009. Early determinants of development: A lipid perspective. *Am J Clin Nutr* 89 (5):1523S–1529S.

Chester, M. A. 1998. IUPAC-IUB Joint Commission on Biochemical Nomenclature (JCBN). Nomenclature of glycolipids–recommendations 1997. *Eur J Biochem* 257 (2):293–8.

Chu, J. W., and F. J. Sharom. 1995. Gangliosides interact with interleukin-4 and inhibit interleukin-4-stimulated helper T-cell proliferation. *Immunology* 84 (3):396–403.

Clarke, G., R. M. Stilling, P. J. Kennedy, et al. 2014. Minireview: Gut microbiota: The neglected endocrine organ. *Mol Endocrinol* 28 (8):1221–38.

Couzin-Frankel, J. 2013. Breakthrough of the year 2013. Cancer immunotherapy. *Science* 342 (6165):1432–3.

Crespo, F. A., X. Sun, J. G. Cripps, and R. Fernandez-Botran. 2006. The immunoregulatory effects of gangliosides involve immune deviation favoring type-2 T cell responses. *J Leukoc Biol* 79 (3):586–95.

Cryan, J. F., and T. G. Dinan. 2012. Mind-altering microorganisms: The impact of the gut microbiota on brain and behaviour. *Nat Rev Neurosci* 13 (10):701–12.

Day, C. J., E. A. Semchenko, and V. Korolik. 2012. Glycoconjugates play a key role in campylobacter jejuni infection: Interactions between host and pathogen. *Front Cell Infect Microbio* 2:9.

Desplats, P. A., C. A. Denny, K. E. Kass, et al. 2007. Glycolipid and ganglioside metabolism imbalances in Huntington's disease. *Neurobiol Dis* 27 (3):265–77.

Dong, Y., K. Ikeda, K. Hamamura, et al. 2010. GM1 / GD1b / GA1 synthase expression results in the reduced cancer phenotypes with modulation of composition and raft-localization of gangliosides in a melanoma cell line. *Cancer Sci* 101 (9):2039–47.

Ebel, F., E. Schmitt, J. Peter-Katalinic, B. Kniep, and P. F. Muhlradt. 1992. Gangliosides: Differentiation markers for murine T helper lymphocyte subpopulations TH1 and TH2. *Biochemistry* 31 (48):12190–7.

Falk, P., L. C. Hoskins, and G. Larson. 1990. Bacteria of the human intestinal microbiota produce glycosidases specific for lacto-series glycosphingolipids. *J Biochem* 108 (3):466–74.

Fleming, F. E., R. Böhm, V. T. Dang, et al. 2014. Relative roles of GM1 ganglioside, N-acylneuraminic acids, and α2B1 integrin in mediating rotavirus infection. *J Virol* 88 (8):4558–71.

Friedman, S. J., S. Cheng, and P. Skehan. 1983. The occurrence of polysialogangliosides in a human trophoblast cell line. *FEBS Lett* 152 (2):175–9.

Fuller, K. L., T. B. Kuhlenschmidt, M. S. Kuhlenschmidt, R. Jimenez-Flores, and S. M. Donovan. 2013. Milk fat globule membrane isolated from buttermilk or whey cream and their lipid components inhibit infectivity of rotavirus in vitro. *J Dairy Sci* 96 (6):3488–97.

Furukawa, K., K. Hamamura, Y. Ohkawa, and Y. Ohmi. 2012. Disialyl gangliosides enhance tumor phenotypes with differential modalities. *Glycoconj J* 29 (8–9):579–84.

Furukawa, K., Y. Ohmi, Y. Kondo, Y. Ohkawa, and O. Tajima. 2015. Regulatory function of glycosphingolipids in the inflammation and degeneration. *Arch Biochem Biophys.* 571:58–65.

Furukawa, K., Y. Ohmi, Y. Ohkawa, et al. 2011. Regulatory mechanisms of nervous systems with glycosphingolipids. *Neurochem Res* 36 (9):1578–86.

Giuffrida, F., I. M. Elmelegy, S. K. Thakkar, C. Marmet, and F. Destaillats. 2014. Longitudinal evolution of the concentration of gangliosides GM3 and GD3 in human milk. *Lipids* 49 (10):997–1004.

Guan, J., A. MacGibbon, B. Fong, et al. 2015. Long-term supplementation with beta serum concentrate (BSC), a complex of milk lipids, during post-natal brain development improves memory in rats. *Nutrients* 7 (6):4526–41.

Guillermo, R. B., P. Yang, M. H. Vickers, P. McJarrow, and J. Guan. 2015. Supplementation with complex milk lipids during brain development promotes neuroplasticity without altering myelination or vascular density. *Food Nutr Res* 59:25765.

Gurnida, D. A., A. M. Rowan, P. Idjradinata, D. Muchtadi, and N. Sekarwana. 2012. Association of complex lipids containing gangliosides with cognitive development of 6-month-old infants. *Early Hum Dev* 88 (8):595–601.

Hakomori, S. I., and K. Handa. 2015. GM3 and cancer. *Glycoconj J* 32 (1–2):1–8.

Hata, Y., M. Murakami, and S. Okabe. 2004. Glycoconjugates with NeuAc-NeuAc-Gal-Glc are more effective at preventing adhesion of helicobacter pylori to gastric epithelial cells than glycoconjugates with NeuAc-Gal-Glc. *J Physiol Pharmacol* 55 (3):607–25.

Huang, Q., X. Zhou, D. Liu, et al. 2014. A new liquid chromatography/tandem mass spectrometry method for quantification of gangliosides in human plasma. *Anal Biochem* 455:26–34.

Idota, T., and H. Kawakami. 1995. Inhibitory effects of milk gangliosides on the adhesion of escherichia coli to human intestinal carcinoma cells. *Biosci Biotechnol Biochem* 59 (1):69–72.

Inokuchi, J. 2014. GM3 and diabetes. *Glycoconj J* 31 (3):193–7.

Inokuchi, J.-I., M. Nagafuku, I. Ohno, and A. Suzuki. 2013. Heterogeneity of gangliosides among T cell subsets. *Cell Mol Life Sci* 70 (17):3067–75.

Inokuchi, J.-I., M. Nagafuku, I. Ohno, and A. Suzuki. 2015. Distinct selectivity of gangliosides required for CD4+ T and CD8+ T cell activation. *Biochim Biophys Acta* 1851:98–106.

Irani, D. N., K. I. Lin, and D. E. Griffin. 1996. Brain-derived gangliosides regulate the cytokine production and proliferation of activated T cells. *J Immunol* 157 (10):4333–40.

Izquierdo-Useros, N., M. Lorizate, P. J. McLaren, et al. 2014. HIV-1 capture and transmission by dendritic cells: The role of viral glycolipids and the cellular receptor Siglec-1. *PLoS Pathog* 10 (7):e1004146.

Jales, A., R. Falahati, E. Mari, et al. 2011. Ganglioside-exposed dendritic cells inhibit T-cell effector function by promoting regulatory cell activity. *Immunology* 132 (1):134–43.

Ji, S., Y. Ohkawa, K. Tokizane, et al. 2015. b-series gangliosides crucially regulate leptin secretion in adipose tissues. *Biochem Biophys Res Commun* 459 (2):189–95.

Kanda, N. 1999. Gangliosides GD1a and GM3 induce interleukin-10 production by human T cells. *Biochem Biophys Res Commun* 256 (1):41–4.

Kanda, N., and K. Tamaki. 1998. Ganglioside GQ1b enhances Ig production by human PBMCs. *J Allergy Clin Immunol* 102 (5):813–20.

Kanda, N., and K. Tamaki. 1999. Ganglioside GT1b suppresses immunoglobulin production by human peripheral blood mononuclear cells. *Immunology* 96 (4):628–33.

Kanda, N., and S. Watanabe. 2000. Ganglioside GD1a enhances immunoglobulin production by human peripheral blood mononuclear cells. *Exp Hematol* 28 (6):672–9.

Keenan, T. W. 1974. Composition and synthesis of gangliosides in mammary gland and milk of the bovine. *Biochim Biophys Acta* 337 (2):255–70.

Kim, K. S., J. Y. Park, I. Jou, and S. M. Park. 2009. Functional implication of BAFF synthesis and release in gangliosides-stimulated microglia. *J Leukoc Biol* 86 (2):349–59.

Kim, S.-J., T.-W. Chung, H.-J. Choi, et al. 2014. Monosialic ganglioside GM3 specifically suppresses the monocyte adhesion to endothelial cells for inflammation. *Int J Biochem Cell Biol* 46:32–8.

Kimata, H. 1994. GM1, a ganglioside that specifically enhances immunoglobulin production and proliferation in human plasma cells. *Eur J Immunol* 24 (11):2910–3.

Kimata, H., and A. Yoshida. 1994. Differential effects of gangliosides on Ig production and proliferation by human B cells. *Blood* 84 (4):1193–200.

Kimata, H., and A. Yoshida. 1996. Inhibition of spontaneous immunoglobulin production by ganglioside GM2 in human B cells. *Clin Immunol Immunopathol* 79 (2):197–202.

Krengel, U., and P. A. Bousquet. 2014. Molecular recognition of gangliosides and their potential for cancer immunotherapies. *Front Immunol* 5:325.

Lacomba, R., J. Salcedo, A. Alegria, et al. 2009. Determination of sialic acid and gangliosides in biological samples and dairy products: A review. *J Pharm Biomed Anal* 51 (2):346–57.

Ladisch, S., B. Gillard, C. Wong, and L. Ulsh. 1983. Shedding and immunoregulatory activity of YAC-1 lymphoma cell gangliosides. *Cancer Res* 43 (8):3808–13.

Laegreid, A., and A. B. Otnaess. 1987. Trace amounts of ganglioside GM1 in human milk inhibit enterotoxins from vibrio cholerae and escherichia coli. *Life Sci* 40 (1):55–62.

Laegreid, A., A. B. Otnaess, and J. Fuglesang. 1986. Human and bovine milk: Comparison of ganglioside composition and enterotoxin-inhibitory activity. *Pediatr Res* 20 (5):416–21.

Langeveld, M., and J. M. F. G. Aerts. 2009. Glycosphingolipids and insulin resistance. *Prog Lipid Res* 48 (3–4):196–205.

Larson, G., P. Falk, and L. C. Hoskins. 1988. Degradation of human intestinal glycosphingolipids by extracellular glycosidases from mucin-degrading bacteria of the human fecal flora. *J Biol Chem* 263 (22):10790–8.

Larson, G., P. Watsfeldt, P. Falk, H. Leffler, and H. Koprowski. 1987. Fecal excretion of intestinal glycosphingolipids by newborns and young children. *FEBS Lett* 214 (1):41–4.

Ledeen, R. W., and G. Wu. 2015. The multi-tasked life of GM1 ganglioside, a true factotum of nature. *Trends Biochem Sci.* 40 (7):407–18.

Lee, H., D. Garrido, D. A. Mills, and D. Barile. 2014. Hydrolysis of milk gangliosides by infant-gut associated bifidobacteria determined by microfluidic chips and high-resolution mass spectrometry. *Electrophoresis* 35 (11):1742–50.

Lee, H., J. B. German, R. Kjelden, C. B. Lebrilla, and D. Barile. 2013. Quantitative analysis of gangliosides in bovine milk and colostrum-based dairy products by ultrahigh performance liquid chromatography-tandem mass spectrometry. *J Agric Food Chem* 61 (40):9689–96.

Li, R. X., and S. Ladisch. 1991. Shedding of human neuroblastoma gangliosides. *Biochim Biophys Acta* 1083 (1):57–64.

Liu, H., E. C. Radlowski, M. S. Conrad, et al. 2014. Early supplementation of phospholipids and gangliosides affects brain and cognitive development in neonatal piglets. *J Nutr* 144 (12):1903–9.

Lopez, P. H. H., and R. L. Schnaar. 2009. Gangliosides in cell recognition and membrane protein regulation. *Curr Opin Struct Biol* 19 (5):549–57.

Lu, P., and F. J. Sharom. 1995. Gangliosides are potent immunosuppressors of IL-2-mediated T-cell proliferation in a low protein environment. *Immunology* 86 (3):356–63.

Maglione, V., P. Marchi, A. Di Pardo, et al. 2010. Impaired ganglioside metabolism in Huntington's disease and neuroprotective role of GM1. *J Neurosci* 30 (11):4072–80.

Martin-Sosa, S., M. J. Martin, M. D. Castro, J. A. Cabezas, and P. Hueso. 2004. Lactational changes in the fatty acid composition of human milk gangliosides. *Lipids* 39 (2):111–6.

Martin, M. J., E. Vazquez, M. Ramirez, M. H. Dohnalek, and R. Rueda. 2008. Sialic acid and ganglioside contents in starter infant formulas. 3rd World Congress of Pediatric Gastroenterology, Hepatology and Nutrition (WCPGHAN), Iguassu Falls, Brazil, 16–20 August 2008.

Martin, M. J., E. Vazquez, and R. Rueda. 2007. Application of a sensitive fluorometric HPLC assay to determine the sialic acid content of infant formulas. *Anal Bioanal Chem* 387 (8):2943–9.

Martinez, M. A., S. Lopez, C. F. Arias, and P. Isa. 2013. Gangliosides have a functional role during rotavirus cell entry. *J Virol* 87 (2):1115–22.

Martinez, Z., M. Zhu, S. Han, and A. L. Fink. 2007. GM1 specifically interacts with alpha-synuclein and inhibits fibrillation. *Biochemistry* 46 (7):1868–77.

Matarrese, P., T. Garofalo, V. Manganelli, et al. 2014. Evidence for the involvement of GD3 ganglioside in autophagosome formation and maturation. *Autophagy* 10 (5):750–65.

McJarrow, P., N. Schnell, J. Jumpsen, and T. Clandinin. 2009. Influence of dietary gangliosides on neonatal brain development. *Nutr Rev* 67 (8):451–63.

McKallip, R., R. Li, and S. Ladisch. 1999. Tumor gangliosides inhibit the tumor-specific immune response. *J Immunol* 163 (7):3718–26.

Miklavcic, J. J., K. L. Schnabl, V. C. Mazurak, A. B. Thomson, and M. T. Clandinin. 2012. Dietary ganglioside reduces proinflammatory signaling in the intestine. *J Nutr Metab* 2012:280286.

Moller, H. K., T. Thymann, L. N. Fink, et al. 2010. Bovine colostrum is superior to enriched formulas in stimulating intestinal function and necrotising enterocolitis resistance in preterm pigs. *Br J Nutr* 105 (1):44–53.

Momoeda, M., K. Momoeda, K. Takamizawa, et al. 1995. Characteristic expression of GD1 alpha-ganglioside during lactation in murine mammary gland. *Biochim Biophys Acta* 1256 (2):151–6.

Nagafuku, M., K. Okuyama, Y. Onimaru, et al. 2012. CD4 and CD8 T cells require different membrane gangliosides for activation. *Proceedings of the National Academy of Sciences of the United States of America* 109 (6):E336–42.

Nakamura, K., H. Suzuki, Y. Hirabayashi, and A. Suzuki. 1995. IV3 alpha (NeuGc alpha 2-8NeuGc)-Gg4Cer is restricted to CD4+ T cells producing interleukin-2 and a small population of mature thymocytes in mice. *J Biol Chem* 270 (8):3876–81.

Nashar, T. O., H. M. Webb, S. Eaglestone, N. A. Williams, and T. R. Hirst. 1996. Potent immunogenicity of the B subunits of Escherichia coli heat-labile enterotoxin: Receptor binding is essential and induces differential modulation of lymphocyte subsets. *Proc Natl Acad Sci U S A* 93 (1):226–30.

Nayak, D., T. L. Roth, and D. B. McGavern. 2014. Microglia development and function. *Annu Rev Immunol* 32:367–402.

Nikolaeva, S., L. Bayunova, T. Sokolova, et al. 2015. GM1 and GD1a gangliosides modulate toxic and inflammatory effects of E. coli lipopolysaccharide by preventing TLR4 translocation into lipid rafts. *Biochim Biophys Acta* 1851 (3):239–47.

Ohmi, Y., Y. Ohkawa, Y. Yamauchi, et al. 2012. Essential roles of gangliosides in the formation and maintenance of membrane microdomains in brain tissues. *Neurochem Res* 37 (6):1185–91.

Ohmi, Y., O. Tajima, Y. Ohkawa, et al. 2009. Gangliosides play pivotal roles in the regulation of complement systems and in the maintenance of integrity in nerve tissues. *Proc Natl Acad Sci U S A* 106 (52):22405–10.

Ohmi, Y., O. Tajima, Y. Ohkawa, et al. 2011. Gangliosides are essential in the protection of inflammation and neurodegeneration via maintenance of lipid rafts: Elucidation by a series of ganglioside-deficient mutant mice. *J Neurochem* 116 (5):926–35.

Ortaldo, J. R., A. T. Mason, D. L. Longo, et al. 1996. T cell activation via the disialoganglioside GD3: Analysis of signal transduction. *J Leukoc Biol* 60 (4):533–9.

Otnaess, A. B., A. Laegreid, and K. Ertresvag. 1983. Inhibition of enterotoxin from Escherichia coli and Vibrio cholerae by gangliosides from human milk. *Infect Immun* 40 (2):563–9.

Palmano, K., A. Rowan, R. Guillermo, J. Guan, and P. McJarrow. 2015. The role of gangliosides in neurodevelopment. *Nutrients* 7 (5):3891–3913.

Pan, X. L., and T. Izumi. 1999. Chronological changes in the ganglioside composition of human milk during lactation. *Early Hum Dev* 55 (1):1–8.

Pan, X. L., and T. Izumi. 2000. Variation of the ganglioside compositions of human milk, cow's milk and infant formulas. *Early Hum Dev* 57 (1):25–31.

Park, E. J., M. Suh, and M. T. Clandinin. 2005a. Dietary ganglioside and long-chain polyunsaturated fatty acids increase ganglioside GD3 content and alter the phospholipid profile in neonatal rat retina. *Invest Ophthalmol Vis Sci* 46 (7):2571–5.

Park, E. J., M. Suh, K. Ramanujam, et al. 2005b. Diet-Induced changes in membrane gangliosides in rat intestinal mucosa, plasma and brain. *J Pediatr Gastroenterol Nutr* 40 (4):487–95.

Park, E. J., M. Suh, B. Thomson, et al. 2007. Dietary ganglioside inhibits acute inflammatory signals in intestinal mucosa and blood induced by systemic inflammation of Escherichia coli lipopolysaccharide. *Shock* 28 (1):112–7.

Park, E. J., A. B. Thomson, and M. T. Clandinin. 2010. Protection of intestinal occludin tight junction protein by dietary gangliosides in lipopolysaccharide-induced acute inflammation. *J Pediatr Gastroenterol Nutr* 50 (3):321–8.

Park, J. Y., H. Y. Kim, I. Jou, and S. M. Park. 2008. GM1 induces p38 and microtubule dependent ramification of rat primary microglia in vitro. *Brain Res* 1244:13–23.

Peguet-Navarro, J., M. Sportouch, I. Popa, et al. 2003. Gangliosides from human melanoma tumors impair dendritic cell differentiation from monocytes and induce their apoptosis. *J Immunol* 170 (7):3488–94.

Pham, P. H., T.-L. Duffy, A. L. Dmytrash, et al. 2011. Estimate of dietary ganglioside intake in a group of healthy Edmontonians based on selected foods. *J Food Compost Anal* 24 (7):1032–7.

Pope-Coleman, A., and J. S. Schneider. 1998. Effects of chronic GM1 ganglioside treatment on cognitieve and motor deficits in a slowly progressing model of parkinsonism in non-human primates. *Restor Neurol Neurosci* 12 (4):255–66.

Pope-Coleman, A., J. P. Tinker, and J. S. Schneider. 2000. Effects of GM1 ganglioside treatment on pre- and postsynaptic dopaminergic markers in the striatum of parkinsonian monkeys. *Synapse* 36 (2):120–8.

Prinetti, A., N. Loberto, V. Chigorno, and S. Sonnino. 2009. Glycosphingolipid behaviour in complex membranes. *Biochim Biophys Acta* 1788 (1):184–93.

Puente, R., L. A. Garcia-Pardo, and P. Hueso. 1992. Gangliosides in bovine milk. Changes in content and distribution of individual ganglioside levels during lactation. *Biol Chem Hoppe Seyler* 373 (5):283–8.

Puente, R., L. A. Garcia-Pardo, R. Rueda, A. Gil, and P. Hueso. 1994. Changes in ganglioside and sialic acid contents of goat milk during lactation. *J Dairy Sci* 77 (1):39–44.

Puente, R., L. A. Garcia-Pardo, R. Rueda, A. Gil, and P. Hueso. 1995. Ewes' milk: Changes in the contents of gangliosides and sialic acid during lactation. *J Dairy Res* 62 (04):651–4.

Puente, R., L. Garcia-Pardo, R. Rueda, A. Gil, and P. Hueso. 1996. Seasonal variations in the concentration of gangliosides and sialic acids in milk from different mammalian species. *Int Dairy J* 6 (3):315–22.

Puryear, W. B., X. Yu, N. P. Ramirez, B. M. Reinhard, and S. Gummuluru. 2012. HIV-1 incorporation of host-cell-derived glycosphingolipid GM3 allows for capture by mature dendritic cells. *Proc Natl Acad Sci U S A* 109 (19):7475–80.

Ramirez, M., E. Vazquez, M. L. Jimenez, et al. 2008. Effect of prototype formulas enriched in sialic acid, gangliosides and phospholipids, and containing fructooligosaccharides on diarrhea and feeding tolerance in piglets. 3rd World Congress of Pediatric Gastroenterology, Hepatology and Nutrition (WCPGHAN), Iguassu Falls, Brazil, 16–20 August.

Rescigno, M. 2011. Dendritic cells in bacteria handling in the gut. *J Leukoc Biol* 90 (4):669–72.

Rueda, R. 2007. The role of dietary gangliosides on immunity and the prevention of infection. *Br J Nutr* 98 (Supplement S1):S68–73.

Rueda, R. 2013. Gangliosides, immunity, infection and inflammation. In *Diet, Immunity and Inflammation*, edited by P. C. Calder and P. Yaqoob, 341–358. Cambridge, UK: Woodhead Publishing Limited.

Rueda, R., J. L. Garcia-Salmeron, J. Maldonado, and A. Gil. 1996. Changes during lactation in ganglioside distribution in human milk from mothers delivering preterm and term infants. *Biol Chem* 377 (9):599–601.

Rueda, R., and A. Gil. 1998. Role of gangliosides in infant nutrition. In *Recent Advances in Roles of Lipids in Infant Nutrition*, edited by Y.-S. Huang and A. J. Sinclair, 213–234. Champaign, Illinois: AOCS Press.

Rueda, R., J. Maldonado, E. Narbona, and A. Gil. 1998a. Neonatal dietary gangliosides. *Early Hum Dev* 53 Suppl:S135–47.

Rueda, R., R. Puente, P. Hueso, J. Maldonado, and A. Gil. 1995. New data on content and distribution of gangliosides in human milk. *Biol Chem Hoppe Seyler* 376 (12):723–7.

Rueda, R., J. L. Sabatel, J. Maldonado, J. A. Molina-Font, and A. Gil. 1998b. Addition of gangliosides to an adapted milk formula modifies levels of fecal escherichia coli in preterm newborn infants. *J Pediatr* 133 (1):90–4.

Rueda, R., K. Tabsh, and S. Ladisch. 1993. Detection of complex gangliosides in human amniotic fluid. *FEBS Lett* 328 (1–2):13–6.

Ryan, J. M., G. E. Rice, and M. D. Mitchell. 2013. The role of gangliosides in brain development and the potential benefits of perinatal supplementation. *Nutrition Research* 33 (11):877–87.

Salcedo, J., R. Barbera, E. Matencio, A. Alegría, and M. J. Lagarda. 2013. Gangliosides and sialic acid effects upon newborn pathogenic bacteria adhesion: An in vitro study. *Food Chem* 136 (2):726–34.

Sanchez-Diaz, A., M. J. Ruano, F. Lorente, and P. Hueso. 1997. A critical analysis of total sialic acid and sialoglycoconjugate contents of bovine milk-based infant formulas. *J Pediatr Gastroenterol Nutr* 24 (4):405–10.

Sanchez-Juanes, F., J. M. Alonso, L. Zancada, and P. Hueso. 2009. Glycosphingolipids from bovine milk and milk fat globule membranes: A comparative study. Adhesion to enterotoxigenic Escherichia coli strains. *Biol Chem* 390 (1):31–40.

Schengrund, C. L. 2010. Lipid rafts: Keys to neurodegeneration. *Brain Res Bull* 82 (1–2):7–17.

Schengrund, C. L. 2015. Gangliosides: Glycosphingolipids essential for normal neural development and function. *Trends Biochem Sci.* 40 (7):397–406.

Schlaak, J. F., C. Claus, K. H. Meyer zum Buschenfelde, and W. Dippold. 1995. Anti-GD3 antibodies are potent activators of human gamma/delta and alpha/beta positive T cells. *Scand J Immunol* 41 (5):475–80.

Schnaar, R. L., R. Gerardy-Schahn, and H. Hildebrandt. 2014. Sialic acids in the brain: Gangliosides and polysialic acid in nervous system development, stability, disease, and regeneration. *Physiol Rev* 94(2): 461–518.

Schnabl, K. L., M. Larcelet, A. B. Thomson, and M. T. Clandinin. 2009a. Uptake and fate of ganglioside GD3 in human intestinal Caco-2 cells. *Am J Physiol Gastrointest Liver Physiol* 297 (1):G52–9.

Schnabl, K. L., B. Larsen, J. E. Van Aerde, et al. 2009b. Gangliosides protect bowel in an infant model of necrotizing enterocolitis by suppressing proinflammatory signals. *J Pediatr Gastroenterol Nutr* 49 (4):382–92.

Schneider, J. S., S. M. Gollomp, S. Sendek, et al. 2013. A randomized, controlled, delayed start trial of GM1 ganglioside in treated Parkinson's disease patients. *J Neurol Sci* 324 (1–2):140–8.

Shen, W., K. Stone, A. Jales, D. Leitenberg, and S. Ladisch. 2008. Inhibition of TLR activation and up-regulation of IL-1R-associated kinase-M expression by exogenous gangliosides. *J Immunol* 180 (7):4425–32.

Shurin, G. V., M. R. Shurin, S. Bykovskaia, et al. 2001. Neuroblastoma-derived gangliosides inhibit dendritic cell generation and function. *Cancer Res* 61 (1):363–9.

Sonnino, S., and A. Prinetti. 2010. Gangliosides as regulators of cell membrane organization and functions. *Adv Exp Med Biol* 688:165–84.

Suh, M., M. Belosevic, and M. T. Clandinin. 2004. Dietary lipids containing gangliosides reduce Giardia muris infection in vivo and survival of Giardia lamblia trophozoites in vitro. *Parasitology* 128 (Pt 6):595–602.

Svennerholm, L. 1963. Chromatographic separation of human brain gangliosides. *J Neurochem* 10:613–23.

Taga, S., C. Tetaud, M. Mangeney, T. Tursz, and J. Wiels. 1995. Sequential changes in glycolipid expression during human B cell differentiation: Enzymatic bases. *Biochim Biophys Acta* 1254 (1):56–65.

Takamizawa, K., M. Iwamori, M. Mutai, and Y. Nagai. 1986. Selective changes in gangliosides of human milk during lactation: A molecular indicator for the period of lactation. *Biochim Biophys Acta* 879 (1):73–7.

Tanabe, A., M. Matsuda, A. Fukuhara, et al. 2009. Obesity causes a shift in metabolic flow of gangliosides in adipose tissues. *Biochem Biophys Res Commun* 379 (2):547–52.

Timby, N., E. Domellof, O. Hernell, B. Lonnerdal, and M. Domellof. 2014. Neurodevelopment, nutrition, and growth until 12 mo of age in infants fed a low-energy, low-protein formula supplemented with bovine milk fat globule membranes: A randomized controlled trial. *Am J Clin Nutr* 99 (4):860–8.

Timby, N., O. Hernell, O. Vaarala, et al. 2015. Infections in infants fed formula supplemented with bovine milk fat globule membranes. *J Pediatr Gastroenterol Nutr* 60 (3):384–9.

Tommasino, C., M. Marconi, L. Ciarlo, P. Matarrese, and W. Malorni. 2015. Autophagic flux and autophagosome morphogenesis require the participation of sphingolipids. *Apoptosis* 20 (5):645–57.

van Echten-Deckert, G., and J. Walter. 2012. Sphingolipids: Critical players in Alzheimer's disease. *Prog Lipid Res* 51 (4):378–93.

Vazquez, E., A. Gil, and R. Rueda. 2000. Dietary gangliosides increase the number of intestinal IgA-secreting cells and the luminal content of secretory IGA in weanling mice. *J Pediatr Gastroenterol Nutr* 31:S133.

Vazquez, E., A. Gil, and R. Rueda. 2001. Dietary gangliosides positively modulate the percentages of Th1 and Th2 lymphocyte subsets in small intestine of mice at weaning. *Biofactors* 15 (1):1–9.

Vazquez, E., A. Gil, and R. Rueda. 2002. Low concentration of gangliosides strongly stimulate DNA synthesis in cultured resting intestinal lymphocytes from young mice. 11th International Congress of Mucosal Immunology, Orlando, FL, 16–20 June.

Vazquez, I., I. A. Gomez-de-Segura, A. G. Grande, et al. 1999. Protective effect of enriched diet plus growth hormone administration on radiation-induced intestinal injury and on its evolutionary pattern in the rat. *Dig Dis Sci* 44 (11):2350–8.

Vesper, H., E. M. Schmelz, M. N. Nikolova-Karakashian, et al. 1999. Sphingolipids in food and the emerging importance of sphingolipids to nutrition. *J Nutr* 129 (7):1239–50.

Vickers, M. H., J. Guan, M. Gustavsson, et al. 2009. Supplementation with a mixture of complex lipids derived from milk to growing rats results in improvements in parameters related to growth and cognition. *Nutr Res* 29 (6):426–35.

Wada, A., M. Hasegawa, P.-F. Wong, et al. 2010. Direct binding of gangliosides to Helicobacter pylori vacuolating cytotoxin (VacA) neutralizes its toxin activity. *Glycobiology* 20 (6):668–78.

Walter, J., and G. van Echten-Deckert. 2013. Cross-talk of membrane lipids and Alzheimer-related proteins. *Mol Neurodegener* 8:34.

Wang, B., J. Brand-Miller, P. McVeagh, and P. Petocz. 2001. Concentration and distribution of sialic acid in human milk and infant formulas. *Am J Clin Nutr* 74 (4):510–5.

Wang, B., B. Yu, M. Karim, et al. 2007. Dietary sialic acid supplementation improves learning and memory in piglets. *Am J Clin Nutr* 85 (2):561–9.

Wang, J., A. Cheng, C. Wakade, and R. K. Yu. 2014. Ganglioside GD3 is required for neurogenesis and long-term maintenance of neural stem cells in the postnatal mouse brain. *J Neurosci* 34 (41):13790–800.

Wershil, B. K., and G. T. Furuta. 2008. Gastrointestinal mucosal immunity. *J Allergy Clin Immunol* 121 (2):S380–3.

Wiegandt, H. 1982. The gangliosides. In *Advances in Neurochemistry*, edited by B. W. Agranof and M. H. Aprison, 149–223. New York, NY: Plenum Press.

Xu, J., V. Anderson, and S. M. Schwarz. 2013. Dietary GD3 ganglioside reduces the incidence and severity of necrotizing enterocolitis by sustaining regulatory immune responses. *J Pediatr Gastroenterol Nutr* 57 (5):550–6.

Yamamoto, N., T. Matsubara, K. Sobue, et al. 2012. Brain insulin resistance accelerates Abeta fibrillogenesis by inducing GM1 ganglioside clustering in the presynaptic membranes. *J Neurochem* 121 (4):619–28.

Yamamoto, N., M. Tanida, R. Kasahara, K. Sobue, and K. Suzuki. 2014. Leptin inhibits amyloid beta-protein fibrillogenesis by decreasing GM1 gangliosides on the neuronal cell surface through PI3K/Akt/mTOR pathway. *J Neurochem* 131 (3):323–32.

Yaqoob, P., and S. R. Shaikh. 2010. The nutritional and clinical significance of lipid rafts. *Curr Opin Clin Nutr Metab Care* 13 (2):156–66.

Yoon, H. J., S. B. Jeon, K. Suk, et al. 2008. Contribution of TLR2 to the initiation of ganglioside-triggered inflammatory signaling. *Mol Cells* 25 (1):99–104.

Yu, R. K., Y. Nakatani, and M. Yanagisawa. 2009. The role of glycosphingolipid metabolism in the developing brain. *J Lipid Res* 50 Suppl:S440–5.

Yuasa, H., D. A. Scheinberg, and A. N. Houghton. 1990. Gangliosides of T lymphocytes: Evidence for a role in T-cell activation. *Tissue Antigens* 36 (2):47–56.

25 AHCC Nutritional Supplement and the Immune Response

Takehito Miura and Anil D. Kulkarni

CONTENTS

25.1 Introduction..427
25.2 Immunoregulatory Effect of AHCC..428
25.3 AHCC and Infection 428
25.4 Anti-Inflammatory Effect of AHCC..431
25.5 Summary 431
References...431

25.1 INTRODUCTION

Active hexose correlated compound (AHCC) is an extract from a liquid mycelia culture of basidiomycetes belonging to the genus Shiitake (*Lentinula edodes*); the extract contains polysaccharides. Many mushrooms, including shiitake mushrooms, are classified as basidiomycetes. When basidiomycetes change with sufficient mycelia growth under certain conditions of light, temperature, humidity, and nutrition, the sexual reproductive organs they form produce basidiospores, which are known as fruiting bodies. However, fruiting bodies are not formed when mycelia are cultured in a liquid medium, and they proliferate by forming spherical hyphae masses in the culture medium [1]. AHCC is the material containing the components that have been assimilated from the culture medium by the various enzymes that are produced by basidiomycete mycelia using this property of the mycelia of basidiomycetes. AHCC is manufactured through enzyme reaction, separation and concentration, sterilization, and freeze-drying.

AHCC may be used as a nutritional supplement and as a component of a functional food. Functional foods using mushrooms as raw materials are expected to have an immunostimulatory effect since they are known to contain polysaccharides, especially β-glucans, as an active ingredient [1]. However, AHCC contains only 0.2% β-glucan but plenty of α-glucan, and so it differs from other mushrooms and extracts derived from mushrooms. The presence of α-1,4-glucan acylated in positions 2 and 3 (Figure 25.1) has been reported, and this is considered to be one of the active ingredients [2]. The partially acetylated α-1,4-glucan cannot be obtained simply from a basidiomycetes culture extraction and is presumed to be formed by the enzymatic modification of the native α-glucan during the AHCC manufacturing process [2].

Many tests have been performed to ensure the safety of AHCC. In the oral single dose toxicity test, LD50 values for rats (50% lethal dose) have been determined to be over 12,500 mg/kg, the maximum dose of AHCC that can be administered [3]. The high safety quotient has been confirmed, since physiological and biochemical changes were not observed in 4-month repeated-oral-dose toxicity studies conducted in rats, where 2% or 5% AHCC was administered into a powder feed diet [3].

Spierings et al. conducted tests corresponding to the first phase safety studies of AHCC in healthy volunteers. Twenty-six healthy male and female volunteers (age 18–61 years) were asked to take 9 g of AHCC per day, three times the normal recommended intake, for 14 days. No serious

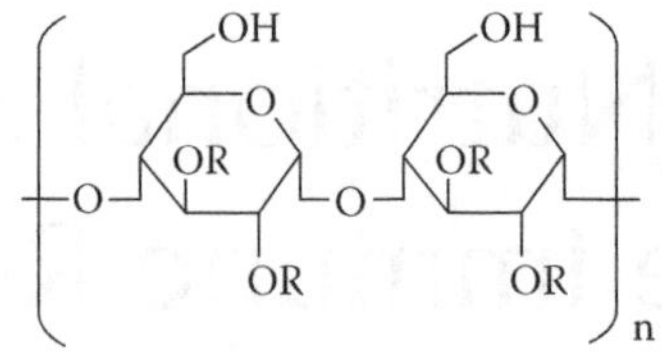

FIGURE 25.1 Structure of an α-1,4-glucan. R indicates the site of acylation.

adverse events were observed, and the authors concluded that AHCC is safe to use as a food in clinical practice [4].

25.2 IMMUNOREGULATORY EFFECT OF AHCC

Matsushita et al. reported that AHCC partly prevents the reduction in the activity of natural killer (NK) cells and the decrease in interleukin (IL)-1β and tumor necrosis factor (TNF)-α expression seen when the chemotherapy drug combination tegafur-uracil (sometimes called UFT) was administered to rats implanted with SST-2 breast cancer [5]. When AHCC was orally administered to C57BL/6 mice that were implanted with B16 melanoma or EL4 lymphoma cells, there was a significant delay in tumor growth, activation, and proliferation of antigen-specific CD4$^+$ and CD8$^+$ T-cells, enhanced interferon (IFN)-γ production, and increased NK cell and $\gamma\delta$T cell numbers [6]. It has been reported that in cancer patients with low NK cell activity before intake, ingestion of AHCC (3 g/day for 2 weeks) increased NK cell activity [7].

Terakawa et al. evaluated dendritic cell count in peripheral blood in a double-blind randomized trial of 21 healthy individuals, with 10 participants in the AHCC treatment group (3 g AHCC per day) and 11 participants in the placebo group [8]. An increase in the total dendritic cell count and in myeloid dendritic cell count (DC1) was observed in the AHCC treatment group (Figure 25.2). DC1 is a cell type that plays an important role in anticancer immunity through its activation of naive T lymphocytes. This suggests that AHCC may improve the immune response of cancer patients. On the other hand, there were no differences observed in cytokine production, such as IFN and interleukins, between the groups. In a study in healthy individuals during the common cold season, AHCC (1 g/day) improved the "SIV" (scoring of immunological vigor) [9], a test used to evaluate the overall immune status using information such as T-cell count, CD8$^+$CD28$^+$ T-cell count, naive T-cell count, B-cell count, NK cell count, CD4/CD8 T-cell ratio, and naive/memory T-cell ratio [10]. These studies suggest that AHCC strengthens immune protection against cancer and has the effect of normalizing a compromised immune system. This suggests that AHCC may have protective effects not only against cancer growth, but also against microbial infection.

Although the partially acetylated α-1,4-glucan mentioned above has been reported to be the active ingredient for the immunoregulatory effect of AHCC [2], other active ingredients may be present. A recent report using cultured intraepithelial lymphocytes suggests that AHCC acts directly on these cells via TLR2 or TLR4 (Figure 25.3) [11], effects which may involve components other than the α-1,4-glucan.

25.3 AHCC AND INFECTION

There are a number of reports on the effectiveness of AHCC in experimental infection models [12–21]. There are reports of a prophylactic effect against *Candida albicans*, *Pseudomonas aeruginosa*, and methicillin-resistant *Staphylococcus aureus* (MRSA) infections in a neutropenia model when cyclophosphamide is administered [12] and a protective effect against *C. albicans* infection in a granulocytopenia model when cyclophosphamide, 5-fluorouracil, doxorubicin, or prednisolone is administered [13]. This suggests that oral intake of AHCC works defensively against opportunistic

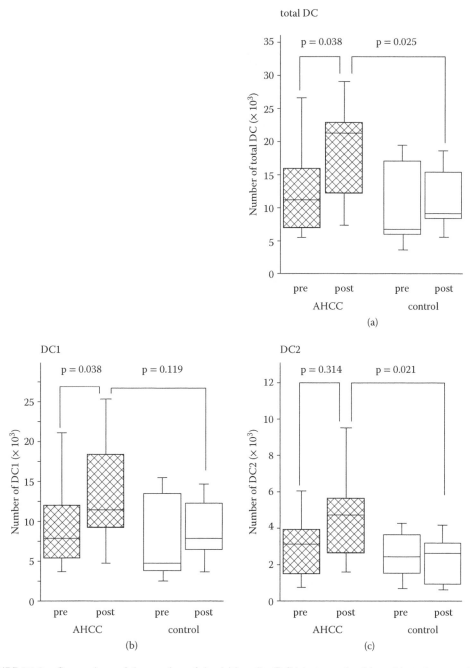

FIGURE 25.2 Comparison of the number of dendritic cells (DCs) between healthy subjects in control and active hexose correlated compound (AHCC) groups. The boxes show the 75th, 50th (median), and 25th percentiles; the horizontal bar shows 90th and 10th percentiles in box plots. (a) identifies total DCs, (b) is DC1s, and (c) is DC2s. (From Terakawa N et al., *Nutr Cancer*, 60, 643–651, 2008.)

infections in an immunosuppressed state caused by chemotherapeutic agents. Aviles et al. reported a protective effect against *Klebsiella pneumoniae* infection in the hindlimb suspension model that is used to reproduce the immunosuppression during spaceflight, along with increased survival rate [14], and improved spleen cell proliferation and cytokine production [15]. Furthermore, Aviles et al. have reported [16,17] an improvement in the survival rate following pneumoniae infection of

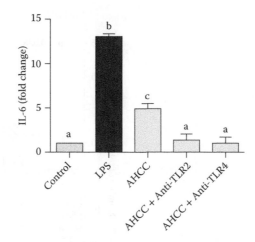

FIGURE 25.3 Effect of AHCC on IL-6 production is mediated via TLRs. Production of IL-6 by murine intraepithelial lymphocytes cultured with complete medium (control), LPS (0.01 μg/mL), AHCC (0.1 mg/mL), or AHCC + anti-TLR2 or anti-TLR4. Values represent mean results from three replicates normalized to fold change ± SEM. Bars that have no letter in common are significantly different from each other ($p \leq 0.05$). (From Mallet JF et al., *Eur J Nutr*, 55, 139–146, 2015.)

surgical wounds by administering AHCC. Thus, the anti-infection role of AHCC may have many applications.

AHCC affects both natural and acquired immunity, and has been reported to be effective not only against fungi and bacteria, but also against viral infections [18–21]. Compared with the infected control group, AHCC caused an increase in lung NK activity in mice 2 days after influenza virus infection and the degree of weight loss after infection was lessened, and recovery was also quicker (Figure 25.4) [18,19]. The protective effect of AHCC has been confirmed with even smaller doses [20]. Studies have been conducted for the H5N1 avian influenza virus, and AHCC caused improvement in the survival rate for lethal infection in mice [21]. Also, a recent report on the infection protective effects of AHCC against West Nile virus (WNV) mentions that the severity of infection is reduced with an improved immune status of the host with increased IgG antibody production and modification of the subset of γδT-cells against WNV [22]. A recent report mentions that administering AHCC to healthy individuals who had received influenza B vaccine increased the number of

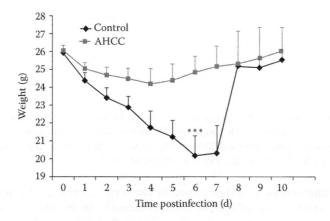

FIGURE 25.4 Body weights of control and AHCC-supplemented young mice following infection with 100 HAU influenza A/PR8 through d 10 postinfection. Values are means ± SEM, $n = 20$. ***Different from AHCC, $p<0.001$.

cytotoxic CD8+ T-cells and NKT-cell activity, and the rise in antibody titer after vaccination was significantly higher, compared with the group where AHCC was not administered [23].

Data from an unpublished study by Judith Smith shows that the virus disappeared in 5 of the 10 subjects who were positive when AHCC was administered to healthy people who tested positive for human papillomavirus (HPV), which is considered to be one of the causes of cervical cancer (paper in preparation). It is expected that this may lead to the prevention of cervical cancer, in addition to protection against HPV.

25.4 ANTI-INFLAMMATORY EFFECT OF AHCC

Studies have been conducted with AHCC investigating its ability to suppress excessive immunity and inflammation. Daddaoua et al. reported that administering 100 or 500 mg/kg AHCC per day in the trinitrobenzene-sulfonic acid (TNBS)-induced colitis model in rats reduced the inflammation score of the large intestine; diminished the production of cytokines such as IL-1β, IL-1ra, MCP-1, and TNF-α; and altered the intestinal bacterial flora [24]. Lactic acid bacteria and bifidobacteria are reduced with TNBS treatment, but by administering AHCC, lactic acid bacteria and bifidobacteria increased, and clostridia decreased. The effect was comparable to sulfasalazine (200 mg/kg), which is used as a therapeutic agent in inflammatory bowel disease [24].

Nitric oxide (NO) is produced in bacterial and viral infections, indicating bactericidal and anti-viral activity (see Chapters 19 and 20). However, inducible nitric oxide synthase (iNOS) is induced along with liver inflammation, injuries, and cancer. This increases NO production and aggravates symptoms. Matsui et al. observed that AHCC treatment reduces the NO produced due to the induced iNOS when rat hepatocytes are stimulated with IL-1β, and they found that AHCC treatment causes decomposition of the iNOS messenger RNA, which is induced by IL-1β [25]. It was revealed with the discovery of the reduction in iNOS mRNA expression in the primary cultured hepatocytes by AHCC that both the sense and antisense strands of the iNOS gene are transcribed and that the antisense strand contributes to the stability of iNOS mRNA [26]. The findings suggest that active ingredients in AHCC might regulate different inflammatory pathways [27].

25.5 SUMMARY

The results achieved so far with AHCC suggest that its effects depend upon the precise physiological or pathophysiological situation. In some settings it enhances the immune response, in others it restores immune homeostasis or reduces inflammation. AHCC has been studied in both cancer and infection. Findings to date suggest that AHCC might prevent carcinogenesis and inhibit cancer growth by enhancing immune surveillance for cancer, and also be effective for the prevention of infectious diseases. It can also be used in combination with chemotherapeutic agents in the field of cancer treatment without concern about drug interactions [28,29], and there are also several reports of reduced side effects [30–32]. AHCC can be expected to have further applications in the future as a safe food that can be used to supplement medical treatments.

REFERENCES

1. Furukawa H, *Mushroom Science*, first edition, Tokyo, Kyoritsu Shuppan Co., 1992, p. 71.
2. Hosokawa M, Yamazaki M and Kamiyama Y (editors). *Fundamentals and Clinical Practice of AHCC*, first edition, Tokyo, Japan: Life Science Inc., 2003, pp. 7–15.
3. Fujii H, Nishioka N, Simon RR, Kaur R, Lynch B and Roberts A. Genotoxicity and subchronic toxicity evaluation of Active Hexose Correlated Compound (AHCC). *Reg Toxicol Pharmacol* 2011;59:237–250.
4. Spierings E, Fujii H, Sun B and Walshe T. A Phase I study of the safety of the nutritional supplement, Active Hexose Correlated Compound, AHCC, in healthy volunteers. *J Nutr Sci Vitaminol* 2007;53:536–539.

5. Matsushita K, Kuramitsu Y, Ohiro Y, Obara M, Kobayashi M, Li YQ and Hosokawa M. Combination therapy of Active Hexose Correlated Compound plus UFT significantly reduces the metastasis of rat mammary adenocarcinoma. *Anti Cancer Drugs* 1998;9:343–350.
6. Gao Y, Zhang D, Sun B, Fujii H, Kosuna K and Yin Z. Active hexose correlated compound enhances tumor surveillance through regulating both innate and adaptive immune responses. *Cancer Immunol Immunother* 2006;55:1258–1266.
7. Ghoneum M, Wimbley M, Salem F, McKlain A, Attallah N and Gill G. Immunomodulatory and anticancer effects of active hemicellulose compound (AHCC). *Int J Immunother* 1995;XI:23–28.
8. Terakawa N, Matsui Y, Satoi S, Yanagimoto H, Takahashi K, Yamamoto T, Yamao J, Takai S, Kwon AH and Kamiyama Y. Immunological effect of active hexose correlated compound (AHCC) in healthy volunteers: A double-blind, placebo-controlled trial. *Nutr Cancer* 2008;60:643–651.
9. Takanari J, Hiarayama Y, Homma K, Miura T, Nishioka H and Maeda T. Effects of active hexose correlated compound on the seasonal variations of immune competence in healthy subjects. *J Evid Based Complementary Altern Med* 2015;20:28–34.
10. Hirokawa K, Utsuyama M, Ishikawa T, Kikuchi Y, Kitagawa M, Fujii Y, Nariuchi H, Uetake H and Sugihara K. Decline of T cell-related immune functions in cancer patients and an attempt to restore them through infusion of activated autologous T cells. *Mech Ageing Dev* 2009;130:86–91.
11. Mallet JF, Graham E, Ritz B, Homma K and Matar C. Active Hexose Correlated Compound (AHCC) promotes an intestinal immune response in BALB/c mice and in primary intestinal epithelial cell culture involving toll-like receptors TLR-2 and TLR-4. *Eur J Nutr* 2016;55:139–146.
12. Ishibashi H, Ikeda T, Tansho S, Ono Y, Yamazaki M, Sato A, Yamaoka K, Yamaguchi H and Abe S. Prophylactic efficacy of a basidiomycetes preparation AHCC against lethal opportunistic infections in mice. *Yakugaku Zasshi* 2000;120:715–719.
13. Ikeda T, Ishibashi H, Tansho S et al. Prophylactic efficacy of a basidiomycetes preparation AHCC against lethal Candida albicans infection in experimental granulocytopenic mice. *Jap J Med Mycol* 2003;44:127–131.
14. Aviles H, Belay T, Fountain K, Vance M, Sun B and Sonnenfeld G. Active Hexose Correlated Compound enhances resistance to Klebsiella pneumoniae infection in mice in the hindlimb-unloading model of spaceflight conditions. *J Appl Physiol* 2003;95:491–496.
15. Aviles H, Belay T, Vance M, Sun B and Sonnenfeld G. Active Hexose Correlated Compound enhances the immune function of mice in the hind-limb-unloading model of spaceflight conditions. *J Appl Physiol* 2004;97:1437–1444.
16. Aviles H, O'Donnell, Sun B and Sonnenfeld G. Active Hexose Correlated Compound (AHCC) enhances resistance to infection in a model of surgical wound infection. *Surg Infect* 2006;7:527–535.
17. Aviles H, O'Donnell P, Orshal J, Fujii H, Sun B and Sonnenfeld G. Active Hexose Correlated Compound activates immune function to decrease bacterial load in a murine model of intramuscular infection. *Am J Surgery* 2008;195:537–545.
18. Ritz B, Nogusa S, Ackerman A and Gardner EM. Supplementation with Active Hexose Correlated Compound increases the innate immune response of young mice to primary influenza infection. *J Nutr* 2006;136:2868–2873.
19. Ritz B. Supplementation with Active Hexose Correlated Compound increases survival following infectious challenge in mice. *Nutr Rev* 2008;66:526–531.
20. Nogusa S, Gerbino J, Ritz B. Low-dose supplementation with active hexose correlated compound (AHCC) improves the immune response to acute influenza infection in C57BL/6 mice. *Nutr Res* 2009;29:139–143.
21. Fujii H, Nishioka H, Wakame K et al. Nutritional food Active Hexose Correlated Compound (AHCC) enhances resistance against bird flu. *Jap J Complement Altern Med* 2007;4:37–40.
22. Wang S, Welte T, Fang H, Chang GJ, Born WK, O'Brien RL, Sun B, Fujii H, Kosuna K and Wang T. Oral administration of Active Hexose Correlated Compound enhances host resistance to West Nile Encephalitis in mice. *J Nutr* 2009;139:598–602.
23. Roman BE, Beli E, Duriancik and Gardner EM. Short-term supplementation with active hexose correlated compound improves the antibody response to influenza B vaccine. *Nutr Res* 2013;33:12–17.
24. Daddaoua A, Martinez-Plata E, Lopez-Posadas R, Vieites JM, González M, Requena P, Zarzuelo A, Suárez MD, de Medina FS and Martínez-Augustin O. Active Hexose Correlated Compound acts as a prebiotic and is anti-inflammatory in rats with hapten-induced colitis. *J Nutr* 2007;137:1222–1228.
25. Matsui K, Kawaguchi Y, Ozaki T, Tokuhara K, Tanaka H, Kaibori M, Matsui Y, Kamiyama Y, Wakame K, Miura T, Nishizawa M and Okumura T. Effect of active hexose correlated compound on the production of nitric oxide in hepatocytes. *J Parent Ent Nutr* 2007;31:373–381.

26. Matsui K, Nishizawa M, Ozaki T, Kimura T, Hashimoto I, Yamada M, Kaibori M, Kamiyama Y, Ito S and Okumura T. Natural antisense transcript stabilizes inducible nitric oxide synthase messenger RNA in rat hepatocytes. *Hepatol* 2008;47:686–697.

27. Matsui K, Ozaki T, Oishi M, Tanaka Y, Kaibori M, Nishizawa M, Okumura T and Kwon AH. Active hexose correlated compound inhibits the expression of proinflammatory biomarker iNOS in hepatocytes. *Eur Surg Res* 2011;47:274–283.

28. Mach C, Fugii H, Wakame K and Smith J Evaluation of active hexose correlated compound hepatic metabolism and potential for drug interactions with chemotherapy agents. *J Soc Integrat Oncol* 2008;6:105–109.

29. Coffer LW, Mathew L, Zhnag X, Owiti NA, Myers AL, Faro J and Smith JA. Evaluation of Active Hexose Correlated Compound (AHCC) on phase II drug metabolism pathways and the implications for supplement-drug interactions. *J Integrat Oncol* 2015;4:142.

30. Hangai S, Iwase S, Kawaguchi T, Kogure Y, Miyaji T, Matsunaga T, Nagumo Y and Yamaguchi T. Effect of active hexose-correlated compound in women receiving adjuvant chemotherapy for breast cancer: A retrospective study. *J Altern Complement Med* 2013;19:905–910.

31. Ito T, Urushima H, Sakaue M, Yukawa S, Honda H, Hirai K, Igura T, Hayashi N, Maeda K, Kitagawa T and Kondo K. Reduction of adverse effects by a mushroom product, active hexose correlated compound (AHCC) in patients with advanced cancer during chemotherapy—the significance of the levels of HHV-6 DNA in saliva as a surrogate biomarker during chemotherapy. *Nutr Cancer* 2014;66:377–382.

32. Yanagimoto H, Satoi S, Yamamoto T, Hirooka S, Yamaki S, Kotsuka M, Ryota H, Michiura T, Inoue K, Matsui Y, Tsuta K and Kon M. Alleviating effect of Active Hexose Correlated Compound (AHCC) on chemotherapy-related adverse events in patients with unresectable pancreatic ductal adenocarcinoma. *Nutr Cancer* 2016;68:234–240.

26 Environmental Stressors, Immunity, and Nutrition

L. Olamigoke, E. Mansoor, D. Grimm,
J. Bauer, V. Mann, and A. Sundaresan

CONTENTS

26.1 Introduction 435
26.2 Microgravity as an Environmental Stressor That Impacts the Immune System 435
     26.2.1 Effects of Microgravity on Muscle and Bone..436
     26.2.2 Effects of Microgravity on the Immune System...436
     26.2.3 Nutrition as a Countermeasure to Protect against the Harmful Effects of
           Microgravity 437
26.3 Space Radiation as an Environmental Stressor 437
     26.3.1 Space Radiation: Introduction 437
     26.3.2 The Risks of Space Radiation...438
     26.3.3 Nutrition as a Countermeasure to Protect against the Harmful Effects of
           Space Radiation 439
26.4 Conclusions..440
References..440

26.1 INTRODUCTION

The immune system benefits from good quality nutrition of the organism (Calder, 2013). Not only does the immune system benefit directly from good nutrition, but indirectly good nutrition will prepare the organism for periods of stress, reducing the adverse effects (e.g., immunosuppression) and enhancing recovery. In this chapter, we will discuss the effects of two environmental stressors of relevance to spaceflight, microgravity and space radiation. Both have major physiological impact and both induce immunosuppression. Although poorly investigated to date, it is likely that nutritional interventions could play a role in enabling the immune system to withstand the effects of such stressors and in promoting recovery.

26.2 MICROGRAVITY AS AN ENVIRONMENTAL STRESSOR THAT IMPACTS THE IMMUNE SYSTEM

The microgravity environment of space presents numerous challenges to the function and well-being of the human body that can potentially compromise health, safety, and performance (Blaber et al., 2010). There are adverse effects on human physiology, impacting on the skeletomuscular, cardiovascular, and sensory motor systems (Clement, 2003; Shackelford, 2008; Blaber et al., 2010). Altered body composition, with loss of muscle and bone, fluid shifts, congestion, altered taste and smell, and space motion sickness all occur (Blaber et al., 2010).

26.2.1 Effects of Microgravity on Muscle and Bone

The major sites of the losses of body mass during spaceflight are the muscles and bones: in space, muscles in the legs, back, spine, and heart weaken and waste away because they no longer are needed to overcome the effect of gravity, just as people lose muscle when they age or are confined to bed rest due to reduced physical activity and reduced use of the postural muscles that maintain the body upright in a gravitational environment. After a 2-week spaceflight, muscle mass is diminished by up to 20% (Clement, 2003) and on longer missions (3–6 months), a 30% loss has been noted (Shackelford, 2008). Bed rest studies on subjects in energy balance have shown that the reduction in muscle size and strength is due to the decreased workload on the muscles. One of the countermeasures for the reductive remodeling of muscle is exercise. If a resistive exercise program is incorporated into a bed rest protocol, the muscle loss can be prevented (Loehr et al., 2011). Hence, exercise is one factor that could mitigate some of the adverse effects of microgravity.

Bone deterioration is a challenge in long-term spaceflight with significant similarities to patients experiencing bone loss. Bone loss will be a problem after return to Earth from very long missions. Recovery of bone is a very slow process, taking longer than the actual duration of the mission (Smith et al., 2012). A recent study, using heavy resistive exercise as a countermeasure to bone loss, for the first time showed that adequate energy, protein, and vitamin D supply are mandatory to maintain bone mineral density after 6 months of spaceflight (Smith et al., 2012).

26.2.2 Effects of Microgravity on the Immune System

Several studies including ground-based models and spaceflight experiments have investigated the effects of microgravity on the immune system (Borchers et al., 2002; Sonnenfeld, 2002; Gridley et al., 2009). The human immune system becomes weaker in space, but, although several hundred cosmonauts and astronauts have flown in space, knowledge about the adaptation of their immune systems to spaceflight is poor. Nevertheless, it has been suggested that an adverse impact of spaceflight on the immune system could limit humanity's ability to explore space (Gueguinou et al., 2009). Immunosuppression and immune dysfunction have been observed in astronauts during space missions (Fitzgerald et al., 2009); effects of spaceflight on immune function include a decrease in natural killer cell number and functionality, changes in T-cell distribution and function, decreases in cell-mediated immunity with altered cytokine production, and an increase in secretion of interleukin (IL)-6 and IL-10 (Baqai et al., 2009; Gridley et al., 2009). The effects of microgravity are seen in altered gene-expression patterns, in particular genes involved in stress, and in glucocorticoid receptor metabolism and T-cell signaling, which are typically linked with immunosuppression (Baqai et al., 2009). A more recent study has shown that the limited activation and proliferation of T-cells because of microgravity can be attributed to the inhibition of the Rel/NF-κB signaling pathway, which in turn affects cell cycle regulation, apoptosis, cytoskeleton functioning, and the expression of several surface molecules and cytokines (Chang et al., 2012). Although short-term spaceflights are associated with known reversible immunological alterations, the effects of long-duration spaceflights on neuroimmune responses are not yet fully understood (Stowe et al., 2011).

The precise mechanisms by which spaceflight and microgravity impact the immune system are not clear. However, among the many factors that could affect immunity during spaceflight, physical and psychological stresses are likely to play a major role (Stowe et al., 2011). Spaceflight is associated with a number of stressful events that can be considered acute (i.e., launch/landing stress) or chronic (prolonged periods of isolation, loneliness, anxiety). Dysregulation of the human immune system has long been known to be present as an acute stress-induced postlanding phenomenon (Levine and Greenleaf, 1998). The duration, intensity, and timing of a physiological stress response are critical factors when determining the impact of stress on immune function and health. A unique characteristic of acute stress is the rapid physiological response that occurs while the stressor is applied, followed by an abrupt shutdown of the response when the stressor is removed. At the other end of the spectrum are the effects of chronic stress. These are persistent or prolonged stressful events (on the order of weeks to months to years) that may result in immune dysregulation or suppression (Dhabhar, 2014).

26.2.3 NUTRITION AS A COUNTERMEASURE TO PROTECT AGAINST THE HARMFUL EFFECTS OF MICROGRAVITY

Adequate nutrient intake is especially important for space travelers because of the length of time they are exposed to a limited, mostly closed food system. Because nutritional status is subject to so many influences, monitoring nutritional status on extended duration space missions is important to ensure crew health and productivity, and ultimately mission success. Many nutrition-related concerns exist, including the potential for inadequate energy intake, macronutrient imbalance, and vitamin and mineral deficiencies or excesses. In addition to nutrient intake, nutrient absorption and metabolism may be altered during spaceflight (Zittermann et al., 2000). Maintaining adequate nutrient intake during spaceflight is important not only to meet nutrient needs of astronauts but also to help counteract negative effects of spaceflight on the human body, including the immunosuppressive effect. Improving the nutrition of cosmonauts and astronauts may, therefore, prove to be an appropriate countermeasure to some of the immunological disturbances observed during and after spaceflight. There may be even greater benefits from targeting the immune system with nutrient interventions: given the considerable interactions between the immune system and bone remodeling, nutritional countermeasures that influence the immune system could also prove beneficial in reducing the significant bone loss occurring during long-term spaceflights.

26.3 SPACE RADIATION AS AN ENVIRONMENTAL STRESSOR

26.3.1 SPACE RADIATION: INTRODUCTION

Radiation that occurs in space (space radiation) is energy in transit in the form of high-speed particles and electromagnetic waves. Electromagnetic radiation is very common in everyday lives in the form of visible light, radio and television waves, and microwaves. Radiation is divided into two categories, ionizing and nonionizing. Ionizing radiation is radiation with sufficient energy to remove electrons from the orbits of atoms resulting in charged particles. Examples of ionizing radiation include γ-rays, protons, and neutrons. If the energy of ionizing radiation is sufficient, electrons other than those in the outermost orbits can be released; this process renders the atom very unstable, and these ions are very chemically reactive. Ionizing radiation travels through living tissues, causing structural damage to DNA and other macromolecules, and altering many cellular processes. Space radiation consists primarily of ionizing radiation that exists in the form of high-energy, charged particles. There are three naturally occurring sources of space radiation: trapped radiation, galactic cosmic radiation (GCR), and solar particle events (SPE) (Figure 26.1). The magnetic field generated by electric currents in the Earth's liquid iron core extends far into space, shielding the planet from 99.9% of harmful radiation. The Earth's atmosphere provides additional protection, equal to a slab of metal about 3 feet (1 m) thick. For people outside the protection of Earth's magnetic field, space radiation becomes a serious hazard. Thus, spaceflight and space exploration greatly enhances exposure to ionizing radiation, including its SPE component. Radiation in space takes the form of subatomic particles from the sun as well as from sources in the Milky Way galaxy and beyond. An instrument aboard the Curiosity Mars rover during its 253-day deep-space cruise revealed that the radiation dose received by an astronaut on even the shortest Earth–Mars round-trip would be about 0.66 sievert. This amount is equivalent to receiving a whole-body CT scan every 5 or 6 days. A dose of 1 sievert is associated with a 5.5% increase in the risk of fatal cancer. The normal daily radiation dose received by the average person living on Earth is 10 microsieverts.

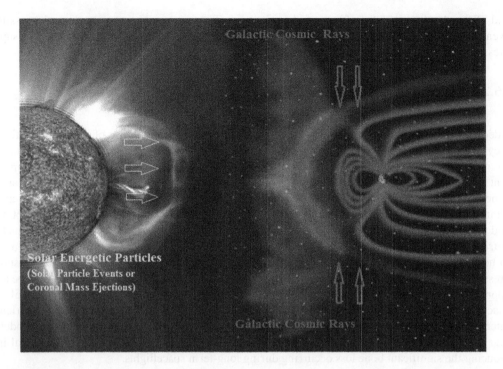

FIGURE 26.1 (See color insert.) The interplanetary space environment showing the toxic combination of galactic cosmic radiation (GCR) and (largely) proton radiation due to solar particle events (SPEs). Figure courtesy of NASA/JPL-Caltech.

26.3.2 THE RISKS OF SPACE RADIATION

There has been major focus recently on the assessment of risks related to exposure to SPE radiation (Kennedy, 2014). Effects related to various types of space radiation exposure that have been evaluated include gene expression changes (primarily associated with programmed cell death and extracellular matrix [ECM] remodeling), increased oxidative stress, increased gastrointestinal tract bacterial translocation and immune system activation, altered peripheral hematopoietic cell counts, emesis, blood coagulation, skin changes, altered behavior, increased fatigue (including social exploration, submaximal exercise treadmill performance, and spontaneous locomotor activity), changed heart functions, and alterations in biological endpoints related to vision (lumbar puncture/intracranial pressure, and ocular ultrasound and histopathology studies); longer-term effects like development of cancer and cataracts have been studied (Kennedy, 2014). The extent and severity of acute effects is determined by the type and amount of radiation exposure. Results from animal experiments show that the biological damage to the central nervous system, which is unique to the high-energy, heavy ions encountered in space, is similar to that associated with aging. There is experimental evidence that radiation encountered in space is more effective at causing the type of biological damage that ultimately leads to cancer than γ- or x-rays commonly encountered on Earth. There are a number of health concerns as a result of space radiation exposure, including increased risk of cancer; changes in motor function and behavior and increased risk of neurological disorders; increased risk of other degenerative tissue defects such as cataracts, circulatory diseases, and digestive diseases; prodromal risks; significant skin injury; or death from a major solar event or combination solar/galactic cosmic ray event. The space radiation risks to the central nervous system (CNS) are considered extremely important. For example, studies suggest that the induction of Alzheimer's disease may be a space radiation risk (Cherry et al., 2012) and attention deficits may arise following exposure to low doses of space radiation (Davis et al., 2014). Many other studies have also indicated that there are major risks to the CNS from space radiation (Limoli et al., 2007; Manda et al., 2007, 2008a,b; Poulose et al., 2011; Lonart et al., 2012; Rivera et al., 2013; Suman et al., 2013; Tseng et al., 2014). Exposure to γ-rays (Hienz et al., 2008) or ^{56}Fe ions (Shukitt-Hale et al., 2000, 2007; Higuchi et al., 2002; Rabin et al., 2002) is also known to have adverse effects on the CNS and neurobehavior of irradiated animals, including reduced performance in motor tasks and deficits in spatial learning and memory.

26.3.3 NUTRITION AS A COUNTERMEASURE TO PROTECT AGAINST THE HARMFUL EFFECTS OF SPACE RADIATION

Nutritional countermeasures to reduce the effects of ionizing radiation can be broadly categorized into two groups. The first group includes specific nutrients (or even foods) that prevent the radiation damage. For example, antioxidants like vitamins C and E may help by soaking up radiation-produced free radicals before they can do any harm. Research has also suggested that pectin fiber from fruits and vegetables, and omega-3–rich fish oils may be beneficial countermeasures to damage from long-term radiation exposure. Other studies have shown that diets rich in strawberries, blueberries, kale, and spinach prevent neurological damage due to radiation. In addition, drugs such as radiogardase (also known as Prussian blue) that contain ferric (III) hexacyanoferrate (II) are designed to increase the rate at which radioactive substances like cesium-137 or thallium are eliminated from the body.

The second group of nutritional countermeasures are those that facilitate a faster recovery from radiation damage. These dietary agents offer protection by stimulating the growth of surviving stem and progenitor cells, or by lengthening the duration of the cell cycle segment that checks for and repairs damaged DNA. These types of agents (called radio-protectants) are used to treat people exposed to radiation contamination on Earth, and may be good candidates for use on long-duration space missions. It is important to note, however, that when administered in effective concentrations, some radioprotectants also have negative side effects such as nausea, hypotension, weakness, and fatigue.

One natural defense system is for an abnormal radiation damaged cell to self-destruct before the cell becomes cancerous; this is achieved by activation of the cell's apoptosis pathways (programmed cell death). Apoptosis can also be triggered intentionally by exposing the cell to enzymes or specific ligands (an ion, an atom, or a molecule) that bind to a cell's death receptors. Other approaches that may also be useful aim to enhance the DNA repair system and immune response by facilitating faster recovery of cell populations damaged by radiation. There are several agents now in clinical trials that may have these effects. Some drugs, for example, stimulate the immune system to "restore and repopulate" bone marrow cells after radiation exposure. Other drugs appear to reduce gene mutations resulting from radiation exposure. Radiation protectants originally developed to protect military personnel in the event of nuclear warfare are now being used to protect cancer patients against the harmful effects of radiation treatment.

Another important countermeasure may be the use of a nutritional supplement called active hexose correlated compound (AHCC) (see Chapter 25). AHCC is a fermented mushroom extract that has been used as a supplement to treat a wide range of health conditions. It helps in augmentation of the natural immune response and affects immune outcomes and immune cell activation (see Chapter 25). Immune suppression in microgravity or due to radiation has been documented for many years. AHCC may be able to counter this (Olamigoke et al., 2015). AHCC is seen to have anticancer action and immunostimulatory effects, and reduces side effects due to chemotherapy, as well as enhancing defense against infection (Olamigoke et al., 2015). Figure 26.2

50µg/ml AHCC, 20x

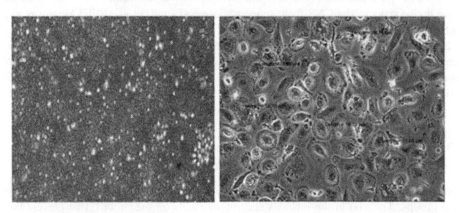

96 hours incubation   360 hours incubation

FIGURE 26.2 (See color insert.)   Representative image of AHCC-treated lymphocytes. Cells were treated with 50 µg/mL AHCC and are shown at 20 × magnification. Note the morphological changes of lymphocytes from 96 hours to 360 hours posttreatment with AHCC. Cells become adherent and phenotypic changes were observed.

shows the immunoproliferative effects of AHCC on normal human lymphocytes mediated via cell adhesion.

26.4   CONCLUSIONS

Stressors of all kinds affect many physiological systems and most adversely influence the immune response. This could be through an altered hormonal milieu that suppresses many immune cell responses or through direct cellular damage. In this chapter, two forms of environmental stressor relevant to space travel—microgravity and ionizing radiation—have been discussed. Both adversely affect the immune response, although more detail on the precise effects and about the mechanisms involved is still required. This is very important since immune impairment has been proposed to be a limitation on further space exploration. Factors that limit the damage caused by space travel or that accelerate the repair process will be important for intervention in the future. Several nutritional factors could play a role in this regard. It is likely that this will become an area ripe for further research.

REFERENCES

Baqai, F.P., Gridley, D.S., Slater, J.M., Luo-Owen, X., Stodieck, L.S., Ferguson, V., Chapes, S.K. and Pecaut, M.J. 2009. Effects of spaceflight on innate immune function and antioxidant gene expression. *J Appl Physiol* 106:1935–42.
Blaber, E., Marcal, H. and Burns B.P. 2010. Bioastronautics: The influence of microgravity on astronaut health. *Astrobiol* 10:463–73.
Borchers, A.T., Keen, C.L. and Gershwin, M.E. 2002. Microgravity and immune responsiveness: Implications for space travel. *Nutrition* 18:889–98.
Calder, P.C. 2013. Feeding the immune system. *Proc Nutr Soc* 72:299–309.
Chang, T.T., Walther, I., Li, C.F., Boonyaratanakornkit, J., Galleri, G., Meloni, M.A., Pippia, P., Cogoli, A. and Hughes-Fulford, M. 2012. The Rel/NF-κB pathway and transcription of immediate early genes in T cell activation are inhibited by microgravity. *J Leuk Biol* 92:1133–45.

Cherry, J.D., Liu, B., Frost, J.L., Lemere, C.A., Williams, J.P., Olschowka, J.A. and O'Banion, M.K. 2012. Galactic cosmic radiation leads to cognitive impairment and increased abeta plaque accumulation in a mouse model of Alzheimer's disease. *PLOS ONE* 7:e53275.

Clement, G. 2003. Musculoskeletal system in space. In: *Fundamentals of Space Medicine*. Dordrecht, the Netherlands: Kluwer Academic Publishers; pp. 173–204.

Davis, C.M., DeCicco-Skinner, K.L., Roma, P.G. and Hienz, R.D. 2014. Individual differences in attentional deficits and dopaminergic protein levels following exposure to proton radiation. *Radiat Res* 181:258–71.

Dhabhar, F.S. 2014. Effects of stress on immune function: The good, the bad, and the beautiful. *Immunol Res* 58:193–210.

Fitzgerald, W., Chen, S., Walz, C., Zimmerberg, J., Margolis, L. and Grivel, J.C. 2009. Immune suppression of human lymphoid tissues and cells in rotating suspension culture and onboard the International Space Station. *In Vitro Cell Dev Biol Anim* 45:622–32.

Gridley, D.S., Slater, J.M., Luo-Owen, X., Rizvi, A., Chapes, S.K., Stodieck, L.S., Ferguson, V.L. and Pecaut, M.J. 2009. Spaceflight effects on T lymphocyte distribution, function and gene expression. *J Appl Physiol* 106:194–202.

Gueguinou, N., Huin-Schohn, C., Bascove, M., Bueb, J.L., Tschirhart, E., Legrand-Frossi, C. and Frippiat, J.P., 2009. Could spaceflight-associated immune system weakening preclude the expansion of human presence beyond Earth's orbit? *J Leuk Biol* 86:1027–38.

Hienz, R.D., Brady, J.V., Gooden, V.L., Vazquez, M.E. and Weed, M.R. 2008. Neurobehavioral effects of head-only gamma-radiation exposure in rats. *Rad Res* 170:292–8.

Higuchi, Y., Nelson, G.A., Vazquez, M., Laskowitz, D.T., Slater, J.M. and Pearlstein, R.D. 2002. Apolipoprotein E expression and behavioral toxicity of high charge, high energy (HZE) particle radiation. *J Radiat Res* 43:S219–24.

Kennedy, A.R. 2014. Biological effects of space radiation and development of effective countermeasures. *Life Sci Space Res (Amst)* 1:10–43.

Levine, D.S. and Greenleaf, J.E. 1998. Immunosuppression during spaceflight deconditioning. *Aviat Space Environ Med* 69:172–7.

Limoli, C.L., Giedzinski, E., Baure, J., Rola, R. and Fike, J.R. 2007. Redox changes induced in hippocampal precursor cells by heavy ion irradiation. *Radiat Environ Biophy* 46:167–72.

Loehr, J.A., Lee, S.M., English, K.L., Sibonga, J., Smith, S.M., Spiering, B.A. and Hagan, R.D. 2011. Musculoskeletal adaptations to training with the advanced resistive exercise device. *Med Sci Sports Exerc* 43:146–56.

Lonart, G., Parris, B., Johnson, A.M., Miles, S., Sanford, L.D., Singletary, S.J. and Britten, R.A. 2012. Executive function in rats is impaired by low (20 cGy) doses of 1 GeV/u (56)Fe particles. *Radiat Res* 178:289–94.

Manda, K., Anzai, K., Kumari, S. and Bhatia, A.L. 2007. Melatonin attenuates radiation-induced learning deficit and brain oxidative stress in mice. *Acta Neurobiol Exp* 67:63–70.

Manda, K., Ueno, M. and Anzai, K. 2008a. Memory impairment, oxidative damage and apoptosis induced by space radiation: Ameliorative potential of alpha-lipoic acid. *Behav Brain Res* 187:387–95.

Manda, K., Ueno, M. and Anzai, K. 2008b. Space radiation-induced inhibition of neurogenesis in the hippocampal dentate gyrus and memory impairment in mice: Ameliorative potential of the melatonin metabolite, AFMK. *J Pineal Res* 45:430–8.

Olamigoke, L, Mansoor, E., Mann, V., Ellis, I., Okoro, E., Wakame, K., Fuji, H., Kulkarni, A., Francoise Doursout, M. and Sundaresan, A. 2015. AHCC activation and selection of human lymphocytes via genotypic and phenotypic changes to an adherent cell type: A possible novel mechanism of T cell activation. *Evid Based Complement Alternat Med* 2015:508746.

Poulose, S.M., Bielinski, D.F., Carrihill-Knoll, K., Rabin, B.M. and Shukitt-Hale, B. 2011. Exposure to ^{16}O-particle radiation causes aging-like decrements in rats through increased oxidative stress, inflammation and loss of autophagy. *Radiat Res* 176:761–9.

Rabin, B.M., Buhler, L.L., Joseph, J.A., Shukitt-Hale, B. and Jenkins, D.G. 2002. Effects of exposure to [56]Fe particles or protons on fixed-ratio operant responding in rats. *J Rad Res* S225–8.

Rivera, P.D., Shih, H.Y., Leblanc, J.A., Cole, M.G., Amaral, W.Z., Mukherjee, S., Zhang, S., Lucero, M.J., Decarolis, N.A., Chen, B.P. and Eisch, A.J. 2013. Acute and fractionated exposure to high-LET (56) Fe HZE-particle radiation both result in similar long-term deficits in adult hippocampal neurogenesis. *Radiat Res* 180:658–67.

Shackelford, L.C. 2008. Musculoskeletal response to space flight. In: Barratt, M.R. and Pool, S.L., editors. *Principles of Clinical Medicine for Space Flight*. New York, NY: Springer Science and Business Media; pp. 293–306.

Shukitt-Hale, B., Carey, A.N., Jenkins, D., Rabin, B.M. and Joseph, J.A. 2007. Beneficial effects of fruit extracts on neuronal function and behavior in a rodent model of accelerated aging. *Neurobiol Aging* 28:1187–94.

Shukitt-Hale, B., Casadesus, G., McEwen, J.J., Rabin, B.M. and Joseph, J.A. 2000. Spatial learning and memory deficits induced by exposure to iron-56-particle radiation. *Rad Res* 154:28–33.

Smith, S.M., Heer, M.A., Shackelford, L., Sibonga, J.D., Ploutz-Snyder, L. and Zwart, S.R. 2012. Benefits for bone from resistance exercise and nutrition in long-duration spaceflight: Evidence from biochemistry and densitometry. *J Bone Miner Res* 27:1896–906.

Sonnenfeld, G. 2002. The immune system in space and micro gravity. *Med Sci Sports Exerc* 34:2021–7.

Stowe, R.P., Sams, C.F. and Pierson, D.L. 2011. Adrenocortical and immune responses following short- and long-duration spaceflight. *Aviat Space Environ Med* 82:627–34.

Suman, S., Rodriguez, O.C., Winters, T.A., Fornace, A.J. Jr., Albanese, C. and Datta, K. 2013. Therapeutic and space radiation exposure of mouse brain causes impaired DNA repair response and premature senescence by chronic oxidant production. *Aging (Albany NY)* 5:607–22.

Tseng, B.P., Giedzinski, E., Izadi, A., Suarez, T., Lan, M.L., Tran, K.K., Acharya, M.M., Nelson, G.A., Raber, J., Parihar, V.K. and Limoli, C.L. 2014. Functional consequences of radiation-induced oxidative stress in cultured neural stem cells and the brain exposed to charged particle irradiation. *Antioxid Redox Signal* 20:1410–22.

Zittermann, A., Heer, M., Caillot-Augusseau, A, Rettberg, P., Scheld, K., Drummer, C., Alexandre, C., Horneck, G., Vorobiev, D. and Stehle, P. 2000. Microgravity inhibits intestinal calcium absorption as shown by a stable strontium test. *Eur J Clin Invest* 30:1036–43.

27 Nutrition, Immunity, and Infection: Ayurvedic and Conventional Perspectives

Kavita D. Chandwani, Shinil K. Shah,
Erik B. Wilson, and Anil D. Kulkarni

CONTENTS

27.1 Introduction 443
27.2 Ayurved—A Science of Healing 444
    27.2.1 Historical Overview 444
    27.2.2 Understanding the Human Body: An Ayurvedic Perspective 445
    27.2.3 Concept of Health and Healing—Ayurved and Modern Medicine 445
    27.2.4 The Place of Nutrition in Healing 446
    27.2.5 Infections in the Ayurvedic Literature 446
27.3 Modern Research and Applications of Ayurved in Infections 446
    27.3.1 Overview 446
    27.3.2 Ayurved and Bacterial and Fungal Infections 447
    27.3.3 Ayurved and Parasitic Infections 447
    27.3.4 Ayurved and Viral Infections 447
27.4 Common Ayurvedic Herbs and Preparations for Possible Use in Infections 447
    27.4.1 General Considerations 447
    27.4.2 Neem 448
    27.4.3 Tulsi 448
    27.4.4 Turmeric 448
    27.4.5 Withania somnifera 448
    27.4.6 Rasayan 449
    27.4.7 Ayurved and Wound Healing 449
    27.4.8 Ayurved and Other Infections 449
27.5 Conclusion and Perspectives 449
References 450

27.1 INTRODUCTION

Infection is defined as the invasion of the body by organisms such as bacteria, viruses, fungi, or parasites; inside the body they may multiply, stay dormant, or be neutralized by the body's defense mechanisms. With the entry of such organisms into the body, immunological processes are aimed at eradicating them and/or stopping their multiplication. The presence of infection is suggested clinically by symptoms and/or signs elicited in those with or without symptoms. Following a confirmatory test or procedure and depending on the body system and the organisms involved, the treatment would include an appropriate anti-infective pharmaceutical agent. However, infection may remain subclinical, resolving on its own, or it could pass into a chronic phase. Use of advanced technology in research has enabled a deeper understanding of the various processes of the point of entry of (micro)organisms into the body, their invasion of tissue, and the various processes at the molecular level leading to the clinical manifestations of infection. In modern conventional or allopathic medicine, treatment of such a condition through the use of pharmaceutical agents is based on evidence of the ability of the agents to kill the organisms, proof of which has been provided in prior laboratory and clinical experiments. Such detailed understanding of these processes has made possible the discovery of antibiotics and anti-infective agents, and also the introduction of newer pharmaceutical agents that include vaccines, antibodies, and immunoglobulins for the prevention and treatment of infectious diseases. However, there are limitations to such a physical systemic approach in understanding of several disease conditions and their treatment. Despite the discovery of newer generations of antibiotics, antibiotic resistance and superinfection by "superbugs" have become major health issues. Thus, both patients and healthcare providers have an increased awareness of and interest complementing their treatment regimen with traditional healing systems, such as Ayurved, and/or nonconventional healing products and techniques. Ayurved has often been perceived as a system of herbal healing. The system is, in fact, a much deeper science that embraces nature and involves a balance of elements between the interior milieu of the human body and its external environment which must undergo constant adjustment. Ayurved also includes the acceptance of plants as life forms and the potential of mutual nourishment among different life-forms (Frawley and Lad 1988). In this chapter, the healing system of Ayurved will be explained, and aspects of its approaches related to resolution of infections and common medical conditions will be discussed.

27.2 AYURVED—A SCIENCE OF HEALING

27.2.1 Historical Overview

The word "Ayurved" literally means "scripture for longevity"; it is derived from two Sanskrit root words—"*ayu*" (life) and "*ved*" (knowledge) (Joshi 1997). Ayurved was the main systematic institution of traditional medical practice for more than 5,000 years in ancient India (Lad 1985; Mishra, Singh, and Dagenais 2001). References to healing of human ailments can also be found in the older Indian texts *Rig Ved* and *Atharva Ved*, especially the latter, which describes diseases and their treatment (Narayanaswamy 1981); Ayurved is said to have originated from *Atharv Ved*. In ancient times, this knowledge was transmitted orally to succeeding generations; later, it was formally written into texts such as *Charak Samhita* by Charak (physician), *Sushrut Samhita* by Sushrut (father of Ayurvedic surgery), *Ashtang Hridayam*, and *Bhavaprakash*. Ayurved was classified as a complementary and alternative medicine (CAM) when the National Center for CAM (renamed as National Center for Complementary and Integrative Health or NCCIH) was formed in the United States; currently, NCCIH classifies it as one of the "Whole Systems".

Ayurved is characterized by thousands of years of experiential observation and acceptance; the unique feature that distinguishes conventional medicine from Ayurved is its association with the comparatively recent inferential system of scientific inquiry. Ayurved existed at a time when the borders of the country went beyond those of the present India. It also spread to the neighboring countries through either the emissaries of King Ashok, a ruler of ancient India, or through traders journeying through different countries such as Egypt, Greece, China, Korea, and Japan; this is the reason that systems very similar to Ayurved can be found in countries like Japan, Tibet, Bhutan, Nepal, Myanmar, Thailand, Sri Lanka, and China. The Buddhist system of medical practice also documents basic concepts of symptom description and diagnostic and therapeutic approaches that are similar to those of Ayurved (Narayana and Lavekar 2005). Similarly, an influence of the Ayurvedic system can be seen in Tibetan medicine. With urbanization, some regional changes in the understanding and practice of Ayurved have been observed. In Sikkim, a state in north India, the practice of traditional Ayurvedic medicine is reported mostly in rural areas. A paucity of interest in continuing with traditional medicine has also been observed among younger generations (Panda and Misra 2010).

27.2.2 Understanding the Human Body: An Ayurvedic Perspective

Ayurved is based on the fundamental theory that the creation, of which a human body is a part, is a combination of, and interplay between, five elements or *panch mahabhutas,* namely, space, air, fire, water, and earth (Joshi 1997). The physical body has seven tissues or *dhatus,* namely, *rasa* (plasma), *rakta* (blood), *mamsa* (muscle), *meda* (fat), *asthi* (bone), *majja* (marrow), and *shukra* and *artav* (reproductive tissues) (Lad 1985). Beginning with *rasa,* the succeeding tissues are formed with the help of *agni* (fire) of the corresponding *dhatu.* The elements of *panch mahabhutas* are present in various combinations in a human body contributing to the three functional constitutions or *prakriti* types or three *doshas: vata, pitta,* and *kapha* (Dey and Pahwa 2014) or combinations of any of the three *doshas.* The combination of the three *doshas* changes with different stages of life and so does the *prakriti* or constitution.

Gunas or the qualities of *prakriti* include *satva, rajas,* and *tamas* indicating the "essence, movement, and inertia," respectively (Lad 1985). A diseased constitution or *prakriti* is reflected in the imbalance of the *doshas.* In modern/conventional medicine, no such classification of the constitution exists, however, research suggests a possibility of association between a person's *prakriti* type and genetics, based on human leucocyte antigen (HLA) typing (Bhushan, Kalpana, and Arvind 2005).

In Ayurved, determining the constitution of a person is the initial step in diagnosis, which subsequently guides treatment. Ayurvedic examination consists of assessment of qualities including physical characteristics of the body as well as the mental alertness, food craving, sleep habits, psychological status among others, and examination of the pulse. After determining a person's *dosha* imbalance, correction of the diseased constitution can be achieved (Joshi 1997), the basic aim of therapy or *cikitsa* being to strengthen the host and to cure the disease (Chopra and Doiphode 2002).

27.2.3 Concept of Health and Healing—Ayurved and Modern Medicine

The understanding of human existence according to modern science is a mere physical modality with various organ systems performing their respective functions. In contrast, according to Ayurved, the understanding of human existence is different: physical body (*sarir*) is habited by a soul (*atma*) and permeated by a vital force (*prana*), and this responds to the nature and environment around it as well as to whatever is perceived through the sense organs and the mental faculty. According to the system of Ayurved, each individual acquires a unique constitution at birth that is critical for his or her body's responses to the environment, a concept that is somewhat similar to genetics and immunity according to conventional medicine.

The common feature of the two systems is the dependence on symptoms and physical signs to arrive at a diagnosis. Yet, the two systems differ on the considerations of the basic treatment approaches. The conventional system decides the treatment based on the physical qualities and laboratory and other tests, while the Ayurvedic treatment approach is based on perceiving and treating a whole person as an individual, which includes a consideration of physical, mental, and spiritual aspects of a person to determine the constitution and reach at a diagnosis. In other words, the Ayurvedic system of healing falls in the modern-day definition of "personalized medicine." With the emergence of the field of complementary and integrative medicine, initial scientific research has begun to validate some of the Ayurvedic principles and approaches. For example, scientific research has shown that the state of mind influences the body processes: psychological distress has been shown to be associated with changes in body processes, including in the immune system (Kiecolt-Glaser et al. 1996).

However, several aspects of Ayurved cannot be verbalized and can only be intuitively discerned on a value-based system that is acquired through traditional training of the Ayurvedic physician or the *Vaidya*. Although with increasing inquiry into "ancient medicine," scientific research could prove to be a way of bridging ancient with modern medicine, but there could be challenges in applying the modern scientific methods of inquiry to aspects of Ayurvedic medicine.

27.2.4 The Place of Nutrition in Healing

Ayurved embraces the concept of nutrition as one of the sources of healthy disease-free living. In a diseased condition, one of the primary approaches to health is through *ahar* or a sound diet. A person with one *prakriti* will be advised to not include certain food and lifestyle practices that might exacerbate a particular *dosha*. Thus, a *dosha*-specific diet is advised in order to restore and maintain a healthy and balanced constitution. In contrast, modern medicine started recognizing nutrition as a part of healing only in the twentieth century (Keusch 2003; Scrimshaw, Taylor, and Gordon 1959). For example, it was observed that the body's resistance to infection was reduced in the presence of one or more nutritional deficiencies (Scrimshaw and SanGiovanni 1997). Examples of such a relation can still be seen in cases of greater morbidity and mortality observed in patients with nutritional deficiencies and in those suffering from diseases such as tuberculosis and human immune deficiency (Scrimshaw 2007).

27.2.5 Infections in the Ayurvedic Literature

Kayachikitsa or internal medicine is one of the eight branches described in Ayurvedic texts (Subbarayappa 2001). Although the term "infection" does not find a place in Ayurvedic medicine, disease descriptions similar to conditions such as tuberculosis can be found in old texts. Reference to *krimi* or "minute organisms or insects" being one of the reasons for disease causation can be found in *Rig Ved* and *Atharv Ved* (Subbarayappa 2001); a mention of *krimi* causing *yakshma* (tuberculosis) and its treatment can found in *Atharv Ved* (Prasad 2002). There is also a description of *ajirna* (indigestion) in Ayurvedic literature; the details of this disease seem similar to that of cholera (Prasad 2005). Furthermore, evidence of infection control related to wound healing has also been found in the ancient texts. Sushrut wrote about the classification of wounds and their treatment, which consisted of either polyherbal application or herbs for internal administration (Bhat et al. 2014; Sushrut 1995).

27.3 MODERN RESEARCH AND APPLICATIONS OF AYURVED IN INFECTIONS

27.3.1 Overview

The basic premise of Ayurved is that the mere presence of microbes in or on the body is not enough to result in infection; the state of the human body is such that it allows for their growth and multiplication. Therefore, the Ayurvedic therapeutic approach strives to create a balanced constitution that is in favor of strengthening the host body rather than killing the microbes. Although no detailed description of (micro)organisms, immunologic processes, or specific antibacterial, antifungal, antiviral, or antiparasitic agents are found in the Ayurvedic texts, the approach worked as a successful healing modality in ancient India. Current Ayurvedic practitioners treating cancer patients have reported that they focus on improving digestion, metabolism, balance, and mental health; reducing toxins; and rejuvenation (Dhruva et al. 2014). Attempts have been made to analyze Ayurved within the framework of modern modes of scientific inquiry. The *dosha* classification represents the mind-body type of the person, and their relation to their biologic characteristics have been shown in a few studies involving enzymes and HLA DRB1 types (Patwardhan and Bodeker

2008). On the other hand, the basis of modern conventional medicine and therapeutics lies in the evidence shown in the form of measurable changes in different levels of physical processes/functions in the human body and, in the context of infection, the associated organism. Yet, its limitations have been revealed through drug resistance and the emergence of superinfections. The inability of modern medicine to control some known common pathogens and the emergence of newer or previously dormant organisms, such as *Staphylococcus aureus*, *Escherichia coli*, and *Pseudomonas aeruginosa*, warrants that the scientific community search for better options. Driven by the ease of self-care options of nonprescription traditional methods/medications/herbs used by some patients who cannot find satisfactory treatment for their chronic disease conditions, empirical evidence of possible efficacy of some nonconventional treatments including Ayurved has been reported in the literature from time to time. This has stimulated greater interest in nonconventional modes of treatment. Some studies of Ayurvedic herbs or mixtures, mostly preclinical, have shown promising results in common infections.

27.3.2 Ayurved and Bacterial and Fungal Infections

Study of a broad range of Indian plants used as a part of Ayurvedic treatment has produced evidence of their efficacy against several bacteria, including *Staphylococcus aureus*, *Staphylococcus epidermidis*, *Escherichia coli*, *Klebsiella pneumoniae*, *Pseudomonas aeruginosa*, *Streptococcus faecalis*, *Candida albicans*, and *Aspergillus niger* (Kumar et al. 2006). Currently, evidence of the possible effectiveness of a wide variety of plant species against *Mycobacterium tuberculosis* has been reported (Gautam, Saklani, and Jachak 2007). Researchers have also examined the efficacy of several Ayurvedic preparations such as *Chandraprabha vati* in urinary tract infections in mice (Christa et al. 2013). In addition to antibacterial effects, *Allium cepa* and *Allium sativum* (garlic juice) have been shown to be effective against some fungi (Srinivasan et al. 2001).

27.3.3 Ayurved and Parasitic Infections

Following unsuccessful attempts at eradicating malaria, a major part of the world population is facing a challenge. Discovery of any effective antimalarial would benefit those populations. In a study of effects of *kutaja* and *neem* in plasmodium-infested mice, the antiplasmodial effect was observed to be similar to that of chloroquine (Priyanka, Hingorani, and Nilima 2013). Patients with other parasitic infestations could also find a treatment or cure through Ayurvedic herbs or preparations as suggested by the results from recent research with *Desmodium gangeticum* (Singh et al. 2005) and *Tinospora sinensis* in visceral Leishmaniasis (Singh et al. 2008).

27.3.4 Ayurved and Viral Infections

Initial results from the study of *Azadirachta indica* or *neem* suggest possible effects against HSV-1 (Tiwari et al. 2010) and the polio virus, where the *neem* polysaccharides showed inhibitory effects when introduced with the polio virus but not when introduced after the virus (Faccin-Galhardi et al. 2012).

27.4 COMMON AYURVEDIC HERBS AND PREPARATIONS FOR POSSIBLE USE IN INFECTIONS

27.4.1 General Considerations

Ayurvedic treatment with herbs could involve administration of a single herb or of a mixture or decoction of multiple herbs; this is usually decided by the *Vaidya* depending on their efficacy in various conditions such as diarrhea, dysentery, abdominal pain, constipation, or infections (Sandhya et al. 2006; Tariq et al. 2015). Scientific evidence of the effects of Ayurvedic preparations in treating infections comes from research studies. One such example is the inhibition of tumor necrosis factor-alpha and nitric oxide production by lipopolysaccharide-stimulated RAW 264.7 mouse macrophages by a mixture of *Withania somnifera, Boswellia serrata, Zingiber officinale*, and *Curcuma longa;* similar beneficial effects were also observed in artificially induced arthritis in rats (Dey et al. 2014).

All traditional medicines are best dispensed by an expert knowledgeable in indigenous practices. Heavy metals such as mercury are known components of some Ayurvedic medicine preparations. An example of safety of Ayurvedic medicine has been reported in a study of mercury-containing *Sidh Makardhwaj,* a preparation used in rheumatoid arthritis and some neurologic disorders, where no toxic effects were reported on rat brain (Kumar et al. 2014). In the current culture of unregulated use of herbs including Ayurvedic medicines, the risk of deleterious side effects is always a possibility. However, treatment taken under the guidance of an experienced *Vaidya* could prevent development of toxicity.

27.4.2 Neem

Neem (Azadirachta indica), a commonly used herb in Ayurvedic practice, is known for its effectiveness in a wide range of conditions. The leaves are most often used, although the *neem* tree has yielded more than 140 biologically active compounds (Subapriya and Nagini 2005). *Neem* has been reported to have antibacterial (Nair, Kalariya, and Chanda 2007), antiplasmodial (with *kutaja*), (Priyanka, Hingorani, and Nilima 2013), antifungal (Khan et al. 1988), and antiviral (Subapriya and Nagini 2005) properties.

27.4.3 Tulsi

Tulsi (Ocimum sanctum) or "holy basil," a shrub, is known in Ayurved as the "elixir of life" (Rastogi et al. 2015). It is traditionally grown and used in religious rituals in Hindu homes. Rich in essential oils, different parts of the plant are used in various disease conditions. It has antibacterial properties (Nair, Kalariya, and Chanda 2007) and traditionally finds use in treatment of upper respiratory infections, earaches, fungal infections, and gastric conditions.

27.4.4 Turmeric

Turmeric *(Curcuma longa)*, a rhizome, is widely used in Ayurvedic practice. It is a commonly used spice in Indian cooking. Its active biologic derivative, curcumin, has been shown to have anti-inflammatory effects (Aggarwal 2010; Deguchi 2015). Studies have shown evidence of its benefits in infection with HIV-1, HSV-2 (Ferreira et al. 2015), *Helicobacter pylori* (Santos et al. 2015), *Klebsiella pueumoniae* (Bansal and Chhibber 2014), cervical human papilloma virus (Basu et al. 2013), and hepatitis C virus (Anggakusuma et al. 2014). Effects of another derivative of curcumin have been reported in HIV-1 infection in cultured lymphoblastoid and peripheral blood mononuclear cells (Kumari et al. 2015).

27.4.5 Withania somnifera

W. somnifera Dunal, belonging to family *Solanaceae,* is also known as *Ashwagandha.* It has been used for a wide range of conditions in Ayurvedic practice as well as by the indigenous populations of South Asian countries. Extracts of its root and leaves are used for treatment purposes. *W. somnifera* has been shown to be have antimicrobial effects against methicillin-resistant *Staphylococcus aureus* and enterococci (Bisht and Rawat 2014). *W. coagulans* is another species that is traditionally used for abdominal pain, constipation, diarrhea, and dysentery (Tariq et al. 2015) and has shown promising results in infections due to *Salmonella* (Owais et al. 2005), aspergillosis (Dhuley 1998), and *Listeria monocytogenes* (Teixeira et al. 2006).

27.4.6 RASAYAN

Rasayan involves a systematic approach toward rejuvenation that reinforces the effects of *Panchakarma*. It is a specialized process of methodical administration of drugs that improve metabolism and immunity, and strengthen the body. During the period of *Rasayan* therapy the subject follows a specialized diet and conduct after undergoing the process of *Panchakarma* (Govindarajan, Vijayakumar, and Pushpangadan 2005). Preliminary results of trials of two different *Rasayan*, *Shilajatu Rasayana* (Gupta et al. 2010) and *Ranahamsa Rasayanaya* (Somarathna et al. 2010), in patients with HIV infection have shown encouraging results in terms of increase in the mean CD4[+] T-cell count.

27.4.7 AYURVED AND WOUND HEALING

Plant-based natural products have been safely used in the past for wound care (Sivamani et al. 2012). According to Ayurvedic texts, honey was used as a means of wound dressing to clean wounds and promote healing (Pecanac et al. 2013). Application of *Panchavalkala*, a preparation made from parts of five trees, has been described in *Sushrut Samhita* (Sushrut 1995); a study of the same has shown a statistically significant reduction in pain, swelling, redness, and tenderness, as well as the microbial load in chronic infected wounds of fifty patients (Bhat et al. 2014). Similarly, an ethanol extract of an *Albizzia lebeck* root, used by Ayurvedic practitioners, has demonstrated wound-healing properties (Joshi et al. 2013).

27.4.8 AYURVED AND OTHER INFECTIONS

A few other examples of research of Ayurvedic medicine in common infections are conjunctivitis (Sharma and Singh 2002) and dental health (Subapriya and Nagini 2005; Telles, Naveen, and Balkrishna 2009). Texts of Ayurved also spell out the type of sticks to use for dental health based on the type of *dosha*—bittersweet for *vatadosha*, bitter for *pitta dosha*, and pungent for *kapha dosha* (Telles, Naveen, and Balkrishna 2009). Oil pulling using different oils or chewing different sticks has been mentioned in old texts for the treatment of gum conditions and plaque formation (Singh and Purohit 2011). Such practices have not been validated, yet this Ayurvedic approach is still followed by a substantial portion of the Indian population (Sharma et al. 2007). A study of a rejuvenating mixture, *Indukantha Ghritha*, reported it to be beneficial in recurrent upper respiratory infections (Nesari et al. 2004; Radhakrishnan et al. 2014).

27.5 CONCLUSION AND PERSPECTIVES

Ayurved has a promising role to play in addressing disease conditions, specifically infections. In a review of new therapeutic agents, it was found that about 50% of the approved new active substances in 2010 were of a natural origin (Newman and Cragg 2012). Although there have been attempts to determine the active component in a plant source, isolating the active molecule or the chemical effective against an organism or receptor and using it to treat a disease condition cannot replace the holistic approach of Ayurvedic treatment. This is because the original Ayurvedic approach involves improving the other faculties of health along with the physical constitution; this removes the imbalance of the elements of the body, a substrate used by the invading organisms to thrive. Continuing to follow the conventional model of drug discovery through isolation of the active components from the agents/herbs used traditionally in Ayurved, and administering those isolates in specific conditions such as infections and avoiding/ignoring the traditional holistic-approach of Ayurved could potentially meet the same fate as the modern drugs; these could include drug resistance and a range of unwanted side effects.

REFERENCES

Aggarwal, B. B. 2010. Targeting inflammation-induced obesity and metabolic diseases by curcumin and other nutraceuticals. *Ann Rev Nutr* 30:173–99.

Anggakusuma, C. C. Colpitts, L. M. Schang, H. Rachmawati, A. Frentzen, S. Pfaender, P. Behrendt, R. J. Brown, D. Bankwitz, J. Steinmann, M. Ott, P. Meuleman, C. M. Rice, A. Ploss, T. Pietschmann, and E. Steinmann. 2014. Turmeric curcumin inhibits entry of all hepatitis C virus genotypes into human liver cells. *Gut* 63:1137–49.

Bansal, S., and S. Chhibber. 2014. Phytochemical-induced reduction of pulmonary inflammation during Klebsiella pneumoniae lung infection in mice. *J Infect Dev Ctries* 8:838–44.

Basu, P., S. Dutta, R. Begum, S. Mittal, P. D. Dutta, A. C. Bharti, C. K. Panda, J. Biswas, B. Dey, G. P. Talwar, and B. C. Das. 2013. Clearance of cervical human papillomavirus infection by topical application of curcumin and curcumin containing polyherbal cream: A phase II randomized controlled study. *Asian Pac J Cancer Prev* 14:5753–9.

Bhat, K. S., B. N. Vishwesh, M. Sahu, and V. K. Shukla. 2014. A clinical study on the efficacy of Panchavalkala cream in Vrana Shodhana w.s.r to its action on microbial load and wound infection. *Ayu* 35:135–40.

Bhushan, P., J. Kalpana, and C. Arvind. 2005. Classification of human population based on HLA gene polymorphism and the concept of Prakriti in Ayurved. *J Altern Complement Med* 11:349–53.

Bisht, P., and V. Rawat. 2014. Antibacterial activity of Withania somnifera against Gram-positive isolates from pus samples. *Ayu* 35:330–2.

Chopra, A., and V. V. Doiphode. 2002. Ayurvedic medicine. Core concept, therapeutic principles, and current relevance. *Med Clin North Am* 86:75–89.

Christa, S. S., A. Swetha, E. Christina, R. Ganesh, and P. Viswanathan. 2013. Modulatory effect of Chandraprabha Vati on antimicrobial peptides and inflammatory markers in kidneys of mice with urinary tract infection. *Iran J Kidney Dis* 7:390–8.

Deguchi, A. 2015. Curcumin targets in inflammation and cancer. *Endocr Metab Immune Disord Drug Targets* 15:88–96.

Dey, D., S. Chaskar, N. Athavale, and D. Chitre. 2014. Inhibition of LPS-induced TNF-alpha and NO production in mouse macrophage and inflammatory response in rat animal models by a novel Ayurvedic formulation, BV-9238. *Phytother Res* 28:1479–85.

Dey, S., and P. Pahwa. 2014. Prakriti and its associations with metabolism, chronic diseases, and genotypes: Possibilities of new born screening and a lifetime of personalized prevention. *J Ayurved Integr Med* 5:15–24.

Dhruva, A., F. M. Hecht, C. Miaskowski, T. J. Kaptchuk, G. Bodeker, D. Abrams, V. Lad, and S. R. Adler. 2014. Correlating traditional Ayurvedic and modern medical perspectives on cancer: Results of a qualitative study. *J Alt Complement Med* 20:364–70.

Dhuley, J. N. 1998. Therapeutic efficacy of Ashwagandha against experimental aspergillosis in mice. *Immunopharmacol Immunotoxicol* 20:191–8.

Faccin-Galhardi, L. C., K. A. Yamamoto, S. Ray, B. Ray, R. E. Carvalho Linhares, and C. Nozawa. 2012. The in vitro antiviral property of Azadirachta indica polysaccharides for poliovirus. *J Ethnopharmacol* 142:86–90.

Ferreira, V. H., A. Nazli, S. E. Dizzell, K. Mueller, and C. Kaushic. 2015. The anti-inflammatory activity of curcumin protects the genital mucosal epithelial barrier from disruption and blocks replication of HIV-1 and HSV-2. *PLOS ONE* 10:e0124903.

Frawley, D., and V. Lad. 1988. *The Yoga of Herbs*. Translated Sanskrit passages to English by David Frawley. Second ed. Twin Lakes, WI: Lotus Press. *Original edition, The Yoga of Herbs by Vasant Lad*.

Gautam, R., A. Saklani, and S. M. Jachak. 2007. Indian medicinal plants as a source of antimycobacterial agents. *J Ethnopharmacol* 110:200–34.

Govindarajan, R., M. Vijayakumar, and P. Pushpangadan. 2005. Antioxidant approach to disease management and the role of 'Rasayana' herbs of Ayurved. *J Ethnopharmacol* 99:165–78.

Gupta, G. D., N. Sujatha, A. Dhanik, and N. P. Rai. 2010. Clinical evaluation of Shilajatu Rasayana in patients with HIV infection. *Ayu* 31:28–32.

Joshi, A., N. Sengar, S. K. Prasad, R. K. Goel, A. Singh, and S. Hemalatha. 2013. Wound-healing potential of the root extract of Albizzia lebbeck. *Planta Med* 79:737–43.

Joshi, S. V. 1997. *Ayurved and Panchakrma*. Twin Lakes, WI: Lotus Press.

Keusch, G. T. 2003. The history of nutrition: Malnutrition, infection and immunity. *J Nutr* 133:336S–40S.

Khan, M., B. Schneider, S. W. Wassilew, and V. Splanemann. 1988. Experimental study of the effect of raw materials of the neem tree and neem extracts on dermatophytes, yeasts and molds. *Z Hautkr* 63:499–502.

Kiecolt-Glaser, J. K., R. Glaser, S. Gravenstein, W. B. Malarkey, and J. Sheridan. 1996. Chronic stress alters the immune response to influenza virus vaccine in older adults. *Proc Natl Acad Sci USA* 93:3043–7.

Kumar, G., A. Srivastava, S. K. Sharma, and Y. K. Gupta. 2014. Safety evaluation of mercury based Ayurvedic formulation (Sidh Makardhwaj) on brain cerebrum, liver & kidney in rats. *Ind J Med Res* 139:610–18.

Kumar, V. P., N. S. Chauhan, H. Padh, and M. Rajani. 2006. Search for antibacterial and antifungal agents from selected Indian medicinal plants. *J Ethnopharmacol* 107:182–8.

Kumari, N., A. A. Kulkarni, X. Lin, C. McLean, T. Ammosova, A. Ivanov, M. Hipolito, S. Nekhai, and E. Nwulia. 2015. Inhibition of HIV-1 by curcumin A, a novel curcumin analog. *Drug Des Devel Ther* 9:5051–60.

Lad, V. 1985. *Ayurved: The Science of Self-Healing—A Practical Guide*. Second ed. Wilmot, WI: Lotus Press.

Mishra, L., B. B. Singh, and S. Dagenais. 2001. Ayurved: A historical perspective and principles of the traditional healthcare system in India. *Altern Ther Health Med* 7:36–42.

Nair, R., T. Kalariya, and S. Chanda. 2007. Antibacterial activity of some plant extracts used in folk medicine. *J Herb Pharmacother* 7:191–201.

Narayana, A., and G. S. Lavekar. 2005. Ayurved gleaned through Buddhism. *Bull Indian Inst Hist Med Hyderabad* 35:131–46.

Narayanaswamy, V. 1981. Origin and development of Ayurved (a brief history). *Anc Sci Life* 1:1–7.

Nesari, T., B. K. Bhagwat, J. Johnson, N. S. Bhatt, and D. Chitre. 2004. Clinical validation of efficacy and safety of herbal cough formula: Study of herbal cough syrup. *J Herb Pharmacother* 4:1–12.

Newman, D. J., and G. M. Cragg. 2012. Natural products as sources of new drugs over the 30 years from 1981 to 2010. *J Nat Prod* 75:311–35.

Owais, M., K. S. Sharad, A. Shehbaz, and M. Saleemuddin. 2005. Antibacterial efficacy of Withania somnifera (ashwagandha) an indigenous medicinal plant against experimental murine salmonellosis. *Phytomedicine* 12:229–35.

Panda, A. K., and S. Misra. 2010. Health traditions of Sikkim Himalaya. *J Ayurved Integr Med* 1:183–9.

Patwardhan, B., and G. Bodeker. 2008. Ayurvedic genomics: Establishing a genetic basis for mind-body typologies. *J Altern Complement Med* 14:571–6.

Pecanac, M., Z. Janjic, A. Komarcevic, M. Pajic, D. Dobanovacki, and S. S. Miskovic. 2013. Burns treatment in ancient times. *Med Pregl* 66:263–7.

Prasad, P. V. 2002. General medicine in Atharvaveda with special reference to Yaksma (consumption/tuberculosis). *Bull Indian Inst Hist Med Hyderabad* 32:1–14.

Prasad, P. V. 2005. Medico—historical study of 'Visucika' (Cholera). *Bull Indian Inst Hist Med Hyderabad* 35:1–20.

Priyanka, J., L. Hingorani, and K. Nilima. 2013. Pharmacodynamic evaluation for antiplasmodial activity of Holarrhena antidysentrica (Kutaja) and Azadirachta indica (Neemb) in Plasmodium berghei infected mice model. *Asian Pac J Trop Med* 6:520–4.

Radhakrishnan, R., S. K. George, S. Kumar, and P. Balaram. 2014. Maintenance of immunological homeostasis by Indukantha ghritha in patients with recurrent upper respiratory tract infections-a pilot study. *Phytother Res* 28:1252–9.

Rastogi, S., A. Kalra, V. Gupta, F. Khan, R. K. Lal, A. K. Tripathi, S. Parameswaran, C. Gopalakrishnan, G. Ramaswamy, and A. K. Shasany. 2015. Unravelling the genome of Holy basil: An 'incomparable' 'elixir of life' of traditional Indian medicine. *BMC Genomics* 16:413.

Sandhya, B., S. Thomas, W. Isabel, and R. Shenbagarathai. 2006. Ethnomedicinal plants used by the Valaiyan community of Piranmalai Hills (reserved forest), Tamilnadu, India—a pilot study. *Afr J Trad CAM* 3:101–4.

Santos, A. M., T. Lopes, M. Oleastro, I. V. Gato, P. Floch, L. Benejat, P. Chaves, T. Pereira, E. Seixas, J. Machado, and A. S. Guerreiro. 2015. Curcumin inhibits gastric inflammation induced by Helicobacter pylori infection in a mouse model. *Nutrients* 7:306–20.

Scrimshaw, N. S. 2007. Prologue: Historical introduction. Immunonutrition in health and disease. *Br J Nutr* 98 Suppl 1:S3–4.

Scrimshaw, N. S., and J. P. SanGiovanni. 1997. Synergism of nutrition, infection, and immunity: An overview. *Am J Clin Nutr* 66:464S–77S.

Scrimshaw, N. S., C. E. Taylor, and J. E. Gordon. 1959. Interactions of nutrition and infection. *Am J Med Sci* 237:367–403.

Sharma, H., H. M. Chandola, G. Singh, and G. Basisht. 2007. Utilization of Ayurved in health care: An approach for prevention, health promotion, and treatment of disease. Part 1–Ayurved, the science of life. *J Altern Complement Med* 13:1011–9.

Sharma, P., and G. Singh. 2002. A review of plant species used to treat conjunctivitis. *Phytother Res* 16:1–22.

Singh, A., and B. Purohit. 2011. Tooth brushing, oil pulling and tissue regeneration: A review of holistic approaches to oral health. *J Ayurved Integr Med* 2:64–8.

Singh, N., A. Kumar, P. Gupta, K. Chand, M. Samant, R. Maurya, and A. Dube. 2008. Evaluation of anti-leishmanial potential of Tinospora sinensis against experimental visceral leishmaniasis. *Parasitol Res* 102:561–5.

Singh, N., P. K. Mishra, A. Kapil, K. R. Arya, R. Maurya, and A. Dube. 2005. Efficacy of Desmodium gangeticum extract and its fractions against experimental visceral leishmaniasis. *J Ethnopharmacol* 98:83–8.

Sivamani, R. K., B. R. Ma, L. N. Wehrli, and E. Maverakis. 2012. Phytochemicals and naturally derived substances for wound healing. *Adv Wound Care (New Rochelle)* 1:213–7.

Somarathna, K. I., H. M. Chandola, B. Ravishankar, K. N. Pandya, and A. M. Attanayake. 2010. A short-term intervention trial on HIV positive patients using a Sri Lankan classical rasayana drug—Ranahamsa Rasayanaya. *Ayu* 31:197–204.

Srinivasan, D., Sangeetha Nathan, T. Suresh, and P. Lakshmana Perumalsamy. 2001. Antimicrobial activity of certain Indian medicinal plants used in folkloric medicine. *J Ethnopharmacol* 74:217–20.

Subapriya, R., and S. Nagini. 2005. Medicinal properties of neem leaves: A review. *Curr Med Chem Anticancer Agents* 5:149–56.

Subbarayappa, B. V. 2001. The roots of ancient medicine: An historical outline. *J Biosci* 26:135–43.

Sushrut. 1995. *Sushrut Samhita*. Translated by Atridev. Edited by Bhaskar Govindji Ghanekar and Pandit Lalchandji Vaidya. Fifth ed. Delhi: Motilal Banarsidas.

Tariq, A., S. Mussarat, M. Adnan, E. F. Abd Allah, A. Hashem, A. A. Alqarawi, and R. Ullah. 2015. Ethnomedicinal evaluation of medicinal plants used against gastrointestinal complaints. *Biomed Res Int* 2015:892947.

Teixeira, S. T., M. C. Valadares, S. A. Goncalves, A. de Melo, and M. L. Queiroz. 2006. Prophylactic administration of Withania somnifera extract increases host resistance in Listeria monocytogenes infected mice. *Int Immunopharmacol* 6:1535–42.

Telles, S., K. V. Naveen, and A. Balkrishna. 2009. Use of Ayurved in promoting dental health and preventing dental caries. *Ind J Dental Res* 20:246.

Tiwari, V., N. A. Darmani, B. Y. Yue, and D. Shukla. 2010. In vitro antiviral activity of neem (Azardirachta indica L.) bark extract against herpes simplex virus type-1 infection. *Phytother Res* 24:1132–40.

28 Poor Maternal Nutritional Status or HIV Infection and Infant Outcomes: Evidence from India and Africa

Sarah Helen Kehoe and Marie-Louise Newell

CONTENTS

28.1 Introduction...453
28.2 Nutritional Status among Indian Women..453
28.3 Mother's Diet in Pregnancy and Infant Outcomes..455
    28.3.1 Dietary Intakes of Indian Women..457
    28.3.2 Maternal Nutrition and Offspring Development...457
    28.3.3 Infant Nutritional Status..458
28.4 The Influence of Maternal HIV Infection on Infant Outcomes 460
28.5 Conclusion 462
References..462

28.1 INTRODUCTION

Nutrition of the mother before and during pregnancy has an impact on the growth and development of her child and exposure to maternal infection, and treatment has been associated with pregnancy outcome and child development. Both maternal nutrition and maternal human immunodeficiency virus (HIV) infection and its treatment could affect the immune development of the fetus and young infant, and as such set the child on a suboptimal path along the life course. Maternal malnutrition at a population level is a significant public health problem in India while HIV infection is especially prevalent in sub-Saharan Africa. In this chapter we present a discussion of these two global regions as case studies to highlight the impact of maternal nutrition and infection, particularly with HIV, on infant development and health.

28.2 NUTRITIONAL STATUS AMONG INDIAN WOMEN

Data from the National Family Health Survey (NFHS) (2006) show that there is variability within India in the proportion of women who are either chronically undernourished (BMI < 18.5 kg/m^2) or overweight (BMI > 25 kg/m^2) (International Institute for Population Sciences 2007). Estimates at the State level range from 11.2% in Sikkim to 45.1% in Bihar for underweight and from 4.6% in Bihar to 29.9% in Punjab for overweight. The double burden of under- and overnutrition within States is a public health problem (Figure 28.1). BMI is an indicator of overall energy intake, but sufficient micro- as well as macronutrients are required for optimal pregnancy outcomes and fetal development. Women may be normal or overweight but still be malnourished in terms of micronutrient balance. This phenomenon has been termed "hidden hunger." The prevalence of various

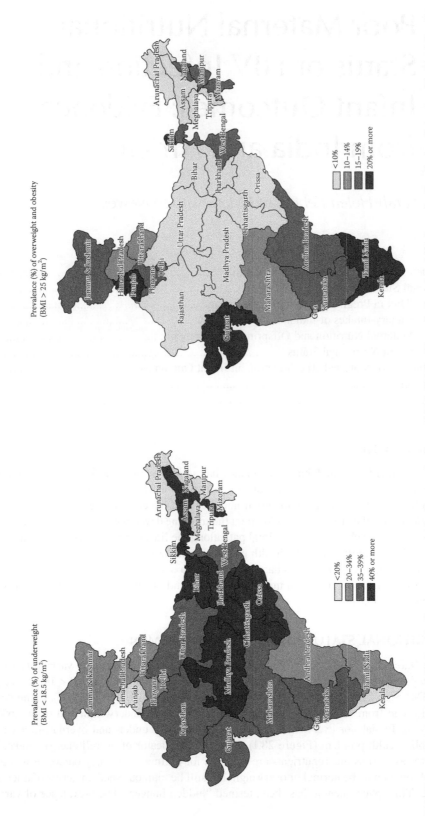

FIGURE 28.1 Mapping of BMI of Indian women aged 15–49 years by State (2005–2006). (From International Institute for Population Sciences. National Family Health Survey (NFHS-3) 2005–06 Volume 1. Mumbai, 2007.)

TABLE 28.1
Summary of Information on Vitamin A Status of Women of Reproductive Age in India

| Date of Study | Sample Size | Xerophthalmia Prevalence (%) | | | Serum or Plasma Retinol Concentration (µmol/L) Prevalence* (%) | | |
		Current Night Blindness[a]	Previous Night Blindness[b]	Bitot's Spots[c]	<0.35	<0.70	<1.05
2003	151 (P)	15.9	–	–	–	–	–
2003	300 (P)	–	–	–	–	33.7	–
2003	220 (NP)	7.0	35.0	5.0	–	–	–
2002	736 (P)	2.9	–	–	3.5	27.3	65.0
2002	1506 (NP)	–	1.46	–	–	–	–
2001–2002	129 (P)	–	–	–	–	17.1	–
2000	1130 (P)	3.21–15.86	–	–	–	–	–
2000	299 (NP)	–	18.3	–	–	–	–
1999–2000	NS (P)	5.2	–	–	–	–	–
1998–2001	5833 (P)	5.5	–	–	–	–	–
1998–2001	5786 (P)	6.1	–	–	–	–	–
1998–1999	32393 (P&NP)	–	12.1	–	–	–	–
1998–1999	300 (P)	–	–	–	–	4.0	14.7

Source: Adapted from the WHO Vitamin and Mineral Nutrition Information System database (World Health Organisation 2012).

P: pregnant; NP: nonpregnant; NS, not stated.

[a] Night blindness experienced at time of assessment.

[b] Night blindness experienced at any time prior to assessment.

[c] Keratin deposits located superficially in the conjunctiva of the eye; a sign of vitamin A deficiency.

* WHO deficiency cutoff = 0.7 µmol/L.

micronutrient deficiencies has been studied differentially. Toward the end of the twentieth-century deficiencies of iron, vitamin A and iodine were of principal concern and most closely studied. Data on specific micronutrient deficiencies (vitamin A and iron) are available in the Vitamin and Mineral Nutrition Information System (VMNIS) database collated by WHO (http://www.who.int/vmnis/database/en/). The most recent Indian data for vitamin A deficiency in young women are presented in Table 28.1. These data show that up to a third of women in India may be vitamin A deficient according to serum concentration measurements. The majority of studies, especially those with larger numbers of participants, used data on clinical signs of deficiency and based on these data it appears that the prevalence of vitamin A deficiency did not decline in India between 1998 and 2003. Vitamin A deficiency is associated with night blindness and this condition is more likely to affect women during pregnancy. Night-blind women tend to have babies of lower birthweight and with increased risk of mortality but interventions to increase retinol intake have not, to date, shown significant effects on these outcomes (Black et al. 2013).

28.3 MOTHER'S DIET IN PREGNANCY AND INFANT OUTCOMES

It is widely accepted that adequate maternal nutrition is required for optimal development of the fetus and a healthy infancy. Several intervention studies and systematic reviews largely based in low- and middle-income countries have assessed the effect of supplementing women during

pregnancy with specific or multiple nutrients on offspring nutritional status. We present a summary of these studies. Secondly, we present data suggesting that a large proportion of Indian
women of reproductive age have suboptimal nutritional status and low intakes of micronutrient-
rich foods.

Data at the national and State level cannot always discriminate between urban and rural dwelling
populations. Furthermore, it is clear that there are limitations to smaller studies in terms of gener-
alizability, and the majority of studies in which more detailed measurement of biochemical indicators of nutritional status are collected are small due to the costs required. Serum retinol concentrations
have been described as the most acceptable measure of vitamin A status (Sommer and Davidson
2002); however, there are more data available on the prevalence of xerophthalmia (a late and irreversible consequence of vitamin A deficiency). Estimates of night blindness among young Indian
women range from 1.5%–35%. Of the four studies in which serum retinol has been measured, two
found that approximately one third of women were deficient, with a concentration below the WHO
cutoff (0.7 µmol/L).

According to NFHS data (International Institute for Population Sciences 2007), the prevalence of anemia among pregnant and nonpregnant women nationwide in India was more than
50% in 2005–2006 in both urban and rural settings (Table 28.2). Of those affected, approximately 39% had mild anemia (Hb, 10–12 g/dL, 10–11 g/dL in pregnancy), 15% had moderate
anemia (Hb 7–9.9 g/dL), and 2% severe anemia (Hb <7 g/dL). Anemia is associated with
increased maternal mortality risk and with adverse birth outcomes including low birth weight
(Black et al. 2013).

In the state of Maharashtra the total prevalence of anemia was lower in nonpregnant and higher in
pregnant women when compared with the national prevalence (Arnold et al. 2009). Interestingly, the
prevalence among urban-dwelling pregnant women was greater than among rural pregnant women,
which was not the case in India as a whole. Although it is not clear as to why this would be the case,
there is a possibility that in Maharashtra there has been a more focused attempt to ensure that pregnant women receive and consume iron-folic acid tablets in rural areas than in the populous urban
slums. Women who had spent more time in education were less likely to be anemic in all settings.

When NFHS data from 2005–2006 (International Institute for Population Sciences 2007) were
compared with those from a previous national survey (1998–1999) (International Institute for Population Sciences 2000), there was a small increase in the prevalence of anemia over time among both
pregnant and nonpregnant women. There was a change to the way the respondents were selected
between the two surveys, which may go some way to explaining this. For the 1998–1999 survey
only married women were recruited to participate, while in the 2005–2006 survey married and
nonmarried women participated. It is possible that there was a greater prevalence of anemia among

TABLE 28.2

Prevalence of Anemia among Pregnant and Nonpregnant Women by Residency and Education; Country Level Compared with Maharashtra State

| | Prevalence of Anemia 2005–2006 (%) | | | | | |
| | By Setting | | By Number of Years of Education | | | |
	Urban	Rural	Uneducated	<5 y	5--9 y	≥10 y
All India						
Nonpregnant	51.5	58.2	60.2	57.9	54.6	46.6
Pregnant women	54.6	59.0	63.0	58.5	56.2	47.4
Maharashtra						
Nonpregnant	46.6	51.1	50.9	52.0	49.6	44.4
Pregnant women	60.1	56.4	61.2	–	61.8	47.9

nonmarried women. There have been calls for research aimed at assessing the micronutrient status of Indian women and the relationship between deficiencies and birth outcomes (Gopalan 2002; Singh, Reddy, and Prabhakaran 2011).

28.3.1 Dietary Intakes of Indian Women

Studies investigating the diets of women of reproductive age living in India have tended to focus on tribal women and those living in rural areas (Agrahar-Murugkar and Pal 2004; Andersen et al. 2003; Mittal and Srivastava 2006; Schmid et al. 2006). This is reflective of poverty and health indicators in rural versus urban areas with greater need perceived in rural areas. Detailed food frequency questionnaires (FFQs) were administered and nutrient composition tables were used to calculate micronutrient intakes. All these studies found that the women were chronically energy deficient and the majority had intakes associated with deficiencies in at least one micronutrient.

Quantitative dietary intake data collected from women living in urban slums indicates very low intake of fruit and vegetables in this population (Anand et al. 2007; Yadav and Krishnan 2008). Anand et al. (2007) found that the mean number of servings per day of fruit and vegetables was only 2.2 among women, with only 5.4% of women consuming the recommended five servings per day.

It is important to consider that intake of nutrient-rich foods may not always lead to improvements in nutritional status; infection (Katona and Katona-Apte 2008) or poor absorption due to antinutrients in the diet (Gibson, Perlas, and Hotz 2006; Gillooly et al. 1983) may interfere with optimal use of nutrients. An example pertinent to India is the inhibitory effect of polyphenols in tea and phytates in cereals on the absorption of nonheme iron from vegetarian foods (Thankachan et al. 2008).

During the pilot phase of the Mumbai Maternal Nutrition Project (a randomized controlled trial of a food-based intervention), a 91-item FFQ was administered to women aged 16–40 years living in a slum area (n = 1651). The data showed that a quarter of the women consumed micronutrient-rich foods including fruit and green leafy vegetables less often than three times per week. Fewer than 50% consumed at least one portion of fruit per day, and only 30% of women ate green leafy vegetables at least once per day. Apart from small quantities in tea, median consumption of milk and milk products was less frequent than twice per week. There was some seasonal variation in intakes of fruit and green leafy vegetables, with the lowest intakes occurring in June and July (the beginning of the wet season) (Chopra et al. 2012).

28.3.2 Maternal Nutrition and Offspring Development

The Institute of Nutrition of Central America and Panama (INCAP) trial was set up in rural Guatemala in 1969 to determine whether increasing protein intake in early life would improve children's mental development (Stein et al. 2008). Several other outcomes including child mortality and growth were also studied. Two pairs of villages were randomized to receive either an intervention drink (atole) or a control drink (fresco); in addition both villages received a health care intervention program. The atole contained 11.5 g of protein, 163 kcal per 180 ml cup and was rich in several micronutrients. The fresco contained no protein, 59 kcal per 180 ml cup and micronutrients were added to the drink such that the concentrations were similar to that of atole. The drinks were freely available to all villagers as per randomization and consumption was recorded for all pregnant women and children younger than 7 years of age, but it was not possible to distinguish between supplementation during pregnancy and in childhood. The village-level infant mortality rate in the atole group was 60/1000 live births compared with 91/1000 in the fresco villages and 113/1000 in villages that did not receive any intervention (Rose, Martorell, and Rivera 1992). There was no significant difference in mean birthweight of children born in the atole versus the fresco villages (Martorell 1995). However there was an effect on children's length at 3 years, with those from the atole villages growing 2.5 cm longer on average (Ruel et al. 1993). The authors point out that the effect of the protein-rich supplement may have been underestimated compared with a scenario in which the drinks would have been given in the absence of the health care intervention (Martorell 1995).

It is important to take into account seasonality when designing an intervention study. A trial in the Gambia studied the effect on birth weight of maternal intake of a protein-rich groundnut biscuit during the last 20 weeks of pregnancy. Women were recruited all year round to the trial. In the Gambia there is a dry (November–June) and a wet (July–October) season; the wet season is also known as the "hungry season," as this is when availability of staple foods is reduced. The control group received no intervention during pregnancy but were given the supplement postnatally, during lactation. The results demonstrated a mean increase in birthweight of 136 g in the intervention group, but there was considerable variability in the difference, with the supplements having the greatest effect on children born following the "hungry season" (Ceesay et al. 1997). Such differences may not be seen in settings where fluctuations in food supply are less common.

The likelihood of a child achieving their genetic potential is highly dependent on the nutritional status of their mother before and during pregnancy and evidence indicates that it may also be dependent on the nutritional status of the child's grandmother (Emanuel, Kimpo, and Moceri 2004). There is a common cycle in India and other low and middle income countries whereby a woman who is born small gives birth to a small baby who is then more likely to be stunted as a child and adult, and herself give birth to a small baby (Scott, Campbell, and Davies 2007). Therefore, young women and those of reproductive age are a group that merit particular attention when designing interventions to reduce the prevalence of undernutrition.

Low birth weight (LBW) is defined as a birth weight of less than 2.5 kg. A meta-analysis of birthweight and neonatal mortality data from India, Pakistan, Nepal, and Brazil published in 2008 calculated that babies born at term and with a birthweight of 1.5 kg–1.99 kg and 2 kg–2.49 kg were respectively eight and three times more likely to die in the neonatal period than those weighing ≥ 2.5 kg (Black et al. 2008). In addition to this there is evidence from a systematic review of studies in India that LBW is associated with a greater risk of neonatal and infant death (Lahariya et al. 2010). Those infants that survive are more likely to be stunted as children and adults and give birth to LBW babies themselves (Scott, Campbell, and Davies 2007). In addition to physical size, birthweight in low and middle income countries was positively associated with formation of human capital highlighting the "vicious cycle" of intergenerational effects of LBW (Victora et al. 2008).

28.3.3 INFANT NUTRITIONAL STATUS

A review by Kramer (Kramer 1987) in the late 1980s focused on randomized controlled trials that assessed the effect of supplementing women's diets during pregnancy on infant birthweight. The review concluded that there was little evidence to suggest that maternal intake of any one particular nutrient had an effect on development of the fetus in terms of birthweight or duration of gestation. Similarly, a more recent small case control study in China found that preconceptional vitamin B status was not associated with LBW or small-for-gestational age (SGA) status (Ronnenberg et al. 2002). It is perhaps unsurprising that this reductionist approach, focusing on single nutrients, has yielded few positive results. It is more conceivable that the intake of a range of vitamins, minerals, and other compounds in foods, and the interactions among them, are required for optimal fetal development (Gluckman and Hanson 2005). An observational study in Nepal found that among pregnant Bhutanese refugees who received food rations, birthweight increased by 116 g and LBW fell from 16% to 8% between 1996 and 1998. The authors concluded that the improvement was due to enhanced diet quality (Shrimpton et al. 2009).

The majority of intervention trials that have investigated the association between micronutrient intake during pregnancy and offspring birthweight have supplemented women's diets with single or multiple micronutrient tablets. A meta-analysis of 12 randomized controlled trials from 10 low income countries was conducted in 2009 (Margetts et al. 2009). Nine of the studies used the United Nations Multiple Micronutrient Preparation (UNIMMAP), which contains one dose of the Recommended Daily Allowance (RDA) of 15 micronutrients (iron, zinc, copper, selenium, iodine, vitamin

A, vitamin B1, vitamin B2, folic acid, niacin, vitamin B6, vitamin B12, vitamin C, vitamin D, and vitamin E); the remaining three studies used a supplement with a similar composition and all contained at least 13 micronutrients. In most studies the control group took iron (60 mg) and folic acid (400 μg) supplements as these were given to women routinely during pregnancy. Women typically started taking the supplements in the first trimester, but in two of the trials, supplementation started in the second or third trimesters. The outcomes investigated included birthweight, proportion of children born SGA, gestational duration, and incidence of preterm deliveries. After adjustment for infant sex, maternal age, weight, parity, and education, there was a small difference in the mean birthweight between control and intervention groups of 22.4 g; the range was 4.9–75 g. There was also a reduction in the prevalence of LBW of about 10% (pooled OR = 0.89 [95% CI, 0.81 to 0.97]; $p = .01$). There was an interaction effect with group allocation of maternal BMI in three of the studies and in the pooled analysis, birthweight was 39 g higher in infants born to mothers with a BMI > 20 kg/m², compared with a negative effect in women with BMI < 20 kg/m², for whom mean birthweight was 6 g lower than the control group. No effects on birth length were observed, nor on duration of gestation or preterm delivery.

As pointed out in the review, an important question is whether the increase in birthweight translates to any developmental benefits for the children (Fall et al. 2009). A follow–up study of one of the Nepali trials in this meta-analysis found that children of mothers who were supplemented with the UNIMMAP were approximately 200 g heavier at 2.5 years than those born to control mothers. Head, mid-upper arm, chest, and hip circumferences, as well as triceps skinfolds, were larger in the intervention children. The differences were modest but statistically significant. There was no difference in mean height, waist circumference, or waist-hip ratio. An explanation put forward by the authors for the modest effect of the intervention was that the iron content of the control supplements was 30 mg higher than that of the UNIMMAP. If the control supplements had contained the same amount of iron as the UNIMMAP, a greater effect may have been observed. They also questioned whether the difference in body weight between the two groups was as a result of increased fetal supply of micronutrients leading to increased lean body mass, or due to greater adiposity as was suggested by the larger triceps skinfold measurements (Vaidya et al. 2008). In the Pune Maternal Nutrition Study (an observational study conducted in a rural area outside the city of Pune), low maternal vitamin B_{12} status as indicated by plasma homocysteine concentrations was associated with LBW after controlling for offspring gender, maternal height, weight, and gestational age (Yajnik et al. 2005). In a randomised trial in Mumbai (Potdar et al. 2014), nonpregnant women (n=6513) were recruited and given a daily micronutrient-rich snack containing green leafy vegetables, fruit, and milk before and during pregnancy. The control group received a snack containing foods of low micronutrient content such as tapioca and potato. Of those recruited, 1962 delivered live singletons and 1360 neonates were measured within 72 hours of birth.

Overall there was no effect on birthweight but per-protocol and subgroup analyses showed a 79-113g difference between groups if the mother was supplemented at least 3 months before conception and was not underweight.

Maternal nutritional status is likely to affect risk of both maternal and infant infection. Women with inadequate macro- or micronutrient intakes are likely to have depressed immune systems and therefore be more susceptible to infection as well as less able to achieve a rapid immune response. Pregnancy is likely to compromise the situation further. The effect of poor maternal nutritional status on infection risk among infants may act via several pathways. Women with poor nutritional status are likely to achieve suboptimal weight gain in pregnancy leading to risk of low birth weight. Babies of lower birth weight have a higher risk of infection. In addition it is likely that maternal nutritional adequacy is necessary for the development of fetal organs and systems required for optimal immune function. Lastly, maternal undernutrition during lactation will affect the quality of breast milk, which may lead to poor micronutrient status of the breastfed infant, impairing immune maturation, and increasing risk of infection.

28.4   THE INFLUENCE OF MATERNAL HIV INFECTION ON INFANT OUTCOMES

HIV infection in the pregnant woman affects pregnancy outcome: in the absence of any interventions, the risk of adverse pregnancy outcomes including stillbirth, miscarriage (Rollins et al. 2007), and SGA infants is increased in HIV-infected women compared with age-matched uninfected women. In a cohort study in which HIV-infected and uninfected pregnant women were enrolled between 2001 and 2004 (before ART availability) in rural South Africa, the prevalence of preterm deliveries was 21.4% while that of SGA was 16.6%, with limited overlap between the two, and maternal HIV infection was associated with a 1.2-fold increased risk of SGA birth (Ndirangu et al. 2012). This significant association was maintained after controlling for water source, delivery place, parity, and maternal height, factors associated with SGA in other studies. However, maternal HIV infection was not significantly associated with preterm delivery before or after adjusting for other confounders. SGA infants were at significantly increased risk of infant mortality compared with those appropriate-for-gestational age (AGA), for both HIV-exposed and unexposed infants, but there was no difference in mortality between the term and preterm births. The risk increased with severity of growth restriction, such that severely growth-restricted infants had a threefold significantly increased risk of death before and after adjusting for other confounders. A plausible mechanism for this may be the increased postnatal morbidity rates. It has been reported that SGA infants are at higher risk of micronutrient deficiency including zinc, which will adversely affect their growth and increase their susceptibility to infections (Duggan 2014; Krebs, Miller, and Hambidge 2014).

In an African cohort of children of HIV-infected women compared to the reference population of infants born to HIV-uninfected women from the same setting, growth of HIV-exposed but uninfected children was as good as that of the reference population. The authors postulated that exclusive breastfeeding for 6 months, which was supported by lay-health workers during home visits, may compensate for vulnerabilities experienced by HIV-exposed, uninfected children (Patel et al. 2010).

Mother-to-child transmission of HIV is the dominant route of acquisition for the child. This can occur during pregnancy, delivery, or breastfeeding, and in settings where breastfeeding is common and prolonged, mother-to-child transmission rates at 18 months can be as high as 35% or more. In recognition of the substantial risk of transmission through breastfeeding, until 2010 WHO recommendations included advice to refrain from breastfeeding where this was safe and affordable and acceptable, or to limit the duration of breastfeeding to 6 months of exclusive breastfeeding. This measure reduced, but did not eliminate the risk (Coovadia et al. 2007). The 2010, 2012, and 2013 WHO recommendations relating to the prevention of mother-to-child transmission recommend the use of antiretroviral drugs from early pregnancy throughout the breastfeeding period; following these changes in guidelines based on new evidence from several large randomized trials, in most settings HIV-infected women are now encouraged to breastfeed, but under the cover of antiretroviral therapy.

HIV-exposed, uninfected children have been reported to be at increased risk of infectious disease morbidity and possibly reduced growth, although methodological issues hinder precise quantification and understanding of this risk. Most of the available evidence predates the widespread availability of antiretroviral treatment to prevent mother-to-child transmission and delay HIV disease progression in the mother, and would have been conducted with limited breastfeeding duration (Fischer Walker et al. 2012, Koyanagi et al. 2011, Muhangi et al. 2013, Rudan et al. 2008).

In a Ugandan study comparing 1380 HIV-unexposed children and 122 HIV-exposed but uninfected children (Muhangi et al. 2013), early weaning was associated with stunting and underweight, while maternal HIV was associated with underweight but not stunting or wasting. In a prevention of mother-to-child transmission (PMTCT) trial in Malawi, morbidity rates in HIV-exposed but uninfected children (overall, pneumonia, diarrhea, by age in the first 48 weeks of life) were lower during breastfeeding (Kourtis et al. 2013). In a study in Tanzania, acute respiratory infection in HIV-exposed but uninfected children was associated with underweight, wasting but not stunting, birthweight, and maternal HIV staging (Mwiru et al. 2013); breastfeeding was protective in the first year of life, halving the incidence of acute respiratory infections. In a study from India, shorter duration of breastfeeding and abrupt weaning were associated with diarrhea; stunting by 6 months of life was found to be more common in HIV-exposed but uninfected infants than in the general population (Singh et al. 2011). In Abidjan, Ivory Coast, both diarrhea and acute respiratory infections were significantly less common in breastfed infant than in formula-fed infants, but malnutrition was equally common in both groups (Becquet et al. 2007). It should be noted that none of these studies examined the impact of maternal nutritional status on the outcomes assessed.

Optimal feeding practices with support for exclusive breastfeeding for 6 months minimized the effect of being born to an HIV-infected mother in rural KwaZulu-Natal, South Africa, with reduced diarrhea episodes in exclusively breastfed infants (Rollins et al. 2013). In Botswana, discontinuation of breastfeeding was the strongest predictor of illness in the infant (Shapiro et al. 2007); this was also the case in the SWEN study in India where shorter duration of breastfeeding and abrupt weaning were associated with serious diarrhea morbidity (Singh et al. 2011).

Overall, these studies provide evidence of reduced diarrhea episodes, fewer acute respiratory infections and incidents of malaria, and improved growth associated with breastfeeding. This was further confirmed in a recent systematic review (Zunza et al. 2013) which summarized the evidence that breastfeeding is protective against diarrhea in early life, and that the effect on diarrhea and respiratory infections carries through to 2 years of age. The evidence regarding protection against malnutrition is less strong, but still suggestive. There was no evidence of statistically significant differences in the rates of non-HIV infections or malnutrition between breastfed infants by duration of ART prophylaxis for the prevention of mother-to-child transmission of HIV.

Cames et al. showed that in 68 nonbreastfed HIV-exposed but uninfected infants between the ages of 6 and 11 months, energy uptake was low despite free access to infant food aid; these findings support the WHO guidelines recommending prolonged breastfeeding under the cover of ART (Cames et al. 2011). Goga et al. present results from a prospective study on infant feeding practices at routine PMTCT sites in South Africa covering ages from birth to 9 months (Goga et al. 2012). Although feeding practices were poor among both infected and uninfected mothers, HIV-positive mothers were more likely to practice safer infant feeding than uninfected mothers.

Concerns have been expressed about whether breastfeeding would affect HIV disease progression in the mother, especially when she is not currently on ART; HIV-infected women, particularly exclusive breastfeeders, could be expected to have lower postpartum weight gain than uninfected women. The effect of chronic HIV stress may trigger lactation energy sparing, including basal metabolic rate changes, caloric intake, physical activity, or tissue store mobilization. However, in a study of breastfeeding ART-naive women, HIV-infected women initially had less weight loss in the first year postpartum than HIV-uninfected women, but both groups experienced similar marginal weight loss by 24 months; further, weight change by 24 months was not associated with breastfeeding modality in the first 5 months after adjusting for sociodemographic, pregnancy, and infant-related factors. In contrast, in Kenya, HIV-infected breastfeeding women experienced more weight loss than formula-feeders from the earliest postnatal visit through 5 to 9 months (Nduati et al. 2001). In Zambia, more women gained than lost weight between 4 and 24 months postpartum, but longer duration breastfeeding was associated with less weight gain (Murnane et al. 2010).

The Kesho Bora trial, carried out in South Africa, Kenya, and Burkina Faso, to evaluate the use of ART during breastfeeding to prevent postnatal transmission of HIV infection, reported morbidity in the infant overall differed only slightly by breastfeeding status in the first 6 months of life, but nonbreastfeeding at any point in early life was associated with significantly increased risk of serious infectious morbidity in HIV-exposed, uninfected infants (Bork et al. 2014). In an earlier paper from the same study, nonbreastfeeding children had a sevenfold increased mortality risk in the first 18 months of life compared with breastfeeding children, with the difference mostly related to lack of breastfeeding in the first 6 months of life (Cournil et al. 2013).

With the current WHO guidelines recommending ART for the prevention of mother-to-child transmission of HIV for all HIV-infected pregnant women irrespective of their HIV disease progression, an increasing number of HIV infected women will now breastfeed. However, there is little data on the nutritional status of her infant under the cover of ART, which then highlights the issue that in public health terms one needs to look at the whole rather than the components only, and leads to a discussion on whether HIV-infected women, like other women, need nutritional supplements during pregnancy to optimize infant health.

28.5 CONCLUSION

It is clear that the relationships between maternal nutritional status, infection exposure in fetal life, pregnancy outcome, infant nutrition, and development are highly complex. Interventions to improve health outcomes that do not take this complex system into account are unlikely to be successful in the long term. It is probable that interventions across the whole lifecourse are required. The challenge for the public health community is to develop such holistic lifecourse interventions that are acceptable to the target communities and populations. The involvement of the target populations in developing such interventions is likely to be very valuable and should be sought.

REFERENCES

Agrahar-Murugkar, D., and P. P. Pal. 2004. Intake of nutrients and food sources of nutrients among the Khasi tribal women of India. *Nutrition* 20:268–273.

Anand, K., B. Shah, K. Yadav, R. Singh, P. Mathur, E. Paul, and S. K. Kapoor. 2007. Are the urban poor vulnerable to non-communicable diseases? A survey of risk factors for non-communicable diseases in urban slums of Faridabad. *Natl. Med. J. India* 20:115–120.

Andersen, L. T., S. H. Thilsted, B. B. Nielsen, and S. Rangasamy. 2003. Food and nutrient intakes among pregnant women in rural Tamil Nadu, South India. *Public Health Nutr.* 6:131–137.

Asbjornsdottir, K. H., J. A. Slyker, N. S. Weiss, D. Mbori-Ngacha, E. Maleche-Obimbo, D. Wamalwa, and G. John-Stewart. 2013. Breastfeeding is associated with decreased pneumonia incidence among HIV-exposed, uninfected Kenyan infants. *AIDS* 27:2809–15.

Becquet, R., L. Bequet, D. K. Ekouevi, I. Viho, C. Sakarovitch, P. Fassinou, G. Bedikou, M. Timite-Konan, F. Dabis, and V. Leroy. 2007. Two-year morbidity-mortality and alternatives to prolonged breast-feeding among children born to HIV-infected mothers in Cote d'Ivoire. *PLoS Med.* 4:e17.

Black, R. E., L. H. Allen, Z. A. Bhutta, L. E. Caulfield, M. de Onis, M. Ezzati, C. Mathers, and J. Rivera. 2008. Maternal and child undernutrition: Global and regional exposures and health consequences. *Lancet* 371:243–260.

Black, R. E., C. G. Cesar, S. P. Walker. Z. A. Bhutta, P. Christian, M. de Onis, M. Ezzati, S. Grantham-McGregor, J. Katz, R. Martorel, R. Uauy, and the Maternal and Child Nutrition Study Group. 2013. Maternal and child undernutrition and overweight in low-income and middle-income countries. *Lancet* 382:427–51

Bork, K. A., A. Cournil, J. S. Read, M. L. Newell, C. Cames, N. Meda, S. Luchters, G. Mbatia, K. Naidu, P. Gaillard, and I. de Vincenzi. 2014. Morbidity in relation to feeding mode in African HIV-exposed, uninfected infants during the first 6 mo of life: The Kesho Bora study. *Am J Clin Nutr.* 100:1559–68.

Cames, C., F. Cassard, A. Cournil, C. Mouquet-Rivier, K. Ayassou, N. Meda, and K. Bork. 2011. Nonbreast-fed HIV-1-exposed Burkinabe infants have low energy intake between 6 and 11 months of age despite free access to infant food aid. *J. Nutr.* 141:674–9.

Ceesay, S. M., A. M. Prentice, T. J. Cole, F. Foord, L. T. Weaver, E. M. Poskitt, and R. G. Whitehead. 1997. Effects on birth weight and perinatal mortality of maternal dietary supplements in rural Gambia: 5 year randomised controlled trial. *BMJ* 315:786–790.

Chopra, H., P. Chheda, S. Kehoe, V. Taskar, N. Brown, D. Shivashankaran, G. Subbulakshmi, S. Rao, M. Gandhi, P. Muley-Lotankar, R. Potdar, B. Margetts, and C. Fall. 2012. Dietary habits of female urban slum-dwellers in Mumbai. *Indian J. Matern. Child Health* 14:1–13.

Coovadia, H. M., N. C. Rollins, R. M. Bland, K. Little, A. Coutsoudis, M. L. Bennish, and M. L. Newell. 2007. Mother-to-child transmission of HIV-1 infection during exclusive breastfeeding in the first 6 months of life: An intervention cohort study. *Lancet* 369:1107–16.

Cournil, A., I. De Vincenzi, P. Gaillard, C. Cames, P. Fao, S. Luchters, N. Rollins, M. L. Newell, K. Bork, and J. S. Read. 2013. Relationship between mortality and feeding modality among children born to HIV-infected mothers in a research setting: The Kesho Bora study. *AIDS* 27:1621–30.

Duggan, M. B. 2014. Prevention of childhood malnutrition: Immensity of the challenge and variety of strategies. *Paediatr. Int. Child Health.* 34:271–8.

Emanuel, I., C. Kimpo, and V. Moceri. 2004. The association of grandmaternal and maternal factors with maternal adult stature. *Int. J. Epidemiol.* 33:1243–8.

Fall, C. H., D. J. Fisher, C. Osmond, and B. M. Margetts. 2009. Multiple micronutrient supplementation during pregnancy in low-income countries: A meta-analysis of effects on birth size and length of gestation. *Food Nutr. Bull.* 30 (4 Suppl):S533–S546.

Fischer Walker, C. L., J. Perin, M. J. Aryee, C. Boschi-Pinto, and R. E. Black. 2012. Diarrhea incidence in low- and middle-income countries in 1990 and 2010: A systematic review. *BMC Public Health* 12:220.

Gibson, R. S., L. Perlas, and C. Hotz. 2006. Improving the bioavailability of nutrients in plant foods at the household level. *Proc. Nutr. Soc.* 65:160–168.

Gillooly, M., T. H. Bothwell, J. D. Torrance, A. P. MacPhail, D. P. Derman, W. R. Bezwoda, W. Mills, R. W. Charlton, and F. Mayet. 1983. The effects of organic acids, phytates and polyphenols on the absorption of iron from vegetables. *Br. J. Nutr.* 49:331–342.

Gluckman, P. D., and M. A. Hanson. 2005. *The Fetal Matrix: Evolution, Development and Disease.* Cambridge: Cambridge University Press.

Goga, A. E., T. Doherty, D. J. Jackson, D. Sanders, M. Colvin, M. Chopra, and L. Kuhn. 2012. Infant feeding practices at routine PMTCT sites, South Africa: Results of a prospective observational study amongst HIV exposed and unexposed infants - birth to 9 months. *Int. Breastfeed J* 7:4.

Gopalan, C. 2002. Multiple micronutrient supplementation in pregnancy. *Nutr. Rev.* 60:S2–S6.

International Institute for Population Sciences. 2000. *National Family Health Survey (NFHS-2) 1998–99.* Mumbai/Washington DC.

International Institute for Population Sciences. 2007. *National Family Health Survey (NFHS-3) 2005–06* Volume 1. Mumbai.

Katona, P., and J. Katona-Apte. 2008. The interaction between nutrition and infection. *Clin. Infect. Dis.* 46:1582–1588.

Kourtis, A. P., J. Wiener, D. Kayira, C. Chasela, S. R. Ellington, L. Hyde, M. Hosseinipour, C.van der Horst, and D. J. Jamieson. 2013. Health outcomes of HIV-exposed uninfected African infants. *AIDS* 27:749–59.

Koyanagi, A., J. H. Humphrey, R. Ntozini, K. Nathoo, L. H. Moulton, P. Iliff, K. Mutasa, A. Ruff, and B. Ward. 2011. Morbidity among human immunodeficiency virus-exposed but uninfected, human immunodeficiency virus-infected, and human immunodeficiency virus-unexposed infants in Zimbabwe before availability of highly active antiretroviral therapy. *Pediatr. Infect. Dis. J.* 30:45–51.

Kramer, M. S. 1987. Determinants of low birth weight: Methodological assessment and meta-analysis. *Bull. World Health Organ.* 65:663–737.

Krebs, N. F., L. V. Miller, and K. M. Hambidge. 2014. Zinc deficiency in infants and children: A review of its complex and synergistic interactions. *Paediatr. Int. Child Health* 34:279–88.

Lahariya, C., C. R. Sudfeld, D. Lahariya, and S. S. Tomar. 2010. Causes of child deaths in India, 1985-2008: A systematic review of literature. *Indian J. Pediatr.* 77:1303–11

Margetts, B. M., C. H. Fall, C. Ronsmans, L. H. Allen, and D. J. Fisher. 2009. Multiple micronutrient supplementation during pregnancy in low-income countries: Review of methods and characteristics of studies included in the meta-analyses. *Food Nutr. Bull.* 30 (4 Suppl):S517–S526.

Martorell, R. 1995. Results and implications of the INCAP follow-up study. *J. Nutr.* 125 (4 Suppl):1127S–1138S.

Mittal, P. C., and S Srivastava. 2006. Diet, nutritional status and food related traditions of Oraon tribes of New Mal (West Bengal), India. *Rural and Remote Health* 6:385.

Muhangi, L., S. A. Lule, H. Mpairwe, J. Ndibazza, M. Kizza, M. Nampijja, E. Nakazibwe, M. Kihembo, A. M. Elliott, and E. L. Webb. 2013. Maternal HIV infection and other factors associated with growth outcomes of HIV-uninfected infants in Entebbe, Uganda. *Public Health Nutr.* 16:1548–57.

Murnane, P. M., S. M. Arpadi, M. Sinkala, C. Kankasa, M. Mwiya, P. Kasonde, D. M. Thea, G. M. Aldrovandi, and L. Kuhn. 2010. Lactation-associated postpartum weight changes among HIV-infected women in Zambia. *Int. J. Epidemiol.* 39:1299–310.

Mwiru, R., D. Spiegelman, E. Hertzmark, C. Duggan, G. Msamanga, S. Aboud, and W. Fawzi. 2013. Nutritional predictors of acute respiratory infections among children born to HIV-infected women in Tanzania. *J. Trop. Pediatr.* 59:203–8.

Ndirangu, J., M. L. Newell, R. M. Bland, and C. Thorne. 2012. Maternal HIV infection associated with small-for-gestational age infants but not preterm births: Evidence from rural South Africa. *Hum. Reprod.* 27:1846–56.

Nduati, R., B. A. Richardson, G. John, D. Mbori-Ngacha, A. Mwatha, J. Ndinya-Achola, J. Bwayo, F. E. Onyango, and J. Kreiss. 2001. Effect of breastfeeding on mortality among HIV-1 infected women: A randomised trial. *Lancet* 357:1651–5.

Patel, D., R. Bland, H. Coovadia, N. Rollins, A. Coutsoudis, and M. L. Newell. 2010. Breastfeeding, HIV status and weights in South African children: A comparison of HIV-exposed and unexposed children. *AIDS* 24:437–45.

Potdar R. D., S. A. Sahariah, M. Gandhi, S. H. Kehoe, N. Brown, H. Sane, M. Dayama, S. Jha, A. Lawande, P. J. Coakley, E. Marley-Zagar, H. Chopra, D. Shivshankaran , P. Chheda-Gala, P. Muley-Lotankar, G. Subbulakshmi, A. K. Wills, V. A. Cox, V. Taskar, D. J. Barker, A. A. Jackson, B. M. Margetts, and C. H. Fall. 2014. Improving women's diet quality preconceptionally and during gestation: Effects on birth weight and prevalence of low birth weight—a randomized controlled efficacy trial in India (Mumbai Maternal Nutrition Project). *Am J Clin Nutr.* 100(5):1257–68.

Rollins, N. C., H. M. Coovadia, R. M. Bland, A. Coutsoudis, M. L. Bennish, D. Patel, and M. L. Newell. 2007. Pregnancy outcomes in HIV-infected and uninfected women in rural and urban South Africa. *J. Acquir. Immune Defic. Syndr.* 44:321–8.

Rollins, N. C., J. Ndirangu, R. M. Bland, A. Coutsoudis, H. M. Coovadia, and M. L. Newell. 2013. Exclusive breastfeeding, diarrhoeal morbidity and all-cause mortality in infants of HIV-infected and HIV unin-fected mothers: An intervention cohort study in KwaZulu Natal, South Africa. *PLOS ONE* 8:e81307.

Ronnenberg, A. G., M. B. Goldman, D. Chen, I. W. Aitken, W. C. Willett, J. Selhub, and X. Xu. 2002. Preconception homocysteine and B vitamin status and birth outcomes in Chinese women. *Am. J. Clin. Nutr.* 76:1385–1391.

Rose, D., R. Martorell, and J. Rivera. 1992. Infant mortality rates before, during, and after a nutrition and health intervention in rural Guatemalan villages. *Food Nutr. Bull.* 14:215–220.

Rudan, I., C. Boschi-Pinto, Z. Biloglav, K. Mulholland, and H. Campbell. 2008. Epidemiology and etiology of childhood pneumonia. *Bull. World Health Organ.* 86:408–16.

Ruel, M. T., J. Rivera, H. Castro, J. P. Habicht, and R. Martorell. 1993. Secular trends in adult and child anthro-pometry in four Guatemalan villages. *Food Nutr. Bull.* 14:246–253.

Schmid, M. A., G. M. Egeland, B. Salomeyesudas, P. V. Satheesh, and H. V. Kuhnlein. 2006. Traditional food consumption and nutritional status of Dalit mothers in rural Andhra Pradesh, South India. *Eur. J. Clin. Nutr.* 60:1277–1283.

Scott, J., D. Campbell, and M. Davies. 2007. Mothers and Infants. In *Public Health Nutrition: From Principles to Practice*, edited by M. Lawrence and T. Worsley, 74–99. Allen and Unwin.

Shapiro, R. L., S. Lockman, S. Kim, L. Smeaton, J. T. Rahkola, I. Thior, C. Wester, C. Moffat, P. Arimi, P. Ndase, A. Asmelash, L. Stevens, M. Montano, J. Makhema, M. Essex, and E. N. Janoff. 2007. Infant morbidity, mortality, and breast milk immunologic profiles among breast-feeding HIV-infected and HIV-uninfected women in Botswana. *J. Infect. Dis.* 196:562–9.

Shrimpton, R., A. Thorne-Lyman, K. Tripp, and A. Tomkins. 2009. Trends in low birthweight among the Bhu-tanese refugee population in Nepal. *Food Nutr. Bull.* 30 (2 Suppl):S197–S206.

Singh, H. K., N. Gupte, A. Kinikar, R. Bharadwaj, J. Sastry, N. Suryavanshi, U. Nayak, S. Tripathy, R. Paranjape, A. Jamkar, R. C. Bollinger, and A. Gupta. 2011. High rates of all-cause and gastroenteritis-related hospi-talization morbidity and mortality among HIV-exposed Indian infants. *BMC Infect. Dis.* 11:193.

Singh, K., K. S. Reddy, and D. Prabhakaran. 2011. What are the evidence based public health interventions for prevention and control of NCDs in relation to india? *Indian J. Community Med.* 36 (Suppl 1):S23–S31.

Sommer, A., and F. R. Davidson. 2002. Assessment and control of vitamin A deficiency: The Annecy accords. *J. Nutr.* 132 (9 Suppl):2845S–2850S.

Stein, A. D., P. Melgar, J. Hoddinott, and R. Martorell. 2008. Cohort profile: The Institute of Nutrition of Cen-tral America and Panama (INCAP) Nutrition Trial Cohort Study. *Int. J. Epidemiol.* 37:716–720.

Thankachan, P., T. Walczyk, S. Muthayya, A. V. Kurpad, and R.F. Hurrell. 2008. Iron absorption in young Indian women: The interaction of iron status with the influence of tea and ascorbic acid. *Am. J. Clin. Nutr.* 87:881–886.

Vaidya, A., N. Saville, B. P. Shrestha, A. M. Costello, D. S. Manandhar, and D. Osrin. 2008. Effects of antena-tal multiple micronutrient supplementation on children's weight and size at 2 years of age in Nepal: Follow-up of a double-blind randomised controlled trial. *Lancet* 371:492–499.

Victora, C. G., L. Adair, C. Fall, P. C. Hallal, R. Martorell, L. Richter, and H. S. Sachdev. 2008. Maternal and child undernutrition: Consequences for adult health and human capital. *Lancet* 371:340–357.

World Health Organisation. 2012. Vitamin and Mineral Nutrition Information System. Last Modified 2012 Accessed 11/15/2012. http://www.who.int/vmnis/en/.

Yadav, K., and A. Krishnan. 2008. Changing patterns of diet, physical activity and obesity among urban, rural and slum populations in North India. *Obes. Rev.* 9:400–408.

Yajnik, C. S., S. S. Deshpande, A. V. Panchanadikar, S. S. Naik, J. A. Deshpande, K. J. Coyaji, C. Fall, and H. Refsum. 2005. Maternal total homocysteine concentration and neonatal size in India. *Asia Pac. J. Clin. Nutr.* 14:179–181.

Zunza, M., G. D. Mercer, L. Thabane, M. Esser, and M. F. Cotton. 2013. Effects of postnatal interventions for the reduction of vertical HIV transmission on infant growth and non-HIV infections: A systematic review. *J. Int. AIDS Soc.* 16:18865.

29 Postpregnancy Ethnic Nutritional Practices in India: A Critical Perspective of Immunity and Infection

P. R. Janci Rani, N. Tharani Devi, and Murali Rangarajan

CONTENTS

29.1 Introduction..465
29.2 Nutrition, Immunity, and Infection after Pregnancy: An Indian Perspective....................468
    29.2.1 Overview...468
    29.2.2 Postpartum Morbidity: An Indian Assessment 468
    29.2.3 Effects of Nutritional History on Postpartum Maternal Health Status.................469
    29.2.4 Nutritional Requirements during Lactation 470
29.3 Postpartum Ethnic Nutritional Practices in India...471
    29.3.1 Traditional Foods and Nutritional Practices in Indian Postpartum Care:
            Beliefs and Health Benefits...472
    29.3.2 Functional Foods in Traditional Indian Postpartum Care.....................................488
29.4 Traditional Food Formulations and Postpartum Menus...491
29.5 An Evaluation of Ethnic Indian Postpartum Nutritional Practices 499
    29.5.1 An Evaluation of Traditional Postpartum Menus Based on RDA 500
    29.5.2 Macro- and Micronutrients in Traditional Indian Postpartum Formulations........502
    29.5.3 Traditional Indian Postpartum Formulations for Immunity
            and Prevention of Infection..502
29.6 Future of Traditional Postpartum Nutritional Practices 505
Acknowledgments..507
References..507

29.1 INTRODUCTION

In modern society, health, medicine, and nutrition are domains where traditional knowledge and beliefs, based on thousands of years of observation and experience, are still preserved and practiced. Ancient India, for instance, was home to about 15%–20% of the world's population due to its abundant natural resources, as well as the traditional bodies of knowledge reflected in its culture. Indian culture has had diverse and rich traditional postpartum nutritional practices that have been beneficial for mothers and children. However, the past two centuries have witnesed significant losses of this traditional wisdom, which has often resulted in people holding on to beliefs without a clear understanding of their origins or relevance. Recent years have seen increased awareness of traditional systems of healthcare (see also Chapter 27). It has been recognized as far back as 1978 by the World Health Organization (WHO, 1978) that traditional medicine can play a significant role in the extension of health services, particularly in remote rural areas, and in the domain of maternal and child health. The World Health Organization has further identified three strategic objectives toward harnessing traditional healthcare systems for health maintenance, disease prevention, and treatment (WHO, 2013):

- Build a knowledge base for effective management of traditional healthcare systems
- Strengthen the quality assurance, safety, proper use, and effectiveness of traditional healthcare systems
- Integrate traditional healthcare systems into healthcare service delivery and self-healthcare

While Ayurveda and Siddha are traditional healthcare systems of Indian origin, these objectives are particularly relevant for traditional postpartum nutritional practices as well.

The postpartum period is noted for traditional practices related to rest, healing, and the consumption of specific nutritive foods, supplements, and drinks. Elders of a family guide the new mother throughout this period to restore her health after childbirth. The circle of people most closely involved with her to enhance her physical and mental health include mothers, grandmothers, sisters, partner, friends, and neighbors. They form her core support system. In the Indian context, this support system is supplemented by the healthcare system in the country, viz., *dais* (*dai*: midwife), community workers, primary healthcare centers, nongovernmental organizations, and government and private hospitals. The Indian healthcare system is based on national programs and policies for healthcare. Relevant Indian programs for maternal and child health include Reproductive and Child Health Programme (RCH), Child Survival and Safe Motherhood Programme (CSSM), Janani Suraksha Yojana (JSY), Vandemateram Scheme (VMS), and many more. These programs are further guided by global health programs and policies, such as those promoted through WHO, UNICEF, and FAO. Thus, while health parameters and nutritional needs are prescribed from a global perspective based on contemporary knowledge of medicine, nutrition, and healthcare, their implementation is significantly influenced and guided by traditional practices at the community level. The different levels of support system, policymaking, and implementation of nutrition and healthcare for a new mother are depicted in Figure 29.1.

There is increasing recognition of the value of traditional postpartum nutritional practices and the strong influence they wield in the delivery of postpartum nutrition and healthcare in India. In this light, it is necessary to develop a contemporary analysis of these practices based on current paradigms of nutrition, immunity, and infection. This chapter is an attempt to provide a review and an evaluation of ethnic postpartum nutritional practices of India from this perspective. It presents a broad overview of selected traditional Indian postpartum foods, their food functions, the special food formulations/supplements through which these foods are consumed, and the nutritive content in them. The scientific literature in this area is vast; on the one hand are surveys of traditional Indian postpartum beliefs and practices concerning nutrition, while on the other hand are analyses of the traditional foods for various active ingredients, and their functions through *in vitro*, *in vivo*, and clinical studies. However, an overall framework for defining *food functions* in a postpartum context is lacking. Also lacking is a framework for evaluating the ethnic postpartum nutritional practices in their ability to nourish the mother and aid in improving her immunity. Among the outcomes of the review of existing literature in this chapter are the identification of eight food functions in postpartum care, and a preliminary evaluation of ethnic Indian nutritional practices from the standpoint of Recommended Dietary Allowances (RDA). Section 29.2 discusses typical postpartum morbidities, and explores possible connections between the nutritional status of a postpartum mother and the morbidities experienced by her. It then lists the special nutritional needs during pre- and postpartum care and analyses of the RDA for pregnant women and lactating mothers. Thus, this section offers a contemporary basis for assessing the traditional postpartum nutritional practices of India. Section 29.3, which discusses the traditional postpartum nutritional practices of India, first presents a preliminary

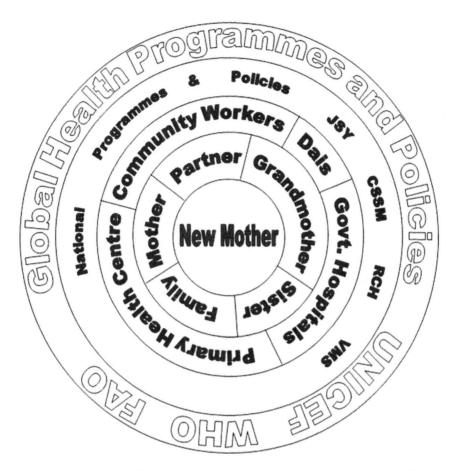

FIGURE 29.1 Postpartum morbidity and potential food functions: A paradigm for classifying traditional foods and functional foods.

list of 56 foods used in traditional Indian postpartum diets and the available scientific evidence for their use as *functional foods*. Traditionally, these foods are classified as hot or cold, and are included or avoided based on this classification. Based on the common postpartum morbidities, eight functions relevant to the health of postpartum women are identified, and the traditional foods are reclassified with regard to the functions they may fulfill. This section then considers traditional food formulations that utilize these foods and presents recipes of selected formulations, including an estimate of their nutrient content. Thus, this section presents a systematic compilation of the ethnic postpartum nutritional practices in India. Section 29.4 presents a critical examination of the impact of Indian ethnic postpartum nutritional practices on maternal health, immunity, and infection. To do so, four sample ethnic postpartum menus are presented using the food formulations discussed in Section 29.3. The amounts of macro- and micronutrients are evaluated for the four sample daily menus. These results are compared against the RDA for lactating mothers, and observations are made on postpartum dietary imbalance in lactating Indian mothers and their nutritional status. The effects of specific foods in the traditional postpartum formulations and their functional food properties with regard to supporting immunity and preventing infection are discussed. In light of this, Section 29.5 proposes strategies for two major efforts in line with the WHO strategic objectives for traditional healthcare systems: to create a more thorough scientific database evaluating postpartum ethnic foods, food formulations, and nutritional practices, and to better adapt traditional postpartum practices into contemporary maternal healthcare systems.

29.2 NUTRITION, IMMUNITY, AND INFECTION AFTER PREGNANCY: AN INDIAN PERSPECTIVE

29.2.1 OVERVIEW

Women undergo remarkable changes during pregnancy, childbirth, and the immediate postpartum period. During pregnancy, these changes enable both the fetus and the placenta to grow, and prepare the mother and baby for childbirth. After childbirth, the changes a new mother undergoes enable her to continue to provide nourishment for the infant even as her body gradually recovers back toward its prepregnancy state. The postpartum period, defined as the time from one hour after the delivery of placenta to 6 weeks after birth, is critical to maternal health as well as to that of the child. However, it is reported that 61% of all maternal deaths occur during the postpartum period (Singh and Kumar, 2014). As WHO (2014) reports, there were an estimated 289,000 maternal deaths across the world in 2013, of which 50,000 (Maternal Mortality Ratio, MMR: 190) were from India. Despite an estimated 65% reduction in maternal mortality from 1990 to 2013, India still had the highest incidence (17%) of maternal mortality in 2013.

Postpartum morbidity, the illnesses and complications borne by women during the postpartum period, presents a much wider challenge. It is estimated that for every maternal death, at least thirty other women suffer serious disabilities (Singh and Kumar, 2014). While the focus of the Indian government's maternal health programs is on pregnancy, skilled birth attendance, institutional delivery, and antenatal care with the aim of reducing maternal mortality, there are no programs dedicated to postpartum maternal health to address morbidity issues in India. Postpartum morbidities, especially those causing long-term health issues for mothers and children alike, have significant impact not only on the physical, mental, and sexual health of the mother but also on the socioeconomic status of the mother and the family. Considering that traditional postpartum care is commonly practiced across India, it is worthwhile to examine these ethnic nutritional practices and determine how they could address postpartum morbidities and mortalities in women.

29.2.2 POSTPARTUM MORBIDITY: AN INDIAN ASSESSMENT

Recently, studies have been initiated on examining postpartum morbidity and its causes in Indian contexts as well as in other parts of the world (Iyengar, 2012; Shriraam et al., 2012; Singh and Kumar, 2014; Yealy et al., 2015; Patra et al., 2008; MacArthur et al., 2003; WHO, 1998; Ronsmans et al, 2008). The most commonly reported morbidity conditions are:

- Body weakness
- Anemia
- Hemorrhage/excessive bleeding
- Infections—urinary tract infection (upper/lower), respiratory tract infection (upper/lower), vaginal tract/uterine infections causing purulent discharge, sepsis, breast infections, fevers, and wounds
- Incontinence—urinal and fecal
- Pains—backache, upper/lower abdominal pain, pelvic pains, lower limb pain, and swelling of feet
- Headache, hypertension, preeclampsia, and eclampsia
- Constipation, hemorrhoids, and rectal bleeding
- Breast-related problems—cracked/sore nipples, engorgements, and abscess

- Agalactorrhea
- Depression, anxiety, and extreme tiredness

Among these, hemorrhage, preeclampsia, postpartum genital infections (sepsis, etc.), and obstructed labor account for nearly 60% of postpartum maternal mortality (Bale et al., 2003). While different studies report similar postpartum morbidities experienced by the mothers interviewed/examined, there are significant variations among the studies as to which morbidities are more commonly experienced. These variations could be due to predisposing factors, such as nutritional status, socioeconomic status, lifestyles, past health history, availability/accessibility of healthcare facilities, and regional/seasonal variations.

29.2.3 Effects of Nutritional History on Postpartum Maternal Health Status

Nutritional status before, during, and after pregnancy often turns out to be a major predisposing factor in determining postpartum morbidity. For instance, anemia before and during pregnancy is known to be a strong predisposing factor for postpartum hemorrhage, the most common cause of maternal mortality. Deficiencies in calcium and protein could slow or prevent the regaining of strength in the pelvic and lower abdominal areas, resulting in chronic aches.

Many studies have examined the effects of nutritional interventions on the prevention/reduction of postpartum morbidity around the world. The ability of iron, folic acid, and zinc supplementations to mitigate postpartum hemorrhage and infections such as sepsis has been demonstrated (Christian et al., 2009). Calcium intake has been shown to reduce hypertension and preeclampsia (Kulier et al., 1998; Ronsmans et al., 2008). In a review, Ronsmans et al. (2008) discussed extensively the relationship between nutritional deficiencies and maternal health, particularly the associations between malnutrition and obstructive labor, calcium deficiency and eclampsia, iron deficiency and anemia, vitamin A deficiency and anemia or infection, and zinc deficiency and hemorrhage or infection. They have reported that preeclampsia has been associated with oxidative stress, and supplementation with antioxidants could improve vascular endothelial function. Supplementations of vitamins C and E have been shown to reduce preeclampsia. The authors have reviewed studies that have indicated that vitamin A or β-carotene deficiency could be correlated with puerperal infections from bacteria and yeast, painful urination, swelling, lower abdominal pain, vaginal discharge, low hemoglobin levels, and preeclampsia. However, they have suggested that the deficiencies could be markers of infections rather than causal agents. They have also reported that there is no direct evidence linking vitamin A or β-carotene deficiency with uterine atony and have concluded that vitamin A is most likely to act by improving the hematological and immune status of the mother.

In an analysis of 250 studies of predominantly randomized control trials, Middleton et al. (2013) have concluded that calcium intervention significantly reduces mortality or morbidity. While magnesium intervention causes a significant reduction in eclampsia, calcium reduces incidence of preeclampsia. Supplementation of iron and folic acid or multiple micronutrients have been highly effective in reducing anemia. Women with anemia are often found to be deficient in other micronutrients, such as iodine, vitamin A, and zinc, which could lead to greater incidence of morbidity and mortality. Villar et al. (2003) found that calcium supplementation reduced the incidence of preeclampsia and hypertension. Bale et al. (2003) have pointed out that preexisting conditions such as malaria and viral hepatitis may exacerbate postpartum morbidity and result in mortality. Brinch et al. (1998) have found that women with poor diets have six times the expected rate of perinatal mortality.

Maternal micronutrient deficiencies during lactation can cause a major reduction in the concentration of some of these nutrients in breast milk, leading to subsequent infant depletion (Allen and Graham, 2003). Allen (1994) identified the priority nutrients for lactating mothers to be thiamine, riboflavin, vitamins B_6 and B_{12}, vitamin A, and iodine. Allen studied the relation between maternal status or intake of each nutrient and its effect on the nutrient concentration in breast milk. Low maternal intake or stores reduced the amount of these nutrients in breast milk, and maternal supplementation reversed this (Astrachan-Fletcher et al., 2008). There is a well-established adverse effect of unchanged or poor dietary intake of mothers on maternal and infant nutritional status, particularly for chronically undernourished women (Gopalan and Kaur, 1989; Rao and Yajnik, 2010).

Historically, malnutrition and growth failure have been treated as a deficiency of protein. However, malnutrition is now recognized as inadequate intake of energy and protein in addition to vital minerals (iron, zinc, and iodine), vitamins (vitamin A), and essential fatty acids. Many of these nutrients are not produced by the human body but are essential for everyday physiological functions. For this reason, supplements with these nutrients are recommended when needs cannot be met through the diet (UNICEF, 2013).

Poor nutrition during the postnatal period can also cause depression. Women's bodies need enough iron and vitamin B_3 (niacin) to convert tryptophan into 5-hydroxy-L-tryptophan (5-HTP). Other B vitamins and magnesium are necessary to convert vitamin B_6 to pyridoxyl-5-phosphate (P5P). Without enough 5-HTP and P5P available in the brain, serotonin cannot be made at adequate levels, which in turn can lead to postpartum depression (Astrachan-Fletcher et al., 2008).

Examining correlations between nutritional imbalances and morbidities is an open and critical problem of research. While there is a growing body of evidence pointing to such correlations, there are many controversies and open questions. For example, whether nutritional imbalances *cause* maternal morbidities or they merely indicate the existence of morbidities is a question that is yet to be answered conclusively. Furthermore, the biological mechanisms of how a nutritional imbalance may induce morbidity often remain to be established. Carefully developed protocols need to be adopted in research studies; particularly, care has to be taken in recognizing what conclusions may be drawn from adopting a specific protocol. A combination of clinical studies (nutritional status, recall of dietary patterns, assessment of nutritive contents of diets, effects of interventions, and analysis of morbidities) and *in vivo* studies (inducing imbalances to examine morbidity outcomes) are necessary to establish correlations between nutritional imbalances and maternal morbidities. The biological mechanisms of these nutritional interventions may further be established through well-designed *in vitro* and *in vivo* studies.

29.2.4 NUTRITIONAL REQUIREMENTS DURING LACTATION

The enhanced nutritional needs of a mother during and after pregnancy are a reflection of the physiological, biochemical, and hormonal changes she undergoes toward ensuring optimal growth of the infant while recovering to her prepregnancy health. Table 29.1 lists the RDA for moderately working expectant and lactating mothers, and compares them with those for a moderately active adult woman in the Indian context (NIN, 2014).

The energy requirement during pregnancy for a moderately active adult woman is 300 kcal more than that for a normal adult woman. It increases to +550 kcal in the first 6 months of lactation before reducing to +400 kcal during 6–12 months. The basis of this recommendation is as follows: mother's milk has about 65 kcal of energy per 100 mL. If one were to assume an optimal output of 750 mL per day of milk from the mother, and that 80% of her energy intake is converted into energy in the milk, approximately 550 kcal per day of additional energy intake is suggested for the mother. The National Institute of Nutrition, India (2014) has not provided any specific recommendations for other vitamins and minerals for lactating mothers. In their absence, dietary reference intakes from the National Academies Press (Otten et al., 2006) may be used, as presented in Table 29.2.

These nutritional needs have to be met through the foods consumed by the postpartum mothers as well as through the supplements they take. Thus, the guidelines presented in Tables 29.1 and 29.2 together form a basis on which ethnic postpartum nutritional practices may be assessed. It is to be noted

TABLE 29.1

Recommended Dietary Allowances for a Nonpregnant, Nonlactating Adult Woman, a Pregnant Woman, and a Lactating Mother of Moderate Activity

Nutrient	Adult Woman	Pregnant Woman	Lactating Woman 0–6 months	6–12 months
Energy (Kcal)	2225	2525	2775	2625
Protein (g)	50	65	75	68
Fat (g)	20	30	45	45
Calcium (mg)	400	1000	1000	1000
Iron (mg)	30	38	30	30
Retinol (IU)	600	600	950	950
β-carotene (μg)	2400	2400	3800	3800
Ascorbic acid (mg)	40	40	80	80
Folic acid (dietary folate) (μg)	100	400	150	150
Fiber (g)	25	28	32	32

Table 29.2

Dietary Reference Intakes for Selected Vitamins and Minerals

Nutrient	Daily Recommendation	Nutrient	Daily Recommendation
Vitamin B_6 (mg)	2.0	Vitamin D (μg)	50
Vitamin B_{12} (μg)	2.8	Vitamin E (mg)	19
Biotin (μg)	35	Iodine (μg)	290
Choline (mg)	550	Magnesium (mg)	310
Vitamin K (μg)	90	Phosphorus (mg)	700
Niacin (mg)	17	Selenium (μg)	70
Pantothenic Acid (mg)	7.0	Potassium (g)	5.1
Riboflavin (mg)	1.6	Sodium (g)	2.3
Thiamine (mg)	1.4	Zinc (mg)	12

that these recommendations are made based on the current understanding of the connections between nutrition and health, particularly in the pregnancy and postpartum periods. As this understanding evolves, so will the RDA, and so will the evaluation of the postpartum ethnic nutritional practices.

29.3   POSTPARTUM ETHNIC NUTRITIONAL PRACTICES IN INDIA

Ethnic foods are traditional foods that originate from a specific heritage and culture. They may include locally available foods, special formulations, and supplements, varying based on the topography of the region, culture, traditions, and religious practices of the country. Ethnic nutritional practices include the traditional food formulations and practices associated with the consumption of ethnic foods. Traditional food formulations are important sources of many nutrients especially for the most vulnerable sections of the society, such as women and children, whether the scientific knowledge is understood by the society or not. Among women, pregnant and lactating mothers are the most targeted group for specific nutritional care.

29.3.1 TRADITIONAL FOODS AND NUTRITIONAL PRACTICES IN INDIAN POSTPARTUM CARE: BELIEFS AND HEALTH BENEFITS

India, being a land of diverse cultures and traditions, has its unique traditional beliefs regarding foods and practices for pre- and postpartum care. Given the range of diversity in soil type, climate, and occupations, the traditions vary significantly. However, each of them uses locally available resources like ethnic cereals and millets, pulses, spices, herbs, greens, vegetables, fruits, nuts, and seafoods in their cuisines and food formulations. Table 29.3 provides a list of 56 traditional Indian postpartum foods, classified according to the food groups they belong to, and summarizes the studies conducted on these foods. These studies are mainly of two kinds: those that analyze the beliefs of people pertaining to the uses of these foods, and those that study their functions and the active ingredients that cause these functions. The former relies primarily on surveys, interviews, and their analyses. The latter includes clinical trials, extraction, and identification of specific ingredients from foods, and *in vitro* and *in vivo* studies seeking to establish links to specific functions. With increasing levels of education and awareness, it is probably inevitable that the traditional beliefs of people are influenced by their awareness of the modern paradigms of nutrition and healthcare.

Some of the key observations, based on the literature reviewed in Table 29.3, are presented below:

- India has rich, diverse, and highly nutritious food resources used especially in ethnic formulations for postpartum women. These foods are abundant in macro- and micronutrients, and also possess many essential molecules that are known to promote health, enable specific postpartum functions, and help mitigate many diseases that postpartum mothers are otherwise vulnerable to.
- Indians have held strong beliefs regarding specific functions that the foods included in postpartum care enable. These functions are enhancing lactation, enabling smooth bowel movement,

---

TABLE 29.3
Traditional Postpartum Foods in India: Beliefs and Scientific Evidence

Number	Foods and Common Beliefs	Potential Functional Properties and Active Components
	Green Leafy Vegetables	
1	*Moringa oleifera†* Drumstick leaves Galactagogue Prevents constipation Rich in nutrients (Ramya and Jose, 2014; Awadesh et al., 2008)	Galactagogue activity (Raguindin et al., 2014); antimicrobial, antioxidant activity (Marrufo et al., 2013); anticancer, antiulcer, antispasmodic, hypotensive, hypocholesterolemic, sympatholytic, antibacterial, and antiviral activity (Asiedu-Gyekye et al., 2014; Jung, 2014; Siddhuraju and Becker, 2003) Active components: calcium, β-carotene, vitamin C, benzyl isothiocyanate, niazimicin, pterygospermin, benzyl isothiocyanate, 4-{a-L-rhamnopyranosyloxy}benzyl glucosinolate (Mahmood et al., 2010)
2	*Murraya koenigii†* Curry leaves Rich in nutrients Blood purifier Antifungal Antidepressant Anti-inflammatory Helps body aches (Jain, 2012)	Wound-healing effect, antimicrobial, antioxidant, anticancer, antimutagenic, anti-inflammatory, cytotoxic, antiulcer, memory enhancing, vasodilating, hypocholestreolemic, antidiabetic, phagocytic, antidiarrheal (Handral et al., 2012) Active components: calcium, β-carotene, crude fiber, folic acid, murrayacine, koenine, koenigine, mukonicine, mahanimbine, mahanine, mahanimbinine, murrayacinine, isomahanimbine, mahanimboline, murrayanine, cyclomahanimbine or curryanine, murrayanol, and glycozoline (Handral et al., 2012); carbazole alkaloids, tannins, and phenolics (Tachibana et al., 2001; Ramsewak et al., 1999; Roy et al., 2004; Khan et al., 1996; Nutan et al., 1998)

(Continued)

TABLE 29.3 (*Continued*)

Traditional Postpartum Foods in India: Beliefs and Scientific Evidence

Number	Foods and Common Beliefs	Potential Functional Properties and Active Components
3	*Sesbania grandiflora†* Agathi leaves Wound healer Immunity booster Contraceptive Helps vagina-related problems (Sudha and Mathanghi, 2012)	Antioxidant, antimicrobial, cytoprotective (Zarena et al., 2014); imunomodulatory (Mallik and Nayak, 2014) Active components: calcium, β-carotene, vitamin C, agathi leaf protein (Zarena et al., 2014; Gowri and Vasantha, 2010; Nataraj et al., 2012)
4	*Trigonellafoenum graecum†* Fenugreek leaves Galactagogue (Gabay, 2002; Alamer and Basiouni, 2005; Nice, 2011)	Galactagogue (Zuppa et al., 2010) induces oxytocin, prolactin (Turkyilmaz et al., 2011; Gabay, 2002); anticancer, antidiabetic, hypoglycemic, hypocholesterolemic (Khalil et al., 2015) Active components: β-carotene; phytoestrogenic molecule—diosgenin (Tabares, et al., 2014); oxytocin, prolactin (Marasco, 2008; Nice, 2011); alkaloids, flavonoids, terpenoids, polyunsaturated fatty acids, steroidal saponogenins, fiber, galactomannans, antioxidants, amino acids such as 4-hydroxyisoleucine (Khalil et al., 2015)
5	*Solanum nigrum* Manathakali leaves and fruit Treats fever Helps urinary diseases Expedites child birth Prevents anemia Laxative (Nisha and Rajeshkumar, 2010)	Wound healer, antioxidant, hepatoprotective, antitumor, cytostatic, anticonvulsant, antiulcer, anti-inflammatory (Atanu and Ajayi, 2011; Kirtikar and Basu, 1935; Saleem et al., 2009; Jain et al., 2011; Shanmugam et al., 2012; Chou et al., 2008) Active components: iron, cuscutin, amarbelin, betasterol, stigmasterol, kaempferol, dulcitol, myricetin, qurecetin, coumarin, and oleanolic acid (Arunachalam et al., 2009)
6	*Spinacia oleracea* Spinach Promotes breast tissue health Galactagogue (Gogoi and Zaman, 2013)	Hepatoprotectant, anticancer, antihelmintic, anti-inflammatory, antihistaminic (Subash et al., 2010); antioxidant and antigenotoxic (Ko et al., 2014) Active components: β-carotene, folic acid; flavonoids and p-coumaric acid (Grossman, 2001)
	Vegetables	
7	*Momordica charantia* Bitter gourd Rectifies hormonal imbalance Galactagogue (Vaidya et al., 2013; Warrier et al., 1995) Cures wounds and infections (Sankaranarayanan and Jolly, 1993)	Antidiabetic and hypoglycemic (Joseph and Jini, 2013); wound-healing activity (Sankaranarayanan and Jolly, 1993); immunomodulatory (Majumdar and Debnath, 2014) Active components: vitamin C; charantin, polypeptide-p, and vicine (Keller et al., 2011)
8	*Lagenaria siceraria†* Bottle gourd Galactagogue (Vaidya et al., 2013; Warrier et al, 1995) Laxative Diuretic Prevents genito-urinary tract infections Aids wound healing (Upaganlawar and Balaraman, 2009)	Antidiabetic (Saha et al., 2011); antioxidant, analgesic, anti-inflammatory, antihyperglycemic, antihyperlipidemic, antimicrobial, anthelmintic, cytotoxic, anticancer, and immunomodulatory (Deshpande et al., 2008); cardioprotective, hepatoprotective, bronchospasm protective, antidiarrheal, and diuretic (Palamthodi and Lele, 2013) Active componets: flavonoid complexes—flavone, glycosides (Jaiswal and Kuhnert, 2014)

(Continued)

TABLE 29.3 (*Continued*)

Traditional Postpartum Foods in India: Beliefs and Scientific Evidence

Number	Foods and Common Beliefs	Potential Functional Properties and Active Components
9	*Moringa oleifera†* Drumstick Improves immunity Antimicrobial Fights infections Helps with urinary tract infections Galactagogue (Fuglie, 1999)	Anti-inflammatory, antiulcer, antispasmodic, diuretic, cardiac and circulatory stimulants, antitumor, antipyretic, antiepileptic, antihypertensive, hypocholesterolemic, antioxidant, antidiabetic, hepatoprotective, antibacterial and antifungal (Anwar and Gilani, 2007) Active components: crude fiber, vitamin C; zeatin, quercetin, β-sitosterol, caffeoylquinic acid and kaempferol, flavanoids, Quercetin (Michel et al., 2008)
10	*Daucus carota* Carrot Considered as a cold food Relieves constipation Treats heat disorders (Etkin, 2007)	Antioxidant and anticancer (Sharma et al., 2012) Active compounds: phosphorous; phenolics (Babic et al., 1993); polyacetylenes (Hansen et al., 2003; Kidmose et al., 2004); carotenoids (Block, 1994); β-carotene and tocopherol (Hashimoto and Nagayama 2004); fiber (Bao and Chang, 1994; Anderson et al., 1994)
11	*Phaseolus vulgaris* L. beans Relieves constipation (Chaudhary and Sharma, 2013)	Cardioprotective, renal protective, and reduces cataract (Bazzano et al., 2001); relieves constipation, improves gastrointestinal integrity, stabilizes blood sugar, brain and immune dysfunction (Bourdon et al., 2001) Active components: protein, fat, starch, fiber (Wang et al., 2009)
12	*Beta vulgaris†* Beetroot Improves blood hemoglobin (Manisha et al., 2012; Rao et al., 2014)	Antioxidant, antimicrobial, anti-inflamatory, anticancer (Ninfali and Angelino, 2013) Active components: essential oils, flavonoids, polyphenols, sugars, anthocyanin pigment, betalain (Ninfali and Angelino, 2013)
	Fruits	
13	*Carica papaya* Papaya (ripe) Galactagogue (Ajesh and Kumuthakalavalli, 2012)	Galactagouge (Marasco, 2008; Nice, 2011); hepatoprotective, immunomodulatory, antioxidant, laxative, diuretic activity, and relieves urinary tract infection (Krishna et al., 2008) Active components: oxytocin (Marasco, 2008; Nice, 2011); amino acids, citric and malic acid (Krishna et al., 2008)
14	*Solanum lycopersicum* Tomato	Antioxidant, anticancer, mitigates neurodegenerative diseases (Valero et al., 2011; Rao and Balachandran, 2002) Active components: lycopene, β-carotene, tocopherols, tocotrienols chlorophyll, anthocyanins (Friedman, 2004)
	Cereals and Millets	
15	*Oryza sativa†* Rice Prevents retention of placenta Nourishment and strength Wound healing Relieves cough (Tiwari and Pande, 2010)	Aphrodisiac, diuretic, and useful in biliousness (Caius, 1986); hypotensive, anticancer prevention, dysentery, skin care, prevents Alzheimer's disease, and immunomodulatory (Gamal et al., 2011) Active components: energy, carbohydrates, low fat, low sodium, no cholesterol, thiamine, niacin, iron, riboflavin, vitamin D, calcium, fiber, low sugar, and insoluble fibers (Umadevi et al., 2012)

(Continued)

TABLE 29.3 (*Continued*)
Traditional Postpartum Foods in India: Beliefs and Scientific Evidence

Number	Foods and Common Beliefs	Potential Functional Properties and Active Components
16	*Triticum spp.*† Wheat, broken wheat, and wheat flour For gaining calories and nourishment (Manisha et al., 2012)	Antioxidant (Zhou and Parry, 2005; Yu et al., 2002; Zieliski and Kozlowska, 2000) Active components: protein, carbohydrates; tocopherols, tocotrienols, phenolic acids, phytic acid, phytosterols, flavonoids, carotenoids (Abdel-Aal et al., 2002; Abdel-Aal et al., 2007); tocopherols (Zhou et al., 2004); phenolic acids (Abdel-Aal et al., 2001) and anthocyanins (Abdel-Aal et al., 2006)
17	Rice (puffed) Stops bleeding Promotes wound healing (Harish and Meghendra, 2006; Bandyopadhyay, 2009)	No scientific evidence available Active components: protein, niacin (NIN, 2014)

Pulses and Lentils

Number	Foods and Common Beliefs	Potential Functional Properties and Active Components
18	*Phaseolus mungo* *Vigna radiata*† Green gram/Mung bean (whole and hulled, split bean) Emollient Thermogenic Diuretic Aphrodisiac Treats anorexia Treats constipation Treats hepatopathy Treats neuropathy Galactagogue Kumar et al., 2011b Internal injury healing (Tiwari and Pande, 2010)	Antioxidant (Silva et al., 2013; Ramesh et al., 2011); improves anemia, recovery of tissues and muscles, improves immunity, improves digestion, antimicrobial, anti-inflammatory, antihypertensive, and antitumor (Tang et al., 2014); antidiabetic and low glycemic index (Madar and Stark, 2002) Active components: minerals (Fe, Mg, Ca, Na, K, Zn, Se, P); phenolics (arbutin, gallic acid, chlorogenic acid, ferulic acid, qurecetin) (Mesallam and Hamza, 1987; Nair et al., 2015); sterols and triterpenes, flavonoids, tannins, organic acids, polyunsaturated fatty acids (Ramesh et al., 2011; Silva et al., 2013); tocopherols, seven essential amino acids (lysine is limiting), crude fiber (Mesallam and Hamza, 1987; Jom et al., 2011); antinutritional factors: phytic acid, however, in much smaller quantities than soybean and pigeon pea (Chitra et al., 1995); proteins and amino acids (Tang et al., 2014)
19	*Lens esculenta Medikus* Red dal Strengthening of muscles Relieves flatulence Removes hyperpigmentation (Manisha et al., 2012)	Antioxidant (Zou et al., 2011); reduces anemia (Thavarajah et al., 2009) Active components: minerals (Fe, Zn, Ca, P, Na, K) (Savage, 1988; Thavarajah et al., 2009); phenolics—benzoic and cinnamic, tartaric esters, flavanols, isoflavanones, anthocyanins (Oomah et al., 2011; Xu and Chang, 2010); phytosterols, alkaloids, bioactive carbohydrates, proteins—all essential amino acids (methionine and cystine are limiting), water-soluble vitamins (niacin, thiamin, riboflavin) (Rochfort and Panozzo, 2007)
20	*Vigna mungo* Black gram Galactagogue (Tiwari and Pande, 2010)	Galactagogue (Zia Ul-Haq et al., 2014); hypocholesterolemic (Indira and Kurup, 1989); antioxidant (Girish et al., 2012); immunestimulatory (Dhumal et al., 2013) Active components: phosphorus, potassium, sulfur, magnesium; fat, protein, phenolic acids like hallic, protocatechuic, gentisic, vanillic, syringic, caffeic, and ferulic acids (Girish et al., 2012)

(Continued)

TABLE 29.3 (*Continued*)
Traditional Postpartum Foods in India: Beliefs and Scientific Evidence

Number	Foods and Common Beliefs	Potential Functional Properties and Active Components
21	*Cicer arietinum* Bengal gram dal Chickpeas Nourishment (Pandey and Enumeratio, 1993) Treats throat problems, blood disorders, bronchitis, skin diseases, biliousness—in traditional medicines (Sastry and Kavathekar, 1990) Blood enrichment; treats ear infections, skin ailments, liver and spleen disorders—in traditional medicines (Warrier et al., 1995)	Hypoglycemic, hypocholesterolemic, reduces malnutrition, smooth bowel movement (Pittaway et al., 2007); antiulcerative, antibacterial, antifungal, anti-inflammatory, anticancer, antiobesity, hypocholesterolemic, hypolipidemic, insulin sensitization (Jukanti et al., 2012, and references therein); uterotonic (Gruber and O'Brien, 2011) Active components: protein, fiber, folate (El-Adawy, 2002); lysine, isoleucine, tryptophan, and aromatic amino acids (Carrillo et al., 2007); all essential amino acids except sulfur-containing, starch, oligosaccharides, polyunsaturated fatty acids, sterols (β-sitosterol, campesterol, stigmasterol), calcium, magnesium, phosphorus, potassium, riboflavin, thiamine, niacin, folate, β-carotene (Jukanti et al., 2012)

Dairy Products

22	Cow's milk† Strengthens muscles and bones Galactagogue (Dietary guidelines for Indian foods, 2010; Awadesh et al., 2008; Rao et al., 2014)	Immunological protection, treatment for diarrhea, antihypertensive, antimicrobial, anticoagulant activity, activates mineral malabsorption, immune booster, and increased bioavailability of calcium (Unal, 2005) Active components: Mill proteins, peptides, whey proteins such as lactoferrin, lysozyme, and immunoglobulins, oligosaccharides, fucosylated oligosaccharides, hormone growth factors, mucin, gangliosides, and endogenous peptides (Severin and Wenshui, 2005)

Animal Foods

23	Fish†(shark, catfish, anchovy, dried fish) Calcium-rich food Galactagogue (Nadkarni, 2007)	Builds up bone mass density (Zalloua et al., 2007); antihypertensive, anticoagulant, antibacterial, antioxidant, anti-inflammatory (Wu et al., 2008); promotes optimum fetal and neonatal cognitive development; reduces obesity risk in children (Muhlhausler et al., 2010) Active components: calcium, protein, omega-3 polyunsaturated fatty acids, ACE inhibitory peptides (Wu et al., 2008)
24	Egg Source of protein, calcium, and fat (Rao et al., 2014)	Antimicrobial, immunomodulatory, antioxidant, anticancer, and antihypersensitive, (Abeyrathne et al., 2013) Active components: essential amino acids, polyunsaturated fatty acids, saturated fat (palmitic, stearic, and myristic acids). Egg white contains protein, riboflavin, pantothenic acid, vitamin B_{12}, choline, and phosphorus (Weggemans et al., 2001)

Sugars

25	*Borassus flabellifer Linn* Jaggery† Body strengthening (Mathur, 1983)	Strengthening and nourishment, hemostatic, expectorant, energy, prevents anemia, and antimicrobial (Nagnur et al., 2006) Active components: calcium, lauric acid, phenolics (Sreeramulu and Raghunath, 2011)

(*Continued*)

TABLE 29.3 (*Continued*)

Traditional Postpartum Foods in India: Beliefs and Scientific Evidence

Number	Foods and Common Beliefs	Potential Functional Properties and Active Components
		Spices
26	*Allium Sativum†* Garlic Galactagogue Wound healing and contraction of uterus (Awadesh et al., 2008; Bandyopadhyay, 2009)	Galactagogue (Srinivas et al., 2014); antibacterial, antifungal, antiviral, and antiprotozoal; wound-healing potential (Harris et al., 2001; Jalali et al., 2009); hypoglycemic, antidyspeptic, antiflatulent, duodenal ulcers, rubefacient in skin diseases (Shi et al., 2011); immunomodulatory (Gammal et al., 2011) Active components: oxytocin (Marasco, 2008; Nice, 2011); disulfide compounds: di (2-propenyl) disulfide and 2-propenylpropyl disulfide (Kumari et al., 1995; Augusti and Sheela, 1996)
27	*Curcuma longa†* Turmeric Heals internal injury Wound healing Galactagogue Treats cough, cold, constipation, hematuria Antibacterial Removes hyperpigmentation (White, 2002; Tiwari and Pande, 2010; Awades et al., 2008)	Antiinflammatory (Suryanarayana et al., 2003; Arun and Nalini, 2002); antibacterial and antifungal (Mahady, 2005; Misra and Sahu, 1977; Chattopadhyay, 2004); diuretic, laxative, hepatoprotective, antidiabetic (Shi et al., 2011); carminative, tonic, antirheumatic, blood purifier, antiseptic, and prevents liver ailments (Luthra et al., 2001) Active components: monoteroene alcohols, flavonoids, and polyphenols (Srinivasan, 2005); essential oils, curcumin (Mukherjee et al., 2011)
28	*Trigonella foenum graecum†* Fenugreek seeds Galactagogue (Awadesh et al., 2008; Rao et al., 2014)	Galactagogue (Sreeja et al., 2010); diuretic, hypoglycemic, emmenagogue, emollient, cardioprotective (Shi et al., 2011); gastroprotective (Pandian et al., 2002); hypolipidemic (Mukherjee, 2003); carminative, gastric stimulant, antidiabetic, galactogogue, hypocholesterolemic, hypolipidemic, antioxidant, hepatoprotective, anti-inflammatory, antibacterial, antifungal, antiulcer, antilithogenic, anticarcinogenic (Yadav and Bacquer, 2014) Active components: protein, choline, folic acid, magnesium, potassium, phytoestrogens (Sreeja et al., 2010); fiber and gum (Sharma, 1986; Sharma et al., 1996; Srinivasan, 2005)
29	*Zingiber officinale†* Ginger and dried ginger Controls cold and cough Heals wound of umbilical cord (Kanwar and Sharma, 2011; Manisha et al., 2012; Ajesh and Kumuthakalavalli, 2012); Controls postpartum bleeding Uterine cleansing agent (Choudhry, 1997)	Anti-inflammatory, antibacterial, prevents urinary tract infection (Mahady, 2005); antidepressant (Lakshmi and Sudhakar, 2010; Felipe et al., 2008); choleretic (Thomas et al., 2007); immunomodulatory (Mishra et al., 2012) Active compounds: magnesium; curcumin (Thomas et al., 2007); phenolics: gingerols and 6-gingerdiol (Ficker, 2003)

(Continued)

TABLE 29.3 (*Continued*)
Traditional Postpartum Foods in India: Beliefs and Scientific Evidence

Number	Foods and Common Beliefs	Potential Functional Properties and Active Components
30	*Foenicum vulgare*† Fennel seed Eases constipation Releases excess gas Galactagogue (Sayed et al., 2007)	Galactagogue (Mills and Bone, 2000; Abascal and Yarnell, 2008; Tomas, 2009); antioxidant (Miguel et al., 2010); hepatoprotective (Hanefi et al., 2004); antispasmodic, antifungal, and hypoglycemic (Dongare et al., 2011); antibacterial, antithrombotic, antimicrobial, oestrogenic, cytoprotective, and antitumor (Rather et al., 2012) Active components: anethole, estragole (Tabares et al., 2014); anethole, fenchone, phenols (Rathore et al., 2012); calcium, potassium, sodium, iron, phosphorus, thiamine, riboflavin, niacin, vitamin C, flavonoids, phenolic compounds, dillapional (Rather et al., 2012)
31	*Pimpinella anisum L.* Anise seed Galactagogue (Zargari, 1996)	Galactagogue (Hosseinzadeh et al., 2013; Eiben et al., 2004); antibacterial, antiviral, antifungal, insecticidal, laxative, antispasmodic, anticonvulsant, muscle relaxant, antiulcer, antidiabetic, hypolipidemic, antioxidant, reduction of pain in dysmenorrhea, digestive, carminative, and relief of gastrointestinal spasms (Shojaii and Fard, 2012) Active components: essential oil (Shojaii and Fard, 2012)
32	*Piper nigrum*† Black pepper Relives constipation Relieves indigestion laxative Improves appetite Aids digestion Stops excessive bleeding (Awadesh et al., 2008; Manisha et al., 2012) Relieves aches and pains (Chaudhry and Tariq, 2006)	Decongestant, relieves digestive problems, anticholera, anti-influenza, antirheumatoid, antiarthritis, antispasmodic, antioxidant, and immunomodulatory (Chaudhry and Tariq, 2006; Damanhouri and Ahmad, 2014; Majdalaweih and Carr, 2010); hypoglycemic (Srinivasan, 2005); hypocholesterolemic (Shirke and Jagtap, 2009) Active components: protein, crude fiber, iron, β-carotene, manganese; alkaloids such as piperine, piperidine, and piperettine (Chaudhry and Tariq, 2006)
33	*Cuminum cyminum*† Cumin seeds Relieves gas Aid digestion Stop excessive bleeding (Manisha et al., 2012)	Antispasmodic, carminative, digestive stimulant (Shi et al., 2011); anti-inflammatory, relieves pain, digestive disorders, purifies blood (Proestos et al., 2006) Active components: protein, fat, crude fiber, calcium, phosphorous, iron, choline, sodium, potassium, zinc; cuminaldehyde, pinene, α-terpinene, and p-cymene, volatile oils (Rathore et al., 2012)
34	*Trachyspermumammi L.* † Bishop's weed Galactagogue Corrects gastric disorder (Shahin and Ahmad, 2014; Awadesh et al., 2008)	Smooth bowel movement, antiasthma, antibronchitis, painkiller, wound healing, antiinfluenza (Silver, 2006) Active components: protein, fat, crude fiber, iron, calcium, phosphorus, magnesium, zinc, essential oil, thymol, α-pinene, p-cymene, limonene, and terpinene. The major components of T. copticum L. oils are piperitone (23.65%), alpha-pinene (14.94%), limonene (14.89%), 1, 8-cineole (7.43%) and thymol (37.2%), p-cymene (32.3%), and gamma-terpinene (27.3%) (Hawrelak et al., 2009)

(Continued)

TABLE 29.3 (*Continued*)
Traditional Postpartum Foods in India: Beliefs and Scientific Evidence

Number	Foods and Common Beliefs	Potential Functional Properties and Active Components
35	*Bunium bulbocastanum* *Nigella sativa* Black cumin seed Cools the stomach Galactagouge (Goodburn and Gazi, 1995) Birth control To start menstruation (Ahmad et al., 2013)	Galactagogue (Hosseinzadeh et al., 2013); antibacterial, antihistamine, antimicrobial, immune booster, antitumor, antifertility, antioxytocic, cytotoxic, hepatoprotective, analgesic, antihelmenthic, (Ahmad et al., 2013); promotes lactation (Elmofty, 1997) Active compounds: oxytocin (Marasco, 2008; Nice, 2011); essential fatty acids, arginine, carotene, calcium, iron, sodium, and potassium.
36	*Anogeissus latofoia* Edible gum Galactagogue (Kuroda et al., 2010) Relieves back pain Wound healing (Katewa et al., 2004)	Wound healing, antiulcer, anti-inflammatory, antidiabetes, controls hemorrhages, hemoptysis, diarrhea, dysentery, hemorrhoids (Maury et al., 2013) Active Compounds: calcium salt, gallic acid, quinic and shikmik acids, quercetin, and myricetin. (Maury et al., 2013)
37	Embelia ribes Vavding Anthelmintic Astringent Carminative Smooth bowel movement (Shahin and Ahmad, 2014)	Antioxidant, antifertility, anthelmintic, anti-inflammatory, antimicrobial, enzyme inhibitory, antispermatazoal, antiandrogenic, wound healing, antihyperlipidemic, anticonvulsant, antitumor, anticancer, chemopreventive, antidiabetic, antiulcer, and antiangiogenesis activity (Radhakrishnan and Gnanamani, 2014) Active components: quinone derivatives, embelin, alkaloids, christembine, volatile oil, vilangin embelin, and embelin (Radhakrishnan and Gnanamani, 2014)
38	*Anethum graveolens* Dill seeds Reduces postpartum hemorrhage Galactagogue (Samira et al., 2012; Saini et al., 2014)	Galactagogue (Marasco, 2008; Nice, 2011); antihyperlipidemic and antihypercholesterolemic (Yazdanparast and Alavi, 2001; Yazdanparast and Bahramikia, 2008); regulation of menstrual cycle, anticancer, antidiabetic, antioxidant, antisecretory, antispasmodic, insecticidal, and diuretic (Monsefi et al., 2006) Active compounds: oxytocin (Marasco, 2008; Nice, 2011); essential oils, proteins, fiber, calcium, potassium, magnesium, phosphorous, sodium, vitamin A, and niacin (Kaur and Arora, 2010)
39	*Papaver somniferum* Poppy seeds Relives abdominal pain Keeps stomach cool Galactagogue (Choudhury and Ahmed, 2011)	Narcotic and analgesic (Kaplan, 1994); antispasmodic, antinociceptive, psychodysleptic, hypnotic, sedative (Malta Wild Plants; Wiart, 2006) Active compounds: protein, fats, fiber, calcium, phosphorous, iron, magnesium, mangenese, zinc, morphine, codeine, thebaine, papaverine, and noscapine (EFSA Panel on Contaminants in the Food Chain, 2011)
40	*Coriandrum sativum* Corriander seeds Anti-inflammatory Galactagogue (The Academy of Breastfeeding Medicine Protocol Committee, 2011)	Antioxidant, hypoglycemic, insecticidal, aflatoxin control, antibacterial, hypolipidemic, relieves mouth ulcers, anticancer, anticonvulsant, antihistaminic, and hypnotic (Rathore et al., 2012) Active V: protein, fat, fiber, phosphorus, iron, choline, magnesium, potassium, zinc; volatile oil-carvone, geraniol, limonene, borneol, camphor, elemol, and linalool (Purseglove et al., 1981)

(Continued)

TABLE 29.3 (*Continued*)

Traditional Postpartum Foods in India: Beliefs and Scientific Evidence

Number	Foods and Common Beliefs	Potential Functional Properties and Active Components
41	*Ferula asafetida†* Asafoietida Antiflatulent Corrects gastric problems Improves digestion Sets hormonal imbalance (Awadesh et al., 2008)	Antihistamic and analgesic (Ballabh and Chaurasia, 2007); possesses anti-influenza A (H1N1) activity, antiviral, and cytotoxic (Lee et al., 2009) Active components: iron; resin, volatile oils, asareninotannols A and B, ferulic acid, and umbelliferone (Lee et al., 2009)
42	*Piper longum* Arisi thippili (dried fruit), kanda thippili (dried bark) Prevents cold (Shahin and Ahmad, 2014)	Antioxidant, cardioprotective (Jagdale et al., 2009); analgesic (Vedhanayaki et al., 2003); insecticidal, acaricidal activity, antifungal, antiamoebic, antimicrobial, antiasthmatic, antidiabetic, immunomodulatory, anti-inflammatory, anticancer, antidepressant, antiulcer, and hepatoprotective activity (Khandhar et al., 2010) Active Components: protein, phosphorus, iron; piperine, alkaloids and amides, lignans, esters, volatile oil (Chauhan et al., 2010)

Fats and Oils

Number	Foods and Common Beliefs	Potential Functional Properties and Active Components
43	Ghee† Galactagogue Improve health Wound healing (Bandyopadhyay, 2009)	Hypocholesterolemic and anticarcinogenic (Shi et al., 2011) Active compounds: conjugated linoleic acid, butyric acid, fat-soluble vitamins A, D, E, and K (Shi et al., 2011)
44	*Sesamum indicum* Sesame oil/Gingelly oil Antidepressant Facilitates recovery Wound healing (Liu-Chiang, 1995)	Wound-healing and antioxidant activity (Kiran and Asad, 2008); antihyperlipidemic (Asgary et al., 2013; Saleem et al., 2012); strengthening of bones and muscles (Serra et al., 2011) Active components: oleic, linoleic, palmitic, and stearic acids (Saydut et al., 2008)
45	*Brassica juncea* Mustard oil Healing of umbilical cord (Deepthi et al., 2010)	Wound healing, carminative, diuretic, anti-inflammatory, antimicrobial, antifungal, antibacterial, hypoglycemic (Oliver et al., 1999; Nadarajah et al., 2005; Grover et al., 2003) Active components: allyl isothiocyanate (Inoue et al., 1997; Simons et al., 2004)

Nuts and Oil Seeds

Number	Foods and Common Beliefs	Potential Functional Properties and Active Components
46	*Amygdalus communis* Almonds Provides energy and nourishment (Manisha et al., 2012)	Antiulcer, anti-HIV, anti-inflammatory, proliferative activities, antidiabetic (Wijeratne et al., 2006; Frison et al., 2002; Shah et al., 2011) Active components: protein, fat, phosphorus, magnesium, zinc, sitosterol, daucosterol, uridine and adenosine, betulinic, oleanic, and ursolic acids (Sang et al., 2002)
47	*Anacardium occidentale* Cashew Galactagogue (Manisha et al., 2012.)	Active components: protein, fats, magnesium, zinc (NIN, 2014)

(Continued)

TABLE 29.3 (*Continued*)

Traditional Postpartum Foods in India: Beliefs and Scientific Evidence

Number	Foods and Common Beliefs	Potential Functional Properties and Active Components
48	*Vitis vinifera* Raisins Reduces body temperature Laxative Provides iron (Manisha et al., 2012.)	Antioxidant (Ghrairi et al., 2012); cardioprotective (Barnes et al., 2011) Active components: iron, flavonoids, fiber (Kaliora et al., 2009)
49	*Cocos nucifera* Coconut Coconut oil Uterine wound healing Increase weight of the mother (Manisha et al., 2012.)	Wound healing (Srivastava and Durgaprasad, 2008); aphrodisiac, controls hemorrhoids, scabies, eczema, freckles, mange, mucolytic, antipsychotic, antiulcers, hypocholesterolemic (Saganuwan, 2010); immunomodulatory (Vigila and Baskaran, 2008); oil strengthens bones and muscles (Hayatullina, 2012); digestive health (Nevin and Rajamohan, 2010) Active components: fat, iron, potassium, magnesium, chlorine, protein, fatty acids, fiber, citric acid (Saganuwan, 2010)
50	*Sesamum indicum* Gingelly/sesame Sesame seeds Recovering from menstrual bleeding and irregular menstrual cycle (Chmielowska and Shih, 2007; Manisha et al., 2012)	Wound healing (Kiran and Asad, 2008); antianalgesic, antidepressant, bone strengthening, muscle strengthening, antihypertensive (Jhon Shi et al., 2011) Active components: folic acid, phosphorus, magnesium, copper, calcium, iron, zinc, vitamin B, vitamin E, polyunsaturated fatty acids, antioxidants (Matsumura et al., 1998; Miyawaki et al., 2009; Jhon Shi et al., 2011)
51	*Areca catechu L.* Betel nut Prevents urinary infections (Manisha et al., 2012)	Antihelmintic (Thomas et al., 2007); antioxidant, anti-inflammatory/antimelanogenisis, hypoglycemic, antihypertensive, α-glucosidase inhibitory and hypoglycemic, hypolipidemic, antihypertensive, vascular-relaxation, antidepressant, wound healing, antimicrobial, antiradical capacity, antiallergic, central nervous system stimulant, anti-HIV activity, molluscicidal activity (Senthilamudhan et al., 2012) Active components: polyphenols, alkaloid, fat (Senthilamudhan et al., 2012); calcium, phosphorus, iron, vitamin B_6 and vitamin C, (Ragavan 1958); arecoline (Thomas et al., 2007); phenolics and antioxidants (Sreeramulu and Raghunath, 2011)
52	*Phoenix dactylifera* Date fruit Prevents hemmorhage Increases iron content in blood (Kanwar and Sharma, 2010)	Antioxidant, antimutagenic, antimicrobial, anti-inflammatory, gastroprotective, hepatoprotective, nephroprotective, anticancer, immunostimulant, strengthens uterus muscles (Baliga et al., 2011); arrests postpartum hemorrhage (Khadeem et al., 2007) Active Components: iron, serotonin, anthocyanins, phenolics, sterols, carotenoids, procyanidins, and flavonols (Baliga et al., 2011)
53	*Lepidium sativum L.* Garden cress Galactagogue Nourishing Regain energy Strengthen bones (Chopra et al., 1996; Pullaiah, 2006)	Hypoglycemic, antioxidants, laxative, mucoprotective, aphrodisiac, carminative, galactagogue, and emmenagogue (Nadkarni, 2007); hypoglycemic activity (Eddouks et al., 2005); antihypertensive and diuretic (Maghrani, 2005) Active components: protein, fat, iron, phosphorus, calcium, fiber, niacin, magnesium, antioxidants, phenolics (Agarwal and Sharma, 2013)

(*Continued*)

TABLE 29.3 (*Continued*)

Traditional Postpartum Foods in India: Beliefs and Scientific Evidence

Number	Foods and Common Beliefs	Potential Functional Properties and Active Components
		Herbs
54	*Asparagus recemosus†* Shathavari Galactagogue Uterine tonic Maintains health Provides energy (Shahin and Ahmad, 2014; Awadesh et al., 2008; Manisha et al., 2012; Ajesh and Kumuthakalavalli, 2012)	Galactagogue (Tabares et al., 2014); antihepatotoxic and immunomodulatory (Goyal et al., 2003); antioxidant (Kamat et al., 2000) Active components: induces prolactin (Gupta and Show,. 2011); shatavarine (Tabares et al., 2014)
55	*Azadirachta indica* Neem leaves Prevents uterine infections Prevents abdominal itching Controls excessive menstrual bleeding (Awadesh et al., 2008; Manisha et al., 2012; Ajesh and Kumuthakalavalli, 2012)	Antipyretic, anti-inflammatory, antiviral, antibacterial, antifungal antimalarial, diuretic (Pant et al., 1986; Biswas et al., 2002); immunomodulatory (Ray et al., 1996; Sen et al., 1992) Active compounds: cyclic trisulphide (Siddiqui, 1942); cyclic tetrasulphide (Mitra, 1963); irodin A (WHO 2008; Anyaehie, 2009); azadiractin, meliantriol, salannin, nimbin, nimbidin (National Research Council, 1992)
56	*Piper betle* Betel leaves Wound healing (Prasad and Aggarwal et al., 2011)	Digestion-stimulating, aromatic, carminative (Shi et al., 2011); antidiabetic, antiproliferative, and antinociceptive (Arambewela et al., 2005); phenolics with antimutagenic, antitumor, and antioxidant activities (Paranjpe et al., 2013) Active components: iron, β-carotene, magnesium, copper, manganese, zinc, phenols, hydroxychavicol, and chavibetol (Paranjpe et al., 2013)

wound healing and prevention of bleeding, preventing infections, improving immunity, strengthening of muscles and bones, and nourishment. They correlate strongly with the most common postpartum morbidity conditions faced by Indian women and women in other parts of the world.

- A large number of studies have been reported in the literature examining the functions of various foods included in ethnic Indian postpartum care. Some of them have helped disprove beliefs held regarding adverse effects of foods leading to their exclusion. However, interestingly, no studies have been found that invalidate a belief regarding a specific potential functional property of a food. This indicates that there was likely a highly evolved understanding of human anatomy, physiology, and healthcare in ancient India, as well as the nature of foods and their compatibility with the body of a lactating mother even as she recovered from pregnancy and delivery.
- Predominantly, the consumed foods are cereals, spices, herbs, pulses, nuts, and dairy products. There is a clear lack of green leafy vegetables and fruits in the consumed foods.
- During postpartum care, some foods are used widely irrespective of geographic diversity in the country (marked by the symbol †). These foods are of two types: staple foods such as rice or wheat, and foods that are specifically included in postpartum care. Examples of the latter are milk and ghee (clarified butter), garlic, fenugreek, turmeric, Bishop's weed, dried ginger, black and long pepper, cumin, betel leaves, areca nut and lime, and jaggery (i.e., brown sugar from sugarcane/palm instead of white sugar). Though these foods are consumed normally, they are consumed in larger quantities during postpartum care due to

strong beliefs that they enable specific functions. On the other hand, many of the consumed foods are used only in specific regions, as seen in Table 29.4 and in the diversity of the sample postpartum menus presented in Section 29.4.

TABLE 29.4
Potential Functional Foods in Traditional Indian Postpartum Care

Functions	Basis	Food	Food Formulations and Supplements
Galactagogue	Clinical studies	*Moringa oleifera*/drumstick leaves (Raguindin et al., 2014)	*Boiled vegetables/soups*
		Trigonella foenum graecum/fenugreek leaves and seeds (Turkyilmaz et al., 2011; Gabay, 2002; Mortel and Mehta, 2013)	*Methi dosa/methi paratha, decoctions, spice in foods*
		Asparagus recemosus/shathavari wild (Gupta and Shaw, 2011)	*In powder form mixed with milk*
	In vivo studies	*Trigonella foenum graecum*/fenugreek seeds (Tabares et al., 2014)	*Methi dosa/methi paratha, decoctions, spice in foods*
		Nigella sativa L./black cumin seeds (Hosseinzadeh et al., 2013)	*Decoction*
		Foenicum vulgare/fennel seed (Mills and Bone, 2000; Shah et al., 1991; Abascal and Yarnell, 2008)	
		Pimpinella anisum L./anise seed (Hosseinzadeh et al., 2014; Eiben et al., 2004)	
		Allium sativum/garlic (Nice, 2011)	*Many food formulations*
	In vitro studies	*Trigonella foenum graecum*/fenugreek seeds (Sreeja et al., 2010)	*Seeds in boiled and powdered form*
Wound Healing, Preventing Infections, and Improving Immunity	Clinical studies	*Momordica charantia*/bitter gourd (Palamthodi and Lele, 2014; Ramalingum and Mahomoodally, 2014; Majumdar and Debnath, 2014)	*Boiled vegetables*
		Nigella sativa/black cumin seeds (Paarkh, 2010)	*Decoction*
	In vivo studies	*Lagenaria siceraria*/bottle gourd (Deshpande et al., 2008)	*Boiled vegetables*
		Sesamum indicum L./sesame seeds and oil (Kiran and Asad 2008; Joshi et al., 2005; Saleem et al., 2012)	*Seasoning and sweets*
		Curcuma longa/turmeric (Suryanarayana et al., 2003; Arun and Nalini, 2002; Mahady, 2002; Chattopadhyay, 2004; Misra and Sahu, 1977; Kurup and Barrios, 2007)	*Seasoning*
		Azadirachta indica/neem leaves (Biswas et al., 2002; Ray et al., 1996; Sen et al., 1992)	*Paste*
		Allium sativum/garlic (Jalali et al., 2009; Harris et al., 2001)	*Many food formulations*

(Continued)

TABLE 29.4 (*Continued*)
Potential Functional Foods in Traditional Indian Postpartum Care

Functions	Basis	Food	Food Formulations and Supplements
		Sesamum indicum L./sesame seeds and oil (Kiran and Asad, 2008; Saleem et al., 2012; Joshi et al., 2005)	*Seasoning and sweets*
		Cocos nucifera/coconut (Srivastava and Durgaprasad, 2008; Vigil and Baskaran, 2008)	*Seasoning*
		Sesbania grandiflora/agathi leaves (Nataraj et al., 2012; Arunabha and Satish, 2014)	*Boiled vegetables/soups*
		Moringa oleifera/drumstick (Ramalingum and Mahomoodally, 2014)	*Boiled vegetables/soups*
		Nigella sativa/black cumin seeds (Ersahin et al., 2011; Alsaif, 2008)	*Decoction*
	In vitro studies	*Murraya koenigii*/curry leaves (Handral et al., 2012; Shah and Juvekar, 2010)	*Seasoning, powder*
		Moringa oleifera/drumstick leaves (Marrufo et al., 2013: Busani et al., 2011; Moyo et al., 2012)	*Boiled vegetables/soups*
		Solanum nigrum/manathakali leaves and fruit (Saleem et al., 2009; Jain et al., 2011; Shanmugam et al., 2012; Chou et al., 2008)	*Boiled vegetables*
		Curcuma longa/turmeric (Mahady, 2002; Chattopadhyay, 2004)	*Many food formulations*
		Sesamum indicum L./sesame seeds and oil (Joshi et al., 2005)	*Seasoning and sweets*
		Oryza sativa/rice (Gammal et al., 2011)	*Staple food*
		Lagenaria siceraria/bottle gourd (Oragwa et al., 2013)	*Boiled vegetables*
		Moringa oleifera/drumstick (Siddhuraju and Becker 2003)	*Boiled vegetables/soups*
		Zingiber officinale/ginger and dried ginger (Mahady, 2005; Mishra et al., 2012)	*Paste, dried powder, seasoning, decoctions*
		Sesbania grandiflora/agathi leaves (Zarena et al., 2014; Nataraj et al., 2012; Gowri and Vasantha, 2010)	*boiled vegetables/soups*
		Piper nigrum/black pepper (Damanhouri and Ahmad, 2014; Majdalaweih and Carr, 2010)	*In rasam, concoctions, gravies*
Preventing Blood Loss and Anemia	Clinical studies	*Cicer arietinum*/chickpeas (Crujeiras et al., 2007)	*Boiled in gravy*
		Phoenix dactylifera/date fruit (Khadeem et al., 2007)	*Sweets*
	In vivo studies	*Murraya koenigii*/curry leaves (Handral et al., 2012)	*Seasoning, powder*

(Continued)

TABLE 29.4 (*Continued*)
Potential Functional Foods in Traditional Indian Postpartum Care

Functions	Basis	Food	Food Formulations and Supplements
		Nigella sativa/black cumin seeds (Erşahin et al., 2010; Asgary et al., 2012)	*Decoction*
		Cicer arietinum/chickpeas (Yang et al., 2007; Wang et al., 1996)	*Boiled in gravy*
	In vitro studies	Cow's milk (Unal, 2005)	*Sweet pudding, fluids*
		Murraya koenigii/curry leaves (Handral et al., 2012)	*Seasoning, powder*
		Moringa oleifera/drumstick leaves (Ilyas et al., 2015)	*Boiled vegetables/soups*
		Allium sativum/garlic (Zhang et al., 2008)	*Many food formulations*
		Piper Betel/betel leaves (Chakroborty and Shah, 2011)	*Betel leaf quid*
		Cicer arietinum/chickpeas (Jukanti et al., 2012)	*Boiled in gravy*
		Zingiber officinale/ginger (Ferri-Lagneau et al., 2012; Geng et al., 2012)	*Paste, dried powder, seasoning, decoction*
Strengthening of Bones and Muscles	Clinical studies	Fish/shark, catfish, anchovy, dried fish (Pierre and Zalloua et al., 2007)	*Steamed or shallow fat-fried pieces*
	In vivo studies	*Sesamum indicum L.*/sesame oil (Serra et al., 2011)	*Seasoning and sweets*
		Nigella sativa/black cumin seeds (Paarkh, 2010)	*Decoction*
		Cocos nucifera/coconut (Hayatullina, 2012)	*Fresh and dried forms*
	In vitro studies	Cow's milk (Unal, 2005)	*Sweet pudding, fluids*
		Gingelly/sesame oil (Serra et al., 2011)	*Seasoning and sweets*
		Cicer arietinum/chickpeas (Gruber and O'Brien, 2011; Jukanti et al., 2012)	*Boiled in gravy*
		Beta vulgaris/beetroot (Ninfali and Angelino, 2013)	*Boiled vegetables*
Enable Smooth Bowel Movement	Clinical studies	*Piper nigrum*/black pepper (Liu et al., 1997; Suseelappan, 1991)	*In rasam, concoctions, gravies*
		Foenicum vulgare/fennel seed (Srinivasjois, 2009)	*Decoctions*
		Cicer arietinum/chickpeas (Murty et al., 2010)	*Boiled in gravy*
	In vivo studies	*Ferula asafetida*/asafetida (Patel and Srinivasan 2006; Patel and Srinivasan 2002)	*Seasonings, powders*
		Trachyspermum ammi L./Bishop's weed (Krishnamoorthi and Madalageri, 1999)	*Decoctions*
		Nigella sativa/black cumin seeds (Paarkh, 2010)	*Decoctions*
		Cuminum cyminum/cumin seeds (Nadkarni, 2007; Chopra et al., 1996)	*Seasonings, decoctions, concoctions*

(Continued)

TABLE 29.4 (*Continued*)
Potential Functional Foods in Traditional Indian Postpartum Care

Functions	Basis	Food	Food Formulations and Supplements
		Piper nigrum/black pepper (Matsuda, 2008)	*Powder, concoctions, cushiness*
	In vitro studies	*Trachyspermum copticum L.*/Bishop's weed (Jabbar et al., 2006)	*Decoctions*
Strengthening the Nervous System	Clinical trial	*Phaseolus vulgaris L.*/beans (Bourdon et al., 2001)	*Soups, boiled vegetables*
		Nigella sativa/black cumin seeds (Leong et al., 2013; Paarkh, 2010)	*Decoctions*
	In vivo studies	*Solanum nigrum*/manathakali leaves and Fruit (Atanu and Ajayi, 2011)	*Boiled vegetables*
		Murraya koenigii/curry leaves (Handral et al., 2012)	*Seasoning, powder*
		Sesbania grandiflora/agathi leaves (Kasture et al., 2002)	*Boiled vegetables/soups*
		Phaseolus mungo; vigna radiata/green gram/mung bean (Tang et al., 2014)	*Gravy*
		Nigella sativa/black cumin seeds (Leong et al., 2013; Paarkh, 2010)	*Decoctions*
		Pimpinella anisum L./anise seed (Shojaii and Fard, 2012)	*Sweet balls*
		Moringa oleifera/drumstick leaves (Bakre et al., 2013)	*Boiled vegetables/soups*
		Lepidium sativum L./garden cress (Maghrani, 2005)	*Sweet balls*
	In vitro studies	*Moringa oleifera*/drumstick seeds (Anwar and Gilani, 2007)	*Boiled vegetables, soups*
		Cow's milk (Unal, 2005)	*Sweet pudding, fluids*
		Fish (Wu et al., 2008)	*Steamed, shallow fat-fried*
		Areca catechu/betel nut (Senthilamudhan et al., 2012)	*Betel leaf quid*
Antidepression and Antinociceptive	*In vivo* studies	*Coriandrum sativum*/corriander seeds (Rathore et al., 2012; Emamghoreishi and Heidari-Hamedani, 2005; Emamghoreishi et al., 2005)	*Boiled, dried, concoction*
		Allium sativum/garlic (Dhingra and Kumar, 2008)	*Many food formulations*
		Oryza sativa/rice (Caius, 1986)	*Staple food*
		Zingiber officinale/ginger and dried ginger (Lakshmi and Sudhakar, 2010; Felipe et al., 2008)	*Paste, dried powder, seasoning, decoctions*
		Papaver somniferum/poppy seeds (Kaplan, 1994)	*Sweet porridge, concoction*
		Nigella sativa/black cumin seeds (Perveen et al., 2009)	*Decoction*

(*Continued*)

TABLE 29.4 (*Continued*)
Potential Functional Foods in Traditional Indian Postpartum Care

Functions	Basis	Food	Food Formulations and Supplements
		Areca catechu/betel nut (Abbas et al., 2013; Dar et al., 1997)	*Betel leaf quid*
		Moringa oleifera/drumstick leaves (Kirisattayakul et al., 2009)	*Boiled vegetables/soups*
		Sesamum indicum/sesame seed oil (Kumar et al., 2011a)	*Many food formulations*
		Trigonella foenum-gracum/fenugreek seeds (Gaur et al., 2012; Khursheed et al., 2014)	*Methi dosa/methi paratha, decoctions, spice in foods*
	In vitro studies	*Moringa oleifera*/drumstick leaves (Asiedu-Gyekye et al., 2014)	*Boiled vegetables/soups*
		Areca catechu L./betel nut (Senthilamudhan et al., 2012)	*Betel leaf quid*
		Curcuma longa/turmeric (Ahmad et al., 2008 and references therein)	*Many food formulations*

- The information in "the "Foods and Common Beliefs" and "Potential Functional Properties and Active Components" columns is not always necessarily from the same sources. This indicates a major gap in the literature that has to be actively filled by future research.
- While the many studies cited in Table 29.3 show clear evidence that traditional foods have significant nutritive value and are useful in promoting health, it remains equally true that more than 50% of women suffer from anemia, one-third of married women have BMI less than 18.5 kg/m^2, and more than 60% of children suffer from food deficiency, which impacts their weight-for-age and height-for-age measurements. This is a major contradiction; it indicates that the traditional knowledge is not practiced sufficiently and that nutritional supplements prescribed for postpartum women are not consumed properly.
- One of the common observations is that certain foods are specifically avoided based on traditional beliefs. This is based on classification of foods as "hot" or "cold." It is believed that pregnancy is a state of hotness and that delivery renders the body in a colder state. Therefore "cold" foods are avoided during postpartum period (Rao et al., 2014). A scientific basis for avoiding specific foods during the postpartum period does not exist currently. Examining if certain foods cause postpartum morbidity is an open problem.
- In the case of some of the avoided foods and practices, probable causes may be found from a historical perspective. In the past, infections from food were most commonly contracted through water and foods that are vulnerable to infestation with worms and insects. The most vulnerable groups for such infections were lactating mothers, infants, and children. This could be one of the reasons why juicy foods such as fruits, and many vegetables including *Abelmoschus esculentus* (okra or ladies finger), *Solanum melongena* (brinjal or eggplant), and *Trichosanthes cucumerina* (snake gourd) are avoided. This could also be a reason to restrict water intake in the postpartum period, a common practice across India. Further, increased consumption of water would fill the bladder quickly resulting in the need for frequent micturition. In the past, given the lack of toilets in households, postpartum women had to walk long distances for micturition and defecation, both of which were

considered risky, especially at night. This was also a cause for giving less food to post-partum women in order to minimize bowel movement. Even today, communities believe that postpartum women may be affected by the evil eye when venturing outside (Rao et al., 2014).

29.3.2 Functional Foods in Traditional Indian Postpartum Care

Based on Table 29.3, it may be seen that many of the traditional foods in Indian postpartum care have been found to possess significant health benefits. For a lactating mother, these foods are used to nourish and strengthen her and the infant. On the other hand, there are common postpartum morbidities. It is possible to mitigate these morbidities by well-designed nutritional interventions, where specific traditional foods serve as functional foods. Recognizing exact roles played by the foods in mitigating morbidities and designing nutritional interventions are open research problems. However, as a first step, based on an analysis of the existing literature on postpartum morbidities and on ethnic postpartum foods, beliefs, and practices, eight food functions in postpartum care are postulated below:

- Nourishment
- Wound healing/preventing infection/improving immunity
- Preventing blood loss and anemia
- Strengthening muscles and bones
- Strengthening nervous system
- Strengthening digestive system
- Galactagogue
- Antidepressant

Through the above functions, a paradigm is sought to be framed for classifying ethnic Indian postpartum foods as functional foods by mapping the needs arising from postpartum morbidity conditions with the various functions that these foods can serve. A schematic depicting this is presented in Figure 29.2. Based on the available clinical studies, *in vivo* studies, *in vitro* studies, and determination of active ingredients, the foods surveyed in Table 29.3 are now classified as functional foods in Table 29.4. A food may be classified as a functional food only when there is a clinical validation of its food function. However, it must be emphasized that a broader definition of functional foods is adopted in this classification. Table 29.4, taken together with Table 29.3, immediately shows the vast potential for research in identifying and establishing food functions, determining the active ingredients that are responsible for the observed food functions, and their biological mechanisms of action. Of the eight food functions, nourishment is the fundamental requirement for a postpartum mother. Some of the main sources of the various macro- and micronutrients in traditional Indian postpartum diets are listed later in the chapter (see Box 29.1, Section 29.4). However, since all foods provide nourishment in some form or the other, studies establishing the function of nourishment have not been specifically sought.

Tables 29.4 also lists some of the traditional postpartum food formulations that use these foods. Recipes of selected formulations are presented in Section 29.4. Based on these formulations, sample menus for the day may be arrived at for regions with rice-based staple foods and wheat-based staple foods. These menus are presented and discussed in Section 29.4. They may be considered as the basis for estimating the average nutritional status available for lactating mothers consuming traditional postpartum diets in India. This is likely to be true especially for urban women and those who work moderately to heavily. An analysis of the nutritive content of the food provides a basis for evaluating the traditional food practices from the perspective of immunity and infection.

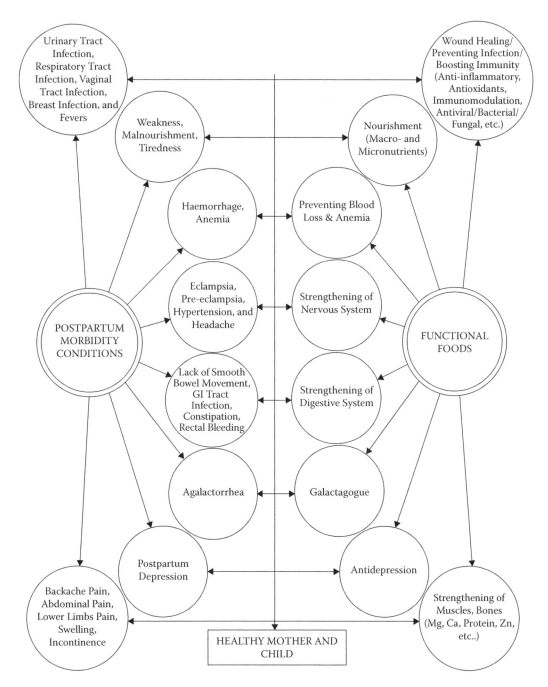

FIGURE 29.2 Different levels of the support system for maternal health care in India. (CSSM, Child Survival and Safe Motherhood Programme; JSY, Janani Suraksha Yojana; RCH, Reproductive and Child Health Programme; VMS, Vandemateram Scheme.)

BOX 29.1   TRADITIONAL INDIAN POSTPARTUM FOOD FORMULATIONS/SUPPLEMENTS

SWEET BALLS: Edible gum sweet balls (*Dink laddu*), Fenugreek sweet balls (*Methi laddu*), **Garden cress seeds (Aliv) sweet balls** (*Aliv laddu*), Ginger powder sweet balls (*Sonth laddu*), **Jaggery cheese sweet balls** (*Jaggery rasagulla*)

PUDDING / PORRIDGE: Wheat flour sweet porridge (*raab*), Rice pudding (*akki payasam*), Rice and chickpea pudding, *Asparagus recemosus* paste (*shathavari gulam herbal jam/ paste*), **Milk sweet pudding (poppy seeds or khas khas kheer)/almonds (badam kheer)** /tapioca sago/finger millet), *Morinda reticulata* thick porridge (neyvallikurukku), Coconut flower thick porridge (*pookkula kurukku*), Pulses and lentils mixed porridge (*navadhaniam kanji*), Condensed milk with dried ginger and nuts (*kharani*)

FLUIDS/CONCOCTIONS: Dill seeds concoction (sepyacha pani), Dill seeds and fenu-greek seeds water (suva methi pani), **Carom seeds (ajwain) water,** Fennel seeds (saunf) water, Carom and fennel seeds water (ajwain aur saunf ka pani), Barley and fennel water (jau aur saunf ka pani), Holy basil (tulsi) water, Cumin (jeera) water, **Black cumin seed concoction**, Indian gooseberry wine with jaggery (nellikka arishtam), Orange peel tea, Mint tea, Ginger tea, Corriander seeds and ginger tea, Bishop—weedtea, Almond (*badaam*) milk, Hot milk with turmeric, Hot milk with dried ginger, Hot milk with ajwain, Black pepper soup (*milagu rasam*), Cumin seeds soup (*jeeraga rasam*), **Long pepper soup (kandathippili rasam), Garlic soup (garlic rasam),** Tomato and pumpkin leaves soup (*tomato and pumpkin leaves rasam*), Neem soup (*neem rasam*), *Solanum nigrum* soup (*manathakali vathal rasam*), Moringa leaves soup (*murangai rasam*), Mutton soup (*Attin kaal soup*), Spice soup (*selavu rasam*)

DESSERTS: Carrom seeds dessert *(ajwain halwa)*, Finger millet dessert *(mandua ka halwa)*, Green gram dal dessert *(mung dal halwa)*, **Postpartum special supplements** (*ullilehyam*, **Prasava lehyam),** Spinach dessert (*amaranth halwa*), Bishop weed dessert (*ajwain halwa*), Lentils dessert (*lentils halwa*), Garlic dessert (*Poondu halwa*), Palm jaggery dessert (*karup-paty lehiyam*), Turmeric and neem leaves paste, Rice pudding, Harira (*Ginger powder, black pepper, nutmeg, turmeric, caraway, betel nut and molasses jam/paste*), **Wheat flour dessert (sheera),** Broken wheat and jaggery dessert (*Dalia kheer*)

MIXTURE/ POWDER: Panjiri (*whole-wheat flour fried in sugar and ghee, heavily laced with dried fruits and herbal gums*), Chutney powder *(bananti podi)*, Balanti kashaya powder (*energy drink powder*), Phakki (*postnatal delivery powder*), **Postnatal special chutney pow-der (angaya podi)** and (*Kalathu powder*), Bananti Podi-Chutney powder

MAIN COURSE RECIPES:

STAPLE FOODS: Boiled rice, Wheat bread (*chapathi*: unleavened wheat bread baked on a griddle, *paratha*: unleavened wheat bread fried on a griddle), Carom seeds fried breads (*ajwain paratha*), Spinach fried bread (*palak paratha*), Milk solids fried bread (*paneer paratha*), **Fenugreek fried breads** (*methi paratha*), Fenugreek leaves fried breads (*methi poori*—deep-fried in hot oil), Green gram dal and rice staple mixture (*mung dal vegetable kitcheri*), Parboiled rice porridge (*puzhungal arisi kanji*), Raw rice pancakes (*akki dosa*), Garlic rice, *Solanum nigrum* dried fruit gravy with rice, **Fenugreek pancake (dosa),** Fermented rice + black gram flour: steamed/pancakes (idli or dosa), Rice flour extrusion (*sevai*)

BOILED VEGETABLES, DAL, AND CURRIES: Black pepper curry (*milahu kozhambu*), Garlic curry (*poondu kuzhambu*), Curry leaves curry (*karuvapellai kozhambu*), Dal chutney (*paruppu thuvayal*), Puffed rice with banana, **Eggplant tender and neem leaves boiled vegetables**, Garlic and cloves salt pickle, Redgram dal, ***Moringa and Sesbania grandiflora* leaves boiled vegetables** (*drumstick leaves and agathi leaves poriyal*), Ivy gourd fry (*Tindora fry*), Dal and vegetable boiled mix (*Poricha kootu*), Tomato sweet chutney, Mung dal, Citron dried pickle (*Narthangai salt pickle*), **Bottle gourd boiled vegetables**, Yam and raw banana boiled and blended with spice (Mulagushiyam)

NON-VEGETARIAN FOODS: Dried anchovy fish, Shark fry, Egg, **Fish curry**, Red meat and liver curry/soup, Mutton soup (*Attin kaal soup*)

29.4   TRADITIONAL FOOD FORMULATIONS AND POSTPARTUM MENUS

The foods listed in Tables 29.3 and 29.4 are mainly consumed through many traditional food formulations/supplements, which form the postpartum menus for new mothers. Some of the common food formulations are listed in Table 29.4. Excluding the staple foods such as boiled rice, wheat breads (e.g., chapathi), boiled vegetables, and raw cut fruits, the remaining formulations may be classified into six types: sweet balls, pudding/porridge, fluids/concoctions, desserts, mixture/powder (dry), and main course recipes. Some of these traditional supplements are listed below in Box 29.1. A collection of standardized recipes for all these formulations and their analysis are beyond the scope of this chapter. However, to provide a sense of the types of formulations, their methods of preparation, and their potential food functions, recipes are presented for selected formulations (bold-faced), for which an estimation of the macro- and micronutrient content is also provided in Box 29.2. Note that the composition of the traditional food supplements in terms of their nutrient content is presented per 100 g of cooked weight. Ingredients whose quantities are less than 5 g have not been included in the estimation of nutritive content. The quantities of ingredients are approximately what are necessary for a daily serving. Unless otherwise specified, all the pulses are hulled and split. Chickpeas are consumed hulled but not split.

From the recipes, it may be seen that the food formulations/supplements involve a blend of spices and herbs, except in the case of sweet balls and porridges. All foods are generally bland with only mild ginger/pepper-based hotness. Oily and deep-fried foods are avoided, though ghee (clarified butter) is used extensively. Most of the foods are steamed, boiled, or grilled with ghee. White sugar is avoided whereas brown sugar or jaggery (from sugarcane or palm) is preferred. Sweets made of jaggery are consumed extensively. From a survey of literature as well as from interviews conducted with elderly Indian women (see Section 29.5), it is clear that many herbs are used extensively in traditional postpartum foods, though a detailed analysis of the same deserves separate studies.

BOX 29.2   RECIPES OF SELECTED TRADITIONAL INDIAN POSTPARTUM FOOD FORMULATIONS/SUPPLEMENTS

Note: *1 cup-60 g; ½ cup-30 g; 1 tsp-5 g; 1 tbsp-1 g:*

BOX 29.2A   RECIPE 1: EDIBLE GUM SWEET BALLS (DINK LADDU)

Origin/Practice: *East and North India*
Potential Food Function: *Wound healing*

Ingredients:

Dates: 12 g
Dried Coconut: 25 g
Cashews: 10 g
Almonds: 5 g
Raisins: 2.5 g
Edible Gum: 5 g
Poppy seeds: 1 tbsp (optional)
Cloves: 3
Nutmeg grated: ¼ tsp
Jaggery (powdered): 10 g
Ghee: 4 g

Procedure:

Deep fry the edible gums in ghee until they are light and puff up, and pound them into a fine paste.

Mix choped dates, raisins, toasted poppy seeds, almonds, cashews, dried coconut, ground cloves and nutmeg with fried edible gum.

Prepare the jaggery syrup; add it to the mixture to make tightly pressed balls.

Nutritive Value: Energy: 154 kcal; Protein: 1.38 g; Fat: 8 g; Calcium: 34 mg; Iron: 1.4 g; β-Carotene: 33 µg; Fiber: 0.5 g; Vit. C: 0.4 mg; Carbohydrates: 19 g.

(Continued)

BOX 29.2 (*Continued*)   RECIPES OF SELECTED TRADITIONAL INDIAN POSTPARTUM FOOD FORMULATIONS/SUPPLEMENTS)

BOX 29.2B   RECIPE 2: GARDEN CRESS SEEDS SWEET BALLS (ALIV LADDU)

Origin/Practice: East and North India
Potential Food Function: Galactagouge and nourishing

Ingredients:	Procedure:
Garden cress (aliv) seeds: 30 g; Grated fresh coconut: 20 g; Jaggery: 40 g; Almonds chopped: 5 g	Soak aliv seeds in coconut water for 2 hours. Add grated fresh coconut and jaggery, saute for a minute, and add soaked aliv seeds in a hot pan.
Cashew nuts chopped: 5 g	Cook over medium heat until thick. Add almonds,
Raisins: 4 g; Ghee: 10 g	cashew nuts, raisins, and cardamom powder and
Cardamom powder: ½ tsp	mix well.
	Stir until the mixture turns thick.
	Let it cool and press tightly into balls.

Nutritive Value: Energy: 324 kcal; Protein: 325 g; Fat: 134 g; Calcium: 156 mg; Iron: 11 g; Folic acid: 2.5 µg; β-Carotene: 11 µg; Fiber: 0.8 g; Vit. C: 0.2 mg; Carbohydrates: 45 g.

BOX 29.2C   RECIPE 3: JAGGERY CHEESE SWEET BALLS (JAGGERY RASAGULLA)

Origin/Practice: West India
Potential Food Function: Strengthning of the body

Ingredients:	Procedure:
Milk: 120 mL;	In a vessel, bring the milk to a boil. Add a tablespoon of lemon juice to it and mix until the milk curdles and separates.
Water: 1¾ cup; Jaggery: 50 g	
Lemon juice: 1½ tbsp	
A pinch of cardamom powder	Strain the paneer (milk solids) in a muslin cloth and squeeze the excess water.
	Kneed the paneer to make smooth pliable and make into small smooth round balls.
	Prepare jaggery syrup with water keep the syrup in medium flame, and add the rasagullas carefully. Serve chilled.

Nutritive Value: Energy: 216 kcal; Protein: 4 g; Fat: 5 g; Calcium: 120 mg; Iron: 2 g; Folic acid: 2.4 µg; β-Carotene: 64 µg; Fiber: 0 g; Vit. C: 2.4 mg; Carbohydrates: 53 g.

BOX 29.2D   RECIPE 4: SWEET MILK PUDDING (KHUS KHUS KHEER)

Origin/Practice: West India and North India
Potential Food Function: Analgesic: relieves abdominal pain

Ingredients:	Procedure:
Poppy seeds soaked: 20 g; Rice soaked: 20 g	Grind poppy seeds, rice, and coconut to a fine paste. Strain this paste. Heat milk, add sugar, while milk boils add the above paste and cardamom powder and stir well.
Grated coconut: 20 g	
Milk: 60 mL; Sugar: 20 g	
Ghee: 20 g; Cashew nuts broken: 4 - 6 nos	
Cardamom powder : ¼ tsp	Cook for 2-3 minutes. When the kheer becomes thick, add fried cashew nuts along with ghee and mix well.

Nutritive Value: Energy: 541 kcal; Protein: 10 g; Fat: 37 g; Calcium: 366 mg; Iron: 4 g; Folic acid: 6 µg; β-Carotene: 155 µg; Fiber: 2 g; Vit. C: 1.4 mg; Carbohydrates: 50 g.

(Continued)

BOX 29.2 (*Continued*)   RECIPES OF SELECTED TRADITIONAL INDIAN POSTPARTUM FOOD FORMULATIONS/SUPPLEMENTS)

BOX 29.2E   RECIPE 5: ALMOND MILK (BADAM MILK)

Origin/Practice: North India and West India
Potential Food Function: Provides energy and nourishment

Ingredients:	*Procedure:*
Almonds: 20 g; Milk: 200 mL; Sugar: 10 g Saffron, few strands; Green cardamom powder: ¼ tsp	Wash and soak almonds in lukewarm water and after 5 minutes peel the skin. Bring 2 cups of milk to a boil; add saffron, sugar, and cardamom powder. Simmer for 2 minutes.

Nutritive Value: Energy: 149 kcal; Protein: 9 g; Fat: 8 g; Calcium: 166 mg; Iron: 1.1 g; Folic acid: 30.4 µg; β-Carotene: 113.6 µg; Fiber: 0.18 g; Vit. C: 4 mg; Carbohydrates: 31 g.

BOX 29.2F   RECIPE 6: CAROM / BLACK CUMIN / DILL SEEDS CONCOCTION

Origin/Practice: All over India
Potential Food Function: Galactagouge, anti-inflammatory and analgesic

Ingredients:	*Procedure:*
Carom: 10 g (or) Black cumin seeds: 10 g (or) Dill seeds: 10 g Water: 200 mL	Clean black cumin seeds and fry the seeds in a pan. After 5 minutes grind it to coarse powder. Add two glasses of water and boil until it becomes one glass. Add a pinch of asafoetida and drink it hot. Same procedure can be followed with dill seeds or ajwain.

Nutritive Value: Energy: 36 kcal; Protein: 2 g; Fat: 1.5 g; Calcium: 108 mg; Iron: 1 g; β-Carotene: 52 µg; Fiber: 1.2 g; Vit. C: 0.3 mg; Carbohydrates: 4 g.

BOX 29.2G   RECIPE 7: (LONG PEPPER SOUP) KANDANTHIPPILI RASAM

Origin/Practice: South India
Potential Food Function: Anti-inflamatory and antioxidant

Ingredients:	*Procedure:*
Tamarind: half the size of a lemon; Salt: to taste; Pepper: 3 g; Cumin seeds: 3 g; Long pepper: 5 g; Red dal: 5 g; Dry red chilis: 1 no; Asafoetida: a pinch; Mustard seeds: ¼ tsp; Curry leaves: few Ghee: 10 g	Fry pepper, cumin seeds, kandathippili, red dal and red chili in a spoon of ghee till golden brown and grind to a powder. In a vessel, pour a cup of water, add tamarind, salt, and asafoetida and allow it to boil till raw smell of the tamarind is lost. Add the ground powder and bring it to a boil. Add 3 more cups of water and bring to a boil until frothy. In a small pan, heat ghee and temper it with mustard seeds and curry leaves and pour it over the rasam.

Nutritive Value: Energy: 136 kcal; Protein: 1.6 g; Fat: 10 g; Calcium: 74 mg; Iron: 4 g; Folic acid: 5 µg; β-Carotene: 70 µg; Fiber: 0.8 g, Vit. C: 0.1 mg; Carbohydrates: 10 g.

(Continued)

BOX 29.2 (*Continued*)   RECIPES OF SELECTED TRADITIONAL INDIAN POSTPARTUM FOOD FORMULATIONS/SUPPLEMENTS)

BOX 29.2H   RECIPES 8: GARLIC SOUP (GARLIC RASAM)

Origin/Practice: South India
Potential Food Function: Wound healing and galactagouge

Ingredients:	*Procedure:*
Tamarind: 5 g; Garlic: 10 g; Tomato juice: 10 mL	Dry grind whole black pepper, cumin seeds, and 1 garlic clove. Take tamarind extract (about 1 cup), add chopped tomatoes, salt, curry leaves, whole peeled garlic, crushed garlic, and the coarsely ground powder. Boil over low flame until it thickens a little and the raw smell of the tamarind goes. Then add 1 ½–1 ¾ cup of water. Boil until it froths at the top. Before removing, add ghee.
Whole black pepper: 1 tsp	
Cumin seeds: 3 g; Red dal: 5 g	
Ghee: 5 g; Mustard: ½ tsp	
Cumin / jeera seeds: ½ tsp; Curry leaves: few	
Coriander leaves: finely chopped	
Salt as required	

Nutritive Value: Energy: 92 kcal; Protein: 2 g; Fat: 5 g; Calcium: 20 mg; Iron: 1.2 g; Folic acid: 8.2 μg; β-Carotene: 75 μg; Fiber: 0.5 g; Vit. C: 20 mg; Carbohydrates: 9.6 g.

BOX 29.2I   RECIPE 9: POSTPARTUM SPECIAL PREPRATION (PRASAVA LEHIYAM)

Origin/Practice: South India
Potential Food Function: Anti-inflamatory, wound healing, and antioxidant

Ingredients:	*Procedure:*
Rice, Long pepper (Arisithippli): 10 sticks	Sieve the powder. Slightly heat it in a frying pan. Mix a little water to form dough.
Dry ginger: small piece; Basil: 100 g Pepper: ½ tablespoon	Take equal quantity of jaggery. Dissolve jaggery in a ladle of water and filter it. Now heat a heavy bottomed pan, add the dough and jaggery and stir well.
Coriander seeds: ½ tablespoon Cardamom: 2 or 3; Jaggery: 100 g; Ghee: 25 g	When half done and thick, add oil and ghee. Stir continuously and make small balls out of it, and consume a ball after the meal.

Nutritive Value: Energy: 608 kcal; Protein: 0.4 g; Fat: 25 g; Calcium: 80 mg; Iron: 3 g; Folic acid: 0 μg; β-Carotene: 150 μg; Fiber: 0 g; Vit. C: 0 mg; Carbohydrates: 95 g.

Note: This is a simple version of the supplement. There are significant variations in the recipe in different cultures and parts of India. This is a supplement where many herbs are added.

(Continued)

BOX 29.2 (*Continued*)   RECIPES OF SELECTED TRADITIONAL INDIAN POSTPARTUM FOOD FORMULATIONS/SUPPLEMENTS)

BOX 29.2J   RECIPE 10: WHEAT FLOUR DESSERT (SHEERA)

Origin/Practice: South, North and West India
Potential Food Function: Nourishment

Ingredients:	*Procedure:*
Wheat flour: 50 g Ghee: 30 g; Sugar: 50 g Milk: 100 mL Almonds: 2 nos chopped; Cashews: 4g Cardamom powder: 1 tsp	Heat ghee and fry almonds and cashews. Set aside. Add the wheat flour in the ghee and fry it on low flame until it changes color to a dull pinkish and becomes fragrant. Add the hot milk slowly while stirring so as to avoid lumps. Add all the milk, stir well, and cover to let it cook for about 5 minutes on very low flame. Add sugar, almonds, cashews, saffron, and cardamom powder, stir well, and cover for a minute or two until cooked.

Nutritive Value: Energy: 707 kcal; Protein: 9 g; Fat: 35 g; Calcium: 150 mg; Iron: 2.7 g; Folic acid: 26 µg; β-Carotene: 248 µg; Fiber: 1 g; Vit. C: 2 mg; Carbohydrates: 89 g.

BOX 29.2K   RECIPE 11: BROKEN WHEAT DESSERT (DALIYA KHEER)

Origin/Practice: Many regions of North and West India
Potential Food Function: Nourishment

Ingredients:	*Procedure:*
Broken wheat: 30 g; Milk: 120 mL; Water: 3-4 cups; Jaggery: 30 g; Powdered cardamom: ½ tsp; Ghee: 10 g; Cashew: 5 g; Raisins: 5 g.	Wash broken wheat with water, pressure cook it thoroughly mash and cool it. Heat 2 cups milk in a saucepan. Add powdered jaggery and cardamom to the milk. Add the wheat, stir and boil continuously until the jaggery has melted. Roast cashews and raisins in ghee and add it to the kheer.

Nutritive Value: Energy: 378 kcal; Protein: 7 g; Fat: 17 g; Calcium: 134 mg; Iron: 2.0 g; Folic acid: 6 µg; β-Carotene: 127 µg; Fiber: 0.2 g; Vit. C: 2.5 mg, Carbohydrates: 63 g.

(Continued)

**BOX 29.2 (*Continued*)   RECIPES OF SELECTED TRADITIONAL
INDIAN POSTPARTUM FOOD FORMULATIONS/SUPPLEMENTS)**

BOX 29.2L   RECIPE 12: FENUGREEK PANCAKE (DOSA)

Origin/Practice: South India
Potential Food Function: Galactagouge and smooth bowel movement

Ingredients:	*Procedure:*
Parboiled rice: 100 g	Wash and soak the rice; wash and soak the black gram dal, red dal, and fenugreek seeds together for 3-4 hrs.
Fenugreek seeds: 20 g	
Black gram dal: 25 g	
Red dal: 10 g	First add black gram dal, red dal, and fenugreek seeds for 10 mins before adding soaked rice. Grind it to smooth batter with required water and salt.
Salt and water as needed	
	Let it ferment for 7 hours or overnight.
	Pour it as pancake.

Nutritive Value: Energy: 533 kcal; Protein: 20 g; Fat: 2.1 g; Calcium: 87 mg; Iron: 3.5 g; Folic acid: 71 µg; β-Carotene: 42 µg; Fiber: 2 g; Vit. C: 0 mg; Carbohydrates: 108.5 g.

BOX 29.2M   RECIPE 13: FENUGREEK FRIED BREADS (PARATHA)

Origin/Practice: North and West India
Potential Food Function: Galactagouge and smooth bowel movement

Ingredients:	*Procedure:*
Wheat Flour: 60 g	Crush garlic and ginger and make it a paste.
Fenugreek leaves: 30 g	Wash and chop the fenugreek leaves and keep them aside. Heat 2 teaspoons of oil in a pan. Add the cumin seeds and fry for a few seconds, add the ginger garlic paste and fry for a few seconds.
Garlic: 5 g	
Cumin seeds: 3 g	
Turmeric powder: 1 g	
Oil; Salt to taste.	Add chopped fenugreek leaves and turmeric powder and turn off the flame and let it cool.
	Take the flour, salt, and fenugreek mixture in a bowl and combine. Make smooth and pliable dough.
	Roll each ball into a circle. Heat a gridle and place the paratha with small quantity of oil until cooked.

Nutritive Value: Energy: 230 kcal; Protein: 9 g; Fat: 1 g; Calcium: 212 mg; Iron: 3 g; Folic acid: 79 µg; β-Carotene: 725 µg; Fiber: 0.9 g; Vit. C: 16 mg; Carbohydrates: 39 g.

(Continued)

BOX 29.2 (*Continued*)   RECIPES OF SELECTED TRADITIONAL INDIAN POSTPARTUM FOOD FORMULATIONS/SUPPLEMENTS)

BOX 29.2N   RECIPE 14: EGGPLANT TENDER NEEM LEAVES BOILED VEGETABLES

Origin/Practice: Many regions of South India
Potential Food Function: Anti-inflammatory

Ingredients:	*Procedure:*
Eggplant: 120 g	Marinate the chopped eggplant cubes with turmeric powder and salt for 8 to 10 minutes. Heat oil in pan and fry the eggplant until turns to brown color and set aside. Fry the neem leaves over low heat until they turn brown. Mix and mash the fried brinjal with neem leaves and serve.
Tender neem leaves: 4 g	
Mustard oil: 1 tbsp; Turmeric powder: 1g Salt to taste	

Nutritive Value: Energy: 378 kcal; Protein: 7 g; Fat: 17 g; Calcium: 134 mg; Iron: 2 g; Folic acid: 5.7 µg; β-Carotene: 127 µg; Fiber: 0.2 g; Vit. C: 2.5 mg; Carbohydrates: 63 g.

BOX 29.2O   RECIPE 15: MORINGA AND SESBANIA GRANDIFLORA BOILED VEGETABLES (PORIYAL)

Origin/Practice: Many regions of South India
Potential Food Function: Nourishmment and galactagogue

Ingredients:	*Procedure:*
Peanut oil: 3 mL; Mustard seeds: 2 g	Heat oil in a pan; add in the mustard seeds, dry red chili, and black gram dal. Wait until the dal turns golden brown. Add in the finely chopped onions and the salt. Saute until the onions are soft and slightly brown. Add in the cleaned, washed, and dried drumstick and agathi leaves. Saute in medium flame until the leaves are cooked and all the moisture has escaped. Add in the shredded coconut and saute briefly.
Hulled and split black gram dal: 4 g;	
Red chili: 1 no (for seasoning)	
Onion: 10 g	
Moringa leaves (drumstick leaves): 50 g	
Agathi leaves (sesbania grandiflora): 50 g	
Salt: to taste	
Shredded coconut: 10 g	

Nutritive Value: Energy: 143 kcal; Protein: 8.2 g; Fat: 5.7 g; Calcium: 790 mg; Iron: 2.7 g; Folic acid: 1.3 µg; β-Carotene: 6091 µg; Fiber: 2 g; Vit. C: 194 mg; Carbohydrates: 15 g.

(Continued)

BOX 29.2 (*Continued*)   RECIPES OF SELECTED TRADITIONAL
INDIAN POSTPARTUM FOOD FORMULATIONS/SUPPLEMENTS)

BOX 29.2P   RECIPE 16: BOTTLE GOURD BOILED VEGETABLES (SABZI)

Origin/Practice: South India
Potential Food Function: Galactagogue

Ingredients:

Bottle gourd: 50 g; Oil: 2 mL
Mustard: 2 g;
Hulled, split bengal gram dal: 10 g
Onion: 20 g
Red chili: 1 no
Curry leaves: 1 strand; Salt to taste

Procedure:

In a pan add oil and heat; when the mustard starts spluttering add chopped onion, and one whole red chili, curry leaves and bengal gram dal, fry until the onion is golden brown color. Add the chopped bottle gourd, turmeric, and salt. Add ¼ cup of water and mix them well. Cook this for about 10 to 15 min until the vegetable is cooked and the water is completely drained.

Nutritive Value: Energy: 77 kcal; Protein: 2 g; Fat: 0.6 g; Calcium: 26 mg; Iron: 1.6 g; Folic acid: 16 µg; β-Carotene: 13 µg; Fiber: 1 g; Vit. C: 2.3 mg; Carbohydrates: 9 g.

BOX 29.2Q   RECIPE 17: FISH CURRY

Origin/Practice: Many parts of South India, East and North India
Potential Food Function: Galactagouge, rich in polyunsaturated fatty acids and proteins

Ingredients:

Fish: 250 g; Lemon juice: 4 mL
Turmeric powder: 2 g; Salt: to taste
Mustard oil: 20 mL; Mustard seeds: 2 g
Black cumin seeds: 4 g; Red chili: 1 no
Bay leaf: 1 no; Ginger paste: 5 g
Garlic paste: 10 g; Onions chopped: 50 g
Mustard paste: 5 g; Coriander powder: 5 g
Fresh coriander leaves chopped: 5 g

Procedure:

Marinate fish fillets with lemon juice, half a teaspoon of turmeric powder, and salt for half an hour. Heat two tablespoons of oil in a pan and shallow fry fish pieces on both sides until slightly browned.

Heat remaining oil in the same pan, add mustard seeds, onion, whole red chili, and bay leaf and add ginger garlic paste. Add chopped onions and cook until slightly brown in color. Add mustard paste and coriander powder. Stir and cook masala until oil starts separating. Add two cups of water and salt bring to a boil and then add shallow fried fish.

Nutritive Value: Energy: 642 kcal; Protein: 46 g; Fat: 37 g; Calcium: 1805 mg; Iron: 4.5 g; Folic acid: 4.5 µg; β-Carotene: 447 µg; Fiber: 4.3 g; Vit. C: 86 mg; Carbohydrates: 28 g.

(*Continued*)

BOX 29.2 (*Continued*)   RECIPES OF SELECTED TRADITIONAL INDIAN POSTPARTUM FOOD FORMULATIONS/SUPPLEMENTS)

BOX 29.2R   RECIPE 18–ANGAYA PODI

Origin: South India
Potential Food Function: Galactagogue, anti-inflammatory

Ingredients:	*Procedure:*
Cumin seeds: 15 g; Coriander seeds: 10 g; Black pepper: 3 g; Dry ginger powder: 4 g; Red dal: 30 g; Bengal gram: 10 g; Black gram: 10 g; Mustard seeds: 2 g; Asafoetida: 2 g; Dried *Solanum thorvum* fruit: 10 g; Dry neem flowers: 10 g; Dried *Solanum nigrum* fruit: 1 cup; Salt as required	Dry roast all the ingredients separately and grind together into a fine powder. Mix with hot rice and serve.

Nutritive Value: Energy: 282 kcal; Protein: 16 g; Fat: 5.3 g; Calcium: 307 mg; Iron: 6.4 g; Folic acid: 62 µg; β-Carotene: 274 µg; Fiber: 7.5 g; Vit. C: 0.6 mg; Carbohydrates: 42.4 g.

BOX 29.2S   RECIPE 19–PANJEERI

Origin: North India
Potential Food Function: Galactagogue

Ingredients:	*Procedure:*
Ghee: 30 mL; Edible gum (gondh) crystals: 10 g; Puffed lotus seeds (makhana): 10 g; Wheat flour: 15 g; Semolina: 4 g; Sugar: 30 g; Almonds: 30 g; Ginger powder/carom seed powder/fennel seed powder/cardamom powder: 4 g (optional)	Heat part of the ghee in a deep pan. Fry the makhana and gondh (separately). Grind the gondh and makhana (separately) to coarse powders. Heat the remaining ghee, add the wholemeal flour and semolina. Stir continuously in medium flame and cook until the mixture is pale golden in color. When the flour and semolina are fully roasted, add all the other ingredients (including the fried and ground gondh and makhana). Mix well and turn off the heat.

Nutritive Value: Energy: 564 kcal; Protein: 14 g; Fat: 32 g; Calcium: 404 mg; Iron: 6 g; Folic acid: 5 µg; β-Carotene: 221 µg; Fiber: 4 g; Vit. C: 0.9 mg; Carbohydrates: 54 g.

29.5   AN EVALUATION OF ETHNIC INDIAN POSTPARTUM NUTRITIONAL PRACTICES

This section analyses the information collated and presented in Section 29.4. A preliminary evaluation of how the foods discussed in Section 29.4 together provide the required nutrition for a lactating mother is presented in Section 29.5.1. This evaluation is based on a comparison with the RDA for Indian mothers (Section 29.2; NIN, 2014). Four sample postpartum menus have been chosen based on interviews of 32 elderly Indian women (age range: 60–80 years) for whom traditional postpartum care was given, and who have given traditional postpartum care to their children. As per the modified Kuppuswamy's socioeconomic scale (Bairwa et al., 2013), all the women interviewed were either in the upper middle or upper class. Section 29.5.2 specifically lists the foods rich in macro- and micronutrients present in these traditional formulations, while Section 29.5.3 discusses how these foods help in improving immunity and preventing infection.

29.5.1 AN EVALUATION OF TRADITIONAL POSTPARTUM MENUS BASED ON RDA

This subsection presents four sample traditional Indian postpartum menus (Table 29.5) using the recipes presented in Section 29.4. Two of the menus are from southern India (Tamil Nadu) and the other two are from western (Maharashtra) and eastern (West Bengal) parts of India, respectively.

TABLE 29.5
Sample Traditional Indian Daily Postpartum Menus

One Day Traditional Postpartum Model Menus

Southern Indian Vegetarian		South Indian Nonvegetarian	
Time	Menu	Time	Menu
Prebreakfast	Cow's milk, postpartum special preparation (prasava lehiyam), black cumin seeds concoction with jaggery	Prebreakfast	Cow's milk, palm jaggery ball, (jaggery, dried ginger, garlic)
Breakfast	Fenugreek dosa with ghee and sugar	Breakfast	Idli, coconut chutney, ghee, and sugar
Lunch	Rice, carrot, and beans boiled vegetables, long pepper rasam, *Solanum nigrum* dried fruit fried in ghee and mixed with rice, fried papad, buttermilk, betel leaf quid (betel leaves, lime and arecanut), citron dry pickle.	Lunch	Rice, mung dal with ghee, garlic rasam, bottle gourd boiled vegetables, drumstick leaves and *Sesbania* leaves boiled, curd, and betel leaf quid
Evening	Tea	Evening	Fried fish/dried fish
Dinner	Cow's milk and rice	Dinner	Milk and rice
Note: The above-mentioned recipes is with reference to vegeterian southern Indian Iyer and Iyengar menu		Note: The above-mentioned recipes is with reference to nonvegeterian southern Indian menu	
Western Indian Vegetarian		**Eastern Indian Nonvegetarian**	
Time	Menu	Time	Menu
Prebreakfast	Tea/coffee/milk, broken wheat porridge and milk with (almonds/ poppy seeds/ garlic/*Asparagus racemosus* powder)	Prebreakfast	Cow's milk
Breakfast	Sheera, garlic chutney powder	Breakfast	Chapathi, carrot, and potato boiled and seasoned vegetables, boiled egg
Lunch	White rice, wheat flour flat breads, red dal (soup of thin consistency), bottlegourd boiled vegetables, mung dal, ghee, and betel leaves quid (leaves, lime, arecanut)	Lunch	White rice, bitter gourd, egg plant fried with ghee and tender neem leaves, ghee, red dal, papaya, payasam rice with milk
Evening	Garden cress seeds/edible gum sweet ball, vavding decoction	Evening	Poori and bengal gram dal, carom seeds decoction
Dinner	Mung dal vegetable kitcheri, ghee, garlic chutney, rice, flattened wheat breads, seasoned, and cooked okra—*Abelmoschus esculentus*, dill seed decoction, boiled fenugreek seeds (after soaking)	Dinner	Rice, fish curry, jaggery rasagulla, tomato sweet chutney, dry nuts, almond milk.
Note: The above-mentioned recipes is with reference to vegeterian Maharashtrian Brahmin menu		Note: The above-mentioned recipes is with reference to nonvegeterian menu from West Bengal	

Similarly, two of the menus are vegetarian (without eggs, meat, and seafood), while the other two menus are nonvegetarian (with eggs and fish). Thus, these menus potentially provide some perspective of the diversity of ethnic postpartum nutritional practices in India. Based on the recipes and using the available data on the nutritive value of Indian foods (NIN, 2014), an estimation of macro- and micronutrients in the menus has been carried out. A comparison of the estimated nutritive content of the menus with the RDA for lactating mothers (0–6 months) is provided in Table 29.6.

It is seen that in all four menus there are five meals, with a prebreakfast and an evening snack in addition to breakfast, lunch, and dinner. Lunch is the heaviest meal, and milk is consumed multiple times in large quantities. Rice is the staple food in the southern Indian diet while wheat-based bread (e.g.,. chapathi, paratha) is in the western and eastern Indian diets. However, both also consume at least a small quantity of rice every day. Some of the commonly consumed foods include fenugreek (methi), garlic, jaggery (brown sugar), mung dal (*Vigna radiata*), and betel leaf quid with leaves, lime, and areca nut. Fish and eggs are the most common nonvegetarian foods consumed. Fruits are avoided significantly and green, leafy vegetables are consumed in lower quantity. Water, when consumed, is taken in the form of decoction with spices such as Bishop's weed (ajwain), dill seeds, cumin seeds, and black cumin seeds.

Fleshy foods are a good source of protein, iron, and other vitamins. Iron from the animal tissues such as meat, fish, and poultry helps to reduce postpartum hemorrhage. Polyunsaturated fatty acids in fish are the building blocks for breast milk, which helps to enhance milk secretion. The essential amino acids in egg and meat repair the damaged tissues. In the menus considered above, the only nonvegetarian menus that have been considered are egg- and fish-based.

Table 29.6 indicates that all the four menus contain excess fat, protein, calcium, and folic acid. Carbohydrate is lower than the recommended amount, except in the East Indian menu. However, the energy needs are met through the excess fat and protein content in the food. All four menus are highly deficient in fiber, for which < 50% of the RDA is met. Along with high consumption of iron (except in the South Indian vegetarian menu), this could be a reason for the constipation problems faced by lactating mothers in India. The southern Indian nonvegetarian (Kongu Nadu) menu emphasizes significant consumption of drumstick (Moringa oleifera) and Agathi leaves (Sesbania grandiflora). This is the reason for the large quantities of calcium, Vitamin C, and β-carotene available in that diet. In the nonvegetarian menus, fish provides a rich source of calcium, protein, and polyunsaturated fatty acids. Eggs are rich in proteins, fat, and folic acid. The vegetarian menus are highly deficient in Vitamin C, while the southern Indian vegetarian menu is also deficient in iron. The eastern and western Indian menus, on the other hand, are deficient in β-carotene. The existence

TABLE 29.6
Macro- and Micronutrients in the Traditional Indian Daily Postpartum Menus and Comparison with RDA

Nutrients	Southern Indian Veg	Western Indian Veg	Southern Indian Nonveg	Eastern Indian Nonveg	RDA (NIN, 2014)
Carbohydrates (g)	428	461	449	594	517
Protein (g)	98	109	150	148	75
Fat (g)	85	120	91	104	45
Fiber (g)	10	17	12	21	32*
Energy (kcal)	2860	2999	3209	3671	2775
Calcium (mg)	1902	1983	3278	1627	1000
Iron (mg)	18	30	28	34	30
β-Carotene (μg)	3794	2401	6393	1969	3800
Vit C (mg)	46	31	161	126	80
Folic Acid (μg)	305	225	301	281	150

* RDA for fiber is not available from NIN, 2014. This value has been adapted from USDA.

of any correlations between these nutritional deficiencies and the maternal and neonatal health status in these regions needs to be explored. To the best of our knowledge, only one study exists (Piers et al., 1995), in which an estimate of macronutrients consumed by 17 lactating mothers has been arrived at by recall method at 12 weeks postpartum. The intakes presented in Table 29.5 compare well with those reported therein.

The menus presented in Table 29.5 are representative of moderately working women from families of upper middle and upper socioeconomic classes (Bairwa et al., 2013) belonging to certain communities in the regions indicated. There exist significant variations in the postpartum food patterns of people belonging to different financial, social, and cultural backgrounds. These variations need to be explored in detail, as they would shed light on the diversity in the postpartum maternal health status of the country. On the other hand, the data presented here indicates the increasing tendency for obesity among new mothers in India. Some of the foods in the menus—particularly the sweet balls and puddings—are likely to be consumed more often only by women belonging to high-income families. However, in all traditions, there are significant differences between the regular and postpartum menus. For instance, tribal populations are known to use excess of long and short peppers, dried ginger, palm sugar, and garlic in their postpartum formulations either as sweet balls or soups. They also consume dried fish and betel leaf quids, and a number of herbs such as shatavari. Together with rice and an increased consumption of milk, such formulations should provide significant quantities of carbohydrates, proteins, and calcium. On the other hand, their menus could be deficient in many micronutrients. This also needs to be examined in further detail.

29.5.2 MACRO- AND MICRONUTRIENTS IN TRADITIONAL INDIAN POSTPARTUM FORMULATIONS

Many of the traditional postpartum formulations are rich in macronutrients, antioxidants, and other micronutrients such as minerals and vitamins. Foods that are particularly rich in energy, protein, and fat, and essential micronutrients such as iron, calcium, folic acid, Vitamin C, and β-carotene are listed below in Box 29.3. The criterion used in arriving at this list is that these foods, at the levels used in the food formulations and sample menus presented earlier, provide at least 10% of RDA of the corresponding nutrient for lactating mothers.

It is apparent from Box 29.3 that some foods are highly rich in both macro- and micronutrients, and are used across the country. These are cow's milk, rice/wheat (in different forms), ghee (clarified butter), betel leaves quid, lentils (mung and urad dal, in particular), fenugreek, and garlic. Cow's milk, in the quantities consumed, provides at least 10% of the RDA of energy, protein, fat, iron, calcium, β-carotene, Vitamin C, and folic acid. Rice and wheat, consumed in different forms such as boiled/puffed rice and wheat flour/broken wheat, provide carbohydrates, energy, protein, iron, and folic acid. Foods such as drumstick and sesbania, even when consumed at 30 grams per day (or two 100 g servings per week), are rich sources of micronutrients such as Vitamin C, β-carotene, and calcium. Long pepper (thippili) is rich in iron and calcium. Betel leaf quids provide calcium and β-carotene. Milk, ghee, and coconut/oils provide fat. Ajwain is a rich source of iron. Chickpeas provide a rich source of iron and folic acid. Fish, when consumed, provides large quantities of protein, iron, and calcium. Based on the analysis of the postpartum menus as well as the information provided above, it is clear that a balanced diet that meets the postpartum nutritional demands of lactating mothers can be constructed using ethnic Indian foods.

29.5.3 TRADITIONAL INDIAN POSTPARTUM FORMULATIONS FOR
IMMUNITY AND PREVENTION OF INFECTION

The use of plant foods can modulate the body's immune system. Studies report that a variety of plant derivatives such as polysaccharides, lectins, peptides, flavonoids, and tannins modulate the immune system in various *in vivo* models (Shivaprasad et al., 2006). Medicinal plants used for immunomodulation can provide potential alternatives to conventional chemotherapies for a variety

BOX 29.3   FOOD SOURCES OF MACRO- AND MICRO-NUTRIENTS FOR LACTATING MOTHERS IN TRADITIONAL INDIAN POSTPARTUM DIETS

Energy	Rice, Wheat, Cow's Milk, Freshly Grated/Dry Coconut, Jaggery, Puffed Rice
Carbohydrates	Rice, Wheat, Cow's Milk, Puffed Rice
Protein	Fish, Cow's Milk, Wheat, Rice, *Vigna radiata* (hulled, split green gram/ mung dal), *Vigna mungo* (hulled, split black gram/urad dal), *Trigonella foenum graecum* (fenugreek), Puffed Rice, Eggs
Fat	Ghee (clarified butter), Cow's Milk, Freshly Grated/Dry Coconut, Cooking Oil (gingelly, mustard, or coconut oil), Almonds, Cashews, *Trachyspermum ammi* (ajwain), Eggs, Wheat Flour, *Prasava Lehiyam*
Fiber	None
Calcium	Betel Leaves Quid (betel leaves + arecanut + lime), Cow's Milk, Fish, *Trachyspermum ammi* (ajwain), *Sesbania grandiflora* (agathi leaves), *Moringa oleifera* (drumstick leaves and fruit), *Piper longum* (thippili), Wheat
Iron	Wheat, *Piper longum* (thippili), Puffed Rice, *Prasava Lehiyam*, *Trachyspermum ammi* (ajwain), Rice, Fish, *Trigonella foenumgraecum* (fenugreek), Cow's Milk, *Cicer arietinum* (chickpeas), Palm sugar (jaggery)
β-Carotene	*Moringa oleifera* (drumstick leaves and fruit), *Sesbania grandiflora* (agathi leaves), Betel Leaves Quid (betel leaves + arecanut + lime), Carrots, *Murraya koneigii* (curry leaves), Cow's Milk
Vitamin C	*Moringa oleifera* (drumstick leaves and fruit), *Momordica charantia* (bitter gourd), *Sesbania grandiflora* (agathi leaves), *Carica papaya* (ripe fruit), Cow's Milk, Tomato
Folic Acid	Cow's Milk, Wheat, *Cicer arietinum* (chickpeas), *Vigna mungo* (hulled, split black gram/urad dal), *Vigna radiata* (hulled, split green gram/ Mung dal), Eggs, *Trigonella foenumgraecum* (fenugreek), Rice

of diseases, especially when the host defense mechanism has to be activated under the conditions of impaired immune response (Mukherjee et al., 2014).

Murraya koenigii (curry) leaves have been found to contain phytochemicals that show excellent potential to boost immunity and prevent infection (Handral et al., 2012). Murraya is one of the oldest traditional foods in India, consumed across the country in the form of dry powders and for seasoning many food formulations. Studies on male albino rats have established wound-healing properties, while evidence has been found on antimicrobial activity to various bacteria, including *Staphylococcus* species that are known to commonly cause postpartum infections. The active ingredients include carbazole alkaloids such as murrayacine, mahanimbine, mahanine, mahanimbinine, murrayacinine, mahanimbicine, mahanimboline, isomahanine, cyclomahanimbine, murrayanol, and glycozoline.

Another green leafy vegetable that is known for its high amounts of calcium, β-carotene, iron, potassium, vitamin C, proteins, manganese, selenium, zinc, amino acids, and polyunsaturated fatty acids is drumstick or *Moringa oleifera* (Moyo et al., 2012; Ramalingum and Mahomoodally, 2014). The leaves are known to possess anti-inflammatory and antimicrobial activities arising from iso-thiocyanates, glucosinolates, niazimicin, and pterygospermin. Strong antimicrobial activity has been established against *Candida albicans*, *Staphylococcus aureus*, and *Enterococcus faecalis*, while weak activity has been found against *Escherichia coli*, *Salmonella typhimurium*, *Klebsiella pneumoniae*, and *Pseudomonas aeruginosa* (Moyo et al., 2012; Marrufo et al., 2013).

Solanum nigrum (fruits and leaves) is found to exhibit dose-dependent antiinflammatory effects in animal studies (Jain et al., 2011 and references therein), which could have arisen from the presence of (E)-ethyl caffeate, a component isolated from *S. nigrum* that shows strong inhibitory effect on leukotrienes.

Curcuma longa (turmeric) has shown antibacterial, antifungal, antiprotozoal, antiviral, and anti-inflammatory activities (Mahady, 2005; Chattopadhyay et al., 2004 and references therein), arising from curcumin as well as other active ingredients such as sesquiterpenes and zingiberene. Many animal (mouse, rat) and *in vitro* studies have been conducted on the wound-healing properties of curcumin as well as the oil extracts containing the other active ingredients. Curcumin has been found to be effective in normal as well as diabetic rats. Curcumin has also shown antibacterial effects against *Streptococcus, Staphylococcus, and Helicobacter pylori*, antifungal activities toward *Aspergillus flavus, A. parasiticus, Fusarium moniliforme,* and *Penicillium digitatum*, and antiprotozoal activities towards *Entamoeba histolytica, Leishmania major,* and *Plasmodium falciparum*.

Zingiber officinale (ginger) has shown strong antibacterial effects against a number of bacteria including *Streptococcus pyogenes* and *pneumoniae, Staphylococcus aureus, Haemophilus influenzae,* and *Helicobacter pylori* (Mahady, 2005).

One of the most common postpartum foods in India is garlic (*Allium sativum*), which has a variety of benefits, mainly due to it being a galactagogue. It is also known for its beneficial effects on cardiovascular and immune systems. The main active ingredients of garlic are allicin, alliin, diallyl disulfide, and other thiosulfinates. These ingredients have shown strong activity (Harris et al., 2001; Jalali et al., 2009; Gammal et al., 2011) towards protozoans such as *Trichomonas vaginalis, Opalina ranarum, Opalina dimidicita, Balantidium entozoon, Entamoeba histolytica, Trypanosomes, Leishmania, Leptomonas,* and *Crithidia*; bacteria such as *Pseudomonas proteus, Staphylococcus aureus, Escherichia coli, Salmonella, Micrococcus, Bacillus subtulis, Clostridium, Mycobacterium,* and *Helicobacter*; fungi such as *Candida albicans, Torulopsis, Trichophyton, Trichosporon, Aspergillus niger, Rhodotorula,* and *Paracoccidiodes*; and viruses such as influenza A and B, viral pneumonia, rotavirus, rhinovirus, and cytomegalovirus.

Black pepper (*Piper nigrum* L.), the most common spice used in all Indian postpartum cuisines, is also known to possess strong activity toward preventing infection. Ahmad et al. (2012, 2016) have demonstrated this effect against *Escherichia coli, Pseudomonas aeroginosa, Salmonella typhi, Bacillus subtilis, Bacillus cereus, Staphylococcus aureus,* and *chcandida albicans with fresh and regenerated tissues of p. nigrum* through *in vitro* studies pepper has also demonstrated antiapoptotic, antifungal, antidiarrheal, anti-inflammatory, antioxidative, immunomodulatory, and antiasthmatic effects (Ahmad et al., 2012 and references therein), primarily arising from the isolate piperine.*Candida albicans* with fresh and regenerated tissues of *P. nigrum* through *in vitro* studies. Pepper has also demonstrated antiapoptotic, antifungal, antidiarrheal, anti-inflammatory, antioxidative, immunomodulatory, and antiasthmatic effects (Ahmad et al., 2012 and references therein), primarily arising from the isolate piperine.

Bottle gourd (*Lagenaria Siceraria*) is a commonly consumed vegetable in India that is rich in many micronutrients including iron, phosphorus, magnesium, and potassium, and a moderate source of Vitamin C (Ramalingum and Mahomoodally, 2014 and references therein). It is also rich in cardiac glycosides, alkaloids, saponins, tannins, flavonoids, choline, and triterpenoids (cucurbitacins). Its antiviral effect is known to arise from the protein lagenin, which is a ribosome-inactivating protein. The antioxidant, anti-inflammatory, and immunomodulatory activity of bottle gourd fruit has been established via *in vitro* and *in vivo* studies (Deshpande et al., 2008).

Sesbania grandiflora L., commonly known as sesbania and agathi, is widely used in Indian traditional medicine for the treatment of a broad spectrum of diseases including leprosy, gout, rheumatism, tumor, and liver disorders (Sreelatha et al., 2011). Zarena et al. (2014) have isolated agathi leaf protein from *Sesbania grandiflora leaves* and demonstrated *in vitro* its antioxidant (scavenging lipid peroxidation, DNA damage), cytoprotective (lymphocyte), and antibacterial activity against *Pseudomonas aeruginosa* and *Staphylococcus aureus*. Antimicrobial properties towards pathogenic bacteria like *Lactobacillus acidophilus* was also identified by Ratna et al. (2012).

Neem (*Azhadiracta indica*) is a well-known Indian medicinal plant with significant activity toward preventing infection and improving immunity. Several compounds have been identified from neem, such as nimbidin, sodium nimbidate, gallic acid, epicatechin, catechin, peptidoglycans (e.g., NB-II), and polysaccharides (e.g., GIIa, GIIIa) that have exhibited anti-inflammatory and immunomodulatory behaviors (Biswas et al., 2002). The aqueous extract of neem leaf has been shown to possess immunostimulant activity based on both humoral and cell-mediated responses (Sen et al., 1992; Ray et al., 1996). An antiulcer effect of neem leaf aqueous extract has been demonstrated in rats (Garg et al., 1993). Antimalarial activity has been shown for neem seed and leaf extracts (Khalid et al., 1986, 1989; Badani et al., 1987). Antifungal activity of neem leaf extract has been shown against *Trichophyton, Epidermophyton, Microsporum, Trichosporon, Geotricum,* and *Candida* (National Research Council, 1992). Neem oil, extracted from its leaves, seeds, and bark, exhibits antibacterial action against *M. tuberculosis, M. pyogenes,* and streptomycin-resistant strains, *Vibrio cholerae,* and *Klebsiella pneumoniae* (Satyavati et al., 1976). Aqueous extract of neem leaves has shown antiviral activity against vaccinia virus, chinkungunya and measles viruses (Gogati and Marathe, 1989). Badam et al. (1999), in an *in vitro* study, have demonstrated antiviral activity of methanolic extracts of neem leaves against group-B Coxsackievirus.

Coconut is another common food consumed in India, especially in the southern regions. Its components present in plants, such as polysaccharides, lectins, proteins, and peptides, have shown immunostimulatory effects (Tzianabos, 2000; Bafna and Mishra, 2005). Vigila and Baskaran (2008) have shown that cyclophosphamide is a potent suppressor of immune function, demonstrating a sustained decrease in both the number and function of T- and B-cells (Cupps et al., 1982). Cocosin, a globular protein in coconut (Osborne et al., 1916), exhibits counteractivity to cyclophosphamide-induced myelosuppression and thrombocytopenia. This immunostimulatory activity of cocosin is through IgE-mediated and cell-mediated hyperreactivity. Also, Shilling et al. (2013), in an *in vitro* study, demonstrate the growth inhibition of *Clostridium difficile* mediated by medium-chain fatty acids derived from virgin coconut oil.

One of the oldest cultivated plants in the world, known for its oil-rich edible seeds, is sesame (*Sesamum indicum L*). Joshi et al. (2005) have shown antioxidant effects of sesame seeds and its ingredient sesamol. Kiran and Asad (2008) have shown in a *in vivo* study that sesame oil is more effective in healing excision and burn wounds. Constituents such as sesamol, sesaminol, and sesamolin, present in both seeds and oil, may be responsible for the wound-healing activity.

Bitter melon (*Momordica charantia*) possesses several phytochemicals such as alpha- and beta-momorcharin, lectin, and *Momordica* anti-HIV protein (MAP30), and these have shown *in vitro* antiviral activity against Epstein-Barr, herpes, HIV, Coxsackievirus B3, and polio viruses (Palamthodi and Lele, 2014). Hexane, ethyl acetate, and ethanol seed extracts have also exhibited antimicrobial activity against *Escherichia coli, Candida albicans, Staphylococcus aureus, Staphylococcus epidermidis,* and *Klebsiella pneumonia* (Oragwa et al., 2013).

29.6 FUTURE OF TRADITIONAL POSTPARTUM NUTRITIONAL PRACTICES

The discussion presented so far in this chapter provides insights into the presence of various active ingredients such as proteins, fatty acids, vitamins, minerals, alkaloids, sterols, tannins, saponins, anthraquinones, glycosides, flavonoids, amin acids, and polyphenols in traditional Indian postpartum foods, the various postpartum food supplements, an estimate of the nutritive content in them, and how ethnic practices provide the required nutrition to new mothers. Numerous studies have shown that these foods play specific functions enabling the new mother to recover from pregnancy and childbirth even as she nurses the infant in a healthy manner.

However, many open research problems exist in this field. There is insufficient data on content of many active substances including many minerals, specific B vitamins, fat-soluble vitamins, amino acids, nucleosides, and nucleotides. *In vivo* and clinical studies have to be conducted to establish the functional properties of ethnic foods and food supplements, while *in vitro* studies have to be conducted to establish their biological mechanisms of action. There is a significant gap in determining the connections between macro- and micronutrient imbalances and postpartum morbidities. Unlike the USDA nutrient databases, NIN's database lacks data on the nutrient content of ethnic Indian foods in their cooked forms as well as the nutrient contents of various ethnic food formulations.

Understanding the value of ethnic nutritional practices in postpartum care is a multidimensional problem that needs to be tackled from various perspectives such as:

• Creating a knowledge base of traditional nutritional practices; their regional, socioeconomic, and cultural diversities; possible historical reasons underlying these practices; and the evolution of these practices
• Standardizing the recipes of the different food formulations that form part of the traditional postpartum practices
• Evaluating the macro- and micronutrients and other active ingredients in these foods in their natural form as well as in the forms they are likely to take after cooking
• Evaluating the macro- and micronutrients in the standardized food formulations, their variations with shelf life, and their modes of preservation
• Developing standardized postpartum menus based on traditional formulations that cover all the food groups and provide the recommended quantities of the nutrients
• Understanding postpartum morbidities, their causes, and connections with lifestyles and nutritional imbalances
• Recognizing food functions that alleviate postpartum morbidities, and functional foods and formulations having those functions
• Determining the functional properties of ethnic foods and food formulations through *in vitro*, *in vivo*, and clinical studies
• Examining the synergistic interactions between the various foods and food formulations in promoting the recovery and health of the new mother and infant
• Identifying the best postpartum lifestyle practices that promote the recovery and health of the new mother and infant
• Developing low-cost, locally available/preparable and functional food formulations for new mothers from different socioeconomic strata
• Developing strategies for effectively creating awareness, counseling, integrating, evaluating, and monitoring traditional postpartum practices into the present-day care delivered through modern governmental and nongovernmental institutions

Postpartum ethnic care is therefore a fertile area of research, development, and implementation. Given the highly rich nutritive values of traditional postpartum foods and given the large number of new mothers in India suffering from morbidities and children suffering from stunting and wasting, transforming postpartum care is a highly challenging task, but one with high potential for success.

As a conclusion to the chapter, based on the survey and analysis of existing literature, the following specific recommendations may be made for the daily postpartum diet that could make an immediate positive impact on the health of the new mothers and the infants:

• Include at least 400 mL of milk in the diet
• Include at least 200 grams of boiled rice or whole wheat (including in the form of wheat breads/chapathi)
• Include at least 50 grams of lentils (such as *Vigna radiata* and *Vigna mungo*)
• Include at least 20 grams of spices that are galactagogues such as *Allium sativum*, *Trigonella foenum-graecum*, and *Piper longum*
• Include at least 50 grams of green, leafy vegetables in the diet, particularly foods like *Moringa oleifera* and *Sesbania grandiflora*, which are rich in iron, calcium, Vitamin C, and folic acid
• Include sweet ball–type ethnic foods of the local variety (at least two sweet balls per day)
• Consume water in large quantities (at least two liters per day) in the form of water-boiled decoctions (with spices such as *Anethum graveolens*, *Zingiber officinale*, *Bunibum bulbocastanum*, *Cuminum cyminum*, and *Trachyspermum copticum L.*)

- Include at least one locally available fresh fruit per day
- Include a fiber-rich diet (such as in the form of whole grain millets—rice/wheat, fiber-rich fruits and vegetables)

ACKNOWLEDGMENTS

The authors would like to acknowledge the kind assistance of P. Manimegalai and B. Balaji in preparing the tables, figures, and references. They would also like to acknowledge Amrita Vishwa Vidyapeetham for the kind support in carrying out this work.

REFERENCES

Aal, A., J. C. Young, I. Rabalski, P. Hucl and J. F. Reid. 2007. Identification and quantification of seed carotenoids in selected wheat species. *J Agric Food Chem* 55:787–794.

Aal, A., J. C. Young, P. J. Wood, I. Rabalski, P. Hucl, D. Falk and J. F. Reid. 2002. Einkorn: A potential candidate for developing high lutein wheat. *Cereal Chem* 79:455–457.

Aal, A., P. Hucl, F. W. Sosulski, R. Graf, C. Gillott and L. Pietrzak. 2001. Screening spring wheat for midge resistance in relation to ferulic acid content. *J Agric Food Chem* 49:3559–3566.

Aal, A., J. C. Young and I. Rabalski. 2006. Anthocyanin composition in black, blue, pink, purple and red cereal grains. *J Agric Food Chem* 54:4696–4704.

Abascal, K. and E. Yarnell. 2008. Botanical galactagogues. *Alternat Complement Ther* 14:288–294.

Abbas, G., S. Naqvi, S. Erum, S. Ahmed, Atta-ur-Rahman and A. Dar. 2013. Potential antidepressant activity of Areca catechu nut via elevation of serotonin and noradrenaline in the hippocampus of rats. *Phytother Res* 27:39–45.

Abeyrathne, E. D. N. S., H. Y. Lee and D. U. Ahn. 2013. Egg white proteins and their potential use in food processing or as nutraceutical and pharmaceutical agents—A review. *Poult Sci* 92:3292–3299.

Agarwal, N. and S. Sharma. 2013. Garden cress (Lepidium sativum L.)—A non-conventional traditional plant item for food product. *Indian J Tradit Know* 12:699–706

Aggarwal, B. B., S. Prasad, S. Reuter, R. Kannappan, V. R. Yadev, B. Park, J. H. Kim, S. C. Gupta, K. Phromnoi, C. Sundaram, S. Prasad, M. M. Chaturvedi and B. Sung. 2011. Identification of novel anti-inflammatory agents from ayurvedic medicine for prevention of chronic diseases. *Curr Drug Targets* 12:1595–1653.

Ahmad, A., A. Husain, M. Mujeeb, S. A. Khan, A. K. Najmi, N. A. Siddique, Z. A. Damanhouri and F. Anwar. 2013. A review of therapeutic potential of Nigella sativa: A miracle herb. *Asian Pac J Trop Biomed* 3:337–352.

Ahmad, I., M. Zahin, F. Aqil, S. Hasan, M. S. A. Khan and M. Owais. 2008. Bioactive compounds from Punica granatum, Curcuma longa and Zingiber officinale and their therapeutic potential. *Drugs Fut* 33:329.

Ahmad, N., H. Fazal, B. H. Abbasi, S. Farooq, M. Ali and M. A. Khan. 2012. Biological role of Piper nigrum L. (Black pepper): A review. *Asian Pac J Trop Biomed* 2:S1945-S1953.

Ahmad, N., B. H. Abbasi, H. Fazal. 2016. Effect of different in vitro culture extracts of black pepper (Piper nigrum L.) on toxic metabolites-producing strains. *Toxicol Ind Health* 32:500–506

Ajesh, T. P. and R. Kumuthakalavalli. 2012. Ethnic herbal practices for gynaecological disorders from Urali tribes of Idukki district of Kerala, India. *Int J Pharm Life Sci* 3:2213–2219.

Alamer, M. and G. Basiouni. 2005. Feeding effects of fenugreek seeds (Trigonella foenum graecum L.) on lactation performance, some plasma constituents and growth hormone level in goats. *Pak J Biol Sci* 25:28–46.

Allen, L. H. 1994. Maternal micronutrient malnutrition: Effects on breast milk and infant nutrition, and priorities for intervention. *SCN News* 11:21–24.

Allen, L. H. and J. M. Graham. 2003. Assuring micronutrient adequacy in the diets of young infants. *In Micronutrient deficiencies in the first six months of life*, ed. F. M. Delange and K. P. J. West, 55–88. Dubai: Nestle Nutrition Institute Workshop Series, Vol. 52. Basel: Karger Medical and Scientific Publishers.

Alsaif, M. A. 2008. Effect of Nigella sativa oil on metabolic responses to prolonged systematic injury to rats. *J Biol Sci* 8:974–983.

Amudhan, M. S., B. V. Hazeena and K. B. Hebbar. 2012. A review on phytochemical and pharmacological potential of Areca catechu L. seed. *Int J Pharm Sci Res* 3:4151–4157.

Anderson, J. W., B. M. Smith and N. J. Gustafson. 1994. Health benefits and practical aspects of high-fiber diets. *Am J Clin Nutr* 59:1242–1247.

Anwar, F., S. Latif, M. Ashraf and A. H. Gilani. 2007. Moringa oleifera: A food plant with multiple medicinal uses. *Phytother Res* 21:17–25.

Anyaehie, U. B. 2009. Medicinal properties of fractionated acetone/water neem (Azadirachta indica) leaf extract from Nigeria: A review. *Niger J Physiol Sci* 24:157–159.

Arambewela, L. S. R., L. D. A. M Arawwawala and W. D. Ratnasooriya. 2005. An antidiabetic activity of aqueous and ethanolic extracts of Piper betel leaves in rats. *J Ethnopharmacol* 102:239–245.

Arun, N. and N. Nalini. 2002. Efficacy of turmeric on blood sugar and polyol pathway in diabetic albino rats. *Plant Foods Hum Nutr* 57:41–52.

Arunabha, M. and N. Satish. 2014. Evaluation of immunomodulatory activity of Sesbania grandiflora flowers extract in mice. *Indonesian J Pharm* 25:277–283.

Arunachalam, G., N. Subramanian, G. P. Pazhani, M. Karunanithi and V. Ravichandran. 2009. Evaluation of anti-inflammatory activity of methanolic extract of Solanum nigrum (Solanaceae). *Iranian J Pharm Sci* 5:151–156.

Asgary, S., M. R. Kopaei, S. Najafi, E. Heidarian and A. Sahebkar. 2013. Antihyperlipidemic effects of Sesamum indicum L. in rabbits fed a high-fat diet. *Sci World J*: 365892.

Asgary, S., S. Najafi, A. Ghannadi, G. Dashti and A. Helalat. 2012. Efficiency of black cumin seeds on hematological factors in normal and hypercholesterolemic rabbits. *ARYA Atheroscler* 7:146–150.

Asiedu-Gyekye, I. J., S. F. Manso, C. Awortwe, D. A. Antwi and A. K. Nyarko. 2014. Micro-and macroelemental composition and safety evaluation of the nutraceutical Moringa oleifera leaves. *J Toxicol* 2014:786979.

Atanu, F. O., U. G. Ebiloma and E. I. Ajayi. 2011. A review of the pharmacological aspects of Solanum nigrum Linn. *Biotech Mol Biol Rev* 6:1–7.

Augusti, K. T. and C. G. Sheela. 1996. Antiperoxide effect of S-allyl cysteine sulfoxide, an insulin secretagogue, in diabetic rats. *Experientia* 52:115–20.

Awadesh, N. S., R. Gautam, A. Ghaeami, R. K. Gautam and A. K. Gharami. 2008. *Indigenous Health Care and Ethno Medicine*. New Delhi: Sarup and Sons Publishing.

Babic, I., M. J. Amiot, C. Ngugen-The and S. Aubert. 1993. Changes in phenolic content in fresh, ready-to-use and shredded carrots during storage. *J Food Sci* 58:351–356.

Badam, L., S. P. Joshi and S. S. Bedekar. 1999. In vitro antiviral activity of neem (Azadirachta indica. A. Juss) leaf extract against group B coxsackie viruses. *J Comm Diseases* 31:79–90.

Badani, L., R. P. Deolankar, M. M. Kulkarni, B. A. Nagsampgi and U. V. Wagh. 1987. In vitro antimalarial activity of neem (Azadirachta indica A. Juss) leaf and seed extracts. *Indian J Malariol* 24:111–117.

Bafna, A. R. and S. H. Mishra. 2005. Immunomodulatory activity of methanol extract of roots of Cissamplelos pareira Linn. Pharmacy Department. *Ars Pharm* 46:253–262.

Bairwa, M., M. Rajput and S. Sachdeva. 2012. Modified Kuppuswamy's socioeconomic scale: Social researcher should include updated income criteria. *Indian J Community Med* 38:85–186.

Bakre, A. G., A. O. Aderibigbe and O. G. Ademowo. 2013. Studies on neuropharmacological profile of ethanol extract of Moringa oleifera leaves in mice. *J Ethnopharmacol* 149:783–789.

Bale, J. R., B. J. Stoll and A. O. Lucas. 2003. *Improving birth outcomes: Meeting the challenge in the developing world*. Washington, DC: National Academies Press.

Baliga, M. S., B. R. V. Baliga, S. M. Kandathil, H. P. Bhat and P. K. Vayalil. 2011. A review of the chemistry and pharmacology of the date fruits (Phoenix dactylifera L.). *Food Res Int* 44:1812–1822.

Ballabh, B. and O. P. Chaurasia. 2007. Traditional medicinal plants of cold desert ladakh. *J Ethnopharmacol* 112:341–349.

Bandyopadhyay, M. 2009. Impact of ritual pollution on lactation and breastfeeding practices in rural West Bengal, India. *Int Breastfeed J* 4:2.

Bao, B. and K. C. Chang. 1994. Carrot pulp chemical composition, colour and water-holding capacity as affected by blanching. *J Food Sci* 59:1159–1161.

Barnes, J. L., D. D. Schramm, C. Keen, J. E. Painter and A. R. Waters. 2011. Raisin consumption may lower circulating oxidized LDL levels, potentially decreasing the risk of coronary heart disease. *J Amer Diet Assoc* 111:46.

Bazzano, L., J. He, L. G. Ogden, C. Loria, S. Vupputuri, L. Myers and P. K. Whelton. 2001. Legume consumption and risk of coronary heart diseases in US men and women. NHANES I Epidemiologic follow-up Study. *Arch Intern Med* 161:2573–2578.

Biswas, K., I. Chattopadhyay, R. K. Banerjee and U. Bandyopadhyay. 2002. Biological activities and medicinal properties of neem (Azadirachta indica). *Curr Sci* 82:1336–1345.

Block, G. 1994. Nutrient sources of provitamin carotenoids in the American diet. *Am J Epidemiol* 139:290–293.

Bourdon, I., B. Olson, R. Backus, B. D. Richter, P. A. Davies and B. O. Schneeman. 2001. Beans as a source of dietary fiber, increase cholecystokinin and apolipoprotein B48 response to test meals in men. *J Nutr* 131:1485–1490.

Brinch, M., T. Isager and K. Tolstrup. 1988. Anorexia nervosa and motherhood: Reproduction pattern and mothering behaviour of 50 women. *Acta Psychiatr Scand* 77:611–617.

Caius, J. F. 1986. *The medicinal and poisonous plants of India* (Reprint). Jodhpur: Scientific Publishers.

Carrillo, M., C. V. Alarcón, R. G. Dorado, O. G. C. Valenzuela, R. M. Escobedo, J. A. G. Tiznado and C. R. Moreno. 2007. Nutritional properties of quality protein maize and chickpea extruded based weaning food. *Plant Foods Hum Nutr* 62:31–37.

Chakroborty, D. and B. Shah. 2011. Antimicrobial, antioxidative and antihemolytic activity of piper betel leaf extracts. *Int J Pharm Pharm Sci* 3:192–199.

Chattopadhyay, I., K. Biswas, U. Bandyopadhyay and R. K. Banerjee. 2004. Turmeric and curcumin: Biological actions and medicinal applications. *Curr Sci* 87:44–53.

Chaudhary, R. and S. Sharma. 2013. Conventional nutrients and antioxidants in red kidney beans (Phaseolus vulgaris L.): An explorative and product development endeavour. *Food Sci Technol* 14:258–275.

Chaudhry, N. M. and P. Tariq. 2006. Bactericidal activity of black pepper, bay leaf, aniseed and coriander against oral isolates. *Pak J Pharm Sci* 19:214–218.

Chauhan, K., L. Parmar, R. Solanki, V. Kagatharaand and D. Madat. 2010. Effect of Piper longum Linn. on histopathological and biochemical changes in isoproterenol induced myocardial infarction in rats. *Res J Pharm Biol Chem Sci* 1:759–766.

Chitra, U., V. Vimala, U. Singh and P. Geervani. 1995. Variability in phytic acid content and protein digestibility of grain legumes. *Plant Food Hum Nutr* 47:163–172.

Chmielowska, E. and F. S. Shih. 2007. Folk customs in modern society: 'Tradition of Zuoyuezi' in Taiwan: A physical anthropology perspective. EATS IV conference. Stockholm. Available at http://www.soas.ac.uk/taiwanstudies/eats/eats2007/file38472.pdf. Accessed on February 26, 2015.

Chopra, R. N., S. L. Nayer and I. C. Chopra. 1996. *Glossary of Indian medicinal plants*. New Delhi: National Institute of Science Communication and Information Resources.

Chou, H. L., H. C. Tseng, J. L. Wang and C. Loa. 2008. Hepatoprotective effects of Solanum nigrum Linn extract against CCl_4-induced oxidative damage in rats. *Chem Biol Interact* 171:283–293.

Choudhry, U. K. 1997. Traditional practices of women from India: Pregnancy, childbirth and newborn care. *J Obstet Gynecol Neonatal Nurs* 26:533–539.

Choudhury, N. and S. M. Ahmed. 2011. Maternal care practices among the ultra-poor households in rural Bangladesh: A qualitative exploratory study. *BMC Pregnancy Childbirth* 11:15.

Christian, P., S. K. Khatry, S. C. LeClerq and S. M. Dali. 2009. Effects of prenatal micronutrient supplementation on complications of labor and delivery and puerperal morbidity in rural Nepal. *Int J Gynecol Obstet* 106:3–7.

Crujeiras, A. B., D. Parra, I. Abete and J. A. Martinez. 2007. A hypocaloric diet enriched in legumes specifically mitigates lipid peroxidation in obese subjects. *Free Radic Res* 41:498–506.

Cupps, T. R., L. C. Edgar and A. S. Fauci. 1982. Suppression of human B lymphocyte function by cyclophosphamide. *J Immunol* 128:2453–2457.

Damanhouri, Z. A., and A. Ahmad. 2014. A review on therapeutic potential of Piper nigrum L. (black pepper): The king of spices. *Med Aromat Plants* 3:161.

Dar, A., S. Khatoon, G. Rahman, Atta-Ur-Rahman. 1997. Anti-depressant activities of Areca catechu fruit extract. *Phytomedicine* 4:41–45.

Deepthi, S., M. Varma, E. Khan and A. Hazra. 2010. Increasing postnatal care of mothers and newborns including follow-up cord care and thermal care in rural Uttar Pradesh. *J Fam Welfare* 56:31–42.

Deshpande, J. R., A. A. Choudhary, M. R. Mishra, V. S. Meghre, S. G. Wadodkhar and A. K. Dorle. 2008. Beneficial effects of Lagenaria siceraria (Mol) Standley fruit epicarp in animal models. *Indian J Exp Biol* 46:234–242.

Dhingra, D. and V. Kumar. 2008. Evidences for the involvement of monoaminergic and GABAergic systems in antidepressant-like activity of garlic extract in mice. *Indian J Pharmacol* 40:175–179.

Dhumal, J. S., S. U. Yele and S. N. Ghodekar. 2013. Evaluation of immunomodulatory activity of Vigna mungo (L) hepper. *J Pharm Phytother* 1:9–14.

Dongare, V., G. Kulkarni, M. Kondawar, C. Magdum, V. Haldarnekar and A. Arvindekar. 2011. Inhibition of aldose reductase and anti-cataractaction of Trans-anethole isolated from Foeniculun vulgare Mill fruits. *Food Chem* 132:385–390.

Efferth, T., P. C. H. Li, V. S. B. Konkimalla and B. Kaina. 2007. From traditional Chinese medicine to rational cancer therapy. *Trends Mol Med* 13:353–361.

EFSA Panel on Contaminants in the Food Chain (CONTAM). 2011. Scientific Opinion on the risks for public health related to the presence of opium alkaloids in poppy seeds. *EFSA Journal* 9(11):2405.

Eiben, C. S., A. A. Rashwan, K. Kustos, K. Godor-Surmann and Z. Szendro. 2004. *Effect of anise and fenugreek supplementation on performance of rabbit does.* In Proceedings of the 8th World Rabbit Congress. Puebla, Mexico: World Rabbit Science Association. Available at http://world-rabbit-science.com/WRSA-Proceedings/Congress-2004-Puebla/Puebla-2004-a.htm. Accessed on January 18, 2015.

El-Adawy, T. A. 2002. Nutritional composition and antinutritional factors of chickpeas (*Cicer arietinum L.*) undergoing different cooking methods and germination. *Plant Foods Hum Nutr* 57:83–97.

Elmofty, M., A. Abdelgalil, M. Shwaireb, M. Eldakhakhny, A. Rizk and E. Hofny. 1997. Prevention of skin tumors induced by 7, 12-dimethylbenz(a)anthracene in mice by black seed oil.*Oncology reports* 4:139–141.

Emamghoreishi, M. and G. Heidari-Hamedani. 2006. Sedative-hypnotic activity of extracts and essential oil of coriander seeds. *Iran J Med Sci* 31:22–27.

Emamghoreishi, M., M. Khasaki, M. F. Aazam. 2005. Coriandrum sativum: Evaluation of its anxiolytic effect in the elevated plus-maze. *J Ethnopharmacol* 96:365–370.

Erşahin, M., H. Z. Toklu, D. Akakin, M. Yuksel, B. Ç. Yeğen and G. Sener. 2011. The effects of Nigella sativa against oxidative injury in a rat model of subarachnoid haemorrhage. *Acta Neurochir* 153:333–341

Etkin, N. L. 2007. *Edible medicines: An ethonopharamacology of foods.* Tucson: University of Arizona Press.

Felipe, C. F. B., K. S. Fonsêca, A. L. dos Reis Barbosa, J. N. S. Bezerra, M. A. Neto, M. M. de França Fonteles and G. S. de Barros Viana. 2008. Alterations in behavior and memory induced by the essential oil of Zingiber officinale Roscoe (ginger) in mice are cholinergic-dependent. *J Med Plants Res* 2:163–170.

Ferreira, P. M. P., D. F. Farias, J. T. Oliveira, A. F. U. Carvalho. 2008. Bioactive compounds and nutritional potential. *Rev Nutr Campinas* 21:431–437.

Ferri-Lagneau, K. F., K. S. Moshal, M. Grimes, B. Zahora, L. V. Lishuang, S. Shengmin and T.-C. Leung. 2012. Ginger stimulates hematopoiesis via Bmp pathway in Zebrafish. *PLoS One* 7:e39327.

Ficker, C., M. L. Smith, K. Akpagana, J. Zhang, T. Durst, R. Assabgui and J. T. Arnason. 2003. Bioassay-guided isolation and identification of antifungal compounds from ginger. *Phytother Res* 17:897–902.

Fletcher, A. E., C. Veldhuis, N. Lively, C. Fowler and B. Marcks. 2008. The reciprocal effects of eating disorders and the postpartum period: A review of the literature and recommendations for clinical care. *J Women Health* 17:227–241.

Frison, S. and P. Sporns. 2002. Variation in the flavonol glycoside composition of almond seed coats as determined by MALDI-TOF mass spectrometry. *J Agric Food Chem* 50:6818–6822.

Fuglie, L. J. 1999. The miracle tree: The multiple attributes of Moringa. Wageningen: CTA Publishing.

Gabay, M. 2002. Galactogouges: Medications that induce lactation. *J Hum Lact* 18:274–279.

Gammal, Y. M. E., O. A. Elmasry, D. H. El-Ghoneimy and I. M. Soliman. 2011. Immunomodulatory effects of food. *Egypt J Pediatr Allergy Immunol* 9:3–13.

Garg, G. P., S. K. Nigam and C. W. Ogle. 1993. The gastric antiulcer effects of the leaves of the neem tree. *Planta Med* 59:215–217.

Gaur, V., S. L. Bodhankar, V. Mohan and P. Thakurdesai. 2012. Antidepressant-like effect of 4-hydroxyisoleucine from Trigonella foenum graecum L. seeds in mice. *Biomed Aging Pathol* 2:121–125.

Geng, Y., X. Du, X. Cao, Y. Chen, H. Zhang, H. Liu, Z. Chen and X. Zeng. 2012. The therapeutic effects of Zingiber officinale extract on mice irradiated by ⁶⁰Co ⊠-ray. *J Med Plants Res* 6:2590–2600.

Ghrairi, F. E., A. Amira, C. Henda, L. Lahouar, L. Achour and S. Said. 2012. Hypoglycemic and hypolipidemic effects of raisin aqueous extract "karkni" in alloxan-induced diabetic rats. *J Diabetes Metab* 3:211.

Girish, T. K., V. M. Pratape and R. U. J. S. Prasada. 2012. Nutrient distribution, phenolic acid composition, antioxidant and alpha-glucosidase inhibitory potentials of black gram (*Vigna mungo L.*) and its milled byproducts. *Food Res Int* 46:370–377.

Gogati, S. S. and A. D. Marathe. 1989. Anti-viral effect of neem leaf (Azadirachta indica) extracts on chinkungunya and measles viruses. *J Res Educ Indian Med* 8:1–5.

Gogoi, B. and K. Zaman. 2013. Phytochemical constituents of some medicinal plant species used in recipe during 'Bohag bihu' in Assam. *J Pharmacogn Phytochem* 2:30–40.

Goodburn, E. A., R. Gazi and M. Chowdhury. 1995. Beliefs and practices regarding delivery and postpartum maternal morbidity in rural Bangladesh. *Stud Fam Planning* 26:22–32.

Gopalan, C. and S. Kaur. 1989. *Women and nutrition in India.* New Delhi: Nutrition Foundation of India.

Gowri, S. and K. Vasantha. 2010. Free radical scavenging and antioxidant activity of leaves from Agathi (Sesbania grandiflora) (L.) Pers. *Am-Eurasian J Sci Res* 5:114–119.

Goyal, R. K., J. Singh and H. Lal. 2003. Asparagus racemosus—An update. *Indian J Med Sci* 57:408

Grossman, S., M. Bergman, L. Varshavsky and H. E. Gottlieb. 2001. The antioxidant activity of aqueous spinach extract: Chemical identification of active fractions. *Phytochem* 58:143–152.

Grover, J. K., S. P. Yadav and V. Vats. 2003. Effect of feeding Murraya koeingii and Brassica juncea diet on
kidney functions and glucose levels in streptozotocin diabetic mice. *J Ethnopharmacol* 85:1–5.

Gruber, C. W. and M. O'Brien. 2011. Uterotonic plants and their bioactive constituents. *Planta Med* 77:207–220.

Gupta, M. and B. Shaw. 2011. A double-blind randomized clinical trial for evaluation of galactogogue activity
of Asparagus racemosus wild. *Iranian J Pharm Res* 10:167–172.

Handral, H. K., A. Pandith and S. D. Shruthi. 2012. A review on Murraya koenigii: Multipotential medicinal
plant. *Asian J Pharm Clin Res* 5:5–14.

Hanefi, O., S. Ugras, I. Bayram, I. Uygan, E. Erdogan, A. Ozturk and Z. Huyut. 2004. Hepatoprotective effect
of Foeniculum vulgare essential oil: A carbon tetrachloride induced liver fibrosis model in rats. *Scand J
Lab Anim Sci* 31:9–17.

Hansen, S. L., S. Purup and L. P. Christensen. 2003. Bioactivity of falcarinol and the influence of processing
and storage on its content in carrots (*Daucus carota* L). *J Sci Food Agric* 83:1010–1017.

Harris, J. C., S. L. Cottrell, S. Plummer and D. Lloyd. 2001. Antimicrobial properties of Allium sativum (garlic). *Appl Microbiol Biotechnol* 57:282–286.

Hashimoto, T. and T. Nagayama. 2004. Chemical composition of ready-to-eat fresh carrot. *J Food Hyg Soc
Japan* 39:324–328.

Hawrelak, J. A., T. Cattley and S. P. Myer. 2009. Essential oils in the treatment of intestinal dysbiosis: A preliminary in vitro study. *Altern Med Rev* 14:380–384.

Hayatullina, Z., N. Muhammad, N. Mohamed and I. N. Soelaiman. 2012. Virgin coconut oil supplementation
prevents bone loss in osteoporosis rat model. *Evid Based Complement Alternat Med* 2012:1–8.

Hosseinzadeh, H., M. Tafaghodi, S. Abedzadeh and E. Taghiabadi. 2014. Effect of aqueous and ethanolic extracts of Pimpinella anisum L. seeds on milk production in rats. *J Acupunct Meridian Stud*
7:211–216.

Hosseinzadeh, H., M. Tafaghodi, S. Abedzadeh and E. Taghiabadi. 2013. Effect of aqueous and ethanolic
extracts of Nigella sativa L. seeds on milk production in rats. *J Acupunct Meridian Stud* 6:8–23.

Malta Wild Plants. Available at http://www.maltawildplants.com/PAPV/Papaver_somniferum_subsp_setigerum.
php; Accessed: 26th June 2015.

Ilyas, M., M. U. Arshad, F. Saeed and M. Iqbal. 2015. Antioxidant potential and nutritional comparison of
Moringa leaf and seed powders and their tea infusions. *J Anim Plant Sci* 25:226–233.

Indira, M. and P. A. Kurup. 1989. Effect of neutral detergent fiber from black gram (Phaseolus mungo) in rats
and rabbits. *J Nutr* 119:1246–1251.

Inoue, H., T. Asaka, N. Nagata and Y. Koshihara. 1997. Mechanism of mustard oil-induced skin inflammation
in mice. *Eur J Pharmacol* 333:231–240.

Iyengar, K. 2012. Early postpartum maternal morbidity among rural women of Rajasthan, India: A community-
based study. *J Health Popul Nutr* 30:213–225.

Jabbar, A., Z. Iqbal and M. N. Khan. 2006. In vitro anthelmintic activity of Trachyspermum ammi seeds.
Pharmacogn Mag 2:126–129.

Jagdale, S. C., B. S. Kuchekar, A. R. Chabukswar, P. D.Lokhande and C. G. Raut.2009. Antioxidant activity of
Piper longum Linn. *Int J Bio Chem* 3:119–125.

Jain, R., A. Sharma, S. Gupta, I. P. Sarethy and R. Gabrani. 2011. Solanum nigrum: Current perspectives on
therapeutic properties. *Altern Med Rev* 16:78–85.

Jain, V. 2012. Murraya koenigii: An updated review. *Int J Ayurvedic and Herbal Med* 2:607–627.

Jaiswal, R. and N. Kuhnert. 2014. Identification and characterization of the phenolic glycosides of Lagenaria
siceraria stand (bottle gourd) fruit by liquid chromatography–tandem mass spectrometry. *J Agric Food
Chem* 62:1261–1271.

Jalali, F. S. S., H. Tajik, S. Javedi, B. H. Mohammadi and S. S. A. Athari. 2009. The efficacy of alcoholic extract
of garlic on the healing process of experimental burn wound in the rabbit. *Int J Anim Vet Adv* 8:655–659.

Jom, K. M., T. Frank, K. H. Engel. 2011. A metabolite profiling approach to follow the sprouting process of
mung beans (Vigna radiata). *Metabolomics* 7:102–117.

Joseph, B. and D. Jini. 2013. Antidiabetic effects of *Momordica charantia* (bitter melon) and its medicinal
potency. *Asian Pac J Trop Dis* 3:93–102.

Joshi, R., M. S. Kumar, K. Satyamoorthy, M. K. Unnikrisnan and T. Mukherjee. 2005. Free radical reactions and antioxidant activities of sesamol: Pulse radiolytic and biochemical studies. J Agric Food Chem
53:2696–2703

Judge, M. P., C. T. Beck, M. M. Mckelvey and C. J. Lammi-Keefe. 2011. Maternal docosahexaenoic acid (DHA, 22: 6n-3) consumption during pregnancy decreases postpartum depression (PPD) symptomatology. *FASEB J* 25:349–357.

Jung, I. L. 2014. Soluble extract of Moringa olifera leaves with a new anticancer activity. *PLoS One* 9:e95492.

Kaliora, A. C., A. M. Kountouri and V. T. Karathanos. 2009. Antioxidant properties of raisins (Vitis vinifera L.). *J Med Food* 12:1302–1309.

Kamat, J. P., K. K. Boloor, T. P. Devasagayam and S.R. Venkatachalam. 2000. Antioxidant properties of Asparagus racemosus against damage induced by gamma-radiation in rat liver mitochondria. *J Ethnopharmacol* 71:425–435.

Kanwar, P. and N. Sharma. 2011. Traditional pre–and postnatal dietary practices prevalent in Kangra district of Himachal Pradesh. *Indian J Tradit Know* 10:339–343.

Kaplan, R.1994. Poppy seed dependence. *Med J Aust* 161:176.

Kasture V. S., V. K. Deshmukh and C. T. Chopde. 2002. Anxiolytic and anticonvulsive activity of Sesbania grandiflora leaves in experimental animals. *Phytother Res* 16:455–460.

Katewa, S. S., B. L. Chaudhary and A. Jain. 2004. Folk herbal medicines from tribal area of Rajasthan. *Indian J Ethnopharmacol* 92:41–46.

Kaur, G. J. and D. S. Arora. 2010. Bioactive potential of Anethum graveolens, Foeniculum vulgare and Trachyspermum ammi belonging to the family Umbelliferae—Current status. *J Med Plants Res* 4:87–94.

Keller, A. C., J. Ma, A. Kavalier, K. He, A. M. Brillantes and E. J. Kennelly. 2011. Saponins from the traditional medicinal plant *Momordica charantia* stimulate insulin secretion *in vitro*. *Phytomedicine* 19:32–37.

Khadem. N., A. Sharaphy, R. Latifnejad, N. Hammod and S. Ibrahimzadeh. 2007. Comparing the efficacy of dates and oxytocin in the management of postpartum hemorrhage. *Shiraz E Med J* 8:64–71.

Khalid, S. A., A. Farouk, T. G. Geary and J. B. Jensen. 1986. Potential antimalarial candidates from African plants: An in vitro approach using Plasmodium falciparum. *J Ethnopharmacol* 15:201–209.

Khalid, S. A., Duddect, H. and M. Gonzalez-Sierra. 1989. Isolation and characterization of an antimalarial agent of the neem tree Azadirachta indica. *J Nat Prod* 52:922–927.

Khalil, M. I. M., M. M. Ibrahim, G. A. El-Gaaly and A. S. Sultan. 2015. Trigonella foenum (Fenugreek)-induced apoptosis in hepatocellular carcinoma cell line, Hepg2, mediated by upregulation of p53 and proliferating cell nuclear antigen. *BioMed Res Int* 2015:914645.

Khan, B. A., A. Abraham and S. Leelamma. 1996. Biochemical response in rats to the addition of curry leaf (Murraya koenigii) and mustard seeds (Brasika juncea) to the diet. *Plant Foods Hum Nutr* 49:295–299.

Khandhar, M. Z., P. Amit, P. Samir and P. Archita. 2010. Chemistry and pharmacology of Piper longum L. *Int J Pharm Sci Rev Res* 5:67–76.

Khursheed, R., G. H. Rizwani, V. Sultana, M. Ahmed and A. Kamil. 2014. Antidepressant effect and categorization of inhibitory activity of monoamine oxidase type A and B of ethanolic extract of seeds of Trigonella foenum graecum Linn. *Pak J Pharm Sci* 27:1419–1425.

Kidmose, U., S. L. Hansen, L. P. Christensen, M. Edelenbos, M. Larsen and R. Norback. 2004. Effects of genotypes, root size, storage and processing on bioactive compounds in organically grown carrots (*Daucus carota* L). *J Food Sci* 69:388–394.

Kiran, K. and M. Asad. 2008. Wound healing activity of Sesamum indicum L seed and oil in rats. *Indian J Exp Biol* 46:777–782.

Kirisattayakul, W., T. Tong-Un, J. Wattanathorn, S. Muchimapura, P. Wannanon and J. Jittiwat. 2009. Evaluation of total phenolic compound, antioxidant effect, and neuropharmacological activities of Moringa oleifera Lam leaves extract. *North-Eastern Thai J Neurosci* 6:80–92.

Kirtikar, K. R. and B. D. Basu. 1935. *Indian medicinal plants*. New Delhi: Saujanya Books.

Ko, S. H., J. H. Park, S. Y. Kim, S. W. Lee, S. S. Chun and E. Park. 2014. Antioxidant effects of spinach (Spinacia oleracea L.) supplementation in hyperlipidemic rats. *Prev Nutr Food Sci* 19:19–26.

Krishna, K. L., M. Paridhavi and J. A. Patel. 2008. Review on nutritional, medicinal and pharmacological properties of papaya (Carica Papaya.Linn). *Indian J Nat Prod Resour* 7:364–373.

Krishnamoorthi, V., M. B. Madalageri. 1999. Bishop's Weed (Trichyspermum ammi), an essential crop for North Karnataka. *J Med Aromat Plants Sci* 21:996–998.

Kulier, R., M. de Onis, A. M. Gulmezoglu and J. Villar. 1998. Nutritional interventions for the prevention of maternal morbidity. *Int J Gynecol Obstet* 63:231–246.

Kumar, B., A. Kuhad and K. Chopra. 2011a. Neuropsychopharmacological effect of sesamol in unpredictable chronic mild stress model of depression: Behavioral and biochemical evidences. *Psychopharmacology* 214:819–828.

Kumar, G., G. S. Banu, T. Rajarajan and G. Sathishkumar. 2011b. Medicinal flora of Palayapalayam, Namakkal district, Tamilnadu. *Indian J Pure and Appl Bio* 26:135–158.

Kumari, K., B. C. Mathew and K. T. Augusti. 1995. Antidiabetic and hypolipidemic effects of s-methyl cysteine sulfoxide isolated from Allium cepa Linn. *Indian J Biochem Biophys* 32:49–54.

Kuroda, S., M. Watanabe, T. Santo, Y. Shimizuishi,T. Takano, Y. Hidaka, T. Kimura and Y. Iwatani. 2010. Postpartum increase of serum thioredoxin concentrations and the relation to CD8 lymphocytes. *Ann Clin Biochem* 47:62–66.

Kurup, V. P. and C. S. Barrios. 2007. Immunomodulatory effects of curcumin in allergy. *Mol Nutr Food Res* 52:1031–1039.

Lakshmi, B.V.S. and M. Sudhakar. 2010. Attenuation of acute and chronic restraint stress-induced perturbations in experimental animals by Zingiber officinale Roscoe. *Food Chem Toxicol* 48:530–535.

Lee, C. L., L. C. Chiang, L. H. Cheng, C. C. Liaw, M. H. Abd El-Razek, F. R. Chang and Y. C. Wu. 2009. Influenza A (H(1)N(1)) antiviral and cytotoxic agents from Ferula asafoetida. *J Nat Prod* 72:1568–1572.

Leong, X. -F., M. R. Mustafa and K. Jaarin. 2013. Nigella sativa and its protective role in oxidative stress and hypertension. *J Evid Based Complementary Altern Med* 2013:120732.

Liu, J. H., G. H. Chen, H. Z. Yeh, C. K. Huang and S. K. Poon. 1997. Enteric-coated peppermint-oil capsules in the treatment of irritable bowel syndrome: A prospective, randomized trial. *J Gastroenterol* 32:765–768.

Liu-Chiang, C. Y. 1995. Postpartum worries: An exploration of Taiwanese primiparas who participate in the Chinese ritual of Tso-Yueh-Tzu. *Matern Child Nurs J* 23:110–122.

Loganayaki, N., N. Suganya and S. Manian. 2012. Evaluation of edible flowers of agathi (Sesbania grandiflora L.Fabaceae) for in vivo anti-inflammatory and analgesic, and in vitro antioxidant potential. *Food Sci Biotechnol* 21:509–517.

Luthra, P. M., R. Singh and R. Chandra. 2001. Therapeutic uses of Curcuma longa (Turmeric). *Indian J Clin Biochem* 16:153–160

MacArthur, C., H. R. Winter, D. E. Bick, R. J. Lilford, R. J. Lancashire, H. Knowles, D. A. Braunholtz, C. Henderson, C. Belfield and H. Gee. 2003. Redesigning postnatal care: A randomised controlled trial of protocol-based midwifery-led care focused on individual women's physical and psychological health needs. *Health Technol Assess* 7:1–98.

Madar, Z. and A. H. Stark. 2002. New legume sources as therapeutic agents. *Br J Nutr* 88:S287–S292.

Maghrani, M., N. A. Zeggwagh, J. B. Michel and M. Eddouks. 2005. Antihypertensive effect of Lepidium sativum L. in spontaneously hypertensive rats. *J Ethnopharmacol* 100:193–197.

Mahady, G. B. 2005. Medicinal plants for the prevention and treatment of bacterial infections. *Curr Pharm Des* 11:2405–2427.

Mahady, G. B., S. L. Pendland, G. Yun and Z. Z. Lu. 2002. Turmeric Curcuma Longa and curcumin inhibit the growth of Helicobacter pylori, A group 1 carcinogen. *Anticancer Res* 22:4179–4181.

Mahmood, K. T., T. Mugal and I. U. Haq. 2010. Moringa oleifera: A natural gift—a review. *J Pharm Sci Res* 2:775–781.

Majdalaweih, A. F. and R. I. Carr. 2010. In vitro investigation of the potential immunomodulatory and anti-cancer activities of black pepper (Piper nigrum) and carrdamon (Eletttaria cardamomum). *J Med Food* 13:371–381.

Majumdar, B. and T. Debnath. 2014. Immunomodulatory activity of ethanolic extract of bitter gourd (Momordica Charantia) in experimental models. *J Biomed Pharm Res* 3:59–63.

Manisha, P. M., M. M. Routh, R. B. Shinde and S. M. Karuppayil. 2012. Ethnic uses of medicinal plants from thirty eight villages in India for gynecological care. *Asian J Tradit Med* 7:292–304.

Marasco, L. 2008. Inside track: Increasing your milk supply with galactogogues. *J Hum Lact* 24:455–456.

Marrufo, T., F. Nazzaro, E. Mancini, F. Fratianni, R. Coppola, L. De Martino, A. B. Agostinho and V. De Feo. 2013. Chemical composition and biological activity of the essential oil from leaves of Moringa oleifera Lam cultivated in Mozambique. *Molecules* 13:10989–11000.

Mathur, H. N., P. N. Sharma and T. P. Tain. 1983. Traditional way of maternal and child health care in Rajasthan, India. *In Primary maternal and neonatal health: A global concern*, ed. F. del Mundo, E. Ines-Cuyegkeng and D. M. Aviado, 473-481. New York: Plenum Press.

Matsuda, H., K. Ninomiya, T. Morikawa, D. Yasuda, I. Yamaguchi and M. Yoshikawa. 2008. Protective effects of amide constituents from the fruit of Piper chaba on D-galactosamine/TNF-alpha-induced cell death in mouse hepatocytes. *Bioorg Med Chem Lett* 18:2038–2042.

Matsumura, Y., S. Kita, Y. Tanida, Y. Taguchi, S. Morimoto, K. Akimoto and T. Tanata. 1998. Antihypertensive effect of sesamin III Protection against development and maintenance of hypertension in stroke-prone spontaneously hypertensive rats. *Biol Pharm Bull* 21:469–473.

Maury, P. K., S. K. Jain, N. Lal and S. Alok. 2013. A review on antiulcer activity. *IJPSR* 3:2487–2493.

Mendel. F. 2004. Analysis of biologically active compounds in potatoes (Solanum tuberosum), tomatoes (Lycopersicon esculentum), and jimson weed (Datura stramonium) seeds. *J Chromatogr* 1054(1):143–155.

Mesallam, A. S. and M. A. Hamza. 1987. Studies on green gram (Phaseolus aureus) protein concentrate and Flour. *Plant Food Hum Nutr* 37:17–27.

Miguel, M. G., C. Cruz, L. Faleiro, M. T. Simoes, A. C. Figueiredo, J. G. Barroso and L.G. Pedro. 2010. Foenicum vulgare essential oils: Chemicals, composition, antioxidant and antimicrobial activities. *Nat Prod Commun* 5:319–328.

Mills, S. and K. Bone. 2000. Principles and practice of phytotherapy: Modern herbal medicine. Edinburgh: Churchill Livingstone.

Mishra, R. K., A. Kumar and A. Kumar. 2012. Pharmacological activity of Zingiber officinale. *IJCPS* 1:1422–1427.

Misra, S. K. and K. C. Sahu. 1977. Screening of some indigenous plants for antifungal activity against dermatophytes. *Indian J Pharmacol* 9:269–272.

Mitra, C. R. 1963. *Neem*. Hyderabad: Indian Central Oilseeds Committee.

Miyawaki, T., H. Aono, Y. Toyoda-Ono, H. Maeda, Y. Kiso and K. Moriyama. 2009. Antihypertensive effects of sesamin in humans. *J Nutr Sci Vitaminol* 55:87–91.

Monsefi, M., M. Ghasemi and A. Bahaoddini. 2006. The effects of Anethum graveolens L. on female reproductive system. *Phytother Res* 20:865–868.

Mortel, M. and S. D. Mehta. 2013. Systematic review of the efficacy of herbal galactogogues. *J Hum Lact* 29:154–62.

Moyo, B., P. J. Masika and V. Muchenje. 2012. Antimicrobial activities of Moringa oleifera lam leaf extract. *Afr J Biotechnol* 11:2797–2802.

Muhlhausler, B. S., A. R. Gibson and M. Makrides. 2010. Effect of long-chain polyunsaturated fatty acid supplementation during pregnancy or lactation on infant and child body composition: A systematic review. *Am J Clin Nutr* 92:857–863.

Mukherjee, P. K. 2003. Plant products with hypocholesterolemic potentials. *Adv Food Nutr Res* 47:277–338

Mukherjee, P. K., N. Maity, N. K. Nema and B. K. Sarkar. 2011. Bioactive compounds from natural resources against skin aging. *Phytomedicine* 19:64–73.

Mukherjee. P. K., N. K. Nema, S. Bhadra, D. Mukherjee, F. C. Braga and M. G. Matsabisa. 2014. Immunomodulatory leads from medicinal plants. *Indian J Tradit Know* 13:235–256.

Murty, C. M., J. K. Pittaway and M. J. Ball. 2010. Chickpea supplementation in an Australian diet affects food choice, satiety and bowel function. *Appetite* 54:282–288.

Nadarajah, D., J. H. Han and R. A. Holley. 2005. Use of mustard flour to inactivate Escherichia coli O157:H7 in ground beef under nitrogen-flushed packaging. Int J Food Microbiol 99:257-267.

Nadkarni, K. M. 2007. *Indian Materia Medica*. Mumbai: Popular Prakashan Pvt Ltd.

Nagnur, S., N. Channammaand, G. Channal. 2006. Indigenous pre-natal and post-delivery care practices of rural women. *Asian Agri Hist* 10:60-73.

Nair, R. M., D. Thavarajah, P. Thavarajah, R. R. Giri, D. Ledesma, R. Y. Yang, P. Hanson, W. Easdown, J. A. Hughes and J. D. H. Keatinge. 2015. Mineral and phenolic concentrations of mungbean (Vigna radiata (L.) R. Wilczek var. radiate) grown in semi-arid tropical India. *J Food Compost Anal* 39:23–32.

National Research Council. 1992. *Neem: A tree for solving global problems*. Washington, DC.: National Academy Press.

Nevin, K. G. and T. Rajamohan. 2010. Effect of topical application of virgin coconut oil on skin components and antioxidant status during dermal wound healing in young rats. *Skin Pharmacol Physiol* 23:290–297.

Nice, F. J. 2011. Common herbs and foods used as galactogogues. *Infant Child Adolesc Nutr* 3:129–132.

NIN. 2010. Dietary guidelines for Indians—A manual. National Institute of Nutrition, Hyderabad: ICMR.

NIN. 2014. Nutritive value of Indian foods. National Institute of Nutrition, Hyderabad: ICMR.

Ninfali, P. and D. Angelino. 2013. Nutritional and functional potential of *Beta vulgaris cicla* and *Rubra*. *Fitoterapia* 89:188-199.

Nisha, M. C. and S. Rajeshkumar. 2010. Survey of crude drugs from Coimbatore city. *Indian J Nat Prod Resour* 1:376–383.

Nutan, M. T. H., A. Hasnat and M. A. Rashid. 1998. Antibacterial and cytotoxic activities of Murrayya koeinigii. *Fitoterapia* 69:173–175.

Olivier, C., S. F. Vaughn, E. S. Mizubuti and R. Loria. 1999. Variation in allyl isothiocyanate production within Brassica species and correlation with fungicidal activity. *J Chem Ecol* 25:2687–2701.

Oomah, D. B., F. Caspar, L. J. Malcolmson and A. S. Bellido. 2011. Phenolics and antioxidant activity of lentil and pea hulls. *Food Res Inter* 44:436–441.

Oragwa, L. N., O. O. Efiom and S. K. Okwute. 2013. Phytochemicals, anti-microbial and free radical scavenging activities of Momordica charantia linn (Palisota Reichb) seeds. *Afr J Pure Appl Chem* 7:405–409.

Osborne, T. B. 1916. *Vegetable proteins*. London: Longmans, Green, and Co.

Otten. J., Hellwig, J. Pitzi and L. D. Meyers. 2006. *Dietary reference intakes: The essential guide to nutrient requirements*. Washington, DC: National Academies Press.

Palamthodi, S. and S. S. Lele. 2014. Nutraceutical applications of gourd family vegetables: *Benincasa hispida*, *Lagenaria siceraria* and *Momordica charantia*. *Biomed Prev Nutr* 4:15–21.

Pandian, R. S., C. V. Anuradha and P. Vishwanathan. 2002. Gastroprotective effect of fenugreek seeds (Trigonella foenum graecum) on experimental gastric ulcer in rats. *J Ethnopharmacol* 81:393–397.

Pant N., H. S. Garg, K. P. Madhusudanan and D. S. Bhakuni. 1986. Sulfurous compounds from Azhadiracta indica leaves. *Fitoterapia* 57:302–304.

Paranjpe, R., S. R. Gundala, N. Lakshminarayana, A. Sagwal, G. Asif, A. Pandey and R. Aneja. 2013. Piper betel leaf extract: Anticancer benefits and bio-guided fractionation to identify active principles for prostate cancer management. *Carcinogenesis* 34:1558–1566.

Patra, S., B. Singh, V. P. Reddaiah. 2008. Maternal morbidity during postpartum period in a village of North India: A prospective study. *Trop Doc* 38:204–208.

Perveen, T., S. Haider, S. Kanwal and D. J. Haleem. 2009. Repeated administration of Nigella sativa decreases 5-HT turnover and produces anxiolytic effects in rats. *Pak J Pharm Sci* 22:139–144.

Philippa, M., C. Crowther, T. Bubner, V. Flenady, Z. Bhutta, T. S. Thach and Z. Lassi. 2013. Nutrition interventions and programs for reducing mortality and morbidity in pregnant and lactating women and women of reproductive age: A systematic review. *ARCH*. Available at https://www.adelaide.edu.au/arch/research/3ie/AUSAID_short_version_May_2013.pdf. Accessed on March 10, 2015.

Pierro, D. F., A. Callegari, D. Carotenuto and M. M. Tapia. 2008. Clinical efficacy, safety and tolerability of BIO-C (micronized Silymarin) as a galactagogue. *Acta Biomed* 79:205–210.

Piers, L. S., S. N. Diggavi, S. Thangam, J. M. Van Raaij, P. S. Shetty and J. G. Hautvast. 1995. Changes in energy expenditure, anthropometry and energy intake during the course of pregnancy and lactation in well-nourished Indian women. *Am J Clin Nutr* 61:501–513.

Pittaway, J. K., K. D. K. Ahuja, I. K. Robertson and M. J. Ball. 2007. Effects of a controlled diet supplemented with chickpeas on serum lipids, glucose tolerance, satiety and bowel function. *J Am Coll Nutr* 26:334–340.

Platel, K. and K. Srinivasan. 2004. Digestive stimulant action of spices: A myth or reality? *Indian J Med Res* 119:167–179.

Proestos, C., I. S. Boziaris, J. E. Nychas and M. Komaitis. 2006. Analysis of flavonoids and phenolic acids in green aromatic plants: Investigation of their antioxidant and antimicrobial activity. *Food Chem* 95:664–671.

Pullaiah, T. 2006. *Encyclopedia of world medicinal plants*. New Delhi: Regency Publications.

Purseglove, J. W., E. G. Brown, C. L. Green and S. R. J. Robbins. 1981. *Spices* Vol II. London and New York: Longman.

Radhakrishnan, N. and A. Gnanamani. 2014. 2, 5-Dihydroxy-3-Undecyl-1, 4-Benzoquinone (Embelin)-A second solid gold of India-A review. *Int J Pharm Pharm Sci* 6:23–30.

Raguindin, P. F., L. F. Dans and J. F. King. 2014. Moringa oleifera as a galactagogue. *Breastfeed Med* 9:323–324.

Ramalingum, N. and M. F. Mahomoodally. 2014. The therapeutic potential of medicinal foods. *Adv Pharmacol Sci* 2014:1–18.

Ramesh, C. K., A. Rehman, B. T. Prabhakar, V. Avin and A. Rao. 2011. Antioxidant potentials in sprouts vs. seeds of Vigna radiata and Macrotyloma uniflorum. *J Appl Pharm Sci* 1:99–103.

Ramsewak, R. S., M. G. Nair, G. M. Strasburg, D. L. DeWitt and J. L. Nitiss. 1999. Biologically active carbazole alkaloids from Murraya koenigii. *J Agric Food Chem* 47:444–447.

Ramya, R. and S. Jose. 2014. Indigenous food formulations of Kerala used in maternal care—An exploratory study. *Int J Pharm Bio Sci* 5:325–331.

Rao, A. V. and B. Balachandran. 2002. Role of oxidative stress and antioxidants in neurodegenerative diseases. *Nutr Neurosci* 5:291–309.

Rao, C. R., S. M. Dhanya, K. Ashok and S. Niroop. 2014. Assessment of cultural beliefs and practices during the postnatal period in a coastal town of South India-A mixed method research study. *GJMEDPH* 3(5): 1-8.

Rao, S. and C. Yajnik. 2010. Maternal diets in the developing world. *In Maternal-fetal nutrition during pregnancy and lactation*, ed. M. E. Symonds and M. M. Ramsay, 44-52. Cambridge: University Press.

Rather, M. A., B. A. Dar, S. N. Sofi, B. A. Bhat and M. A. Qurishi. 2012. Foeniculum vulgare: A comprehensive review of its traditional use, phytochemistry, pharmacology and safety. *Arabian J Chem* 9(2) S1574–1583

Rathore, S. S., S. N. Saxena and S. Balraj. 2012. Potential health benefits of major seed spices. Int J Seed Spices 3:1–12.

Ratna, C., S. Mukherjee, S. Sen, S. Bosea, S. Datta, H. Koley, S. Ghosh, P. Dhar. 2012. Antimicrobial activity of Sesbania grandiflora flower polyphenol extracts on some pathogenic bacteria and growth stimulatory effect on the probiotic organism Lactobacillus acidophilus. *Micro Resear* 167: 500–506.

Ray, A., B. D. Banerjee and P. Sen. 1996. Modulation of humoral and cell-mediated immune responses by *Azadirachta indica* (Neem) in mice. *Indian J Exp Biol* 34:698–701.

Rochfort, S. and J. Panozzo. 2007. Phytochemicals for health, the role of pulses. *J Agric Food Chem* 55:7981–7994.

Ronsmans, C., S. Collin and V. Filippi. 2008. Maternal mortality in developing countries. *Nutrition and health in developing countries*, ed. R. D. Semba and M. W. Bloem, 33-62. New Jersey: Humana Press.

Roy, M. K., V. N. Thalang, G. Trakoontivakorn and K. Nakahara. 2004. Mechanism of mahanine-induced apoptosis in human leukemia cells (HL-60). *Biochem pharmacol* 67:41–51.

Saganuwan, A. 2010. Some medicinal plants of Arabian Pennisula. J Med Plant Res 4:766–788.

Saha, P., U. K. Mazumder, P. K. Haldar, A. Islam and R. B. Sureshkumar. 2011. Evaluation of acute and sub-chronic toxicity of Lagenaria siceraria aerial parts. *IJPSR* 2:1507–1512.

Saini, N., G. K. Singh and B. P. Nagori. 2014. Spasmolytic potential of some medicinal plants belonging to family Umbelliferae: A review. *Int J Res Ayurveda Pharm* 5:74–83.

Saleem, M. T. S, C. M. Chetty, S. Ramkanth, M. Alagusundaram, K. Gnanaprakash, V. S. T. Rajan and S. Angalaparameswari. 2009. Solanum nigrum Linn—A review. *Phcog Rev* 3:342–345.

Saleem, T. S. M., C. M. Chetty and S. Kavimani. 2012. Sesame oil enhances endogenous antioxidants in ischemic myocardium of rat. *Braz J Pharmacogn* 22:669–675.

Saleem, T. S. M., S. D. Basha, G. Mahesh, P. V. S. Rani, N. S. Kumarand, C. M. Chetty. 2011. Analgesic, anti-pyretic and anti-inflammatory activity of dietary sesame oil in experimental animal models. *Pharmacologia* 2:172–177.

Sang, S., K. Lapsley, W. S. Jeong, P. A. Lachence, C. T. Ho and R. T. Rosen. 2002. Antioxidative phenolic compounds isolated from almond skins (Prunus amygdalus Batsch). *J Agri Food Chem* 50:2459–2463.

Sankaranarayanan, J. and C. I. Jolly. 1993. Phytochemical, antibacterial, and pharmacological investigations on Momordica charantia Linn. Emblica offidnalis Gaertn and Curcuma longa Linn. *Indian J Pharm Sci* 55:95–100.

Sastry, C. S. T. and K. Y. Kavathekar. 1990. *Plants for reclamation of wastelands*. New Delhi: Council of Scientific and Industrial Research.

Satyavati, G. V., M. K. Raina and M. Sharma. 1976. *Medicinal plants of India*. New Delhi: Indian Council of Medical Research.

Savage, G. P. 1988. The composition and nutritive value of lentils (Lens culinaris). *Nutr Abs Rev Ser A* 58:320–343.

Saydut, A, M. Z. Duz, C. Kaya, A. B. Kafadar and C. Hamamci 2008. Trans-esterified sesame (Sesamum indicum L.) seed oil as a biodiesel fuel. *Bioresour Techol* 99:6656–6660.

Sayed, N. Z., R. Deo and U. Mukundan. 2007. Herbal remedies used by Warlis of Dahanu to induce lactation in nursing mothers. *Indian J Tradit Know* 6:602–605.

Sen, P., P. K. Medinata and A. Ray. 1992. Effects of Azadirachta Indica on some biochemical, immunological and visceral parameters in normal and stressed rats. *Indian J Exp Biol* 30:1170–1175.

Serra, C., S. Bhasin, F. Tangherlini, E. R. Barton, M. Ganno, A. Zhang, J. Shansky, H. H. Vandenburgh, T. G. Travison, R. Jasuja and C. Morris. 2011. The role of GH and IGF-I in mediating anabolic effects of testosterone on androgen-responsive muscle. *Endocrinology* 152:193–206.

Severin, S. X. Wenshui. 2005. Milk biologically active components as nutraceuticals: Review. *Crit Rev Food Sci Nutr* 45:645–656.

Shah, A. H., S. Qureshi and A. M. Ageel. 1991. Toxicity studies in mice of ethanol extracts of Foeniculum vulgare fruit and Ruta chalepensis aerial parts. *J Ethnopharmacol* 34:167–172.

Shah, A. S., A. S. Wakade and A. R. Juvekar. 2011a. Immunomodulatory activity of methanolic extracts of Murraya koenigii (L) Spreng leaves. *Indian J Exp Biol* 46:505–509.

Shah, K. H., J. B. Patel, V. J. Sharma, R. M. Shrma, R. P. Patel and U. M. Chaunhan. 2011b. Evaluation of antidiabetic activity of Prunus amygdalus batsch in streptozotocin-induced diabetic mice. *Res J Pharm Biol Chem Sci* 2:429–434

Shahin, S. and N. Ahmad. 2014. Herbs used during pregnancy and postpartum in a group of women in Patna district. *Int J Phytotherapy* 4:58–62.

Shanmugam, S., K. Rajendran and K. Suresh. 2012. Traditional uses of medicinal plants among the rural people of Sivagangai district of Tamil Nadu, Southern India. *Asian Pac J Trop Biomed* 2:429–434.

Sharma, K. D., S. Karki, N. S. Thakur and S. Attri. 2012. Chemical composition, functional properties and processing of carrot—A review. *J Food Sci Technol* 49:22–32.

Sharma, R. D. 1986. Effect of fenugreek seeds and leaves on blood glucose and serum insulin responses in human subjects. *Nutr Res* 6:1353–1364.

Sharma, R. D., A. Sarkar and Hazra, D. K. 1996. Hypolipidemic effect of fenugreek seeds: A chronic study in non-insulin dependent diabetic patients. *Phytother Res* 10:332–334.

Shi, J., C. T. Ho, F. Shahidi. 2011. *Functional foods of the east.* Boca Raton, FL: CRC Press/Taylor & Francis.

Shilling, M., L. Matt, E. Rubin, M. P. Visitacion, N. A. Haller, S. F. Grey and C. J. Woolverton. 2013. Antimicrobial effects of virgin coconut oil and its medium-chain fatty acids on Clostridium difficile. *J Med Food* 16:1079–1085.

Shirke, S. S. and A. G. Jagtap. 2009. Effects of methanolic extract of Cuminum cyminumon total serum cholesterol in ovariectomized rats. *Indian J Pharmacol* 41:92–93.

Shivaprasad, H. N., M. D. Kharya, A. C. Rana and S. Mohan. 2006. Preliminary immunomodulatory activities of aqueous extract of Terminalia chebula. *Pharm Biol* 44:32–34.

Shojaii, A. and M. A. Fard. 2012. Review of pharmacological properties and chemical constituents of *Pimpinella anisum. ISRN Pharm* 2012:1–8.

Shriraam, V., P. B. Shah, M. A. Rani, G. Palani and B. W. Sathiyasekaran. 2012. Postpartum morbidity and health seeking pattern in a rural community in South India: Population-based study, *Indian J Matern Child Health* 14:1–10.

Siddhuraju, P. and K. Becker. 2003. Antioxidant properties of various solvent extracts of total phenolic constituents from three different agroclimatic origins of drumstick tree (Moringa oleifera Lam.) leaves. *J Agric Food Chem* 51:2144–2155.

Siddiqui, S. 1942. A note on the isolation of three new bitter principles from the neem oil. *Curr Sci* 11:278–279.

Silver, R. J. 2006. Ayurvedic veterinary medicine: Principles and practices. *In Veterinary herbal medicine*, ed. S. G. Wynn and B. J. Fougère, 59-83. St. Louis: Mosby Elsevier.

Simons, C. T., S. Sudo, M. Sudo and E. Carstens. 2004. Mustard oil has differential effects on the response of Trigeminal caudalis neurons to heat and acidity. *Pain* 110:64–71.

Singh, A. and Kumar, A. 2014. Factors associated with seeking treatment for postpartum morbidities in rural India. *Epidemiol Health* 36:e2014026.

Sreeja, S., V. S. Anju and S. Sreeja. 2010. In vitro estrogenic activities of fenugreek Trigonella foenum graecum seeds. *Indian J Med Res* 131:814–819.

Sreelatha, S., P. R. Padma and E. Umasankari. 2011. Evaluation of anticancer activity of ethanol extract of Sesbania grandiflora (Agati Sesban) against Ehrlich ascites carcinoma in Swiss albino mice. *J Ethnopharmacol* 134:984–987.

Sreeramulu, D. and M. Raghunath. 2011. Antioxidant and phenolic content of nuts, oil seeds, milk and milk products commonly consumed in India. *Food Nutr Sci* 2:422–427.

Srinivas, R., K. Eagappan and S. Sasikumar. 2014. The effect of naturally formulated galactagogue mix on breast milk production, prolactin level and short-term catch-up of birth weight in the first week of life. *Int J Health Sci Res* 4:242–253.

Srinivasan, K. 2005. Plant foods in the management of diabetes mellitus: Spices as beneficial antidiabetic food adjuncts. *Int J Food Sci Nutr* 56:399–414.

Srinivasjois, R., S. Rao and S. Patole. 2009. Prebiotic supplementation of formula in preterm neonates: A systematic review and meta-analysis of randomised controlled trials. *Clin Nutr* 28:237–242.

Srivastava, P. and S. Durgaprasad. 2008. Burn wound healing property of Cocos nucifera: An appraisal. *Indian J Pharmacol* 40:144–146.

Subash, G. P., S. R. Virbhadrappa and O. K. Vasant. 2010. Spinacia oleracea Linn: A pharmacognostic and pharmacological overview. *Int J Res Ayurveda Phar* 1:78–84.

Sudha, K. and S. K. Mathanghi. 2012. Traditional underutilized green leafy vegetables and its curative properties. *Int J Pharm* 2:786–793.

Suryanarayana, P., K. Krishnaswamy and G. B. Reddy. 2003. Effect of curcumin on galactose-induced cataractogenesis in rats. *Mol Vis* 9:223–230.

Suseelappan, M. S. 1991. Medicinal uses of pepper in ayurveda. *Int Pepper News* 15:6–7.

Tabares, F. P., V. B. J. Juliana and T. R. C. Zulma. 2014. Pharmacological overview of galactogogues. *Vet Med Int* 2014:1–18.

Tachibana, Y., H. Kikuzaki, N. H. Lajis and N. Nakatani. 2001. Antioxidative activity of carbazoles from Murraya koenigii leaves. *J Agri Food Chem* 49:5589–5594.

Tang. D., Y. Dong, H. Ren, L. Liand and C. He. 2014. A review of phytochemistry, metabolite changes, and medicinal uses of the common food mung bean and its sprouts (*Vigna radiata*). *Chem Cent J* 8:4.

Thavarajah, D., P. Thavarajah, A. Sarker and A. Vandenberg. 2009. Lentils (Lens culinaris Medikus Subspecies culinaris): A whole food for increased iron and zinc intake. *J Agric Food Chem* 57:5413–5419.

The Academy of Breastfeeding Medicine Protocol Committee. 2011. ABM clinical protocol: Use of galactogogues in initiating or augmenting the rate of maternal milk secretion (First revision January 2011). *Breastfeed Med* 6:41–49.

Tiwari, L. and P. C. Pande. 2010. Ethnoveterinary medicines in Indian perspective: Reference to Uttarakhand, Himalaya. *Indian J Tradit Know* 9:611–617.

Tomas, L. 2009. Best breastfeeding and formulas. *J Complement Med* 8:32–40.

Turkyilmaz, C., E. Onal, I. M. Hirfanoglu, O. Turan, E. Koç, E. Ergenekon and Y. Atalay. 2011. The effect of galactagogue herbal tea on breast milk production and short-term catch-up of birth weight in the first week of life. *J Altern Complement Med* 17:139–142.

Tzianabos, A. O. 2000. Polysaccharide immunomodulators as therapeutic agents: Structural aspects and biologic functions. *Clin Microbid Rev* 13:523–533.

Umadevi, M., R. Pushpa, K. P. Sampathkumar and B. Debjit. 2012. Rice—Traditional medicinal plant in India. *J Pharmacogn Phytochem* 1:6–12.

Unal, G., S. N. Eland, S. Kilic. 2005. In vitro determination of calcium bioavailability of milk, dairy products and infant formulas. *Int J Food Sci Nutr* 56:13–22.

UNICEF. 2013. Improving child nutrition. The achievable imperative for global progress. Available at http://www.unicef.org/publications/index_68661.html.

Upaganlawar, A. and R. Balaraman. 2009. Bottle Gourd (Lagenaria Siceraria) "A vegetable food for human health"—A comprehensive review. *Pharmacologyonline* 1:209–226.

Vaidya, D., N. Rana, S. Sharma and V. Mishra. 2013. Development and quality evaluation of beverages from bottle gourd, Lagenaria siceraria (mol.) Standl. *Indian J Nat Prod Resour* 4:219–222.

Valero, M. A., A. Vidal, R. Burgos, F. L. Calvo, C. Martínez, L. M. Luengo and C. Cuerda. 2011. Meta-analysis on the role of lycopene in type 2 diabetes mellitus. *Nutr Hosp* 26:1236–1241.

Vedhanayaki, G., G. V. Shastri and A. Kuruvilla. 2003. Analgesic activity of Piper longum Linn. root. *Ind J Exp Biol* 41:649–651.

Vigila, G. A. and X. Baskaran. 2008. Immunomodulatory effect of coconut protein on cyclophosphamide induced immune suppressed Swiss albino mice. *Ethnobot Leaflets* 12:1206–1212.

Villar, J., M. Merialdi, A. M. Gulmezoglu, E. Abalos, G. Carroli, R. Kulier and M. D. Onis. 2003. Nutritional interventions during pregnancy for the prevention or treatment of maternal morbidity and preterm delivery: An overview of randomized controlled trials. *J Nutr* 133:S1606-S1625.

Wang, X., W. Gao, J. Zhang, H. Zhang, Z. Hua, J. Li, X. He and H. Ma. 2009. Subunit, amino acid composition and in vitro digestibility of protein isolate from Chinese kabuli and desi chickpea (Cicer arietinum L.) cultivars. *Food Res Int* 43:567–572.

Wang, Y. H. A. and G. H. McIntosh. 1996. Extrusion and boiling improves rat body weight gain and plasma cholesterol lowering ability of peas and chickpea. *J Nutr* 126:3054–3062.

Warrier, P. K., V. P. K. Nambiar and C. Ramankutty1995. *Indian medicinal plants*,Volume 3. Madras: Orient Longman Limited.

Weggemans, R. M., P. L. Zock and M. B. Katan. 2001. Dietary cholesterol from eggs increases the ratio of total cholesterol to high-density lipoprotein cholesterol in humans: A meta-analysis. *Am J Clin Nutr* 73:885–891.

White, P. M. 2002. Crossing the river: Khmer women's perception of pregnancy and postpartum. *J Midwifery Womens Health* 47:4.

WHO. 1978. *The promotion and development of traditional medicine*. Geneva: World Health Organization.

WHO. 1998. *Postpartum care of the mother and newborn: A practical guide*. Geneva: World Health Organization.

WHO. 2008. *World malaria report*. Geneva: World Health Organization.

WHO. 2013. *WHO traditional medicine strategy: 2013-2014*. Geneva: World Health Organization.

WHO. 2014. *Trends in maternal mortality: 1990 to 2013. Estimates by WHO, UNICEF, UNFPA, the World Bank and the United Nations Population Division*. Geneva: World Health Organization.

Wiart, C. 2006. *Ethnopharmacology of medicinal plants: Asia and the Pacific*, Boca Raton, FL: CRC Press.

Wijeratne, S. S., M. M. Abou-Zaid and F. Shahidi. 2006. Antioxidant polyphenols in almond and its co-products. *J Agric Food Chem* 54:312–318.

Wu, H., H. L. He, X. L. Chen, C. Y. Sun, Y. Z. Zhang and B. C. Zhou. 2008. Purification and identification of novel angiotensin-I-converting enzyme inhibitory peptides from shark meat hydrolysate. *Process Biochem* 43:457–461.

Xu, B. and S. K. Chang. 2010. Phenolic substance characterization and chemical and cell-based antioxidant activities of 11 lentils grown in the northern United States. *J Agric Food Chem* 58:1509–1517.

Yadav, U. C. and N. Z. Baquer. 2014. Pharmacological effects of Trigonella foenum graecum L. in health and disease. *Pharm Biol* 52:243–254.

Yang, Y., L. Zhou, Y. Gu, Y. Zhang, J. Tang, F. Li, W. Shang, B. Jiang, X. Yue and M. Chen. 2007. Dietary chickpeas reverse visceral adiposity, dyslipidaemia and insulin resistance in rats induced by a chronic high-fat diet. *Br J Nutr* 98:720–726.

Yazdanparast, R. and M. Alavi. 2001. Antihyperlipidaemic and antihypercholesterolemic effects of Aethum graveolens leaves after the removal of furocoumarins. *Cytobios* 105:185–191.

Yazdanparast, R. and S. Bahramikia. 2008. Evaluation of the effect of Anethum graveolens L. crude extracts on serum lipids and lipo-proteins profiles in hypercholesterolemic rats. *DARU J Pharm Sci* 16:88–94.

Yealy, D. M., D. T. Huang, A. Delaney, M. Knight, A. G. Randolph, R. Daniels and T. Nutbeam. 2015. Recognizing and managing sepsis: What needs to be done? *BMC Medicine* 13:98.

Yu, L., K. Zhou and J. W. Parry. 2005. Inhibitory effects of wheat bran extracts on human LDL oxidation and free radicals. *LWT-Food Sci Technol* 38:463–470.

Yu, L., S. Haley, J. Perret and M. Harris. 2002. Antioxidant properties of hard wheat extracts. *Food Chem* 78:457–461.

Zagami, S. E., N. Golmakani, M. Kabirian and M. T. Shakeri. 2012. Effect of Dill (Anethum graveolens Linn.) seed on uterus contractions pattern in active phase of labor. *Indian J Tradit Know* 11:602–606.

Zalloua, P. A., Y. H. Hsu, H. Terwedow, T. Zang, D. Wu, G. Tang, Z. Li, X. Hong, S. T. Azar, B. Wang, M. L. Bouxsein, J. Brain, S. R. Cummings, C. J. Rosen and X. Xu. 2007. Impact of seafood and fruit consumption on bone mineral density. *Maturitas* 56:1–11.

Zapantis, A., J. G. Steinberg and L. Schilit. 2012. Use of herbals as galactagogues. *J Pharm Pract* 25:222–231.

Zarena, A. S., S. Gopal and R. Vineeth. 2014. Antioxidant, antibacterial, and cytoprotective activity of agathi leaf protein. *J Anal Meth Chem* 2014:1–8.

Zargari, A. 1996. *Medicinal plants*. Tehran: University Press.

Zhang, Y., H. P. Yao, F. F. Huang, W. Wu, Y. Gao, Z.-B. Chen, Z.-Y. Liang and T.-B. Liang. 2008. Allicin, a major component of garlic, inhibits apoptosis in vital organs in rats with trauma/hemorrhagic shock. *Crit Care Med* 36:3226–3232.

Zhou, K., L. Su and L. Yu. 2004. Phytochemicals and antioxidant properties in wheat bran. *J Agric Food Chem* 52:6108–6114.

Zia-Ul-Haq, M., S. Ahmad, S. A. Bukhari, R. Amarowicz, S. Ercisli and H. Z. Jaafar. 2014. Compositional studies and biological activities of some mash bean (*Vigna mungo* (L.) Hepper) cultivars commonly consumed in Pakistan. *Biol Res* 47:23.

Zieliski, H. and H. Kozlowska. 2000. Antioxidant activity and total phenolics in selected cereal grains and their different morphological fractions. *J Agric Food Chem* 48:2008–2016.

Zou, Y., S. K. C. Chang, Y. Gu and S. Y. Qian. 2011. Antioxidant activity and phenolic compositions of lentil (Lens culinaris var. Morton) extract and its fractions. *J Agric Food Chem* 59:2268–2276.

Zuppa, A. A., P. Sindico, C. Orchi, C. Carducci, V. Cardiello, C. Romagnoli and P. Catenazzi. 2010. Safety and efficacy of galactogogues: Substances that induce maintain and increase breast milk supply. *J Pharm Pharmaceut Sci* 13:162–174.TABLE 29.3

Index

A

AA, *see* Arachidonic acid
ACAD, *see* Activated T-cell autonomous death
ACD, *see* Anemia of chronic infection
Acrodermatitis enteropathica (AE), 246
Activated T-cell autonomous death (ACAD), 168
Activation-induced cell death (AICD), 168
Active hexose correlated compound (AHCC), 427,
        439–440
    anti-inflammatory effect, 431
    immunoregulatory effect, 428
    and infection, 428–431
Acute phase proteins (APP), 7, 60
Ad-36, *see* Adenovirus 36
Adaptation mechanisms, adipocytokine involvement in
    adipokines role, 117–118
    cytokines role, 114–117
Adaptive immunity, 9–10, 36–37, 336, 337
    B-cells, 169–172, 190, 260
    B-lymphocytes, 13–14
    human immunodeficiency virus infection, 381–382
    response, 2
    T-cells, *see* T-cells
    T helper cells, 381
    thymic function, 188–189
    T-lymphocytes, recognition by, 10–11
    Tregs, 382
    in tuberculosis, 382–383
    type II diabetes mellitus, 383
Addressins, 7
Adenovirus 36 (Ad-36), 39
Adhesion molecules, 7–8
Adipocytes, immune-like phenotypes for, 45
Adipocytokine involvement, in eating disorders, 114–118
Adipokines, 35–36
    regulation of, immune function, 46–48
    role of, 117–118
Adiponectin, 35, 47, 117
Adiponectin receptor (Adipo-R), 35
Adipose tissue, 43–44
    adipokine regulation, of immune function, 46–48
    developmental origin, 44–45
    and immune cells, 45
    resident immune cells, *see* Resident immune cells
    types of, 46
AE, *see* Acrodermatitis enteropathica
Agathi, see Sesbania grandiflora L.
Age-related macular degeneration (AMD), 74
Agglutination, 22
AHCC, *see* Active hexose correlated compound
AICD, *see* Activation-induced cell death
Allium sativum, see Garlic
Allograft, nucleotides modulation of, 395
Alpha-Tocopherol Beta-Carotene Cancer Prevention
        (ATBC) study, 204
AMD, *see* Age-related macular degeneration
Amino acids, direct anabolic influences of, 88–89

AN, *see* Anorexia nervosa
Anemia of chronic infection (ACD), 75
Animal source foods (ASFs)
    meat, 98
    milk, 98–101
Anorexia nervosa (AN)
    adipokines, 117–118
    cytokines, 114–117
    eating disorder, 111
    immune system characteristics in, 111–112
    lymphocyte subsets, 112–113
    perinatal immune factors, in disease etiology, 119
    refractory to infections, 113–114
    restrictive behavior of, 118–119
Antibody responses, 190
Antigen receptor complex, 12
Anti-inflammatory effect
    active hexose correlated compound, 431
    retinoic acid, 167
Antimicrobial peptides, *see* Host defense peptides
Anti-rotavirus activity, of human milk oligosaccharides, 149
Antiviral immunity, 238
Apoptosis, 254, 321–323
APP, *see* Acute phase proteins
Arachidonic acid (AA), 300
Arginine, 335–336
    cell-mediated immunity, *see* Cell-mediated immunity
    follicular helper T-cells, 341–342
    humoral immunity, 342
    immune response, 336–337
Ascorbic acid, *see* Vitamin C
ASFs, *see* Animal source foods
Ashwagandha, 448
Aspirin, 318
Asthma, 240
ATBC study, *see* Alpha-Tocopherol Beta-Carotene Cancer
        Prevention study
Autoimmune diseases
    nitric oxide in, 352
    n-3 polyunsaturated fatty acids and, 302–303
    zinc and, 265–266
Autoimmunity, development of, 151
Autophagy, 172
    gangliosides and, 414
Ayurvedic perspective, 443–444
    healing, nutrition in, 446
    herbs and preparations, 447–449
    history, 444–445
    human body, 445
    in infections, 446–447
    modern medicine, 445–446
Azhadiracta indica, see Neem

B

Bacterial infections, 38–39, 239, 447
BAFF, *see* B-cell activating factor
Basophils, 6

B-cell activating factor (BAFF), 411
B-cells, 2, 172
    adaptive immunity, 260
    development, 13–14, 169, 190
    in vitro activation of, 171–172
    proliferation of, 169–170
    repertoire, 14
    retinoic acid, *see* Retinoic acid
    zones, 15
Beta-defensins, 217
Bifidobacteria, 418
Bifidogenic effect, of gangliosides, 417
Bitter melon, 505
Black pepper, 504
B lymphocytes, 13–14, 51
BMP, *see* Bone morphogenetic protein
BN, *see* Bulimia nervosa
Body mass index (BMI), 95, 96, 453
Bone deterioration, 436
Bone growth regulation, 85–86
    amino acids and zinc, 88–89
    endochondral ossification, 86–87
    endocrine regulation, 87
    paracrine signaling, 87–88
Bone morphogenetic protein (BMP), 217
Breast cancer, 268–269
Breastfeeding, 95
    allergy development, lowers risk of, 150–151
    autoimmunity and, 151
    infection, risk for, 147–149
    on vaccination-induced immune responses, 149–150
Bulimia nervosa (BN), 111

C

cAMP, *see* Cyclic adenosine monophosphate
cAMP response element-binding protein (CREB), 261
Cancer
    gangliosides and, 410–411
    selenium and, 238
Cardiovascular risk, 52–53
Carotenoids, 74, 161
Cationic amino acid transporter 2 (CAT2), 338
CC-chemokine receptor 9 (CCR9), 190
CD8+ T-cells, 341
Cecal ligation and puncture (CLP), 327
Cell-mediated immunity
    CD8+ T-cells, 341
    follicular helper T-cells, 341–342
    regulatory T-cells, 340–341
    Th1 cells, 338
    Th2 cells, 338–339
    Th9 cells, 339
    Th17 cells, 340
Cellular communication, 15
Cellular iron homeostasis, 214–216
cGMP, *see* Cyclic guanosine monophosphate
Chemerin, 48
Chemokines, 7
α-Chemokines, 8
β-Chemokines, 8
Chemotaxis, 321
Cholecalciferol, *see* Vitamin D
Chylomicron remnants (CR), 161

CLP, *see* Cecal ligation and puncture
CLS, *see* Crown-like structure
Colony-stimulating factors, 7
Common cold, 268
Common variable immunodeficiency (CVID), 173
Complement system, 47–48
Copper, 77
C1q- and TNF-related protein (CTRP), 45
CR, *see* Chylomicron remnants
CREB, *see* cAMP response element-binding protein
Crown-like structure (CLS), 36
CTRP, *see* C1q- and TNF-related protein
Curcuma longa, see Turmeric
CVID, *see* Common variable immunodeficiency
Cyanocobalamin, *see* Vitamin B$_{12}$
Cyclic adenosine monophosphate (cAMP), 257
Cyclic guanosine monophosphate (cGMP), 257
Cytokines, 7, 114–117

D

DC1, *see* Dendritic cell count
DCs, *see* Dendritic cells
Death by neglect, 167, 168
Defense against infection, 398
Delayed hypersensitivity, 395
Dendritic cell count (DC1), 428
Dendritic cells (DCs), 163–164, 237, 259
    development, 186–187
    function of, 284
    glutathione and, 379
Dextran sulfate sodium (DSS), 340
Diabetes mellitus type I, 265
Diarrhea, 267
Dietary intake data, 457
Dietary nucleotides, 387–388
    absorption of, 388–389
    defense against infection, 398
    degradation, 389–391
    delayed hypersensitivity, 395
    immunoglobulin production by, 395–398
    intestinal inflammation, 398–399
    lymphocyte maturation, effects on, 392–393
    and lymphocyte subpopulations, 394
    potential mechanism of, 399–400
    sources of, 388
Disease etiology, perinatal immune factors in, 119
DSS, *see* Dextran sulfate sodium

E

EAA, *see* Essential AA
Early life immune development, 146
Eating disorder (ED)
    anorexia nervosa, *see* Anorexia nervosa
    bulimia nervosa, 111
    etiology, adipocytokine involvement in, 114–118
Ectosomes, *see* Microparticles
ED, *see* Eating disorder
EED, *see* Environmental enteric dysfunction
eEFSec, *see* Eukaryotic elongation factor
Eicosanoids, 300–301
Electromagnetic radiation, 437
Endochondral ossification, 86–87, 103–104

Endocrine regulation, 87
Endothelial cells, of vascular diseases, 352–353
Endothelial nitric oxide synthase (eNOS), 350
Energy intake, 93–95
eNOS, *see* Endothelial nitric oxide synthase
Environmental enteric dysfunction (EED), 102–103
Environmental stressor, 435
    microgravity of, 435–437
    space radiation, 437–440
Eosinophils, 6, 50, 184
Epicardial fat, 52–53
Epithelial surfaces, 182–183
ERK activation, *see* Extracellular signal-related kinase
Erythropoiesis, 218
Essential AA (EAA), 335
Ethnic indian postpartum nutritional practices,
      499–500
    traditional postpartum formulations, 502–505
    traditional postpartum menus, 500–502
Eukaryotic elongation factor (eEFSec), 233
Exogenous nucleotides, 388
Extracellular signal-related kinase (ERK) activation, 263

F

Fat-soluble vitamins
    vitamin A, 62–64
    vitamin D, 64–66
    vitamin E, 66–68
    vitamin K, 68
Fe, *see* Iron
Ferroportin, 217
FFAR2, *see* Free fatty acid receptor-2
FFAR3, *see* Free fatty acid receptor-3
FF infants, *see* Formula fed infants
FFQs, *see* Food frequency questionnaires
Folic acid, 72–73
Follicular helper T-cells (Tfh), 341–342
Food frequency questionnaires (FFQs), 457
Formula fed (FF) infants, 95
Free fatty acid receptor-2 (FFAR2), 281
Free fatty acid receptor-3 (FFAR3), 281
Fungal infections, 447

G

GALT, *see* Gut-associated lymphoid tissue
Gambian infants, 102
Gangliosides, 405
    bifidogenic effect of, 417
    and cancer, 410–411
    definition of, 406
    effects on, 414–417
    in immunity, 414
    inflammation, 413
    lipid raft constituents, 409–410
    neural development, 411–412
    neurodegenerative disorders, 412–413
    potential role of, 418
    quantification of, 406–409
Garlic, 504
Gastrointestinal (GI) tract, 146
GATA-6, 186
GCL, *see* Glutamate cysteine ligase

Germinal center (GC) reaction, 171
GGT, *see* γ-glutamyltranspeptidase 1
Ghrelin, 118
GI tract, *see* Gastrointestinal tract
Glucocorticoids, 167–168
Glutamate cysteine ligase (GCL), 376
Glutamine, 357
    in context of exercise, 363–366
    lymphocyte metabolic requirements, 362–363
    macrophage metabolic requirements, 361–362
    metabolism, 358–360
    neutrophil metabolic requirements, 360–361
    provision of, 366–369
Glutamine synthetase (GS), 358
γ-Glutamyltranspeptidase 1 (GGT), 377
Glutathione (GSH), 375–376
    adaptive immune system, *see* Adaptive immunity
    bacteria, 383
    dendritic cells, 379
    immune system, 377
    macrophages, 378
    natural killer cells, 380
    synthesis of, 376–377
Glutathione disulfide (GSSG), 376
Glutathione synthetase (GSS), 376
GPCRs, *see* G protein-coupled receptors
GPR109A, 281, 282
G protein-coupled receptors (GPCRs), 281–282, 319
Granulocytes, 183–184, 255–256
GS, *see* Glutamine synthetase
GSH, *see* Glutathione
GSNO, 378
GSS, *see* Glutathione synthetase
GSSG, *see* Glutathione disulfide
Guanine nucleotides, 389
Gut-associated lymphoid tissue (GALT), 19, 415
    effector sites, 21–22
    immune cell trafficking, 25–26
    inductor sites, 19–21
    intestinal microbiota, 26
    nonlymphoid tissues, antigen presentation in, 24
    oral tolerance, 22–24
Gut microbiota, 153
Gut permeability, 153

H

HD, *see* Huntington's disease
HDACs, *see* Histone deacetylases
HDPs, *see* Host defense peptides
Hepatic synthesis, 119
Hepcidin synthesis, 217–218
High endothelial venules (HEVs), 25, 163
Histological techniques, 25
Histone deacetylases (HDACs), 281
HIV infection, *see* Human immunodeficiency virus
      infection
HLAs, *see* Human leukocyte antigens
HMOs, *see* Human milk oligosaccharides
Host control, of inflammation, 315–316
Host defense peptides (HDPs), 283
Human immunodeficiency virus (HIV) infection, 267,
      381–382, 460–462
Human leukocyte antigens (HLAs), 10, 11

Human milk, 145
   breastfeeding, *see* Breastfeeding
   early life immune development, 146
   gut microbiota, 153
   human milk oligosaccharides, 146–147, 149, 151–153
   infant formula, oligosaccharides in, 153–154
Human milk oligosaccharides (HMOs), 146–147, 149,
      151–153
Humoral immunity, 336, 342
Hungry season, 458
Huntington's disease (HD), 412
Hydroxycarboxylic acid receptor-2 (HCA2), *see* Niacin
      receptor-1
Hydroxyl radical, 69

I

IBDs, *see* Inflammatory bowel diseases
IFNs, *see* Interferons
IgA, *see* Immunoglobulin A
IGF-1 activity, 87
IL-6, *see* Interleukin-6
IL-1β, *see* Interleukin-1β
ILCs, *see* Innate lymphoid cells
ILFs, *see* Isolated lymphoid follicles
Immune modulation by oligosaccharides, 152–153
Immune response, 336–337
Immune tolerance, 15–16
Immunoglobulin A (IgA), 22, 190
Immunoglobulin production, 395–398
Immunological synapse (IS), 298
Immunomodulatory endocrine organ, 33–36
INCAP, *see* Institute of Nutrition of Central America and
      Panama
Inducible nitric oxide synthase (iNOS), 350, 431
Infant formula, oligosaccharides in, 153–154
Infant nutritional status, 458–459
Infant outcomes
   human immunodeficiency virus infection on,
      460–462
   mother's diet in, 455–459
Infectious diseases
   common cold, 268
   diarrhea, 267
   malaria, 267–268
   n-3 polyunsaturated fatty acids, 303
Inflammatory bowel diseases (IBDs), 239–240, 302, 303
Inflammatory response, 59–60, 315–316
Influenza virus, 38
Innate immune cells, 36
Innate immune response
   cellular components of, 3–6
   chemokines, 8–9
   pattern recognition receptors, 2–3
   soluble factors involved in, 6–7
Innate immunity, 162
   dendritic cells, 186–187, 259
   granulocytes, 183–184, 255–256
   innate lymphoid cells, 164–165, 187–188
   macrophage development, 184–186
   monocytes/macrophages, 256–259
   mucosal barriers, 163–164
   toll-like receptors, 165
Innate lymphoid cells (ILCs), 164–165, 187–188

iNOS, *see* Inducible nitric oxide synthase
Institute of Nutrition of Central America and Panama
      (INCAP), 457
Interferon regulatory factor-1 (IRF-1), 264–265
Interferons (IFNs), 7
Interleukin-6 (IL-6), 47
Interleukin-1β (IL-1β), 47
Interleukins, 7
Intestinal inflammation, 398–399
Intestinal microbiota, 26
Intracellular proteins, zinc regulation by, 247–253
Intracellular zinc pools, 255
In vitro activation, of B-cells, 171–172
In vitro supplementation, 202
In vivo antibody responses, 171
Iodine intake, 97–98
Ionizing radiation, 437
IREs, *see* Iron Response Elements
IRF-1, *see* Interferon regulatory factor-1
Iron
   by acute-phase response, 218–219
   experimental evidence, 221
   genetic evidence, 219–220
   impacts immune cell function, 223–224
   requirement for, 213–214
   supplementation, on infections, 221–223
   trafficking, in mammals, 214–218
Iron (Fe), 74–75
Iron-malaria-anemia conundrum, 222–223
Iron Regulatory Proteins-1 (IRP-1), 214
Iron Response Elements (IREs), 214
IRP-1, *see* Iron Regulatory Proteins-1
IS, *see* Immunological synapse
Isolated lymphoid follicles (ILFs), 19, 21

K

Kayachikitsa medicine, 446
Killer-cell immunoglobulin-like receptors (KIR), 380
Krüppel-like factor 10 (Klf-10), 264–265

L

LAA, *see* Leukocytes
Lactase persistence (LP), 100–101
Lactation, nutritional requirements during, 470–471
Lagenaria Siceraria, 504
L-arginine, 362
LBW, *see* Low birth weight
Leptin, 34–35, 46–47, 117
Leukocytes (LAA), 69, 282–285
L-glutamine, 366
Lipid
   mediators, 316–318
   peroxidation, 201–202
   raft constituents, 409–410
Lipocalin-2, 219
Low birth weight (LBW), 458
LP, *see* Lactase persistence
LTi, *see* Lymphocyte tissue inducer
Lymphocytes
   maturation, effects on, 392–393
   metabolic requirements, 362–363
   mucosal targeting of, 190

subpopulations, 394
subsets, 112–113
Lymphocyte tissue inducer (LTi), 164–165
Lymphoid stem cells, 3
Lymphoid tissue, 15

M

Macrobiotic diet, 93
Macronutrients, in postpartum formulations, 502
Macrophage inhibitory cytokine (MIC-1), 116
Macrophage phagocytic activity, 394
Macrophages, 5–6, 48–49, 378
    development, 184–186
    metabolic requirements, 361–362
    proresolving lipids on, 323–326
Major histocompatibility complex (MHC), 6, 10, 11
Malaria, 267–268
Mammalian target of rapamycin (mTOR), 340, 341
Mammals, iron trafficking in
    cellular iron homeostasis, 214–216
    hepcidin synthesis, 217–218
    systemic iron homeostasis, 218
    systemic iron trafficking, 216–217
MAMPs, see Microbial-associated molecular patterns
MAP-kinase phosphatases (MKPs), 259
MAPKs, see Mitogen-activated protein kinases
Mast cells, 6, 49, 237
Master regulators, 13
Maternal nutrition, 457–458
Mature T-cells, retinoic acid of, 168–169
Mesenteric lymph nodes (MLNs), 19, 21
Meta-analysis, adjustment factors, 60–62
Metabolic syndrome, 52, 413
Metallothionein (MT), 253
Metal regulatory transcription factor-1 (MTF-1), 248
MHC, see Major histocompatibility complex
MIC-1, see Macrophage inhibitory cytokine
Microbial-associated molecular patterns (MAMPs), 2, 4
Microbial killing, 321
Microbiota, in immune development, 26
Microgravity, 435
    harmful effects of, 437
    on immune system, 436–437
    on muscle, 436
Micronutrients, in postpartum formulations, 502
Microparticles, 318–319
Microvesicles, see Microparticles
Milk-fat globule membrane (MFGM), 406, 414, 418–419
Mitogen-activated protein kinases (MAPKs), 258–259
Mixed lymphocyte culture (MLC), 263, 264, 265
MKPs, see MAP-kinase phosphatases
MLC, see Mixed lymphocyte culture
MLNs, see Mesenteric lymph nodes
M1 macrophages, 36, 351
M2 macrophages, 36, 351
Momordica charantia, see Bitter melon
Monocytes, 5–6, 48–49, 256–259
Mother's diet, in infant outcomes, 455–457
    dietary intakes, of Indian women, 457
    infant nutritional status, 458–459
    maternal nutrition, 457–458
MS, see Multiple sclerosis
MT, see Metallothionein

MTF-1, see Metal regulatory transcription factor-1
mTOR, see Mammalian target of rapamycin
Mucosal immunity, 163–164
Multiple sclerosis (MS), 266
Murraya koenigii, 503
Muscle, microgravity on, 436
Myeloid stem cells, 3, 183

N

N-acetylglutamate (NAG) synthase, 336
National Family Health Survey (NFHS), 456
Natural killer (NK) cells, 6, 50, 187, 259, 351–352
    activity of, 395
    and glutathione, 380
Natural killer T (NKT) cells, 50, 341–342
Natural Treg cells, 15–16
NE, see Neutrophil elastase
NEAA, see Nonessential AA
Neem, 448, 504
Neoplasia
    breast cancer, 268–269
    p53, 269
NETs, see Neutrophil extracellular traps
Neural development, 411–412
Neurodegenerative disorders, 412–413
Neuronal nitric oxide synthase (nNOS), 349
Neutrophil elastase (NE), 361
Neutrophil extracellular traps (NETs), 256, 361
Neutrophils, 3–5, 183
    in adaptive immunity, 50
    apoptosis, 321–323
    chemotaxis, 321
    metabolic requirements, 360–361
    phagocytosis, 255–256
    recruitment, 320–321
NFHS, see National Family Health Survey
Niacin, 71
Niacin receptor-1, 281
Nicotinic acid, see Niacin; Vitamin B_3
Nitric oxide (NO), 349–350, 378, 431
    in autoimmune diseases, 352
    diet and, 353–354
    and immune system, 350–352
    pharmaceutical agents, 354
    vascular diseases, 352–353
Nitric oxide synthase (NOS), 343, 349–350
NK cells, see Natural killer cells
NKT cells, see Natural killer T cells
nNOS, see Neuronal nitric oxide synthase
NO, see Nitric oxide
Non-α-tocopherol vitamin E, 205–206
Nonessential AA (NEAA), 335
Nongenetic mechanisms, 86
Nonlymphoid tissues, antigen presentation in, 24
Nontransferrin-bound iron (NTBI), 221
NOS, see Nitric oxide synthase
n-3 polyunsaturated fatty acids (PUFAs), 295, 296–297
    autoimmune diseases, 302–303
    eicosanoids, 300–301
    infection diseases, 303
    nuclear receptors, 302
    phospholipids, 297–300
    pro-resolving lipid mediators, 301–302

NTBI, *see* Nontransferrin-bound iron
Nutrient status, 57–58, 197, 453–455
    fat-soluble vitamins, *see* Fat-soluble vitamins
    inflammatory response, 59–60
    meta-analysis, 60–62
    minerals, 74–77
    water-soluble vitamins, *see* Water-soluble vitamins
Nutritional countermeasures, of space radiation, 439–440

O

Obesity, 33
    adaptive immune system, 36–37
    bacterial infections in, 38–39
    hypothesis, infectious origin of, 39
    immunomodulatory endocrine organ, 33–36
    innate immune cells, 36
    viral infection in, 37–38
Ocimum sanctum, see Tulsi
Offspring development, 457–458
Oligosaccharides
    immune modulation by, 152–153
    in infant formula, 153–154
Omentin, 48
Oral tolerance, 22–24
Ovalbumin (OVA), 23

P

p53, 269
Panch mahabhutas, 445
Paracrine signaling, within growth plate, 87–88
Parasitic infections, 239, 447
Parkinson's disease (PD), 412
Pattern recognition receptors (PRRs), 2–3
PBMCs, *see* Peripheral blood mononuclear cells
P5C synthase, *see* Pyrroline-5-carboxylate synthase
PD, *see* Parkinson's disease
PD1, *see* Protectin D1
Perinatal immune factors, in disease etiology, 119
Periodontitis, 38, 286
Peripheral blood mononuclear cells (PBMCs), 168, 265
Peroxisome proliferatoractivated receptor-g (PPARg), 302
Peyer's patches (PPs), 19–21
Phagocytosis, 321
Pharmaceutical agents, 354
Phosphatase and tensin homolog deleted on chromosome 10 (PTEN), 263
Phospholipids, 297–300
Phylloquinone, *see* Vitamin K
Plasmodium infection, liver stage of, 221
PLP, *see* Pyridoxal-5'-phosphate
Postpartum ethnic care, 506
Postpartum maternal health status, 469–470
Postpartum menus, 491
Postpartum morbidities, 468–469
Postpartum nutritional practices, 471
    beliefs and scientific evidence, 472–482
    ethnic Indian, *see* Ethnic Indian postpartum nutritional
        practices
    functional foods, 483–487
    traditional Indian postpartum care, 488–489
Postpartum period, 468
Postpregnancy ethnic nutritional practices, 465–468

ethnic Indian postpartum nutritional practices,
        499–505
    nutrition, after pregnancy, 468–471
    postpartum ethnic nutritional practices,
        see Postpartum nutritional practices
    traditional food formulations, 491
    traditional postpartum nutritional practices, 505–507
PPARg, *see* Peroxisome proliferatoractivated receptor-g
PPs, *see* Peyer's patches
Preadipocytes, immune-like phenotypes for, 45
Prebiotics
    definition, 125
    and vaccine responses, 135–138
Pregnancy, mother's diet in, 455–459
Probiotics, 125, *See also* Vaccine responses
Pro-inflammatory cytokines, 114–115
Pro-inflammatory roles, of retinoic acid, 167
Propionate, 279
Pro-resolving lipid mediators, 301–302
Prostate cancer, 269
Protectin D1 (PD1), 316, 320
Protein, 89–91
    intake, 95–96
PRRs, *see* Pattern recognition receptors
Pseudomembranous colitis, 287
PTEN, *see* Phosphatase and tensin homolog deleted on
        chromosome 10
PUFAs, *see* n-3 polyunsaturated fatty acids
Purine
    base, 390–391
    nucleotide catabolism, 389
Pyridoxal-5'-phosphate (PLP), 71
Pyridoxine, 71–72
Pyrimidine
    base, 390–391
    nucleotide catabolism, 389–390
Pyrroline-5-carboxylate (P5C) synthase, 336

Q

Quality Protein Maize (QPM), 96

R

RA, *see* Retinoic acid; Rheumatoid arthritis
RALDH, *see* Retinal dehydrogenases
RAREs, *see* Retinoic acid response elements
RARs, *see* Retinoic acid receptors
Rasayan, 449
RBP, *see* Retinol binding protein
RDA, *see* Recommended Dietary Allowances
Reactive oxygen species (ROS), 283, 361, 377
Recommended Dietary Allowances (RDA), 471,
        500–502
Regulatory T-cells (Tregs), 340–341, 382
Resident immune cells
    B lymphocytes, 51
    mast cells, 49
    monocytes, 48–49
    neutrophils, 50
    in pathological states, 51–53
    T lymphocytes, 50–51
Resistin, 118
Resolvins, 317

Retinal dehydrogenases (RALDH), 161–162
Retinoic acid (RA)
  in antibody production, 171–172
  anti-*versus* pro-inflammatory roles of, 167
  and B-cells development, 169
  in lymphocyte functions, 172
  on macrophage gene expression, 185
  of mature T-cells, 168–169
  mode of action, 162
  and T-cells, 166–167
  of thymocytes, 167–168
  vitamin A, 162
Retinoic acid receptors (RARs), 162, 185
Retinoic acid response elements (RAREs), 162
Retinoids, 160–161
Retinoid X response elements (RXREs), *see* Retinoic acid
    response elements
Retinol binding protein (RBP), 161
Retro-retinoids, 172
Rheumatoid arthritis (RA), 266
Riboflavin, 70–71
ROS, *see* Reactive oxygen species

S

SAs, *see* Sialic acids
SCFAs, *see* Short-chain fatty acids
Se, *see* Selenium
Seasonal influenza vaccine composition, 141–142
Secretory IgA (sIgA), 150
Selenium, 231
  asthma, 240
  and cancer, 238
  dietary sources of, 232–233
  on different immune cells, 235–237
  inflammatory bowel diseases, 239–240
  parasitic infections, 239
  selenoproteins, family of, 233
  status, 233–235
  and viral infections, 238–239
Selenium (Se), 76–77
Selenocysteine, 233
Selenoproteins, 233
Serum iron, 75
Serum nutrients, 57, 59–60
Sesbania grandiflora L., 504
SGA infants, *see* Small-for-gestational age infants
Short-chain fatty acids (SCFAs), 151, 279–280
  in epithelial cells, 282–285
  G protein-coupled receptors, 281–282
  and infection, 286–288
  inflammation by, 285–286
Sialic-acid-binding immunoglobulin-like lectins
    (Siglecs), 409
Sialic acids (SAs), 409
Siderophores, 219
Siglecs, *see* Sialic-acid-binding immunoglobulin-like
    lectins
Signal transducer and activator of transcription (STAT)
    proteins, 13
Skeletal muscle, growth of, 91
Small-for-gestational age (SGA) infants, 460
Solanum nigrum, 503
Space radiation, 437–438

harmful effects of, 439–440
  risks of, 438–439
Specialized proresolving mediators (SPMs)
  active termination, of inflammation, 320–323
  infection, 327–328
  signal, 319
Squamous metaplasia, 182
STAT proteins, *see* Signal transducer and activator of
    transcription proteins
Superoxide anion, 256
Synbiotics, 125
  and vaccine responses, 138–140
Systemic iron homeostasis, 218
Systemic iron trafficking, 216–217

T

T-cells, 2, 165–169, 237
  adaptive immunity, 260–265
  antigen receptor complex, 12
  anti-*versus* pro-inflammatory roles, of retinoic
      acid, 167
  death, 167–169
  dependent, 14
  development, 11–12, 189–190
  and immune tolerance, 15–16
  inflammation, 295–296
  retinoic acid, 166–167
  subpopulations, 12–13
  Th1 cells, 166
TCJ, *see* Tight cell junction
T1D, *see* Type 1 diabetes
T2DM, *see* Type II diabetes mellitus
Terminal deoxynucleotidyl transferase (TdT), 392
Tfh, *see* follicular helper T-cells
Th1 cells, 166, 338
Th2 cells, 166, 338–339
Th9 cells, 339
Th17 cells, 340
Th22 cells, 340
T helper cells, 381
Thiamin, 70
Thymic function, 188–189
Thymocytes, retinoic acid and, 167–168
Tight cell junction (TCJ), 19
TLRs, *see* Toll-like receptors
T-lymphocytes, 11–13, 296
  in adaptive immunity, 50–51
  recognition by, 10–11
TNF-α, *see* Tumor necrosis factor alpha
TNF-α receptor II (TNFRII), 118
α-Tocopherol, *see* Vitamin E
Tocopherols, 205–206
Tocotrienols, 206
Toll-like receptors (TLRs), 2, 4, 45, 165
Traditional postpartum foods
  beliefs and scientific evidence, 472–482
  formulations and postpartum menus, 491–499,
      500–502
  functional foods, 483–487, 488–490
  for immunity, 502–505
  macro-and micronutrients in, 502
Transferrin, 220
Tregs, *see* Regulatory T-cells

Tryptophan, 101
Tuberculosis, glutathione in, 382–383
Tulsi, 448
Tumor necrosis factor alpha (TNF-α), 47
Tumor responses, nucleotides modulation of, 395
Turmeric, 448, 503–504
Type 1 diabetes (T1D), 151
Type II diabetes mellitus (T2DM), 383

U

Undernutrition, in children, 83–85
    animal models, observed in, 89–92
    animal source foods, 98–101
    bone growth regulation, 85–89
    energy intake, 93–95
    infection and, 101–104
    iodine intake, 97–98
    protein intake, 95–96
    zinc intake, 96–97

V

Vaccination-induced immune responses, 149–150
Vaccine responses, 125–127
    in adults, 128–133
    in infants, 127–128
    in older adults, 133–135
    prebiotics and, 135–138
    synbiotics and, 138–140
Vascular diseases
    endothelial dysfunction, 352–353
    inflammation, 353
VDBP, *see* Vitamin D-binding protein
Vibrio vulnificus, 221
Viral infections, 238–239, 447
    in obesity, 37–38
Vitamin A, 62–64, 159–160
    and adaptive immunity, *see* Adaptive immunity
    B-cells development, 190
    deficiency, 455
    dendritic cell development, 186–187
    dietary intake of, 160–161
    epithelial surfaces, 182–183
    granulocyte development, 183–184
    in immune-related diseases, 172–173
    and innate immunity, 162–165
    innate lymphoid cell development, 187–188
    macrophage development, 184–186
    metabolism, 161–162
    retinoic acid, 162
    T-cell development, 189–190
    thymic function, 188–189
    in twentieth century, 181–182
Vitamin B$_1$, *see* Thiamin

Vitamin B$_2$, *see* Riboflavin
Vitamin B$_3$, 71
Vitamin B$_6$, *see* Pyridoxine
Vitamin B$_{12}$, 73
Vitamin C, 68–70
Vitamin D, 64–66
Vitamin D-binding protein (VDBP), 64
Vitamin E, 66–68, 197–199
    animal models, 203
    deficiency, 199–200
    effect of, 201–202
    human studies, 203–204
    natural source, 198–199
    non-α-tocopherol, 205–206
    supplementation, 200–201
Vitamin K, 68

W

Water-soluble vitamins
    carotenoids, 74
    folic acid, 72–73
    niacin, 71
    pyridoxine, 71–72
    riboflavin, 70–71
    thiamin, 70
    vitamin B$_{12}$, 73
    vitamin C, 68–70
Withania somnifera, 448–449

X

Xanthine oxidase, 389
Xerophthalmia, 182

Z

Zinc (Zn), 75–76, 91–92, 245–246
    absorption, 254
    adaptive immunity, *see* Adaptive immunity
    allergic reactions, 265
    autoimmune diseases, 265–266
    deficiency, 253–254
    direct anabolic influences of, 88–89
    homeostasis, 246–247
    infectious diseases, 267–268
    innate immunity, *see* Innate immunity
    intake, 96–97
    intracellular proteins, 247–253
    neoplasia, 268–269
    status, assessment of, 255
Zingiber officinale, 504
ZIP family (ZIP1-14), 88–89
Zip transporters, 247
Zn, *see* Zinc

#0006 - 190917 - C8 - 254/178/29 [31] - CB - 9781482253979